PELVIC PAIN
DIAGNOSIS AND MANAGEMENT

PELVIC PAIN

DIAGNOSIS AND MANAGEMENT

Senior Editor

FRED M. HOWARD, MS, MD

*Director of Gynecology and Associate Chair
Department of Obstetrics and Gynecology
University of Rochester School of Medicine and Dentistry
Rochester, New York*

Editors

C. PAUL PERRY, MD, FACOG

*Director, Pelvic Pain Center
Department of Gynecology
Brookwood Women's Medical Center
Birmingham, Alabama*

JAMES E. CARTER, MD, PHD, FACOG

*Medical Director
Women's Health Center of South Orange County, Inc.
Mission Viejo, California*

AHMED M. EL-MINAWI, MD, MSC, PHD

*Assistant Professor
Department of Gynecology and Obstetrics
Kasr El-Aini School of Medicine
Cairo University, Cairo, Egypt*

RONG-ZENG LI, MD, MAMS, CMI

*Senior Medical Illustrator
UMDNJ-Robert Wood Johnson Medical School*

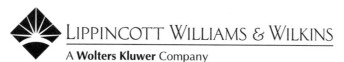

LIPPINCOTT WILLIAMS & WILKINS

A **Wolters Kluwer** Company

Philadelphia • Baltimore • New York • London
Buenos Aires • Hong Kong • Sydney • Tokyo

Acquisitions Editor: Lisa McAllister
Developmental Editor: Pamela Sutton
Production Editor: Rakesh Rampertab
Manufacturing Manager: Kevin Watt
Cover Designer: Mark Lerner
Compositor: Lippincott Williams & Wilkins Desktop Division
Printer: Edwards Brothers

© 2000 by LIPPINCOTT WILLIAMS & WILKINS
530 Walnut Street
Philadelphia, PA 19106 USA
LWW.com

Printed in the USA

Library of Congress Cataloging-in-Publication Data

Pelvic pain: diagnosis and management / edited by Fred M. Howard, senior editor ... [et al.]; illustrations by Rong-Zeng Li.
    p.; cm.
  Includes bibliographical references and index.
  ISBN 0-7817-1724-8
    1. Pelvic pain. 2. Generative organs, Female—Diagnosis. I. Howard, Fred M.
  [DNLM: 1. Pelvic Pain—diagnosis. 2. Pelvic Pain—therapy. WP 155 P3934 2000]
RG483.P44 P45 2000
617.5'5'0082—dc21
                                                                    00-027378

10 9 8 7 6 5 4 3 2 1

To
our patients who have taught us so much,
though we have so much more to learn.

And
our families who have been our constant support
with their love and patience.

ACKNOWLEDGEMENT

Many people deserve acknowledgement for their role in making this book possible. First I wish to thank my coeditors and contributors for jobs well done. They worked tirelessly on this project. It would not have been possible without them. Especially, I want to acknowledge the work of Dr. Ahmed El-Minawi. He started his work on this book while a research fellow with me in Rochester, New York, and brought an international flavor to this publication. His work in caring for women with pelvic pain in Cairo, Egypt, carries on that started by his father, Professor Mahmoud El-Minawi, and I am pleased that I have been able to influence him, too, in some small measure. I wish to thank his wife Meral, and son, Jousef, for their sacrifice in allowing him the time to study with me and work on this book.

Several people at Lippincott Williams & Wilkins deserve to be acknowledged also. This was not an easy book for them to bring to press. Lisa McAllister believed in the merit of this project and supported it even when we were behind schedule—many thanks to her from my coeditors and me. Pamela Sutton and Rakesh Rampertab worked enthusiastically to assure the quality of this book and we thank them, too, for their energetic assistance. Dr. Li is recognized for his superb illustrations.

I wish to acknowledge some of the people have taught me what I know of pelvic pain. Drs. John Slocumb and John Steege from Colorado and North Carolina respectively, have both been personal mentors and friends. Drs. Richard Beard and Philip Reginald, both from England, through their writing and personal communication have also taught me much. To paraphrase Isaac Newton, what I have seen has been possible only because I have stood on the shoulders of giants.

I must thank my students and, especially, my patients, all of whom have taught me so much, enduring my inadequacies of knowledge with patience and love. I know that with their help we will learn better and safer ways to alleviate the suffering of women with chronic pelvic pain. Above all else, this book is dedicated to them.

Finally, I wish to acknowledge the support and patience of my wife, Dr. Cynthia Roy Howard, and youngest daughter, Laurel Roy Howard. They sacrificed much during the preparation of this book, while constantly supporting me in my work. I could not have completed this without their love and encouragement. My grown children, Shon Tucker Howard and Kelly Leigh Howard, also deserve acknowledgement. Although they were not at home during the writing of this book, I would like to thank them for their invaluable sacrifices to my career.

Fred M. Howard, M.S., M.D.
Senior Editor
Rochester, New York

ACKNOWLEDGEMENT

Sufferers from chronic pelvic pain are the medical "lepers" of our patients. They face misdiagnosis, unhelpful surgeries, and prejudice as drug seekers. I wish to dedicate this book to our patients who have taught us love and compassion, how to rise above our own prejudices and that we must learn from other disciplines in order to deliver hope and relief. Our aim is to educate other medical professionals and to encourage the public to seek out those who have been called to their care. I would also like to express appreciation to my wife and children who have given me up so I may pursue this mission.

C. Paul Perry, M.D., F.A.C.O.G.
Coeditor
Birmingham, Alabama

ACKNOWLEDGEMENT

I dedicate this book to my mother, Eleanor Higgins Carter, and in memory of my father, Alpha George Carter for their tireless dedication to my education, and their encouragement for all of my work. I dedicate this book also to my wife, Grace Change Carter, for her patience and encouragement and loving support during all of my educational efforts. I also give thanks to my patients who have taught me so much about the trauma that chronic pelvic pain can inflict on an individual's life. My thanks also to Dr. David Simons for his support, suggestions, and especially his leadership and teachings on myofascial pain and dysfunction. In any book of this magnitude there are usually many to whom gratitude should be shown—to all who have contributed toward this book, I am grateful. I would like to thank, in memory, Dr. Arnold J. Kresch for his dedication to the subject of chronic pelvic pain and on whose work and teachings we have all relied.

James E. Carter, M.D., Ph.D., F.A.C.O.G.
Coeditor
Mission Viejo, California

CONTENTS

CONTRIBUTING AUTHORS

Joan S. Brown, PT Owner and Director, Marguerite Physical Therapy Clinic, 27401 Los Altos, Suite 488, Mission Viejo, California 92691

Charles W. Butrick, MD Clinical Assistant Professor, Department of Obstetrics and Gynecology, Kansas University, 39th Street and Rainbow, Kansas City; and Director, The Urogynecology Center, Kansas City Women's Clinic, 10600 Quivira Road, Overland Park, Kansas 66215

James E. Carter, MD, PhD, FACOG Associate Clinical Professor, Department of Obstetrics and Gynecology, University of California, Irvine College of Medicine, 101 The City Drive South, Orange, California 92868; and Medical Director, Women's Health Center of South Orange County Inc., 26732 Crown Valley Parkway, Mission Viejo, California 92691

Daniel M. Doleys, PhD Director, Department of Clinical Psychology, Pain & Rehabilitation Institute, 720 Montclair Road, Suite 204, Birmingham, Alabama 35213

Ahmed M. El-Minawi, MD, MSc, PhD Assistant Professor, Department of Gynecology and Obstetrics, Kasr El-Aini School of Medicine, Cairo University, Cairo, Egypt; and former Visiting Associate Professor and Post-Doctoral Fellow, Department of Obstetrics and Gynecology, University of Rochester, School of Medicine and Dentistry, 601 Elmwood Avenue, Rochester, New York 14642

Fred M. Howard, MS, MD Director of Gynecology and Associate Chair, Department of Obstetrics and Gynecology, University of Rochester, School of Medicine and Dentistry, 601 Elmwood Avenue, Rochester, New York 14642

Kevin M. Kinback, MD Assistant Clinical Professor, Department of Psychiatry, Loma Linda University, School of Medicine; and Assistant Clinical Professor, Department of Psychiatry, University of California, Irvine School of Medicine, Orange, California 92868

Daniel C. Lowery Research Assistant, Pain & Rehabilitation Institute, 720 Montclair Road, Suite 204, Birmingham, Alabama 35213

C. Paul Perry, MD, FACOG Clinical Instructor, Department of Obstetrics and Gynecology, University of Alabama, Medical College at Birmingham, 619 South 19th Street, Birmingham, Alabama 35233; and Director, Pelvic Pain Center, Department of Gynecology, Brookwood Women's Medical Center, 2006 Brookwood Medical Center Drive, Birmingham, Alabama 35209

PREFACE

For the diagnosis and treatment of women with acute abdominopelvic pain, the clinician has many sources of information. Many women, however, suffer with recurrent, persistent, or chronic pelvic pain and few sources of information are available to assist with the diagnosis and treatment of these unfortunate women. This text is offered with the hope that it will meet this need.

To facilitate use of this textbook, it is divided into three major sections. In the first section the chapters present information basic to the care of women with pelvic pain, covering the scope of the problem, the essentials of the history and physical examination, an overview of diagnostic laboratory and imaging tests, and the role of endoscopic evaluations.

The second section, encompassing the bulk of the book, uses an organ system approach to present chapters on diagnosis and treatment of disorders of the reproductive, gastrointestinal, urinary, and musculoskeletal system. Also in this section are chapters on a number of systemic, psychiatric, and metabolic disorders that may cause or contribute to pelvic pain. Each chapter in this section is similarly organized to simplify its use by the clinician. Each starts with a mini-glossary of key terms and definitions. This is followed by a general introduction, including discussions of etiology and pathology if appropriate to the disorder and if sufficient knowledge is available. The organization of the chapters then follows the sequence that a clinician would assume in evaluating a patient, going through the history (symptoms), the physical examination (signs), diagnostic tests (laboratory and imaging), the differential diagnosis, and finally making a diagnosis. Next, treatment or management of the disorder is presented, with subdivisions into medical and surgical treatment as appropriate. Each chapter concludes with key points presented in a bulleted format, subdivided into differential diagnoses, most important questions a clinician should ask a patient, most important physical examination findings, most important diagnostic studies, and treatments. It is our hope that this organization will aid the clinician not only in the use of this book as a creditable read for basic education, but also to find it useful as a reference source in the clinical setting.

The final section includes chapters covering general topics pertinent specifically to chronic pain, including one which regards chronic pain as a diagnosis. This represents a significant change of mindset for most clinicians, as we tend to think of pain as a symptom and not as a disease. Also, it is important in the care of many women with pelvic pain that pain be considered as a disease or diagnosis in itself, not as a symptom of some other disorder. This permits treatment to be directed specifically toward pain, in an approach that is essential for many women who are hopeful of returning to an active and fulfilling life.

Although edited by obstetrician/gynecologists, this book reflects our interests as primary care physicians for women in the diagnosis and treatment of women with pelvic pain, not a denial of the importance of multiple disciplines in the care of women with chronic pelvic pain. *Pelvic Pain* is directed especially to obstetrician/gynecologists, with our prayers that it will lead to improved care for women. Additionally, we hope that it will also be of immense use to any clinician who attends to women with pelvic pain. We all have much to learn together if we are to provide the best possible care to our patients (to whom the quality of our care is all that matters, not the medical specialty we practice).

Thankfully, knowledge about recurrent, persistent, and chronic pain is expanding rapidly. While this is critical if we are to ever achieve the ability to fully assure patients of effectively alleviating their suffering, it also means that some of the information presented in this textbook may, in time, become outdated or even inaccurate. Thus, we welcome your help with corrections, additions, and constructive comments.

Fred M. Howard, M.S., M.D.
Senior Editor

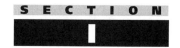

SECTION

I

APPROACH TO THE PATIENT
WITH CHRONIC PELVIC PAIN

1

INTRODUCTION

FRED M. HOWARD

Through love all pain is turned to healing.
Rumi

Pelvic pain is an important part of clinical practice for any clinician who provides health care for women. Pelvic pain may be acute, recurrent, or chronic. The distinction is not simply semantic or academic. Most authorities agree that if a woman has pain of more than 3 or 6 months' duration that is located primarily in the pelvis, she should be diagnosed with *chronic pelvic pain* (1,2). Some consider the cyclic pain of dysmenorrhea or the episodic pain of dyspareunia as a criterion for chronic pelvic pain, but it is probably better classified as *recurrent pelvic pain,* because it almost always represents symptoms of a disease. Also, the diagnosis and treatment of dysmenorrhea or dyspareunia frequently differ from chronic pelvic pain. However, women with chronic pelvic pain may also have dysmenorrhea or dyspareunia as part of their symptom complex (3). The 3- or 6-month criterion is an arbitrary convention. *Acute pelvic pain* rarely lasts more than 1 month without crisis, resolution, or cure; therefore, any pain lasting more than 1 month could easily be considered chronic (4). Part of the rationale for a 3- or 6-month criterion is that after months of pelvic pain, pain itself can become an illness rather than a symptomatic manifestation of some other disease (5).

This leads to the several premises about pelvic pain that form the foundations of this book. One is that although acute and chronic pelvic pain may share many of the same etiologies, acute pelvic pain is best thought of as a symptom of disease, whereas chronic pelvic pain is best viewed as a disease in itself. There are many books that sufficiently cover the diagnosis and treatment of acute abdominopelvic pain, but few that similarly cover chronic pelvic pain. For that reason this book is directed mostly to the care of women with chronic pelvic pain. A second premise of this book is that the diagnostic evaluation and the treatment of the woman with chronic pelvic pain should be approached from a biopsychosocial perspective. Using only a biological, psychological, or social approach to such a woman is inadequate and leads to less than ideal care. All are important to varying degrees in all women with chronic pelvic pain.

Although this book has a bent toward the biological aspects of chronic pelvic pain, this is not meant to downplay the importance of psychological and social factors. A third premise of this book is that ideal care of the woman with chronic pelvic pain is delivered with a multidisciplinary approach. Sometimes this is best accomplished via a multidisciplinary clinic, but that is not always necessary or possible. The woman's internist, urologist, family physician, gynecologist, or gastroenterologist, for example, may provide a multidisciplinary approach to diagnosis and treatment, using consultants as indicated, and thereby provide better continuity, confidence, and personal attention than can occur in many pain clinics, without any loss of efficacy. This requires sufficient time, interest, and knowledge. Our hope is that this book will serve as a venue to acquiring the requisite knowledge, serving both as a textbook and a reference.

Chronic pelvic pain is a significant problem. In a study of women in primary care offices (nongynecologic) in a university setting, 12% of women reported chronic pelvic pain currently and 33% related a past history of chronic pelvic pain (6). In another study of reproductive-age women in primary care private practices, 39% had pelvic pain at least some of the time and 12% had more than 5 days of pain per month or pain that lasted a full day or more each month (7). A Gallup poll found that 16% of women reported pelvic pain problems, 11% limited home activity because of it, 16% took medications for it, and 4% missed at least 1 day of work per month because of it (8).

Chronic pelvic pain may lead to years of disability and suffering, with loss of employment, marital discord and divorce, as well as numerous untoward and unsuccessful medical misadventures. Often the woman suffering with chronic pelvic pain has been told that there is nothing wrong, the pain is in her head, and has been referred to a psychiatrist; or that there is nothing that can be done and she must learn to live with the pain. Not unexpectedly, a history of such turmoil often causes women with chronic pelvic pain to be difficult patients. They may distrust health care providers, and may be uncooperative and noncompliant. Often they move from physician to physician in an attempt to find one they can trust, one with a promise of cure.

Chronic pelvic pain, unfortunately, is an affliction of women during the peak of their productive years, at a mean age of about 30 years (Fig. 1.1). It accounts for a significant volume of medical care. It is impossible to estimate the number of radiologic, laboratory, and invasive diagnostic tests that are performed in the evaluation of pelvic pain. Pelvic pain is estimated to account for 10% of all referrals to a gynecologist (9). It is the indication for 12% of all hysterectomies performed in the United States. Of women with irritable bowel syndrome, a common cause of chronic pelvic pain, 21% aged 18 to 40 years have undergone hysterectomies. This is significantly higher than the national average of about 6% (10). Pelvic pain is the indication for over 40% of gynecologic diagnostic laparoscopies (11). It is estimated that direct and indirect costs of chronic pelvic pain in the United States are over two billion dollars per year.

Chronic pelvic pain is a frustrating problem for most physicians, partially because the majority thinks of pain within the context of the classic Cartesian model. This model postulates that pain is the direct result of tissue trauma that activates specific neuroreceptors and neural pain fibers, and that the severity of pain is directly proportional to the severity of the traumatic insult. As a corollary, pain that is unassociated with identifiable tissue injury is regarded as spurious or as psychogenic. Although this model is fairly useful in acute pain, it is not applicable to chronic pain. Attempts to find enough organic pathology to explain chronic pelvic pain have routinely been frustrating; somatic pathologies, such as endometriosis, adhesions, or leiomyomata, have at best an uncertain relationship to chronic pelvic pain if the scientific evidence is closely scrutinized. Considering chronic pain solely a psychiatric disor-

der has also been frustrating and not supported by available scientific evidence. Workers in chronic pain currently believe that a biopsychosocial model must be used to grapple with this problem and that any culpable theory can only be useful if it takes into account the influences of nociceptive stimulation, individual psychological characteristics, and social determinants of pain.

Melzack's and Wall's gate control theory is the model most frequently utilized in trying to understand chronic pain. In oversimplified terms, this theory states that afferent neural impulses from the periphery may be modulated by spinal and cortical signals ("gates"). The modulation may be either enhancement or diminution of the afferent impulse. The neurophysiologic events that gate or modulate the pain impulse are influenced by numerous factors, both peripheral and central. The gates may be affected by (a) the level of firing of the visceral afferent nerves, (b) afferent input from cutaneous and deep somatic structures, (c) endogenous opioid and nonopioid analgesic systems, and (d) various central excitatory and inhibitory influences from the brainstem, hypothalamus, and cortex (12). This theory provides a neurologic basis for the influence or both somatic and psychogenic factors on pain (i.e., anxiety, depression, physical activity, mental concentration, marital discord, etc., may increase or decrease the perception of pain). Although neurophysiologic and biochemical research have resulted in significant modifications of this theory since its original proposal, it still works as a good (but not only) model for the clinical observations in chronic pain patients and provides a more productive approach to therapy than the classic Cartesian model.

The common association of depression and chronic pelvic pain, for example, may be explained by the gate theory as being caused by the dysregulation of neurotransmitters associated with depression, which "opens" the central nervous system (CNS) gate, increasing sensitivity to nociception (13). Conversely, this model allows an explanation of chronic pain as a cause of depression: Chronic somatic nociception may deplete the descending CNS modulators of pain (e.g., endogenous opioids), and this depletion may biochemically lead to depression. Thus, potential mechanisms for depression leading to chronic pelvic pain and for chronic pelvic pain leading to depression can be postulated; there is neurophysiologic evidence to support both (13,14).

Such theoretical concepts may have clinical relevance. For example, Steege has found depression to be a significant indicator of the clinical responsiveness of chronic pelvic pain patients and has included it as one of the major criteria for diagnosing "chronic pain syndrome" (15). Patients with chronic pain syndrome have a much poorer response to traditional treatment for pelvic pain, such as surgical lysis of abdominopelvic adhesions, than do pain patients without chronic pain syndrome (16). Furthermore, it has been clinically noted that major depressive illness is sometimes seen in chronic pain patients, via a cycle of pain, depression, and withdrawal.

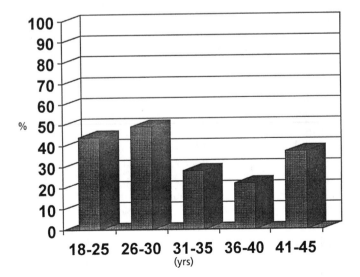

FIGURE 1.1. Ages of 65 women with chronic pelvic pain.

Such observations have led to a search for identifiable psychosocial characteristics of chronic pelvic pain patients. Psychological interviews suggest these patients are anxious and depressed, and have low self-esteem and high dependency. Psychometric testing, for example with the Minnesota Multiphasic Personality Inventory, shows that chronic pelvic pain patients have a characteristic personality profile, with high scores on the hysteria, hypochondriasis, and depression scales. These personality profiles are noted in patients in whom organic pathology can be found and in those in whom no such pathology is noted (17). Such psychological changes tend to maintain or increase the level of pain, regardless of the degree of physical disease. Additionally, when pain treatment is successful, the high scores on hysteria, hypochondriasis, and depression revert to normal.

The clinical relevance of current pain theories is that diagnosis and treatment must integrate many influences; the patient's personality and affect, cultural influences, stress, organic changes that may trigger nociceptive signals, sensory thresholds or gates, and the patient's cognition about pain. Clearly, for chronic pelvic pain no clear distinction between psychological and physical causes of pain can be made, nor are attempts to make such a distinction useful. Rather than trying to establish organic versus functional etiologies, it is more useful to ask in each patient: (a) Is there any physical disease or abnormality that requires medical or surgical treatment? and (b) Is there emotional or psychological distress that requires treatment?

The women suffering from chronic pelvic pain are a heterogeneous group, and the contributing factors and possible diagnoses in addition to chronic pelvic pain are numerous and varied (Table 1.1). There are few large series of patients with thorough evaluation of chronic pelvic pain available for review. Table 5.10 summarizes the final diagnoses in

TABLE 1.1. DISEASES THAT MAY CAUSE OR CONTRIBUTE TO CHRONIC PELVIC PAIN IN WOMEN

Gynecologic—Extrauterine
    Adhesions
    Adnexal cysts
    Chronic ectopic pregnancy
    Chlamydial endometritis or salpingitis
    Endometriosis
    Endosalpingiosis
    Ovarian retention syndrome (residual ovary syndrome)
    Ovarian remnant syndrome
    Ovarian dystrophy or ovulatory pain
    Pelvic congestion syndrome
    Postoperative peritoneal cysts
    Residual accessory ovary
    Subacute salpingooophoritis
    Tuberculous salpingitis
Gynecologic—Uterine
    Adenomyosis
    Atypical dysmenorrhea or ovulatory pain
    Cervical stenosis
    Chronic endometritis
    Endometrial or cervical polyps
    Intrauterine contraceptive device
    Leiomyomata
    Symptomatic pelvic relaxation (genital prolapse)
Urologic
    Bladder neoplasm
    Chronic urinary tract infection
    Interstitial cystitis
    Radiation cystitis
    Recurrent, acute cystitis
    Recurrent, acute urethritis
    Stone/urolithiasis
    Uninhibited bladder contractions
        (detrusor-sphincter dyssynergia)
    Urethral diverticulum
    Urethral syndrome
    Urethral caruncle
Gastrointestinal
    Carcinoma of the colon
    Chronic intermittent bowel obstruction

Colitis
Constipation
Diverticular disease
Hernias
Inflammatory bowel disease
Irritable bowel syndrome
Musculoskeletal
    Abdominal wall myofascial pain (trigger points)
    Chronic coccygeal pain
    Compression of lumbar vertebrae
    Degenerative joint disease
    Disk
    Faulty or poor posture
    Fibromyositis
    Hernias: ventral, inguinal, femoral, Spigelian
    Low back pain
    Muscular strains and sprains
    Neoplasia of spinal cord or sacral nerve
    Neuralgia of iliohypogastric, ilioinguinal, and/or
genitofemoral nerves
    Pelvic floor myalgia (levator ani spasm)
    Piriformis syndrome
    Rectus tendon strain
    Spondylosis
Other
    Abdominal cutaneous nerve entrapment in surgical scar
    Abdominal epilepsy
    Abdominal migraine
    Bipolar personality disorders
    Depression
    Familial Mediterranean fever
    Neurologic dysfunction
    Porphyria
    Shingles
    Sleep disturbances
    Somatic referral

one small series, but includes only patients with a negative laparoscopy and referral to a chronic pelvic pain clinic (18). In my experience patients commonly have more than one problem or diagnosis. For example, bladder irritability, irritable bowel syndrome, poor posture, and emotional stresses may all be contributing factors in a single patient, with the need for simultaneous urologic, gastroenterologic, and psychological treatment, and physical therapy.

Treatment or management of pelvic pain in patients with multiple problems is complex and goals of treatment must be realistic. Scientific research on treatment has been difficult because of the heterogeneity of patients with chronic pelvic pain (19). We have tried to reflect such complexity in this book. Although we have sectioned the chapters into reproductive, gastrointestinal, urologic, and neuromuscular diseases, we realize that such divisions are artificial. A full appreciation of the complexity of evaluation and treatment of women with chronic pelvic pain undoubtedly requires an integration of understanding and knowledge of all pelvic organ systems, as well as psychosocial medicine. Furthermore, it requires a complete and compassionate clinician dedicated to the care of such women. We hope this book will provide the impetus for others to further our knowledge and skill in the care of women afflicted with this disabling disorder.

REFERENCES

1. Reiter RC, Gambone JC. Nongynecologic somatic pathology in women with chronic pelvic pain and negative laparoscopy. *J Reprod Med* 1991;36:253–259.
2. Steege JF, Stout AL. Resolution of chronic pelvic pain after laparoscopic lysis of adhesions. *Am J Obstet Gynecol* 1991;165:278–281.
3. Reiter RC, Shakerin LR, Gambone JC, et al. Correlation between sexual abuse and somatization in women with somatic and nonsomatic chronic pelvic pain. *Am J Obstet Gynecol* 1991;165:104–109.
4. Howard FM. The role of laparoscopy in the evaluation of chronic pelvic pain: promise and pitfalls. *Obstet Gynecol Survey* 1993;48:10–46.
5. Steege JF. Assessment and treatment of chronic pelvic pain. *Telinde's Operative Gynecol Updates* 1992;1:1–10.
6. Walker EA, Katon WJ, Jemelka RP, et al. The prevalence of chronic pelvic pain and irritable bowel syndrome in two university clinics. *J Psychosom Obstet Gynecol* 1991;12(Suppl):65–75.
7. Jamieson DJ, Steege JF. The prevalence of dysmenorrhea, dyspareunia, pelvic pain, and irritable bowel syndrome in primary care practices. *Obstet Gynecol* 1996;87:55–58.
8. Mathias SD, Kuppermann M, Liberman RF, et al. Chronic pelvic pain: prevalence, health-related quality of life, and economic correlates. *Obstet Gynecol* 1996;87:321–327.
9. Reiter RC. A profile of women with chronic pelvic pain. *Clin Obstet Gynecol* 1990;33:130–136.
10. Prior A, Whorwell PJ. Gynaecological consultation in patients with the irritable bowel syndrome. *Gut* 1989;30:996–998.
11. Howard FM. The role of laparoscopy in chronic pelvic pain: promise and pitfalls. *Obstet Gynecol Survey* 1993;48:357–87.
12. Rapkin AJ. Neuroanatomy, neurophysiology, and neuropharmacology of pelvic pain. *Clin Obstet Gynecol* 1990;33:119–129.
13. Rosenthal RH. Psychology of chronic pelvic pain. *Obstet Gynecol Clinics NA* 1993;20:627–642.
14. Walker EA, Sullivan MD, Stenchever MA. Use of antidepressants in the management of women with chronic pelvic pain. *Obstet Gynecol Clin NA* 1993;20:743–751.
15. Steege JF, Stout AL, Somkuti SG. Chronic pelvic pain in women: toward an integrative model. *Obstet Gynecol Surv* 1993;48:95–110.
16. Steege JF, Stout AL. Resolution of chronic pelvic pain after laparoscopic lysis of adhesions. *Amer J Obstet Gynecol* 1991;165:278–281.
17. Rapkin AJ, Kames LD. The pain management approach to chronic pelvic pain. *J Reprod Med* 1987;32:323–327.
18. Reiter RC, Gambone JC. Nongynecologic somatic pathology in women with chronic pelvic pain and negative laparoscopy. *J Reprod Med* 1991;36:253–259.
19. Peters AAW, van Dorst E, Jellis B, et al. A randomized clinical trial to compare two different approaches in women with chronic pelvic pain. *Obstet Gynecol* 1991;77:740–744.

2

TAKING A HISTORY

FRED M. HOWARD
AHMED M. EL-MINAWI

INTRODUCTION

The patient history represents a powerful diagnostic and therapeutic tool. As a diagnostic tool, a thorough history often leads to an accurate diagnosis that further evaluations by physical examination and laboratory testing serve primarily to confirm. As a therapeutic tool, a compassionately taken history, during which the patient talks and the physician listens, establishes rapport and allows the patient to leave the physician's office feeling better.

Unfortunately, the diagnostic approach to the woman with chronic pelvic pain (CPP) often is directed as much by the specialty of the evaluating physician as by the woman's clinical characteristics. Clearly, the diversity of potential etiologic or associated diagnoses demands a more general approach with a thorough, explorative history that directs further evaluation and requisite referrals and consultations. Although the history is directed to the patient's pain, a thorough review of systems, with particular attention to the gastrointestinal, reproductive, urologic, and musculoskeletal systems, must not be neglected. This chapter goes through the basic questions about pain and the basic questions from the review of systems that are important in obtaining the history of any woman with CPP. More detailed questions may be needed in individual patients depending on their associated diseases; that information is included in the chapters on specific disorders associated with CPP.

THE INITIAL VISIT

Ideally the physician's initial interview of the woman with CPP should accomplish the following:

- A thorough biopsychosocial history should be obtained.
- The patient's expectations and needs should be made apparent to the physician.
- The patient should be oriented to the physician's philosophy of care of patients with chronic pelvic pain and the physician's expectations.

- Fears or misunderstandings should be addressed with appropriate re-education of the patient about her illness and her role in its treatment.
- A relationship between the physician (and the clinical team) and patient should be established (i.e., rapport established).
- The patient should be motivated to continued involvement and collaboration in her evaluation and treatment (1–3).

A biopsychosocial approach seems essential because the physician has two separate but interrelated tasks in the diagnostic evaluation: first, to evaluate the *pain,* with the patient as a carrier of the pathophysiologic mechanisms that result in pain; and second, to assess the *patient as a person* with a unique and complex history, who has pain as a primary complaint (4). Another way of expressing these two interrelated tasks is with the two questions: "Is there physical disease that requires medical or surgical treatment?" and "Is there emotional or psychological distress that requires treatment?" It is important to recognize that the precise connection between these two questions cannot usually be determined (5).

Accomplishing all the ideals of the initial visit may be impractical at the time of the first encounter, especially in a busy practice with time constraints. However, the importance of establishing rapport with the patient at the initial visit cannot be overstated—it may well be the most important objective of the initial encounter (3). It is crucial that the patient be taken seriously. Nothing she relates in her history should be dismissed as ridiculous, impossible, or unimportant, because stating such things to the patient is counterproductive and only creates mistrust. The woman with CPP needs to have a chance to tell her story in her own words and to have someone listen. Tolerance is important in listening to the patient's telling and interpretation of her history. This is a major step in establishing rapport and in obtaining the patient's perspective about her pain.

Thus, although pain questionnaires are useful in evaluating women with CPP, they must be used to supplement, not replace, allowing the patient to tell her story. The physician should personally go through at least the most critical portions of the history with the patient. Not only does this allow the chance to obtain more detail about the patient's history, but it also allows observation of her emotional reaction to critical aspects of the history and enhances establishment of rapport and trust between the patient and physician. It is important that this initial interview occur while the patient is fully clothed, because personal and intimate questions about psychosocial issues such as abuse or dyspareunia need to be asked (3).

PAIN HISTORY

Pain is "an unpleasant sensory and emotional experience primarily associated with tissue damage or described in terms of such damage, or both" (6). Pain is defined in this way to make it clear that pain is a personal subjective experience, not an objective physiological event. This subjectivity makes a detailed pain history vital in evaluating the woman with CPP. There are no objective tests that allow measurement, characterization, or confirmation of the patient's pain. The history should be used to characterize the patient's pain as completely as possible, with the goal of obtaining diagnostic and therapeutic direction.

At a minimum, the clinical assessment of pain should include its location, severity, timing and frequency characteristics, provocative and palliative factors, chronology, emotional response (affective and semantic components), and psychological characteristics (4).

Where does it hurt? The location of pain is a crucial part of the history. A useful technique at the initial interview and at subsequent intervals during care is to have the patient to do a "pain map" on a human anatomy diagram (Fig. 2.1). (This has historical precedent in the centuries-

old use of ivory models of the female figure that patients used to localize symptoms in traditional Chinese medicine.) The patient is asked to fill in the areas where she has pain. Some authorities suggest that the patient label the areas of pain with a pain severity score, for example, using a 1 to 10 rating system (7). However, we have found this to be difficult and confusing for many patients.

Pain maps often reveal more than the patient's pelvic pain. For example, up to 60% of women with chronic pelvic pain also have headaches, and up to 90% have backaches (8). Sometimes the pain map may also be useful in showing a distribution of pain, suggesting a dermatomal distribution or a myotomal pattern, thus directing the subsequent evaluation toward the musculoskeletal system (4). Table 2.1 shows areas of referred pain for musculoskeletal disorders that may be associated with pelvic pain.

The location of CPP is useful in differential diagnosis, but by itself is rarely diagnostic. One major reason for this is that true visceral pain is not as well localized as somatic or dermatomal pain; therefore, patients with chronic pain and visceral pathology may have trouble localizing their pain. Furthermore, because the cervix, uterus, and adnexae have the same metameric innervation as the bladder, distal ureter, lower ileum, colon, and rectosigmoid, it is often difficult to determine if visceral abdominopelvic pain is of gynecologic, urologic, or intestinal origin (9).

About 60% of women with CPP have unilateral pain and about 40% have bilateral or diffuse pain (10). Lateral pelvic pain is commonly of adnexal or sigmoid colonic origin (11). However, because of the long mesentery of the sigmoid colon, pain associated with it may be variable in location and be right, left, or even midline lower abdominal pain. Severe distention of the left hemicolon usually localizes to the left lower quadrant. Similarly, pain associated with distention of the right hemicolon is periumbilical or

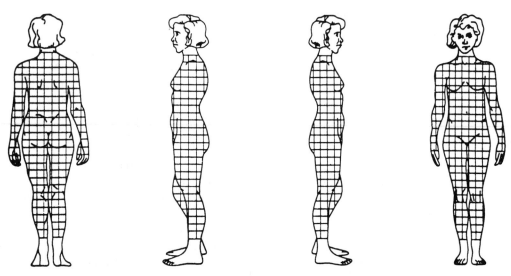

FIGURE 2.1. Example of a human figure on which the patient may "map" her areas of pain.

TABLE 2.1. MUSCULOSKELETAL ORIGINS OF PELVIC PAIN AND REFERRED PAIN SITES

Structure	Innervation	Referred Pain Sites	Common Disorders
Hip	T12–S1	Lower abdomen; anterior medial thigh; knee	Degenerative joint disease; capsular stiffness or inflammation; bursitis
Lumbar ligaments, facets, discs	T12–S1	Low back; posterior thigh and calf; lower abdomen; lateral trunk; buttock	Degenerative joint disease; capsular entrapments; instability; herniation; capsular stiffness or inflammation
Sacroiliac joints	L4–S3	Posterior thigh; buttock; pelvic floor	Acute strain; laxity; displacement
Abdominal muscles	T5–L1	Abdomen; anteromedial thigh; sternum	Weakness; strain; diastasis; trigger points
Iliopsoas	L1–L4	Lateral trunk; lower abdomen; low back; anterior thigh	Adaptive shortening; trigger points; protective guarding
Piriformis	L5–S3	Low back; buttock; pelvic floor	Adaptive shortening; trigger points; protective guarding
Pubococcygeus	S1–S4	Pelvic floor, vagina; rectum; buttock	Adaptive shortening; weakness; lengthening strain; trigger points
Obturator internus and externus	L3–S2	Pelvic floor; buttock; anterior thigh	Adaptive shortening; protective guarding; weakness
Quadratus lumborum	T12–L3	Anterior lateral trunk; anterior thigh; lower abdomen	Adaptive shortening; weakness

From Baker PK. Musculoskeletal origins of chronic pelvic pain. *Obstet Gynecol Clin NA* 1993;20:719–742, with permission.

midline suprapubic, but with severe distention localizes to the right lower quadrant (9). Midline or central infraumbilical pain may be secondary to the uterus, uterosacral ligaments, posterior cul-de-sac, or cervix, but may also be caused by mild distention of either the left or right hemicolon. Pain associated with pathology of the small bowel is usually localized to the periumbilical area, but this clearly may be confused with pain from the reproductive or urinary tract. Pain from the bladder or vagina may localize over the mons pubis, public bone, or groin. Back pain in the lower sacral and midline areas may be from the uterosacral ligaments, posterior cul-de-sac, or cervix. Complaints of pain both ventrally and dorsally often suggest intrapelvic pathology, whereas only dorsal low back pain suggest an orthopedic or musculoskeletal origin (Fig. 2.2).

Pain located in the distribution of a cutaneous nerve may suggest an entrapped nerve. With the iliohypogastric or ilioinguinal nerve this pain radiation runs medially along

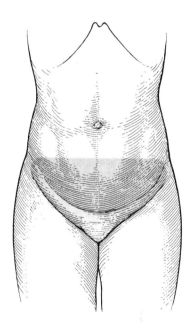
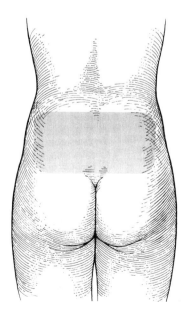

FIGURE 2.2. Pain of gynecologic origin is usually referred to both the anterior abdomen and the posterior low back.

the lower abdomen into the labia or upper inner aspect of the thigh.

It is common to obtain a history of a progressively larger anatomic area of involvement of pain over time. Although the reasons for this are not completely clear, a simplistic explanation may be that it represents a breakdown or "wearing out" of the physiologic systems that deal with pain.

Radiation of pain should also be asked about. It is common for the lateral pain of adnexal origin to radiate down the anterior or anteromedial thigh (11). Pain of uterine or cervical origin, including dysmenorrhea, may also radiate down the anteromedial thigh. Radiation down the posterior thigh is often associated with musculoskeletal problems. Sciatica associated with lumbosacral disease is a classic example of this.

The location of pain is not predictive of positive or negative findings at the time of laparoscopic evaluation. For example, in Baker and Symonds' series of 60 women with CPP and a negative laparoscopy, 45% had unilateral pain, 20% bilateral pain, and 35% generalized pain (12). However, consistent description of pain in the same location for more than 6 months correlates with laparoscopically visualized abnormalities. In a series of such CPP patients reported by Kresch, 83% had abnormal findings (13).

How severe is your pain? Because of pain's subjectivity, the patient should use some type of rating system to evaluate its severity or intensity with a degree of objectivity and reproducibility. In clinical practice, a simple rating system of no pain, mild pain, moderate pain, severe pain is often used. This simple rating system is not very sensitive to smaller changes in pain severity and, therefore, may be less useful in following patients' responses during treatment. The American Fertility Society (now the Society of Reproductive Medicine, Birmingham, AL) has suggested for endometriosis-associated pain the rating system used in the McGill Pain Questionnaire that uses mild, discomforting, distressing, horrible, and excruciating as descriptors of pain severity. In the American Fertility Society system these descriptors are noted as A through E, respectively, whereas in the McGill Pain Questionnaire they are given numeric values of 1 through 5 (Fig. 2.3).

Numerical scales are more useful and reliable for research and in chronic pain clinics (4). The best studied numerical scale is the visual analog scale (VAS), which uses a 10-cm line with descriptive labels of pain severity at the ends. The patient marks the line at the point that best represents the severity of her pain (Fig. 2.4). The distance in centimeters from the beginning of the line to the patient's mark is a measure of her pain severity on a 0 to 10 scale. Slide "algometers" are also available that use a VAS measurement (Fig. 2.5). One of many commonly used adaptations of the VAS, which simplifies the measurement and the scale, is shown in Figure 2.6. This type of adaptation allows the patient to directly give a numerical rating to her pain and facilitates conversion to a verbal numerical rating system. Clear definitions of the end

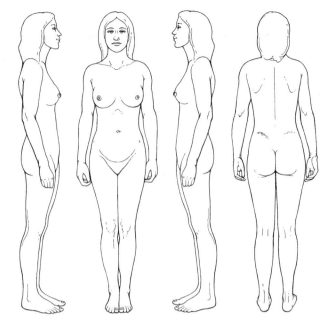

FIGURE 2.3. The pain map and pain rating system suggested by The American Fertility Society (now The Society of Reproductive Medicine) as "a clinical instrument to document the extent of endometriosis and pelvic pain." Describe the patient's symptoms of pain quality and position, and any limitation caused by these symptoms. Abbreviate quality of pain as: A, mild; B, discomforting; C, distressing; D, horrible; and E, excruciating. On these anatomic drawings, draw a *solid line* around the area(s) of pain described by the patient, and mark the most intense area(s) with an X.

points of the scale are of particular importance with the traditional VAS or its modifications, especially if used verbally. For verbal ratings, a 0 to 10 scale is most commonly used, with end points and scaling explained as 0 representing no pain, and 10 the worst pain imaginable. Some systems also add the rating of 4–5 as moderate pain (3). Although based on experimental evaluations, visual analog scales that use graphic representations seem superior to verbal scales. Verbal pain scores are usually easier to incorporate into clinical practice (4). Some have suggested visual and verbal scales with more detailed descriptors of pain severity assigned to each numerical value. An example of one such scale uses ratings of 0 as no pain, 1 as mild pain, 5 as moderate pain, 9 as severe pain requiring prescription pain medications but with ability to work, and 10 as incapacitating severe pain requiring bedrest and inability to work (14).

Another approach to quantifying pain severity is to utilize the effect of pain on ability to function as a measure of severity or intensity. An example of such a multidimensional pain score is shown in Table 2.2 (15).

Whatever pain severity scale is used, it is important to be consistent. The patient should be asked to rate her pain at the first visit, both as an indicator of her pain severity and as a baseline to evaluate her response to any treatments. Accurate records of pain levels and other symptoms in the patient's medical chart, as well as in a diary kept by the

Pain severity at its <u>WORST</u>

No
Pain

Worst Possible Pain
You Can Imagine

Pain severity at its <u>LEAST</u>

No
Pain

Worst Possible Pain
You Can Imagine

Pain severity at its <u>AVERAGE</u> level

No
Pain

Worst Possible Pain
You Can Imagine

FIGURE 2.4. Example of a visual analog scale that may be used to evaluate the severity of chronic pain. (The line should measure 10 cm in length.)

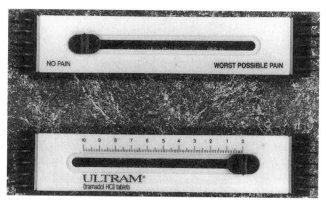

FIGURE 2.5. Example of a slide algometer that can be used to assess pain severity via a visual analog scale.

Pain severity at its <u>WORST</u>

0   1   2   3   4   5   6   7   8   9   10
No
Pain

Worst Possible Pain
You Can Imagine

Pain severity at its <u>LEAST</u>

0   1   2   3   4   5   6   7   8   9   10
No
Pain

Worst Possible Pain
You Can Imagine

Pain severity at its <u>AVERAGE</u> level

0   1   2   3   4   5   6   7   8   9   10
No
Pain

Worst Possible Pain
You Can Imagine

FIGURE 2.6. Example of a modification of the traditional visual analog scale that may be used to evaluate the severity of chronic pain.

patient, can be important (Fig. 2.7). Often as improvement occurs the patient may forget the severity of her previous symptoms (3).

Is your pain the same 24 hours a day, 7-days a week? Is your pain constant or intermittent? Determining the temporal pattern of pain is useful. Accurate records are useful during the initial history as well as during follow-up and treatment evaluations. Asking the patient to keep a diary of symptoms is sometimes helpful, with timing and severity of pain, medication use, and other potentially related factors noted (16). Doing this for 2 weeks prior to an office visit is often useful and yet not overly onerous for the patient.

TABLE 2.2. EXAMPLE OF A MULTIDIMENSIONAL PAIN SCORE THAT CAN BE USED TO INDICATE PAIN SEVERITY

Working ability	Unaffected = 0
	Rarely affected = 1
	Moderately affected = 2
	Clearly inhibited = 3
Coexistent symptoms	Absent = 0
	Present = 1
Need for analgesics	No = 0
	Rarely = 1
	Regularly = 2
	Ineffective = 3
Sum of scores	Mild = 0–3, Moderate = 4–5,
	Severe = 6–7

From Candiani GR, Fedele L, Vercellini P, et al. Presacral neurectomy for the treatment of pelvic pain associated with endometriosis: a controlled study. *Am J Obstet Gynecol* 1992;167:100–103, with permission.

Temporal characteristics that should be sought are whether the pain is constant, waxing and waning, intermittent, cyclic, or irregular (4). In one published series of women with CPP, 55% had acyclic pain and 45% had cyclic pain (12). Stress-related and musculoskeletal-associated pain may differ depending on the day of the week, corresponding with work or activity level. Muscular pain may have episodes of spasms. Often such musculoskeletal pain follows but does not accompany physical activity. Although pelvic pain of musculoskeletal origin may be constant, similar to the pain of musculoskeletal headaches, it is not characteristically constant. Rather it usually varies, even during the course of the day (4,17). For example, although arthritic conditions of the pelvis only occasionally present as CPP, in such cases pain improves during the course of the day. In contrast, pain associated with pelvic floor relaxation (prolapse problems) worsens during the course of the day as the woman is on her feet.

Vascular pain characteristically is periodic, lasting a few days or weeks (4). Vascular pain caused by ischemic bowel disease may present as abdominopelvic pain, but it is usually only in older women (over 70 years) with arteriosclerotic disease of more than one of the mesenteric vessels. It classically occurs 15 to 30 minutes after eating and lasts for several hours (9). Nerve injury pain may also be irregular, but is often in periods of short duration (Table 2.3). Chronic pain associated with abdominal wall hernias is usually intermittent, with associated abdominal distention (9).

What increases your pain? What decreases your pain? The patient should be asked about factors that provoke, intensify, and palliate her pain. The amount, type, and effectiveness of pain medications may be included in this part of the history, too. Examples of factors that may alter pain intensity include work, exercise, sitting, standing, lifting, lying down, heat or heating pad, ice packs, eating, menses, intercourse, urination, or defecation. After the patient answers an open-ended question about factors that affect her pain, it is important to ask specific questions about potential factors that the patient did not mention, especially bowel function, bladder function, and intercourse.

Activities that increase or decrease pain sometimes give clues as to possible etiologies or associated diseases. For example, rest often decreases pain of musculoskeletal or adnexal origin, but has no effect on pain of mostly psychological origin. The pain of pelvic congestion syndrome, which is related to posture, is least on arising from sleep or rest and worsens during the day or the longer the woman is on her feet. In contrast, pain associated with adenomyosis or endometriosis is not influenced as much by rest or time of day. Certain spicy foods or alcohol may worsen the pain associated with inter-

---

Name_____   Date Started_____

	Morning	Noon	Dinner	Bedtime
M				
Tu				
W				
Th				
F				
Sa				
Su				

Please Record
1. Pain intensity number:
    0 - No pain
    1 - Mild
    2 - Discomforting
    3 - Distressing
    4 - Horrible
    5 - Excruciating
2. Number of analgesics you have taken.
3. Please note any unusual symptoms, pains, or activities on back
4. Record hours slept in morning column

FIGURE 2.7. McGill Home Recording Card that can be used for the patient's diary of her pain.

TABLE 2.3. TEMPORAL CHARACTERISTICS OF PAIN CORRELATED WITH POSSIBLE SOURCES

Characteristics	Potential Sources
Both steady and intermittent	Visceral
Steady ache with periodic sharp superimposed pain	
Spasms	Muscular
Following physical activity	Musculoskeletal
Constant	Musculoskeletal
Throbbing	Vascular
Short shooting or jabbing	Nerve injury
Cramping, colicky, bloating	Small bowel

From Sternbach RA. Clinical aspects of pain. In: Sternbach RA, ed. *The psychology of pain*, 2nd ed. New York: Raven Press, 1986:223–237; Rapkin AJ, Mayer EA. Gastroenterologic causes of chronic pelvic pain. *Obstet Gynecol Clin NA* 1993;20:663–683, with permission.

stitial cystitis, but foods rarely affect pain associated with reproductive tract diseases. Similarly, certain foods, for example, fatty foods, may intensify pain associated with irritable bowel syndrome. Prolonged standing may particularly exacerbate pain associated with pelvic congestion syndrome or pelvic floor relaxation, as well as musculoskeletal diseases. Pain that is particularly increased by straining or lifting may suggest a hernia (9). Pain that is focal and positional may suggest association with adhesive disease.

The effect of menses on pain should be ascertained. Menstrual exacerbation has been reported to occur in more than one in four women with chronic pelvic pain (10). Although characteristically pain of gynecologic origin has premenstrual and menstrual exacerbation, the same may occasionally be true with pain of intestinal, urologic, or musculoskeletal origin, also (17). Menstrual exacerbation may occur with several different pain origins, not just those of the reproductive system.

A history of pain or increased pain with coitus is frequently sought during the history and varyingly interpreted as pathognomonic of psychological disease, marital problems, endometriosis, vulvodynia, and so on. In fact, dyspareunia is present in about 50% of women with chronic pelvic pain, but may not be revealed without directed questioning (10). It occurs with all of the noted problems as well as with irritable bowel disease, inflammatory bowel disease, interstitial cystitis, adhesions, and pelvic floor defects, and is not specific for any particular disease. If intercourse is painful, it is important to find out if pain is with entry at the outermost part of the vagina or if it is with deeper penetration high in the vagina or pelvis, or both. Per se, diseases associated with CPP do not generally cause entry dyspareunia, except as vaginismus secondary to deep dyspareunia. Dyspareunia occurring with deep penetration, lasting for several hours or more after coitus, or precipitating pelvic or abdominal pain may suggest endometriosis, abdominopelvic adhesions, or pelvic congestion syndrome. At laparoscopy, women with these complaints are significantly more likely to have endometriosis or

pelvic adhesions than women without such complaints (18). However, this type of dyspareunia is also common with lower urinary tract hypersensitivity, and visual laparoscopic findings are negative in these women (Chapter 31).

What is the quality or character of your pain? The quality or nature of pain should be sought, because such descriptors may have diagnostic value (4). Patients sometimes have difficulty with this part of the history and the physician may need to supply possible descriptive terms for the nature of the pain. The terms used in the McGill Pain Questionnaire are listed in Table 2.4; these may be useful. For example, the pain of cutaneous nerve entrapment is often described as sharp, piercing, or burning. Of course, location in the distribution of a specific nerve is further suggestion of this eti-

TABLE 2.4. MCGILL PAIN QUESTIONNAIRE DESCRIPTORS USED IN THE PAIN RATING INDEX (PRI)

From the following list of descriptive terms, please circle only one from each group that applies to your pain. (If none of the descriptive terms in a group applies to your pain, do not circle any in that group.)

1. Flickering
   Quivering
   Pulsing
   Throbbing
   Beating
   Pounding

2. Jumping
   Flashing
   Shooting

3. Pricking
   Boring
   Drilling
   Stabbing
   Lancinating

4. Sharp
   Cutting
   Lacerating

5. Pinching
   Pressing
   Gnawing
   Cramping
   Crushing

6. Tugging
   Pulling
   Wrenching

7. Hot
   Burning
   Scalding
   Searing

8. Tingling
   Itchy
   Smarting
   Stinging

9. Dull
   Sore
   Hurting
   Aching
   Heavy

10. Tender
    Taut
    Rasping
    Splitting

11. Tiring
    Exhausting

12. Sickening
    Suffocating

13. Fearful
    Frightful
    Terrifying

14. Punishing
    Grueling
    Cruel
    Vicious
    Killing

15. Wretched
    Blinding

16. Annoying
    Troublesome
    Miserable
    Intense
    Unbearable

17. Spreading
    Radiating
    Penetrating
    Piercing

18. Tight
    Numb
    Drawing
    Squeezing
    Tearing

19. Cool
    Cold
    Freezing

20. Nagging
    Nauseating
    Agonizing
    Dreadful
    Torturing

Groups 1 to 10 are sensory descriptors, groups 11 to 15 are affective descriptors, group 16 is evaluative, and groups 17 to 20 are supplementary.

ology. Nerve injury pain is often shooting, jabbing, or electric shocklike in quality. It may also be burning in nature or have associated skin hyperesthesia. Muscular pain may be aching in quality, worsening by remaining in one position for too long and with sharp, lancinating pain with changes in positions. Similar qualities of aching with occasional intermittent sharp and radiating pains may also be described with visceral pain. Visceral pain is usually described as being a "deep" or internal pain (4). With small bowel involvement, pain may be described as crampy, colicky, or bloating (9). Vascular pain, in nonpelvic pain syndromes, may be throbbing with vasodilation, as in migraine, or cramping with vasoconstriction, as in Raynaud's. Similar qualities may be observed with pelvic pain of vascular origin. The description of the sensation of pelvic pressure or "that everything is falling out" is classically associated with pelvic floor relaxation defects. However, the same description is also often given by women with contraction or spasm of the pelvic floor muscles (levator ani), whether in response to pelvic pain from some other source (e.g., endometriosis) or primarily from the levator ani owing to trigger points or to postural or musculoskeletal abnormalities.

When and how did your pain start and how has it changed? Many of the published series of CPP patients show median pain duration of 2 to 5 years when medical help is sought (19). Although the duration of pain probably has little diagnostic value, it may have prognostic value. In many patients with chronic pain the pain worsens in intensity, changes in nature, and expands to involve larger areas of the body over time. The prognosis is worse in patients whose pain has significantly expanded to involve areas not originally involved in pain.

If a specific precipitating factor(s) can be found, it may aid in diagnosis. For example, an immediately antecedent trauma, such as a fall, surgery, or motor vehicle accident, suggests a musculoskeletal cause. Pain that started with a pregnancy or immediately postpartum may suggest peripartum pelvic pain syndrome (PPPPS). This syndrome is thought to be owing to strain of the ligaments in the pelvis and lower spine from a combination of factors, including specific hormonal changes, damage to pelvic ligaments, muscle weakness, and the weight of the fetus and gravid uterus (20). Pain that started at or soon after menarche as dysmenorrhea, progressed to premenstrual pain, and then became constant suggests endometriosis. If pain started soon after a physical or sexual assault, it may have significant musculoskeletal or psychological components.

What prior evaluations or treatments have you had for your pain? Have any of the previous treatments helped? A thorough history about prior treatments or evaluations can be time-consuming in women with chronic pelvic pain, because they have often been through extensive prior evaluations and treatments. An accurate compilation of this record may be extremely useful in suggesting associated or etiologic diseases. If nothing else, it avoids repeating invasive and expensive diagnostic and therapeutic procedures. For example, the randomized trial of Peters et al. showed quite clearly that performing a laparoscopy in women who had prior negative laparoscopies or laparotomies did nothing to improve the outcome of patients compared to multidisciplinary pain therapy without laparoscopy (21).

Patients should be asked to evaluate their response to prior treatments, including the duration of any positive responses. For example, a good response to gonadotropin-releasing hormone agonist (GnRH-a), that was followed by a pregnancy and 2 to 3 years of pain relief, suggests that GnRH-a therapy is a good option for the treatment of recurrent CPP. Similarly, a good response to surgery may suggest repeat surgery is an option for recurrent pain. An example of a rating scale that may be used to evaluate response to surgical treatment is shown in Table 2.5.

Prior medical and psychiatric treatments without response may suggest musculoskeletal problems associated with the pain. Because of the medical and psychological bias of most physicians and the fact that pain associated with musculoskeletal disorders is similar in many ways to that of reproductive or gastrointestinal origin, musculoskeletal problems as major contributors to CPP are often not considered during the primary evaluation (17). Thus, it not uncommon to learn that many medical and psychological interventions have been attempted without a full evaluation of the musculoskeletal system by a physical therapist. Musculoskeletal problems are believed to be of paramount importance in the pathophysiology of CPP by many clinicians who care for women with CPP.

How has the pain affected your quality of life? Although including an evaluation of the effect of pain on the woman's quality of life is not always helpful in differential diagnosis, it certainly aids in the evaluation of the severity of pain, as well as helping in setting goals for treatment. Many women with CPP have had their lives totally disrupted by their pain, resulting in job loss, marital discord and divorce, isolation from friends and family, and so on. Although distressing, it is important to elicit such information.

An example of a screening tool for evaluating quality of life in women with CPP is shown in Figure 2.8.

TABLE 2.5. A SELF-RATING QUESTIONNAIRE FOR POSTOPERATIVE FOLLOW-UP

0. I am completely relieved of my pain.
1. The operation has helped a great deal, but every now and then I have some pain. It does not influence my life.
2. The operation has helped somewhat, but I still have pain and it influences my life.
3. The operation was of no help of me; the pain has continued unchanged.
4. The pain has been worse since the operation.

Rate your overall quality of life?

0   1   2   3   4   5   6   7   8   9   10
Very Poor   Excellent
(As bad as it can get)   (As good as it can get)

How much does pain specifically affect your quality of life?

0   1   2   3   4   5   6   7   8   9   10
No impact   Very large impact

Rate how much your pain interferes with each of the following:

General Activity:

0   1   2   3   4   5   6   7   8   9   10
Does Not   Completely
Interfere   Interferes

Ability to Work or Go to School:

0   1   2   3   4   5   6   7   8   9   10
Does Not   Completely
Interfere   Interferes

Normal Family Activities:

0   1   2   3   4   5   6   7   8   9   10
Does Not   Completely
Interfere   Interferes

Sleep:

0   1   2   3   4   5   6   7   8   9   10
Does Not   Completely
Interfere   Interferes

Ability to Enjoy Life:

0   1   2   3   4   5   6   7   8   9   10
Does Not   Completely
Interfere   Interferes

Mood:

0   1   2   3   4   5   6   7   8   9   10
Does Not   Completely
Interfere   Interferes

FIGURE 2.8. Example of a screening tool for evaluating the effect of chronic pelvic pain on quality of life and usual daily activities.

MEASURING PAIN

The measurement of pain in man is essential for the evaluation of methods to control pain.

Melzack, 1975 (22).

In pain centers or practices specializing in the care of women with chronic pelvic pain, it seems crucial that pain be evaluated as fully and completely as possible. For example, much of the published work on endometriosis-associated pelvic pain is flawed by its very limited evaluation of pain. Hence, its relevance in trying to characterize the response of CPP to various therapies is also quite limited.

Particularly in centers specializing in pelvic pain or doing research on CPP, an instrument like the McGill Pain Questionnaire (MPQ) should be used. Assessments with all five of the components of the MPQ are useful in the evaluation and follow-up of pain. This instrument or others similar to it may overcome the limitations imposed by our simpler measuring tools for pain. These simple tools, like the VAS, invariably treat pain as though it were a specific sensory quality that only varies in intensity. Such a unifocal assessment of pain ignores the affective and semantic components of pain and ignores the recognized fact that emotional responses to pain significantly influence the intensity of pain. The MPQ addresses this concern by including descriptors to assess the affective, evaluative, and sensory components of pain experience.

The McGill Pain Questionnaire has five components: the Pain Rating Index (PRI), the Present Pain Index (PPI), a temporal evaluation, a pain map, and a listing of pain medications used (22). The PRI of the MPQ consists of descriptors of pain and may be used to more formally quantify the patient's interpretation of her pain according to sensory, affective, evaluative, and supplementary terms (Table 2.4). These descriptors are attempts to evaluate the sensory (temporal, spatial, pressure, and thermal), affective (tension, fear, and autonomic), and evaluative (subjective overall intensity of the pain experience) aspects of pain.

The first ten groups of the PRI are *sensory* descriptors, the next five are *affective* descriptors, the sixteenth group is *evaluative,* and the last four are *supplementary* descriptors. Although there are a number of ways to score the PRI, the simplest that still maintains correlation is the rank score (PRI(r)), calculated by giving each selected term in each group a numerical value based on its rank (first term = 1, second term = 2, etc.), then totaling the values for each category and for all the groups. Patients only choose applicable descriptors and need not select a descriptor from each group. However, they are not to select more than one descriptor from a group. In an early evaluation of these descriptors, Melzack found that of 248 patients with various pain syndromes (only 25 had "menstrual pain"), the percentage choosing a group of descriptors ranged from a low of 13% (group 19-cool, cold, freezing) to a high of 94% (group 16-annoying, troublesome, miserable, intense, unbearable).

A second component of the MPQ is the evaluation of the severity of pain (PPI). This questionnaire utilizes the descriptive terms mild, discomforting, distressing, horrible, and

TABLE 2.6. PAIN SEVERITY RATING ON THE MCGILL PAIN QUESTIONNAIRE (PPI)

People agree that the following five words represent pain of increasing intensity:

1	2	3	4	5
Mild	Discomforting	Distressing	Horrible	Excruciating

To answer the questions below, write the number of the most appropriate word in the space beside the question.

1. Which word describes your pain right now? ———
2. Which word describes it at its worst? ———
3. Which word describes it when it is least? ———
4. Which word describes the worst toothache you ever had? ———
5. Which word describes the worst headache you ever had? ———
6. Which word describes the worst stomachache you ever had? ———

TABLE 2.7. MCGILL PAIN QUESTIONNAIRE: TEMPORAL QUALITIES AND FACTORS THAT AFFECT PAIN

1. Which word or words would you use to describe the pattern of your pain?

(1)	(2)	(3)
Continuous	Rhythmic	Brief
Steady	Periodic	Momentary
Constant	Intermittent	Transient

2. What kind of things relieve your pain?
3. What kind of things increase your pain?

excruciating, giving them numerical values of 1, 2, 3, 4, and 5, respectively (Table 2.6). Melzack found that patients' ratings of changes of pain on both the descriptor ratings (PRI) and severity ratings (PPI) were very consistent (22).

The next of the five components of the MPQ is an evaluation of the temporal properties of pain. This asks the patient to choose descriptors from three different groups of three terms each describing duration and patterns of pain. Table 2.7 is an example of the MPQ for temporal qualities of pain.

The other two components of the MPQ ask the patient to do a pain map on a unisex diagram, similar to the pain mapping already discussed, and to tell of any pain medications that have been used for treatment (Fig. 2.9). The amount, type, and effectiveness of pain medications are included in this part of the history.

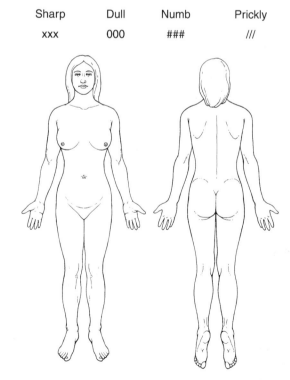

Sharp	Dull	Numb	Prickly
xxx	000	###	///

FIGURE 2.9. The pain map and symbols used in the McGill Pain Questionnaire (modified for use in women).

TABLE 2.8. CRITERIA FOR CHRONIC PAIN SYNDROME

1. Chronic pain (usually pain of 6 or more months' duration)
2. Pain out of proportion to pathology
3. Altered physical activities at home or work (e.g., stopping running or playing tennis, stopping working)
4. At least one vegetative sign of depression, usually early morning awakening not caused by pain
5. Significantly altered emotional roles within the family, or identification of the patient's illness as the most significant problem the family faces. Examples of alterations of emotional roles are:
   a. Family decision-making
   b. Supervision and discipline of children
   c. Nurturing of children and partner

CHRONIC PAIN SYNDROME

Pain perception is the final result of a complex series of events: physical stimulation, sensory perception, neuroregulatory modulation, and psychological processes. Some chronic pain sufferers seem to maintain a good level of physical and psychological function despite significant pain, whereas others develop a set of emotional and behavioral characteristics that is called chronic pain syndrome (CPS) (Table 2.8). The diagnosis and treatment of CPS can be critical to the successful treatment of CPP. Although not well studied, it seems reasonable to include psychological evaluation and treatment from the outset in women with CPS. An algorithm, suggested by Steege, utilizing the presence of CPS as a determinant of evaluation pathway is shown in Figure 2.10.

When the history clearly reveals evidence of CPS, it is important to directly discuss this with the patient. The syndrome should be explained in terms that she can understand. In doing this it is important to maintain good rapport. Discussing CPS in the framework of pain theory, such as the gate theory, is sometimes helpful. It is not helpful to attempt to determine the relative contribution to CPS of physical versus psychological factors; the patient is best served if she understands the importance of both factors in causing CPS.

GYNECOLOGIC AND OBSTETRIC HISTORY

How old are you? The woman's age may be a helpful part of the history in regard to reproductive system involvement in CPP. Women with CPP associated with reproductive system disease tend to be of reproductive age (i.e., 15 to 50 years of age). Reports of series of women with chronic pelvic pain show that most women with CPP are of reproductive age, with mean and median ages of 27 to 34 years; therefore, the possibility of reproductive disease must usually be considered (12,23–25).

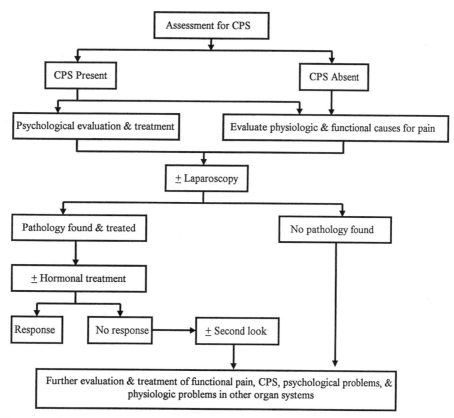

FIGURE 2.10. An algorithm for the evaluation of chronic pelvic pain based on the presence or absence of CPS.

Women older than reproductive age are much less likely to have abnormalities of the reproductive tract as etiologic factors for their pain. However, there are reports of endometriosis in postmenopausal women, with or without estrogen replacement therapy; therefore, although rare, this diagnosis must still be considered (26–28).

How many pregnancies have you had? Did you have problems with pelvic pain or low back pain during or right after any of your pregnancies? Pregnancy and childbirth may be traumatic events to the musculoskeletal system, especially of the pelvis and back, and are possible causes or contributors to CPP. There is clear evidence that hormonal changes of pregnancy cause laxity of ligaments and this may lead to pain associated with insufficiency of pelvic ligaments. Historical risk factors associated with pregnancy and pain include lumbar lordosis, delivery of a large infant, muscle weakness and poor physical conditioning, a difficult delivery, vacuum or forceps delivery, and use of gynecologic stirrups for delivery. These factors are believed to increase the chance of severe stretching with subsequent strain and damage to the ligaments and joints of the pelvis and lower spine, resulting in *peripartum pelvic pain syndrome* (PPPPS).

PPPPS may be defined as pain in the pelvic region, with or without radiation, that started during pregnancy or within the first 3 months after delivery, and for which no clear diagnosis is available to explain the pain (20). It is characterized by pain predominantly around the sacroiliac joints and the pubic symphysis, but may also extend to other parts of the pelvis, upper legs, and occasionally the lower legs. Figure 2.11 shows the distribution of pain in a series of women with PPPPS (20).

PPPPS is suggested by a history of onset of pain during pregnancy or the postpartum period (Fig. 2.12). The pain may be of continuous or disabling quality, particularly when turning in bed, walking, lifting, getting up from a chair, standing for 30 minutes or more, or climbing stairs (20,39). However, it should be noted that 15% to 25% of gravid women have symptoms suggestive of PPPPS and about 50% have low back pain at some time during pregnancy (this is three to eight times the frequency of low back pain in nonpregnant women) (20,39). Thus, women with CPP may coincidentally have a history of pain during pregnancy and not have PPPPS.

Pelvic floor relaxation may occasionally be a cause of CPP. A history of prior pregnancy, especially multiparity, is a risk factor for pelvic floor relaxation with cystocele, rectocele, enterocele, or uterine descensus. Parity may also be a contributor or cause of pelvic congestion syndrome.

Do you have pain with your periods? Does your pain occur only with your menses? Does your pain change with your menstrual cycle? Three of the more common gynecologic diagnoses associated with CPP, endometriosis, adenomyosis, and pelvic congestion, correlate with the menstrual cycle and have similar premenstrual patterns of pain or pain severity (Fig. 2.13). Dysmenorrhea is generally more severe with endometriosis, although it may occur with adenomyosis as well. Dysmenorrhea is not characteristic of pelvic congestion.

With adenomyosis, dysmenorrhea is usually the first type of pain present, but with time the pain gradually becomes present in the mid- to late-luteal phase of the menstrual cycle, as well. It is unusual for the pain associated with adenomyosis to occur in the proliferative phase of the cycle. Endometriosis-associated pain also starts as menstrual pain, then progresses to include more and more of the luteal phase, but in many women progresses to constant pain with premenstrual and menstrual exacerbation. Pain associated with pelvic congestion is typically worst premenstrually,

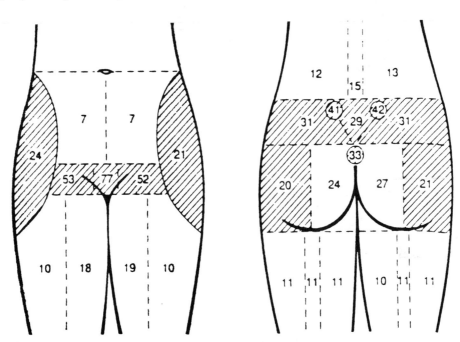

FIGURE 2.11. Location of pain in 394 women with PPPPS. Numbers represent percentages of women experiencing pain in the specific area. The shaded area represents the required pain locations to diagnose PPPPS.

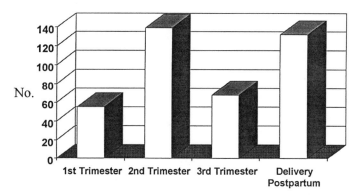

FIGURE 2.12. Timing during pregnancy of the onset of pelvic pain in women with PPPPS. Based on a retrospective study of 394 women with PPPPS.

and although menstrual pain may be present, menses are not usually the time of most severe pain.

Mittleschmerz, as described by Fehling in 1881, is the lower abdominal pain that occurs at midcycle associated with ovulation. It is believed to be owing to the release of fluid and blood from the ovarian follicle with ovulation. It is self-limiting and rarely lasts longer than 12 to 24 hours (30). However, it may recur on a monthly basis and present as CPP.

Although it is gynecologic pain that is characteristically thought of with premenstrual and menstrual exacerbations, the same may also be true with pain of intestinal or musculoskeletal origin. For example, about three-fourths of women with PPPPS report increased pain around the time of their menses (20). Irritable bowel syndrome symptom severity may also be exacerbated premenstrually in some women, with a cyclic pattern of pain that may be confused with pain of gynecologic origin (9).

Have you ever been diagnosed with or treated for a sexually transmitted disease or pelvic inflammatory disease? It is pertinent to ask about prior sexually transmitted diseases (STD) or pelvic inflammatory disease (PID) because it is estimated that 18% to 27% of all women with acute PID will develop CPP (31). Epidemiologic studies suggest that PID is most frequent among teenagers and women less than 25 years of age, which is about a decade younger than the mean age of women with CPP (32).

Clinically, the pain of chronic PID is usually related to coitus and physical activity and is acyclic, although there may be premenstrual or menstrual exacerbation. Little has been written about the actual mechanisms by which CPP results from PID. No clear explanations have been found to explain why most women with reproductive organ damage secondary to acute PID do not develop CPP (33).

A history of HIV infection or AIDS may be important to consider. There is a report of Burkitt's lymphoma presenting as ovarian disease with severe pelvic and rectal pain (34).

Although neither a sexually transmitted disease nor a common diagnosis in the United States, tuberculous PID must be remembered as a potential diagnosis in patients with CPP, especially because the incidence of tuberculosis (TB) has increased in association with human immunodeficiency virus (HIV) and acquired immunodeficiency syndrome (AIDS). As many as 25% of women with pulmonary TB have pelvic TB, and about 25% of women with pelvic tuberculosis will have CPP (35,36).

What form of birth control do you use or have you used in the past? Hormonal contraceptive therapy may have masked gynecologic pain associated with diseases such as endometriosis or adenomyosis. Asking about prior use may reveal the onset or exacerbation of pain to have correlated with discontinuation of hormonal contraception. This is not an unusual history that may lead women to attribute their pain to tubal sterilization, because they stop their contraception after the sterilization. Also, if hormonal contraception is currently being used, then it is less likely that these medications will offer a therapeutic option for CPP.

A history of other contraceptive methods may also be relevant. There is a report of an intrauterine device (IUD) fragment as the cause of pain in the one of 122 CPP patients reported by Reiter et al (37). After removal and doxycycline therapy the patient had pain relief.

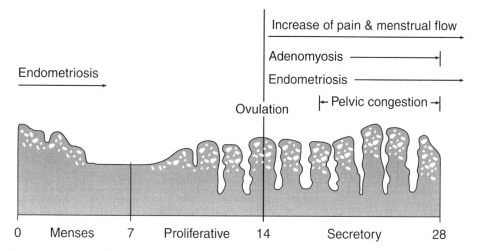

FIGURE 2.13. Characteristic patterns of pain with endometriosis, pelvic congestion, and adenomyosis.

Have you ever had any kind of surgery? Obviously, a past history of surgery for pain may lead to the consideration of recurrence or inadequate surgery of the specific disease that was treated. Past surgical history, however, may be pertinent other than for the specific diagnosis for which the surgery was performed. For example, spillage of gallstones at the time of laparoscopic and open cholecystectomy is believed to have been the cause of CPP of 3 years' duration in a 23-year-old woman and of 1 year's duration in a 39-year-old woman. Multiple stones, with significant pelvic inflammatory reaction, were found and removed in these two cases. Pain was relieved at 6 and 12 month follow-up, respectively, in these two women (38,39).

Past history of a Marshall-Marchietti-Kranz procedure for urinary incontinence may also be significant. CPP with localization to the pubic symphysis may suggest osteitis pubis or even osteomyelitis. Several cases have been reported of osteomyelitis long after surgery presenting without fever but with altered gait and significant pelvic pain. In suspected cases aggressive diagnostic evaluation with biopsy and needle aspiration guided by computer-assisted tomography is advised (40).

A prior history of cervical surgery for dysplasia may be relevant. There is a report of cervical stenosis after cold knife conization, with resultant hematometra and CPP. The patient had relief of pain after cervical dilation and uterine evacuation (37).

A history of a prior hysterectomy is common in women with CPP of more than 1 year's duration. One published series of CPP patients showed that 58% of women with more than 1 year of CPP had undergone a hysterectomy, compared to only 26% of women with less than 1 year's duration of pain (41). If the patient did not have pain prior to the hysterectomy, then ovarian retention syndrome (residual ovary syndrome) or pelvic adhesive disease may be considered. In women treated with hysterectomy for CPP without any extrauterine pathology, about 25% have persistence or recurrence of pain (42).

More generically, any past history of a laparotomy may be pertinent because of the possibility of an incisional hernia. Although not a common contributor to CPP, an incisional or ventral hernia may occasionally result in chronic abdominopelvic pain (37). This is more likely if the surgery was complicated by a postoperative wound infection or if the incision was vertical (9).

Also, neuropathies of surgical nerve entrapments may present with abdominopelvic pain, particularly of the iliohypogastric and ilioinguinal nerves with Pfannenstiel incisions.

NEUROMUSCULOSKELETAL HISTORY

Have you noticed any weakness or numbness? Neuropathies and nerve injuries, for example, from a herniated disc, do not generally result in pelvic pain that suggests pelvic pathology. However, occasionally patients presenting with severe low back pain and pelvic pain of several months' duration, on complete evaluation are found to have a herniated disc. Additionally, patients with multiple sclerosis have pain problems and occasionally may present with abdominopelvic pain as part of their symptom complex. Significant symptoms of weakness or numbness suggest the need for neurological evaluation.

Have you ever had any major injuries, severe falls or slips? Prior to the onset of your pain did you suffer any trauma, falls, or slips? Questions such as these should be asked because a history of prior low back pain or injury, a motor vehicle accident, or a fall preceding the onset of CPP may suggest the pain is associated with musculoskeletal pathology or injury (43).

Is your pain only in the front or only in the back? Pelvic pain of musculoskeletal origin may occur in both the anterior abdominopelvis and low back, or only in the low back. However, it is unusual for musculoskeletal pain to occur only in the anterior abdominopelvic area. For example, in one series of cases of musculoskeletal pain only 18% presented with only anterior pelvic pain without low back pain (20).

Are their specific physical activities that aggravate or ease your pain? Musculoskeletal pain is often aggravated by specific positional changes, physical activities, movements, prolonged standing, or prolonged sitting (43). For example, in one study of musculoskeletal pain owing to pelvic joint and ligament relaxation, 90% of women noted worsening of pain on standing for 30 minutes (Table 2.9) (20). However, pain associated with pelvic relaxation, pelvic congestion syndrome, or adhesions may also change with physical

TABLE 2.9. SOME ACTIVITIES OF DAILY LIVING THAT PROVOKED PAIN IN 394 WOMEN WITH PELVIC PAIN OF MUSCULOSKELETAL ORIGIN THAT STARTED DURING PREGNANCY OR DELIVERY

Activity	Percent
Standing for 30 minutes	90
Carrying a full shopping bag	86
Standing on one leg (e.g., to put on pants)	81
Walking for 30 minutes	81
Climbing stairs	79
Turning over in bed	74
Sexual intercourse	68
Riding a bicycle for 30 minutes	63
Bending forward	62
Stepping into and out of bed	62
Driving a car for 30 minutes	52
Swimming	51
Sitting on a favorite chair for 30 minutes	49
Traveling by public transport	46
Lying in bed for 30 minutes	8

From Mens JMA, Vleeming A, Stoeckart R, et al. Understanding peripartum pelvic pain: implications of a patient survey. *Spine* 1996;21:1363–1370, with permission.

activity; therefore, such a correlation is not specific to musculoskeletal disease.

GASTROINTESTINAL HISTORY

How often do you have a bowel movement? The number of potential gastrointestinal symptoms that can be explored in women with chronic pelvic pain is long. A thorough review often eliminates wasted radiologic evaluations; most women with gastrointestinal-associated pelvic pain have normal upper gastrointestinal and barium enema x-ray studies. The frequency of bowel movements is important to ask. Simply asking about constipation or diarrhea is insufficient. Some women have bowel movements once a week and think it is normal, but only rarely is this so. Bowel movements less than once every 3 days represent a form of constipation in most women, especially if the appearance and character of the stool is abnormal. This may be the result of poor diet, social factors, inadequate fluid intake, irritable bowel syndrome, or megacolon. Constipation may be a cause or contributor to CPP. It is also important to know if laxatives are used chronically to have bowel movements.

Bowel movements may also occur too frequently. Three or more times per day is almost always abnormal, especially if the appearance and character of the stool is abnormal. This may be associated with irritable bowel syndrome, inflammatory bowel disease, malignancy, or enterocolitis, and may cause or contribute to CPP.

What is the appearance of your bowel movements? Some patients have trouble describing their bowel movements and may be embarrassed to do so. Directed questions may be helpful: "Are they small and hard, loose and runny, formed and soft, formed and hard? What color are your bowel movements? Are they bloody or tarry or mucus-like?" Abnormal stools aid in determining if the patient has constipation, irritable bowel syndrome, gastrointestinal bleeding, inflammatory bowel disease, diverticulitis, and so on.

Does your pain increase or decrease with bowel movements? Although pain associated with diseases other than those of the gastrointestinal tract can vary with bowel movements (e.g., endometriosis and ovarian cancer), such increases or decreases with the need to defecate or with passage of bowel movements or flatus are characteristic of gastrointestinal disease. Decreased pain associated with defecation is a characteristic of irritable bowel syndrome. Pain may be increased with diverticulitis.

Do you have to strain to have a bowel movement? Patients with constipation and with irritable bowel syndrome characteristically have this symptom. Obstruction caused by endometriosis or malignancy may also cause this symptom.

Do you have urgency of bowel movements? Urgency of defecation is most characteristic of inflammatory bowel disease, irritable bowel syndrome, and enterocolitis. How often this symptom occurs, when present, is also important

to ascertain. It tends to be more constant with inflammatory bowel disease and enterocolitis.

Do you feel like you completely empty with bowel movements? The sensation of fullness and incomplete emptying is a diagnostic characteristic of irritable bowel disease (9). Patients with inflammatory bowel disease or diverticulitis may also have this symptom.

Do you have bloating or abdominal distention? Although these symptoms are not specific to gastrointestinal disease, their presence, particularly if the previous questions elicited gastrointestinal symptoms, leads the physician to consider irritable bowel syndrome, inflammatory bowel disease, diverticulitis, or chronic constipation as likely diagnoses. Gynecologic malignancies, with or without ascites, as well as gastrointestinal cancer may also cause these symptoms.

UROLOGIC HISTORY

How often do you usually urinate during the daytime? A 24-hour voiding diary is useful in women with chronic pelvic pain and any suggestion of voiding or urinary tract symptoms (44). Voiding five or more times in 12 hours may be considered increased or abnormal frequency (45). Almost all women with interstitial cystitis (greater than 95%) have chronic urinary frequency, and these women average voiding about every 60 minutes during the daytime (46). More than 50% of women with chronic urethral syndrome complain of frequency (47). Bladder tumors, especially carcinoma *in situ,* may cause symptoms similar to those of interstitial cystitis and chronic urethral syndrome (48).

How often do you usually get up at nighttime to urinate? Urinating two or more times per night is considered abnormal unless the patient is on medications that may account for nocturia (45). Early nighttime frequency may be owing to sensory disorders of the urethra or bladder, such as chronic urethral syndrome, acute urethritis, or cystitis. For example, patients with chronic urethral syndrome usually only get up once or, at most, twice at night to void and this is usually early nighttime voiding (49). Constant voiding throughout the night suggests a limited bladder capacity owing to intrinsic disease of the bladder wall, such as occurs with interstitial cystitis (44). In fact, the absence of significant nocturia makes the diagnosis of interstitial cystitis suspect, because greater than 95% of women with interstitial cystitis have nocturia (44,50). Again, bladder tumors may cause similar symptoms.

Do you have urgency when you need to urinate? Urgency is a characteristic symptom of bladder inflammation, whether owing to urinary tract infection, chronic urethral syndrome, interstitial cystitis, or tumor (47). About 70% of women with interstitial cystitis and about 60% with chronic urethral syndrome have urgency (47,50). Irritable bladder syndrome and unstable bladder (detrusor instability) may also cause urgency.

Do you have pain during urination? Pain with urination occurs with chronic urethral syndrome, recurrent urinary tract infections, and interstitial cystitis (50,51). It may also occur acutely with numerous disorders, such as urinary tract infection, vaginitis, and herpes simplex. Previoiding and postvoiding exacerbation of pain suggest possible urologic contributions to CPP (37).

Do you feel like you completely empty your bladder when you urinate? Incomplete emptying, often with hesitancy, may suggest chronic urethral syndrome, pelvic floor relaxation, pelvic floor pain syndrome, lower urinary tract hyperesthesia, or obstructive disorders of the urethra or vesical neck (44).

Do you have problems urinating after intercourse? In addition to dyspareunia, patients with chronic urethral syndrome often experience difficulty voiding after coitus (44). Patients with interstitial cystitis may also complain of this symptom, but less prominently (3).

Have you frequently been treated for urinary tract infections? A history of recurrent urinary tract infections associated with negative urine cultures, or no cultures, may suggest chronic urethral syndrome or interstitial cystitis (44). In fact, most women with interstitial cystitis have had their symptoms for 3 to 7 years and have been treated for recurrent urinary tract infections repetitively prior to the diagnosis being established (48). A history of any procedures such as meatotomy, urethrotomy, or urethral dilations may also be significant (3).

PSYCHOSOCIAL HISTORY

A complete psychosocial evaluation involves extensive interviews of the patient and her family or partner, questionnaires, behavioral observation, and psychological testing evaluations with instruments such as the Minnesota Multiphasic Personality Inventory and Beck Depression Inventory. Clearly, this usually requires a psychologist, or similarly educated professional, and cannot always be done initially, nor is it always necessary. However, some degree of psychosocial history is always an important part of the history in the woman with CPP. The following questions represent a minimal evaluation.

Are you depressed or anxious? The relationship of depression and chronic pain is complex and confusing. For example, the common association of depression and chronic pelvic pain may be explained by the gate theory as owing to the dysregulation of neurotransmitters associated with depression, which "opens" the CNS gate, increasing sensitivity to nociception (2). Conversely, this model allows an explanation of chronic pain as a cause of depression: Chronic somatic nociception may deplete the descending CNS modulators of pain (e.g., endogenous opioids), and this depletion may biochemically lead to depression. Thus, potential mechanisms for depression leading to chronic

pelvic pain and for chronic pelvic pain leading to depression can be postulated, and there is neurophysiologic evidence to support both (2,52).

Such theoretical concepts may have clinical relevance. For example, depression is one of the predictors of pain severity identified in evaluating women with CPP (Table 2.10) (1). Also, Steege has found depression to be a significant indicator of the clinical responsiveness to treatment of chronic pelvic pain patients and has included it as one of the major criteria for diagnosing "chronic pain syndrome" (see preceding discussion) (5). Patients with chronic pain syndrome have a much poorer response to traditional treatment for pelvic pain, such as surgical lysis of abdominopelvic adhesions, than do pain patients without chronic pain syndrome. Furthermore, it has been clinically noted that major depressive illness is sometimes seen in chronic pain patients, via a cycle of pain, depression, and withdrawal.

Such observations have led to a search for identifiable psychosocial characteristics of chronic pelvic pain patients. Psychological interviews suggest these patients are anxious and depressed, and have low self-esteem and high dependency. Psychometric testing, for example, with the Minnesota Multiphasic Personality Inventory, shows that chronic pelvic pain patients have a characteristic personality profile, with high scores on the hysteria, hypochondriasis, and depression scales. These personality profiles are noted in patients in whom organic pathology can be found and in those in whom no such pathology is noted (53). Such psychological changes tend to maintain or increase the level of pain, regardless of the degree of physical disease. When pain treatment is successful, the high scores on hysteria, hypochondriasis, and depression revert to normal. However, scientific research on these patients has been difficult owing to the heterogeneity of patients with chronic pelvic pain (21).

Thus, it is important to seek evidence of depression in women with CPP. In addition to simply asking if the patient is depressed, the following symptoms that may suggest depression may be sought: (a) consistently depressed or

TABLE 2.10. PREDICTORS OF PAIN SEVERITY IN WOMEN WITH CHRONIC PELVIC PAIN

Predictor	Statistical Significance
Depression	<0.01
Prior abuse	<0.01
Spouse responses	—
Solicitous	<0.03
Punishing	<0.05
Marital adjustment	NS
Employment status	NS
Laparoscopic findings	—
Adhesions	NS
Endometriosis	NS

From Milburn A, Reiter RE, Rhamberg AT. Multidisciplinary approach to chronic pelvic pain. *Obstet Gynecol Clin NA* 1993;20:643–661, with permission.

irritable mood, (b) diminished interest in or pleasure from daily activities, (c) poor appetite, (d) weight loss, (e) overeating, (f) weight gain, (g) insomnia, (h) trouble falling asleep, (i) awakening during the night with inability to fall back to sleep, (j) sleeping too much or much more than usual, (k) feeling tired or having little energy, (l) feeling bad about oneself, (m) feelings of letting oneself or one's family down, (n) feelings of worthlessness, (o) feelings of excessive guilt, (p) inability to concentrate normally, (q) inability to make decisions, and (r) thoughts about death or committing suicide.

Are you taking any drugs? It is important to find out about medication use, as well as self-medication with street or illegal drugs. Alcohol use should also be included in this questioning. It is important that the patient understand that this information is important in trying to seek medical ways to control or alleviate pain, while avoiding untoward drug and medication interactions. A past history of substance abuse prior to a history of CPP may be particularly useful in planning treatment. Such women have a significant risk of noncompliant, overuse of prescription opioid pain medication if this is part of their treatment. Furthermore, the history of drug abuse frequently precedes any history of CPP. For example, in 13 women with a history of ever abusing drugs, nine had a history prior to their onset of CPP.

In the past have you been or are you now being abused physically or sexually? Are you safe? It has been suggested that sexual abuse might in some way be specifically related to the development of chronic pelvic pain. Although it is mechanistically tempting to etiologically link sexual abuse with pelvic pain, current data do not support an association with major sexual abuse any more specifically than they do an association with major physical (nonsexual) abuse. In other words, there appears to be an association between physical or sexual abuse and chronic pelvic pain. It may be that a history of both physical and sexual abuse serves as a marker for a greater magnitude of abuse, and that the greater the magnitude of abuse, the stronger the correlation with chronic pelvic pain (54,55).

With the correlation of abuse and chronic pain, and with the high prevalence of domestic violence, it is important to ask women with CPP if they are in a safe environment. It is important that this question be asked in a private setting without the spouse or significant other present. Satisfaction or dissatisfaction with marital or family relationships may be explored at this time, also (56).

What other symptoms or health problems do you have? Although certainly this question is a part of every patient's past history and review of systems, in this context it is included as a guide or clue to somatization disorders. Table 2.11 gives an example of series of symptoms that can sought and then used as a way to evaluate somatization. In a small study of this "somatization scale," women with CPP and a nonsomatic diagnosis had on average two more symptoms

TABLE 2.11. EXAMPLE OF A SOMATIZATION SCALE THAT HAS BEEN USED TO EVALUATE WOMEN WITH CHRONIC PELVIC PAIN

A—Headache
B—Low back pain
C—Pain with urination
D—Sleeplessness
E—Weight loss or gain
F—Dizziness
G—Passing out
H—Depression
I—Premenstrual syndrome
J—Shortness of breath
K—Joint pain
L—Nausea
M—Bloating
N—Vomiting
O—Diarrhea
P—Constipation
Q—Fatigue

High score is eight or more symptoms.

than those with a somatic diagnosis for their pain (8.9 versus 6.8, $p < 0.02$) (57). If the patient had eight or more symptoms and also had a history of sexual abuse, there was a 78% chance of a nonsomatic diagnosis after thorough evaluation of her pain. Somatization represents a common psychologic diagnosis in women with CPP. It is important to seek evidence of somatization during the history, because its presence complicates treatment and suggests that psychological evaluation and treatment are needed (57).

What do you believe or do you fear is the cause of your pain? The patient's cognitive perspectives on her pain can be explored by asking for her ideas of the cause of her pain. A goal of this exploration is especially to evaluate and discern fears the patient may have about the etiology of her pain, such as cancer, pelvic infection owing to remote past sexual acts, arguments with her spouse, divine retribution, and so on (5). This question may also include an exploration of the patient's concerns about what will happen to her during the evaluation and treatment of her pain.

CONCLUSION

The requisite detail of history that needs to be obtained in women with CPP is demonstrated by the unfortunate case of a 19-year-old woman who had undergone a right salpingo-oophorectomy at 16 years owing to a pelvic infection with a 8-cm mass, then a left salpingo-oophorectomy at 17 years owing to repeated pelvic infections and a chronic tuboovarian abscess. Her pain continued until at 19 years she was noted to have a nontender cauliflower-like mass at the upper left vagina, a tender 4-cm rectovaginal nodule, and an ultrasound finding of a 5-cm fluid-filled encapsulated abscess. At laparotomy, exploration of the left retroperitoneum revealed a 4 × 4 cm bottle cap, which the patient subsequently freely admitted inserting into the vagina when she was 12 years old. She was unable to remove it, developed a foul discharge and pain, but after multiple physician visits became convinced that it must have come out (as all the physicians insisted). Prior to her eventual accurate diagnosis, not only did she lose both ovaries, but also dropped out of school and became socially isolated (58).

A thorough history also may provide the physician with a "proceed with caution sign," suggesting that a slow, deliberate evaluation, including thorough consultation with a psychologist or other specialists, is valuable—especially before considering invasive or aggressive treatments. Some of the caution signs include:

- Excessive pain behavior (e.g., moaning or splinting movement)
- Poor response to previous appropriate treatment
- Immediate relief after a prior treatment followed by worsening or moving pain
- Unusual reaction to specific treatment modalities
- Withdrawal from normal life activities, such as work, school, or relationships
- Spending significant time lying down
- Severe depression
- Severe anxiety
- History of physician shopping (having seen several other doctors over a short time period)
- Unwillingness to admit to any stress or upset whatsoever
- Blaming all problems on the pain, believing life would be perfect if her pain were gone
- Extreme unassertiveness
- Noncompliance with a prior treatment regimen
- Excess medication use or drug dependence
- Significant family, marital, or sexual problems
- History of incest or onset of pain associated with physical or sexual abuse (53)

Finally, it is worth reiterating that the patient history represents a powerful diagnostic and therapeutic tool. It is a vital and crucial component of the care of the woman with CPP. And it is an endeavor to which the physician challenged with the care of the woman with CPP can never devote too much time or intensity.

REFERENCES

1. Milburn A, Reiter RC, Rhamberg AT. Multidisciplinary approach to chronic pelvic pain. *Obstet Gynecol Clin NA* 1993;20:643–661.
2. Rosenthal RH. Psychology of chronic pelvic pain. *Obstet Gynecol Clin NA* 1993;20:627–642.
3. Bavendam TG. Irritable bladder—a commonsense approach. *Contemp Ob/Gyn* 1993;April:70–77.
4. Sternbach RA. Clinical aspects of pain. In: Sternbach RA, ed. *The psychology of pain,* 2nd ed. New York: Raven Press, 1986:223–237.
5. Steege JF. Assessment and treatment of chronic pelvic pain. *Telinde's Op Gynecol Updates* 1992;1:1–10.
6. IASP Subcommittee on Taxonomy. Pain terms: a list with definitions and notes on usage. *Pain* 1979;6:249.
7. Kresch AJ, Seifer DB, Steege JF. How to manage patients with chronic pelvic pain. *Contemp Ob/Gyn* 1985;26:213–220.
8. Reiter RC. Chronic pelvic pain. *Clin Obstet Gynecol* 1990;33:117–118.
9. Rapkin AJ, Mayer EA. Gastroenterologic causes of chronic pelvic pain. *Obstet Gynecol Clin NA* 1993;20:663–683.
10. Rapkin AJ. Adhesions and pelvic pain: a retrospective study. *Obstet Gynecol* 1986;68:13–15.
11. Malinak LR. Pelvic pain—when is surgery indicated? *Contemp Ob/Gyn* 1985;26:43–50.
12. Baker PB, Symonds EM. The resolution of chronic pelvic pain after normal laparoscopic findings. *Am J Obstet Gynecol* 1992;166:835–856.
13. Kresch AJ, Seifer DB, Sachs LB, et al. Laparoscopy in 100 women with chronic pelvic pain. *Obstet Gynecol* 1984;64:672–674.
14. Lee RB, Stone K, Magelssen D, et al. Presacral neurectomy for chronic pelvic pain. *Obstet Gynecol* 1986;68:517–521.
15. Candiani GB, Fedele L, Vercellini P, et al. Presacral neurectomy for the treatment of pelvic pain associated with endometriosis: a controlled study. *Am J Obstet Gynecol* 1992;167:100–103.
16. Rapkin AJ, Karnes LD. New hope for patients with chronic pelvic pain. *Female Patient* 1988;31:100–173.
17. Baker PK. Muscoskeletal origins of chronic pelvic pain. *Obstet Gynecol Clin NA* 1993;20:719–742.
18. Mahmood TA, Templeton AA, Thomson L, et al. Menstrual symptoms in women with pelvic endometriosis. *Br J Obstet Gynaecol* 1991;98:558–563.
19. Low WY, Edelmann RJ, Sutton C. Short term psychological outcome of surgical intervention for endometriosis. *Br J Obstet Gynaecol* 1993;100:191–192.
20. Mens JMA, Vleeming A, Stoeckart R, et al. Understanding peripartum pelvic pain: implications of a patient survey. *Spine* 1996;21:1363–1370.
21. Peters AAW, van Dorst E, Jellis B, et al. A randomized clinical trial to compare two different approaches in women with chronic pelvic pain. *Obstet Gynecol* 1991;77:740–744.
22. Melzack R. The McGill Pain Questionnaire: major properties and scoring methods. *Pain* 1975;1:277–299.
23. Howard FM. Laparoscopic evaluation and treatment of women with chronic pelvic pain. *J Amer Assoc Gynecol Laparoscopists* 1994;1:325–331.
24. Walker E, Katon W, Harrop-Griffiths J, et al. Relationship of chronic pelvic pain to psychiatric diagnoses and childhood sexual abuse. *Am J Psychiatry* 1988;145:75–80.
25. Longstreth GF, Preskill DB, Youkeles L. Irritable bowel syndrome in women having diagnostic laparoscopy or hysterectomy. Relation to gynecologic features and outcome. *Dig Dis Sci* 1990;35:1285–1290.
26. Hajjar LR, Kim WS, Nolan GH, et al. Intestinal and pelvic endometriosis presenting as a tumor and associated with tamoxifen therapy: report of a case. *Obstet Gynecol* 1993;82:642–644.
27. Redwine DB. Endometriosis persisting after castration: clinical characteristics and results of surgical management. *Obstet Gynecol* 1994;83:405–413.
28. Kempers RD, Dockerty MB, Hunt AB, et al. Significant postmenopausal endometriosis. *Surg Gynecol Obstet* 1960;3:348–356.
29. Hansen A, Jensen DV, Larsen E, et al. Relaxin is not related to symptom-giving pelvic girdle relaxation in pregnant women. *Acta Obstet et Gynecol Scand* 1996;75:245–249.
30. Hann LE, Hall DA, Black EB, et al. Mittelschmerz: sonographic demonstration. *JAMA* 1979;241:2731–2732.

31. Westrom L. Effect of acute pelvic inflammatory disease on fertility. *Am J Obstet Gynecol* 1975;121:707–713.
32. Reiter RC. A profile of women with chronic pelvic pain. *Clin Obstet Gynecol* 1990;33:130–136.
33. Ranaer M, ed. *Chronic pelvic pain in women.* New York: Springer-Verlag, 1981:93.
34. Neary B, Young SB, Reuter KL, et al. Ovarian Burkitt lymphoma: pelvic pain in a woman with AIDS. *Obstet Gynecol* 1996; 88:706–708.
35. Charles D. Pelvic tuberculosis: not gone, but sometimes forgotten. *Contemp Ob/Gyn* July 1991;35:97.
36. Ranaer M, ed. *Chronic pelvic pain in women.* New York: Springer-Verlag, 1981:91.
37. Reiter RC, Gambone JC. Nongynecologic somatic pathology in women with chronic pelvic pain and negative laparoscopy. *J Reprod Med* 1991;36:253–259.
38. Dulemba JF. Spilled gallstones causing pelvic pain. *J Amer Assoc Gynecol Laparoscopists* 1996;3:309–311.
39. Pfeifer ME, Hansen KA, Tho SPT, et al. Ovarian cholelithiasis after laparoscopic cholecystectomy associated with chronic pelvic pain. *Fertil Steril* 1996;66:1031–1032.
40. Sexton DJ, Heskestad L, Lambeth WR, et al. Postoperative pubic osteomyelitis misdiagnosed as osteitis pubis—report of 4 cases and review. *Clin Infect Dis* 1993;17:695–700.
41. Carlson KJ, Miller BA, Fowler FJ. The Maine women's health study: II. Outcomes of nonsurgical management of leiomyommas, abnormal bleeding, and chronic pelvic pain. *Obstet Gynecol* 1994;83:566–572.
42. Stovall TG, Ling FW, Crawford DA. Hysterectomy for chronic pelvic pain of presumed uterine etiology. *Obstet Gynecol* 1990;75: 676–679.
43. Baker PK. Musculoskeletal origins of chronic pelvic pain. *Obstet Gynecol Clin NA* 1993;20:719–742.
44. Summit Jr RL. Urogynecologic causes of chronic pelvic pain. *Obstet Gynecol Clin NA* 1993;20:685–698.
45. Gillenwater JY, Wein AJ. Summary of the National Institute of Arthritis, Diabetes, Digestive and Kidney Disease workshop on interstitial cystitis, National Institute of Health, Bethesda, Maryland, August 28–29, 1987. *J Urol* 1988;140:203–206.
46. Hanno PM, Buehler J, Wein AJ. Use of amitriptyline in the treatment of interstitial cystitis. *J Urol* 1989;141:846–848.
47. Barbalias GA, Meares EM. Female urethral syndrome: clinical and urodynamic perspectives. *Urology* 1984;23:208–215.
48. Messing EM. The diagnosis of interstitial cystitis. *Urology* 1989; 29(Suppl):4–21.
49. Summit RL, Ling FW. Urethral syndrome presenting as chronic pelvic pain. *J Psychosom Obstet Gynecol* 1991;12(Suppl):77–86.
50. Holm-Bentzen M, Jacobsen F, Nerstrom B, et al. Painful bladder disease: clinical and pathoanatomical differences in 115 patients. *J Urol* 1987;138:500–502.
51. Kaplan WE, Firlit CF, Schoenberg HW. The female urethral syndrome: external sphincter spasm as etiology. *J Urol* 1980;124: 48–49.
52. Walker EA, Sullivan, Stenchever MA. Use of antidepressants in the management of women with chronic pelvic pain. *Obstet Gynecol Clin NA* 1993;20:743–751.
53. Rapkin AJ, Kames LD. The pain management approach to chronic pelvic pain. *J Reprod Med* 1987;32:323–327.
54. Rapkin AJ, Kames LD, Darke LL, et al. History of physical and sexual abuse in women with chronic pelvic pain. *Obstet Gynecol* 1990;76:92–96.
55. Walling MK, Reiter RC, O'Hara MW, et al. Abuse history and chronic pain in women: I. Prevalences of sexual abuse and physical abuse. *Obstet Gynecol* 1994;84:193–199.
56. Stout AL, Steege JF, Dodson WC, et al. Relationship of laparoscopic findings to self-report of pelvic pain. *Am J Obstet Gynecol* 1991;164:73–79.
57. Reiter RC, Shakerin LR, Gambone JC, et al. Correlation between sexual abuse and somatization in women with somatic and nonsomatic chronic pelvic pain. *Am J Obstet Gynecol* 1991;165:104–109.
58. O'Hanlan KA, Westphal LM. First report of a vaginal foreign body perforating into the retroperitoneum. *Am J Obstet Gynecol* 1995;173:962–964.

3

PHYSICAL EXAMINATION

FRED M. HOWARD

INTRODUCTION

The physical examination is comparable to the patient history as a powerful diagnostic and therapeutic tool. As a diagnostic tool, a systematic examination, guided by a thorough history, frequently leads to an accurate diagnosis that directs therapy or further evaluations by laboratory and imaging testing. As a therapeutic tool, a gently and meticulously performed physical examination, especially if it follows a compassionately taken complete history, establishes trust that the physician is caring and competent. Because the examination is often uncomfortable and painful for the patient with chronic pelvic pain (CPP), it is important that the physician go slowly enough to allow the patient to recover and relax between various portions of the examination. In some cases this can be quite time-consuming and, as was pointed out in the discussion about taking a history (Chapter 2), may preclude accomplishing all of the essential components of the examination at the time of the initial visit—especially in a busy practice with time constraints. Additionally, during the physical examination it is not uncommon for the patient to remember aspects of her history that she previously omitted, and time must be allowed for her to relate these additions to the history. Patience and kindness go a long way in establishing rapport with the patient, especially during the initial evaluation. The importance of establishing rapport with the patient at the initial visit cannot be overstated—it may well be the most important objective of the initial encounter.

During the examination a patient with CPP sometimes exhibits behavior that seems exaggerated or even hysterical, or she may relate sensations or pain distributions that seem nonanatomic or nonphysiologic. In spite of this, it is crucial that the patient be taken seriously and her behavior and descriptions not be dismissed as ridiculous, impossible, or unimportant. Such reactions by the physician are counterproductive and only create mistrust and anger. Tolerance and an open mind are important in evaluating the woman with CPP and go a long way in establishing rapport. It is important to remember that even a "routine" pelvic examination is very emotionally stressful for many patients with CPP (1).

Another major goal of the examination is to detect, inasmuch as possible, the exact anatomic locations of tenderness and correlate these with areas of pain. At each tender or painful area palpated, the patient should be asked whether this pain reproduces the complaint for which she is being evaluated. This requires a systematic and methodical attempt to duplicate the pain by palpation or positioning. The physician may find it useful to record these findings on a human anatomy diagram similar to that used by the patient for recording her pain locations or one that can be easily sketched in the medical record (Fig. 2.1 and 3.1). Some physicians find that a schematic representation of their findings is more useful than an anatomic diagram (Fig. 3.2) (2).

STANDING EXAMINATION

Ideally, the examination starts as the patient enters the office or examination room. Gait and posture are observed, especially noting limp or lurch, altered or asymmetric gait, lordosis, kyphosis-lordosis, scoliosis, or one-leg standing. One-leg standing refers to a posture characterized by consistently standing with all or most of the body weight shifted so as to be on one leg. In this posture there is a tendency to stand with one knee flexed or one leg externally rotated as the patient leans her weight onto the opposite leg. This posture, as well as slouching or generally poor posture hint at a musculoskeletal cause of or contribution to pain (3).

A "typical pelvic pain posture" (TPPP), consisting of marked thoracic kyphosis and lumbar lordosis, has been described in women with CPP (Fig. 3.3). This is best observed by viewing from the side with the middle and low back exposed. Obesity may exaggerate this posture. It causes or results from shortening of the thoracolumbar fascia and decreased flexibility of the posterior lumbar myofascia and joints. Evaluation of forward bending may be helpful. Normally this causes a reversal of the concave lumbar lordotic curve to a slightly convex curve, but in patients with TPPP or lordosis this reversal does not occur

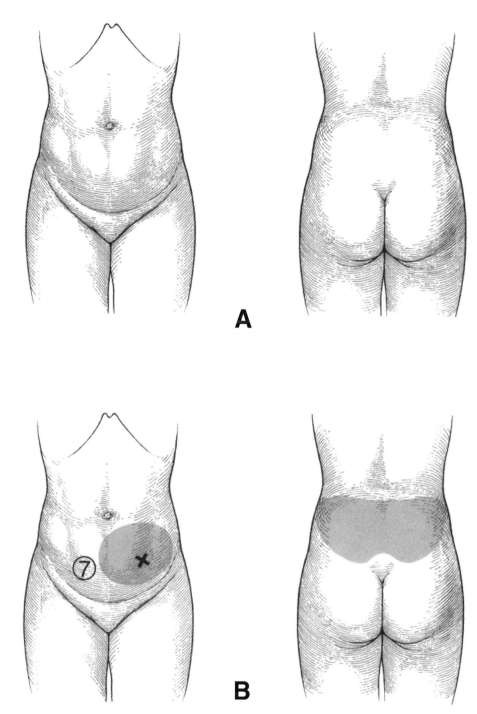

FIGURE 3.1. A: Example of a human anatomy diagram that can be used to record findings at the time of standing and supine examinations. **B:** In this example, shading indicates general areas of tenderness, "X" marks an area of particular or maximal tenderness, and "O" marks areas of trigger points with intensity indicated by the enclosed number "7" (0 to 10 scale).

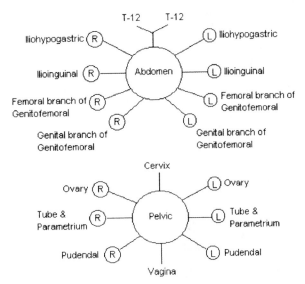

(diagram labels)

T-12   T-12

Iliohypogastric (R) — Abdomen — (L) Iliohypogastric

Ilioinguinal (R) — (L) Ilioinguinal

Femoral branch of (R) — (L) Femoral branch of
Genitofemoral   Genitofemoral

Genital branch of (R) — (L) Genital branch of
Genitofemoral   Genitofemoral

Cervix

Ovary (R) — Pelvic — (L) Ovary

Tube & (R) — (L) Tube &
Parametrium   Parametrium

Pudendal (R) — (L) Pudendal

Vagina

FIGURE 3.2. A schematic representation to document physical examination findings that some physicians find is more useful than an anatomic diagram.

and the curvature remains concave with forward bending (Fig. 3.4) (4).

Scoliosis should also be noted. This is best observed from behind the patient with the entire spine exposed. It leads to pelvic asymmetry, as well as trunk and lower extremity muscle imbalances, and may thereby contribute to pelvic pain.

The patient should be asked to stand on one leg to see if it causes pain at the pubic symphysis. If not, she should flex the hip of the raised leg to 90 degrees to see if symphysis pain occurs (Fig. 3.5). This suggests laxity of the pubic symphysis and pelvic girdle (5). Inability to stand on one leg without abnormal wobbling, reaching for support or dropping of the iliac crest suggests weakness of the hip and pelvis (Fig. 3.6) (4). Rotation of the trunk in both directions should be observed to see if this motion produces pain.

The clinician can also evaluate unequal iliac crest heights by placing the flattened palms on the superior aspects of the iliac crests and noting asymmetry; more than a one-quarter inch difference is significant and may occur with short leg syndrome or unilateral standing habit (Fig. 3.7). The asymmetric pelvic posture caused by an *anatomic short leg* may cause traction forces on the abdominal, paravertebral, and gluteal muscles, resulting in muscular strain and pain that may present as chronic pelvic pain. Treatment with a heel lift to the short limb is indicated. Most primary care physi-

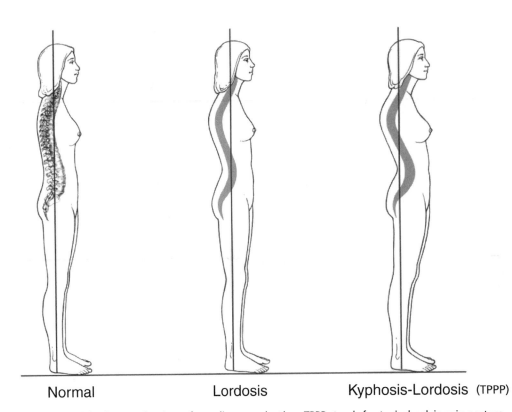

Normal   Lordosis   Kyphosis-Lordosis (TPPP)

FIGURE 3.3. Postural findings at the time of standing examination. TPPP stands for typical pelvic pain posture.

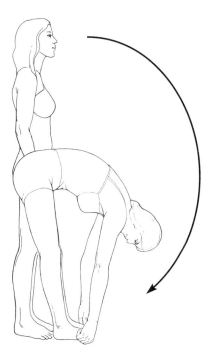

FIGURE 3.4. Illustration of the normal reversal of the concave lumbar lordotic curve to a slightly convex curve with forward bending. In patients with TPPP or with abnormal lordosis this reversal does not occur and the curvature remains concave with forward bending.

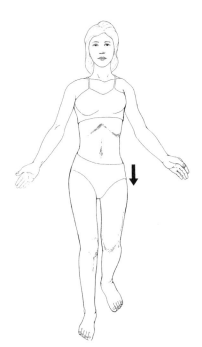

FIGURE 3.6. Illustration of dropping of the left iliac crest at the time of left hip flexion during standing examination. This finding suggests weakness of the hip and pelvis.

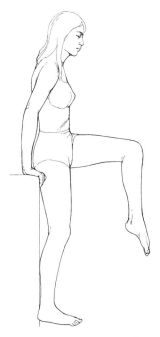

FIGURE 3.5. Illustration of hip flexion to about 90 degrees during the standing examination. Standing on one leg may elicit pubic symphysis pain at the pubic symphysis in some women with chronic pelvic pain.

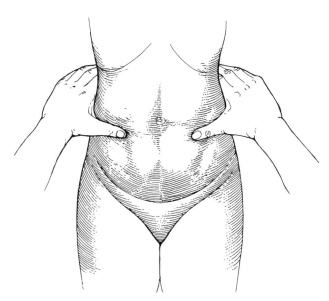

FIGURE 3.7. The clinician can evaluate unequal iliac crest heights by placing the flattened palms on the superior aspects of the iliac crests and noting asymmetry; more than a one-quarter inch difference is significant and may occur with short leg syndrome or unilateral standing habit.

cians need orthopedic and physical therapy consultation for the diagnosis and treatment of such patients.

Also in the standing position, evaluation for incisional, femoral, and inguinal hernias is done by palpation both with and without Valsalva maneuvers (Fig. 3.8). Groin hernias are relatively uncommon in women, or at least relatively uncommonly diagnosed. Indirect are more common than direct inguinal hernias in women. They represent a congenital failure of closure of the processus vaginalis and may allow intraabdominal contents to protrude through the internal inguinal ring into the inguinal canal (6). Femoral hernias are four times more common in women than men and account for up to one-third of abdominal wall hernias in women. They are almost as frequent as inguinal hernias in women. Surgical scars should be carefully palpated so as not to miss small incisional hernias. Palpation for tenderness at the pubic symphysis should be performed. Tenderness may suggest symptomatic pelvic girdle relaxation (5,6). Palpation bilaterally for generalized tenderness and for trigger points of the sacroiliac joints and both hips should be performed, especially in women with associated buttocks or sciatic pain (4). Figure 3.9 shows the three most common trigger points associated with buttocks pain. If buttocks or hip trigger or tender points are found, it is appropriate to perform an evaluation of the sites of tender points that characterize fibomyalgia (Fig. 3.10).

The standing position is also useful for evaluation of pelvic floor relaxation defects, by placing the index finger of one hand in the vagina and the index finger of the other hand in the rectum while the patient bears down (Fig. 3.11). Occult enterocele, rectocele, cystocele, and uterine

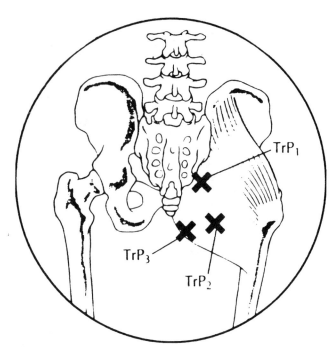

FIGURE 3.9. Illustration that shows the three most common trigger points associated with buttocks pain.

prolapse may be diagnosed with this procedure more accurately than when the patient is in the lithotomy position. However, this standing evaluation is usually performed after the pelvic examination and only if findings suggestive of pelvic floor relaxation were noted.

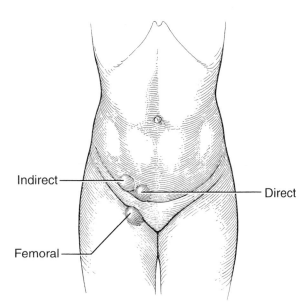

FIGURE 3.8. Illustration showing the general areas where inguinal and femoral hernias occur and that should be evaluated at the time of both standing and supine examinations.

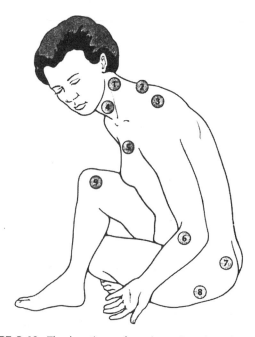

FIGURE 3.10. The locations of tender points that characterize fibromyalgia.

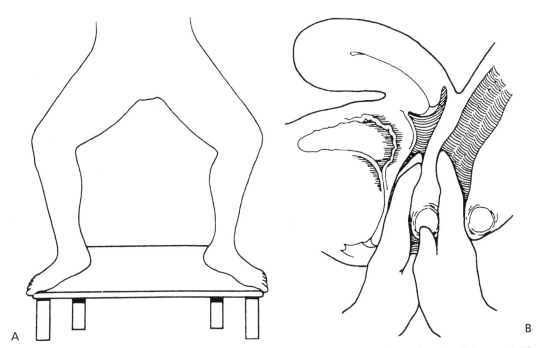

FIGURE 3.11. A: The standing position is often useful for evaluation of pelvic floor relaxation defects and differentiation of enterocele, rectocele, cystocele, and uterine descensus. **B:** The index finger of one hand is placed in the vagina and the index finger of the other hand in the rectum while the patient bears down.

SITTING EXAMINATION

Posture should also be observed in the sitting position. How the patient sits during the history should be noted, as well as on the examination table. For example, sitting asymmetrically with all the weight on one buttocks or consistently sitting forward in the chair may suggest levator muscle spasm and pelvic floor pain syndrome (7).

Palpation for tenderness of the upper and lower back and sacrum should be repeated, including single digit palpation for trigger points, especially along the sacrum, gluteal muscles, and piriformis muscles. Palpation for tenderness of the posterior superior iliac crests should be performed also. If any foci are noted that appear consistent with trigger points, it is valuable to block them with 0.25% to 0.5% bupivicaine to evaluate the contribution of the trigger points to the patient's pain. Figure 3.12 illustrates a technique to block the piriformis.

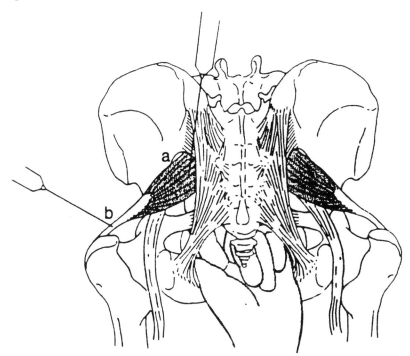

FIGURE 3.12. Illustration of a technique to block the piriformis in patients with piriformis syndrome. Usually this is performed with the patient in the lateral decubitus position.

Basic sensory testing to sharpness, dullness, and light touch may be indicated, as well as muscle strength testing and deep tendon reflexes of the trunk and lower extremities. A cursory neurologic examination of the lower extremities should be performed to assess the lower lumbar and upper sacral nerve roots, including pinprick and touch sensation, and deep tendon and Babinski reflexes (8).

SUPINE EXAMINATION

After the patient lies down, inspection and palpation for lordosis or pelvic tilt are performed again. Inability to lower the legs completely without arching the low back suggests abdominal weakness and stiffness of the lumbar spine (4). Active leg flexion, knee to chest, can be done to elicit low back dysfunction, low back pain, and abdominal muscle weakness. Obturator and psoas signs, usually performed in the evaluation of patients with an acute abdomen, are also often useful in women with CPP to look for shortening, dysfunction, or spasm of the obturator or iliopsoas muscles or fascia (Figs. 3.13 and 3.14). Head raise and leg raise can also be useful. Pain on straight leg raising may suggest a possible herniated disc, especially if there are also abnormal reflexes or sensory function associated with this finding (3). Positive findings with any of the preceding may suggest the

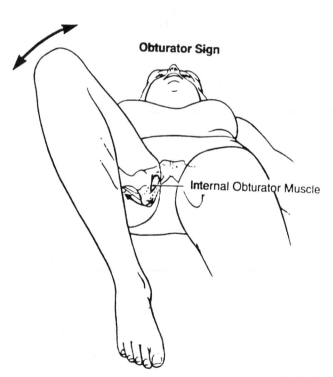

Obturator Sign

Internal Obturator Muscle

FIGURE 3.13. Examination for the obturator sign. If pain is elicited in a patient with chronic pelvic pain (not acute pelvic pain), this may suggest shortening, dysfunction, or spasm of the obturator muscles or fascia.

need for full physical therapy or orthopedic evaluation. Any of the following muscles or muscle groups may cause or contribute to CPP: rectus abdominis, external obliques, internal obliques, transversus abdominis, quadratus lumborum, pyramidalis, iliopsoas, coccygeus, levator ani, obturator internus, adductor magnus, and piriformis.

The patient should be asked to point to the area of pain using one finger, then she should show the whole area of pain using one or both hands. Another technique is to have her draw a circle around the area of pain using a single finger (7). Next she is asked to demonstrate how hard one must press at the area of maximal pain to elicit tenderness. Abdominal palpation by the physician then starts and should initially be superficial, noting hyperesthesias or hypersensitivity (hyperalgesia) of the skin and checking superficial abdominal reflexes. Gentle pinching in each dermatomal area is one technique that is useful. Head's maneuver is also quite useful. In this technique a simple syringe needle is scratched in concentric or parallel lines while held at a 25-degree angle with constant pressure so as not to be painful on normal tissue. The patient will exhibit a painful reaction in areas of hyperalgesia. Evaluation for dermographism may also be helpful. In this evaluation the physician's thumbnail is used to scratch the skin in longitudinal parallel lines 2 cm apart. Normal skin undergoes a vasodilation reaction causing red lines to appear. In hyperalgesic skin this reaction does not persist, because the ischemic phase of dermographism takes precedence and the lines turn white (9). These findings of hyperalgesia may be present with nerve entrapment or with visceral referred pain. These evaluations should particularly be performed in the T-10 to L-1 dermatomes (Fig. 3.15).

Next single digit palpation for trigger points is carefully and systematically done, including the inguinal areas. Gentle single fingertip pressure is applied to the abdomen, starting at the area identified by the patient as the location of her pain. This is followed by systematically checking the whole abdomen in the same manner. It is useful to have the patient rate any focal tender points on a 1 to 10 scale of severity. The physician should mark each elicited tender point. This technique is also useful for localizing cutaneous nerve entrapment. At each point of tenderness the patient should be asked if this palpation duplicates or is similar to her pain (10). The abdominal wall tenderness test may then be used to distinguish abdominal wall (myofascial) tenderness or trigger points from visceral tenderness. (The abdominal wall tenderness test is also known by the eponym "Carnett's test.") (14) In this test, while the area of abdominal tenderness is palpated, the patient voluntarily tenses the abdominal muscles, which is readily accomplished by having her raise her head or legs. If the pain is increased, it suggests that the pain is of myofascial origin. If the pain is decreased or unchanged, it suggests that the pain is not of myofascial origin and that intraabdominal disease is likely. Myofascial pain suggested by the abdominal wall

Psoas Sign

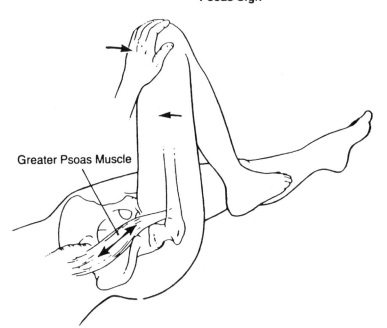

Greater Psoas Muscle

FIGURE 3.14. Examination for the psoas sign. If pain is elicited in a patient with chronic pelvic pain (not acute pelvic pain), this may suggest shortening, dysfunction, or spasm of the psoas muscles or fascia.

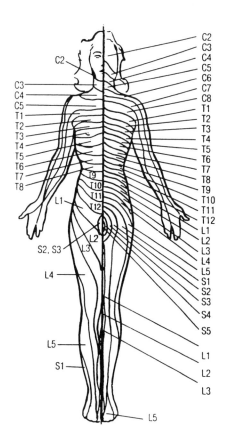

FIGURE 3.15. Illustration of the distribution of dermatomes anteriorly and posteriorly.

tenderness test may be owing to muscular strain, nerve entrapment, viral myositis, trauma, epigastric artery rupture, or an abdominal wall hernia, as well as myofascial trigger points (11).

Myofascial or *trigger point pain syndrome* is a not uncommon finding in chronic pelvic pain patients. In this syndrome there are discrete, 1- to 2-cm, hyperpathic areas deep to the subcutaneous fat. These focal areas of marked tenderness are generally found on the anterior abdomen within the T11, T12, and L1 dermatomes, but sometimes are also noted posteriorly over the same dermatomes on the midback or in the dermatomes of S2, S3, and S4 over the sacrum (Fig. 3.15). Slocumb suggests that any trigger points be blocked with local anesthetic 5 min prior to performing the pelvic examination to help differentiate between abdominal and vaginal pain components (14). The technique he recommends is injection of the trigger points with a 22-gauge, 1½ inch needle inserted until it just penetrates Camper's fascia, is superficial to the abdominal muscular fascia and elicits the patient's pain. Two to five milliliters of 0.25% bupivicaine are injected below and above Camper's fascia, which causes sharp and severe pain in true trigger points, followed within 5 to 10 min by pain relief. Up to 50 mL can be injected per patient. It is important to aspirate before each infiltration to avoid intravascular injection. After 5 minutes re-examination is performed to document improvement and elicit any trigger points that may have been missed. In Slocumb's experience, 90% of patients with trigger points had abdominal wall points (70% had paracervical-vaginal and 25% had sacral). It is important to remember that neither the presence of trigger points nor a

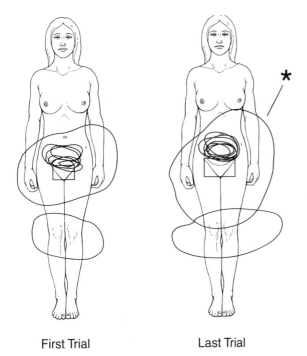

First Trial   Last Trial

FIGURE 3.16. Illustration showing areas of referral of discomfort from bladder distention to the lower abdomen. The two figures demonstrate the increased sensitivity and increased area of distribution with repeated distention of the bladder.

therapeutic response to trigger point treatment rules out intraabdominal disease.

Abdominal wall trigger points appear to occur in some patients as areas of referral from visceral pain. For example, the discomfort of bladder distention is referred to the lower abdomen, but shows an increased sensitivity and area of distribution with repeated distention (Fig. 3.16). Trigger points

are believed to show similar distribution properties. Figure 3.17 shows the distribution and correlation of trigger points and referred pain to pelvic viscera as observed by Slocumb.

Surgical scars should be noted. Palpation for hernial defects should be done, including careful repalpation of any surgical scars even if the standing examination for hernial defects was negative. Abdominal wall hernias may sometimes be appreciated as an abdominal mass (6). Palpation for Spigelian hernias should be done just lateral to the lateral margin of the rectus sheath feeling for tenderness or a weakness in the fascia. Spigelian hernias are small, spontaneous, lateral ventral hernias that protrude through the transversus abdominis aponeurosis lateral to the edge of the rectus muscle, but medial to the "Spigelian line." The Spigelian line is the point of transition of the transversus abdominis muscle to its aponeurotic tendon. Spigelian hernias are most likely just below the level of the umbilicus, because this is the location where the fascial tendon is the widest. Spigelian hernias have been reported as potential causes of abdominopelvic pain, but are difficult to diagnose. There may be tenderness at the location, but these fascial defects are small and hard to palpate. Sometimes there is a small tender mass palpable owing to herniation of a fatty plug, and this may help to lead the physician to consider this diagnosis and perform further evaluations (Chapter 42).

The pubic symphysis should be palpated for tenderness. This finding may suggest symptomatic pelvic girdle relaxation, rectus muscle inflammation, or injury at its fascial insertion, osteitis pubis, or osteomyelitis (5).

The usual components of the abdominal examination should not be neglected. Examination for distention, abdominal masses, ascites, bowel sounds, shifting dullness, vascular bruits, and palpation for deep tenderness, guard-

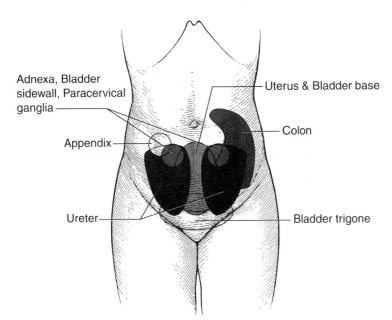

Adnexa, Bladder sidewall, Paracervical ganglia

Appendix

Ureter

Uterus & Bladder base

Colon

Bladder trigone

FIGURE 3.17. Abdominal and pelvic areas of referred tenderness associated with visceral pain suggested by Slocumb.

ing, or rigidity are essential. Visceral pain may cause local tenderness to pressure, with aching or sharp and radiating tenderness. A palpable, tender sigmoid colon may suggest irritable bowel syndrome. A tender left lower quadrant mass may suggest diverticulosis, subacute diverticulitis, or acute diverticulitis. Vascular bruits may suggest vascular disease and ischemic bowel disease. It is essential to rule out acute processes superimposed on chronic pain—CPP patients develop acute diseases at least as often as women without CPP. The physician must remember to rule out distention, tympany, generalized tenderness, and high-pitched bowel sounds suggestive of bowel obstruction or abdominal rigidity, rebound tenderness, and decreased bowel sounds suggestive of peritonitis, for example. The abdominal wall tenderness test is also useful in distinguishing between abdominal wall tenderness and acute intraabdominal pathology. In one reported series, only one of 24 patients with a positive test had intraabdominal pathology and that patient had a gangrenous appendix that was adherent to the anterior abdominal wall with secondary inflammation of the internal oblique and transversus abdominus muscles as the reason for the positive test. Of 96 patients with a negative test, 94 had significant intraabdominal pathology (68 with appendicitis). One of the two with a false test had constipation and the other had vomiting and diarrhea of undetermined etiology (11). The value of the abdominal wall tenderness test is diminished in patients with abdominal rigidity and obvious signs of peritonitis.

Lithotomy Examination

Visual inspection of the external genitalia should be performed noting redness, discharge, abscess formation, excoriation, perineal fistula, ulcerations, pigment changes, condylomata, atrophic changes (thinning, paleness, loss of vaginal rugae, protruding urethral mucosa), or signs of trauma. Fistulas and fissures should be noted and may occasionally be the first objective evidence of inflammatory bowel disease.

Basic sensory testing to sharpness, dullness, and light touch, as well as bulbocarvenosus and anal wink reflexes, should be done. A cotton-tipped swab may be used to evaluate the vestibule for localized tenderness of vulvar vestibulitis. The labia are held apart gently while the vestibule, vulva, hymen, and the area of the minor vestibular glands are palpated gently with the cotton-tipped swab. Patients with vulvar vestibulitis demonstrate exquisite tenderness in localized areas at the minor vestibular glands just external to the hymen, with normal sensation in adjacent vestibular and vulvar areas (Fig. 3.18). This technique or single-digit palpation should also be used to evaluate the vulva and pubic arch for trigger points, or for skin or mucosal lesions that reproduce the patient's symptoms. Areas of previous vulvar or vaginal trauma, or scars from surgeries or deliveries should be given particular attention.

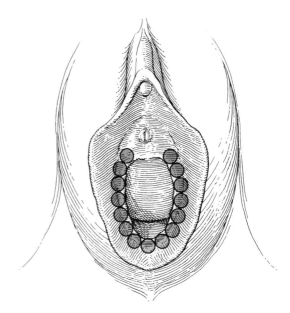

FIGURE 3.18. Examination of the vulva for vulvar vestibulitis. The circles illustrate the characteristic areas of tenderness to cotton-tipped swab palpation with this syndrome.

If any areas of abnormality are noted during the examination of the external genitalia, they should be shown to the patient. This is best done by having her sit more upright and use a hand mirror to visualize the genitalia while the physician demonstrates the lesions or areas of tenderness. This not only educates the patient as to the findings, but may also allow her a sense of increased control during the examination. This technique also allows the patient to guide the physician in localizing areas of tenderness during the examination when there is entrance dyspareunia or vulvar pain (12).

Colposcopic evaluation of the vulva and vestibule is sometimes helpful in further delineating any abnormal findings. Acetowhite areas, punctation, and papillary lesions at areas of tenderness or pigment change may require biopsies. Generally this evaluation is best reserved to follow-up, not the initial visit.

Pain or tension in the pelvic floor muscles can be assessed by insertion of a Sims retractor or a single blade of the speculum into the posterior vagina (8). While the patient is asked to relax, the resistance to downward or posterior pressure can be evaluated to reveal increased muscle tone, tension, or spasm (13). This maneuver may also reproduce part of the patient's symptom complex. Single speculum blade or Sims type retractor examination may also reveal evidence of pelvic relaxation. Although not a common diagnosis in women with CPP, pelvic floor defects may be associated with pain (Chapter 20). During the pelvic examination evidence of a cystocele, enterocele, or rectocele should be sought.

Of course, the traditional speculum examination is done for full visual inspection and to obtain requisite cytologic and bacteriologic specimens. Also a cotton-tipped swab should be used to evaluate the cervical os and the paracervical and cervical tissues for tenderness, especially at 1, 3, 6, and 9 o'clock. In posthysterectomy patients the full vaginal cuff should be similarly palpated for tenderness with a cotton-tipped applicator. If localized tender points are elicited, it is worthwhile to block them with 0.25% bupivicaine and re-evaluate for tenderness after 5 minutes (14).

The manual portion of the pelvic examination should always be initiated with a single index finger, first noting any introital tenderness or spasm. Vaginismus can be identified by involuntary introital spasm at this point in the examination in 75% of patients with the diagnosis (12). Vaginismus is dyspareunia or inability to have coitus owing to the involuntary spasm of primarily the bulbocavernosus muscles, but sometimes the levator ani muscles, too. The bulbocavernosus muscles lie distal to the hymeneal ring, allowing them to be easily differentiated from the levators (15). Next the levator ani muscles are directly palpated for tone and tenderness, especially at the 4:30 and 7:30 o'clock positions. The levator ani muscles are easily palpated during vaginal or rectal examination. They lie adjacent to the lateral vaginal walls just above the hymeneal ring (Fig. 3.19). The medial margins of the muscles are slightly thicker than a standard pencil, running in an anteroposterior direction. Identification may be confirmed by having the patient contract her pelvic muscles. The anus simultaneously elevates when the levators are contracted. Normally this palpation causes only a pressure sensation, but in patients with pelvic floor pain syndrome (PFPS) it may cause pain consistent with at least part of the patient's clin-

ical pain symptoms. PFPS is often a form of tension myalgia that mechanistically is thought to produce pain much as tension headaches cause pain. The tension or spasm involves the musculature of the pelvic floor and causes pain in these muscles or in their areas of attachment to the sacrum, coccyx, ischial tuberosities, and pubic rami. Several names have been used for syndromes that appear to be similar: pelvic floor myalgia, piriformis syndrome, levator ani spasm syndrome, diaphragma pelvis spastica, and coccydynia. PFPS may also result from trigger points of one or more of the muscles of the pelvis. The most common finding with PFPS is tenderness and spasm of one or more of the levator muscles of the pelvic floor (puborectalis, pubococcygeus, and iliococcygeus) (Fig. 3.20). In some patients with PFPS, there will also be tenderness of the coccyx, lateral sacrum, or sacrococcygeal ligaments. Digital pressure on the involved muscle characteristically reproduces or intensifies the patient's pain symptoms. It is not unusual for the tenderness to be unilateral. The insertion of the levators should also be palpated if possible, both laterally at the arcus tendinei and anteriorly at the pubic rami. Levator ani spasm or PFPS may be a primary problem or it may be secondary to other diseases such as interstitial cystitis or urethral syndrome.

The piriformis, coccygeus, and obturator internus muscles should be gently palpated bilaterally seeking tenderness that reproduces the patient's pain (4). The piriformis muscles are somewhat more difficult to palpate than the levators. Rectal examination may allow an easier evaluation than vaginal examination. As illustrated in Figure 3.21, the piriformis originates from the anterior surface of the sacrum and passes from the pelvis via the greater sciatic notch, and may be palpated along this portion of its course. Transvaginally or transrectally the examining finger is pressed posteriolaterally just superiorly to the ischial spine. In the lithotomy position, if the patient is asked to abduct the thigh against resistance (hold the patient's knee on the same side being examined) as the piriformis is palpated, the muscle may be more easily palpated and there is exquisite tenderness of the muscle if there is spasm or tension myalgia involving the piriformis (piriformis syndrome).

The anterior vaginal urethral and trigonal areas should be gently palpated to elicit any areas of tenderness, induration, or thickening. The urethra should also be massaged to elicit any secretions. Urethral tenderness with or without discharge is consistent with chronic urethritis or chronic urethral syndrome. Next the "gutter" on either side of the urethra should be evaluated for any fullness, fluctuance, or discomfort that might suggest a urethral diverticulum or vaginal wall cyst (13). The bladder base is also evaluated for tenderness. Its presence is consistent with trigonitis or interstitial cystitis.

With deeper palpation the cervix, paracervical areas, and vaginal fornices should be palpated with the single

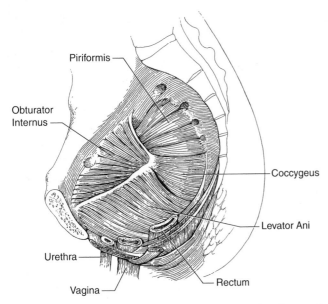

FIGURE 3.19. Illustration of the muscles of the pelvic floor and sidewall, demonstrating their proximity to the vagina and rectum, which allows easy palpation either vaginally or rectally.

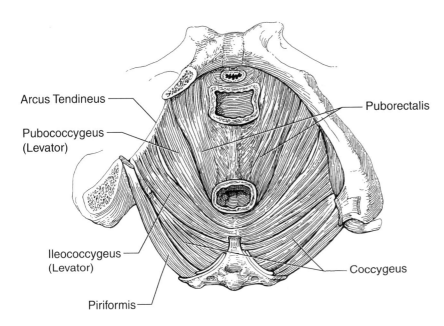

FIGURE 3.20. A view of the pelvic floor muscles from below. Levator ani muscles are the puborectalis, pubococcygeus, and ileococcygeus. The coccygeus is usually considered a muscle of the pelvic floor as well.

digit for tenderness or trigger points. Cervical tenderness may suggest problems such as cervicitis, repeated cervical trauma (usually from intercourse), or pelvic infection. Vaginal forniceal tenderness may suggest problems such as pelvic infection, endometriosis, ureteral tenderness, or trigger points.

The uterus should be compressed against the sacrum to evaluate uterine tenderness (Fig. 3.22). Uterine tenderness may be consistent with diseases such as adenomyosis, pelvic congestion syndrome, pelvic infection, or premenstrual syndrome. A uterus that is immobile and fixed in position, especially a retroflexed position, may suggest endometriosis or adhesions. The coccyx should also be palpated with the single digit and attempt should be made to move it 30

degrees or less. This part of the examination may also be done during the bimanual or rectovaginal examination. Normally the coccyx moves 30 degrees without eliciting pain, but in patients with coccydynia this movement elicits pain.

The adnexal areas should be palpated next, still using a single digit without the use of the abdominal hand. This is often a more accurate manner of assessing intrinsic tenderness of the ovaries or tube than the traditional bimanual examination, especially in patients with abdominal wall tenderness or trigger points. All ovaries are normally tender; therefore, it is the degree of tenderness and the similarity to the chief pain complaint that are clinically useful.

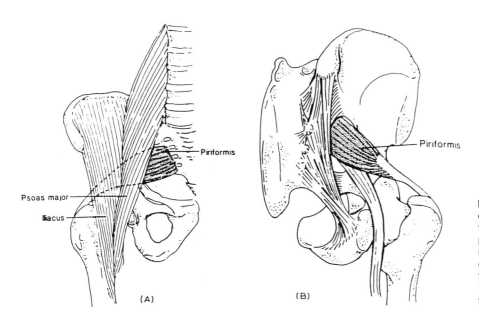

FIGURE 3.21. A,B: The piriformis muscle. It originates from the anterior surface of the sacrum and passes from the pelvis via the greater sciatic notch, and may be palpated along this portion of its course. Transvaginally or transrectally the examining finger is pressed posteriolaterally just superiorly to the ischial spine.

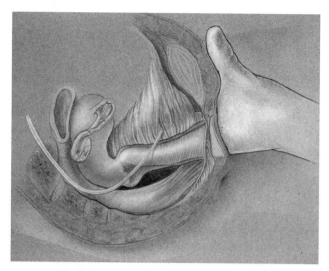

FIGURE 3.22. Illustration of a technique to evaluate uterine tenderness by compressing the uterus against the sacrum with the vaginal examining finger. (Illustration, courtesy of John Slocumb, MD, Denver, CO.)

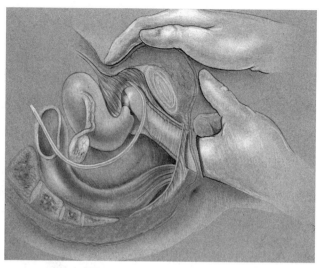

FIGURE 3.23. Illustration of bimanual examination of the bladder showing how all the layers of the abdominal wall, the parietal peritoneum, and the palpated organ or organs are palpated with the bimanual examination. (Illustration, courtesy of John Slocumb, MD, Denver, CO.)

All of the preceding are "monomanual-monodigital" evaluations, that is, only one finger of one hand is used. No abdominal palpation with the other hand is involved. Some have suggested that the single speculum blade or Sim's retractor evaluation be delayed until after the single-handed digital and bimanual examinations to avoid producing pelvic floor muscle spasm and obscuring findings on digital examination (16). An argument against this is that the use of lubricant with the digital or bimanual examination may cause inaccuracies of any cytologies or cultures that are obtained during the speculum examination. The author has not found it to be a problem to perform the speculum examinations first.

The traditional bimanual examination is the last portion of the pelvic examination in the pelvic pain patient. It is the least sensitive portion of the evaluation because it involves stimulation of all layers of the abdominal wall, the parietal peritoneum, and the palpated organ or organs (Fig. 3.23) (11). The uterus should be evaluated for size, shape, tenderness, and mobility. A fixed, retroverted uterus may suggest endometriosis or cul-de-sac adhesions. Endometriosis is also suggested by tenderness of the posterior uterus, nodularity of the uterosacral ligaments and cul-de-sac, and narrowing of the posterior vaginal fornix. Pelvic nodularity is however not diagnostic of endometriosis and may occur with other conditions, particularly ovarian carcinoma.

Adnexae are evaluated for thickening, mobility, or enlargement. Asymmetric, enlarged ovaries, particularly if fixed to the broad ligament or pelvic sidewall, may imply the presence of endometriosis. Bilateral or unilateral ovarian tenderness almost always occurs with pelvic congestion syndrome.

The ureters should be palpated for abnormal tenderness and possible reproduction of pain complaints, particularly at the uterovesical junctions. They are not infrequently a source of pain and tenderness. Figure 3.24 illustrates the technique used to examine the uterers.

On the right the cecum should be carefully palpated and on the left the rectosigmoid for masses, hard feces, and tenderness. Either or both may be abnormally tender with irri-

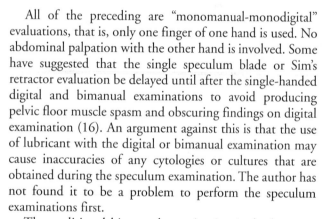

FIGURE 3.24. Illustration of the technique used to examine the uterers for abnormal tenderness and possible reproduction of pain complaints, particularly at the uterovesical junctions. The ureters are not infrequently a source of pain and tenderness. (Illustration, courtesy of John Slocumb, MD, Denver, CO.)

table bowel syndrome, but more commonly the rectosigmoid is tender.

Rectal or rectovaginal examination should usually be performed last. Marked discomfort with digital rectal examination often accompanies irritable bowel syndrome or chronic constipation, as may hard feces in the rectum. Function of the internal and external anal sphincter should be evaluated by reflex "wink" and voluntary constriction. The rectovaginal septum should be carefully examined for nodularity and tenderness, suggesting endometriosis, especially if done while the patient is menstruating. Much of the previously described examinations performed vaginally can be re-evaluated at the time of the rectovaginal examination. In particular it is useful to re-examine the pelvic floor muuscles. With rectal examination, as one starts in the posterior midline and sweeps laterally and anteriorly, the rectal finger passes over the piriformis, the coccygeus, and then the levator ani muscles. Rectal examination should also include evaluation for rectal masses because many colorectal carcinomas are palpable this way. Tenderness of the anal canal may suggest

abscess or fissures in the canal. Testing for occult blood should be performed.

CONCLUSION

Although findings can be briefly explained during the physical examination, after completion the physician should fully explain any positive or negative findings. Often the physician will have one or more tentative diagnoses after the examination and these should be explained as well. Any further testing or evaluations needed should be discussed, described, and justified. If there is time, the physician's philosophy of care of patients with CPP should be reviewed again within the context of the patient's history and physical examination findings. Finally, any questions should be answered.

The clinician can obtain a great deal of information by performing a thorough pelvic pain-directed examination (Tables 3.1 to 3.4). It is well worth the diligence and time required to do it well.

TABLE 3.1. COMPONENTS OF THE STANDING PHYSICAL EXAMINATION

Standing Examination	Possible Problems Diagnosed
Gait	Short leg syndrome Herniated disc General musculoskeletal problems
Posture with and without forward bending	Typical pelvic pain posture Scoliosis One-leg standing
Standing on one leg with and without hip flexion	Laxity of the pubic symphysis Laxity of pelvic girdle Weakness of the hip and pelvis
Iliac crest symmetry	Short leg syndrome One leg standing
Groin evaluation with and without Valsalva	Inguinal hernia Femoral hernia
(Incisional evaluation with and without Valsalva)	Incisional hernia
Pubic symphysis evaluation, including trigger points	Peripartum pelvic pain syndrome Trigger points Osteitis pubis Osteomyelitis pubis
Hip and sacroiliac evaluation, including trigger points	Arthritis of hip Trigger points
Buttocks (gluteus and piriformis) evaluation, including trigger points	Piriformis syndrome Pelvic floor pain syndrome Gluteal trigger points
Fibromyalgia tender point evaluation	Fibromyalgia
Pelvic floor relaxation evaluation	Enterocele Rectocele Cystocele Uterine descensus

Examination of the woman with chronic pelvic pain and general problems or diagnoses that may be suggested based on these components of the examination.

TABLE 3.2. COMPONENTS OF THE SITTING PHYSICAL EXAMINATION

Sitting Examination	Possible Problems Diagnosed
Posture	Levator ani spasm Pelvic floor pain syndrome
Palpation of the upper and lower back	Trigger points Myalgia Arthritis
Palpation of sacrum	Trigger points Sacroiliitis
Palpation of gluteal and piriformis muscles	Trigger points Myalgia
Palpation of the posterior superior iliac crests	Peripartum pelvic pain syndrome
Basic sensory testing to sharpness, dullness, and light touch	Herniated disc
Muscle strength testing and deep tendon	Herniated disc

Examination of the woman with chronic pelvic pain and general problems or diagnoses that may be suggested based on these components of the examination.

TABLE 3.3. COMPONENTS OF THE SUPINE PHYSICAL EXAMINATION

Supine Examination	Possible Problems Diagnosed
Posture for lordosis or pelvic tilt	Lordosis Pelvic tilt Abdominal weakness Stiffness of the lumbar spine
Active leg flexion, knee to chest	Low back dysfunction Low back pain Abdominal muscle weakness Deconditioning
Obturator and psoas sign testing	Shortening, dysfunction, or spasm of the obturator or iliopsoas muscles or fascia
Head raise and leg raise	Herniated disc Abdominal muscle weakness Deconditioning
Light abdominal palpation	Referred visceral pain Nerve entrapment Neuropathy
Gentle pinching	Referred visceral pain Nerve entrapment Neuropathy
Head's maneuver	Referred visceral pain Nerve entrapment Neuropathy
Dermographism evaluation	Referred visceral pain Nerve entrapment Neuropathy
Single digit palpation	Trigger points Myofascial pain Hernias Nerve entrapments
Abdominal wall tenderness test	Abdominal wall pain Visceral pain
Groin and abdominal evaluation with and without Valsalva	Inguinal hernia Spigelian hernia Epigastric hernia Diastasis recti
Incisional evaluation with and without Valsalva	Incisional hernia
Pubic symphysis evaluation	Trigger points Osteitis pubis Osteomyelitis pubis
Traditional abdominal examination for distention, masses, ascites, bowel sounds, shifting dullness, vascular bruits, deep tenderness, guarding, or rigidity	Acute disease

Examination of the woman with chronic pelvic pain and general problems or diagnoses that may be suggested based on these components of the examination.

TABLE 3.4. COMPONENTS OF THE LITHOTOMY PHYSICAL EXAMINATION

Lithotomy Examination	Possible Problems Diagnosed
Visual inspection of the external genitalia	Inflammatory and infectious diseases Vulvar abscess Trauma Fistula Ulcerative disease Pigmented lesions (neoplasias) Condylomata Atrophic changes Fissure
Basic sensory testing to sharpness, dullness, and light touch	Nerve entrapment Neuropathy Spinal cord lesion
Cotton-tipped swab evaluation of the vestibule	Vulvar vestibulitis
Single digit palpation of vulva and pubic arch	Trigger points
Colposcopic evaluation of the vulva and vestibule	Neoplasia
Sims retractor or single blade speculum examination of vagina and pelvic muscles	Enterocele Cystocele Rectocele Uterine descensus
Cotton-tipped swab evaluation of cervical os, paracervical and cervical tissues	Trigger points
Cotton-tipped swab evaluation vaginal cuff	Trigger points Neuroma
Single digit pelvic examination of introitus	Vulvar vestibulitis Vaginismus Trigger points
Single digit pelvic examination of levator ani	Pelvic floor pain syndrome Trigger points
Single digit pelvic examination of coccygeus	Pelvic floor pain syndrome Trigger points
Single digit pelvic examination of piriformis with and without abduction	Piriformis syndrome
Single digit pelvic examination of anterior vaginal urethral and trigonal evaluation	Chronic urethral syndrome Urethritis Cystitis Interstitial cystitis Trigonitis Urethral diverticulum Vaginal wall cyst
Single digit pelvic examination of cervix, paracervical areas, and vaginal fornices	Trigger points Endometriosis Cervicitis Repeated cervical trauma Pelvic infection Ureteral pain
Single digit pelvic examination of uterus	Adenomyosis Pelvic congestion syndrome Pelvic infection Premenstrual syndrome Adhesions
Single digit pelvic examination of coccyx	Coccydynia
Single digit pelvic examination of adnexa	Pelvic congestion syndrome Endometriosis
Bimanual pelvic examination	See text
Rectovaginal examination	See text

Examination of the woman with chronic pelvic pain and general problems or diagnoses that may be suggested based on these components of the examination.

REFERENCES

1. Thompson TL. Managing the "difficult" ob/gyn patient. *Female Patient* 1990;15:81–92.
2. McDonald JS. Management of chronic pelvic pain. *Obstet Gynecol Clin NA* 1993;20:817–838.
3. Lipscomb GH, Ling FW. Relationship of pelvic infection and chronic pelvic pain. *Obstet Gynecol Clin NA* 1993;20:699–708.
4. Baker PK. Musculoskeletal origins of chronic pelvic pain. *Obstet Gynecol Clin NA* 1993;20:719–742.
5. Hansen A, Jensen DV, Larsen E, et al. Relaxin is not related to symptom-giving pelvic girdle relaxation in pregnant women. *Acta Obstet et Gynecol Scand* 1996;75:245–249.
6. Rapkin AJ, Mayer EA. Gastroenterologic causes of chronic pelvic pain. *Obstet Gynecol Clin NA* 1993;20:663–683.
7. Steege JF. Office assessment of chronic pelvic pain. *Clin Obstet Gynecol* 1997;40:554–563.
8. Summit RL Jr. Urogynecologic causes of chronic pelvic pain. *Obstet Gynecol Clin NA* 1993;20:685–698.
9. Giamberardino MA, Vecchiet L. Pathophysiology of visceral pain. *Curr Rev Pain* 1996;1:23–33.
10. Applegate WV. Abdominal cutaneous nerve entrapment syndrome. *Surgery* 1972;71:118–124.
11. Thomson H, Francis DMA. Abdominal wall tenderness: a useful sign in the acute abdomen. *Lancet* 1977;2:1053–1054.
12. Steege JF, Ling FW. Dyspareunia: a special type of chronic pelvic pain. *Obstet Gynecol Clin NA* 1993;20:779–793.
13. Bavendam TG. Irritable bladder—a commonsense approach. *Contemp Ob/Gyn* 1993;April:70–77.
14. Slocumb JC. Neurologic factors in chronic pelvic pain: trigger points and the abdominal pelvic pain syndrome. *Am J Obstet Gynecol* 1984;149:536–543.
15. DeLancey JO, Sampselle CM, Punch MR. Kegel dyspareunia: levator ani myalgia occurred by overexertion. *Obstet Gynecol* 1993;82:658–659.
16. Summit RL Jr. Urogynecologic causes of chronic pelvic pain. *Obstet Gynecol Clin NA* 1993;20:685–698.

4

LABORATORY AND IMAGING EVALUATION

FRED M. HOWARD

INTRODUCTION

The history and physical examination are indispensable in the evaluation of the woman with pelvic pain. Often a thorough history, with confirmatory physical findings, is diagnostic. The decision to perform any laboratory or imaging evaluations is based on the need for confirmation of the diagnosis, to rule out other potentially life-threatening illnesses, in preparation for medical or surgical treatment, or when, in spite of careful and meticulous history taking and physical examination, the diagnosis is unclear.

The use of "routine" tests in women with chronic pelvic pain (CPP) is discouraged. All too often all women with CPP are routinely put through a barium enema and upper gastrointestinal series to "rule out" gastrointestinal disease, an intravenous pyelogram to "rule out" urinary tract disease, a pelvic ultrasound to "rule out" gynecologic disease, a complete blood count and sedimentation rate to "rule out" infection, and so on. Such algorithmic approaches are not worthwhile, especially because such general tests rarely accomplish their intended purpose of "ruling out" the involvement of organ systems or inflammatory or infectious processes.

Laboratory tests should be obtained when the results will change the diagnosis, change the further evaluation, or change the treatment. The clinician should know what she will do with the results before she orders them. This is important because the list of potential diagnostic tests is extensive (Table 4.1).

This chapter is meant to be an overview of potential laboratory and imaging tests. A more thorough discussion of the utilization of diagnostic tests in specific disorders is found in Section Two in the chapters that discuss specific disorders important in CPP.

STD TESTING

It is reasonable to test for sexually transmitted diseases in women with CPP as you would test any other woman in your practice. Cervical cultures or smears for gonorrhea and chlamydia, syphilis serology, hepatitis B surface antigen screening, and HIV testing are all appropriate as part of primary health care for the patient. Obviously the need for such testing depends on the patient's history and her history of prior testing for sexually transmitted diseases.

In patients with dyspareunia, testing for sexually transmitted diseases, especially with urethral and cervical gonorrhea cultures and chlamydial PCR testing (which can also be done on urine) is advisable regardless of risk factors or prior history. Other specific infectious causes of painful intercourse should also be ruled out. This requires vaginal cultures, urine cultures, vaginal wet preps, and vaginal pH. These tests for infectious etiologies are advisable in almost all cases of dyspareunia.

URINE TESTING

Urinalysis and urine culture are usually performed in the initial evaluation of the woman with pelvic pain. Although they are relatively inexpensive and noninvasive, they are not always necessary. However, in the woman with any urinary tract symptoms or who is to undergo invasive procedures that include bladder catheterization, it seems advisable to perform them routinely. Persistent irritative bladder symptoms of frequency and urgency associated with chronic pelvic pain may suggest interstitial cystitis, but neoplasia must also be ruled out, especially if the woman is a smoker. Urine cytology should be done is such cases, in addition to urinalysis and culture.

Women with CPP and hematuria need particular attention. Although most women with bladder cancer do not present with pain or irritable bladder symptoms, 80% present with hematuria. Thus, hematuria must be carefully investigated with history, physical examination, urine culture, urine cytology, cystourethroscopy, and intravenous pyelography or CT scan. If the urine culture is positive, treatment should be initiated and then urine re-evaluated to determine if hematuria is persistent.

TABLE 4.1. LABORATORY TESTS AND IMAGING STUDIES USEFUL WITH DIFFERENT DISORDERS ASSOCIATED WITH CPP

Symptom, Finding, or Suspected Diagnosis	Potentially Useful Tests
Abdominal epilepsy	Electroencephalography
Adenomyosis	Ultrasonography Hysterosalpingography Magnetic resonance imaging
Chronic intermittent bowel obstruction	Flat and upright abdominal radiographs Computerized tomography
Chronic pelvic pain—general	Complete blood cell count Sedimentation rate
Chronic urethral syndrome	Urodynamic testing
Colorectal cancer	Barium enema radiography Computerized tomography
Compression or entrapment neuropathy	Nerve conducting velocities Needle electromyographic studies
Constipation	Anorectal balloon manometry Colonic transit time
Depression	Thyroid stimulating hormone Thyroxine Triiodothyronine levels Antithyroid antibody Complete blood count Renal function tests Hepatic function tests Electrolytes Rapid plasma reagen Human immunodeficiency virus testing
Diarrhea	Stool specimens for ova and parasites Stool polymorponuclear leukocytes and red blood cells Stool cultures Stool for *C. difficile* toxin Stool guiaic testing Barium enema radiography
Diverticular disease	Barium enema radiography
Dyspareunia	Urethral and cervical gonorrhea cultures Chlamydial PCR testing Vaginal cultures Urine cultures Vaginal wet preps Vaginal pH
Endometrial polyps	Ultrasonography Sonohysterography Hysterosalpingography
Endometriosis	Ca-125 Ultrasonography Barium enema radiography Hysterolsapingography Computerized tomography Magnetic resonance imaging
Hematuria	Urine culture Urine cytology Cystourethroscopy Computerized tomography

(continued)

TABLE 4.1. *(continued)*

Symptom, Finding, or Suspected Diagnosis	Potentially Useful Tests
Hernia of the linea alba	Abdominal wall ultrasonography Computerized tomography
Inflammatory bowel disease	Barium enema radiography Upper gastrointestinal series with follow through Computerized tomography
Inguinal hernia	Herniography
Internal supravesical hernia	Ultrasonography Computerized tomography
Interstitial cystitis	Urine cytologies Urodynamic testing
Leiomyoma uteri	Ultrasonography Hysterosalpingography
Musculoskeletal disorders (some)	Plain film radiography Computerized tomography
Obstructive cervical stenosis	Ultrasonography
Obturator hernia	Herniography Computerized tomography
Osteomyelitis	Bone scan
Ovarian cancer	Ca-125 Ultrasonography Computerized tomography
Ovarian remnant syndrome	Follicle-stimulating hormone Estradiol Gonadotropin releasing hormone agonist stimulation test Ultrasonography ± clomiphene stimulation Barium enema radiography Computerized tomography
Ovarian retention syndrome	Ultrasonography Computerized tomography
Pelvic congestion syndrome	Pelvic venography Ultrasonongraphy ± Doppler
Pelvic floor relaxation	Vaginal sonography Perineal ultrasound Introital sonography Rectosonography Colporectocystourethrography Magnetic resonance imaging Anal electromyography Pudendal nerve terminal latency
Pelvic mass	Ultrasonography Computerized tomography
Pelvic tuberculosis	Chest x-ray
Perineal hernia	Herniography
Porphyria	Urine porphobilinogen
Richter hernia	Computerized tomography
Sciatic hernia	Computerized tomography
Spigelian hernia	Abdominal wall ultrasonography Computerized tomography Herniography

(continued)

TABLE 4.1. *(continued)*

Symptom, Finding, or Suspected Diagnosis	Potentially Useful Tests
Spinal disc pathology	Magnetic resonance imaging
Stress fracture	Bone scan
Substance abuse	Drug screen
Umbilical hernia	Abdominal wall ultrasonography Computerized tomography Herniography
Uncertain intrauterine device	Ultrasonography
Urethral diverticulum	Vaginal sonography Voiding cystourethrography Double balloon cystourethrography Magnetic resonance imaging
Urinary tract infection	Urinalysis Urine culture
Uterine anomalies	Hysterosalpingography
Vesical-sphincter dyssynergia	Urodynamic testing
Vulvar vestibulitis	Urinary oxalate

Urinary oxalate levels are often measured in women with vulvar vestibulitis, because oxalate crystals are the most commonly mentioned irritant in association with vulvar vestibulitis (1). Although the usefulness of urinary oxalate testing has been seriously questioned by many investigators, it may still be worthwhile in certain cases.

Sometimes a urine drug screen is indicated in the woman with CPP, especially if there is a past history of substance abuse or significant psychological symptoms. Testing to rule out illegal street, as well as prescription, drug abuse should be done.

Porphyria is a rare diagnosis in women with CPP. Diagnosis depends on the history, symptoms, and measurement of porphyrins or precursors in urine or stool specimens. The Watson-Schwartz test is a qualitative screening test for porphobilinogen (PBG) in urine. Ideally, this should be done between attacks. With porphyria, PBG levels are twice normal.

STOOL TESTING

In patients with diarrhea and pelvic pain, possible infection with *Giardia,* amoeba, and other parasites should be evaluated by testing three stool specimens for ova and parasites (O&P). Microscopic examination of stool samples for polymorponuclear leukocytes and red blood cells, as well as stool cultures, are indicated if symptoms suggest that infectious enterocolitis is possible. If pseudomembranous colitis is suspected, then stool for *C. difficile* is indicated, but may not be diagnostic because only 75% of isolates produce toxins. With pseudomembranous colitis, testing for fecal

leukocytes has a sensitivity of 30% to 50% and a positive test rules out benign or simple antibiotic diarrhea. Stool guiaic testing should be done in any woman with gastrointestinal symptoms and any woman over 50 years of age.

BLOOD TESTING

Most women with chronic pelvic pain should have a complete blood cell count and sedimentation rate done, because they are relatively inexpensive, noninvasive, and informative. They allow a general determination regarding the presence of an infectious or inflammatory process, and the hematocrit and hemoglobin detect the presence of anemia. There are many causes of anemia, but in CPP patients malignancy (e.g., colon, ovarian, or bladder cancer) can be a life-threatening etiology. Measurement of liver enzymes sometimes may be indicated for similar concerns.

Hormonal Assays

In suspected cases of ovarian remnant syndrome, evidence of continuing ovarian activity helps to establish the diagnosis. Ovarian activity is suggested by premenopausal levels of follicle-stimulating hormone (less than 40 mIU/mL) or estradiol (30 pg/mL or more), provided there is no exogenous hormonal replacement. Premenopausal FSH levels are present in 50% to 75% of women with an ovarian remnant. A postmenopausal level of FSH is not absolute proof of the absence of an ovarian remnant.

In addition to the determination of a random estradiol level, measuring estradiol after the administration of a gonadotropin releasing hormone agonist (GnRH-a stimulation test) can be a useful method for diagnosing ovarian remnant syndrome. A significant rise in estradiol levels within the first 7 days after depot-leuprolide injection, in the absence of exogenous hormonal replacement, confirms that hormonally responsive ovarian tissue is present.

In women with depression, thyroid stimulating hormone, thyroxine, triiodothyronine levels (TSH, T4, T3), and sometimes antithyroid antibody assays should be measured to rule out thyroid conditions that may manifest as depression. Other tests that may be indicated in the depressed woman include blood counts to rule out anemia and infection, renal and hepatic function tests, electrolytes, rapid plasma reagen (RPR) to rule out neurosyphilis, and human immunodeficiency virus (HIV) testing to rule out autoimmune deficiency syndrome.

Ca-125

Ca-125 levels may be elevated with diseases associated with pelvic pain, such as endometriosis or leiomyomata, but there are also many other causes of Ca-125 elevation that are not related to pelvic pain. Ca-125 levels have been evaluated as aids to diagnosis and follow-up of patients with endometriosis, in particular. However, as a diagnostic test Ca-125 has a low sensitivity and specificity, although it is more reliable for advanced stage disease (Table 14.7) (2). A major concern with the use of Ca-125 levels for diagnosis of endometriosis is that levels are also elevated with cancers of the ovary, endometrium, gastrointestinal tract, fallopian tube, and breast. They are also increased with pelvic inflammatory disease, pregnancy, menses, and leiomyomata (3).

ABDOMINOPELVIC ULTRASOUND

Ultrasonography is a noninvasive diagnostic tool that may be helpful in many women with either acute or chronic pelvic pain. In patients with a pelvic mass, it may help to identify the origin of the mass as uterine, adnexal, gastrointestinal, or bladder.

In cases of suspected uterine pathology, ultrasonography can be valuable in women with leiomyomata, both to confirm the diagnosis and to document the number of fibroids, their location, degree of calcification, and rate of growth. Transvaginal sonography, in particular, may identify and distinguish leiomyomas from adenomyomas. An adenomyoma usually appears as a disharmonious, circumscribed area in the myometrium with indistinct margins and anechoic lacunae of various diameters. A leiomyoma is diagnosed when a nodular formation with well-defined margins, heterogeneous structure, and variable echogenicity is detected in the myometrium. Using these criteria for distinguishing adenomyomas and leiomyomas, transvaginal sonography

has a sensitivity of 87%, a specificity of 98%, and a negative predictive value of 99% (4). Ultrasound is not as reliable for the diagnosis of adenomyosis without adenomyoma formation. In general, patients who have adenomyosis sonographically have an enlarged uterus, irregular vascular spaces within the myometrium, and an acoustically enlarged posterior wall (5).

In some cases ultrasonography may detect endometrial polyps or an unsuspected intrauterine device. However, conventional transvaginal sonography will sometimes miss an endometrial polyp (6). In such cases, hysterosonography is usually effective in distinguishing endometrial thickening from endometrial polyps (7).

When performed transvaginally, ultrasonography may allow the diagnosis of cervical stenosis, if it is obstructive. Sonography may show fluid or debris, or a fluid–debris level in the endometrial cavity (8). A lobulated or distorted cervix may suggest an occult carcinoma or fibroids as the cause.

Pelvic ultrasonography is also helpful if an adnexal cyst or mass is suspected. Location, size, and solid or cystic components may be determined sonographically and may aid in nonoperative or preoperative diagnosis. If endometriosis is suspected, ultrasonography is especially useful to identify possible endometriomas prior to laparoscopic evaluation and treatment. It can also be used to follow patients after treatment and identify any recurrence of the endometriomas.

Ultrasonography can also be useful in the diagnosis of ovarian retention syndrome and ovarian remnant syndrome. Vaginal ultrasound shows a pelvic mass in 50% to 85% of cases of ovarian remnant syndrome. The mass is usually cystic or multiseptated with a well defined solid tissue ring surrounding it. The diagnostic accuracy of ultrasound may be improved by pretreatment with clomiphene citrate (9). Not all ovarian remnants have functional follicles that respond and enlarge with clomiphene; therefore, this technique is not invariably helpful.

Ultrasound can be used to identify pelvic varicosities and suggest a diagnosis of pelvic congestion syndrome (10,11). Although Doppler and color Doppler have been suggested as possible techniques to diagnose decreased venous flow and congestion, the technology has not yet reached the stage where it can be applied in the diagnosis of pelvic congestion syndrome (12). Its use in the pelvis has been limited mainly to identification of arterial flow disturbances associated with the condition and not actual measurement of venous flow patterns (13,14).

If pelvic floor relaxation defects are believed to contribute to pelvic pain, vaginal sonography, perineal ultrasound, introital sonography, and rectosonography can all be used to evaluate pelvic floor muscle function, particularly at the urethrovesical junction and bladder base. Coughing results in fast, caudally oriented movement of the bladder and the urethra. The extent of movement increases with insufficiency of the urethrovesical attachments. Perineal and introital applications of linear array and mechanical sector scanners have been found to be most suitable for patients with lower urinary tract disorders.

Abdominal wall ultrasound or CT scan may assist if the diagnosis of hernias of the linea alba and umbilical hernias, but both of these types of hernias can usually be diagnosed by physical examination. Spigelian hernias, however, are more difficult to diagnose by examination. Ultrasound diagnosis is accurate in about 80% of cases of Spigelian hernias. A combination of ultrasound and tangential radiographs can improve the accuracy. If the hernia is reduced and no mass is palpable, ultrasound scanning will show a break in the echogenic shadow of the semilunar line corresponding to the fascial defect. Whether or not the hernia is palpable, if it is not reduced, the hernial sac and contents will be demonstrated passing through the defect in the Spigelian fascia and lying in an interstitial or subcutaneous plane. Scanning by thin section CT can also confirm the presence of a Spigelian hernia. Ultrasound can also be helpful in confirming the existence of an internal supravesical hernia.

RADIOGRAPHY

Plain Film Radiography

Musculoskeletal causes of CPP can sometimes be evaluated with plain film radiography to rule out problems such as fractures, infections, ankylosing spondylitis, tumors, and so on. Occasionally they may identify other structural abnormalities, as well as bony changes in density or texture. Plain radiographs will adequately illustrate gross bony abnormalities such as vertebral fractures, osteophytes, or severe osteoporosis, which may themselves cause pain or may lead to pain through nerve entrapment or compression.

If pelvic tuberculosis is suspected as a cause of pelvic pain, a chest radiograph showing active disease provides presumptive supportive evidence of tuberculosis. Pelvic tuberculosis is uncommon in the United States and Western Europe. Its prevalence may increase with the increase of HIV infections.

If chronic intermittent bowel obstruction is considered, then flat and upright abdominal radiographs may be useful to distinguish complete versus partial bowel obstructions by the presence of dilated loops of small bowel and the absence or presence of gas in the colon.

Barium Enema

In patients in whom intestinal endometriosis is suspected, evaluation of the intestinal tract is usually normal, as most patients have involvement of the serosa or muscularis, not the mucosa. Sigmoidoscopy may show a bluish submucosal mass in some of these cases. Mucosal lesions may be diagnosed by sigmoidoscopy, colonoscopy, or barium enema studies, but these evaluations are certainly not necessary on a routine basis (15).

Barium enema radiography to evaluate the lower gastrointestinal tract may be advisable in cases of ovarian remnant syndrome if there is any suspicion of involvement or stricture of the colon.

If inflammatory bowel disease is possible, then barium enema, as well as small bowel follow through radiographs, are often diagnostic. Barium enema or gastrografin study is indicated if diverticular disease is considered. This is an uncommon diagnosis in women less than 50 years of age.

Hysterosalpingography

Hysterosalpingography (HSG) is not a commonly performed test in women with CPP, but it may detect uterine anomalies, endometrial polyps, or Asherman syndrome. It also may be useful in women suspected of having adenomyosis, because the contrast medium may reveal short, spiculelike structures extending 1 to 4 mm deep perpendicularly from the borders of the uterine cavity (16). Another HSG finding consistent with adenomyosis is localized contrast material in the myometrium appearing as small rounded ponds with an almost honeycombed appearance. Areas of adenomyosis that do not communicate with the endometrial surface will not be revealed on HSG. Large localized adenomyomas can distort and enlarge the cavity, causing a radiographic shadow indistinguishable from a submucous myoma.

Adolescents with endometriosis should be evaluated by HSG for obstructive anomalies, because about 10% will have such an anomaly.

Herniography

Inguinal and abdominal wall hernias may play a more important role in CPP than generally recognized. As they are not always easy to diagnose, herniography can be a useful adjunct in diagnosis. To perform a herniogram, radiopaque contrast material is injected intraperitoneally and the patient is maneuvered through various positions in an attempt to introduce the material into an actual or potential hernial sac to demonstrate the sac radiographically. This technique reveals true or potential hernial sacs, but it has failed to gain popularity because of the general reliance on physical examination to diagnose most hernias. It may be of use in specially selected or difficult cases, for instance, to confirm or exclude the presence of an inguinal hernia in a patient complaining of unexplained groin pain. Herniography also has been shown to identify obturator hernias and perineal hernias that may or may not be symptomatic.

Colporectocystourethrography

Colporectocystourethrography (CRCU) is a radiological technique that uses radiopaque media in the urethra and bladder neck, vagina, rectum, and anal canal to visualize dynamic changes of the pelvic organs caused by pelvic floor muscle activity. The technique is relatively painless and easy to perform. The patient ingests barium 2 hours prior to the procedure to opacify the small bowel. The vagina and rectum are filled with barium paste, whereas the bladder is filled via a small catheter with 200 mL of a water-soluble contrast. Additionally, radiopaque markers are placed on specific areas on the perineum. These permit assessment of structures in relation to the perineal body (17). Nonrelaxing puborectalis syndrome can be evaluated with this technique, also (18).

The patient is seated on a radiologic commode and resting images are obtained during squeezing and straining. The contraction of the puborectalis may be observed during the squeezing frame. Indentation of the posterior rectum is noted. The dynamic portion of the examination follows as the patient empties her rectum completely. This form of study has excellent clinical value and is the best study and most practical technique for radiographic evaluation of women with prolapse. It is of use in women with CPP believed related to pelvic floor relaxation and possibly pelvic floor pain syndromes. However, CRCU requires a significant radiation dose and significant effort and preparation. Therefore, it is not a method that is useful in routine clinical evaluation.

Cystograms, Viscerograms, Colpocystograms, and Defecography

These studies are similar to CRCU, but involve visualization of only portions of the pelvic floor or pelvic viscera. As with CRCU, their primary use is to evaluate pelvic floor defects and function, and they have limited use in women with CPP. *Cystourethrograms* allow analysis of the posterior urethrovesical angle. *Dynamic pelvic viscerograms* with injection of the levator muscles with contrast solution (levator myography) allow evaluations of vaginal and rectal positions with increases in abdominal pressure, and evaluation of the levator hiatus. A *colpocystogram* adds opacification with contrast medium of the bladder, urethra, rectum and vagina and allows a dynamic study of pelvic support and function. *Defecography* or *dynamic proctography*, similar to colpocystography but done with fluoroscopy during defecation, is particularly helpful in evaluating rectoceles, enteroceles, sigmoidoceles, rectal prolapse, occult prolapse, or idiopathic incontinence. No bowel preparation is needed. The rectum is filled with a radiopaque paste using a special applicator and the patient seated on a radiolucent toilet seat. Evacuation should be done as quickly and completely as possible (19).

Pelvic Venography

Pelvic venography is performed in women with possible pelvic congestion syndrome, and currently is the only reliable way to diagnose this syndrome. *Transuterine venography* has been the most commonly employed method owing to its relative ease, low risk of complications, and relatively low cost (20,21). Water soluble contrast medium is introduced into the uterine venous system via injection into the myometrium of the uterine fundus with a special single-lumen needle (Rocket Needle, Rocket Co., London, England). Images are taken for 1 min after injection (22). The images are scored based on the maximum diameter of the ovarian veins, time of disappearance of contrast, and the degree of congestion of the ovarian plexus (see Table 18.2). The score can range from 3 to 9, with 3 or 4 being normal and 5 to 9 suggesting increasingly severe pelvic congestion. This method has a sensitivity of 91% and specificity of 89%, and a likelihood ratio of 8.3 for a positive test and a likelihood ratio 0.1 for a negative test.

Selective ovarian venography has also been used to diagnose pelvic congestion syndrome and can either be performed via a jugular venous approach or via the much more commonly used transfemoral approach (23). Special teflon catheters are passed under fluoroscopic guidance into the ovarian veins and nonionic water-soluble contrast medium injected. Because the right ovarian vein drains directly into the inferior vena cava, it is more difficult to cannulate and usually involves using a different type or size catheter than the left side. Some consider this invasive technique to be the method of choice for diagnosis of pelvic varicosities. Criteria that suggest venous congestion are maximum ovarian vein diameter of 10 mm, congestion of the ovarian venous plexus, filling of veins across the midline, or filling of vulvar and thigh varicosities (24).

Other much less commonly used techniques of venography are vulvar phlebography, in which contrast medium is injected via vulvar vein injection, and selective ovarian venography via vulvar vein puncture (25,26).

COMPUTERIZED TOMOGRAPHY

Computerized tomography (CT) may be diagnostically helpful in many women with acute or chronic pelvic pain. It is of particular use in women with pelvic masses and may be helpful in distinguishing ovarian from uterine masses, but it is more expensive than sonography and not always necessary. It may also be useful in cases of suspected ovarian remnant syndrome, especially if ultrasonography is negative (27).

In patients with suspected urinary tract involvement by endometriosis, ovarian remnant syndrome, ovarian retention syndrome, pelvic masses, and so on, intravenous pyelography has traditionally been used, but CT with intravenous contrast is a more accurate and informational technique, and is preferable in most cases. In addition to evaluating for possible obstruction of the ureters, CT should be done to identify any effects that previous operations or the current condition have had on ureteral location. This is of importance because dense pelvic adhesions are usually encountered in these cases and may distort the anatomy and make the ureters difficult to identify during surgery (28). Serum urea nitrogen and creatinine levels should be obtained if there is evidence of ureteral dilation, hydronephrosis, or ureteral deviation.

Urinary tract calculi are rare causes of chronic abdominopelvic pain, but if suspected a CT scan with intravenous contrast or an intravenous pyelogram should be done. The most common areas of identification of calculi associated with pelvic pain are illustrated in Fig. 34.2.

CT with intravenous contrast medium can sometimes help with the diagnosis of sciatic hernia. In some cases of sciatic hernia the ureter herniates into the sciatic foramen and gives a pathognomonic urographic appearance of a redundant, horizontally oriented ureter within a hernia sac that has been called a "curlicue ureter" (29,30).

Patients with tuberculosis may present with CPP and rarely may have stenosis or fistula formation of the gastrointestinal tract. Abdominal CT with oral or enema radiographic contrast material will generally demonstrate these findings if they are present.

Abdominal wall CT scan may assist if the diagnosis of hernias. Hernias of the linea alba and umbilical hernias are usually diagnosed by physical examination, but CT can sometimes be helpful. Spigelian hernias are more difficult to diagnose by examination. Ultrasound diagnosis is fairly accurate, but in some cases scanning by thin section CT can confirm the presence of a Spigelian hernia.

The diagnosis of herniation into an incision site also can be made by CT scan or ultrasonography. In patients with intermittent symptoms in whom a Richter's hernia is suspected, CT scan will very accurately demonstrate the loop of small bowel above the fascia. Omental herniations have also occurred, especially in laparoscopic procedures with their smaller incision sites. These can also be detected by CT scan (31). Other hernias, such as internal supravesical hernias, may also be confirmed with CT scan.

Potential musculoskeletal sources of pelvic pain, such as fractures, infections, ankylosing spondylitis, tumors, and so on, can be evaluated with plain film radiographs, but computerized tomography gives higher resolution and may often be more appropriate than plain radiographs to evaluate for structural abnormalities.

MAGNETIC RESONANCE IMAGING

Magnetic resonance imaging (MRI) has not been extensively used in women with CPP, but it holds great promise because of the superb anatomic images it provides. For the preopera-

tive diagnosis of adenomyosis, MRI provides excellent soft tissue contrast, is minimally invasive, and avoids ionizing radiation. On T2-weighted images, diffuse adenomyosis distorts normal zonal anatomy of the uterus, causing enlargement of the functional zone, seen as a wide band with low signal intensity adjacent to the endometrium. The endometrium maintains its normal, high intensity signal. The endometrium also shows high intensity signals and adenomatous signs in the myometrium. Adenomyosis has irregular and indistinct margins because of its more invasive nature, as compared to leiomyomata, which have well-encapsulated margins. In one study assessing the capability of MRI to differentiate adenomyosis and leiomyomas, all cases of adenomyosis were diagnosed correctly, 10 of 12 leiomyomata were diagnosed correctly, but two cases of leiomyomata could not be differentiated from focal adenomyosis. Microscopic foci of adenomyosis were not seen with MRI (32).

Magnetic resonance imaging is also be helpful in the evaluation for obstructive uterine anomalies in adolescents with endometriosis. MRI has been investigated as a noninvasive diagnostic modality for pelvic congestion syndrome (33). It is not as yet clear if it will be of diagnostic value (34). Theoretically, magnetic resonance imaging should be very accurate in detecting an ovarian remnant, but as with pelvic congestion, there have not been published reports to allow an evaluation of its utility.

MRI, because of its ability to provide soft tissue contrast resolution and distinguish the various fascial and muscular layers of the pelvis, may aid in the evaluation of pelvic support. However, the supine position that currently is required is not a gravity dependent position and therefore is not the best position for the evaluation of a pelvic floor dysfunction. With advancing technology, dynamic MRI imaging in the sitting and standing positions may make MRI the primary method of clinically evaluating patients with prolapse, incontinence, suspected enterocele, anorectal defects, and multicompartment prolapse.

Bone scans with radioactive tracers are sometimes useful in cases of suspected infection, fractures (especially stress fractures), and tumors, but MRI is better at visualizing soft tissue and may soon supplant bone scans and other imaging modalities for diagnostic evaluation. It is now commonly used to evaluate possible spinal disc pathology, ligamentous tears, spinal cord tumors, osteochondritis, and many central nervous system (CNS) disorders. CT scans and MRI studies along with myelogram or discography may be needed to diagnose more subtle areas of nerve root compression or tumors.

URODYNAMIC TESTING

Urodynamic testing is indicated in the woman with CPP if chronic urethral syndrome is suspected. These studies can identify patients with abnormal voiding patterns owing to dyssynergic voiding. Voiding and electromyographic studies reveal prolonged or intermittent voiding patterns and hyperactivity of the pelvic floor or external urethral sphincter. Mean urinary flow rates are notably decreased and mean flow times are increased with intermittent and prolonged flow rate patterns (Fig. 37.1) (35). Maximal urethral closure pressure is increased by twofold over normal in women with chronic urethral syndrome. In spite of the common symptom of incomplete emptying, women with chronic urethral syndrome do not have an increase in residual volume. Maximal intravesical pressure is normal, as is functional bladder capacity. Not all patients with clinical evidence of chronic urethral syndrome have urodynamic abnormalities.

Urodynamics may reveal uninhibited bladder contractions. Uroflowmetry when the patient experiences stranguria demonstrates the erratic prolonged flow characteristic of vesical-sphincter dyssynergia (36). Pelvic floor electromyography and pressure studies can also objectively document muscle spasm and inability to relax during voiding.

GASTROINTESTINAL FUNCTION TESTING

In some patients with CPP and intractable constipation, anorectal manometry is indicated. For example, patients with Hirschsprung disease or intestinal neuronal dysplasia may have loss of the recto-anal inhibitory reflex. Anorectal balloon manometry is one method that detects this loss. It uses a manometer attached to a balloon that is placed through the anus and into the rectum. Patients with poor rectal sensation may need more than the normal volume of 60 cc of air to initiate a reflex, those with Hirschsprung have absence of an inhibitory reflex, and patients with sphincter hypertonia have excessively high pressure coupled with the inhibitory reflex (37).

Testing colonic transit time may also be helpful in the evaluation of chronic constipation. There are a number of methods available, such as radiopaque markers, scintigraphy, breath hydrogen concentration, and liquid transit (38). Radiopaque marker ingestion is the most commonly utilized technique. An abnormal transit time is usually more than 72 hours.

ELECTROENCEPHALOGRAPHY

Electroencephalography (EEG) is not a normal test in the woman with CPP. However, it is indicated if abdominal epilepsy is in the differential diagnosis, as most patients with this syndrome have an abnormal EEG. Although there is no stereotypical pattern of EEG abnormalities, the two most common patterns are:

- Paroxysmal generalized dysrhythmia of slow activity. This usually occurs episodically throughout the EEG record.

- Paroxysmal spike-wave activity. The spikes or sharp waves are most commonly localized over one or both temporal regions.

NERVE CONDUCTION AND ELECTROMYOGRAPHIC STUDIES

Occasionally pelvic pain is secondary to compression or entrapment neuropathy. Electrophysiologic studies of nerve function may help in the localization and assessment of the severity of compression or entrapment neuropathies. Studies include determination of nerve conducting velocities of the sensory and motor fibers and needle electromyographic (EMG) studies. Conduction tests are more applicable in the study of motor neurons than sensory neurons. They are not very sensitive in detecting degeneration of small fibers or of a few large fibers in association with preservation of a great number of large fibers. They may be of value in documenting the existence of a generalized neuropathy that may predispose to compressive neuropathy. EMG studies may be helpful in determining whether muscular atrophy, if present, is owing to a neuropathic or myopathic disorder. Generally speaking they are of relatively low value in the neuropathies of the smaller branches of the lumbosacral plexus.

Anal electromyography (EMG) and measurement of pudendal nerve terminal latency (PNTML) are of value in assessing the electrical activity of the pelvic floor. Anal EMG is particularly useful in diagnosing paradoxical puborectalis contraction and in revealing neuromuscular damage related to chronic straining. The technique uses an anal plug electrode to measure electrical activity of the anal sphincter apparatus. EMG recording of the external anal sphincter muscle shows a paradoxical increase in activity during evacuation efforts in cases of paradoxical puborectalis contraction or anismus (39). The technique of measuring PNTML is of use in assessing pudendal nerve injury and discovering intrinsic neurologic injury to the striated sphincter muscles of the pelvic floor. It involves a glove-mounted nerve stimulating and recording device that is introduced through the rectum and brought into contact with the ischial spine on each side. A PNTML value greater than 2.2 ms is considered abnormal. Thus, in patients with chronic pelvic pain, injury to the pudendal nerve may be the cause of both their pain and the accompanying constipation. Additional diagnostic procedures include the balloon expulsion test and scintigraphic defecography.

REFERENCES

1. Solomons CC, Melmed MH, Heitler SM. Calcium citrate for vulvar vestibulitis: a case report. *J Reprod Med* 1991;36:879–882.
2. Lanzone A, Marane R, Muscatello R, et al. Serum Ca-125 levels in the diagnosis and management of endometriosis. *J Reprod Med* 1991;36:603–607.

3. Adamson GD. Diagnosis and clinical presentation of endometriosis. *Am J Obstet Gynecol* 1990;162:568–569.

4. Fedelle L, Bianchi S, Dorta M. Transvaginal ultrasonography in the differential diagnosis of adenomyoma versus leiomyoma. *Am J Obstet Gynecol* 1992;167:603–606.

5. Bohlman Me, Ensor RE, Saunders RC. Sonographic findings in adenomyosis of the uterus. *Am J Roentgenol* 1987;148:765–766.

6. Bonilla-Musoles F, Raga F, Osborne NG, et al. Three-dimensional hysterosonography for the study of endometrial tumors: comparison with conventional transvaginal sonography, hysterosalpingo-sonography, and hysteroscopy. *Gynecol Oncol* 1997; 65:245–252.

7. Cohen JR, Luxman D, Sagi J, et al. Sonohysterography for distinguishing endometrial thickening from endometrial polyps in postmenopausal bleeding. *Ultrasound Obstet Gynecol* 1994;4: 227–230.

8. Hall DA, Yoder IC. Ultrasound evaluation of the uterus. In: Callin PW, ed. *Ultrasonography in obstetrics and gynecology.* Philadelphia: WB Saunders, 1994:586–614.

9. Kaminski PF, Sorosky JI, Mandell MJ, et al. Clomiphene citrate as an adjunct in locating ovarian tissue in ovarian remnant syndrome. *Obstet Gynecol* 1990;76(5 Part 2):924–926.

10. Montanari GD, Alfieri G, Grella P, et al. Ultrasonic tomography in the diagnosis of pelvic congestion. *Minerva Ginecologica* 1975; 27(3):219–223.

11. Frede TE. Ultrasonic visualization of varicosities in the female genital tract. *J Ultrasound Med* 1984;3(8):365–369.

12. Taylor KJW, Burms PN, Woodcock JP. Blood flow in deep abdominal and pelvic vessels: ultrasonic and pulsed Doppler analysis. *Radiology* 1985;154:487–493.

13. Fleischer AC, Kepple DM. Transvaginal color duplex sonography: clinical potentials and limitations. *Semin Ultrasound, CT MR* 1992;13(1):69–80.

14. Smith MR. Pulsatile pelvic masses: options for evaluation and management of pelvic arteriovenous malformations. *Am J Obstet Gynecol* 1995;172(6):1857–1863.

15. Rapkin AJ, Mayer EA. Gastroenterologic causes of chronic pelvic pain. *Obstet Gynecol Clin NA* 1993;20:663–683.

16. Hunt RB, Siegler AM. *Hysterosalpingography: techniques and interpretation.* Chicago: Yearbook Publishers, 1990:75.

17. Kelvin FM, Maglinte D, Hornback JA, et al. Pelvic prolapse: assessment with evacuation proctography (defecography). *Radiology* 1992;184:547–551.

18. Blatchford GJ, Cali RL, Christensen MA. Surgical treatment of rectocele. In: Wexner SD, Bartolo DCC, eds. *Constipation. Etiology, evaluation and management.* Oxford: Butterworth-Heinemann, 1995:199–209.

19. Kuijpers HC. Defaecography. In: Wexner SD, Bartolo DCC, eds. *Constipation. Etiology, evaluation and management.* Oxford: Butterworth-Heinemann, 1995:75–77.

20. Hammen R. The technique of pelvic phlebography. *Acta Obstet Gynecol Scand* 1965;44:370–374.

21. Bellina JH, Dougherty C, Michal A. Transmyometrial pelvic venography. *Obstet Gynecol* 1969;34(2):194–199.

22. Murray E, Comparato MR. Uterine phlebography. *Am J Obstet Gynecol* 1968;102(8):1088–1093.

23. Tarazov PG, Prozorovskij KV, Ryzhkov VK. Pelvic pain syndrome caused by ovarian varices. Treatment by transcatheter embolization. *Acta Radiologica* 1997;38:1023–1025.

24. Kennedy A, Hemmingway A. Radiology of ovarian varices. *Br J Hosp Med* 1990;44:38–43.

25. Craig O, Hobbs JT. Vulval phlebography in the pelvic congestion syndrome. *Clin Radiol* 1974;25:517–525.

26. Grabham JA, Barrie WW. Laparoscopic approach to pelvic congestion syndrome. *Br J Surg* 1997;84:1264–1267.

27. Price FV, Edwards R, Buchsbaum HJ. Ovarian remnant syndrome: difficulties in diagnosis and management. *Obstet Gynecol Surv* 1990;45(3):151–156.

28. Berek JS, Darney PD, Lopkin C, et al. Avoiding ureteral damage in pelvic surgery for ovarian remnant syndrome. *Am J Obstet Gynecol* 1979;133:221–222.

29. Beck WC, Baurys W, Brochu J, et al. Herniation of the ureter into the sciatic foramen ("curlicue ureter"). *JAMA* 1952;149: 441–442.

30. Spring DB, Vandeman F, Watson RA. Computed tomographic demonstration of ureterosciatic hernia. *AJR* 1983;141:579–580.

31. Boike GM, Miller CE, Spirtos NM, et al. Incisional bowel herniations after operative laparoscopy: a series of 19 cases and review of the literature. *Am J Obstet Gynecol* 1995;172:1726–1733.

32. Mark AS, Hricak H, Heinrich LW. Adenomyosis and leiomyoma: differential diagnosis with MR imaging. *Radiology* 1987; 168:527–529.

33. Gupta A, McCarthy S. Pelvic varices as a cause for pelvic pain, MRI appearance. *MRI* 1994;12(4):679–681.

34. Joja I, Asakawa M, Motoyama K, et al. Uterine cirsoid aneurysm: MRI and MRA. *J Assist Tomogr* 1996;20(2):290–294.

35. Summit RL Jr. Urogynecologic causes of chronic pelvic pain. *Obstet Gynecol Clin NA* 1993;20:685–698.

36. Kaplan WE, Firlit CF, Schoenberg HW. The female urethral syndrome: external sphincter spasm as etiology. *J Urol* 1980;124: 48–49.

37. Stein BL, Roberts PL. Manometry and the rectoanal inhibitory reflex. In: Wexner SD, Bartolo DCC, eds. *Constipation. Etiology, evaluation and management.* Oxford: Butterworth-Heinemann, 1995:63–76.

38. von der Ohe M, Camilleri M. Measurement of small bowel and colonic transit: indications and methods. *Mayo Clin Proc* 1992; 67:1169–1179.

39. Preston DM, Lennard-Jones JE. Anismus in chronic constipation. *Dig Dis Sci* 1985;30:413–418.

5

ENDOSCOPY

FRED M. HOWARD

INTRODUCTION

The endoscopic procedures most often used in the evaluation and treatment of women with CPP are laparoscopy, cystourethroscopy, hysteroscopy, sigmoidoscopy, and colonoscopy. Although endoscopic evaluations, particularly laparoscopy, sometimes have been considered a routine part of the evaluation, ideally the decision about any endoscopic procedure should be based on the patient's history and physical examination findings. This approach avoids unnecessary risks, expense, and false expectations for the patient.

This chapter covers laparoscopy, hysteroscopy, and cystourethroscopy in general terms. More information related to endoscopy and specific diagnoses are in the relevant chapters about each disease.

CYSTOURETHROSCOPY

Diseases associated with CPP that are best diagnosed via cystourethroscopy are bladder neoplasia, interstitial cystitis, radiation cystitis, urethral diverticulum, and urethral syndrome. Also, cystourethroscopy is often necessary when the following diseases are considered in the differential diagnosis: chronic urinary tract infections, urolithiasis, and uninhibited bladder contractions. In regions where schistosomiasis occurs, schistosomiasis of the bladder may also be a source of pain (1).

The visual findings are generally characteristic with bladder neoplasms; however, biopsies for histological confirmation are mandatory. When cystourethroscopy is performed for suspected urethral diverticulum, great scrutiny during the urethral part of the procedure is crucial. The opening of the diverticulum in the urethral mucosa can usually, but not always, be visualized. Voiding cystography may be helpful in confirming the diagnosis. Cystourethroscopic evaluations in women with suspected chronic urethral syndrome may show erythema, exudate, cystic dilation of periurethral glands, and inflammatory fronds throughout the urethra (2). It may also demonstrate incomplete funneling of the

bladder neck and distal urethral narrowing. In patients with CPP and chronic urethral syndrome, urethroscopy invariably reproduces their pain symptoms. Passing a urethral catheter may often produce similar excessive pain. Cystoscopy is normal, with no increase of bladder trabeculations (3).

Of the urologic diagnoses, interstitial cystitis (IC) appears to be the most common in women with CPP. It occurs predominantly in women at 30 to 59 years of age. The estimated incidence in the United States is 36 cases per 100,000 women (3,4). Pelvic pain is an inconsistent finding, occurring in 50% to 70% of women with IC. Occasionally it is the presenting symptom or chief complaint. In a series of 57 women with CPP and negative laparoscopies, only one (1.8%) was found to have IC (5). In a consecutive series of 197 women that I have cared for with CPP as a presenting complaint, four (2%) were diagnosed with IC. Although IC is an infrequent diagnosis, physicians caring for women with CPP still must be familiar with it. In many cases the diagnosis is not made until the patient has undergone numerous operative procedures such as laparoscopies, neurolytic procedures, hysterectomy, and salpingo-oophorectomy (3).

Cystoscopic findings are one of the three generally accepted diagnostic criteria of IC (Chapter 32).Because significant bladder distention is needed and this is very painful in women with IC, general or spinal anesthesia should be used. Cystoscopy for the diagnosis of IC is best performed in a somewhat standardized manner. After urethroscopy is completed the bladder is not allowed to collapse around the cystoscope, as this may traumatize the bladder mucosa and cause iatrogenic artifacts. The bladder is distended to 70 to 80 cm water pressure for 1 min or more. This may require compression of the urethra by upward digital compression of the anterior vaginal wall against the urethroscope to prevent leakage. Although the risk is low, it is possible to rupture the bladder in IC patients during this distention. Findings during this first filling are usually normal, although occasionally faint trabeculation may be noted. When maximal capacity is reached, the volume is noted and the irrigant drained. The terminal portion of this drainage may be

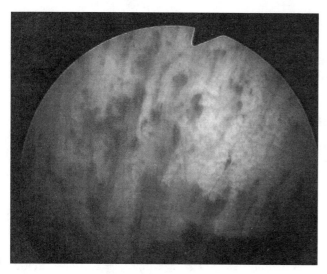 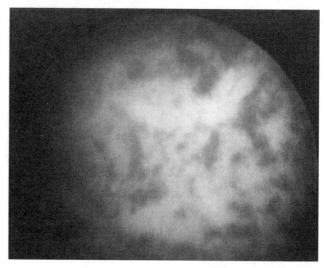

A   B

FIGURE 5.1. A: Hemorrhage from the bladder mucosa during emptying after first fill. **B:** Glomerulations at the time of second filling of the bladder.

blood-tinged. If videocystourethosocpy is performed and observation is continued during the emptying phase of the procedure, uniformly distributed focal areas of hemorrhage are noted. Mean cystoscopic bladder capacity in IC patients is 545 mL with a range of 150 to 950 mL (6). The bladder is then refilled and with IC reveals splotchy, submucosal hemorrhages throughout the bladder. These hemorrhages are called glomerulations (Fig. 5.1). Glomerulations do not occur in a normal bladder. A Hunner's ulcer may rarely be seen and when noted is diagnostic. Patients with markedly decreased bladder capacity are more likely to show Hunner's ulcer. Bladder biopsies are not mandatory, but may be useful. Any suspicious lesions must be biopsied to rule out carcinoma or carcinoma in situ. Also, the histologic finding of increased mast cells (special fixation and staining required) has been reported to be useful for confirmation of IC. Histologic findings of nonspecific inflammation in the bladder submucosa and muscularis, as well as vasodilation and edema in the submucosa, are characteristic but not pathonigmonic of IC.

It is important that any infection be cleared several weeks before cystoscopy, not only because of infection con-

cerns, but also specifically because current or recent infection may cause cystoscopic findings similar to those of IC.

The mainstay of urologic treatment of IC for more than 50 years has been hydrodistension of the bladder. This procedure can be performed at the time of diagnostic cystoscopy if general or spinal anesthesia is used. After diagnostic evaluation is completed the bladder is filled to maximal capacity at 80 to 100 cm water pressure for 2 min. There is some risk of bladder rupture with this procedure, estimated at less than 15% (4). Patients complain of increased pain immediately postoperatively and it is generally several weeks until they note a remission of symptoms. About 50% of patients have a successful response to hydrodistension.

HYSTEROSCOPY

At least two recognized authorities in the evaluation and treatment of CPP have reported hysteroscopic findings in a large series of women with CPP (Table 5.1) (7,8). Together their series suggest that about one-third of women with

TABLE 5.1. HYSTEROSCOPIC FINDINGS AT THE TIME OF COMBINED LAPAROSCOPIC AND HYSTEROSCOPIC EVALUATIONS IN WOMEN WITH CPP

Diagnoses	Carter (*n* = 140)	Nezhat et al. (*n* = 499)	Total (*n* = 639)
Submucuous leiomyomas	25 (18%)	32 (6.4%)	57 (8.9%)
Intrauterine polyps	9 (6.4%)	35 (7.0%)	44 (6.9%)
Cervical stenosis	4 (2.9%)	55 (11%)	59 (9.2%)
Intrauterine scarring	3 (2.1%)	—	3 (0.5%)
Hyperplasia	2 (1.4%)	7 (1.4%)	9 (1.4%)
Uterine septum	—	7 (1.4%)	7 (1.1%)
Other	—	26 (5.2%)	26 (4.1%)
Total	43 (30%)	162 (32%)	205 (32%)

CPP have a uterine abnormality at the time of hysteroscopy. These authors recognized that their findings did not equate to cause and effect. They also found significant abnormalities laparoscopically in almost all of these patients.

Interestingly, neither of these series reported a diagnosis of adenomyosis, even though hystersoscopy had been suggested as a possible way to diagnosis adenomyosis. This is probably because only diagnostic hysteroscopy was performed and it is now clear that diagnostic hysteroscopy alone is not sufficient for the diagnosis of adenomyosis. Although sometimes examination of the uterine cavity reveals small diverticulae when there is a connection between the ectopic sites of adenomyosis and the endometrial cavity, such findings are often absent. A normal appearing cavity at hysteroscopy does not rule out adenomyosis. In symptomatic patients with a normal appearing endometrial cavity, an endomyometrial biopsy may be helpful (9). One study of 90 patients with menorrhagia showed 50 had normal appearing cavities, 27 had gross endometrial polyps and 13 had submucous myomas. At the time of the hysteroscopy a 1.5- to 3-cm biopsy specimen was obtained with a 5-mm Loop electrode, mostly from the posterior wall near the fundus using 70 W of cutting current. Of the 50 women with normal appearing cavities, 66% had significant adenomyosis (10). A hysteroscopic myometrial biopsy may be one way to confirm the diagnosis of adenomyosis without performing a hysterectomy.

The role of hysteroscopy in the evaluations of a women with CPP is not established. Although up to one-third may have uterine or cervical pathology, it is not clear that treatment of the hysteroscopically found disease will affect their pain. Carter and Nezhat believe that because the incidence of abnormalities is high and the procedure is quick and safe in the hands of an experienced surgeon, hysteroscopy should be done routinely at the time of laparoscopy for CPP. Although this seems a resonable suggestion, it does not address the issue of treatment versus no treatment of non–life-threatening diseases found at the time of hysteroscopy. Realistically, routine hysteroscopy with laparoscopy could easily lead to unnecessary treatments of incidental abnormalities in this unlucky group of women who are already exposed to too many unsuccessful operative procedures. The same concerns also apply to the use of hysteroscopic myometrial biopsies as a routine part of the evaluation for adenomyosis. Before a recommendation can be made regarding the role of hysteroscopy in the evaluation and treatment of women with CPP, more research is clearly needed.

LAPAROSCOPY

Because laparoscopy allows a minimally invasive evaluation of the reproductive organs, often with concurrent operative laparoscopic treatment of any abnormalities detected, it is liberally used by gynecologists in a comprehensive evaluation of the patient with pelvic pain (11). A survey of published laparoscopy series suggests that over 40% of gynecologic diagnostic laparoscopies are done for CPP (Table 5.2) (12). Although an abnormal examination correlates in 70% to 90% of cases with abnormal laparoscopic findings, still more than half of those with abnormal laparoscopic findings have a normal preoperative pelvic examination (Table 5.3) (13–15). Thus, the use of laparoscopy allows the detection of potentially treatable pathology not detected by examination (16). Conversely, in other cases it may prevent inappropriate major surgical evaluation or treatment. Some of the other advantages of laparoscopy in the evaluation of women with CPP are given in Table 5.4.

Published series show that no visible pathology is detected in 35% of patients (Table 5.5) (17). Endometriosis is the most common pathologic diagnosis (33%), followed by adhesive disease (24%). These three account for about 92% of all laparoscopic diagnoses in women with CPP. Overall, about 65% of women with CPP have at least one diagnosis detectable by laparoscopy and it is common to attribute causality to this diagnosis. However, it is not that simple, nor that clear. Data from studies of patients without CPP show that these women have a significant incidence of abnormal laparoscopic findings: 28% had abnormalities, with endometriosis (5%) and adhesions (17%) accounting for most of the diagnoses (Table 5.6) (14). Comparing these results to those from women with CPP shows that CPP patients have approximately twice the incidence of laparoscopically detected pathologies as do "normal" women. Although such data suggest that endometriosis, adhesions, chronic pelvic inflammatory dis-

TABLE 5.2. CPP AS THE INDICATION FOR LAPAROSCOPY

Study	Total No. of Laparoscopies	No. for CPP	Percent for CPP
Renaer, 1981	200	108	54
Royal College of Ob-Gyn, c. 1980	21,000	10,857	51
Cunanan et al., 1983	3,831	1,268	33
Liston et al., 1972	1,215	134	11
Bahary and Gorodeski, 1987	433	130	30
Mahmood et al., 1991	1,200	156	13
Total	28,679	12,653	44

TABLE 5.3. CORRELATION BETWEEN LAPAROSCOPY FINDINGS AND PREOPERATIVE PHYSICAL EXAMINATION IN PATIENTS WITH ACUTE OR CHRONIC PELVIC PAIN

Preoperative Examination	No. with Normal Laparoscopic Findings	No. with Abnormal Laparoscopic Findings
Normal	300 (76%)	496 (56%)
Abnormal	94 (24%)	397 (44%)
Total	394 (100%)	893 (100%)

TABLE 5.4. ADVANTAGES OF LAPAROSCOPY OVER CLINICAL, LABORATORY, RADIOLOGY, AND LAPAROTOMY EVALUTION OF WOMEN WITH CPP

Patient reassurance
Differentiation between gynecologic and nongynecologic etiology
Rule out serious or malignant disease
Increased accuracy of diagnoses
   Best diagnostic method for endometriosis, adhesions, and PID
   Six- to eightfold magnification possible
   Better view of cul-de-sac, ovarian fossae, and upper abdomen
   Allows histologic documentation of diagnoses
Immediate surgical treatment is often possible
   May prevent need for a laparotomy
   Decreases *de novo* adhesion formation
   May avert need for hospitalization

TABLE 5.5. LAPAROSCOPIC FINDINGS IN WOMEN WITH CHRONIC PELVIC PAIN

	No. of Patients	No Visible Pathology (%)	Endometriosis (%)	Adhesions (%)	Chronic PID (%)	Ovarian Cysts (%)	Pelvic Varicosities (%)	Myomas (%)	Other (%)
Renaer, 1981	108	58	20	0	21	0	0	0	0
Kresch et al., 1984	100	9	32	51	0	0	3	0	5
Rosenthal et al., 1984	60	25	17	40	—	—	—	—	18
Levitan et al., 1985	186	92	2	3	4	0	0	0	0
Rapkin, 1986	100	36	37	26	0	1	0	0	0
Bahary et al., 1987	130	18	5	2	29	15	1	4	25
Longstreth et al., 1990	76	36	20	36	4	17	0	5	7
Vercellini et al., 1990	126	37	32	18	6	2	0	0	3
Koninckx et al., 1991	227	3	74	52	2	0	0	0	0
Peters et al., 1991	49	65	8	18	0	4	2	2	0
Mahmood et al., 1991	156	57	15	28	0	0	0	0	0
Howard, 1994	65	8	38	34	3	6	0	2	9
Carter, 1994	141	0	80	13	0	0	0	3	2
Totals	1,524	35	33	24	5	3	<1	<1	4

TABLE 5.6. LAPAROSCOPIC FINDINGS IN WOMEN WITHOUT CPP AND COMPARISON TO FINDINGS IN WOMEN WITH CPP

	No. of Patients	No Visible Pathology (%)	Endometriosis (%)	Adhesions (%)	Myomas (%)	Ovarian Cysts (%)	Chronic PID (%)	Pelvic Varicosities (%)	Other (%)
Drake and Grunert, 1980	43	76	5	12	7	—	—	—	—
Strathy et al., 1982	200	74	2	7	6	—	2	—	9
Kresch et al., 1984	50	56	15	14	—	—	—	(15)[a]	—
Trimbos et al., 1990	200	74	3	14	5	2	2	—	—
Stout et al., 1991	12	42	25	25	8	—	—	—	—
Mahmood et al., 1991	598	72	6	22	—	—	—	—	—
Totals, Without CPP	1,103	72	5	17	2	—	1	—	2
Totals, With CPP	1,524	35	33	24	<1	3	5	<1	4

[a]Pelvic varicosities were not considered in analysis of "normal" patients because no other authors made the diagnosis in any patients.

ease, and ovarian cysts are each *associated* with CPP, but are insufficient to prove *causation*.

Laparoscopy and Endometriosis

Sampson, who is generally credited with coining the term "endometriosis" in about 1921, defined it as "the presence of ectopic tissue which possesses the histological structure and function of the uterine mucosa", and this remains the currently accepted definition (18–23). Thus, endometriosis is a histologically defined disease; that is, it *clearly requires histologic confirmation before the diagnosis can be made.* To confirm endometriosis histologically, one must see both endometrial glands and stroma (24,25). Before the introduction of diagnostic laparoscopy, this required an exploratory laparotomy, which was not done without extreme symptoms (26). Because of its advantages (Table 5.4), laparoscopy, not laparotomy, is the diagnostic procedure currently recommended for any patient suspected of having endometriosis (27).

Many gynecologists believe it appropriate to exclude or diagnose endometriosis solely of the basis of visual findings at the time of laparoscopy (28). However, endometriosis presents with a variety of appearances, which may make visual diagnosis difficult and inaccurate (Fig. 5.2) (29–31). Some of the descriptive terms that have been aptly applied to endometriosis are red raspberries, purple raspberries, blueberries, blebs, peritoneal pockets, whitish scar tissue, stellate scar tissue, strawberry-colored lesions, red vesicles, white vesicles, clear vesicles, powder burns, peritoneal win-

dows, yellow-brown patches, brown-black patches, adhesions, clear polypoid lesions, red polypoid lesions, red flame-like lesions, black puckered spots, white plaques with black puckers, and chocolate cysts (19,29,32–35). Sometimes endometriosis is classified into *atypical* versus *typical* lesions. Atypical or "subtle" generally applies to red, yellow, white, or clear lesions. Typical or "classical" refers to black-brown, black, or puckered black stellate scar lesions. Typical lesions have the appearances classically recognized as endometriosis, whereas the atypical lesions have often been overlooked or gone unnoticed (30). This can lead to significant underdiagnosis, as it has been reported that up to one-third of patients with endometriosis have only lesions of the atypical type (25,36). Martin has found that increased awareness of atypical lesions and the liberal use of biopsies increase the frequency of laparoscopic diagnosis of endometriosis from 42% to 72% (38).

Conversely, solely visual diagnosis can lead to overdiagnosis of endometriosis. By appearance alone the following lesions may be misdiagnosed as endometriosis: hemangiomas, old suture, ovarian carcinoma, residual carbon deposits from prior surgery, ectopic pregnancy, adrenal rest, Walthard rest, breast carcinoma, epithelial inclusions, reaction to oil-based hysterosalpingogram medium, inflammatory cystic inclusions, inflammation with or without Psammoma bodies, splenosis, endosalpingiosis, submesothelial microbleeding, and normal peritoneum (25,29,37). Table 5.7 shows the correlation between visual and biopsy diagnoses with some of the various appearances possible with endometriosis (25,29,33). Obviously, the wide variety of

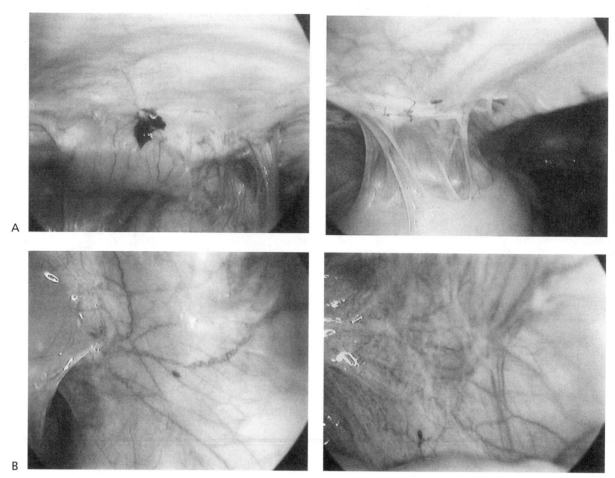

FIGURE 5.2. A: Pigmented lesions at herniorrhaphy site; not endometriosis. **B:** Pigmented lesions over the right ureter; histologically confirmed endometriosis. Both lesions were in the same patient.

TABLE 5.7. RATES OF HISTOLOGIC CONFIRMATION WITH VARIOUS APPEARANCES OF ENDOMETRIOSIS

	Confirmation of Diagnosis		
Description of Lesion	No. of Biopsies	No.	Percent
Black lesions	48	43	90
Brown lesions	63	49	78
White lesions	91	69	76
Red lesions	49	33	67
Clear papules	27	18	67
Glandular	21	14	67
Peritoneal defects	49	20	41
Superficial yellow-brown patches	53	21	40
Adhesions (ovarian)	40	16	40
Carbon	6	1	17
Adhesions (nonovarian)	33	4	12
Cribriform peritoneal defects	11	1	9

appearances can prove deceptive. For example, in one study of 132 cases of endometriosis diagnosed laparoscopically, biopsies were sent in only 15 cases (11%) and in all 15 the diagnoses were not confirmed by histology (38). Furthermore, when all cases surgically diagnosed as endometriosis were evaluated, including those diagnosed by laparotomy and hysterectomy, histologic findings confirmed the diagnoses of endometriosis in only two-thirds of the cases. In another study of 142 patients diagnosed by laparoscopic appearances as having endometriosis, 110 had biopsies taken and in only 60% did the histologic findings confirm the diagnoses (39). Clearly the potential for misdiagnosis is high enough that visual diagnosis is insufficient. Before CPP is attributed to endometriosis, any lesion believed consistent with endometriosis should be biopsied and the diagnosis confirmed by the histologic finding of endometrial glands and stroma.

The variety of possible appearances of endometriosis also mandates that laparoscopic evaluation be thorough and complete. Atypical endometriosis may result in missed diagnoses in 7% of cases and underestimated extent of disease in up to 50% of patients. Thus, a thorough knowledge of the various possible appearances of endometriosis, a thorough evaluation of the pelvis, and the liberal use of excisional biopsies are essential at the time of diagnostic laparoscopy for CPP if we are to avoid incorrectly labeling findings as normal or underestimating the extent of endometriosis present.

The common sites in the pelvis and abdomen that must be closely inspected include the ovaries (all surfaces) and ovarian fossae, pelvic peritoneum (particularly the cul-de-sac, periureteral, and bladder peritoneum), uterine ligaments, sigmoid colon, appendix, fallopian tubes, and rectovaginal septum. Koninckx et al., in a study of 716 women with endometriosis, found the following anatomic distributions: cul-de-sac and uterosacrals, 69%; ovaries, 45%; fossa ovaricae, 33%; and vesicouterine fold, 24% (40). Perez found that endometriosis involved the appendix in one of 25 patients with pelvic endometriosis (41). To adequately evaluate all of these anatomic sites, it is necessary to use at least a double-puncture technique and perform biopsies liberally. "Near-contact" laparoscopy, which results in up to an eightfold magnification, may be helpful in searching for atypical, nonpigmented endometriosis, as well as peritoneal lesions as small as 400 μ. Redwine has suggested that "painting" the peritoneal surfaces with blood may also be helpful for visualizing nonpigmented lesions (42). Needle puncture of the ovaries has also been suggested to detect occult endometriomas and properly stage endometriosis (43). If an ultrasound is done preoperatively, cysts and endometiomas can be visualized. Thus, a preoperative ultrasound seems prudent before a laparoscopic evaluation for CPP, in case endometriosis and ovarian enlargement are found. When endometriosis has not been visualized anywhere else in the pelvis and a preoperative ultrasound shows normal ovaries, there is no role for ovarian needle puncture in the laparoscopic evaluation of patients with CPP.

It is important to fully describe the extent and appearance of endometriosis. Traditionally, the AFS staging system has been used, but this scoring system has little relevance to either the presence or severity of CPP (Chapter 14, Endometriosis and Endosalpingiosis). Thus documenting only the AFS score seems insufficient. It may be important to note and record the depth of infiltration of lesions, in addition to size and distribution, as there is some evidence that depth of invasion of lesions may correlate with pain severity. The ability to document findings with photographs or videotape is helpful.

One of the advantages of laparoscopic evaluation for endometriosis is the potential to treat it at the same time as the diagnostic evaluation. This is discussed more fully in Chapter 14, but a brief review is pertinent here. The technical objectives of surgery are (a) to restore normal pelvic anatomy, and (b) to resect, coagulate, or vaporize all endometriosis implants. These objectives can be accomplished with mechanical, thermal, electrical, or laser energy,

and there are no objective data that one is better than the other. The surgeon's knowledge, familiarity, and competence with the energy sources are far more important than any differences between them. It seems important for best results, to insure complete, full-depth resection of all implants, including atypical lesions (44). Usually the border between normal tissue and endometriosis is fairly obvious during resection, coagulation, or vaporization, but it can be difficult at times with deep lesions. Davis and Brooks suggest that any peritoneal lesion 5 mm or more in size should be excisionally biopsied, rather than ablated, which may aid in insuring complete removal of larger and deeper disease, as well as giving histologic confirmation of the diagnosis (44). Again, my opinion is that histologic confirmation is essential before CPP is attributed to endometriosis.

Laparoscopy and Adhesions

The physical appearances of adhesions are not specific to the underlying cause, so etiology is usually assigned based on the associated history or surgical diagnosis of PID, endometriosis, perforated appendix, prior surgery, or inflammatory bowel disease (45). A preoperative history of at least one of these etiologies is present in about 50% of women with pelvic adhesions (46). However, one-half of women with adhesions have no historical reason for them; furthermore, one-fourth of women with adhesions have no preoperative findings by either history or physical examination (cervical, uterine, or adnexal tenderness, adnexal mass, or uterine immobility) that suggest the presence of adhesions. Thus, although nonsurgical methods may suggest the presence of adhesions, presently the only definitive way to diagnose them is by surgical visualization. This is usually done via laparoscopy instead of laparotomy.

The presence of pelvic adhesions is not a reliable predictor of pelvic pain (Chapter 8). Laparoscopic studies reveal adhesions in 24% of CPP patients and 17% of non-CPP patients (Table 5.6). Also, it has not been possible to demonstrate a relationship between the duration and severity of pain and the extent or location of adhesions (47). Similarly to the case with endometriosis and CPP, attempts to use the AFS classification of adhesions in women with CPP have not been beneficial. For example, in a prospective, laparoscopy study by Stout et al., the AFS scores did not correlate with duration of pain, severity of pain, limitation of activity, or medication use (47). Thus, documenting the locations, vascularity, thickness, sizes, and density of adhesions is more useful than simply recording a score.

Chronic PID, in which adhesive disease has a significant role, has not been a common laparoscopic diagnosis in CPP patients, accounting for 5% of all diagnoses. Apparently, the primary usefulness of laparoscopy in chronic PID is to disprove the clinical diagnosis. However, this negative utility should not be denigrated because it avoids the social stigma and "pelvic cripple" syndrome

TABLE 5.8. PAIN RELIEF AFTER LAPAROSCOPIC ADHESIOLYSIS

Study	No. of Patients	Pain Better (%)	Pain Not Better (%)	Study
Sutton and Macdonald, 1990	65	53 (82%)	10 (15%)	Retrospective/Uncontrolled
Goldstein et al., 1980	18	16 (89%)	2 (11%)	Prospective/Uncontrolled
Steege and Stout, 1991	30	19 (63%)	11 (37%)	Prospective/Uncontrolled
Total	103	88 (85%)	23 (22%)	

that have been associated with the diagnosis of chronic PID. Additionally, in the patient with a clinical diagnosis of chronic PID there is frequently a suspected adnexal mass (assumed to be a tuboovarian postinflammatory complex), and in this setting laparoscopy is useful to definitively make a diagnosis and eliminate worry of malignant disease or active infection.

As it has been difficult to definitively demonstrate that adhesions cause CPP, so it has also been difficult to show that adhesiolysis relieves CPP. Most of the published studies of adhesiolysis address infertility or adhesion reformation, but Table 5.8 summarizes three studies on adhesiolysis and relief of CPP (17). These studies (a) used laparoscopic adhesiolysis, (b) had 1 year of follow-up, and (c) excluded patients with other diseases, such as endometriosis or PID. Together they show an 85% efficacy rate, but in all three the evaluations of pain were observational, not blinded, and no control groups were included. The only randomized clinical trial of adhesiolysis used laparotomy, not laparoscopy. That study showed efficacy for the treatment of CPP by adhesiolysis only in patients with dense and severe adhesions (48).

Although the available data on adhesions and CPP are not straightforward, they still suggest that adhesions may cause CPP (and infertility), and therefore are best prevented if possible (49). Barrier materials, such as Interceed, have been shown to decrease postoperative adhesions, and can be used at the time of laparotomy or laparoscopy (50,51). Although fairly easy to apply during laparotomy, these are somewhat more difficult to use during laparoscopy. Azziz et al. suggest the following ten recommendations for the use of Interceed laparoscopically (51):

1. Insure that the placement channel is completely dry.
2. Obtain meticulous hemostasis at the site of placement.
3. Remove excess irrigation fluid or blood.
4. Place the barrier immediately prior to terminating the procedure to avoid inadvertently moving it.
5. The sigmoid colon or the uterus may be used as a shelf to initially place and unfold the barrier.
6. Avoid dropping the barrier into the cul-de-sac, especially if there is fluid in it.
7. After placement of the barrier, moisten it with 1 to 3 mL of irrigation to increase its adherence.
8. Place the barrier between two peritoneal surfaces, using the pressure between the pelvic organs to keep it in place.
9. Place the barrier into the entry ports by grasping the cut piece at a corner or by folding the fabric unevenly, which aids in causing it to spontaneously unfold.
10. Select the port for introducing the barrier based on the size of the piece.

Of course, adherence to classically taught meticulous surgical technique is important to decrease adhesion formation. This consists mostly of things that the surgeon should try to avoid, including peritoneal drying, residual blood or clots, unnecessary tissue trauma and handling, unneeded bowel manipulation, and unnecessary suture material (52). These guidelines are more easily adhered to during laparoscopy than during laparotomy and, consistent with this, there are good animal and human data suggesting that primary surgical procedures performed laparoscopically cause significantly less postoperative adhesions than the same procedures done by laparotomy (53,54). These data support the primary use of operative laparoscopy rather than laparotomy whenever feasible (55–57).

Laparoscopy and Ovarian Cysts

Laparoscopic evaluations of patients with CPP reveal ovarian cysts in only 3% of all cases (Table 5.5). This is not surprising as most ovarian cysts capable of causing pelvic pain, such as hemorrhagic corpora lutea or follicle cysts, are usually asymptomatic, and when they cause pain it is almost always acute. These cysts generally resolve spontaneously within one or two cycles and are rarely, if ever, a cause of CPP. Occasionally functional cysts may cause recurrent cyclic pain, but this is generally responsive to oral contraceptive therapy (58). Thus, except in the case of endometriomas, ovarian cysts are not a common cause of CPP.

However, this does not mean that ovarian cysts never cause CPP. Stone and Swartz reported four cases of young women with recurrent functional cysts and CPP in whom prolonged ovarian suppression with oral contraceptives and repeated surgical interventions with laparotomy were necessary (59). I have also cared for several young women with similar histories. The issue of when or if ovarian cysts are a cause of CPP is clinically important because the ovaries tend to form significant adhesions when surgically manipulated and such adhesions may cause CPP (or infertility) (60). Clearly, surgery on the ovary is best avoided unless benefits are likely, a judgment that is not always easy.

Another uncommon cause of ovarian cysts and CPP is residual ovary syndrome. Residual ovary syndrome refers to the occurrence of pain secondary to one or both ovaries in a woman with a previous hysterectomy with preservation of one or both ovaries (Chapter 16). Salpingo-oophorectomy is the definitive treatment and can sometimes be performed laparoscopically. Perry and Upchurch have reported their experience with 17 patients, of whom 14 probably had CPP associated with residual ovary syndrome (61). After laparoscopic adnexectomy, they reported that all patients were pain free at 5 to 22 months follow-up. One case was complicated by postoperative hemorrhage requiring transfusion of two units of blood and exploratory laparotomy. Although ureteral complications did not occur in this series, the authors pointed out the importance of ureteral identification before laparoscopic oophorectomy.

A predicament that not uncommonly occurs is what should be done when a significant or persistent ovarian cyst is found by examination or sonography during the evaluation of a patient with pelvic pain. Although observation is often indicated, histologic diagnosis is sometimes necessary, which requires surgical excision or biopsy. Operative laparoscopy for excision or biopsy offers lower morbidity, reduced postoperative adhesions, faster return to functional activity, lower cost, and better cosmetic results than laparotomy (62). However, a major concern whenever laparoscopic removal of an ovary or ovarian cyst is considered is the exclusion of malignancy (63). If laparoscopic treatment of ovarian pathology is to be performed safely, then it should be performed with the intention of excluding ovarian cancer at every step. Preoperative sonography is recommended and has been reported to exclude malignancy in ovarian masses with a 91% accuracy (64). If sonographic findings and Ca-125 levels suggest an increased chance of malignancy, then either a laparotomy or a closed extirpative laparoscopic technique is indicated (Table 5.9) (65). If all preoperative evaluations suggest benign disease, then laparoscopic treatment is appropriate.

Even when the preoperative evaluation suggests benign ovarian disease, it is essential that cul-de-sac peritoneal washings be obtained or any cul-de-sac peritoneal fluid be aspirated for cytology (66). Next, careful visual inspection of the

involved ovary, pelvic peritoneum, contralateral ovary, paracolic gutters, omentum, diaphragm, liver, and intestines should be done. If there are ovarian or peritoneal excrescences, papillary projections, or nodules, or any suspicion of possible ovarian metastases or ascites noted at this time, the ovarian capsule should not be violated and an immediate laparotomy should be performed. If no worrisome visible findings are noted, then the next step should be a fine needle aspiration of the cyst, taking care to minimize spillage and to copiously irrigate and aspirate any spillage that does occur. The aspirated fluid should be visually inspected. The nature of the fluid has been shown to be characteristically diagnostic when chocolate (usually endometrioma or hemorrhagic corpus luteum), sebaceous (teratoma), or mucinous (mucinous cystoma), but contrary to popular opinion, it is not diagnostic when clear, yellow, or hemorrhagic. In fact, in Mage et al.'s large laparoscopic series, the two cancers not grossly diagnosed had yellow and hemorrhagic fluid, respectively (66). The aspirated fluid may also be sent for cytology. The next step is to open the cyst and do an inspection of the lining for papillary structures or excrescences. If these are noted, then a laparotomy should be done immediately. Finally, a generous biopsy of the lining for histologic evaluation should be an integral part of the laparoscopic management of ovarian cysts if the cyst or ovary is not being completely removed. Even when the surgeon is "certain" at laparoscopy that the ovary is benign, it is essential that tissue be sent for histologic evaluation.

Using an intraoperative protocol similar to this, Mage et al. operated on 481 women with 508 ovarian cysts and diagnosed seven of nine cancers during gross visual inspection and the other two after opening the cysts (66). They were incorrectly suspicious of cancer in another 10 women, resulting in 19 laparotomies for cancer or suspected cancer. Overall, they were able to remove the cysts laparoscopically in 420 of 481 patients, with laparotomies necessary in only 61; furthermore, of 230 women with 1 to 6 years of follow-up, only three had recurrences of nonendometriosis cysts.

A controversial issue regarding laparoscopic treatment of ovarian cysts, even with a careful protocol as in the preceding, is that spillage from a malignancy may still occur, with a resulting change in staging. However, the significance of this is debatable (67). Sometimes it is possible for the skilled laparoscopic surgeon to perform an ovarian cystectomy without rupture of the cyst. When feasible, this probably represents the ideal way to avoid concerns of spill of malignant fluid.

TABLE 5.9. PREOPERATIVE CRITERIA FOR OPERATIVE LAPAROSCOPIC TREATMENT OF ADNEXAL MASSES

Sonographic characteristics
  Size less than 10 cm
  Cystic
  Distinct, smooth borders
  No irregular solid parts
  No thick septa
  No evidence of multiple septations
  No evidence of ascites
  No evidence of matted bowel
Serum CA-125 less than 35 U/mL

Laparoscopy and Pelvic Varicosities

Although the diagnosis of pelvic varicosities is mentioned in some studies of laparoscopy for CPP, laparoscopy is not the recommended method for making the diagnosis of pelvic congestion syndrome (Chapter 18). Retrograde ovarian venography and transuterine pelvic venography that demonstrate increased ovarian or uterine venous diameters, venous stasis, and venous congestion are the recognized techniques of diagnosis (68,69). However, in our experience it has been possible to visualize pelvic varicosities by decreasing the intraabdominal pressure and gradually placing the patient in a reverse Trendelenburg position. This technique has been reported by El-Minawi and El-Minawi in 83 patients in whom suspected varicosities at laparoscopy were later confirmed by venography or ultrasound (70). It should also be noted that some investigators have shown that in women with CPP and negative laparoscopies, up to 91% had dilated veins and pelvic congestion on venography (71). This suggests that it may be worthwhile to perform an evaluation in reverse Trendelenburg with decreased intraabdominal pressure.

Some of the clinical characteristics of pelvic congestion syndrome are pertinent to this discussion, because they correlate with the likelihood of positive laparoscopic fingings (68). Pelvic congestion patients tend to have episodes of severe, acute pelvic pain in addition to their underlying chronic pain (94% of patients with pelvic congestion versus 41% of patients with other pathology). They tend to complain of moving pelvic pain locations, whereas patients with other pelvic pathology tend to complain of consistent pain locations (moving pain in 63% of pelvic congestion patients versus 23% of patients with other pathology). Pelvic congestion patients have exacerbation of pain by walking, standing, lifting, bending, and stress, whereas patients with other pathology tend to less aggravation of pain by activity (86% versus 50%, respectively). On physical examination pelvic congestion patients usually have bilateral ovarian tenderness (86%), but patients with other pathology have similar tenderness just 32% of the time. Finally, the finding of ovarian tenderness combined with a history of postcoital aching is present in 94% of pelvic congestion patients; however, this combination is present in only 23% of women with other pelvic pathology. Although none of these clinical clues is specific enough to be diagnostic, they may still be useful to the clinician in planning the diagnostic evaluation. For example, if a woman with CPP gives a history of moving pelvic pain that is increased by most normal activities, has episodes of severe and acute pelvic pain, has aching pain after intercourse, has "congestive" dysmenorrhea, and has tenderness over both ovaries, then the likelihood of finding a pathologic abnormality at laparoscopy is less than 1%. In such a case evaluations other than laparoscopy, especially pelvic venography, may be more appropriate.

Appropriate therapy for pelvic congestion is uncertain. The British research group led by Beard has shown that bilateral oophorectomy with hysterectomy is an effective therapy for women with pelvic congestion syndrome (72). However, it is important to note that they used transuterine pelvic venography to make the diagnosis, not a subjective

visual diagnosis of dilated pelvic veins. The use of objective diagnostic criteria is crucial if we are to avoid the experience of the 1950s when, after Taylor popularized the diagnosis, many women had hysterectomies for "pelvic congestion syndrome" that did not result in relief of CPP (73–75). Semm has pelviscopically ligated varicosities in the broad and infundibulopelvic ligaments and stated that results in patients with pelvic pain have been good (personal communication, 1991). However, he has not studied this in a controlled manner, nor has he published his results. Both Metzger (personal communication, 1998) and I have ligated and transected the infundibulopelvic ligaments in women with venographically documented pelvic congestion, with preliminary results that suggest good responses. However, until controlled studies of these technique have been performed they should not be routinely applied to women with CPP and pelvic varicosities.

Laparoscopy in Women With No Uterus and No Ovaries

Women who have had prior hysterectomy and bilateral oophorectomies and have CPP are difficult diagnostic dilemmas. Often it is assumed that such patients cannot have pelvic pathology associated with their pain. However, if laparoscopic evaluation is done, not unexpectedly, adhesions are often present, which may or may not have a potential role in their pain. It is not clear whether or not it is worthwhile to lyse pelvic adhesions noted at laparoscopy in such patients.

A specific form of adhesive disease that may occur in patients with prior surgical procedures is postoperative peritoneal cyst (76–79). It appears that these cysts may also rarely occur in women with previous PID without any prior surgery. Postoperative peritoneal cysts, at least symptomatic ones, are rare, with apparently only 16 published cases. They have been reported 6 weeks to 13 years after surgery and, interestingly, only in women. These patients present with CPP or chronic abdominal pain and sometimes with constipation, abdominal swelling, or dysuria. No other particular symptoms have been noted. All laboratory and radiologic studies are normal except for sonographic demonstration of a large septated cyst. Histology shows cuboidal or flat mesothelial cells, occasionally with minimal inflammation. There are no reports of laparoscopic diagnosis or treatment of such patients; the three patients that I have operated on had such severe adhesive disease that the surgery would not have been amenable to laparoscopic diagnosis or treatment.

Another treatable cause of CPP in women with prior hysterectomy-bilateral salpingo-oophorectomy is ovarian remnant syndrome. Ovarian remnant syndrome refers to the presence of painful, histologically documented ovarian tissue in a patient who has undergone a previous bilateral oophorectomy (Chapter 17). Steege has suggested that it may be a more common cause of CPP than is generally recognized (80). Although laparoscopy may in some cases have a role in diagnosis and treatment, these remnants are often embedded in dense scar tissue over the ureter and the surgery is difficult, tedious, and complicated (81). Even when laparotomy is done for excision, there is a resulting subsequent recurrence rate of 20% (80). Ureteral, bladder, or bowel injury and the need to perform bowel or bladder resections are not infrequent (82). Although skilled operative laparoscopists have successfully diagnosed and treated cases of ovarian remnant, laparoscopy is not appropriate in many cases.

Finally, it should be remembered that endometriosis may occur, albeit rarely, after bilateral oophorectomy and hysterectomy (83,84). Such cases have usually been recurrences and have occurred both with and without estrogen replacement therapy.

Laparoscopy and No Apparent Pathology

About 35% of women with CPP will have no apparent pathology laparoscopically (Table 5.5). Unfortunately, many physicians consider laparoscopy the ultimate or definitive diagnostic evaluation of CPP and, when the findings are negative, may make one or more of the following statements to their patients.

1. There is nothing wrong.
2. The pain is in your head and you should see a psychiatrist or psychologist.
3. You should have a neurolytic procedure, such as uterine nerve transection or presacral neurectomy.
4. The only thing that is left to do is a hysterectomy.
5. Nothing can be done and you must learn to live with the pain.

Although statements 2, 3, and 4 may at times be appropriate, generally speaking all five statements are inappropriate without significant knowledge about the patient and evaluations other than a laparoscopy. It is worthwhile to consider the ramifications of each of these statements in more detail.

There is nothing wrong. A negative laparoscopy is not synonymous with no diagnosis or no disease: Laparoscopy must not be viewed as a final, definitive test. Realistically, the major role of laparoscopy for CPP is to diagnose endometriosis or adhesive disease. A meticulously performed negative laparoscopy means that a woman does not have endometriosis-associated or adhesion-associated pain; it does not mean that a woman has no physical basis for her pain.

Many other diseases may contribute to CPP and laparoscopy is usually not necessary to diagnose them. For example, even though published series list leiomyomas, ovarian cysts, or pelvic varicosities as laparoscopic diagnoses (Table 5.5), other less invasive modalities can be used to make these diagnoses. Other diseases, particularly nongynecological diseases such as irritable bowel syndrome or interstitial cystitis, are not diagnosable via laparoscopy. Clearly a negative laparoscopy does not rule out an organic disease that may contribute to or cause CPP. For example, Reiter and Gambone have reported that with thorough evaluation, occult somatic pathology was diagnosed in 47% of women with negative laparoscopies (5). Their diagnoses in 57 of 122 women with CPP and a negative laparoscopy are summarized in Table 5.10.

There is evidence that telling the patient she does not have a life-threatening disease (e.g., ovarian cancer) or a serious gynecological disease (e.g., endometriosis or apparent sterility) may be helpful, resulting in a decrease of subsequent pain in some women (85). However, this aspect of a negative laparoscopy is probably of limited benefit in most CPP patients. Indeed in a randomized clinical trial, Peters et al. showed that omitting laparoscopy from the

TABLE 5.10. DIAGNOSES IN 57 OF 122 WOMEN WITH CHRONIC PELVIC PAIN AND NEGATIVE LAPAROSCOPIES

Diagnosis	Number	Percent	Response to Therapy
Myofascial pain	17	14	65%
Atypical menstrual pain	10	9	82%
Gastrointestinal disease	8	7	88%
Urologic disease	6	7	67%
Infectious disease	4	3	100%
Pelvic congestion syndrome	3	2	67%
Cervical stenosis	1	0.8	Yes
Abdominal hernia	1	0.8	Yes
Retroperitoneal fibrosis	1	0.8	Yes
Coccygeal trauma	1	0.8	No
Uterine descensus	1	0.8	Yes
Uterine retroversion	1	0.8	Improved
Adenomyosis	1	0.8	Yes
Residual accessory ovary	1	0.8	No

No somatic diagnosis was made in the remaining 65 patients.

evaluation of women with long-standing CPP neither improves nor worsens their outcomes (86).

More appropriate than postoperatively telling a woman with a negative laparoscopy that "nothing is wrong," is to explain *preoperatively* that many causes of CPP cannot be found laparoscopically and that about one-third of women will not have an abnormality found. Questions and concerns about diseases other than endometriosis and adhesions are best discussed preoperatively with all patients, and then discussed again with those women with a "negative laparoscopy." With this approach a patient is more likely to understand that if she is told that the laparoscopy was negative, it does not mean "nothing is wrong." Also, she is far more likely to understand the need for further evaluations and diagnostic tests.

Such preoperative counseling is also important in women with positive laparoscopic findings, because a significant number of women with adhesions or endometriosis do not respond adequately to surgical treatment. In these cases the need to do further investigations and other treatments is better understood by patients who have been counseled preoperatively about other diseases and problems not amenable to laparoscopic diagnosis and treatment. When this is not done, it makes the management even more frustrating for those patients not adequately helped by laparoscopy.

The pain is in your head and you should see a psychiatrist or psychologist. It must be remembered that the neural activity induced by the stimulation of nociceptors and nociceptive pathways is not pain; pain is the psychologic state that may (or may not) result from this neural activity. Pain is a subjective experience, regardless of etiology, and pain of supposed somatic etiology is not more real than pain of supposed psychologic etiology (87). Thus we must not, because of a normal laparoscopy and assumed psychologic etiology, ourselves believe, nor imply to our patient that we believe that her pain is inconsequential and not worthy of further evaluation or treatment. Indeed, the separation of CPP into somatic and psychological categories is probably artificial anyway. For example, many investigators have found that psychological test scores and profiles are not significantly different in CPP patients without and with apparent pathology (2,10,23,88). Several interpretations of these data are possible. It may be interpreted as suggesting that there is not a significant psychosomatic origin to CPP in patients without pathology. It may also mean that a psychosomatic origin for CPP is present in all CPP patients and is just as important in those with pathology as in those without apparent pathology. It may also be interpreted as evidence that CPP is a disease that causes a certain psychologic profile as one of the end points of the disease process. And of course, these data may simply reflect the limitations of the diagnostic abilities of the psychologic tests used. So far only one study has attempted to compare in a controlled manner the effectiveness of psychologic treatment to that of

treatment without psychologic interventions in patients with histories of negative laparoscopies; the authors concluded that psychologic interventions as part of a holistic treatment gave better results than traditional treatment without psychologic methods (86). At this point it can only be stated that more objective evaluations are needed before psychotherapy can be stated to be effective in the treatment of women with CPP without obvious pathology.

You should have a neurolytic procedure, such as uterine nerve transection or presacral neurectomy. The efficacy of presacral neurectomy (PSN) or of uterosacral neurectomy (USN) in women with CPP and a negative laparoscopy is unproved. PSN is better studied, with a history of almost 100 years of utilization. From observational studies, it appears to be an effective procedure for the relief of central dysmenorrhea. The results of 633 published cases suggests a 74% "success" rate for relief of pain (89). However, PSN is most often performed as part of conservative surgery for endometriosis, not in cases with no visible pathology, and it is not clear how many of the 633 patients reported in these publications had no evidence of pathology at the time of surgery. For example, in the series reported by Lee et al., of 45 patients treated with PSN, only four had no apparent pathology and nondysmenorrheic pain (dyspareunia). All four had significant pain relief after PSN (89). In all of the more recent other series regarding PSN for CPP, significant pathology, usually endometriosis, was present at the time of PSN (90). There is simply not sufficient information to allow a statement regarding the use of PSN for the treatment of CPP in women with a negative laparoscopy. PSN can be performed laparoscopically, although extensive data on its success and complications performed this way are not available (91,92).

It has been suggested that performing superior hypogastric nerve blocks prior to considering a presacral neurectomy might be predictive of surgical success. In a report by Bourke et al., 10 of 11 patients with pain relief after superior hypogastric plexus nerve blocks had greater than 50% pain relief with subsequent presacral neurectomies (93). As will be discussed later in this chapter, superior hypogastric plexus nerve block at the time of conscious pain mapping has also been suggested as possibly predictive of success of presacral neurectomy (94).

This uncertainty is even greater with USN, a procedure with a much shorter history. Essentially, this is a laparoscopic modification of Doyle's transvaginal procedure, a procedure that consists of transection of both uterosacral ligaments and, before the advent of nonsteroidal antiinflammatory drugs and oral contraceptives, was used to treat acquired dysmenorrhea with 85% to 90% efficacy (95). This procedure was not particularly popular until the advent of operative laparoscopy. Done laparoscopically it is commonly referred to as laparoscopic uterine nerve ablation (LUNA) and is a relatively simple procedure that is frequently performed in clinical practice. However, little is published regarding the efficacy of laparoscopic USN. Lichten has presented data on the treatment of women with severe incapacitating dysmenorrhea not responsive to oral contraceptives or nonsteroidal antiinflammatory drugs and without visible pathology. He reports "significant relief" in 22 of 34 such patients (96). Other reports of USN relate to cases with pathology, such as endometriosis (97). As is the case for PSN, there is simply not sufficient information to allow a statement regarding the use of USN for the treatment of CPP in women with a negative laparoscopy. Malinak has suggested that USN might be useful in the following situations (98):

1. When a nodule of endometriosis or a myoma is present at the base of the uterosacral ligament, necessitating excision of part of the ligament
2. When exposure of the presacral nerve is inadequate to allow presacral neurectomy
3. When pain recurs after a presacral neurectomy

However, the efficacy of laparoscopic USN clearly needs to be established through well-designed randomized trials before it is widely used in women with CPP. It seems wisest currently to only perform PSN or USN as part of an approved research protocol in cases of CPP and negative laparoscopy.

The only thing that is left to do is a hysterectomy. It is tempting for the caring physician, desperate to help his or her patient, to consider nonspecific surgical therapy for CPP, in spite of being trained that surgery should always be restricted to patients with an appropriate specific diagnosis, with established efficacy of operative therapy. Hysterectomy, with or without bilateral oophorectomy, has been the most frequent surgical treatment considered in this situation. Indeed, it has been estimated that 12% of all hysterectomies performed in the United States are for CPP (16). This amounts to about 70,000 hysterectomies per year that, with an estimated mortality rate of 0.1%, could account for 70 deaths each year. Clearly the anticipated benefit must justify this risk. Despite the prevalence of hysterectomies for chronic pelvic pain, no study to date has clearly defined those patients for whom the procedure is efficacious, nor the generally anticipated results after hysterectomy for CPP. As laparoscopic hysterectomy can and is being performed more frequently, undoubtedly this technology will be applied to the treatment of CPP patients (99). A tabulation of some of the earlier series of laparoscopic hysterectomies suggests that CPP may be a primary indication for surgery in 24% of cases (Table 5.11).

Although hysterectomy as a procedure for CPP is frequently criticized, few studies of the outcome after hysterectomy for CPP have actually been published. Stovall et al. retrospectively evaluated the outcomes after hysterectomy for CPP with no extrauterine pathology by analyzing 500 hysterectomy cases over 5 years (1982–1987) (100). Of these, 104 (21%) had hysterectomies for CPP and met the study criteria of 6 months or more of pelvic pain, and no

TABLE 5.11. CPP AS AN INDICATION FOR LAVHS

Study	Number of LAVHs	Number[a] for CPP	Percent[a] for CPP
Liu	72	48	67
Daniell et al.	68	27	40
Johns and Diamond	119	67	56
Casey et al.	220	20	9
Ou et al.	839	159	19
Total	1,318	321	24

[a]Represents an estimate based on information in published series.

extrauterine diagnosis preoperatively or postoperatively to explain the pain (e.g., endometriosis or adhesions). Only 99 had follow-up for more than 12 months. Seventy-seven (75%) of these 99 were pain free and 22 (25%) had persistent pain. However, only 57 of these patients had pelvic pain other than dysmenorrhea or dyspareunia. Of these 57, 43 (78%) were pain free. Interestingly, of the 99 patients with pain and 12 months of follow-up, only 18 had prior surgery that also might have been related to the diagnosis or treatment of CPP: 12 with laparoscopies, two with appendectomies, two with uterine suspensions, and two with oophorectomies. Thus, this retrospective study of women with CPP and no extrauterine disease such as endometriosis or adhesive disease (i.e., they would have had a negative laparoscopy) suggests that about three-fourths are relieved of CPP by hysterectomy. Although this sounds like a "good" outcome, note that it suggests than one out of four women who has a hysterectomy for CPP without a preoperative extrauterine diagnosis continues to have pain.

The Maine Women's Health Study prospectively assessed outcomes after 311 hysterectomies from June, 1989, to January, 1991, and compared the outcomes at a year to those of a medically treated cohort of 380 women (101). This was an observational study, not a randomized trial. Follow-up was available on 65 women treated with hysterectomy for moderate to severe CPP, and only two (3%) continued to have moderate to severe pelvic pain. In the comparison group of 42 patients with significant CPP treated medically, 24 (49%) continued to have moderate to severe CPP. It is not clear from the published data how many of these patients had negative laparoscopic findings, but it appears that about 50% had evidence of endometriosis, leiomyomas, or adhesions. Thus, this study had about 32 women with CPP and no specific pathologic findings, and showed that pain relief after hysterectomy occurred in about 90% of cases.

Although the only two published studies that allow an assessment of the efficacy of hysterectomy for CPP in women who would have a negative laparoscopy suggest that it is 75% to 95%, both studies have significant methodologic flaws. Some caution before performing a hysterectomy in such circumstances seems advisable.

Reiter et al. suggest that hysterectomy is not indicated for treatment of chronic pelvic pain before thorough medical and psychologic evaluation and then only when gross anatomic uterine pathology sufficient to explain the degree of disability has been documented, such as leiomyomata or adenomyosis (5). In their series of CPP patients, only six of 122 with a negative laparoscopy had indications for hysterectomy. Although imaging studies are quite accurate in diagnosing leiomyomata, they are less accurate for adenomyosis. Thus, a preoperative diagnosis of adenomyosis is usually made clinically and generally cannot be confirmed without a hysterectomy. The error rate reported when adenomyosis was used as a clinical preoperative diagnosis is 60%, suggesting a high failure rate might be expected if this were the presumptive diagnosis for a hysterectomy for CPP treatment (102). Reiter and Gambone suggested that the diagnosis of adenomyosis may be confirmed preoperatively by pain relief with local anesthetic injection of the uterosacrals, but reported only one case.

Nothing can be done and you must learn to live with the pain. There are patients whom the clinician is not going to cure with operative or medical treatment, despite the best of intentions, medical knowledge, and surgical skills. This realistically reflects the inadequate knowledge about pain in general, and specifically about chronic pain. This is not a reason to discharge the patient from further care and leave her to a solitary attempt to "live with the pain."

Throughout much of medical history, physicians had little to offer in the way of effective treatment for any illness, yet patients sought out the physician's care. The placebo effect of an encounter with a compassionate physician should not be denigrated (Chapter 56). Indeed, much of what is believed to be effective treatment may in fact be placebo effect (43,44). The physician can always offer support and caring. Rather than say that nothing can be done, it may be better to say, "I don't have an explanation or specific treatment now, but I will continue to work with you to see if we can find ways to improve your pain." Continued visits with reassurance and encouragement may help.

Although not a panacea, referral to a multidisciplinary chronic pain clinic can be beneficial, if one is available. Multidisciplinary pain clinics can obtain significant improvements in pain levels and functional abilities for patients. If a clinic dedicated to CPP is available, it may give optimal results (16). If a multidisciplinary pain clinic is not available, or if the patient is unwilling or unable to go to such a clinic, there are a number of good self-help books available that can be suggested to improve control of her pain and function.

LAPAROSCOPIC TREATMENT OF CPP

In addition to the previously described operative laparoscopic procedures, there are a number of other procedures that have been used to treat women with CPP with varying

TABLE 5.12. SURGICAL PROCEDURES FOR THE TREATMENT OF CPP

Ablation of endometriosis
Adhesiolysis
Appendectomy
Hysterectomy
Ovarian cystectomy
Oophorectomy
Presacral neurectomy
Resection or excision of endometriosis
Resection of persistent omphalomesenteric ligament (one case report)
Salpingectomy
Uterosacral nerve resection or ablation
Uterine suspension

success, particularly uterine suspensions and appendectomies (Table 5.12).

Gilliam-type uterine suspensions have a mixed history of usefulness in patients with CPP. These procedures can be performed laparoscopically, either by shortening the round ligaments with falope rings or by pulling the round ligaments up through second and third puncture sites and suturing them to the rectus sheath (103). The suggested indications are for pain owing to uterine retrofixation or excessive retrodisplacement. These are probably rare causes of CPP. Most who have recommended this procedure suggest a preoperative 4- to 6-week trial of a pessary to antevert the uterus and, if there is relief of the pain while the pessary is in place and pain returns after the pessary is removed, predict a good result with surgical suspension. However, a retrospective review by Yoong of laparoscopic uterine suspensions on 43 patients with CPP and no apparent pathology other than retroversion suggested a success rate between 19% and 46% (104).

Laparoscopic appendectomy has been reported by Bryson in 55 women with CPP localized to the right lower quadrant or flank: five had endometriosis, 38 had entrapping adhesions, and 12 had histories compatible with chronic appendicitis (105). Of the 55 women, at a mean follow-up time of 2 years, 44 were pain free, nine were improved, and two (with severe endometriosis) were not better. These results reinforce that in CPP patients the appendix must be carefully evaluated and suggest that a laparoscopic appendectomy may sometimes be a useful procedure with persistent right lower quadrant pain.

COMPLICATIONS OF OPERATIVE LAPAROSCOPY

Although the surgical principles that apply to laparotomy also apply to operative laparoscopy, operative laparoscopy is technically quite different. Some of the technical limitations of laparoscopic surgery include: loss of depth perception, inability to directly palpate tissue, limitation of the number of instruments that can simultaneously be used, restriction of the angles available to approach the surgical field, and increased distance from the surgical field to the surgeons' hands that amplifies motion, making fine movements more difficult (106). All of these factors may contribute to surgical complications of operative laparoscopy.

The complication rates associated with operative laparoscopy for CPP have not been extensively evaluated or carefully monitored. The complication rate in our series of 65 patients with combined diagnostic and operative laparoscopy was 9% (six complications) (107). However, not unexpectedly, there have been numerous case reports of various complications with laparoscopy. The following is a sampling of some of the injuries described in published case reports:

Sciatic nerve injury (108)
Femoral nerve injury (109)
Perforation of a patent urachal sinus (110)
Bladder injuries (111)
Bowel injuries (related to electrosurgery, trocar insertion, laser injury, adhesiolysis, etc.) (112)
Ureteral injury (113)
Hemorrhage, intraoperatively and postoperatively (61,114)

LAPAROSCOPIC CONSCIOUS PAIN MAPPING

Laparoscopic conscious pain mapping (CPM) is a diagnostic laparoscopy under local anesthesia, with or without conscious sedation, directed at the identification of sources of pain in women with CPP. Laparoscopy under local anesthesia is not new, but its use to identify lesions that replicate the pain of which a patient chronically complains is a recent development (115). CPM has been reported to lead to the treatment of subtle or atypical areas of disease that might have been overlooked if the procedure had been performed under general anesthesia (116). However, scant data have been presented to confirm this claim. Demco suggests that the advantages of conscious pain mapping, which he prefers calling "Patient-Assisted Laparoscopy" or "PAL," are:

1. The patient is able to show the surgeon and herself the "cause" of the pain.
2. Findings can be demonstrated and explained to the patient.
3. Treatment can be determined and explained to the patient.
4. The patient can be shown potential complications of treatment.
5. The patient can confirm the results of treatment, for example, by release of adhesions.
6. The negative laparoscopy rate can be reduced (117).

Procedure

Proper patient selection is important. Exclusion of morbidly obese patients (BMI greater than 30), and patients with ASA class greater than 2, anxiety disorders, psychiatric disease, and known or suspected severe adhesive disease is wise. Patients with prior laparoscopies are not excluded. Demco, Almeida and Val-Gallas, Palter and Olive, and Reginald (personal communication, 1998) did not include patients with prior laparotomies (116–118). Demco states specifically that this is an exclusion criterion. We have not excluded patients with prior laparotomies from our cases. Ten of our 30 cases had a prior laparotomy, eight of whom had prior hysterectomies.

Counseling and preparation of the patient are crucial. The patient must be informed as to the details of the procedure, and especially what she should expect to experience. Preoperative medication regimens differ. Some premedicate with atropine (0.2 mg) to avoid parasympathetic reactions, and ondansetron (4 mg) to decrease nausea (116). Most surgeons premedicate with a narcotic, such as fentanyl (50 µg), and then given intermittent doses during the procedure as needed (fentanyl, 50–500 µg; dosage may need to be limited in an office setting). The use of amnestics or anxiolytics, such as midazolam (2–4 mg) is controversial; however, many surgeons report it is useful and give preoperative and intraoperative doses as needed.

After the patient is placed in lithotomy position, prepped, and draped, it is helpful to insert an indwelling transurethral catheter. This is done after the urethral mucosa is anesthetized with topical lidocaine gel. Most surgeons also insert a uterine manipulator, and use a paracervical block to do this. There is a concern that this explains the absence of uterine tenderness reported by some, because a properly performed paracervical block results in uterine anesthesia (117,119). I use a local cervical block, directly into the cervix at four points (12, 3, 6, and 9 o'clock) and find this adequate for insertion of the manipulator. Reginald does not use a uterine manipulator, finding that digital or sponge stick manipulation vaginally allows adequate uterine manipulation in most cases. Most surgeons use lidocaine 1% at the incision and trocar sites. Variations have been the presence or absence of epinephrine (1:100,000) and whether or not the lidocaine is buffered with sodium bicarbonate (0.9% diluted 1:10 to lidocaine). Bupivicaine or a combination of 50:50 bupivicaine and lidocaine may be used instead of lidocaine. This should be done as a field block, not simply a subcutaneous injection. The needle should be fanned out after skin infiltration to anesthetize the subcutaneous, fascial, and peritoneal tissues in a relatively wide area. EMLA has been used to decrease the discomfort of injecting local anesthesia at the umbilical and suprapubic areas (117). It should be placed about 2 hours prior to the procedure to optimize efficacy. After local anesthesia is obtained, a Veress needle is inserted. Some find it helpful to have the patient voluntarily protrude her abdomen during Veress needle insertion. We have found lifting the abdomen to be easier. Lifting the patient's abdomen during an office visit to demonstrate tolerance ("abdominal lift test") anecdotally seems a reliable indicator of the patient's ability to tolerate this insertion technique. When carbon dioxide is used the volume should be kept to 600 cc or less. Some believe that nitrous oxide is less irritating to the peritoneum and better tolerated, but a randomized trial comparing carbon dioxide and nitrous oxide showed no difference (120). The sizes of laparoscopes and secondary trocars and instruments used have been 1.7 to 5 mm.

The technique used to map the pelvis is a gentle probing or tractioning of tissues and organs with a blunt probe or forceps passed through the secondary trocar site. There should be a systematic evaluation in this manner of the entire pelvis, seeking the presence or absence of tenderness and pain. A rating system, such as 0 to 10, with 0 for no tenderness and 10 for worst possible tenderness, should be used. A second evaluation, especially of tender areas, should be performed to insure reliability. One systematic way to ensure a complete evaluation is summarized in Table 5.13. Normal bowel and peritoneum should be probed first to establish a baseline or control level of tenderness. Diagnosis of an etiologic lesion or organ should be based on the severity of pain elicited and on replication of the pain that is the patient's presenting symptom. That is, the pain produced by probing should reproduce the pain that the patient usually has. Although Demco has argued vigorously for the importance of the patient viewing the videomonitor during the procedure, others (including this author) have concerns that this may lead to significant bias by both the patient and the surgeon, and suggest that at least the initial mapping not be viewed by the patient (117). I have anecdotally noted great variations in patients' pain ratings between their ratings viewing versus not viewing the video monitor. This is an area that needs further study.

Applying or injecting local anesthetic to sites of focal tenderness may block the pain response, and possibly improve the predictability that surgical excision will be therapeutic. Steege has also reported performance of superior hypogastric plexus block (SHPB) at the time of CPM in two cases with central pelvic pain (94). In one case this led him to perform a presacral neurectomy and in the other to simply excise uterosacral endometriosis, with subsequent good postoperative pain relief in both cases. He used a 15 cm, 22-gauge spinal needle inserted 4 cm inferior to the umbilical cannula to inject 10 mL of 1% lidocaine below the peritoneum of the presacral space.

CPM is not always successful. A successful CPM is when all areas of the pelvis can be systematically inspected, including the base of the cul-de-sac, both fallopian tubes, and bilateral ovarian fossae, allowing for limitations owing to adhesions (118). In Demco's series the success rate was 88% (Table 5.14). Failures in his series were owing to inability to access the peritoneal cavity (3%), reaction to the carbon dioxide with shoulder pain (5%), inability to visualize the pelvis because of adhesions (3%), and inability of the patient to tolerate the procedure (2%) (117). The two failures in Palter and Olive's series were caused by disorientation and an anxiety attack during the procedure (118). Unsuccessful procedures in Reginald's series numbered three, with one caused by withdrawal from the study and two caused by inability to antevert the uterus and visualize the cul-de-sac. We had nine failures, with eight caused by inability of the patient to tolerate the procedure and one caused by dense adhesions that obscured any visualization.

Pain is significant for CPP patients during CPM. They experience significantly more pain than infertility patients undergoing similar diagnostic laparoscopies under local anesthesia, with intraoperative VAS pain ratings of 7.0 versus 5.0 and postoperative ratings of 3.2 versus 0.5, respectively (118). Patients with CPP appear to have generalized visceral hypersensitivity to probing in all areas of the pelvis and abdominal cavity. This was observed in 10 of 11

TABLE 5.13. ONE SYSTEMATIVE METHODOLOGY TO ENSURE COMPLETE EVALUATION DURING LAPAROSCOPIC CONSCIOUS PAIN MAPPING

1. Have the patient rate all areas that are evaluated by probing or stretching on a 0 to 10 rating scale, with 0 as no pain and 10 as the worst pain possible.
2. Probe one or two areas of normal-appearing peritoneum on the abdominal and pelvic sidewall to establish a baseline or control level of pain or tenderness.
3. Probe and stretch a segment of small bowel and large bowel to establish a baseline or control level of pain or tenderness.
4. Inspect and probe the left round ligament, including the internal inguinal ring.
5. Inspect and probe the anterior cul-de-sac peritoneum, including the bladder peritoneum.
6. Inspect and probe the right round ligament, including the internal inguinal ring.
7. Inspect and probe the right fallopian tube.
8. Inspect and probe the right paracolic gutter and appendix.
9. Inspect and probe the right ovary and fossa ovarica.
10. Inspect and probe the uterine fundus.
11. Inspect and probe the right uterosacral ligament, cul-de-sac, and left uterosacral ligament.
12. Inspect and probe the left ovary and the fossa ovarica.
13. Inspect and probe the left fallopian tube.
14. Inspect and probe any abnormalities, lesions, or pathologies.
15. Repeat steps 4 through 14, but in reverse order.

TABLE 5.14. VISUAL ANALOG SCORES OF VARIOUS ANATOMIC STRUCTURES AT THE TIME OF CONSCIOUS PAIN MAPPING

Anatomic Structure	Median VAS When Structure Is Not Site of Pain	Range of VAS When Structure Is Not Site of Pain	Median VAS When Structure Is Site of Pain	Medain VAS When Structure Is Site of Pain
Uterus	2	1–4	9	8–10
Ovaries	3	1–5	8	7–10
Fallopian tubes	2	1–2	—	—
Round ligaments	1	1–2	—	—
Uterosacral ligaments and cul-de-sac	1	1–2	9	8–10
Intestines	1	1–2	—	—

patients reported by Palter and Olive, but was not seen in any of the 16 comparable patients evaluated for infertility. Three types of pain or tenderness seem to occur during CPM of CPP patients.

1. Sharp, stabbing pain related to visceral manipulation or areas of pathology. This pain is decreased by local anesthesia.
2. Crampy, dull pain or a feeling of fullness. This pain is decreased by decreasing the intraabdominal carbon dioxide pressure.
3. Immediate sharp, burning pain with the start of insufflation. This pain is thought to be caused by peritoneal irritation by carbon dioxide.

Reginald noted the VAS ratings of normal viscera and peritoneum in patients with CPP, and found that reproductive viscera tended to be more tender than peritoneum or intestines (Table 5.14).

Results of CPM

The results of five series of CPM procedures, three published and two unpublished, are summarized in Table 5.15. The data are presented in the table so as to highlight the differences between the two series by Demco and by Almeida and Val-Gallas compared to the three series by Palter and Olive, Reginald, and Howard and El-Minawi. Of 88 successful procedures, Demco made a diagnosis of endometriosis in 61. Of 50 successful procedures, Almeida and Val-Gallas diagnosed endometriosis in 42. Thus, in these two series, endometriosis was diagnosed in 102, or 74% of patients with successful CPMs. In contrast, the three other series found endometriosis accountable for pain in only six of 54 successful cases, or 11%. Also there were four cases with no diagnosis in the two series from Demco and from Almeida and Val-Gallas. In only 3% did they not elicit a diagnostic painful lesion. In the other three series there were 18 cases with no diagnosis at the time of CPM, or 33% with no painful lesions detected to account for the CPP. These are striking differences, and may reflect differences in populations, because the latter three series are from clini-

cians with primarily referral practices, or may reflect differences in procedural techniques.

Regardless, it is clear from these series that many endometriotic lesions are not tender to probing at the time of CPM and these findings raise important questions about the role of endometriosis in CPP. In the series by Howard and El-Minawi, 12 of the patients had endometriotic lesions, but in only three (25%) were any of the lesions tender and reproductive of CPP symptoms. Table 5.15 summarizes the lesions diagnosed in these 12 patients. In Reginald's series, of two cases with endometriosis, one mapped to the endometriotic lesion and the other mapped to the uterus and a normal-appearing ovary. In the series of Almeida and Val-Gallas, even though 42 (84%) of their patients were found to have endometriosis, they state that, "reproduction of pelvic pain by probing the lesions was inconsistent, regardless of lesion size or location, with some being entirely nontender." Unfortunately, they give no numerical data as to the tenderness of endometriotic lesions. Palter and Olive observed focal areas of dramatically increased tenderness in only three of their 11 patients and in two these were endometriotic lesions. However, both of these patients had other endometriotic lesions that were not focally tender.

In the previously described series Demco does not give much information about the tenderness of endometriotic lesions. However, in another published series of 50 cases he reports that 19% to 93% of endometriotic lesions are not tender at the time of CPM and that endometriotic lesions involving viscera, in particular, are nontender more than 50% of the time (119). Although peritoneal endometriotic lesions were more likely to be tender (80%), up to as much as a 3-cm area of normal peritoneum surrounding the endometriotic lesions was also tender in about 80% of cases (Table 5.17). Although it is possible that, as Demco suggests, there is "microscopic" endometriosis surrounding the lesion that is not visible, or that whatever chemical irritant is generated by endometriosis may generate a field effect to involve surrounding normal peritoneum, it is just as likely an explanation that the peritoneum is abnormally tender because of a mechanism totally unrelated to the presence or absence of endometriosis. This uncertainty is further compounded by Demco's data regarding tenderness of various

TABLE 5.15. RESULTS OF CONSCIOUS PAIN MAPPING IN WOMEN WITH CPP

Series	No. of Patients	No. of Successful Procedures	Endometriosis	Pelvic Adhesions	Congestion	Hernia	Appendiceal Pathology	Adnexal Myoma	Cysts	Other	No. of Diagnosis	Total No. of Diagnoses
Demco, 1997[a]	100	88 (88%)	61 (69%)	16 (18%)	0	5 (6%)	0	0	0	4 (4%)[a]	2 (2%)	88
Almeida and Val-Gallas, 1997	50	50 (100%)	42 (84%)	31 (62%)	0	0	13 (26%)	1 (2%)	13 (26%)	1 (2%)	2 (4%)	101
Subtotal	150	138 (92%)	103 (74%)	47 (34%)	0	5 (4%)	13 (9%)	1 (1%)	13 (9%)	5 (4%)	4 (3%)	189
Palter and Olive, 1996	11	9 (82%)	2 (22%)	1 (11%)	0	0	0	0	0	0	8 (89%)	3
Reginald 1998	27	24 (89%)	1 (4%)	4 (17%)	7 (29%)	0	0	1 (4%)	0	8 (33%)[b]	3 (12%)	21
Howard and El-Minawi, 1998	30	21 (70%)	3 (14%)	7 (33%)	0	2 (9%)	0	1 (5%)	2 (9%)	11 (52%)[c]	7 (33%)	26
Subtotal	68	54 (79%)	6 (11%)	12 (22%)	7 (13%)	2 (4%)	0	2 (4%)	2 (4%)	19 (35%)	18 (33%)	50
Total	218	192 (88%)	109 (56%)	59 (31%)	7 (4%)	7 (4%)	13 (7%)	3 (2%)	15 (8%)	24 (14%)	22 (11%)	239

[a]One with colon carcinoma, one with chronic ileal disease, one with staple at ureter, and one with pseudostone secondary to gallbladder spillage.
[b]Two with peritoneal puckering, two with ovary, one with tubal cornu, one with uterus and ovary, and two with peritoneal scarring or puckering mapped as painful foci.
[c]One with trigger point, three with bladder pain, three with vaginal apex pain, and four with diffuse peritoneal pain.

TABLE 5.16. THE POSITIVE OR PAINFUL LESIONS IDENTIFIED IN TWELVE PATIENTS WITH ENDOMETRIOSIS AT THE TIME OF CONSCIOUS PAIN MAPPING

Positive Lesions Mapped	Number	Percent
Endometriosis	3	25
Adhesions	2	17
Ovarian/cyst	2	17
Obturator hernia	1	8
Leiomyoma	1	8
Trigger point	1	8
Peritoneum	1	8
Unsuccessful	3	25
Total	14	117

Some patients had more than one positive or painful lesion; therefore, the number of positive lesions is greater than 12.

TABLE 5.17. DISTANCE FROM ENDOMETRIOTIC LESIONS THAT PERITONEUM WAS ABNORMALLY TENDER TO PROBING AT THE TIME OF CONSCIOUS PAIN MAPPING

Distance (mm)	Number	Percent
0	9	21
1–4	3	7
5–8	6	14
9–12	10	23
13–16	10	23
17–20	1	2
21–24	3	7
25–28	1	2

types of endometriotic lesions. At the time of CPM he noted that red vascular lesions were the most likely to be tender (84%), whereas black lesions were least likely to be tender (12%). Demco did not obtain histologic confirmation of the diagnosis of endometriosis at the time of CPM, and it is well-established that black lesions are the most reliably diagnosed as endometriosis based on visual appearance, whereas red lesions are correctly diagnosed visually only 67% of the time (Table 5.18).

Adhesions were the next most common diagnosis after endometriosis in these CPM series (Table 5.15). In the report of Almeida and Val-Gallas, 31 (62%) of their patients were found to have adhesions, but in only 25 of these cases did any of the adhesions exhibit tenderness to manipulation. Palter and Olive found that one of the three patients in their series had an adhesion of small bowel to anterior abdominal wall as the focal area of tenderness. They do not state how many other patients had adhesions. In our series seven of 21 patients with adhesions had focal dramatic tenderness of any of their adhesions. Reginald found that of six patients with adhesions, four mapped to the adhesions. Thus, for the cases with data available, 36 (62%) of 58 patients with adhesions and CPP localized their pain to adhesions at CPM.

Reginald is the only one to diagnose pelvic congestion at the time of CPM. He diagnosed this condition in seven patients, based on the visual appearance of uterine congestion and bilateral broad ligament varicosities. Three of these patients had tenderness of the uterus and one or both ovaries, two had isolated uterine tenderness, one had tenderness of the uterus and uterosacral ligament, and one had tenderness of both ovaries. Thus, six of seven had uterine tenderness, but only four of seven had any ovarian tenderness.

Almeida and Val-Gallas were the only ones to report pain mapping to the appendix. In 13 patients they detected either a tender or an anatomically abnormal appendix. They did not report how many patients were in each group.

One concern with CPM is there are little data confirming its accuracy diagnostically compared to laparoscopy under general anesthesia, especially with microlaparoscopes. One study that attempted to address this compared laparoscopy under local anesthesia with a 2-mm laparoscope to laparoscopy under general anesthesia with a 10-mm laparoscope (Table 5.19) (121). This was a reasonable study of comparison of intersurgeon reliability because the two surgeons involved were blinded to one another's scoring, but was not an ideal evaluation of microlaparoscopic-local anesthesia versus macrolaparoscopic-general anesthesia because each surgeon knew his results from the microlaparoscopy before doing the macrolaparoscopic evaluation. Another concern is

TABLE 5.18. CORRELATION OF TYPE OF ENDOMETRIOTIC LESION AND TENDERNESS AT THE TIME OF CONSCIOUS PAIN MAPPING

Type of Lesion	Lesion More Tender than Normal Peritoneum (%)	Lesion Tenderness the Same as Normal Lesion Peritoneum (%)	Not Tender (%)	Total Cases
Red, vascular	42 (84%)	6 (12%)	2 (4%)	50
Clear	38 (76%)	8 (16%)	4 (8%)	50
White, scar	22 (44%)	9 (18%)	19 (38%)	50
Black	11 (22%)	5 (10%)	34 (68%)	50

TABLE 5.19. RESULTS OF AN EVALUATION OF COMPARABILITY OF DIAGNOSTIC FINDINGS BETWEEN LAPAROSCOPY WITH A 2-MM LAPAROSCOPE UNDER LOCAL ANESTHESIA AND LAPAROSCOPY WITH A 10-MM LAPAROSCOPE UNDER GENERAL ANESTHESIA

	Surgeons Agreed with Each Other's Microlaparoscopic Diagnoses (%)	Surgeons Agreed with Each Other's Macrolaparoscopic Diagnoses (%)	Surgeon A's Macrolaparoscopic Diagnosis Agreed with Own Microlaparoscopic Diagnosis (%)	Surgeon B's Macrolaparoscopic Diagnosis Agreed with Own Microlaparoscopic Diagnosis (%)
Presence or absence of endometriosis (n = 10)	80	90	90	80
Diagnosis of endometriosis when present (n = 5)	60	80	80	60
AFS endometriosis score within two points (n = 5)	60	80	100	80
Presence or absence of adhesions (n = 10)	100	100	100	100
AFS adhesion score within two points (n = 5)	100	100	100	100

The study was done with two surgeons and ten patients.

that the study included only 10 patients, and of that 10, only four or five had endometriosis (there was disagreement between the surgeons in one case) and only six had adhesions.

Another concern regarding CPM is the fact that the tenderness elicited by probing or traction is in response to a mechanical stimulus and hence is nonphysiological. This raises the question of whether the findings at CPM using this methodology have any relevance to the patient's CPP. Furthermore, it remains to be seen whether the source of pain as identified at CPM is indeed responsible for the symptom. In Almeida and Val-Gallas' series, 45 of 48 patients had "significant amelioration" of their pain at 11 to 17 months follow-up after CPM and operative laparoscopy. However, they treated all endometriotic and adhesive lesions at the time of operative laparoscopy, regardless of the findings at the time of CPM.

Finally, it should be noted that it is possible to successfully treat some of the lesions found at the time of CPM under local anesthesia (personal communication, Larry Demco, Alberta, Canada, 1997). This may have the benefit of confirming adequate treatment. It may also result in significant financial savings. For example, in the series from Palter and Olive at Yale University, the costs in 1995 of outpatient laparoscopic CPM versus operating room diagnostic laparoscopy were $1,700 versus $7,500, respectively.

REFERENCES

1. Krolikowski A, Jahowski K, Larsen JV. Laparoscopic and cystopic findings in patients with chronic pelvic pain in Eshowe, South Africa. *Central African J Med* 1995;41:225–226.
2. Barbalias GA, Meares EM. Female urethral syndrome: clinical and urodynamic perspectives. *Urology* 1984;23:208–212.
3. Summit RL. Urogynecologic causes of chronic pelvic pain. *Obstet Gynecol Clinics NA* 1993;20:685–698.
4. Ramahi AJ, Richardson DA. A practical approach to the painful bladder syndrome. *J Reprod Med* 1990;35:805–809.
5. Reiter RC, Gambone JC. Nongynecologic somatic pathology in women with chronic pelvic pain and negative laparoscopy. *J Reprod Med* 1991;36:253–259.
6. Parsons CL. Interstitial cystitis: what options? *Contemp Ob/Gyn* 1992;August:23–28.
7. Carter JE. Combined hysteroscopic and laproscopic findings in patients with chronic pelvic pain. *J Am Assoc Gynecol Laparosc* 1994;2:43–47.
8. Neshat F, Nezhat C, Nezhat CH, et al. Use of hysteroscopy in addition to laparoscopy in evaluating chronic pelvic pain. *J Reprod Med* 1995;40:431–434.
9. Popp LW, Schwiederessen JP, Gaetje R. Myometrial biopsy in the diagnosis of adenomyosis uteri. *Am J Obstet Gynecol* 1993;169:546–548.
10. McCausland AM. Hysteroscopic myometrial biopsy: its use in diagnosing adenomyosis and its clinical applications. *Am J Obstet Gynecol* 1992;166:1619–1628.
11. Roseff SJ, Murphy AA. Laparoscopy in the diagnosis and therapy of chronic pelvic pain. *Clin Obstet Gynecol* 1990;33:137.
12. Howard FM. The role of laparoscopy in chronic pelvic pain: promise and pitfalls. *Obstet Gynecol Survey* 1993;48:357–387.
13. Ripps BA, Martin DC. Focal pelvic tenderness, pelvic pain, and dysmenorrhea in endometriosis. *J Reprod Med* 1991;36:470–472.
14. Kresch AJ, Seifer DB, Sachs LB, et al. Laparoscopy in 100 women with chronic pelvic pain. *Obstet Gynecol* 1984;64:672–674.
15. Cunanan RG, Courey MG, Lippes J. Laparoscopic findings in patients with pelvic pain. *Am J Obstet Gynecol* 1983;146:589–591.
16. Rapkin AJ, Kames LD. The pain management approach to chronic pelvic pain. *J Reprod Med* 1987;32:323–327.
17. Howard FM. The role of laparoscopy in the evaluation of chronic pelvic pain: pitfalls with a negative laparoscopy. *J Am Assoc Gynecol Laparoscop* 1996;4:85–94.
18. Sampson JA. Peritoneal endometriosis due to dissemination of endometrial tissue into the peritoneal cavity. *Am J Obstet Gynecol* 1927;14:422.
19. Sampson JA. Benign and malignant endometrial implants in

the peritoneal cavity and their relationship to certain ovarian tumors. *Surg Gynecol Obstet* 1924;38:287.

20. Sampson JA. Perforating hemorrhagic (chocolate) cysts of the ovary. *Arch Surg* 1921;3:245.

21. Nunley WC. Medical management of endometriosis: a review. *Hosp Formul* 1985;20:704.

22. Droegemueller W, Herbst AL, Mishell DR, et al. *Comprehensive gynecology.* St. Louis: CV Mosby 1987:493.

23. Barbieri RL. Etiology and epidemiology of endometriosis. *Am J Obstet Gynecol* 1990;162:565.

24. Martin DC, Berry JD. Histology of chocolate cysts. *J Gynecol Surg* 1990;6:43.

25. Jansen RP, Russell P. Nonpigmented endometriosis: clinical, laparoscopic, and pathologic definition. *Am J Obstet Gynecol* 1986;155:1154.

26. Muse K. Clinical manifestations and classification of endometriosis. *Clin Obstet Gynecol* 1988;31:813.

27. Israel R. Endometriosis: diagnostic evaluation. In: Mishell DR, Brenner PL, eds. *Common problems in ob/gyn.* Montvale, NJ: Medical Economics, 1988:589.

28. Chatman DL, Zbella EA. Biopsy in laparoscopically diagnosed endometriosis. *J Reprod Med* 1987;32:855.

29. Martin DC, Hubert GD, VanderZwaag R, et al. Laparoscopic appearances of peritoneal endometriosis. *Fertil Steril* 1989;51:63–67.

30. Stripling MC, Martin DC, Chatman DL, et al. Subtle appearance of pelvic endometriosis. *Fertil Steril* 1998;49:427–431.

31. Redwine DB. Age-related evolution in color appearance of endometriosis. *Fertil Steril* 1987;48:1062.

32. Cook AS, Rock JA. The role of laparoscopy in the treatment of endometriosis. *Fertil Steril* 1991;55:663.

33. Vercellini P, Bocciolone L, Vendola N, et al. Peritoneal endometriosis: morphologic appearance in women with chronic pelvic pain. *J Reprod Med* 1991;36:533.

34. Chatman DL. Pelvic peritoneal defects and endometriosis: Allen-Masters syndrome revisited. *Fertil Steril* 1981;36:751.

35. Chatman DL, Zbella EA. Pelvic peritoneal defects and endometriosis: further observations. *Fertil Steril* 1986;46:711.

36. Vercellini P, Bocciolone L, Vendola N, et al. Peritoneal endometriosis: morphologic appearance in women with chronic pelvic pain. *J Reprod Med* 1991;36:533.

37. Adamson GD. Diagnosis and clinical presentation of endometriosis. *Am J Obstet Gynecol* 1990;162:568.

38. Martin DC, Ahmic R, El-Zeky FA, et al. Increased histologic confirmation of endometriosis. *J Gynecol Surg* 1990;6:275.

39. Cornillie FJ, Oosterlynck D, Lauweryns JM, et al. Deeply infiltrating pelvic endometriosis: Histology and clinical significance. *Fertil Steril* 1990;53:978.

40. Koninckx PR, D'Hooghe TD, Oosterlynck D. Response to letter to the editor. *Fertil Steril* 1991;56:590.

41. Perez JJ. Laparoscopic presacral neurectomy: results of the first 25 cases. *J Reprod Med* 1990;35:625.

42. Redwine DB. Peritoneal blood painting: an aid in the diagnosis of endometriosis. *Am J Obstet Gynecol* 1989;161:865.

43. Candiani GB, Vercellini P, Fedele L. Laparoscopic ovarian puncture for correct staging of endometriosis. *Fertil Steril* 1990;53:994.

44. Davis GD, Brooks RA. Excision of pelvic endometriosis with the carbon dioxide laser laparoscope. *Obstet Gynecol* 1988;72:816.

45. Reich H. Laparoscopic adhesiolysis techniques. *Female Patient* 1990;15:85.

46. Stovall TG, Elder RF, Ling FW. Predictors of pelvic adhesions. *J Reprod Med* 1989;34:345.

47. Stout AL, Steege JF, Dodson WC, et al. Relationship of laparoscopic findings to self-report of pelvic pain. *Am J Obstet Gynecol* 1991;164:73.

48. Peters AAW, Trimbos-Kemper GCM, Admiraal C, et al. A randomized clinical trial on the benefit of adhesiolysis in patients with intraperitoneal adhesions and chronic pelvic pain. *Br J Obstet Gynaecol* 1992;99:59–62.

49. Hulka J. Adnexal adhesions: a prognostic staging and classification system based on a five-year survey of fertility surgery at Chapel Hill, North Carolina. *Am J Obstet Gynecol* 1982;144:141–148.

50. Interceed (TC7) Adhesion Barrier Study Group. Prevention of postsurgical adhesions by Interceed (TC7), an absorbable adhesion barrier: a prospective, randomized multicenter clinical study. *Fertil Steril* 1989;51:933.

51. Azziz R, Murphy AA, Rosenberg SM, et al. Use of an oxidized regenerated cellulose absorbable adhesion barrier at laparoscopy. *J Reprod Med* 1991;36:479.

52. Ellis H. The cause and prevention of postoperative intraperitoneal adhesions. *Surg Gynecol Obstet* 1971;133:497.

53. Lundorff P, Hahlin M, Kallfelt B, et al. Adhesion formation after laparoscopic surgery in tubal pregnancy: a randomized trial versus laparotomy. *Fertil Steril* 1991;55:911.

54. Luciano AA, Maier DB, Koch EI, et al. A comparative study of postoperative adhesions following laser surgery by laparoscopy versus laparotomy in the rabbit model. *Obstet Gynecol* 1989;74:220.

55. Nezhat CR, Nezhat FR, Metzger DA, et al. Adhesion reformation after reproductive surgery by videolaseroscopy. *Fertil Steril* 1990;53:1008.

56. Perez RJ. Second-look laparoscopy adhesiolysis: the procedure of choice for preventing adhesion recurrence. *J Reprod Med* 1991;36:700.

57. Diamond MP, Daniell JF, Johns DA, et al. Postoperative adhesion development after operative laparoscopy: evaluation at early second-look procedures. *Fertil Steril* 1991;55:700.

58. Malinak LR. Pelvic pain—when is surgery indicated? *Contemp Ob/Gyn* 1985;26:43.

59. Stone SC, Swartz WJ. A syndrome characterized by recurrent symptomatic functional cysts in young women. *Am J Obstet Gynecol* 1979;134:310.

60. Wiskind AK, Toledo AA, Dudley G, et al. Adhesion formation after ovarian wound repair in New Zealand white rabbits: a comparison of ovarian microsurgical closure with ovarian nonclosure. *Am J Obstet Gynecol* 1990;163:1674.

61. Perry CP, Upchurch JC. Pelviscopic adnexectomy. *Am J Obstet Gynecol* 1990;162:79.

62. Hasson HH. Laparoscopic management of ovarian cysts. *J Reprod Med* 1990;35:863.

63. Maiman M, Seltzer V, Boyce J. Laparoscopic excision of ovarian neoplasms subsequently found to be malignant. *Obstet Gynecol* 1991;77:563.

64. Benacerraf BR, Finkler NJ, Wojciechowski C, et al. Sonographic accuracy in the diagnosis of ovarian masses. *J Reprod Med* 1990;35:491.

65. Levine RL. Pelviscopic surgery in women over 40. *J Reprod Med* 1990;35:597.

66. Mage G, Canis M, Manhes H, et al. Laparoscopic management of adnexal cystic masses. *J Gynecol Surg* 1990;6:71.

67. Webb M, Decker D, Mussey E, et al. Factors inluencing survival in stage I ovarian cancer. *Am J Obstet Gynecol* 1973;116:227.

68. Beard RW, Reginald PW, Wadsworth J. Clinical features of women with chronic lower abdominal pain and pelvic congestion. *Br J Obstet Gynaecol* 1988;95:153.

69. Beard RW, Highman JH, Pearce S, et al. Diagnosis of pelvic varicosities in women with chronic pelvic pain. *Lancet* 1984;2:946.

70. El-Minawi MF, El-Minawi AM. Laparoscopy in chronic pelvic pain: 25 years experience. Presented at the International Congress of Gynecologic Endoscopy, AAGL 26th Annual Meeting. Seattle, Washington, Sept. 23–28, 1997.

71. Osman MI, Din Shafeek MA, Abdalla MI, et al. Chronic pelvic pain in Lippes IUD users. Laparoscopic and venographic evaluation. *Contracept Deliv Syst* 1981;2:41–51.

72. Beard RW, Kennedy RG, Gangar KF, et al. Bilateral oophorectomy and hysterectomy in the treatment of intractable pelvic pain associated with pelvic congestion. *Br J Obstet Gynaecol* 1991;98:988–992.

73. Taylor HC. Vascular congestion and hyperemial: their effect on structure and function in the female areproductive system. *Am J Obstet Gynecol* 1949;57:211.

74. Taylor HC. The clinical aspects of the congestion-fibrosis syndrome. *Am J Obstet Gynecol* 1949;57:637.

75. Schaupp JB. Pelvic varicose veins and varicocele. *Surg Clin NA* 1962;42:975.

76. Gussman D, Thickman D, Wheeler JE. Postoperative peritoneal cysts. *Obstet Gynecol* 1986;68:535.

77. Monafo W, Goldfarb W. Postoperative peritoneal cysts. *Surgery* 1963;53:470.

78. Falk HC, Bunkin IA. Intraperitoneal cysts simulating ovarian cysts. *Obstet Gynecol* 1953;1:181.

79. Lees RF, Feldman PS, Brenbridge ANAG, et al. Inflammatory cysts of the pelvic peritoneum. *Am J Roentgenol* 1978;131:633.

80. Steege JF. Ovarian remnant syndrome. *Obstet Gynecol* 1987;70:64.

81. Nezhat F, Nezhat C. Operative laparoscopy for the treatment of ovarian remnant syndrome. *Fertil Steril* 1992;57:1003–1007.

82. Webb MJ. Ovarian remnant syndrome. *Aust NZ J Obstet Gynaecol* 1989;29:433–435.

83. Metzger DA, Lessey BA, Soper JT, et al. Hormone-resistant endometriosis following total abdominal hysterectomy and bilateral salpingo-oophorectomy: correlation with histology and steroid receptor content. *Obstet Gynecol* 1991;78:946–950.

84. Redwine DB. Endometriosis persisting after castration: clinical characteristics and results of surgical management. *Obstet Gynecol* 1994;83:405–413.

85. Baker PB, Symonds EM. The resolution of chronic pelvic pain after normal laparoscopic findings. *Am J Obstet Gynecol* 1992;166:835–856.

86. Peters AAW, van Dorst E, Jellis B, et al. A randomized clinical trial to compare two different approaches in women with chronic pelvic pain. *Obstet Gynecol* 1991;77:740–000.

87. Bonica JJ. *The management of pain.* Philadelphia: Lea & Febiger, 1989:180.

88. Renaer M, Vertommen H, Nijs P, et al. Psychological aspects of chronic pelvic pain in women. *Am J Obstet Gynecol* 1979;134:75.

89. Lee RB, Stone K, Magelssen D, et al. Presacral neurectomy for chronic pelvic pain. *Obstet Gynecol* 1986;68:517–521.

90. Candiani GB, Fedele L, Vercellini P, et al. Presacral neurectomy for the treatment of pelvic pain associated with endometriosis: a controlled study. *Am J Obstet Gynecol* 1992;167:100–103.

91. Chen F-P, Soong Y-K. The efficacy and complications of laparoscopic presacral neurectomy in pelvic pain. *Obstet Gynecol* 1997;90:974–977.

92. Zulu F, Pellicano M, DeStafano R, et al. Efficacy of laparoscopic denervation in central-type chronic pelvic pain: a multicenter study. *J Gynecol Surg* 1996;12:35–40.

93. Bourke DL, Foster DC, Valley MA, et al. Superior hypogastric nerve block as predictive of presacral neurectomy success: a preliminary report. *Am J Pain Manag* 1996;6:9–12.

94. Steege JF. Superior hypogastric block during microlaparoscopic pain mapping. *J Am Assoc Gynecol Laparoscop* 1998;5:265–267.

95. Doyle JB, Des Rosiers JJ. Paracervical uterine denervation for relief of pelvic pain. *Clin Obstet Gynecol* 1963;6:742–753.

96. Lichten E, Bombard J. Surgical treatment of primary dysmenorrhea with laparoscopic uterine nerve ablation. *J Reprod Med* 1987;32:37–41.

97. Sutton CJG, Ewen SP, Whitelaw N, et al. Prospective, randomized, double-blind trial of laser laparoscopy in the treatment of pelvic pain associated with minimal, mild, and moderate endometriosis. *Fertil Steril* 1994;62:696–700.

98. Malinak LR. Pelvic pain—when is surgery indicated? *Contemp Ob/Gyn* 1985;26:43.

99. Reich H, De Capria J, McGlynn F. Laparoscopic hysterectomy. *J Gynecol Surg* 1989;5:213

100. Stovall TG, Ling FW, Crawford DA. Hysterectomy for chronic pelvic pain of presumed uterine etiology. *Obstet Gynecol* 1990;75:676–679.

101. Carlson KJ, Miller BA, Fowler FJ. The Maine women's health study: II. Outcomes of nonsurgical management of leiomyomas, abnormal bleeding, and chronic pelvic pain. *Obstet Gynecol* 1994;83:566–572.

102. Gambone JC, Reiter RC, Lench JB, et al. The impact of a quality assurance process on the frequency and confirmation rate of hysterectomy. *Am J Obstet Gynecol* 1990;163:545–550.

103. Candy JW. Modified Gilliam uterine suspension using laparoscopic ventrosuspension. *Obstet Gynecol* 1976;47:242.

104. Yoong AFE. Laparoscopic ventrosuspensions. *Am J Obstet Gynecol* 1990;163:1151.

105. Bryson K. Laparoscopic appendectomy. *J Gynecol Surg* 1991;7:93.

106. Cook AS, Rock JA. The role of laparoscopy in the treatment of endometriosis. *Fertil Steril* 1991;55:663.

107. Howard FM. Laparoscopic evaluation and treatment of women with chronic pelvic pain. *J Am Assoc Gynecol Laparosc* 1994;1:325–331.

108. Loffer FD, Pent D, Goodkin R. Sciatic nerve injury in a patient undergoing laparoscopy. *J Reprod Med* 1978;21:371–372.

109. Hershlag A, Loy RA, Lavy G, et al. Femoral neuropathy after laparoscopy: a case report. *J Reprod Med* 1990;35:575.

110. McLucas B, March C. Urachal sinus perforation during laparoscopy: a case report. *J Reprod Med* 1990;35:573.

111. Reich H, McGlynn F. Laparoscopic repair of bladder injury. *Obstet Gynecol* 1990;76:909.

112. Soderstrom RM, Levy BS. Bowel injuries during laparoscopy: causes and medicolegal questions. *Contemp Ob/Gyn* 1986;(March):41.

113. Gomel V, James C. Intraoperative management of ureteral injury during operative laparoscopy. *Fertil Steril* 1991;55:416.

114. Perez JJ. Laparoscopic presacral neurectomy: results of the first 25 cases. *J Reprod Med* 1990;35:625.

115. Metha PV. A total of 250,136 laparoscopic sterilizations by a single operator. *Br J Obstet Gynaecol* 1989;96:1024–134.

116. Almeida Jr OD, Val-Gallas JM. Conscious pain mapping. *J Am Assoc Gynecol Laparosc* 1997;4:587–590.

117. Demco LA. Effect on negative laparoscopy rate in chronic pelvic pain patients using patient assisted laparoscopy. *J Soc Laparoendoscop Surg* 1997;1:319–321.

118. Palter SF, Olive DL. Office microlaparoscopy under local anesthesia for chronic pelvic pain. *J Am Assoc Gynecol Laparoscop* 1996;3:359–364.

119. Demco L. Mapping the source and character of pain due to endometriosis by patient-assisted laparoscopy. *J Am Assoc Gynecol Laparoscop* 1998;5:241–245.

120. Lipscomb GH, Summitt RL Jr, McCord ML, et al. The effect of nitrous oxide and carbon dioxide pneumoperitoneum on operative and postoperative pain during laparoscopic sterilization under local anesthesia. *J Am Assoc Gynecol Laparoscop* 1994;2:57–60.

121. Faber BM, Coddington III CC. Microlaparoscopy: a comparative study of diagnostic accuracy. *Fertil Steril* 1997;67:952–954.

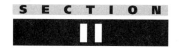

SECTION

II

DIAGNOSES AND TREATMENTS

6

ACCESSORY AND SUPERNUMERARY OVARIES

AHMED M. EL-MINAWI

KEY TERMS AND DEFINITIONS

Accessory ovary: Extra ovarian tissue that is invariably situated near a normally placed ovary, may be connected to it, and seems to have developed from it as tissue that was split from the embryonic ovary during early development.

Ectopic ovary: Extra ovarian tissue; may be a supernumerary or accessory ovary; the tissue must contain ovarian follicles.

Supernumerary ovary: Extra ovary that is entirely separate from the normally placed ovaries and apparently arises from a separate primordium or anlage.

INTRODUCTION

Ectopic ovaries, either accessory or supernumerary, are exceedingly rare. They normally produce no symptoms (1), but can occasionally be associated with chronic abdominopelvic pain (CPP) if they undergo cystic or neoplastic transformation. Since Grohe (2), in 1863, and Winckel (3), in 1890, described the first authentic cases of accessory and supernumerary ovaries, respectively, these anomalies have been reported only sporadically.

The terminology of these conditions is confusing to physicians not familiar with the classifications and definitions (1,4). Wharton's classification distinguishes the two types of ectopic ovaries based on their relationship to a normal ovary (Table 6.1). A supernumerary ovary contains ovarian follicular material and is entirely separate from the normally placed ovaries. It has no connections with the infundibulopelvic, uteroovarian, or broad ligaments. It is believed to be derived from a separate primordium. An accessory ovary is always situated near or connected to a normally placed ovary and is thought to originate from a separated fragment from the developing embryonic ovary (5).

Another classification has been proposed by Lachmann and Berman (4) to attempt to clarify the nomenclature and origin of these ovarian anomalies. They suggest that proper identification of a true extra ovary requires a pelvis free of endometriosis, pelvic inflammatory disease, ectopic pregnancy, adhesions, and prior surgery. Their preferred nomenclature is *ectopic ovary*. Ectopic ovary then can be classified into (a) postsurgical implant, (b) postinflammatory implant, or (c) true or embryologic. Later in this chapter the embryological development of the ovaries and the possible mechanisms whereby these conditions can come about is reviewed, and this may give a better understanding as to why different sets of criteria coexist.

The incidence of these conditions is not known. Wharton (1) reported one case of accessory ovary among 93,000 gynecological admissions to the Johns Hopkins hospital. Supernumerary ovary was reported once in 400,000 admissions. Among the difficulties in determining incidences is the fact that some are only found at autopsy. Wharton mentions finding only one supernumerary ovary among 29,000 autopsies performed at Johns Hopkins Hospital. Older texts (6,7) mention frequencies varying from 2% to 4%, which seem far too high. In particular, one early report (7) of 23 cases of accessory ovary in 500 autopsies was largely discredited by earlier investigators due to lack of histologic confirmation.

A review of the literature reveals that about 30 histologically confirmed cases of supernumerary ovary have been reported since 1891 (Table 6.2) and about 22 cases of acces-

TABLE 6.1. WHARTON'S ORIGINAL DEFINING CHARACTERISTICS OF SUPERNUMERARY OVARY AND ACCESSORY OVARY

■ *Supernumerary ovary* (ueberzachliges ovarium, ovaire supernuméraire) applies to cases in which the extra ovary is entirely separate from the normally placed ovaries and apparently arises from a separate primordium or anlage.

■ *Accessory ovary* is applied to those cases in which the excess ovarian tissue is invariably situated near a normally placed ovary, may be connected to it, and seems to have developed from it as tissue that was split from the embryonic ovary during its early development.

■ To be a supernumerary or accessory ovary, the tissue must contain ovarian follicles.

TABLE 6.2. PUBLISHED CASES OF SUPERNUMERARY OVARIES

Case	Author(s)	Year	Age	Location	Diagnosis	Clinical History[a]
1	Winckel (3)	1890	77	Anterior uterine wall, attached by band	Autopsy	G0P0, liver cirrhosis
2	Falk (25)	1891	37	Omentum	Pathology	P0, recurring pelvic pain, menstrual irregularities
3	Nichols and Postoloff (26)	1951	36	Inferior to liver, at level of gall bladder, attached by a broad pedicle to posterior peritoneum in location of congenitally absent right kidney	Pathology	G1P1, acute pain in RUQ
4a	Wharton (1)	1956	37	Right pelvic wall. Retroperitoneal	Pathology	G0P0, irregular menses, chronic salpingitis
4b	Wharton (1)	1957	39	Sigmoid mesentry. Retroperitoneal	Pathology	Enlarging pelvic mass (same patient as above, new location)
5	Wharton (1)	1959	20	Left of aorta	Autopsy	G2,P2,A2; choriocarcinoma with cerebral metastases
6	Burnett (27)	1961	—	Between left ureter and rectosigmoid. Retroperitoneal	Pathology	G1P1, severe chronic pelvic pain; prior BS for pyosalpinx
7	Pearl and Plotz (5)	1963	34	In cul-de-sac attached by a pedicle to the posterior peritoneum inferolateral to left uterosacral ligament	Pathology	Persistent menses 3 months after BO.
8	Hogan et al. (28)	1967	21	Omentum, not related to either of the adnexa	Pathology	G5,P4,A0; acute pelvic pain, LLQ
9	Williams et al. (16)	1971	26	Right iliac fossa, retroperitoneal, displacing cecum	Pathology	G2,P2; enlarging painless abdominopelvic mass
10	Printz et al. (29)	1973	23	Omentum	Pathology	G4P4; menorrhagia and anemia
11	Arzapalo et al. (30)	1974	19	Left adnexal area	Pathology	Sterility, mosaic; 46XX/45XY
12	Huhn (15)	1975		Omentum	Pathology	
13	Abrego and Ibrahim (31)	1975	38	Mesentry of distal ileum 10 inches proximal to ileocecal valve	Pathology	Chronic pelviabdominal pain
14	Kosasa et al. (23)	1976	31	Left pelvic sidewall overlying left ureter, lateral to left uterosacral ligament, retroperitoneal	Preop disease	G3P3; irregular menses 2 months after BO

15	Roth and Ehrlich (14)	1977	48	Left retroperitoneal space, displacing rectosigmoid colon	Pathology	Enlarging asymptomatic abdominal mass
16	Cruikshank and Van Drie (32)	1982	33	Separate pelvic mass adherent to the descending colon	Laparoscopy	G1P1, recurrent LLQ pain, painful pelvic mass
17	Cruikshank and Van Drie (32)	1982	36	Left retroperitoneal, level of kidney, bound by ovarian vessels medially, descending colon laterally	Pathology	G2P2, Asymptomatic mass, deep dyspareunia
18	Poma (33)	1982	50	Left infundibulopelvic ligament	Pathology	G3P2A11, asymptomatic pelvic mass
19	Lee and Gore (34)	1984	30	Attached between left tubal fimbria and rectosigmoid	Laparoscopy	G1P1, 2ry infertility, dysmenorrhea, left adnexal mass
20	Hahn-Pederson and Larsen (35)	1984	20	At level of L2–3, connected by fibrous string to left ovary	Laparoscopy	G1P0A1, Secondary infertility
21	Mercer et al. (36)	1987	36	Broad ligament, 2 cm caudad to right ovary	Pathology	G3P3, enlarging asymptomatic pelvic mass
22	Mercer et al. (36)	1987	34	Omentum	Preop disease	G8P6, pregnant 8 weeks
23	Harlass et al. (37)	1987	37	Anterior descending colon, projecting from beneath taenia coli	Pathology	G1P0, chronic pelvic pain, rectal mass
24	Navarro et al. (38)	1990	38	Left paracolic gutter above the pelvic brim	Surgery	G1P0A1, LLQ pain radiating to left leg, dysmennorhea, history of endometriosis
25	Alpern (39)	1990	40	Right pelvic sidewall, retroperitoneal	Pathology	G2P2, menorrhagia, severe dysmenorrhea
26	Cruikshank (40)	1990	37	Left pelvic sidewall, retroperitoneal	Pathology	G1P1, acute LLQ pain, tender pelvic mass
27	McCullough et al. (41)	1992	27	External serosal surface at junction of uterus and cervix	Pathology	G3P1A2, metrorrhagia, intermittent abdominal pain, deep dyspareunia
28	Badawy et al. (19)	1995	32	Left pelvic sidewall, overlying iliopsoas muscle and iliac vessels	Pathology	G1P0A1, LUQ, LLQ pain, radiating down to buttocks and back of left leg, history of endometriosis
29	Levy et al. (42)	1997	51	Intrarenal; intraparenchymal in superior role of right kidney	Pathology	G?P2, RUQ mass, weight loss
30	Kini et al. (43)	1998	5		Pathology	G0P0, Wilm's tumor

[a]BO, Bilateral-phorectomy; BS, Bilateral salpinsectomy; LLQ, Left lower quadrant; LUQ,Left upper quadrant; RUQ,..

sory ovaries. There probably are more reports of supernumerary ovary because it is much rarer and generates more interest in publishing than does accessory ovary. One other confusing point in assessing incidence is that some of the cases in the literature are actually tumors that are ovarian in origin, but do not actually contain ovarian tissue. Some investigators have classified these as supernumerary or accessory ovarian neoplasms, whereas others have not. Because retroperitoneal tumors of possible ovarian origin are not uncommonly removed by surgeons, classifying them all as ectopic neoplastic ovaries would greatly (and falsely) increase the incidence. Wharton reviewed 26 reports of ectopic ovarian tumors and found only four containing ovarian tissue. As a result of an opinion that only if there were histologic evidence of ovarian tissue would it be proper to classify neoplasms as ectopic ovarian neoplasms, he classified only these four as accessory ovaries. In reviewing publications in the years subsequent to Wharton's report, there are instances where such cases have not been considered ectopic ovaries and vice versa.

EMBRYOLOGY AND ETIOLOGY

The classic work of Witschi (8) on the migration of germ cells in the human embryo, along with the histochemical study of ovarian development by Pinkerton et al. (9), have provided us with a clear picture of normal ovarian development. The ovary arises from two independent primordia: (a) gonadocytes or germ cells that originate from the caudal–dorsal yolk sac endoderm and (b) the germinal ridge in the medial segment of the intermediate somatic mesoderm. The germ cells are transferred to the hind gut from which they migrate by amoebic movement via the dorsal mesentry into the germinal ridge, all the while increasing through mitotic divisions. They normally reach their positions in the cortex of the primitive gonad by the end of the sixth week, having traversed a maximal distance of 0.5 mm.

Accessory ovaries are thought to arise from a separation or splitting of small fragments of tissue from the developing ovarian primordium (1,5). Because they arise from the same primordium, their blood supply will be derived from that of the normally placed ovary and will be continuous with it. And because they are fragments of the original, accessory ovaries are invariably small in size, rarely reaching 1 cm in diameter (5,10). Early investigators hypothesized about the factors leading to separation of portions of the developing ovary. Their theories included (a) fetal peritonitis-induced adhesions causing ovarian division (6), (b) ovarian pedicle torsion leading to separation of a part, and (c) pressure-induced separation from surrounding organs (1).

Many opinions have been presented to explain the development of supernumerary ovaries, but the three main schools of thought center around either a developmental ovarian mishap or a later mechanistic theory.

The first theory is that there is a *migratory arrest of the gonadocytes* during their migration from the hind gut to the genital ridge. Germ cells are normally found in the early embryo in the same locations where supernumerary ovaries have been found. A supernumerary ovary will develop if the surrounding primitive mesenchyme undergoes differentiation to ovarian stroma. Depending on the ultimate arrest point, the ovary may develop in the future mesentry, bowel, or peritoneum. The totipotential quality of the gonadocyte may also explain the occasional dermoid cyst reported in the omentum (11,12).

The second theory is that there is *detachment and physical transplantation of a part of the genital ridge* onto the dorsal mesentry. Because the distance of gonadocyte migration does not exceed 0.5 mm, this mechanism is feasible because the detachment–reattachment would not involve a much greater distance.

The third theory, the *mechanistic theory* (11), is similar to that previously mentioned in regard to the accessory ovary (12,13). This proposes that secondary peritoneal adhesions or cicatrizations could trap or cut off portions of a differentiated gonad during early development *in utero*. Proponents (6,14) note that the ectopic tissue is most often located along the line of ovarian descent. On a variation of this theme, one author (15) reports a case in which a supernumerary ovarian dermoid became implanted in the omentum following peduncle torsion and "autoamputation" of the ovary.

Other, less-subscribed-to theories exist to explain the cases of retroperitoneal tumors of ovarian origin that have been reported and in which, oftentimes, no frank ovarian tissue is found accompanying the neoplasm. *Coelomic metaplasia* is widely accepted to explain the histogenesis of epithelial neoplasms (14,16,17). In early embryonic life, the germinal epithelium of the ovary appears to arise from an invagination of the coelomic epithelium; an invagination of the same coelomic or peritoneal epithelial layer with concurrent or subsequent metaplasia could account for retroperitoneal ovarian neoplasms. Other investigators (17) find it more plausible that small clusters of coelomic epithelial cells could be deposited along the course of the embryonic ovarian descent. These cells, with or without formation of an ovary, could develop into tumors via metaplasia or proliferation. Theories abound; in all instances a supernumerary ovary will have a blood supply independent of the normally placed ovaries due to its having arisen from a separate anlage (18).

Of importance from the embryologic viewpoint is the increased incidence of associated congenital malformations with supernumerary and accessory ovary. Most of these abnormalities are of organs formed from the urogenital ridge. Some examples are renal and ureteral agenesis, accessory fallopian tube, bladder diverticulum, and double

TABLE 6.3. CONGENITAL MALFORMATIONS ASSOCIATED WITH ECTOPIC OVARIES

Author(s)	Year	Type of Ovary	Associated Malformation(s)
Winckel (3)	1890	Supernumerary	Diverticulum of the bladder, accessory fallopian tube
Falk (25)	1891	Supernumerary	Accessory fallopian tube
Nichols and Postoloff (26)	1951	Supernumerary	Agenesis of right kidney, right ureter, right round ligament, and right fallopian tube
Wharton (1)	1959	Supernumerary	Agenesis of left kidney, left ureter, left renal artery, and left renal vein
Wharton reporting on five cases (1)	1959	Accessory	Accessory fallopian tube (×2), bifid fallopian tube (×1) Accessory tubal ostium (×1), lobulated liver (×1) Septate uterus (×1)
Granat et al. (47)	1981	Accessory	Uterus unicornis
Poma (33)	1982	Supernumerary	Bilateral duplication of the renal collecting systems
Cruikshank and Van Drie (32)	1982	Supernumerary	Left-sided duplication of the renal collecting system
Hahn-Pederson and Larsen (35)	1984	Supernumerary	Uterus unicornis

ureteral collecting systems. The frequency varies, but anomalies are more often described with supernumerary ovaries than with accessory ovaries. Wharton (1) reported finding malformations of the genitourinary system in three out of the four supernumerary ovarian cases he presented. On the other hand, similar malformations were present in only 5 out of 19 cases of accessory ovary. Table 6.3 lists the associated malformations in published cases of ectopic ovaries (3). From the available data (Tables 6.2 and 6.3), the estimated incidence of anomalies is about 23% in cases of supernumerary ovary.

PATHOLOGY

There is great variation in the pathologic diagnoses reported in supernumerary and accessory ovaries. Apart from normal ovarian stroma or follicles, many of these ovaries contain functional cysts of various types or have undergone benign or malignant transformation. Taking into account the high association of these ectopic ovaries with congenital malformations and the fact that many of them are discovered accidentally, it is important to be acquainted with the various histopathologic variations seen in these cases. Table 6.4 lists the various histopathological diagnoses reported.

Corpora lutei are the most commonly reported histopathologic findings, particularly with supernumerary ovary, being found in 30% of reported cases. Ovarian neoplastic diseases have been noted in 7 (23%) of 31 cases of supernumerary ovary and in 2 (40%) of 5 cases of accessory ovary. Benign cystic teratomas (5 cases) and mucinous cystadenomas (3 cases) are the most common. There was only one malignancy, a papillary mucinous cystadenocarcinoma, among the cases of ectopic ovary. Other findings include one case of endometrioma (19). In this case the supernumerary ovary may have been invaded by preexisting pelvic endometriosis. The same patient also demonstrated abundant osseous metaplasia within the ectopic ovarian tissue, possibly a result of stimulation of undifferentiated stromal mesenchymal cells by the neighboring endometriosis.

There exist interesting reports of retroperitoneal tumors of ovarian origin in which no ovarian tissue has been identified. These have included both benign and malignant cystadenomas as well as cystadenofibromas (17,20). These cases, in accordance with the previously mentioned criteria, have not been listed as supernumerary or accessory ovarian tumors despite its use by Barik et al. (20) Truly rare are cases of bilateral agenesis of the normal ovaries with a single ectopic ovary. In two such cases the pathology showed normal ovarian tissue in one and a dermoid cyst in the other (21,22). The fact that in both these cases only one ovary was found, far from the normal site, suggests that these were "true" ectopic ovaries.

SYMPTOMS

Supernumerary and accessory ovaries are usually asymptomatic, which explains why most are found only at autopsy or during surgery for other reasons. Despite the uncertain nature of their origin, they merit attention due to their functional capability as a normal ovary, allowing them to develop the same range of potential pathologic conditions and accompanying symptoms.

The ability to produce ovarian hormones may cause symptoms in some cases. Examples are two cases where menses resumed following bilateral oophorectomy (5,23). In the first case the patient underwent bilateral oophorectomy following a diagnosis of mammary carcinoma. She experienced scant menstrual periods over a period of 11 months following an immediate postsurgical amenorrhea of only two months. This case is the first where a tentative preoperative diagnosis of supernumerary ovary was made, based on the surgeon's interpretation of the evidence,

TABLE 6.4. HISTOPATHOLOGIC DESCRIPTION OF ECTOPIC OVARY CASES

Investigator(s)	Type of Ovary	Histopathologic Disease and Picture
Winckel (3)	Supernumerary	Normal ovarian tissue in normal-sized ovary
Falk (25)	Supernumerary	Normal ovarian tissue in normal-sized ovary
Nichols and Postoloff (26)	Supernumerary	Cystic mass 10 × 5 × 3 cm. Normal ovarian stroma + scattered follicular cysts + hemorrhagic lutein cyst
Wharton (1)	Supernumerary	Case 1: normal ovarian tissue in irregular mass 2 × 2.5 cm Case 2: 10-cm mass containing normal ovarian tissue + corpus luteum + follicular cyst
Wharton (1)	Accessory	4-mm structure, containing normal ovarian tissue + corpus albicans
Burnett (27)	Supernumerary	2 × 1.4 × 1.2-cm mass containing normal ovarian tissue + hemorrhagic corpus luteum + endometriosis
Pearl and Plotz (5)	Supernumerary	1.5 × 0.5-cm mass containing normal ovarian tissue + corpora lutei + corpora albicanti
Hogan et al. (28)	Supernumerary	11 × 7 × 4.5-cm cystic mass containing dark blood and sebaceous material. Benign cystic teratoma + ovarian stroma
Williams et al. (16)	Heterotopic ovary	22 × 16 × 10-cm unilocular cystic mass. Pseudomucinous cystadenoma
Printz et al. (29)	Supernumerary	3.5 × 4.5-cm cystic mass containing yellow caseous material and hair. Benign cystic teratoma + normal ovarian tissue
Huhn (15)	Supernumerary	Cystic mass, benign cystic teratoma + ovarian stroma
Abrego and Ibrahim (31)	Supernumerary	2.5 × 2.5 × 1.5-cm mass containing follicular cysts + normal ovarian tissue
Kosasa et al. (23)	Supernumerary	4 × 3-cm cystic mass containing normal ovarian tissue + hemorrhagic corpus luteum
Roth and Ehrlich (14)	Supernumerary	Papillary mucinous cystadenocarcinoma + ovarian-like stroma
Dillon and Dewey (44)	Accessory	Normal-sized ovary containing normal ovarian tissue
Gabbay-Moore et al. (45)	Accessory (×2)	7 × 7 cm and 5 × 4 cm, bilateral benign cystic teratomas
Poma (33)	Supernumerary	Normal ovarian tissue + corpus luteum
Cruikshank and Van Drie (32)	Supernumerary	Case 1: 3 × 4.5 × 5.3-cm mass containing normal ovarian tissue + hemorrhagic corpus luteum Case 2: 11 × 7 × 6-cm multicystic mass. Mucinous cystadenoma + normal ovarian tissue
Lee and Gore (34)	Supernumerary	3 × 4-cm mass containing normal ovarian tissue + corpus luteum
Hahn-Pederson and Larsen (35)	Supernumerary	1 × 1 × 2-cm ovary containing normal ovarian tissue
Schultze and Fenger (10)	Accessory	4-mm structure containing normal ovarian tissue + corpus albicans
Heller et al. (46)	Accessory	Brenner tumor and ovarian stroma
Harlass et al. (37)	Supernumerary	4-cm ovary with hemorrhagic corpus luteum
Navarro et al. (38)	Supernumerary	3 × 3-cm cystic nodule containing normal ovarian tissue + endometriosis
Alpern (39)	Supernumerary	5 × 3 × 3-mm nodule of normal ovarian stroma
Cruikshank (40)	Supernumerary	6 × 5 × 4-cm cystic mass, hemorrhagic corpus luteum
Lachmann and Bermann (4)	Supernumerary	Normal ovarian tissue
McCullough et al. (41)	Supernumerary	18 × 8 × 5-mm nodule containing normal ovarian tissue + corpora albicantes
Badawy et al. (19)	Supernumerary	5 × 4 × 3-cm cystic mass containing normal ovarian tissue + endometriosis + osseous metaplasia
Roth and Ehrlich (14)	Accessory	Normal ovarian stroma + steroid cell tumor (polygonal cells with eosinopholic cytoplasm)
Granat et al. (47)	Accessory	Ovarian hyperstimulation syndrome
Scalia and Sironi (48)	Supernumerary	Benign cystic teratoma
Levy et al. (42)	Supernumerary	5-cm multicystic mass, ovarian tissue + follicular cysts + corpora albicantia
Kini et al. (43)	Supernumerary	

including an endometrial biopsy showing progestational effects (5). Irregularities of the menstrual cycle have been reported in five of the published cases (Table 6.1), with menorrhagia being the most common complaint. More data are needed before concluding that hormonal production by an ectopic ovary could have a role in abnormal menstrual function.

Pelvic and lower abdominal pain are reported in 40% of cases of supernumerary ovary (Table 6.1). The complaints range from dyspareunia to deep-seated chronic pelvic pain. Acute pain is sometimes a symptom and has been reported in three cases of hemorrhage within a cyst. Histology showed corpora lutei in two and benign cystic teratoma in the third. Chronic and recurrent abdominopelvic pain have been reported in 30% of cases of supernumerary ovary. In 5 of the 10 cases there were cysts (4 corpora lutei and 1 mucinous cystadenoma), and in two there was endometriosis.

Of interest is that the location of pain appears to be related to the site of the ectopic ovary. In 3 of the 10 cases with abdominopelvic pain of long duration the ectopic ovary was adherent to the descending colon in 2 cases and within the mesentery of the distal ileum in one case. In two cases where patients complained of pain radiating to the leg or buttock the supernumerary ovary was found on the pelvic sidewall overlying the iliopsoas muscle on the ipsilateral side; both showed histologic endometriosis.

With accessory ovary the symptoms are somewhat vague, including dysmenorrhea, metrorrhagia, and pelvic tenderness. Acute abdominopelvic pain occurred in one patient as a result of accessory ovarian torsion. In one interesting case, an accessory ovary was the source of an ovum that led to a tubal pregnancy (24). The ectopic ovary was discovered on laparotomy and labeled originally as supernumerary, but was later reclassified as accessory.

SIGNS

There are no cardinal signs for the presence of an ectopic ovary. Each case is unique. Whereas most are asymptomatic, others may present with pain or as painless enlarging masses detected by the patient or by examination. Signs of recurrence or persistence of endometriosis following bilateral oophorectomy should lead the physician to search for evidence of ovarian function. Although ovarian remnant syndrome is usually the culprit, presence of an accessory ovary should be kept in mind. In the more than a century since ectopic ovaries were first detected, only two cases have ever been tentatively diagnosed preoperatively, and both of these were in women who had persistent vaginal bleeding following bilateral oophorectomy for breast carcinoma. In addition, three others have been diagnosed at the time of diagnostic laparoscopy (Table 6.2). Many of these masses

are missed at laparotomy because they are mistaken for benign lymph nodes or are not noticed at all.

The sizes of these masses have ranged from 2 to 22 cm. The majority of the masses presenting abdominally have been neoplasias, such as mucinous cystadenomas and benign cystic teratomas. In most cases they are painless and nontender and have been located in the omentum. Those presenting as pelvic masses usually are tender on bimanual examination, and the majority contains corpora lutei or follicular cysts. They are also smaller in size, usually not exceeding 7 cm. The majority of pelvic supernumerary ovaries are felt separately from the adnexa, toward the pelvic sidewalls or attached to the rectum. Accessory ovaries are usually felt in the vicinity of the adnexa and are often difficult to distinguish. In many cases, asymptomatic pelvic masses are detected on routine pelvic examinations following pelvic surgical procedures. They are sometimes mistaken for hematomas, and they only undergo further investigation after being found to increase in size on subsequent examinations despite treatment.

DIAGNOSTIC STUDIES

Ultrasonography is a noninvasive diagnostic tool that may be helpful in cases with a mass, but no cases have actually been diagnosed sonographically. Laparoscopic findings have directed the surgeons to the diagnosis in three cases. In suspected cases, a thorough examination of the pelvis and peritoneal cavity may locate the ectopic ovary. In particular, accessory ovaries are usually very small in size and are easily missed. The use of diagnostic laparoscopy in suspected cases may lead to more diagnoses.

A novel approach to diagnosis was attempted via the use of human chorionic gonadotropin (HCG) stimulation to confirm the suspicion of an ectopic ovary (23). This was in a patient complaining of recurrent menses following bilateral oophorectomy for breast carcinoma. Following elimination of the adrenal source of estrogen, the patient was stimulated using 10,000 units of HCG intramuscularly. A rise in plasma estrogen levels indicated an ovarian source. After diagnosis, hyperstimulation was done using daily injections of human menopausal gonadotropin to facilitate its location at laparotomy.

TREATMENT

The proper management for symptomatic ectopic ovaries is oophorectomy. There are no reports of any trials of medical treatment. Obviously, extirpation is indicated in the cases with abdominal or pelvic masses. If found incidently at surgery, the recommendation is still removal due to the potential for subsequent pathologic changes.

Because many of the pelvic ectopic ovaries are retroperitoneal, precautions should be taken to properly identify the major pelvic sidewall vessels and the ureters. Some authors (19) suggest catheterizing the ureters prior to dissection of the mass.

KEY POINTS

Differential Diagnoses

- Supernumerary ovary
- Accessory ovaries
- Ovarian remnant syndrome
- Lymph node

Most Important Questions to Ask

- Have you had any prior abdominal or pelvic surgery?

Most Important Physical Examination Findings

- Abdominal or pelvic mass that may or may not be tender

Most Important Diagnostic Studies

- Ultrasound or computerized tomography of the abdomen and pelvis
- Laparoscopy
- HCG stimulation

Treatments

- Surgical treatment is recommended.
- Preoperative diagnosis is quite rare.

REFERENCES

1. Wharton LR. Two cases of supernumerary ovary and one of accessory ovary, with an analysis of previously reported cases. *Am J Obstet Gynecol* 1959;78(5):1101–1118.
2. Grohe F. Ueber den bau und des Wachsthum des menschlichen Eierstocks, und uber einige Krankhafte Storungen desselben. *Virchows Arch Pathol Anat* 1863;26:271–306.
3. Winckel F. *Lehrbuch der Frauenkrankhheiten,* 2nd ed. Leipzig: S Hirzel, 1890:617–220.
4. Lachmann MF, Berman MM. The ectopic ovary. A case report and review of the literature. *Arch Pathol Lab Med* 1991;115:233–235.
5. Pearl M, Plotz EJ. Supernumerary ovary. *Obstet Gynecol* 1963;21(2):253–256.
6. Piersol GA, ed. *Human anatomy. Including structure and development and practical considerations,* vol II, *The ovary.* Philadelphia: JB Lippincott, 1923:1995.
7. Biegel H. *Wien Med Wochnschr* 1877;27:266.
8. Witschi E. Migration of the germ cells of human embryos from the yolk sac to the primitive gonadal folds. *Contrib Embryol* 1948;32:68.
9. Pinkerton JHM, McKay DG, Adams EC, et al. Development of the human ovary—a study using histochemical techniques. *Obstet Gynecol* 1961;18(2):152–181.
10. Schultze H, Fenger C. Accessory ovary. *Acta Obstet Gynecol Scand* 1986;65:503–504.
11. Mobius VW, Carol W. Retroperitoneal gelengenes pseudo muzinkystom, von ektopischem ovarialgewebe ausgehend. *Zentralbl Gynakol* 1964;86:133–136.
12. Angervall L, Knutson H. Heterotopic ovarian tissue. *Acta Obstet Gynecol Scand* 1959;38:275–278.
13. Hansmann GH, Budd JW. Massive unattached retroperitoneal tumours. *Am J Pathol* 1931;7:631–673.
14. Roth LM, Ehrlich CE. Mucinous cystadenoma of the retroperitoneum. *Obstet Gynecol* 1977;49(4):486–488.
15. Huhn FO. Dermoid cysts of the greater omentum. *Arch Gynakol* 1975;220:99–103.
16. Williams PP, Gall SA, Prem KA. Ectopic mucinous cystadenoma. A case report. *Obstet Gynecol* 1971;38(6):831–837.
17. Pennell TC, Gusdon JP Jr. Retroperitoneal mucinous cystadenoma. *Am J Obstet Gynecol* 1989;160(5), Part 1:1229–1231.
18. Mercer LJ, Toub DB, Cibils LA. Tumors originating in supernumerary ovaries. A report of two cases. *J Reprod Med* 1987;32(12):932–934.
19. Badawy SZA, Kasello DJ, Powers C, et al. Supernumerary ovary with an endometrium and osseous metaplasia: a case report. *Am J Obstet Gynecol* 1995;173(5):1623–1624.
20. Barik S, Dhaliwal LK, Gopalan S, et al. Adenocarcinoma of the supernumerary ovary. *Int J Gynecol Obstet* 1990;34:75–77.
21. Peer E, Kerner H, Peretz BA, et al. Bilateral adnexal agenesis with an ectopic ovary—case report and review of the literature. *Eur J Obstet Gynecol Reprod Biol* 1981;12:37–42.
22. Kriplani A, Takkar D, Karak AK, et al. Unexplained absence of both fallopian tubes with ovary in the omentum. *Archives Gynecol Obstet* 1995;256:111–113.
23. Kosasa TS, Griffiths CT, Shane JM, et al. Diagnosis of a supernumerary ovary with human chorionic gonadotropin. *Obstet Gynecol* 1976;47(2):236–238.
24. Swynghedar MP, Houch ME. Un cas d'ovair surnumeraire. *Bull Soc Obstet Gynecol Paris* 1925;14:530.
25. Falk E. Uber uberzahlige Eileiter und Eierstocke. *Berlin Klin Wochnschr* 1891;28:1069–1071.
26. Nichols DH, Postoloff AV. Congenital ectopic ovary. *Am J Obstet Gynecol* 1951;62(1):195–198.
27. Burnett JE. Supernumerary ovary. *Am J Obstet Gynecol* 1961;82:929–930.
28. Hogan ML, Barber DB, Kaufman RH. Dermoid cyst in supernumerary ovary of the greater omentum. *Obstet Gynecol* 1967;29(3):405–408.
29. Printz JL, Choate JW, Townes PL, et al. The embryology of supernumerary ovaries. *Obstet Gynecol* 1973;41(2):246–252.
30. Arzpalo EG, Meneses AC, Garay ME, et al. Ovario supernumerario: reporte de un caso con estudio citogenetico. *Ginecol Obstet Mex* 1974;36:291–300.
31. Abrego D, Ibrahim AA. Mesenteric supernumerary ovary. *Obstet Gynecol* 1975;45:352–353.
32. Cruikshank SH, Van Drie DM. Supernumerary ovaries: update and review. *Obstet Gynecol* 1982;60:126–129.
33. Poma PA. Supernumerary ovary. *Ill Med J* 1982;162:34–35.
34. Lee B, Gore BZ. A case of supernumerary ovary. *Obstet Gynecol* 1984;64(5):738–739.
35. Hahn-Pederson J, Larsen PM. Supernumerary ovary. *Acta Obstet Gynecol Scand* 1984;63:365–366.
36. Mercer LJ, Toub DB, Cibils LA. Tumors originating in supernumerary ovaries. A report of two cases. *J Reprod Med* 1987;32(12):932–934.
37. Harlass F, Magelssen D, Soisson AP. Supernumerary ovary. A case report. *J Reprod Med* 1987;32(6):459–461.

38. Navarro C, Franklin RR, Valdes CT. Supernumerary ovary in association with endometriosis. *Fertil Steril* 1990;54(1): 164–165.

39. Alpern H. Supernumerary ovary. A case report. *J Reprod Med* 1990;35(3):283–285.

40. Cruikshank S. Supernumerary ovary: embryology. *Int J Gynecol Obstet* 1990;34:175–178.

41. McCullough JB, Evans AT, Holley MP. Supernumerary or ectopic ovary: a case report. *Histopathology* 1992;21:582–583.

42. Levy B, DeFranco J, Parra R, et al. Intrarenal supernumerary ovary. *J Urol* 1997;157:2240–2241.

43. Kini H, Baliga PB, Pai KG. Supernumerary ovary associated with Wilm's tumor. *Pediatr Surg Int* 1998;13(1):67–68.

44. Dillon WP, Dewey MD. A case of accessory ovary. *Obstet Gynecol* 1981;58(5):660–661.

45. Gabbay-Moore M, Ovadia Y, Neri A. Accessory ovaries with bilateral dermoid cysts. *Eur J Obstet Gynecol Reprod Biol* 1982;14: 171–173.

46. Heller DS, Harpaz N, Breakstone B. Neoplasms arising in ectopic ovaries: a case of Brenner tumour in an accessory ovary. *Int J Gynecol Pathol* 1990;9(2):185–190.

47. Granat M, Evron S, Navot D. Pregnancy in heterotopic fallopian tube and unilateral ovarian hyperstimulation. *Acta Obstet Gynecol Scand* 1981;60(2):215–217.

48. Scalia L, Sironi I. Benign teratoma in a supernumerary ovary [Italian]. *Pathologica* 1984;76(1045):627–630.

7

ADENOMYOSIS

JAMES E. CARTER

KEY TERMS AND DEFINITIONS

Adenomyosis: An ingrowth of endometrial glands and stroma into the myometrium at least one or two low-power fields from the endometrium. Ectopic glands and stroma of adenomyosis should be located at least 2 to 3 mm below the endometrial surface (45).

Adenomyoma: A nodule of hypertrophic myometrium and ectopic endometrium. Adenomyomas may be confused with intramural leiomyomas, although they are darker in color and not quite as firm.

INTRODUCTION

Adenomyosis was first described by Rokitansky in 1860 (1). The continuity between the basal layer of endometrium and the adenomyotic tissue was not demonstrated until 1908 (2). The reported incidence of adenomyosis ranges from 5% to 70% (3–9), varying with the scrutiny of histologic evaluation and the patient's symptoms, age, and parity. For example, the diagnosis of adenomyosis doubles from 31% to 62% when six blocks rather than the routine three blocks are taken from hysterectomy specimens (5), has been reported in 54% of women in one necropsy study (10), and was found in 19% of uteri removed at the time of surgery for pelvic relaxation (11).

About 80% of cases of adenomyosis are reported in women in their fourth and fifth decades of life (4,5,10). Women less than 30 years of age account for about 17% of cases. Most cases of adenomyosis in younger women are discovered incidentally and are of mild degree (4). Women older than 60 years account for less than 10% of cases (12,13). In postmenopausal women the adenomyotic foci usually demonstrate an atrophic pattern consistent with their hypoestrogenic state (4). Also, the severity of adenomyosis appears to correlate with the patient's age (12).

Eighty percent to 90% of cases of adenomyosis are found in parous patients. Infertility is reported in only 5% of women with adenomyosis, which is not significantly different from the general population (12).

Additional pelvic pathology is found in 60% to 80% of cases of adenomyosis. The most frequent finding, leiomyomata uteri, is present in 35% to 55% of cases (4–6,8,10). Peritoneal endometriosis is noted in 6% to 20% of women with adenomyosis (4–6,8,10). Endometrial polyps occur in 2% of adenomyotic uteri (5,8,10). Endometrial hyperplasia may be more common in patients with adenomyosis than in the general population; estimates range from 7% to 100% (5–7,14).

ETIOLOGY

Adenomyosis occurs when the normal boundary between the basal layer of the endometrium and the myometrium is breached. It has been suggested that uterine trauma of childbirth (12) or postpartum endometritis might cause the initial break in the normal boundary (15). The statistical correlation between adenomyosis and prior dilatation and curettage is supportive of this "trauma" hypothesis (15). The experimental observation that vigorously curetting one horn in a pregnant rabbit while allowing the pregnancy to continue in the opposite horn results in experimentally produced adenomyotic lesions is also supportive of this theory of etiology (3). Subsequent reactive hyperplasia of the basalis endometrium is thought to lead to an invasion of the myometrium and resultant adenomyosis. An early sign of adenomyosis is the marked invasion of stromal fibroblast into the myometrium along the branches of blood vessels (16). Thereafter, uterine glands invade the myometrium following these fibroblasts and producing areas of adenomyosis. Presence of endometrial tissue in myometrial vessels can be found primarily in association with menses. The presence of intravascular endometrial tissue may explain the origin of adenomyotic foci deep in the myometrium without connection to the endometrium (17).

Tubal ligation may also be a risk factor for adenomyosis. Of 93 patients requiring a hysterectomy for chronic pelvic pain, 45% with adenomyosis had a previous bilateral tubal ligation compared to 15% without adenomyosis. It is postulated that increased pressure within the uterine cavity resulting from closure of the tubal openings may explain this finding (15). Prior cesarean section does not appear to be a risk factor for adenomyosis because it was not found to be correlated with development of adenomyosis in one study of 485 cases (18).

Hyperestrogenemia has also been proposed as an initiating factor of adenomyosis (19). The placement of intrauterine isografts of anterior pituitary in mice leads to development of adenomyosis (17). The development of adenomyosis was prevented by oophorectomy but stimulated by estradiol benzoate. It can also be induced in various strains of mice by the prenatal administration of high doses of diethylstilbestrol (DES) (20). Adenomyosis can also be produced by the postnatal administration of high doses of estrogen and progesterone or progesterone alone (21). It appears that high levels of prolactin, estrogen, and progesterone are conducive to the development of the adenomyosis.

Another possible etiology of adenomyosis is an arrest of müllerian cells in the myometrium and the later development into endometrial glands and stroma.

Adenomyosis does not appear to be due to invasion of the uterine serosa by intrapelvic endometriosis. Endometriosis is present in only 6% to 20% of all women with an adenomyotic uterus. Adenomyosis and endometriosis probably are entirely distinct disorders (12).

PATHOLOGY

Adenomyosis is the presence of endometrial glands and stroma deep within the myometrium. Histopathologic criteria for diagnosis range from the presence of glands and stroma at greater than one high-power field from the endometrial surface to as deep as two low-power fields. Most pathologists believe that the ectopic glands and stroma of adenomyosis should be located at least 2 to 3 mm below the endometrial surface (12). Adenomyosis is characterized by the presence of a diffusely enlarged uterus caused by the benign invasion of the myometrium by endometrial glands and stroma. This ectopic tissue is associated with hypertrophy and hyperplasia of the myometrium. The myometrial fibers surrounding the foci of ectopic endometrium display grossly visible whorls that are less organized than those with leiomyomata.

The uterus is enlarged in 60% to 80% of cases. It rarely exceeds that of 12 weeks' gestation. The uterus is diffusely boggy to palpation or it may have a nodular consistency, reminiscent of multiple small intramural fibroids. The color suggests hyperemia or congestion. When cut open the myometrium will bulge outward, displaying a granular or trabeculated appearance. The posterior wall of the uterus is involved to a greater degree by the adenomyotic process, and consequently it is thicker in these uteri.

Microscopically, the glands of adenomyosis are lined by cells similar to those of the basalis layer of normal endometrium (12). Frequently, a continuity may be noted between the basalis layer and adenomyotic foci. Smooth muscle fibers surround the areas of ectopic endometrium. The presence of blood or hemosiderin within the ectopic glandular lumen is rare.

The adenomyotic foci may be diffusely distributed throughout the myometrium or can be well-localized, leading to the formation of adenomyomas (12). Adenomyoma is a nodule of hypertrophic myometrium and ectopic endometrium. Adenomyomas may be confused with intramural leiomyomas, although they are darker in color and not quite as firm. On surgical removal it is evident that there is no plane of dissection as in myomas. Adenomyomas may present as a polypoid mass within the endometrial cavity and have been known to undergo malignant transformations (22). These nodules can become cystic, lined by endometrial tissue, with subsequent ectopic pregnancy implantation or spontaneous rupture (23,24).

Ectopic endometrial glands and stroma appear to respond to cyclic estrogen and progesterone stimuli, depending upon the location of the glands in the myometrium. The ectopic sites closest to the basal area have the smallest response to gonadal steroids (16). For example, in a series of 151 cases of cesarean hysterectomy, 17% of which had adenomyosis, two histological patterns were noted (23). Minimal decidualization similar to that of basal endometrium was noted in superficial foci at a depth of one or two low-power fields. Significant decidualization was found in the deep foci of adenomyosis.

Adenomyosis has been noted in association with endometrial carcinoma in 19% of cases and with endometrial hyperplasia in 20% of cases. A 17% incidence of adenomyosis was found in cases with neither of the above two conditions (25). Malignant transformation of an adenomyoma is rare. Adenocarcinoma in adenomyosis does not suggest a more ominous prognosis (16).

SYMPTOMS AND HISTORY

Although the usual profile of a patient with adenomyosis is a middle-aged, parous woman with menorrhagia and dysmenorrhea, the presence of associated pelvic pathology in 60% to 80% of cases makes accurate diagnosis based only on symptoms and history very difficult. The classic description of abnormal uterine bleeding associated with dysmenorrhea in a parous woman who has a regularly enlarged, slightly tender uterus is not specific to adenomyosis. In patients with these signs and symptoms, the diagnosis is confirmed histologically in only 20% of cases (16). Forty-eight percent of women diagnosed with adenomyosis are 30 to 39 years of age (13), and 80% to 90% are parous (12).

Not all women with adenomyosis are symptomatic. It has been reported as an incidental finding in 19% to 35% of women undergoing hysterectomy (4,11). Of women preoperatively diagnosed as having adenomyosis, 40% demonstrated other pelvic pathology at surgery (11). In women complaining of menstrual bleeding disorders or pelvic pain, 22% and 24%, respectively, were found to have adenomyosis, frequencies not different from that of incidental adenomyosis (12).

In symptomatic patients in whom the only pelvic pathology is adenomyosis, complaints are of menorrhagia in 40% to 50%, dysmenorrhea in 15% to 30%, and metrorrhagia in 10% to 12% (4–6,8). Both menorrhagia and dysmenorrhea are found in about 20% of patients (5).

Women with adenomyosis have greater amounts of blood loss. The mechanism for the development of menorrhagia in patients with adenomyosis is unclear (12). The uterus may be unable to contract properly during menses, permitting a greater degree of blood loss. The greater endometrial surface that accompanies an enlarged uterus with a cavity distorted by submucous adenomyomas may contribute to the increased blood flow. Direct bleeding from the adenomyotic foci apparently occurs infrequently and probably does not contribute to the hemorrhage (12). Blood loss is reduced by mefemic acid, suggesting that prostaglandin may play a role in the menorrhagia of adenomyosis (26).

Dysmenorrhea probably occurs when the volume of adenomyotic lesions exceeds a certain threwhold percentage of the total uterine volume. It has been noted when the glandular invasion of adenomyosis exceeds 80% or more of the myometrium (27). Dysmenorrhea appears to be the result of tonic stimulation of the entire uterus by adenomyosis.

SIGNS AND EXAMINATION

The physical examination of the woman with adenomyosis who is symptomatic with pelvic pain, dysmenorrhea, and menorrhagia usually shows a symmetrically enlarged, tender uterus less than 14 weeks' size when an exam is performed just prior to or during menses (12). The uterus is enlarged in 60% to 80% of cases, but it rarely exceeds a size of 12 weeks' gestation. The uterus is diffusely boggy to palpation or it may have a nodular consistency, reminiscent of multiple small intramural fibroids. Unfortunately, these findings are not consistently present or specific to adenomyosis. Only 2% to 26% of cases are diagnosed preoperatively (3,4,6,8,10), and the preoperative diagnosis of adenomyosis is confirmed only 48% of the time at hysterectomy (11). When adenomyosis is the diagnosis preoperatively the pelvis is found to be normal in 12% and demonstrates other pathology in 40% of women.

The most common variant of adenomyosis is diffuse involvement of the anterior and posterior walls, with the posterior aspect of the uterus involved more often. Essential adenomyosis is diagnosed most consistently when uterine enlargement is noted during the menstrual period (28). Uterine leiomyoma alone and adenomyosis with associated uterine leiomyoma may cause the same tender enlargement. Because the definitive treatment for adenomyosis is hysterectomy, whereas leiomyoma can be treated with myomectomy, an exact preoperative distinction between these conditions is important (29). However, examination alone does not differentiate between adenomyosis and leiomyomas, so further investigations are required.

DIAGNOSTIC STUDIES

Hysterosalpingography

On hysterosalpingography (HSG) some contrast material may fill short, spicule-like structures extending perpendicularly from the borders of the uterine cavity 1 to 4 mm deep in patients with adenomyosis (30). Another radiologic picture is localized contrast material in the myometrium appearing as small rounded ponds with an almost honeycombed appearance. The areas seem to be connected with the uterine cavity by a small channel, but the latter cannot always be seen. Areas of adenomyosis that do not communicate with the endometrial surface will not be revealed on HSG. Large localized adenomyomas can distort and enlarge the cavity, causing a radiographic shadow indistinguishable from a submucous myoma. Adenomyosis can be differentiated from salpingitis isthmica nodosa because the latter is confined more or less to the isthmic part of the tube. Vascular intravasation initially can resemble adenomyosis, but the subsequent outlines of the ovarian and uterine vessels or lymph nodes become evident on later films (16).

Transvaginal Sonography

Sonography cannot always distinguish between adenomyosis and myomata (16). On transvaginal sonography (TVS), adenomyoma is diagnosed as a disharmonious, circumscribed area in the myometrium with indistinct margins and anechoic lacunae of various diameters. On TVS a leiomyoma is diagnosed when a nodular formation with well-defined margins, heterogeneous structure, and variable echogenicity is detected in the myometrium. Using these criteria for distinguishing adenomyoma and lieomyoma, TVS has a sensitivity of 87%, a specificity of 98%, and a negative predictive value of 99% (31).

In an effort to distinguish adenomyosis from leiomyoma, a retrospective study on 80 patients was performed. Sonographically a leiomyoma was characterized by focal or globular uterine enlargement with abnormal echo texture and contour, as well as nonvisualization or displacement of the central cavity complex. The most suggestive sonographic findings of adenomyosis was generalized uterine enlargement with conservation of normal myometrial architecture. In 10 of 11 cases where myomata and adenomyosis were combined, the sonographic diagnosis was myomata, suggesting that in the presence of myomata, adenomyosis cannot be identified. In this study, ultrasound had a sensitivity of only 63%, with a specificity of 97% and a positive predictive value of 71% (28).

In general, patients who have adenomyosis show ultrasound patterns of an enlarged uterus, irregular vascular spaces within the myometrium, and an acoustically enlarged posterior wall. All three ultrasonic characteristics are useful in making the preoperative diagnosis of this entity (16). On TVS a thick anechoic posterior uterine wall with cystic eyelets in the myometrium also suggests adenomyosis (32).

Magnetic Resonance Imaging

Magnetic resonance imaging (MRI) scans of normal uteri show three distinct zones: a central high-intensity zone; a junctional, low-intensity band; and a peripheral, medium-intensity area. Whereas the endometrium (basalis and functionalis) corresponds to a high-intensity zone, the myometrium correlates best with areas of low and medium signal intensity (16).

The use of MRI for the preoperative diagnosis of adenomyosis provides excellent soft tissue contrast, is minimally invasive, and avoids ionizing radiation (16). On T2-weighted images, diffuse adenomyosis distorts normal zonal anatomy of the uterus, causing enlargement of the functional zone, seen as a wide band with low signal intensity adjacent to the endometrium. The endometrium maintains its normal, high-intensity signal. The endometrium also shows high-intensity signals and adenomatous signs in the myometrium. Adenomyosis has irregular and indistinct margins because of its more invasive nature compared to leiomyomata, which have well-encapsulated margins (16).

A prospective study of MRI conducted on 93 women with a mean age of 41 years and enlarged uteri that were clinically suspect for leiomyoma or adenomyosis showed an accurate diagnosis in 92 women. Surgery was performed within 2 weeks of MRI for an enlarged uterus, hypermenorrhea and dysmenorrhea (42%), pressure or pain consistent with a mass lesion (23%), or miscellaneous indications (35%). All 71 cases of leiomyoma, 15 of 16 cases of adenomyosis, and all six cases of simultaneous involvement of both conditions were correctly diagnosed by MRI. On T2-weighted images, all leiomyomas were characteristically well-circumscribed masses, sharply demarcated from surrounding myometrium, although their signal intensity varied from homogeneously low to homogeneously high. In contrast to leiomyomas, adenomyosis appeared as a diffuse, ill-defined lesion extending adjacent to the endometrium. T2-weighted images showed a relatively homogeneous low-intensity lesion embedded with sparse tiny high-intensity spots (32). In one case of nodular adenomyosis MRI could not distinguish this from a degenerating myoma.

The histopathologic explanation for the low signal intensity of adenomyosis might be attributable to less vascularity and lack of edema in the hypertrophic muscle, or the entire lesion might be considered as clusters of miniature low-intensity bands surrounding numerous tiny foci of endometrial tissue. High-intensity spots seen within the lesion are hemorrhagic areas and nonbleeding ectopic tissue, both of which represent exactly the characteristics of adenomyosis on gross pathologic and microscopic studies. Shaggy or irregular interface between endometrium and adenomyosis reflects the histopathologic nature of the lesion in which endometrial islands result from downward growth of the endometrium (32).

In another study assessing the capability of MRI to differentiate adenomyosis and leiomyomas, all cases of adenomyosis were diagnosed correctly and 10 of 12 leiomyomata were diagnosed correctly, but two cases of leiomyomata could not be differentiated from focal adenomyosis. Microscopic foci of adenomyosis were not seen with MRI (33).

Hysteroscopy, Dilatation and Curettage, and Myometrial Biopsy

Dilatation and curettage rarely establishes a diagnosis of adenomyosis. In 8,460 curettage specimens, adenomyosis was diagnosed in only six (34).

Diagnostic hysteroscopy alone is not sufficient for the diagnosis of adenomyosis. A normal-appearing cavity at hysteroscopy does not rule out adenomyosis. One study of 90 patients with menorrhagia showed that 50 had normal-appearing cavities, 27 had gross endometrial polyps, and 13 had submucous myomas. Then at the time of the hysteroscopy a 1.5- to 3-cm biopsy specimen was obtained with a 5-mm loop electrode, mostly from the posterior wall near the fundus using 70 watts of cutting current. Of the 50 women with normal-appearing cavities hysteroscopically, 66% had significant adenomyosis (greater than 1-mm depth). In this study the depth of the adenomyosis correlated with the severity of the menorrhagia (35).

At times on hysteroscopic examination of the uterine cavity, small diverticula can be detected when there is a connection between the ectopic sites of adenomyosis in the endometrial cavity. However, hysteroscopic myometrial biopsy is required in order to confirm the diagnosis of adenomyosis. In symptomatic patients with a normal-appearing endometrial cavity, a myometrial biopsy may be helpful at the time of hysteroscopy (36).

Myometrial biopsies have also been performed during laparoscopy and during vaginal ultrasonography. Prevention of myometrial bleeding is achieved by prophylactic injection of vasopressin into the biopsy cannula (37). The sensitivity of a single myometrial sample for diagnosing adenomyosis uteri ranges from 8% to 19%. The specificity is 100%. Performing 10 or more biopsies from the uterus results in a sensitivity of 40% to 70%, depending on the grade of adenomyosis. Biopsy specimens are 0.9 to 2.0 mm in diameter and 1.7 cm in length. This type of core myometrial biopsy has a relatively low sensitivity in the diagnosis of adenomyosis (38).

DIFFERENTIAL DIAGNOSES

The classic patient with adenomyosis is a multiparous woman in her late forties with menorrhagia and dysmenorrhea, who on physical examination has a slightly enlarged symmetric and somewhat tender uterus. Her past surgical history may include a previous dilatation and curettage or a tubal ligation. However, these signs and symptoms may also indicate chronic endometritis, leiomyomatous uterus, intracavitary lesions including uterine polyps, and endometrial cancer. Other carcinomas of the uterus, including adenocarcinoma and leiomyosarcoma, must also be included in the differential. Although many of these differential diagnoses can be made with dilatation and curettage and diagnostic hysteroscopy, these techniques are not sensitive or specific enough for the diagnosis of adenomyosis. Myometrial biopsy whether by core specimen or by hysteroscopic loop excision (36,38) has a 100% specificity, but sensitivity of the core specimen is low and the sensitivity of the myometrial loop resection is not known. Transvaginal sonography has moderate sensitivity and specificity, but is unable to distinguish accurately between leiomyoma and adenomyosis. MRI demonstrated high sensitivity and specificity. Because dysmenorrhea occurs when the glandular invasion exceeds 80% of the myometrium (30), MRI in patients with severe dysmenorrhea and menorrhagia may be highly accurate in diagnosing adenomyosis.

MANAGEMENT AND TREATMENT
Medical Treatment

Adenomyotic foci contain estrogen and progesterone receptors and undergo decidualization under the influence of progesterone (36,39,40). The hormonal responsiveness of this disease suggests that dysmenorrhea and menorrhagia due to adenomyosis will not respond to treatment with either progestational or combined estrogen and progestin medications. In fact, such medications may make the symptoms more apparent. Exacerbation of symptoms of adenomyosis including growth and decidualization after administration of estrogen–progestin has been reported (41).

Gonadotropin suppression with gonadotropin-releasing hormone (GnRH) agonists may give temporary relief of symptoms, as exemplified by the following published cases. The patient was a 34-year-old nulligravida with infertility, menorrhagia, and severe dysmenorrhea, with a soft and

markedly enlarged posterior uterine wall. Multiple biopsy specimens demonstrated deep adenomyosis. Uterine volume at initiation of therapy was 440 cm^3 (consistent with 10 weeks' size uterus). Treatment consisted of daily 1-mg subcutaneous injections of leuprolide acetate (Lupron, Abbott Laboratories, North Chicago, IL) for 6 months. After 4 months of treatment, ultrasound revealed a 65% reduction of uterine volume to 140 cm^3, which was maintained through the remaining 2 months of therapy. Both menorrhagia and dysmenorrhea recurred 6 months post therapy, gradually worsening to pretreatment severity, and the uterus returned to its originally determined volume of 420 cm (2,38). In another reported case following an adenomyomectomy a 19-year-old woman was treated with GnRH agonist. Several courses of therapy were required because during the intervals without medication, cyclic menstrual pain and uterine enlargement returned. Shortly after her last course of treatment the patient conceived without having had an intervening menses (42). In another case a wedge-shaped biopsy of the uterine fundus was performed at laparotomy and a subsequent 6 month course of GnRH agonists was given. The patient became pregnant 4 months after completing therapy (43). Although medical therapy with GnRH agonists does not provide a definitive cure for adenomyosis, the judicious application of medical intervention in conjunction with conservative operations such as wedge resection of myometrial areas suspicious for adenomyosis may improve the opportunity for childbearing.

Because estrogen synthesis is higher in adenomatous tissue than in normal myometrium and endometrium, danocrine can be used to suppress symptoms of adenomyosis. Danocrine blocks aromatase activity in adenomyosis in cell cultures. This is similar to the activity of danocrine in inhibiting steroidogenesis in the gonads (24). Danocrine also has an inhibitory effect on the autoimmunologic response associated with adenomyosis (44).

RU 486 suppresses the development of adenomyosis in mice (24), suggesting that it may have a role to play in the suppression of symptoms resulting from adenomyosis.

Surgical Therapy for Adenomyosis

There may be a role for conservative surgical treatment with endometrial ablation or resection in some patients with adenomyosis. Adenomyosis penetrating to a depth of 3 mm may be adequately treated with such uterine-preserving therapies, but more deeply penetrating disease may be left under a scar and may cause recurrent bleeding and pain. Furthermore, if the glands become malignant, the scar could delay bleeding and the diagnosis of endometrial cancer. Because uterine-preserving therapies such as endometrial resection and endometrial ablation will likely fail in patients with adenomyotic invasion deeper than 3 to 5 mm, MRI diagnosis of adenomyosis may prevent an inappropriate therapeutic intervention in these patients (32,36).

However, the principal method of diagnosis and therapy of adenomyosis is still hysterectomy (12). Conservative surgical interventions (49,50) combined with medical treatment, as illustrated in the previously described case reports, have been applied in specific instances to improve chances for fertility.

KEY POINTS

Most Important Questions to Ask

- Do you bleed heavily or excessively with menses? How many pads do you use? (Pad count)
- Do you have pain? If so, where does it hurt and when? (Central and at the time of periods)
- Have you been pregnant? How many children have you delivered?
- Have you had a previous tubal ligation?
- Have you had a previous dilatation and curettage?
- What are your plans regarding future fertility?

Most Important Physical Examination Findings

- Enlarged uterus especially at time of menses
- Uterine tenderness at time of menses

Most Important Diagnostic Studies

- MRI is most accurate in specificity and sensitivity, but cost inhibits its use.
- Ultrasound is of value but does not differentiate well between adenomyosis and leiomyoma.
- Hysteroscopy is not helpful.
- D&C is not helpful.
- Hysteroscopic endometrial biopsy is specific, but sensitivity is not known.

Treatments

- Hysterectomy is therapeutic and diagnostic.
- Presacral neurectomy will reduce pain.
- Endometrial ablation and endometrial resection will treat superficial adenomyosis to 3 mm.
- GnRH agonists and danazol can reduce symptoms of bleeding and pain.

REFERENCES

1. Rokitansky K. Ueber uterus-neubildung. *Z Gesellshaft Wien* 1860;16:577.
2. Cullen TS. *Adenomyoma of the uterus.* Philadelphia: WB Saunders, 1908.
3. Benson RC, Sneeden VD. Adenomyosis: a reappraisal of symptomatology. *Am J Obstet Gynecol* 1958;76:1044.
4. Bird CC, McElin TW, Manalo-Estrella P. The elusive adenomyosis of the uterus revisited. *Am J Obstet Gynecol* 1972;112:582–593.
5. Israel SL, Woutersz T. Adenomyosis a neglected diagnosis. *Obstet Gynecol* 1959;13:168.
6. Mathur BBL, Shah RS, Bhende YM. Adenomyosis uteri: a pathologic study of 290 cases. *Am J Obstet Gynecol* 1962;84:1820.
7. Molitor JJ. Adenomyosis: a clinical and pathologic appraisal. *Am J Obstet Gynecol* 1971;110:275.
8. Nikkanen V, Punnonen R. Clinical significance of adenomyosis. *Ann Chir Gynaecol* 1980;69:278.
9. Owolabi TO, Strickler RC. Adenomyosis: a neglected diagnosis. *Obstet Gynecol* 1977;50:424.
10. Lewinski H, Emge LA. The elusive adenomyosis of the uterus. *Am J Obstet Gynecol* 1962;83:1541–1563.
11. Lee NC, Dicker RC, Reuben GL. Confirmation of the preoperative diagnosis for hysterectomy. *Am J Obstet Gynecol* 1984;150:283.
12. Azziz R. Adenomyosis: current perspectives. *Obstet Gynecol Clin North Am* 1989;16:221–235.
13. Thompson JR, Davion RJ. Adenomyosis of the uterus: an enigma. *J Natl Med Assoc* 1986;78:305–307.
14. Marcus CC. Relationship of adenomyosis uteri to endometrial hyperplasia and endometrial carcinoma. *Am J Obstet Gynecol* 1961;82:408.
15. Siegler AM, Camilien L. Adenomyosis. *J Reprod Med* 1994;39:841–853.
16. Mori T, Nagasawa H. Mechanisms of a development of prolactin-induced adenomyosis in mice. *Acta Anat* 1983;116:46.
17. Sahin AA, Silva EG, Landon G. Endometrial tissue in myometrial vessels not associated with menstruation. *Int J Gynecol Pathol* 1989;8:139–146.
18. Harris JW, Daniell JF, Baxter JW. Prior cesarean section: a risk factor for adenomyosis? *J Reprod Med* 1985;30:173–175.
19. Jefcoate TNA, Potter AL. Endometriosis as a manifestation of ovarian dysfunction. *Br J Obstet Gynaecol* 1934;41:684.
20. Walker BE. Uterine tumors in old female mice exposed prenatally to diethylstilbestrol. *J Natl Cancer Inst* 1983;70:477.
21. Ostrander PL, Mills KT, Bern HA. Long-term responses of the musculoskeletal uterus to neonatal diethylstilbestrol treatment and to later sex hormone exposure. *J Natl Cancer Inst* 1985;74:121.
22. Young RH, Treger T, Scully RE. Atypical polypoid adenomyoma of the uterus: a report of 27 cases. *Am J Clin Pathol* 1986;86:139.
23. Azziz R. Adenomyosis in pregnancy: a review. *J Reprod Med* 1986;31:224.
24. Keating S, Quendille NF, Korn GW. Ruptured adenomyotic cyst of the uterus: a case report. *Arch Gynecol* 1986;237:169.
25. Ingrid SM. The relation of adenomyosis to coexistent endometrial carcinoma and endometrial hyperplasia. *Obstet Gynecol* 1976;48:68–72.
26. Fraser IS, McCarron G, Markam R. Measured menstrual blood loss in woman with menorrhagia associated with pelvic disease or coagulation disorder. *Obstet Gynecol* 1986;69:630–640.
27. Nishida M. Relationship between onset of dysmenorrhea and histologic findings in adenomyosis. *Am J Obstet Gynecol* 1991;165:229–232.
28. Siedler D, Laing FC, Jeffrey RB Jr. Uterine adenomyosis: a difficult sonographic diagnosis. *J Ultrasound Med* 1987;6:345–349.
29. Togashi K, Ozasa H, Konishi I. Enlarged uterus: differentiation between adenomyosis and leiomyoma with MR imaging. *Radiology* 1988;166:111–114.
30. Hunt RB, Siegler AM. *Hysterosalpingography: techniques and interpretation.* Chicago: Year Book Medical publishers, 1990:75.
31. Fedelle L, Bianchi S, Dorta M. Transvaginal ultrasonography in

the differential diagnosis of adenomyoma versus leiomyoma. *Am J Obstet Gynecol* 1992;167:603–606.

32. Bohlman Me, Ensor RE, Saunders RC. Sonographic findings in adenomyosis of the uterus. *Am J Roentgenol* 1987;148:765–766.

33. Mark AS, Hricak H, Heinrich LW. Adenomyosis and leiomyoma: differential diagnosis with MR imaging. *Radiology* 1987; 168:527–529.

34. Israel SL, Woutersz TB. Adenomyosis—a neglected diagnosis. *Obstet Gynecol* 1959;14:168–173.

35. McCausland AM. Hysteroscopic myometrial biopsy: its use in diagnosing adenomyosis and its clinical applications. *Am J Obstet Gynecol* 1992;166:1619–1628.

36. Mathur BBL, Shah BS, Bhende YM. Adenomyosis uteri: a pathological study of 290 cases. *Am J Obstet Gynecol* 1962;84: 1820–1828.

37. Popp LW, Schwiederessen JP, Gaetje R. Myometrial biopsy in the diagnosis of adenomyosis uteri. *Am J Obstet Gynecol* 1993;169: 546–548.

38. Grow DR, Filer RB. Treatment of adenomyosis with long-term GnRH analogues: a case report. *Obstet Gynecol* 1991;78:538–539.

39. van der Walt LA, san Fillipo JS, Siegel JC, et al. Estrogen and progestin receptors in human uterus: reference ranges of clinical conditions. *Clin Physiol Biochem* 1986;4:217–218.

40. Casper BJ. Progestational changes in areas of adenomyosis. *Obstet Gynecol* 1964;24:111–115.

41. Falk RJ, Mullin BR. Exacerbation of adenomyosis symptomatology by estrogen–progestin therapy: a case report and histopathological observation. *Int J Fertil* 1989;34:386–389.

42. Nelson JR, Corson SL. Long-term management of adenomyosis with gonadotropin releasing hormone agonist: a case report. *Fertil Steril* 1993;39:441–443.

43. Hirata JD, Moghissi KS, Ginsburg KA. Pregnancy after medical therapy of adenomyosis with gonadotropin releasing hormone agonist. *Fertil Steril* 1993;59:444–445.

44. Ota H, Maki M, Shidara Y. Effects of danazol at the immunological level in patients with adenomyosis with special reference to autoantibodies: a multicenter cooperative study. *Am J Obstet Gynecol* 1971;110:275–284.

45. Azziz R. Adenomyosis: current perspectives. *Obstet Gynecol Clin North Am* 1989;16:221–235.

8

ADHESIONS

C. PAUL PERRY
FRED M. HOWARD

KEY TERMS AND DEFINITIONS

Adhesion: A fibrous tissue by which anatomic structures abnormally adhere to one another.

Nociceptors: A nerve receptor for pain.

Pain mapping: The tactile stimulation of internal structures to elicit a response during laparoscopy under conscious sedation.

INTRODUCTION

Adhesions are well-accepted as causes of intestinal obstruction (1,2) and infertility (3). However, their role as a cause of chronic pelvic pain (CPP) is controversial. Intraabdominal and pelvic adhesions are found at laparoscopy in about 25% of women with CPP (4). This is a higher incidence than generally reported in women without CPP (25% versus 17%, from combined series of 1,318 and 1,103 patients, respectively) (4), suggesting an association between adhesions and CPP. The association from these observational studies is not overly strong, nor does association equate with causation. This association is thought to be coincidental by some investigators; that is, they believe that adhesions do not cause CPP. For example, Rapkin (5) found that women with infertility were as likely to have adhesions as were women with CPP (39% versus 26%, respectively; $p = 0.06$). She also found no difference in the sites or density of adhesions between these two groups of patients. She concluded that "the results of this study seriously question the role of pelvic adhesions as a common cause of pelvic pain." If adhesions cause CPP, then adhesiolysis might be expected to relieve pain. However, the only randomized trial of adhesiolysis failed to show any significant improvement in pain symptoms after lysis of adhesions by laparotomy, compared to a control group that did not undergo adhesiolysis (Table 8.1) (6). Only when a subgroup analysis of the 15 women with severe, stage IV adhesions was done was there any detectable improvement in pain that could be attributed to adhesiolysis. However, a number of observational studies have shown

TABLE 8.1. RESULTS OF A RANDOMIZED TRIAL OF ADHESIOLYSIS VERSUS OBSERVATION IN 48 WOMEN WITH CHRONIC PELVIC PAIN WHO WERE DIAGNOSED WITH ABDOMINOPELVIC ADHESIONS BY LAPAROSCOPY

Pain assessment	Adhesiolysis	Observation
Mean change in McGill score	–5.7	–5.5
Number with a change in McGill score of ≥5 points	11	10
Number with subjective improvement of pain	10	9
Number with less disturbance of daily activities	12	14

Note: In the treatment group, adhesiolysis was done by laparotomy. Pain assessments were done at about 11 months after randomization in both groups. From Peters AAW, Trimbos-Kemper GCM, Admiral C, et al. A randomized clinical trial on the benefit of adhesiolysis in patients with intraperitoneal adhesions and chronic pelvic pain. *Br J Obstet Gynaecol* 1992;99:59–62, with permission.

significant improvement in pain in women with CPP after adhesiolysis, suggesting that adhesions may contribute to CPP (7–9). Also, some investigators have been able to show a correlation between the location of pain or tenderness and adhesions in women with CPP (10,11). Thus, at the current time the best that can be stated is that these abnormal tissue adherences are thought to produce chronic pain by some investigators, but to be coincidental by others. Possibly a more accurate opinion might be that some adhesions produce pain sometimes, but not all adhesions produce pain all the time. As will be discussed later in this chapter, this is an area where conscious pain mapping may prove to be especially valuable in diagnostic evaluation and treatment.

ETIOLOGY

Adhesion formation is a tissue surface event decided in the first 5 days after injury. Immediately following a peritoneal wound, a cascade of events is unleashed, which ultimately determines whether adhesions develop or an adhesion-free reepithelialization occurs. Coagulation, release of chemical messengers, and fibrin matrix deposition are the initial steps. Macrophages recruit new mesothelial cells onto the surface of the injury. These form small islands, which proliferate into sheets of mesothelial cells thereby reepithelializing the peritoneal surfaces. If two injured surfaces coated with fibrin matrix come into apposition, a band or bridge may result. The two pivotal events of adhesion formation are apposition of damaged surfaces and fibrinolysis. Prevention, therefore, focuses on protective barriers to tissue apposition and acceleration of fibrin degradation.

Unfortunately, surgery reduces fibrinolytic activity in two ways: first, by increasing levels of plasminogen activator inhibitors and, second, by decreasing levels of tissue plasminogen activator. Surgeons should be aware of the potential adhesive complications of their procedures. They should minimize the invasiveness of the procedures by reducing tissue trauma, preventing tissue ischemia, and avoiding exposure to intestinal contents. Care should be taken to not introduce foreign bodies into the surgical site (12).

Appendectomy and gynecologic surgery by laparotomy are the two most common procedures likely to produce adhesions in women. Intestinal obstruction may occur many years following laparotomy. The incidence of obstruction may increase with increasing age because of reduced tissue elasticity (13). Postmortem studies reveal that 67% of all patients develop adhesions postoperatively (14). In a study of 33 patients with bowel obstruction following abdominal hysterectomy, 100% were caused by surgical reperitonealization of the anterior abdominal wall. This results in tension on the suture line and tissue ischemia (15).

SYMPTOMS AND SIGNS

As previously discussed, some authorities believe that adhesions do not produce chronic pelvic pain, based mainly on the observations that (a) many patients have adhesions without complaints of pain (5) and (b) lysis of adhesions by laparotomy has yielded mixed results (6). This has fostered the belief by some that any benefit reported in pain reduction may be placebo effect (16).

However, there appears to be sufficient evidence to suggest that adhesions have at least a contributory role in the etiology of pain in at least some women with CPP (7–11). Indirect, supportive evidence that adhesions might be a source of pain comes from the demonstration that adhesions contain nerve fibers, suggesting that pain might originate not just in the parietal peritoneum, but also in the adhesions themselves (17). This observation is consistent with the suggestion by Kresch et al. (11) that the adhesions most likely to be symptomatic are those under tension or those restricting normal organ mobility, presumably resulting in stretching that stimulates the nociceptors in the adhesions or peritoneum. However, in the small series of patients in whom the study of nerve fibers in adhesions was performed, there was no difference in the prevalence of nerve fibers in adhesions of patients with CPP compared to those without pain (17).

Adhesions are generally believed to cause pelvic pain that is exacerbated by sudden movements, intercourse, or certain physical activities. Often the pain is consistent in its location (10,11), although over time the area of involvement may expand. A history of one of the classic causes of adhesions—pelvic inflammatory disease, endometriosis, perforated appendix, prior abdominopelvic surgery, or inflammatory bowel disease—makes this a more likely diagnosis. At least one of these historic factors is present in 50% of women with adhesions (18). Yet about one-half of women with adhesions have no historic reason for them. Also, one-fourth of women with adhesions have no historic risk factors nor any physical findings (such as cervical, uterine, or adnexal tenderness, adnexal mass, or uterine immobility) that suggest the presence of adhesions.

Although it is always important to try to differentiate musculoskeletal from visceral components in women with chronic pelvic pain, it is especially important (and difficult) in patients with adhesions, because of the characteristics of pain that may be associated with adhesions. Piriformis, rectus abdominis, quadratus lumborum, and psoas muscles are frequent sources of pain with either spasms or trigger points. At the time of physical examination these muscle groups should be routinely checked for tenderness, spasm, and trigger points in every chronic pelvic pain patient.

DIAGNOSIS

Although nonsurgical methods such as computerized tomography, magnetic resonance imaging, or ultrasound may suggest the presence of adhesions, presently the only definitive way to diagnose them is by surgical visualization. Laparoscopy, not laparotomy, is the gold standard for diagnosing pelvic adhesive disease.

It is our opinion that patients suspected of having pain associated with adhesive disease should undergo pain mapping whenever possible. This could determine not only the presence of adhesions but also whether they are likely to be responsible for the pain (Chapter 5). Unfortunately, the very patients who might benefit from conscious pain mapping may be those with multiple abdominal incisions and an increased risk for puncture injuries of small or large bowel. Office laparoscopic pain mapping may not be advisable in these patients, and an operating room suite is the more appropriate setting.

At the time of diagnostic laparoscopy or pain mapping, it is crucial that the adhesions be fully described in the operative note. This may be important not just in documentation, but also in the future care of the patient. Many experts believe that adhesions should also be scored or classified. Probably the most commonly used system in published articles on adhesions is the American Fertility Society classification (Table 8.2). This classification was designed for use in the evaluation, treatment, and prognosis of infertility, not for pain.

Because of this, others have proposed a system that is based more on the severity of the adhesions, such as: 0, no adhesions; 1, filmy adhesions that are easily separated with blunt dissection or traction; 2, dense or vascular adhesions; and 3, dense and vascular. In this type of system, dense refers to adhesions that are opaque and vascular to adhesions that bleed significantly on severing. A numerical score is obtained by totaling the severity scores for each area of adhesions—for example, right ovary, left ovary, left tube, right tube, omentum, large bowel, small bowel, pelvic sidewalls, cul-de-sac, and abdominal wall (7).

Finally, one other example of a scoring system for adhesions is the one used by Peters et al. (6) in their study of adhesiolysis, which "stages" the severity of adhesive disease (Table 8.3). This appears clinically to be a particularly useful staging system for adhesive disease. Although there is a fair degree of subjectivity in the classification, it allows a simple and rapid summary of the severity of the patient's adhesions.

TREATMENT

Laparoscopy is not only the gold standard for the diagnosis of adhesion, but in the hands of a skilled laparoscopic sur-

geon is also the preferred method of treatment. Some of the advantages of laparoscopic adhesiolysis over laparotomy are listed in Table 8.4.

Because many patients undergoing laparoscopy for treatment of adhesions have histories of prior abdominopelvic surgery, the risk of periumbilical bowel or omental adhesions is significant (20). Because of this, many experts recommend open laparoscopy in such cases. This may not necessarily prevent injury to any bowel adherent at the umbilicus, however (21,22). Because of this we recommend a left-upper-quadrant Verress needle and 5-mm trocar placement insertion. This allows insertion of the umbilical trocar under direct vision. Occasion-

TABLE 8.3. A STAGING SYSTEM FOR ABDOMINOPELVIC ADHESIONS

Stage I: Some filmy adhesions, not vascularized. Easy to release during laparoscopy.
Stage II: Extensive, nonvascularized, filmy adhesions involving one or more intraabdominal organs (uterus, adnexa, small bowel, colon, bladder) or the mesentery, mesocolon, or omentum.
Stage III: Numerous, partly vascularized adhesions involving one or more intraperitoneal organs, possibly leading to impairment of the function of these organs.
Stage IV: As for stage III, but with dense vascularized adhesions involving the serosa of the small bowel or colon fixed to the outer peritoneum.

From Peters AAW, Trimbos-Kemper GCM, Admiral C, et al. A randomized clinical trial on the benefit of adhesiolysis in patients with intraperitoneal adhesions and chronic pelvic pain. *Br J Obstet Gynecol* 1991;165:278–283, with permission.

TABLE 8.2. THE CLASSIFICATION SYSTEM PROPOSED BY THE AMERICAN FERTILITY SOCIETY FOR ADNEXAL ADHESIONS (29)

Adhesions	<1/3 Enclosure	1/3–2/3 Enclosure	>2/3 Enclosure
Ovary			
R Filmy	1	2	4
R Dense	4	8	16
L Filmy	1	2	4
L Dense	4	8	16
Tube			
R Filmy	1	2	4
R Dense	4[a]	8[a]	16
L Filmy	1	2	4
L Dense	4[a]	8[a]	16

Note: This system allows assignment of a numerical score and classification of adhesive disease as minimal (0–5), mild (6–10), moderate (11–20), or severe (21–32) adhesive disease.
[a]If the fimbriated end of the fallopian tube is completely enclosed, change the point assignment to 16. From the American Fertility Society. The American Fertility Socity classifications of adnexal adhesions, distal tubal occlusion, tubal occlusion secondary to tubal ligation, tubal pregnancies, Mullerian anomalies, and intrauterine adhesions. *Fertil Steril* 1988;49:944–55, with permission.

TABLE 8.4. ADVANTAGES OF ADHESIOLYSIS VIA LAPAROSCOPY RATHER THAN LAPAROTOMY (30)

1. Videotape or photographic records of the findings and procedure can be made easily.
2. Diagnostic and operative procedures can be combined during the same anesthetic.
3. Visualization of the upper abdomen and cul-de-sac is better.
4. Incision time is decreased, both opening and closing.
5. The surgical field is less bloody due to the intraabdominal pressure generated by the pneumoperitoneum.
6. Intraoperative blood loss is decreased due to enhanced visualization with the magnification by the optics and due the pneumoperitoneum.
7. There may be less tissue trauma and less *de novo* adhesion formation.
8. Overall, fewer instruments are needed.
9. Cosmetic results are better.
10. Morbidity is lower due to the smaller incisions.
11. Postoperative recovery is faster.
12. Cost is lower due to the faster postoperative recovery, which allows outpatient surgery in most cases.

From Gomel V, Urman B, Gurgan T. Pathophysiology of adhesion formation and strategies for prevention. *J Reprod Med* 1996;41:35–41, with permission.

ally, adhesions will have to be cleared from the anterior abdominal wall or alternate insertion sites selected before other trocars can be inserted. Additionally, it is possible to safely perform direct trocar insertion at the left upper quadrant and carry out the surgical procedure without placing an umbilical trocar (24).

Adhesiolysis may be accomplished with laser, electrocautery, or sharp scissors dissection. Preoperative bowel preparation is recommended for all patients undergoing this procedure. Gentle traction on the bowel is necessary to prevent unintentional enterotomy. Hemostasis should be meticulous with bipolar desiccation. One of the authors (C.P.P.) strongly prefers the Nd:YAG contact tip laser (SLT, Malvern, PA) through the operating channel of the laparoscope due to its superior hemostasis and precision by line-of-site dissection. For dense bowel adhesions, both of us prefer to use sharp scissors dissection due to the absence of potential thermal injury. If extensive removal of the parietal peritoneum is necessary, the patient should be observed intraoperatively for subcutaneous emphysema. Retroperitoneal dissection of the pneumoperitoneum might produce compromise of the airway or impaired chest wall excursion postoperatively.

Bowel injuries should be immediately repaired. This can be safely performed laparoscopically by surgeons experienced in laparoscopic suturing and stapling techniques. Broad-spectrum antibiotic coverage and conservative diet progression is necessary. Nasogastric suction is no longer considered mandatory.

After surgical adhesiolysis, strategies for preventing recurrence should be employed. Although no completely effective method is currently available, consideration may be given to placing barriers in localized areas of tissue injury. Oxidized regenerated cellulose (Interceed, Johnson & Johnson Medical Inc., Arlington, TX), Gore-tex surgical membrane (W. L. Gore Co., Flagstaff, AZ), and hyaluronic acid–methylcellulose (Seprafilm, Genzyme Corp., Cambridge, MA) are currently available. Crystalloid fluid such as Ringer's solution is easy to use laparoscopically, but its effectiveness is limited by rapid absorption. Colloid fluid such as Dextran 70 can cause rapid fluid shifts and anaphylactic reactions.

Pharmaceutical agents have produced conflicting results. Corticosteroids, nonsteroidal antiinflammatories, plasminogen activators, and calcium channel blockers have been evaluated. To date, no adjuvant has proven uniformly effective (25). Adhesions will likely remain a cause for some cases of chronic pelvic pain until abnormal healing is conquered. Meanwhile, good surgical technique is required to minimize *de novo* and recurrent adhesive disease. Prevention of injured tissue apposition and promotion of fibrinolysis will remain fruitful areas of future investigations.

Uncontrolled, observational studies show that laparoscopic lysis of adhesions is beneficial in reducing the pain level in 60% to 90% of patients with chronic pelvic pain

(4,26). However, the mere presence of adhesions does not correlate with the perception or level of pain. Current pain models incorporating both physical and psychological factors are adequate to explain most of these discrepancies (7).

Pain mapping under conscious sedation may better select those patients who will benefit most from adhesiolysis. Clinical studies are currently underway to establish the role of duplicating pain by touching or tugging on adhesions during conscious laparoscopy (27,28). Until means that are more accurate are available, we are dependent upon traditional and less precise methods of patient selection. It seems best to avoid surgery if possible due to the recurrence of adhesions after lysis in up to 51% of patients regardless of what techniques are used (29,30).

Also, if other contributors to pain are discovered, particularly musculoskeletal disorders, then physical therapy, trigger point injections, and nonsteroidal antiinflammatories should be tried before a surgical procedure is undertaken. Many patients will have a mixed visceral and somatic pelvic pain complex and may benefit most from multidisciplinary treatment in a pain center. Such treatment should be continued until satisfactory relief is obtained or until incomplete symptomatic relief requires surgical intervention.

KEY POINTS

Differential Diagnosis

- Rule out musculoskeletal pain.
- Rule out trigger point formation.
- Rule out irritable bowel syndrome.

Most Important Questions to Ask

- Is there a history of previous surgery, pelvic inflammatory disease, inflammatory bowel disease, or endometriosis?
- Does the pain vary with movement or activity level?
- Is the pain sharp and intermittent or dull and constant?
- Does the pain vary with menstrual cycle?
- Is deep dyspareunia present?

Most Important Physical Examination Findings

- No trigger points or their elimination by local anesthetics does not affect pain
- Presence of abdominal scars

Most Important Diagnostic Studies

- Diagnostic laparoscopy
- Conscious pain mapping

Treatments

- Lysis of adhesions laparoscopically
- Liberal use of adhesion barriers

REFERENCES

1. Miller EM, Winfield JM. Acute intestinal obstruction secondary to postoperative adhesions. *Arch Surg* 1959;78:148–153.
2. Stricker B, Blanco J, Fox HE. The gynecologic contribution to intestinal obstruction in females. *J Am Coll Surg* 1994;178:617–620.
3. Drake TS, Grunert GM. The unsuspected pelvic factor in the infertility investigation. *Fertil Steril* 1980;34:27–31.
4. Howard FM. The role of laparoscopy in chronic pelvic pain: promise and pitfalls. *Obstet Gynecol Survey* 1993;48:357–387.
5. Rapkin AJ. Adhesions and pelvic pain: a retrospective study. *Obstet Gynecol* 1986;68:13–15.
6. Peters AAW, Trimbos-Kemper GCM, Admiraal C, et al. A randomized clinical trial on the benefit of adhesiolysis in patients with intraperitoneal adhesions and chronic pelvic pain. *Br J Obstet Gynaecol* 1992;99:59–62.
7. Steege JF, Stout A. Resolution of chronic pelvic pain after laparoscopic lysis of adhesions. *Am J Obstet Gynecol* 1991;165:278–283.
8. Sutton C, MacDonald R. Laser laparoscopic adhesiolysis. *J Gynecol Surg* 1990;6:155–159.
9. Fayez JA, Clark RR. Operative laparoscopy for the treatment of localized chronic pelvic–abdominal pain caused by postoperative adhesions. *J Gynecol Surg* 1994;10:79–83.
10. Stout AL, Steege JF, Dodson WC, et al. Relationship of laparoscopic findings to self-report of pelvic pain. *Am J Obstet Gynecol* 1991;164:73–77.
11. Kresch AJ, Seifer DB, Sachs LB, et al. Laparoscopy in 100 women with chronic pelvic pain. *Obstet Gynecol* 1984;64:672–674.
12. Holmdahl L, Risberg B, Beck DE, et al. Adhesions: pathogenesis and prevention-panel discussion and summary. *Eur J Surg* 1997;Suppl 577:56–62.
13. Raf LE. Causes of abdominal adhesions in cases of intestinal obstruction. *Acta Chir Scand* 1969;135:73–76.
14. Weibel MA, Majno G. Peritoneal adhesions and their relation to abdominal surgery. *Am J Surg* 1973;126:345–353.
15. Ratcliff JB, Kapernick P, Brooks GG, et al. Small bowel obstruction and previous gynecologic surgery. *South Med J* 1983;76:1349–1350.
16. Beecher HK. Surgery as placebo. *JAMA* 1961;July 1:1102–1107.
17. Kligman I, Drachenberg C, Papadimitriou J, et al. Immunohistochemical demonstration on nerve fibers in pelvic adhesions. *Obstet Gynecol* 1993;82:566–568.
18. Stovall TG, Elder RF, Ling FW. Predictors of pelvic adhesions. *J Reprod Med* 1989;34:345–348.
19. The American Fertility Society. The American Fertility Society classifications of adnexal adhesions, distal tubal occlusion, tubal occlusion secondary to tubal ligation, tubal pregnancies, Mullerian anomalies and intrauterine adhesions. *Fertil Steril* 1988;49:944–955.
20. Brill AI, Nezhat FR, Nezhat CH, et al. The incidence of adhesions after prior laparotomy: a laparoscopic appraisal. *Obstet Gynecol* 1995;85:269–272.
21. Hasson HM. Open laparoscopy versus closed laparoscopy; a comparison of complication rates. *Adv Plan Parent* 1978;13:41–50.
22. Penfield AJ. How to prevent complications of open laparoscopy. *J Reprod Med* 1985;30:660–663.
23. Howard FM. Breaking new ground or just digging a hole? An evaluation of gynecologic operative laparoscopy. *J Gynecol Surg* 1992;8:143–158.
24. Howard FM, El-Minawi AM, DeLoach VE. Direct laparoscopic cannula insertion at the left upper quadrant. *J Am Assoc Gynecol Laparosc* 1997;4:595–600.
25. Gomel V, Urman B, Gurgan T. Pathophysiology of adhesion formation and strategies for prevention. *J Reprod Med* 1996;41:35–41.
26. Duffy DM, diZerega GS. Adhesion controversies pelvic pain as a cause of adhesions, crystalloids in preventing them. *J Reprod Med* 1996;41:19–26.
27. Palter SF, Olive DL. Office microlaparoscopy under local anesthesia for chronic pelvic pain. *J Am Assoc Gynecol Laparosc* 1996;3:359–364.
28. Demco L. Mapping the source and character of pain due to endometriosis by patient-assisted laparoscopy. *J Am Assoc Gynecol Laparosc* 1998;5:241–245.
29. Diamond MP, Daniell JF, Surrey MW, et al. Adhesion reformation and *de novo* adhesion formation after reproductive pelvic surgery. *Fertil Steril* 1987;47:864–866.
30. Filmar S, Jetha N, McComb P, et al. A comparative histologic study on the healing process after tissue transection II carbon dioxide laser and surgical microscissors. *Am J Obstet Gynecol* 1989;160:1068–1072.

9

ADNEXAL CYSTS

C. PAUL PERRY

KEY TERMS AND DEFINITIONS

Cyst: An encapsulated sac of liquid or semisolid fluid.
Nociceptive: A painful perception.
Torsion: Twisting about an axis.

INTRODUCTION

Numerous conditions, such as spastic colon, diverticulitis, adhesions, and abdominal wall trigger points, commonly produce chronic pelvic pain of unilateral or bilateral location. However, lateral pelvic pain is usually assumed to be from the ovary (or fallopian tube) by patients and physicians alike. This assumption not infrequently leads to a mistaken diagnosis.

Adnexal pathology may produce nociceptive stimulation and pain by chemical, mechanical, or hypoxic tissue changes. Ruptured ovarian cyst, ectopic pregnancy, adnexal torsion, or pelvic inflammatory disease are acutely painful based upon the above mechanisms. The production of chronic pelvic pain by adnexal cysts is more complex and less common. Adnexal cysts are enclosed sacs of liquid or semisolid material and may be derived from the ovaries, fallopian tubes, mesonephric remnants, or encapsulated adhesions.

ETIOLOGY

Chronic ovarian cysts usually do not produce pain. Slow distention of the ovary can be completely asymptomatic despite rich visceral innervation. Patients with painlessly advancing ovarian cancer are testimony to this phenomenon. However, anecdotal reports of functional ovarian cysts producing chronic pelvic pain have been published (1,2). Hasson (3), for example, reported laparoscopic treatment of 35 women with chronic pelvic pain (CPP) attributed to ovarian cysts, with pain resolution in 32 at 3 months' follow-up. Unfortunately, the definition of CPP, details of the procedures, and histologic diagnoses were not reported.

Mechanical pressure on adjacent organs and the development of adhesions are likely responsible for any pain associated with adnexal cysts. While many clinicians believe that capsular distention from polycystic ovarian syndrome is painful, little evidence for this exists in the literature.

SYMPTOMS

Recurrent pelvic pain can be produced by entrapment of ruptured ovarian cyst fluid by dense periovarian adhesions. This forms a peritoneal inclusion cyst (Chapter 29). These tight adhesions may have an impaired ability to absorb the released fluid producing prolonged mechanical pressure and pain. Recurrent, cyclic unilateral pelvic pain also may occur rarely due to recurrent functional ovarian cysts. This syndrome has been reported in young women in their twenties (2). The amount of distention in both of these syndromes varies depending upon production–absorption dynamics. Ultrasonography and pelvic examinations may reveal the change in diameter as the patient's symptoms wax and wane (4).

Adnexal torsion with resultant hypoxia and pain is usually an acute surgical emergency. Intermittent partial adnexal torsion can produce chronic pain in the lower abdomen localized to one side. The diagnosis may be obscured by the intermittent and partial nature of the torsion or the lack of a pelvic mass. The right side is almost three times more likely to be involved (5). Pain may be described as sharp, grabbing, or pinching. It may occur daily with no relationship to cycle and may be especially severe during intercourse. Previous tubal desiccation for sterilization has been associated with this condition. Laparoscopic observation may fail to reveal any cyanosis of edema. Only careful inspection of the adnexal structures reveals its hypermobility and tendency to twist on its blood supply. Loss of adnexal stability may be related to the presence of cysts of Morgagni and the amount of the tube destroyed (5). In addition to torsion of the entire adnexa, isolated twisting of the fallopian tube or parovarian cysts has been reported (6,7).

When a remnant of ovarian tissue is left behind while performing oophorectomy, chronic pain will often result (Chapter 17). The majority of these patients experience cyst formation. Constant, lateral pelvic pain with variable periods of exacerbation may be accompanied by dyspareunia (8). Patients usually have a history of a difficult previous surgery due to adhesions or endometriosis. Their pain may be exacerbated by constipation or full bladder. Symptoms may be cyclic. Similar symptoms may also occur with ovarian retention syndrome, which is the development of pelvic pain associated with the retention of one or both ovaries at the time of hysterectomy (Chapter 16). Most of these patients also have cyst formation.

DIAGNOSIS

Bimanual pelvic examination usually establishes the location and size of adnexal cysts. However, the more uncomfortable the examination, the less likely it is to be diagnostic. Colonic stool may obscure the pelvic pathology and also make the diagnosis more difficult. Pelvic ultrasonography is a valuable and cost-effective diagnostic tool if an adnexal cyst is suspected. Location, size, and solid or cystic components may be determined sonographically. Computerized tomography may also be diagnostically helpful in some cases, but is more expensive and not always necessary.

If ovarian remnant is suspected, clomiphene citrate stimulation can be helpful. Patients are administered 50 mg per day for 5 days and ultrasound performed 5 days later. If a previously unseen cyst visualizes or the patient's pain exacerbates with stimulation, an ovarian remnant is likely.

TREATMENT

Hormonal suppression of chronic pelvic cysts is generally unsuccessful. In the uncommon circumstance of cyclical, recurrent pelvic pain associated with functional ovarian cysts, hormonal suppression may be successful (2). Aspiration of adnexal cysts guided by ultrasound is possible, but the recurrence rate is almost 100% if they are of ovarian origin. Therefore, surgical extirpation or cystectomy remains the treatment of choice. Unless contraindicated by sonographic evidence of malignancy, either procedure may be performed laparoscopically. Patients who are candidates for laparoscopic treatment of adnexal cysts experience a more rapid recovery, less postoperative pain, and decreased adhesion formation. Laparotomy is indicated for patients when laparoscopy is contraindicated (9).

Although acute torsion may be treated by reduction of the torsion and stabilization, if torsion is believed the cause of chronic pelvic pain detorsion is not appropriate due to compromised blood supply (10). Color doppler sonography may be beneficial to determine tissue viability (11).

KEY POINTS

Differential Diagnosis

- Musculoskeletal pain
- Trigger points
- Irritable bowel syndrome
- Painful adhesions

Most Important Questions to Ask

- Was pain of gradual or rapid onset?
- Is pain unilateral or bilateral?
- Does the pain change with menstrual cycle?
- Is there dyspareunia?
- Is pain aggravated by constipation or a full bladder?

Most Important Physical Examination Findings

- Palpable pelvic mass
- Absence of abdominal wall trigger points or no change in pain after blocking with local anesthetic
- Abdominal wall tensing diminishes tenderness to abdominal palpation

Most Important Diagnostic Study

- Pelvic ultrasound

Treatments

- Surgical extirpation, oophorectomy, or adnexectomy
- Cystectomy
- Detorsion and tissue fixation, with cystectomy

REFERENCES

1. Howard FM. The role of laparoscopy in chronic pelvic pain: promise and pitfalls. *Obstet Gynecol Survey* 1993;48:357–387.
2. Stone SC, Swartz WJ. A syndrome characterized by recurrent symptomatic functional ovarian cysts in young women. *Am J Obstet Gynecol* 1979;134:310–314.
3. Hasson HH. Laparoscopic management of ovarian cysts. *J Reprod Med* 1990;35:863–867.
4. Hederstrom E, Forsberg L. Entrapped ovarian cyst. *Acta Radiol* 1990;31:285–286.
5. Sasso RA. Intermittent partial adnexal torsion after electrosurgical tubal ligation. *J Am Assoc Gynecol Laparosc* 1996;3:427–430.
6. Blair CR. Torsion of the fallopian tube. *Surg Gynecol Obstet* 1962;June:727–30.
7. Hasuo Y, Higashijima T, Mitamura T. Torsion of parovarian cyst. *Kurume Med J* 1991;38:39–43.
8. Webb MJ. Ovarian remnant syndrome. *Aust N Z J Obstet Gynaecol* 1989;29:433–435.
9. Perry CP, Upchurch JC. Pelviscopic adnexectomy. *Am J Obstet Gynecol* 1990;162:70–81.
10. Righi RV, Fluker MR, McComb PF. Laparoscopic oophoropexy for recurrent adnexal torsion. *Hum Reprod* 1995;10:3136–3138.
11. Chang KH, Hwang KJ, Kwon HC, et al. Conservative therapy of adnexal torsion employing color doppler sonography. *J Am Assoc Gynecol Laparosc* 1998;5:13–17.

10

DYSMENORRHEA

AHMED M. EL-MINAWI
FRED M. HOWARD

KEY TERMS AND DEFINITIONS

Cervical stenosis: A condition, most often acquired, leading to excessive narrowing of the cervical canal to the extent of obstructing the menstrual flow and increasing intrauterine pressure.

Cyclooxygenase pathway: One of the two major pathways of synthesis of prostaglandins; in this pathway, arachidonic acid is converted into cyclic endoperoxides, then into PGE_2, $PGF_{2\alpha}$, prostacyclin, or thromboxane A_2; most nonsteroidal antiinflammatory drugs block the cyclooxygenase pathway.

Dysmenorrhea: Severe, cramping pain in the lower abdomen, lower back, and upper thighs that occurs during menses and may also occur prior to the onset of menses.

Leukotrienes: Class of prostanglandins that cause uterine muscle contractions and are potent vasoconstrictors and bronchoconstrictors.

Lipoxygenase pathway: One of the two major pathways of synthesis of prostaglandins; this pathway leads to the formation of leukotrienes; many nonsteroidal antiinflammatory drugs do not block the lipoxygenase pathway.

Nonsteroidal antiinflammatory drugs (NSAIDs): These block the activity of prostaglandin on tissue by inhibiting prostaglandin synthetase. Also known as *prostaglandin synthetase inhibitors.*

Primary dysmenorrhea: Severe menstrual pain with no identifiable pelvic pathology that accounts for painful menstruation.

Prostaglandins: Unsaturated fatty acids with a cyclopentane ring and two side chains; prostanglandin $F_{2\alpha}$ ($PGF_{2\alpha}$) is particularly associated with dysmenorrhea.

Secondary dysmenorrhea: Severe menstural pain associated with pelvic pathology that is believed to cause the pain with menstruation.

INTRODUCTION

Dysmenorrhea is the term applied to severe, cramping pain in the lower abdomen, lower back, and upper thighs that occurs during menses and is derived from Greek roots meaning bad or difficult monthly flow (1). There is mention by the ancient Egyptians in the Ebers papyrus of a condition that sounds like dysmenorrhea, and Hippocrates and Galen both commented upon it.

Although attitudes and beliefs about dysmenorrhea have changed greatly in recent years, it is still not uncommon for it to be viewed by patients and professionals alike as normal. Serious scientific work on its etiology and treatment over the past 30 years suggest severe dysmenorrhea should not be tolerated as a normal part of femininity. As we end the twentieth century, the syndrome has become a well-recognized and researched entity; gone are the days when it was considered solely a psychologically induced symptom.

Dysmenorrhea represents a significant personal and public health problem. Dysmenorrhea is a common complaint of both adolescent and adult women. In the United States, work absenteeism due to dysmenorrhea is estimated to be 600 million work hours per year, and the economic consequences are estimated at $2 billion dollars per year. Although the incidence in the general population has not been formally assessed, it is estimated that greater than 50% of menstruating women are symptomatic. A large survey done in Sweden revealed a greater than 72% affliction rate of primary dysmenorrhea among a cohort of 586 19-year-old women (2). Mild symptoms were reported by 34%, moderate by 23%, and severe by 15% of the women surveyed. Of course the subjective nature of the disorder makes it difficult to clearly define and diagnose. In an attempt to gain more objective data on the prevalence of dysmenorrhea, Cox and Santirocco (3) used the Virginia Inventory of Premenstrual and Menstrual symptoms to collect data from a cohort of 847 college volunteers and found that 16% of the population had dysmenorrhea.

Dysmenorrhea is classified as primary dysmenorrhea when no pelvic pathology is found that accounts for painful menstruation. It is a diagnosis of exclusion that is generally made in young women, with onset at less than 20 years of age. Improvement of primary dysmenorrhea after age 25 is more common in married women and after pregnancy; however, pregnancies and vaginal deliveries do not necessarily cure primary dysmenorrhea (4). Secondary dysmenorrhea is diagnosed when there is pelvic pathology that is believed to cause pain with menstruation. It is more common in women over age 20.

ETIOLOGY

Hippocrates believed that stagnation of menstrual blood caused by cervical obstruction led to painful menstrual periods. Cervical stenosis can cause increased intrauterine pressure and increased retrograde menstrual flow, and via these mechanisms it can lead to lower abdominal discomfort, dysmenorrhea, and even endometriosis (5,6). However, cervical stenosis is not the cause of primary dysmenorrhea, although occasionally it may be the cause of secondary dysmenorrhea. There is no difference in tightness of the cervical canal in women with primary dysmenorrhea compared to those without dysmenorrhea (7).

Primary dysmenorrhea appears to be due principally to prostaglandins, in particular $F_{2\alpha}$ and E_2, released from the endometrium at menses. The relation between dysmenorrhea and menstrual prostaglandins can be traced back to the 1940s and 1950s when work by pioneers, such as Pickles, identified extracts of menstrual discharge that caused severe vasoconstriction, fibrinolysis, and inflammatory reactions, and were powerful muscle stimulants (8–10). Subsequently these extracts were shown to contain prostaglandins E and F. Few substances have commanded more widespread interest in biological circles than did the prostaglandins. The event leading to their discovery was the observation, made by two American gynecologists, Kurzok and Lieb (11) in 1930, that strips of human uterus relax or contract when exposed to human semen. A few years later Goldblatt (12) in England and Euler (13) in Sweden independently reported smooth-muscle contractor and vasodepressor activity in seminal fluid. Euler identified the active material as a lipid-soluble acid, which he named "prostaglandin" (13,14). Prostaglandins are unsaturated fatty acids with a cyclopentane ring and two side chains. Of the several compounds in this group, prostaglandin E_2 (PGE_2) and prostaglandin $F_{2\alpha}$ ($PGF_{2\alpha}$) have been extensively evaluated. They are synthesized from arachidonic acid via a pathway controlled by microsomal enzymes called prostaglandin synthetase. There are two major pathways of synthesis of prostaglandins (Fig. 10.1). In the cyclooxygenase pathway, arachidonic acid is converted into cyclic endoperoxides, then into PGE_2, $PGF_{2\alpha}$, prostacyclin, or thromboxane A_2. It has been shown that both estradiol and progesterone levels influence the synthesis and levels of endometrial $PGF_{2\alpha}$ (15–17). The other metabolic pathway for arachidonic acid metabolism, the lipoxygenase pathway, leads to the formation of leukotrienes. Leukotrienes cause uterine muscle contractions and are potent vasoconstrictors and bronchoconstrictors. Many nonsteroidal antiinflammatory drugs (NSAIDs) block the cyclooxygenase pathway, but they do not block the lipoxygenase pathway.

The association between increased uterine prostaglandins $F_{2\alpha}$ ($PGF_{2\alpha}$), increased myometrial activity, and dysmenorrhea is now well established. $PGF_{2\alpha}$ is present in higher concentrations in the menstrual fluid of dysmenorrheic women (18,19). In anovulatory cycles in which there is no dysmenorrhea, there are low progesterone levels and no rise in endometrial prostaglandin levels. The intravenous injection of $PGF_{2\alpha}$ reproduces uterine cramps and pain. $PGF_{2\alpha}$ can also produce diarrhea, vomiting, headache, and syncope, symptoms common with primary dysmenorrhea. Also, NSAIDs relieve dysmenorrhea and decrease menstrual flow and uterine contractility. However, the observation that NSAIDs block the cyclooxygenase pathway, but not the lipoxygenase pathway, may explain why these drugs do not relieve primary dysmenorrhea in all patients.

A widely accepted theory is that in women suffering from primary dysmenorrhea there is an abnormal increase in prostaglandin levels that leads to excessive, abnormal uterine contractions. These colicky, spasmodic, and labor-like contractions produce some of the pain of dysmenorrhea. These contractions may last for a relatively long time, with increased intrauterine pressure leading to uterine ischemia and accumulation of anaerobic metabolite (i.e., uterine angina). Investigators have found the most intense pain to occur during this phase of decreased flow, when contraction amplitude often exceeds 200 mmHg (20,21).

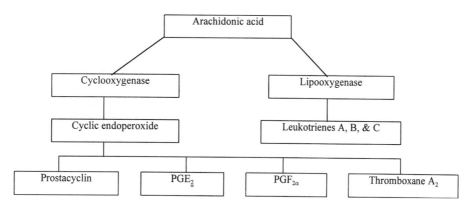

FIGURE 10.1. Schematic of the biosynthetic pathway of prostaglandins and leukotrienes.

Additionally, intermediate products in prostaglandin synthesis, namely cyclic endoperoxides, have direct pain-producing properties (22).

In addition to prostaglandins, several other factors may play a role in the etiology of dysmenorrhea. One is vasopressin, a powerful stimulant of the uterus, particularly at the onset of menstruation. There is a fourfold increase in circulating vasopressin levels during menstruation in women with dysmenorrhea over the levels in asymptomatic women. The effect of vasopressin is not thought to be mediated by prostaglandins because vasopressin levels are not decreased when dysmenorrhea is relieved by prostaglandin synthetase inhibitors (23).

Other etiologic factors may include a familial tendency, because it is common to find that women with dysmenorrhea have daughters with dysmenorrhea. Also, dysmenorrhea is more prevalent among women who have early menarche, women who have increased duration of menses, and women who smoke cigarettes. Pregnancy does not seem to affect its prevalence.

Much has been written about psychological factors and dysmenorrhea. It now seems that purely psychological factors are rarely if ever the cause of dysmenorrhea. However, psychological factors may significantly affect dysmenorrhea by either intensifying or diminishing the severity of pain.

By definition secondary dysmenorrhea is due to a pathologic condition within the pelvis. A variety of conditions may lead to secondary dysmenorrhea (Table 10.1). Cervical stenosis may be congenital, secondary to infection, or iatrogenic due to conization or cryocautery (Chapter 11). The resultant narrowing impedes menstrual flow and increases intrauterine pressure at menses. Because it may be associated with retrograde menstruation, it could be a cause of endometriosis (6).

Imperforate hymen is a cause of obstructive dysmenorrhea associated with failure of canalization of the urogenital

sinus. This also can lead to retrograde menstruation and development of endometriosis. Similarly, blind rudimentary horns may present with dysmenorrhea and may lead to subsequent endometriosis.

Pelvic infections also cause secondary dysmenorrhea, possibly due to the infection and resultant tissue destruction (Chapter 19) (24). Pelvic tuberculosis can lead to dysmenorrhea and is often seen in Middle Eastern countries.

Endometriosis is also a cause of secondary dysmenorrhea (Chapter 14). The prostaglandins in endometriosis are believed to cause the increased pain. Investigators have shown that endometriotic implants have significantly higher levels of prostaglandins compared to other pelvic structures. Adenomyotic implants in severely dysmenorrheic patients were also shown to produce larger amounts of 6-keto-PGF (25). Pelvic congestion syndrome and Allen–Master's syndrome have also been suggested to cause secondary dysmenorrhea (Chapter 18).

Other reported causes of secondary dysmenorrhea include small intracavitary leiomyomas or polyps that can become engorged and painful at time of menstruation. Other investigators have found a significant relation between functional bowel disorder and dysmenorrhea (26).

ANATOMY

The afferent sensory innervation of the uterus runs primarily with the autonomic sympathetic nerves. Transecting the sympathetic autonomic nerves (e.g., in presacral neurectomy) promotes vasodilatation, interrupts sensory input from the uterus, and relieves the pain of dysmenorrhea. Also, relief of primary dysmenorrhea in some women after childbirth may be explained by the fact that short adrenergic neurons in the myometrium tend to be destroyed in pregnancy and do not regenerate afterward.

SYMPTOMS

Primary dysmenorrhea usually begins 6 to 12 months after menarche and coincides with the onset of ovulatory cycles. However, a large percentage of patients also complain of pain from the first cycle (27). A survey by Andersch and Milsom (2) reported that 38% of females experienced dysmenorrhea in the first year after menarche, while 21% experienced it only 4 years later.

Patients complain of spasmodic or cramping lower abdominal pain that may radiate suprapubically, to the low back, and to the anteromedial aspect of the thighs. The pain may also be of continuous dull aching character. Other symptoms, such as headache, nausea, vomiting, diarrhea, and fatigue, often accompany the menstrual pain. Symptoms typically last 48 hours or less, but sometimes may last up to 72 hours. They may also start 1 or 2 days prior to the

TABLE 10.1. COMMON CAUSES OF SECONDARY DYSMENORRHEA

Uterine
Adenomyosis
Leiomyomata
Endometrial polyps
Congenital malformation
Cervical stenosis

Extrauterine
Endometriosis
Pelvic inflammatory disease
Pelvic tuberculosis
Pelvic congestion syndrome
Allen–Masters syndrome
Imperforate hymen

Iatrogenic
Intrauterine contraception device

onset of menses. Occasionally, the accompanying vasoconstriction in the acute phase may be so marked that the patient appears in shock.

Family history is important, because dysmenorrhea has been found to run in families. The overall demeanor of the patient is sometimes helpful in assessing whether there is a psychiatric component to the pain. The psychosocial history should be ascertained. Sexual history should be elicited; often this requires the absence of the parents during questioning. It should be noted that history of a prior pregnancy does not negate the possibility of primary dysmenorrhea. Almost 20% of primary dysmenorrhea patients in a study by Chan and Dawood (28) had resumption of their pain following vaginal delivery.

Secondary dysmenorrhea, caused by identifiable pathologic conditions acting on the internal genital organs or pelvic peritoneum (Table 10.1), has pain symptoms identical to primary dysmenorrhea. It tends, though, to start at a later age than primary dysmenorrhea. However, endometriosis is more common in adolescents than is generally recognized and may be the cause of more cases of "primary" dysmenorrhea than generally recognized (29). Patients with secondary dysmenorrhea may have a history of menorrhagia, past pelvic inflammatory disease, infertility, dyspareunia, or use of an intrauterine contraceptive device.

The onset of the pain in relation to the cycle can be helpful. Pain starting before menstruation is often due to pelvic inflammatory disease, pelvic congestion syndrome, endometriosis, or premenstrual syndrome (30). On the other hand, pain starting with menstruation is sometimes associated with uterine pathology such as submucous leiomyomas or endometrial polyps.

There may be other pain symptoms or gynecological symptoms in patients with secondary dysmenorrhea. For example, menstrual disturbances such as menorrhagia or excessive vaginal discharge may suggest leiomyomas or endometrial polyps.

History of previous surgical procedures involving the cervix may point to cervical stenosis. Intrauterine contraceptive devices are another cause; therefore contraceptive history should be brought up with the patient.

SIGNS

A careful pelvic examination should be performed to look for uterine enlargement or irregularity, pelvic masses, or pelvic tenderness. A rectal examination should be done to assess nodularity and tenderness along the uterosacral ligaments and cul-de-sac, findings suggestive of endometriosis. The presence of an intrauterine device may be confirmed by finding its string at the cervix. The physical examination may reveal findings consistent with anemia secondary to heavy menstruation. Abnormal findings suggest dysmenorrhea is secondary.

In the young woman with suspected primary dysmenorrhea the pelvic examination can be difficult due to anxiety and discomfort. The clinician must be sensitive to this. If a vaginal examination is not feasible, sometimes a rectal exam can be performed and will suffice in many cases.

Primary dysmenorrhea is a diagnosis of exclusion. The general physical examination and pelvic examination reveal no abnormalities. Sometimes a laparoscopy may have to be performed to rule out pelvic pathology, particularly endometriosis.

DIAGNOSTIC STUDIES

No laboratory tests are diagnostic or specific to primary or secondary dysmenorrhea. Ca-125 levels may be elevated with endometriosis or leiomyomata, but there are several other causes of Ca-125 elevation that are not related to dysmenorrhea. Although prostaglandin levels have been measured experimentally in menstrual fluid, this is not a clinically useful test.

Ultrasonography, especially when performed transvaginally, may be useful to look for uterine leiomyomata, uterine enlargement, adnexal masses, endometrial polyps, or an unsuspected intrauterine device. It may also be useful for the nonoperative diagnosis of adenomyosis, but further investigation is needed. Hysterosalpingography often detects uterine anomalies, endometrial polyps, or Asherman syndrome. Cervical cultures for gonorrhea and cervical chlamydial antigen testing may be positive and helpful if pelvic inflammatory disease is suspected. Computerized tomography and magnetic resonance imaging may be useful, but further experience with these modalities is needed to determine their role in the evaluation of dysmenorrhea. In patients with uterine anomalies, intravenous pyelograms and magnetic resonance imaging are indicated to rule out other genitourinary anomilies.

Laparoscopy remains the most important diagnostic procedure to assess the pelvis for any pathology. The role of conscious pain mapping in these patients is not yet established. Simultaneous hysteroscopy to evaluate the uterine cavity may also be useful.

TREATMENT

Medical Treatment

Over the ages, women with dysmenorrhea have received little true sympathy and even less help. A variety of bizarre treatments have been prescribed over the centuries by physicians and nonphysicians alike. During the late nineteenth and early twentieth centuries it was managed with rest, seclusion, refraining from all activities, and a hot bath followed by a good dose of gin (31)!

Successful management of dysmenorrhea can be challenging. A healthy lifestyle, including nutritional supplements and aerobic exercise (such as walking, swimming, and bicycling), may produce an overall benefit and decrease the impact of dysmenorrhea on the patient's daily activities. For appropriate selection of treatment, it is usually helpful to determine is dysmenorrhea is primary or secondary.

Oral contraceptives provide significant relief of primary dysmenorrhea. They suppress ovulation, resulting in lower levels of prostaglandins, and also markedly reduce spontaneous uterine activity. Oral contraceptives are a good first-line therapy for many young women, especially if contraception is also needed.

The NSAIDs that inhibit prostaglandin synthetase have had a pivotal role in treating primary dysmenorrhea for the last 20 years (Table 10.2) (32). Various studies have looked at the effect of NSAIDs on primary dysmenorrhea (33–36). In a review of 51 published trials of primary dysmenorrhea treated with NSAIDs, Owen (37) found that 72% of patients had significant relief with NSAIDs compared to 15% with placebo. Unlike oral contraceptives, NSAIDs need to be taken only 2 to 5 days per month and do not suppress the hypothalamic–pituitary–ovarian axis. Their primary therapeutic benefit is inhibition of prostaglandin formation. They provide relief in up to 80% of patients. It is hypothesized that patients whose pain is not relieved by NSAIDs have increased activity of the alternate lipoxygenase pathway of prostaglandin production.

The choice of a particular NSAID depends on the clinical efficacy, side effects, patient acceptance, and individual clinical experience. NSAIDs should be started at or just before the onset of pain and continued regularly during the symptomatic period. They should be taken on an as-needed basis initially. If pain control with an as-needed regimen is insufficient, it is sometimes worth a trial of scheduled, regular dosing. Also, when pain is inadequately controlled, the initial or loading dose may be increased by up to 50% during the next cycle, but the maintenance dose should be kept the same. A trial of up to 3 to 6 months may be needed to demonstrate effective relief of symptoms. If a particular NSAID is ineffective, it is worth trying a different one, because there is significant variability of individual responsiveness to the NSAIDs. The side effects of NSAIDs include gastric irritation, heartburn, abdominal pain, nausea, vomiting, headache, occasional visual disturbances, allergic reactions, and blood disorders. However, these are unusual when these drugs are used on an intermittent basis for dysmenorrhea. The NSAIDs are contraindicated in patients with asthma or hypersensitivity to aspirin.

Calcium antagonists such as verapamil and nifedipine reduce uterine activity and contractility. They have produced relief in some resistant cases of dysmenorrhea. They may provide a different approach by decreasing the severity of myometrial contractions, thereby decreasing intrauterine pressure and the resultant pain (38). They have no effect on other symptoms such as vomiting or diarrhea (39).

Transcutaneous electrical nerve stimulation (TENS) effectively relieves pain in various conditions, including dysmenorrhea. It seems to act by blocking the transmission of pain impulses through the dorsal nerve horns and by its antiischemic effects. It relieves primary dysmenorrhea without any significant reduction of uterine activity and represents a nonpharmacologic treatment option (40). One study using TENS in two consecutive cycles in 61 sufferers reported 30% marked relief, 60% moderate relief, and 10% no relief of pain (41). Acupuncture also effectively treats primary dysmenorrhea, probably via a similar mechanism (42).

With secondary dysmenorrhea, therapy should be directed at the underlying condition. Women using intrauterine devices can be treated with NSAIDs or can have the device removed. NSAIDs may also offer an added benefit of reduced menstrual flow. Naproxen, mefenamic acid, and ibuprofen are used most commonly. It is important to rule out pelvic inflammatory disease in women with intrauterine devices.

Endometriosis may be treated medically with danazol, medroxyprogesterone acetate, or gonadotropin-releasing hormone analogs. This is discussed in depth in the chapter on endometriosis (Chapter 14). Pelvic inflammatory disease (PID) is best treated medically with aggressive antibiotic therapy, and this is also discussed elsewhere (Chapter 19).

Surgical Treatment

Surgical interruption of neural pathways from the uterus may be done to decrease the pain of primary or secondary dysmenorrhea. Presacral neurectomy consists of transection of the sympathetic nerves of the superior hypogastric plexus at the sacral promontory (Fig. 10.2). It has an efficacy of about 75% in relieving midline dysmenorrhea (Table 10.3). Uterine nerve ablation by transecting the uterosacral ligaments (Fig. 10.3) may be more easily performed than a presacral neurectomy, but there are less reliable data regarding its efficacy. Cervical dilatation has been historically used to relieve dysmenorrhea thought to be secondary to cervical stenosis. Its value is debatable, but it may act by promoting blood flow, by disrupting sensory nerves from the cervix, or

TABLE 10.2. THE NONSTEROIDAL ANTIINFLAMMATORY DRUGS MOST COMMONLY USED FOR DYSMENORRHEA

Drug	Brand Names	Recommended Doses
Ibuprofen	Motrin, Advil	400–800 mg q6–8h
Naproxen	Naprosyn	250–500 mg q6–8h
Mefenamic acid	Ponstel	250–500 mg q6–8h
Naproxen sodium	Anaprox, Aleve	275–500 mg q6–8h

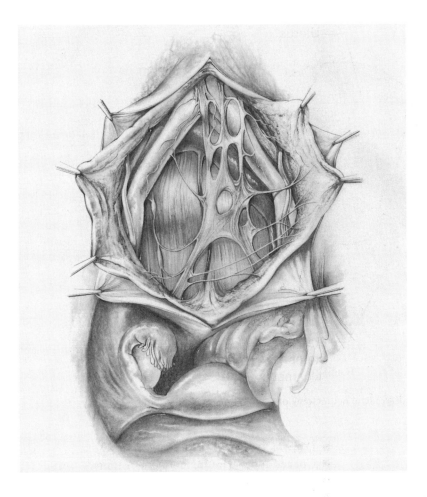

FIGURE 10.2. Anatomy at the site of presacral neurectomy.

by decreasing intrauterine pressure secondary to obstruction.

Endometriosis may be treated surgically, either conservatively by resection or destruction of all lesions or radically by hysterectomy and bilateral salpingoophorectomy, depending on the severity of the symptoms and the patient's age and parity. Leiomyomata uteri may be treated with conservative or radical surgery, with myomectomy or hysterectomy, respectively, again depending on the patient's age, parity, and symptom severity. Adenomyosis is usually treated by hysterectomy but may respond to conservative treatment with NSAIDs or endometrial resection or ablation. Endometrial polyps may be removed via hysteroscopic polypectomy.

TABLE 10.3. RESULTS OF PRESACRAL NEURECTOMY FOR DYSMENORRHEA

Author	Number of Cases	Number with Pain Relief	Percentage with Pain Relief
Meigs (1939)	20	15	75
Phaneuf (1947)	67	40	60
Tucker (1947)	118	59	50
Ingersoll (1949)	108	73	68
Browne (1949)	34	25	74
Counseller (1955)	14	9	64
Doyle (1955)	73	63	86
Blake (1963)	66	59	89
Frier (1965)	20	15	75
Polan (1980)	20	15	75
Lee (1986)	40	29	73
Chen (1997)	392	284	72
Total	**972**	**686**	**71**

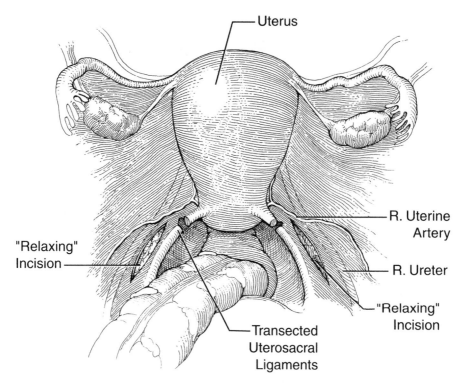

FIGURE 10.3. Illustration of uterosacral neurectomy or uterosacral nerve ablation.

KEY POINTS

Most Important Questions to Ask

- Is pain cyclical or associated only with menses?
- Are there symptoms other than pain at menses or just before the onset of menses?
- Is there a history of sexually transmitted diseases?
- At what age did dysmenorrhea start?

Most Important Physical Examination Findings

- Irregular and/or enlarged uterus
- Adnexal mass or masses
- Uterosacral or cul-de-sac nodularity or tenderness
- Uterine or adnexal tenderness

Most Important Diagnostic Studies

- Laparoscopy
- Ultrasound
- Hysterosalpingography
- Hysteroscopy
- Magnetic resonance imaging

Treatments

- Nonsteroidal antiinflammatory drugs
- Oral contraceptives
- Danazol
- Gonadotropin-releasing hormone agonists
- Medroxyprogesterone acetate
- Presacral neurectomy
- Uterosacral neurectomy
- Transcutaneous electrical nerve stimulation or acupuncture

REFERENCES

1. Smith RP. Cyclic pain and dysmenorrhea. *Obstet Gynecol NA* 1993;20:753–764.
2. Andersch B, Milsom I. An epidemiological study of young women with dysmenorrhea. *Am J Obstet Gynecol* 1982;144: 655–657.
3. Cox DJ, Santirocco LL. Psychological and behavioral factors in dysmenorrhea. In: Dawood MY, ed. *Dysmenorrhea.* Baltimore: Williams & Wilkins, 1981:75–77.
4. Sundell G, Milson I, Andersch B. Factors influencing the prevalence and severity of dysmenorrhea in young women. *Br J Obstet Gynaecol* 1990;97:588–594.
5. Cibils LA. Contractibility of the non-pregnant human uterus. *Obstet Gynecol* 1967;30:441–461.
6. Barbieri RL. Stenosis of the external cervical os: an association with endometriosis in women with chronic pelvic pain. *Fertil Steril* 1998;70:571–573.
7. Aspland J. The uterine cervix and isthmus under normal and pathological conditions. *Acta Radiol (Suppl)* 1952;91:1.
8. Pickles VR. A plain-muscle stimulant in the menstruum. *Nature* 1957;180:1198–1199.
9. Pickles VR, Hall WJ, Best FA, et al. Prostaglandin in endome-

trium and menstrual fluid from normal and dysmenorrheic subjects. *Br J Obstet Gynecol* 1965;72:185–187.

10. Smith OW, Mass B. Menstrual toxin. *Am J Obstet Gynecol* 1947; 54:201.

11. Kurzok R, Lieb CC. Biochemical studies of human semen. II. The action of semen on the human uterus. *Proc Soc Exp Biol Med* 1930;28:268–272.

12. Goldblatt MW. Properties of human seminal fluid. *J Physiol* 1935;84:208–218.

13. Euler US von. On the specific vasodilating and plain muscle stimulating substance from accessory genital glands in man and certain animals (prostaglandin and vesiglandin). *J Physiol* 1936; 88:213–234.

14. Euler US von. Some aspects of the actions of prostaglandins. The first Heymans Memorial lecture. *Arch Int Pharmacodyn Ther* 1973;202(Suppl):295–307.

15. Jordan VC, Pokoly TB. Steroid and prostaglandin relations during the menstrual cycle. *Obstet Gynecol* 1971;49:449–451.

16. Wilson L, Cendella RJ, Butcher RL, et al. Levels of prostaglandins in the uterine endometrium during the ovine estrous cycle. *J Anim Sci* 1972;34:93–96.

17. Pickles VR. Prostaglandin in the human endometrium. *Int J Fertil* 1967;12:335–337.

18. Chan WY, Dawood MY, Fuchs F. Relief of dysmenorrhea with the prostaglandin synthetase inhibitor Ibuprofen: effect on prostaglandin levels in menstrual fluid. *Am J Obstet Gynecol* 1979;135:102–104.

19. Pickles VR, Hall WJ, Bes FA, et al. Prostaglandins in endometriosis and menstrual fluid from normal and dysmenorrheic subjects. *Br J Obstet Gynaecol* 1965;72:185.

20. Akerlund M, Andersson K-E, Ingemarsson I. Effects of terbutaline on myometrial activity, uterine blood flow and lower abdominal pain in women with primary dysmenorrhea. *Br J Obstet Gynaecol* 1976;83:673.

21. Ulmsten U, Anderson K-E. Multichannel intrauterine pressure recording by means of microtransducers. *Acta Obstet Gynecol Scand* 1979;58:115–117.

22. Ferreira SH, Moncada S, Vane JR. Prostaglandins and signs and symptoms of inflammations. In Robinson HJ, Vane JR, eds. *Prostaglandin synthetase inhibitors.* New York: Raven Press, 1974:175–187.

23. Akerlund M, Stromberg P, Forselin MD. Primary dysmenorrhea and vasopressin. *Br J Obstet Gynaecol* 1979;86:484–487.

24. Roy S. Surgery for dysmenorrhea. In Dawood MY, ed. *Dysmenorrhea.* Baltimore: Williams & Wilkins, 1981:165–186.

25. Koike H, Ikenoue T, Mori N. Studies on prostaglandin production relating to the mechanism of dysmenorrhea in endometriosis. *Nippon Naibunpi Gakkai Zasshi. Folia Endocrinol Jpn* 1994;20:43.

26. Crowell MD, Dubin NH, Robinson JC, et al. Functional bowel disorders in women with dysmenorrhea. *Am J Gastroenterol* 1994;89(11):1973–1977.

27. Widholm OM, Kantero RA. A statistical analysis of the menstrual patterns of Finnish girls and their mothers. *Acta Obstet Gynecol Scand (Suppl)* 1971;14:1–2.

28. Chan WY, Dawood MY. Prostaglandin levels in menstrual fluid of nondysmenorrheic and dysmenorrheic subjects with and without oral contraceptive or ibuprofen therapy. *Adv Prostaglandin Thromboxanes Res* 1980;8:1443–446.

29. Goldstein DP, Cholkony C, Emanus JS. Adolescent endometriosis. *J Adolesc Health Care* 1980;1:37–41.

30. Wood C, Larsen L, Williams R. Menstrual characteristics of 2,343 women attending the Shepherd Foundation. *Aust N Z J Obstet Gynaecol* 1979;19:107–110.

31. Kinch RAH. Dysmenorrhea: a historical perspective. In Dawood MY, McGuire JL, Demers LM, eds. Premenstrual syndrome and dysmenorrhea. Baltimore: Urban & Schwarzenberg, 1985: 79–80.

32. Dawood MY. Ibuprofen and dysmenorrhea. *Am J Med* 1984; 87–94.

33. Kajanoja P, Tuulikki V. Naproxen and indomethacin in the treatment of primary dysmenorrhea. *Acta Obstet Gynecol Scand* 1979; 87(Suppl):87–90.

34. Corson SL, Bolognese RJ. Ibuprofen therapy for dysmenorrhea. *J Reprod Med* 1978;20:246–248.

35. Kapadia L, Elder MD. Flufenamic acid in treatment of primary spasmodic dysmenorrhea; a double-blind crossover study. *Lancet* 1978;1:348–349.

36. Smith RP. The dynamics of nonsteroidal antiinflammatory therapy for primary dysmenorrhea. *Obstet Gynecol* 1987;70:785–787.

37. Owen PR. Prostaglandin synthetase inhibitors in the treatment of primary dysmenorrhea: outcome trials reviewed. *Am J Obstet Gynecol* 1984;148:96–99.

38. Anderson KE, Ulmsten U. Effects on nifedipine on myometrial activity and lower abdominal pain in women with primary dysmenorrhea. *Br J Obstet Gynaecol* 1978;85:142–144.

39. Forman A, Anderson KE, Ulmsten U. Combined effects of diflunisal and nifedipine on uterine contractility in dysmenorrheic patients. *Prostaglandins* 1982;23(2):237–239.

40. Milsom I, Hedner N, Mannheimer C. A comparative study of the effect of high-intensity transcutaneous nerve stimulation and oral naproxen on intrauterine pressure and menstrual pain in patients with primary dysmenorrhea. *Am J Obstet Gynecol* 1994; 170:123–126.

41. Kaplan B, Peled Y, Pardo J, et al. Transcutaneous electrical nerve stimulation (TENS) as a relief for dysmenorrhea. *Clin Exp Obstet Gynecol* 1994;21:87–90.

42. Helms JM. Acupuncture in the management of primary dysmenorrhea. *Obstet Gynecol* 1987;69:51–56.

11

CERVICAL STENOSIS

JAMES E. CARTER

KEY TERMS AND DEFINITIONS

Cervical stenosis: Cervical narrowing that prevents insertion of a 2.5-mm Hegar dilator.

Hematometra: Distention of the uterus with blood, due to uterine bleeding with obstruction of the uterine cervix.

Pyometra: Distention of the uterus with exudate or purulent material associated with obstruction of the uterine cervix.

Hydrometra: Distention of the uterus with fluid associated with obstruction of the uterine cervix.

INTRODUCTION

Congenital stenosis of the endocervical canal is an uncommon finding occasionally encountered in the diagnostic investigation of a woman with chronic pelvic pain (CPP) (1). It is also sometimes found in the evaluation of an infertile couple. The diagnosis is made by exclusion and is heralded by failure in attempts to pass a small catheter or probe into the endocervical canal. Acquired stenosis of the cervix may follow chronic cervical infection, treatment of endocervicitis, cauterization of the cervix, cryosurgery or laser surgery of the cervix, radium therapy or senile atrophy (2). It may also follow conization or large loop excision for treatment of cervical dysplasia (3).

Cervical stenosis was found by Carter in 2.9% of women with CPP at time of hysteroscopy (1). Nagele et al. (2) found that passage of a 5-mm diagnostic sheath required cervical dilation in 19.5% of patients undergoing hysteroscopy and that local anesthetics and cervical dilation were required significantly more often by nulligravid, nulliparous, and postmenopausal women. The incidence of cervical stenosis so severe that cervical dilation could not be performed under local anesthesia occurred in 1% of patient's for whom outpatient diagnostic hysteroscopy was planned.

ETIOLOGY

Cervical stenosis may follow chronic cervical infection, treatment of endocervicitis, cauterization of the cervix,

cryosurgery, laser conization or large loop excision of the cervix, radium therapy, or senile atrophy (4). Cervical stenosis may also occur after endometrial ablation or resection, which results in uterine synechiae or is carried out into the endocervical canal (5).

Ten percent of laser conization patients and 4% of large-loop surgical excision patients experience cervical stenosis. However, the type of excision procedure is not independently associated with postoperative surgical stenosis. Rather, the patients who develop postoperative stenosis had significantly higher excisions (20.7 ± 7.0 mm versus 16.8 ± 6.0 mm; $p < 0.001$). The only independent factors associated with the risk of stenosis are the height of the excision and a totally endocervical lesion. When an excision is performed under colposcopic control at a mean height of 22 mm, the overall cervical stenosis rate is 12%. When the excision is performed without colposcopic control at a mean height of 28 mm, 28% of patients develop cervical stenosis. The risk of postoperative stenosis is not found to be significantly different after a second excision than after a single one (6).

In 915 cases of cone biopsy a 17% incidence of cervical stenosis was found (7). The incidence of cervical stenosis was statistically significantly greater in women who had cones greater than 25 mm, but not in those with a base greater than 25 mm. When amenorrhea occurs several months after conization it is likely there is progressive stenosis and finally total obliteration of the external cervical os (8–10).

ANATOMY AND PATHOLOGY

The cervix is cylindrical in shape and measures 2.5 to 3 cm in length and width. The vaginal portion of the cervix projects into the vaginal canal and is surrounded by four vaginal fornices. The terminus of the cervix is rounded and is punctuated with a circular or transverse opening, the external os. Two lips are identified; these are termed the anterior, which is shorter and thicker, and the posterior, which is longer and thinner. Nearly half of the cervix lies within the vagina. The *portio vaginalis* cervix usually enters the vagina obliquely from ventral to dorsal, pointing to the posterior wall of the vagina. The canal of the cervix is, for all practical purposes, spindle-shaped. Longitudinal crests of endocervical mucosa protrude into the cavity anteriorly and posteriorly as the *plicae palmatae*. Secondary oblique branching of the mucosa give the appearance of a tree and constitutes the *arbor vitae*. The endocervical mucosa is whitish pink in color and is thrown into numerous folds interspersed with clefts (11).

The lumen of the cervix ranges between 3 and 10 mm in diameter, depending on individual variation and parity. There is some resilience to light pressure that may allow 1- to 2-mm additional space with stretching. During stretching, the mucosal folds appear flat and white. The *portio vaginalis* (cervical lips) is covered with squamous epithelium, but the endocervix is covered with columnar epithelium. The transition from columnar epithelium to squamous epithelium is abrupt and usually occurs at the level of the external os. The point of juncture of the cervix in the body of the uterus is called the isthmus and corresponds to the level of the internal os. The isthmus is marked by a constriction at the internal os, where it meets the cervix. The cervical canal extends from the anatomic external os through the internal os, where it joins the uterine cavity (12).

Histologically, the uterine cervix is composed predominantly of dense fibrous connective tissue with scanty peripheral smooth muscle. The stroma of the cervix is composed of connective tissue with stratified muscle fibers and elastic tissue. The elastic tissue is primarily found around the wall of the larger blood vessels. The cervix undergoes anatomic changes during the menstrual cycle. The external os progressively widens during the proliferative phase, reaching maximal width just before or at ovulation. At the time of maximal widening, cervical mucous usually exudes from the external os. After ovulation, the cervical os returns to a smaller diameter and the profuse mucous becomes scant and viscid.

Cervical stenosis is generally an acquired condition with obstruction of the cervical canal at the internal or external os. The stenosis is usually caused by iatrogenic manipulation such as conizations, cryotherapy, obstetric trauma, or radiation, or the cervix may simply atrophy after menopause. Rarely, a cervical or uterine fibroid or polyp may obstruct the canal. The most serious cause to be excluded is cervical carcinoma, or less likely endometrial carcinoma (2).

SYMPTOMS OR HISTORY

Stenosis is usually asymptomatic, but it may cause abnormal genital bleeding, dysmenorrhea, or infertility. Observational studies of CPP suggest that it may occasionally cause pain (13). If stenosis is complete or nearly complete, the accumulation of cervical or uterine secretions may cause distention of the uterine cavity, resulting in distention of

the uterus with blood (hematometra), fluid (hydrometra), or exudate (pyometra). These conditions, which produce a distended endometrial cavity, may be asymptomatic for prolonged periods (2). When pain occurs it is typically described as crampy, spasmodic, labor-like, and localized over the lower abdomen in the suprapubic region. It sometimes may be described as a dull ache or a stabbing feeling (14).

Premenopausal patients may experience oligomenorrhea or amenorrhea with cramping or dysmenorrhea. The symptoms are less frequent in postmenopausal patients in whom the uterus slowly enlarges with the accumulation of blood and secretions (12).

SIGNS AND EXAMINATION

Direct visualization of the cervix may be unrevealing as the stenosis is generally found within the canal and detected only by direct probing with a uterine sound or cervical dilator. However the cervix may appear to have a very narrow external os and if the stenosis is a result of previous conization the squamocolumnar junction may be well within the cervical os. Bimanual examination may be normal. However, if the stenosis is complete or nearly complete, the accumulation of cervical or uterine secretions may cause distention of the uterine cavity which on bimanual examination often appears to be cystic. In addition, the uterus may be tender.

DIAGNOSTIC STUDIES

The diagnosis of cervical stenosis is confirmed by failure to pass a 2.5 mm or smaller probe into the endocervical canal (3). Ultrasonography can readily diagnose obstructive cervical stenosis. Either transabdominal or endovaginal sonography will show fluid or debris or a fluid–debris level in the endometrial cavity (4). A lobulated or distorted cervix may suggest carcinoma or fibroids as the cause. Clinically, the obstructed cervical os may be difficult to find, especially in postmenopausal patients after pelvic irradiation. Transabdominal ultrasound guidance may help by directing the probe or sound during gynecologic procedures to drain the uterus.

DIFFERENTIAL DIAGNOSIS

In premenopausal women, all causes of dysmenorrhea such as endometriosis, pelvic inflammatory disease, adenomyosis, pelvic adhesions, ovarian cysts, and obstructive uterine polyps, myomas, or müllerian malformations must be considered. If oligomenorrhea has resulted from severe stenosis, other causes of oligomenorrhea must be considered such as (a) dysfunction of the hypothalamic–pituitary–ovarian axis or (b) uterine synechiae. In post-menopausal women, all causes of accumulation of uterine secretions and debris must be considered such as endometrial cancer, endometrial polyps, and endometritis. Criteria for definitive diagnosis is the inability to pass a probe 2.5 mm or less into the endocervical canal.

SURGICAL TREATMENT

Most patients are treated with endocervical dilatation. One may consider the use of laminaria to facilitate cervical dilatation. The advantage of the laminaria is that it can be placed easily without significant discomfort and may be removed in 24 hours after facilitating cervical dilatation in a slow, controlled fashion. Laminaria dilation significantly reduces the risk of perforation when compared to dilation with Hegar dilators (15). The use or prophylactic antibiotics to reduce the chance of contamination of the endometrial cavity with endogenous pelvic flora is recommended (16). In some cases maintenance of a patent endocervical canal with an indwelling drain is useful (2). The possible adverse impact of an indwelling device that is sutured into the cervix is that it presents a much higher risk for uterine contamination (17).

Hysterectomy may occasionally be indicated. It was required on one patient in whom a laser cone biopsy was performed for severe dysplasia involving the endocervix. The specimen was 4.1 × 2.4 × 2.3 cm. The patient had three normal monthly menses, then became amenorrheic and developed progressive lower abdominal pain. Ultrasound revealed a well-circumscribed midline mass with normal echogenicity and 14 weeks' gestational size. An attempt at cervical dilatation under ultrasound guidance failed. Magnetic resonance imaging demonstrated contents of the endometrial cavity which were homogeneously bright on T1 (slightly less bright than fat) and T2, with a smooth endometrial surface suggestive of hematometra. Because there was no way to extract blood from the lower uterine segment, a hysterectomy was performed. No endocervix or ectocervix was found on the specimen (18). A hysterectomy was also performed for a case of hematocervix following cone biopsy of the cervix (8).

KEY POINTS
Differential Diagnosis

- Endometriosis
- Pelvic inflammatory disease
- Adenomyosis
- Uterine polyps
- Myomas
- Genital obstructive müllerian malformations
- Ovarian cysts
- Pelvic adhesions
- Endometrial cancer
- Endometrial polyps
- Endometritis

Most Important Questions to Ask

- Is there a history of treatment with cryosurgery, laser surgery, loop excision, or endometrial resection or ablation?
- Is there a history of pelvic inflammatory disease?
- Is the pain typically crampy, spasmodic, labor-like, and localized over the lower abdomen in the suprapubic region?
- Is the pain periodic or cyclic, or associated with bleeding?

Most Important Physical Examination Findings

- Inability to pass a 2.5 mm or less probe into the cervical canal.

Most Important Diagnostic Studies

- Ultrasound of the uterus revealing a finding of increased endometrial contents.

Treatments

- Cervical dilatation by laminaria tent or physical dilation with dilators (under ultrasound control).

REFERENCES

1. Carter JE. Combined hysteroscopic and laparoscopic findings in patients with chronic pelvic pain. *J Am Assoc Gynecol Laparosc* 1994;2:43–47.
2. Nagele F, O'Connor H, Davies A, et al. 2500 outpatient diagnostic hysteroscopies. *Obstet Gynecol* 1996;88:87–92.
3. Baldauf J, Dreyfuss M, Ritter J, et al. Risk of cervical stenosis after large loop excision or laser conization. *Obstet Gynecol* 1996; 88:933–938.
4. Hall DA, Yoder IC. Ultrasound evaluation of the uterus. In: Callen PW, ed. *Ultrasonography in obstetrics and gynecology.* Philadelphia: WB Saunders, 1994:586–614.
5. Dwyer N, Hutton J, Stirrat GM. Randomized controlled trial comparing endometrial resection with abdominal hysterectomy for the surgical treatment of menorrhagia. *Br J Obstet Gynaecol* 1993;100:237–243.
6. Hallam NF, West J, Harper C, et al. Large loop excision of the transformation zone (LLETZ) as an alternative to both local ablative and cone biopsy treatment: a series of 1000 patients. *J Gynecol Surg* 1993;9:77–82.
7. Luesley DM, McCrum A, Terry PB, et al. Complications of cone biopsy related to the dimensions of the cone and the influence of prior colposcopic assessment. *Br J Obstet Gynaecol* 1985;92:158–164.

8. Clark A, Hart DM, McCune G. Hematocervix following cone biopsy of the cervix. *J Obstet Gynaecol Br Commonw* 1973;80: 858–861.

9. Pschera H, Kjaeldgaard A. Haematocervix after conization diagnosed by ultrasonography. *Gynecol Obstet Invest* 1990;29:304–310.

10. Ohel G. Complications of cone biopsy of the cervix. *S Afr Med J* 1981;59:382–383.

11. Baggish MS, Barbot J, Valle R. Anatomy of the uterus. In: Baggish MS, Barbot J, Valle R, eds. *Diagnostic and operative hysteroscopy: a text and atlas.* Chicago: Year Book Medical Publishers, 1989:18–25.

12. DiSaia PJ. Disorders of the uterine cervix. In: Scott JR, DiSaia PJ, Hammond CB, et al, eds. *Danforth's obstetrics and gynecology,* 7th ed. Philadelphia: Lippincott, 1994:893–924.

13. Nezhat F, Nezhat C, Nezhat CH, et al. Use of hysteroscopy in addition to laparoscopy for evaluating chronic pelvic pain. *J Reprod Med* 1995;40:431–434.

14. Gidwani GP, Kay M. Dysmenorrhea and pelvic pain. In: Sanfilippo JS, ed. *Pediatric and adolescent gynecology,* Philadelphia: WB Saunders, 1994:233–249.

15. Jonasson A, Larsson B, Bygdeman S, et al. The influence of cervical dilatation by laminaria tent and with Hegar dilators on the intrauterine microflora and the rate of postabortal pelvic inflammatory disease. *Acta Obstet Gynecol Scand* 1989;68: 405–410.

16. Glatstein IZ, Pang SC, McShane PM. Successful pregnancies with the use of laminaria tents before embryo transfer for refractory cervical stenosis. *Fertil Steril* 1997;67:1172–1174.

17. Frishman GN. The use of a stem pessary to facilitate transcervical embryo transfer in women with cervical stenosis. *J Assist Reprod Genet* 1994;11:225–228.

18. Reuter KL, Young SB, Daly B. Hematometra complicating conization with radiologic correlation: a case report. *J Reprod Med* 1994;39:408–410.

12

DYSPAREUNIA

FRED M. HOWARD

KEY TERMS AND DEFINITIONS

Deep dyspareunia: Pain during intercourse at the time of deep vaginal penetration.

Dyspareunia: Pain that occurs immediately before, during, or soon after intercourse.

Entry dyspareunia: Pain with initial penetration or attempts at penetration of the vaginal introitus; also called *introital dyspareunia.*

Generalized dyspareunia: Painful coitus that is not limited to a specific partner or situation.

Primary dyspareunia: Painful coitus that has been present from initial intercourse.

Secondary dyspareunia: Pain with coitus that is acquired after a period of pain-free intercourse.

Situational dyspareunia: Painful coitus with a specific situation, position, or possibly a particular partner.

INTRODUCTION

Dyspareunia is recurrent or persistent pain that occurs with intercourse and is often a component of the symptom complex of women with chronic pelvic pain (1). The etymology of the term stems from roots that mean difficult mating or badly mated. It is one of the most common sexual dysfunctions seen by clinicians and is estimated to affect about two-thirds of women at some point in their lifetime. Dyspareunia may be classified as generalized or situational and as primary or secondary. *Generalized dyspareunia* refers to painful coitus that is not limited to a specific partner or situation—in contrast to *situational,* which refers to dyspareunia with a specific situation, position, or possibly a particular partner. *Primary dyspareunia* refers to pain that has been present from initial intercourse, whereas *secondary dyspareunia* is pain that is acquired after a period of pain-free intercourse. Secondary dyspareunia occurs, on average, about 10 years after the onset of sexual activity. *Entry dyspareunia,* also termed introital dyspareunia, refers to pain with initial penetration of the vaginal introitus. *Deep dyspareunia* is painful intercourse with deep vaginal penetration. It is possible to have both entry and deep dyspareunia.

Dyspareunia is a biopsychosocial condition, so it is important that social, psychologic, and physical factors be considered when caring for women with this plight. It is important that the clinician not attempt to categorize dyspareunia into solely psychologic or physical etiologies. Even when a specific physical cause is identified, it is important for the clinician to remember that sexual response is a complex process that does not lend itself to quick fixes or oversimplification. Even when diagnosis and treatment are flawless, fear of pain and the presence of anxiety before and during intercourse can inhibit arousal and, due to lack of vaginal lubrication, lead to discomfort, such that the patient views the physician's efforts as having failed.

Although it is certainly possible to lead a healthy life and to have a successful and satisfying relationship as a couple without sexual intercourse, sex culminating with coitus is a basic part of the human experience of love and relationship for most individuals. Repetitive pain during intercourse can lead to anticipation of a negative sexual experience and eventually to markedly decreased sexual frequency or even sexual avoidance. It may also cause significant distress, anxiety, and interpersonal difficulties. Those clinicians who care for women with dyspareunia often observe that it is a significant component in the dissolution of the woman's marriage or relationship.

ETIOLOGY

There are a number of disorders that may cause or contribute to dyspareunia (Table 12.1). Many of these disorders are discussed in detail in other chapters of this text. Infection of the Bartholin gland, with or without abscess formation, may cause entry dyspareunia. Vulvovaginitis due to any of the many common vaginal pathogens, such as *Candida, Trichomonas, Herpes,* or *Gardnerella,* or due to contact dermatitis from to a topical irritant, such as over-the-counter vaginal sprays, douches, or contraceptive

TABLE 12.1.   CAUSES OF DYSPAREUNIA

Entry Dyspareunia	Deep Dyspareunia
Anal fissure	Adenomyosis
Bartholin gland infection or tumor	Endometriosis
	Fixed uterine retroversion
Bartholin duct obstruction	Inflammatory bowel disease
Chronic vulvitis	Interstitial cystitis
Contact vulvovaginitis	Irritable bowel syndrome
Episiotomy scar	Leiomyomas
Hemorrhoids	Ovarian pathology
Inadequate sexual arousal and lubrication	Pelvic adhesions
	Pelvic floor relaxation
Müllerian abnormality	Pelvic inflammatory disease
Posttraumatic pubic symphysis pain	Radiation-induced vaginal scarring
Rigid hymeneal ring	Shortened vagina
Urethral caruncle	Urethral syndrome
Urethral diverticulum	
Urethritis	
Vaginal atrophy	
Vaginismus	
Vulvar dystrophy	
Vulvar vestibulitis	
Vulvodynia	
Vulvovaginitis	

creams, are common causes of transient entry dyspareunia. Acute urethritis due to *Chlamydia* or *Gonorrhea* may also cause transient entry dyspareunia.

One of the most common causes of either primary or secondary, generalized dyspareunia is friction due to inadequate sexual arousal and lack of vaginal lubrication. Of course this becomes a vicious cycle as anticipated pain leads to lack of arousal, thus ensuring pain, and so on (Fig. 12.1). Another fairly common cause of chronic or generalized entry dyspareunia is vulvar vestibulitis syndrome. This is particularly common in women with chronic pelvic pain. It is a constellation of symptoms consisting of severe pain or burning on vestibular touch and attempted vaginal entry. In addition to dyspareunia, these patients may have pain with tampon insertion or with pressure, as, for example, from a bicycle seat. On examination, diffuse or focal vulvar erythema sometimes is noted around the orifices of the Bartholin, Skene, periurethral, or vestibular glands. In general, the cause of this syndrome is unknown, although it occasionally may be caused by an infection [subclinical human papillomavirus (HPV), bacterial vaginosis, chronic candidiasis] (2,3), irritants (soaps, detergents, douches, or vaginal sprays), or altered vaginal pH secondary to a decrease of lactobacilli. Vulvar vestibulitis may be iatrogenic secondary to treatment of HPV with podophyllin, trichloroacetic acid, or laser.

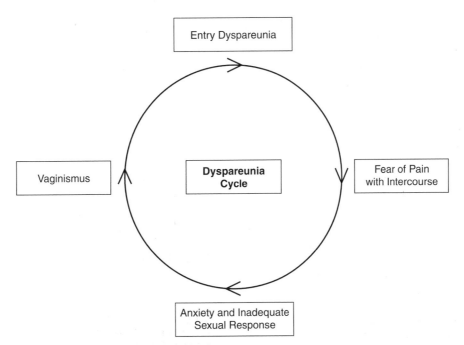

FIGURE 12.1. A simplified diagram of the type of cycle that can occur and result in persistent vaginismus and entry dyspareunia. Entry dyspareunia due to several possible organic or functional factors, many of them transient, can be the entry point to this cycle. Fear, anxiety, interpersonal conflicts, psychologic problems, and so on, may lead to inadequate sexual response, which may also lead to entry dyspareunia and be an entry point. Breaking this cycle with treatment may require interventions at all of the points in the cycle.

Pain secondary to episiotomy scar is another not infrequent cause of entry dyspareunia. It is not clear why in some women the episiotomy scar becomes hyperesthetic. Rigidity of the hymeneal ring may be similar in some ways, as in some women after initial disruption the hymen becomes taught and hyperesthetic. In postmenopausal women especially, atrophic changes of the vulva and vagina may lead to entry dyspareunia. Occasionally a similar process occurs postpartum. Vulvar and vaginal atrophy may also occur after radiation therapy and lead to dyspareunia.

Vaginismus is probably the most common cause of entry dyspareunia, affecting about 1% of women. It is characterized by recurrent or persistent involuntary contraction of the lower third of the vagina which prevents sexual intercourse when vaginal penetration is attempted. It can be global or situational. Vaginismus is an involuntary reflex precipitated by real or imagined attempts at vaginal penetration. Many women with vaginismus have normal sexual desire, experience normal vaginal lubrication, and are orgasmic, but cannot have intercourse. Vaginismus can be primary (the women has never been able to have intercourse) or secondary (often due to acquired dyspareunia). Some couples may cope with this difficulty for years before they decide to seek help. They usually seek treatment because they desire children or decide they would like to consummate their relationship. Vaginismus can be a conditioned response to an unpleasant experience such as past sexual abuse, a painful first pelvic examination, or a painful first attempt at intercourse, or it may be secondary to religious orthodoxy or sexual orientation concerns. Many women with vaginismus have an extreme fear of penetration and misconceptions about their anatomy and about the size of their vagina. They may believe that their vagina is too small to accommodate a tampon or penis, and that great physical harm will result from placing anything inside of them.

Medical conditions are rarely the cause of vaginismus, but conditions such as endometriosis, chronic pelvic inflammatory disease, partially imperforate hymen, and vaginal stenosis must be ruled out by a careful pelvic examination. The pelvic examination, which should be done if possible in the presence of the women's partner, allows the physician to help educate the couple about normal female anatomy and may help dispel misconceptions about the size of the introitus and vagina. Providing the patient with a mirror so she can observe the examination is helpful. Because the etiology of vaginismus is usually psychophysiologic, patients with this condition should not have surgery to enlarge their introitus unless they have a partially imperforate hymen or another valid indication for surgery.

Causes of midvaginal pain include a congenitally shortened vagina and interstitial cystitis, a chronic idiopathic inflammatory condition of the bladder. Midvaginal pain or deep dyspareunia may occasionally be due to stenosis or stricture after vaginal reconstructive surgery, especially combined anterior and posterior colporrhaphies.

Pain with orgasm may be associated with painful uterine contractions, which may in some patients be associated with adenomyosis, pelvic congestion syndrome, or endometriosis.

Dyspareunia with deep vaginal penetration can be associated with inadequate vaginal lengthening and lubrication secondary to inadequate sexual arousal, pregnancy, menopause, or the use of oral contraceptives. Chronic pelvic inflammatory disease, endometriosis, a fixed retroverted uterus, a pelvic mass, an enlarged uterus secondary to myomata or adenomyosis, inflammatory bowel disease, irritable bowel syndrome, or pelvic relaxation are also possible causes of deep dyspareunia.

Psychological factors contributing to dyspareunia include developmental factors, such as an upbringing that invested sex with guilt and shame; traumatic factors such as rape, childhood sexual abuse, or other sexual assault; and relationship factors such as anger or resentment toward a sexual partner or fear of pregnancy.

SYMPTOMS AND HISTORY

It is important to ask all women, including those with chronic pelvic pain (CPP), about their sexual activity (Table 12.2) (4,5). As a minimum the following three questions should be a routine part of the history: "Are you sexually active?"; "Are you having pain with intercourse?"; and "Do you have any problems or questions regarding your sexual activity?" These questions should be asked well into the interview, after some rapport has been established, so the woman will be comfortable talking about any problems she may be experiencing. Women often discuss their pain with their sexual partner, but fewer than half consult a physician about their dyspareunia. Many women with dyspareunia will not bring up the subject if not asked by the clinician.

As with all pain problems, in women with dyspareunia a thorough and extensive history, particularly directed to details about the pain symptom, is crucial. Information about onset, location, duration, severity, nature or quality of pain, particular positions or timing that cause it, any precipitating factors, any prior treatments, and any ameliorative factors should be sought. General, open-ended questions often are insufficient, and directed detailed questions must be asked. For example, it may be necessary to ask for the specific location on the vulva or in the vagina where the pain occurs, to ask if the pain occurs during foreplay, on

TABLE 12.2. THREE BASIC QUESTIONS REGARDING SEXUALITY THAT SHOULD BE ASKED FOR EVERY WOMAN WITH CHRONIC PELVIC PAIN

1. Are you sexually active?
2. Are you having pain with intercourse?
3. Do you have any problems or questions regarding your sexual activity?

penile entry, throughout intercourse, after intercourse, or only on deep thrusting, and to ask if the pain is always present or if there are times when intercourse is not painful. A complete chronology of the discomfort and an assessment of the impact of the dyspareunia on the patient and her partner should be obtained. Trying to make an accurate diagnosis as to the cause or causes of dyspareunia can be time-consuming.

The patient's understanding of sexual physiology and sexual behavior should also be assessed and any myths or misinformation addressed. Patients who are anxious about sexuality because of sexual misconceptions, guilt, fear of pregnancy or sexually transmitted disease, or prior unpleasant sexual experiences may be unable to relax during lovemaking, leading to impaired arousal and lubrication. Patients must be carefully and sensitively asked about a history of childhood sexual or physical abuse or adult sexual assault.

Significant problems in the couple's relationship or communication may also contribute to dyspareunia, so it is often helpful to interview the couple together. It can be useful to think of dyspareunia as a couple's problem, and couples often can provide useful clues about the etiology of the dysfunction. The patient's partner may pick an inconvenient time or may not spend enough time on foreplay for the patient to become adequately sexually aroused and lubricated. Or there may be conflicts about family size, contraception, sexual frequency, and sexual technique that may lead to anger, distrust, misunderstanding, depression, and ultimately pain.

Entry pain that involves the entire vulvar and introital area may suggest vulvitis, vulvar dystrophies, or vulvodynia. Usually there is associated pruritus or burning discomfort, even without coitus, with these problems. Entry dyspareunia that is concentrated only at the vaginal opening may suggest vulvar vestibulitis, vaginismus, inadequate lubrication, or vulvovaginitis. There may also be burning on vestibular touch and attempted vaginal entry. In addition to dyspareunia, patients with vestibulitis may have pain with tampon insertion or with pressure, as, for example, from a bicycle seat. With vaginismus, in addition to entry dyspareunia, there may be pelvic aching after intercourse and aggravation of this aching with prolonged sitting.

Dyspareunia related to chronic urethral syndrome, urethral diverticulitis, or interstitial cystitis is often difficult for the patient to localize by history. Dyspareunia associated with endometriosis, adhesive disease, or pelvic congestion syndrome is usually deep secondary dyspareunia and not infrequently is characterized by continued aching for hours or days after coitus. Postcoital aching pain is a particular characteristic of pelvic congestion syndrome (6). Women with pelvic floor pain syndrome often describe a tightness with coitus or a very uncomfortable pressure. The description that it feels like something is being run into or bumped with deep thrusting is often given by women with endometriosis, adhesive disease, symptomatic uterine retroversion, or adnexal pathology.

SIGNS AND PHYSICAL EXAMINATION

A careful and thorough physical examination to identify any possible factors contributing to the dyspareunia, no matter how subtle, is vital (Chapter 3) for a full description of the examination. It is important to rule out, insofar as possible, conditions such as endometriosis, chronic pelvic inflammatory disease, partially imperforate hymen, and vaginal stenosis by a thorough pelvic examination. However, sensitivity and gentleness are vital to obtaining meaningful information. Physiologic changes that occur during sexual arousal may account for pain that is present during intercourse, but absent during a pelvic examination. For example, a Bartholin gland cyst may swell during intercourse and cause pain but may be difficult or impossible to detect during the examination.

The physical examination should be done so as to educate the patient and also allow her to direct the evaluation. She should be examined while sitting slightly upright and should be given a hand mirror to observe the pelvic examination and to allow her to indicate the location of her pain. While performing the pelvic examination the physician should be sure the patient is instructed to report if pain is elicited and especially if the pain of intercourse is replicated by any of the portions of the examination. If possible, the pelvic examination should be done in the presence of the women's partner because this allows the physician to help educate the couple about normal female anatomy and may help dispel misconceptions about the size of the introitus and vagina.

Inspection of the external genitalia can identify ulcerations, erythema, or pigment changes. Diffuse or focal vulvar erythema sometimes is noted around the orifices of the Bartholin, Skene, periurethral, or vestibular glands. In general, the cause of this syndrome is unknown, although it occasionally may be caused by an infection (subclinical HPV, bacterial vaginosis, chronic candidiasis), irritants (soaps, detergents, douches, or vaginal sprays), or altered vaginal pH secondary to a decrease of lactobacilli. Erythema at the vestibular glands is sometimes observed with vulvar vestibulitis, which is usually iatrogenic, but can be secondary to treatment of HPV with podophyllin, trichloracetic acid, or laser. Palpation with a moist cotton-tipped swab can identify exquisitely tender sites at the vestibule in patients with vulvar vestibulitis. This simple "Q-tip test" should be performed on all patients with dyspareunia (Fig. 12.2). Biopsy of these lesions are not helpful as yet, and they cause these patients unnecessary emotional and physical trauma.

Colposcopy with application of 5% acetic acid may help identify abnormal areas on the vulva and introitus, particu-

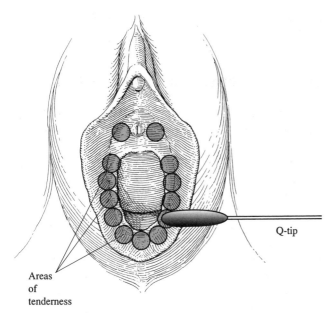

Areas
of
tenderness

FIGURE 12.2. The "Q-tip test" is a valuable component of the physical evaluation for vulvar vestibulitis and should be a routine part of the examination in women with dyspareunia. A moistened or dry cotton-tipped applicator is used to gently palpate the entire vulva and vestibule. In patients with vulvar vestibulitis syndrome the areas of the openings of the minor vestibular glands, illustrated in this figure by the circles, are very tender with a burning or painful sensation when palpated with the applicator, whereas the remainder of the vulva is not abnormally tender. Skene's glands are also tender in many women (represented in this diagram by the upper circles that are lateral to the urethra).

larly condylomas, papillary areas, punctation, and acetowhite changes, but is not necessary routinely.

The vagina should be gently and carefully examined with one finger, checking for any scars from previous surgery or an episiotomy, any specific areas of tenderness at hymeneal remnants, and any involuntary spasm of the muscles of the introitus or the levator sling. Having the patient contract the muscles of her pelvic floor (Kegel exercises) while the examiner places a finger inside her vagina helps assess the tone of the pelvic floor and helps identify these muscles as a possible source of the dyspareunia. Stroking the anterior vagina under the bladder base and urethra may reproduce pain caused by trigonitis, interstitial cystitis, chronic urethritis, or a urethral diverticulum.

A speculum examination should be done, at which time cervical cultures and smear, along with vaginal secretions for wet-mount examination, are obtained. If cervical cytology is needed, it is important to remember to not use any lubricant in the vagina prior to the speculum examination. The vagina and cervix should be visually assessed for atrophy or ulcers. Also the vagina, cervix, and paracervical areas should be evaluated for tenderness. This can be readily done using a cotton-tip applicator (Q-tip) to carefully palpate all areas for tenderness, particularly any that produce pain that is similar to the patient's dyspareunia.

A careful, thorough, and systematic abdominal, low back, and pelvic examination should be carried out seeking evidence of any pelvic pathology that may be contributing to CPP and dyspareunia. This is fully described in Chapter 3.

LABORATORY AND IMAGING STUDIES

It is essential that specific infectious causes of painful intercourse be ruled out. This requires vaginal cultures, urine cultures, vaginal wet preps, and vaginal pH. Testing for sexually transmitted diseases should also be done with urethral and cervical gonorrhea cultures and chlamydial polymerase chain reaction (PCR) testing (which can also be done on urine). These tests for infectious etiologies are advisable in almost all cases. Biopsies of the vulva are indicated if vulvar dystrophy is suspected.

Other laboratory and imaging tests are dependent on the historic and physical findings. For example, if chronic urethral syndrome is suspected, then urodynamic testing and urethroscopy are indicated. If an endometrioma or endometriosis is suspected, then ultrasonography and laparoscopy may be indicated. Cystoscopy is needed if interstitial cystitis is possible.

MANAGEMENT AND TREATMENT
Medical Treatment

Details of treatment of many of the diseases that cause or contribute to dyspareunia are given in the appropriate chapters elsewhere in this text, so only some general points about treatment will be discussed in this chapter. An important component of the treatment of the patient with dyspareunia is providing her and her partner information about sexual physiology and behavior. This may involve specific reeducation regarding the couple's sexual attitudes and practices. A common example of this is the woman with dyspareunia secondary to inadequate vaginal lubrication because of inhibited sexual desire or inadequate time of foreplay. For both of these problems the couple can be given general information about the genital anatomy and the physiology of the sexual response. Consistent with cultural sensitivies, specific suggestions can be offered about prolonging foreplay, improving communication, using water-soluble lubricants during intercourse, having the patient and her partner stimulate her clitoris before and during intercourse, and using fantasy to improve desire and response.

Vaginismus, in many cases, represents a conditioned response with no other direct etiology for the dyspareunia. Behavioral treatment of this type of vaginismus is directed toward extinguishing the conditioned involuntary vaginal spasm. This is initiated by helping the woman become more familiar with her anatomy and by demonstrating to her (and her partner) the vaginal muscular contraction at the time of pelvic examination. She is then instructed in the use of Kegel exercises to gain control over the muscles surrounding her introitus and is specifically taught to relax the bulbocavernosus and levator ani muscles. She is specifically instructed to use these techniques to help her relax when she anticipates vaginal penetration. Next she is instructed on the use of graduated vaginal dilators (fingers can also be used as dilators).

The protocol for use of the dilators is explained to the patient while she is in the office, but the actual placement of the dilators is done by the patient at home. It is important for the patient to maintain total control over the use of the dilators and to use them in an environment that is comfortable and safe. Best results seem to be obtained if intercourse is forbidden during this portion of the treatment. The dilators should be covered with a warm, water-soluble lubricant such as K-Y Jelly. She should initially try to place the dilators (or her finger) in her vagina when she is alone and relaxed. If she cannot relax enough to place the smallest dilator in her vagina, she may be able to reduce her anxiety by learning relaxation or self-hypnosis techniques. Medications such as propranolol or alprazolam may occasionally be needed to help reduce anxiety. Once she has been able to place the smallest dilator in her vagina, she can progressively insert the larger dilators, practicing Kegel exercises while they are in place. When she is comfortable inserting the larger dilators, she can instruct her partner how to place the dilators in her vagina while she maintains control over how quickly they are placed. She may then be ready to proceed to intercourse. Again, this must be under her control, with her sitting or kneeling over her partner and inserting his penis herself. The majority of couples who follow this protocol are successful and able to have intercourse (7,8). As part of this therapy the patient should be helped to be more comfortable with her sexuality. In some cases there may be unresolved conflicts involving sexuality or relationships that must be addressed before successful treatment can be accomplished (9).

The treatment of dyspareunia due to *pelvic floor myalgia* is twofold. First find and treat any persistent tissue injury that may be triggering the spasm (for example, endometriosis or interstitial cystitis). Second, begin muscle retraining with physical therapy. Patients can be instructed to perform pubococcygeus and piriformis stretching. Biofeedback may be useful in alleviating painful vestibulitis and vaginismus. Heat, exercise, and trigger point injections are also helpful adjuncts to full recovery. In addition to treating physical problems, the physician can assign the patient and her partner behavior therapy exercises they can practice at home. These exercises can help desensitize the patient to the discomfort she may anticipate with vaginal penetration and help her extinguish the learned pain response to intercourse. Suggested exercises might include assigned readings, progressive sexual fantasies, instruction in deep muscle relaxation, and couple pleasuring exercises ("sensate focus"). As in the treatment of vaginismus, Kegel exercises and the use of graduated vaginal dilators can help the patient overcome her discomfort. Once the patient has gained voluntary control over her levator muscles, she may want to proceed to intercourse, eventually incorporating sexual responsiveness and a variety of coital positions into lovemaking.

Vaginal atrophy secondary to natural or surgical menopause responds to systemic or vaginal estrogen replacement. Also, Kegel exercises may be beneficial with this condition, because they help the patient improve control of her vaginal muscles and increase the elasticity of the vaginal canal. *Vaginal strictures* or *vaginal shortening* following surgery or radiation therapy can be treated with estrogen vaginal cream and progressive dilatation of the vagina with vaginal dilators.

Treatment of the *vulvar dystrophies* is based on diagnosis by biopsy. They are generally responsive to long-term treatment with potent topical corticosteroids, such as clobetasol cream. Testosterone ointment, a long-standing treatment for lichen sclerosus, has been shown in randomized clinical trials to be no more efficacious than the ointment base alone and not as effective as clobetasol, and it is no longer recommended for treatment (10–12).

Patients with dyspareunia related to *chronic or recurrent vulvovaginitis* should be thoroughly and accurately evaluated, and any specific pathogens or etiologic agents should be identified using vaginal cultures, wet preps, and vaginal pH. Treatment should then be specifically directed to the etiologic agent. In many cases, a specific organism is not found, but the patient may often be able to decrease symptoms or recurrences by changing some hygienic habits. Perfumed soap for baths or showers, use of soap in her vaginal area, douches, vaginal sprays, or scented tampons should be avoided. Wearing cotton underwear and loose-fitting clothing may help. Because many chemicals can be irritating to the vulvar skin, it may take some detective work to identify an inciting agent, especially with cases of vulvitis.

Treating *vulvar vestibulitis* can be difficult (13). Patients often have other types of pelvic pain such as severe dysmenorrhea, endometriosis, interstitial cystitis, vaginismus, abdominal wall trigger points, or painful adhesions. This lends credence to the belief of a neuropathic etiology of vestibulitis with central nervous system sensitization of peripheral nerve endings. In this case, segmental hyperesthesia of the pudendal nerve (S_{2-4}), which is the main innervation of the vestibule, may be produced by the other chronic pelvic pain. This may be at least a partial explanation for the difficulty of obtaining ideal results from treatment. Treatments of vestibulitis may be oral, topical, injectable, or surgical. Treatment should start with the least invasive, with least adverse effects, and progress to more invasive only as needed.

Based on the belief that vestibulitis is associated with calcium oxalate crystals, many women try dietary supplementation with calcium citrate and avoidance of dietary oxalate (14). While calcium citrate and dietary modification can reduce urinary oxalate absorption and excretion, the theory of sharp oxalate crystals causing severe burning on contact with the vestibule cannot be scientifically verified, despite numerous patient testimonials (15,16). There are no apparent adverse effects from this treatment, however, so a 3-month trial seems reasonable if this is what the patient wishes.

Medical treatment protocols usually begin with low-dose tricyclic antidepressants. Amitriptyline doses as low as 10 mg per day may be sufficient to give good relief. Doses may be increased if response is inadequate, but patients often cannot tolerate the dry mouth, constipation, drowsiness, and weight gain of higher doses. Many patients with vestibulitis are depressed, and it is important to treat this aggressively when present. The selective serotonin reuptake inhibitors seem well-tolerated and can be used in addition to low-dose tricyclic antidepressant therapy.

Topical treatment is sometimes helpful. Acyclovir ointment is a safe initial topical treatment. It is massaged into the tender vestibular areas by the patient twice a day for a month. If there is improvement, then acyclovir is continued with frequent reevaluations until cure or failure is apparent. Second-line topical treatment is with corticosteroids. Sometimes a combination, with a compounded gel of ketoprofen, carbamazepine, 5% lidocaine, and amitriptyline, used four to six times a day, is a better alternative than corticosteroid alone. Topical 5-flurouracil has also been tried, but it has significant potential for adverse reactions. One tablespoonful is left on the vestibule for 2 hours twice a week. Patients must be instructed to not leave it on the vestibule for more than 2 hours, to wash thoroughly after the 2-hour application, and to skip doses if soap and water begin to burn. They should set a timer so as not to exceed 2 hours. Follow-up is the same as for acyclovir. Topical capsaicin has also been used, but it also has the potential to cause significant topical vulvitis (17).

If topical therapy proves ineffective, intralesional injection of 20 mg of triamcinolone (0.5 mL of triamcinolone solution mixed with 0.5 mL of 0.5% bupivicane) may be tried. Before all vestibular injections, benzocaine ointment is applied for 15 minutes to decrease the pain of injections as much as possible. Patients are asked to return in 2 weeks to evaluate response. If improvement is noted injections may be repeated up to three times every 2 weeks for maximum resolution. Another injectable therapy is alpha-interferon. It may be injected at 1, 3, 4, 8, 9, and 11 o'clock at a total dose of 2.5 million units (1 mL) in divided doses twice a week for 4 weeks. Remapping of the vestibule is done before the eighth injection. If improvement is noted, the treatment is repeated once a week for 4 weeks. It seems wisest to reserve surgical treatment for vestibulitis to those

patients with severe dyspareunia who do not respond to medical management.

Complicated patients, those with marital problems, those with signficant psychosocial difficulties, and those who do not respond to basic interventions may require intensive individual or couple therapy with a therapist who specializes in sexual dysfunction. Patients who are sexual abuse survivors and those who have significant anxiety or depression, sexual aversion, or significant marital dysfunction should also be treated by an appropriate specialist and therapist.

Surgical Treatment

Surgical treatment specific to diseases that may be the cause of deep dyspareunia, such as endometriosis, adhesions, symptomatic uterine retroversion, or pelvic congestion syndrome, is sometimes appropriate and therapeutic. The surgical treatment of endometriosis is described elsewhere, but improvement or worsening of dyspareunia can be a guide to the success or failure of treatment. With laparoscopic lysis of pelvic adhesions, many patients note improvement in chronic pelvic pain and dyspareunia. Laparoscopy can also be used to diagnose and treat adnexal masses and to suspend a fixed, retroverted uterus. These surgical procedures are discussed elsewhere in this text. However, a technically elegant technique for laparoscopic uterine suspension, developed by Carter and used to treat patients with deep dyspareunia that appears to be secondary to a retroverted uterus, is illustrated in Fig. 12.3.

Vulvar surgery is occasionally appropriate in the treatment of entry or introital dyspareunia. For example, perineoplasty to release stenosis of the introitus due to *postoperative stricture* after posterior colpoperineorrhaphy or episiotomy is sometimes beneficial. Rarely, excision of one or both *Bartholin glands* may be appropriate in cases of dyspareunia secondary to tenderness localized to these glands (18,19). Dyspareunia due to scarring or rigidity and tenderness of the *hymenal remnants* may justify surgical excision of part or all of the hymenal ring in rare circumstances (20). Surgery to treat vulvar vestibulitis syndrome is also indicated in appropriately selected cases.

The most common surgical treatment of *vulvar vestibulitis* is vestibulectomy, in which the vestibule is excised and the vaginal tissue is advanced to cover the defect (Fig. 12.4) (21,22). In observational studies, success rates as high as 95% have been reported, but with long-term follow-up success rates are 70% to 90% (23,24). Baggish has suggested that the Bartholin glands be removed at the time of vestibulectomy and that the CO_2 laser may be used for excision of the vestibule and Bartholins (25). However, anecdotal experience with pudendal neuralgia after laser application to the vulva has caused concern. Bornstein and Abramovici (26) has suggested that long-term failures can be decreased by either extending the excision of vestibular tissue above the urethra or by injecting this area with alpha-

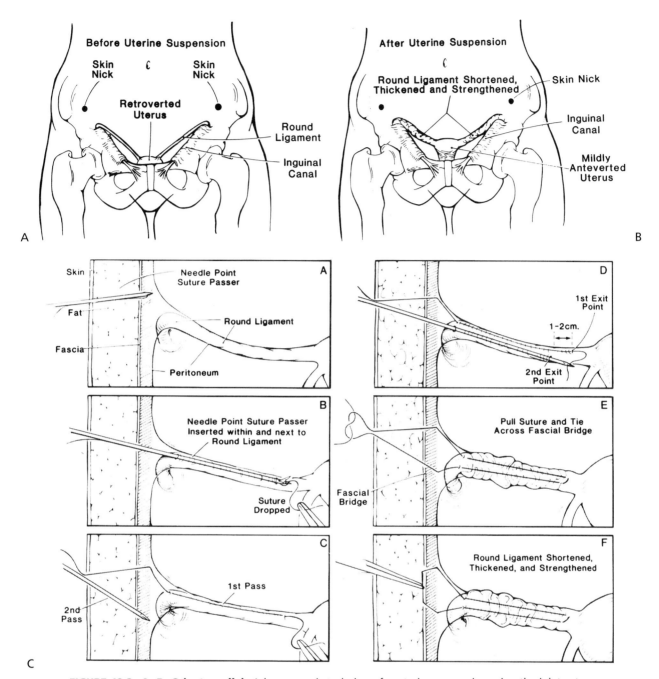

FIGURE 12.3. A, B, C (externally): A laparoscopic technique for uterine suspension using the inlet suture passer and referred to by the acronym UPLIFT (*u*terine suspension and *p*ositioning by *li*gament *i*nvestment, *f*ix-ation, and *t*runcation).

interferon. It is clear that vestibulectomy is effective, but should probably be a treatment of last resort. At least two characteristics appear to be predictive of higher failure rates with vestibulectomy: (a) If there is constant vulvar pain, not just pain with intercourse, and (b) if dyspareunia has been present since the first episode of coitus (23). If the patient is so unfortunate as to fail vestibulectomy, few options remain (27). Neuroma formation is a feared complication

of this procedure and remains one of the most difficult challenges.

Finally, it is worth restating that when evaluating and treating patients with dyspareunia, clinicians should be aware that psychologic, physical, and relationship factors all contribute to this condition. After a careful and systemic physical examination, developmental, personal, interpersonal, and relationship issues should be explored. It is

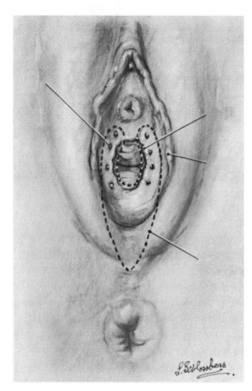

FIGURE 12.4. The minor vestibular glands exit lateral to the hymenal ring. They are very superficial and thus seldom produce definable "nodules," even when chronically infected.

important to help the patient set realistic goals and expectations for treatment and to realize that treatment is an ongoing process that may require more than one treatment approach. Most patients with primary and secondary dyspareunia improve when treated by an interested, empathetic, and knowledgeable clinician.

KEY POINTS

Most Important Questions to Ask

- Are you sexually active?
- Are you having pain with intercourse?
- Do you have any problems or questions regarding your sexual activity?
- When did pain with intercourse start?
- Where does it hurt?
- When during sexual activity does it hurt? Before? At entry? During? With deep thrusting? After?
- How much does it hurt?
- What type of pain do you have? Describe how it feels?
- Are there particular positions or particular times that intercourse hurts?
- Are there any specific factors that seem to consistently cause pain?
- Are there any things you can do that decrease the pain?

- What treatments, whether self-treatments or prescribed by a healthcare provider, have you tried? What was the result of the treatment?
- Are there any significant problems in your relationship with your partner?
- Have you ever or are you now being abused, physically or sexually?

Most Important Physical Examination Findings

- Hand mirror evaluation by patient during the pelvic examination, especially external examination
- Tender sites that replicate the pain with intercourse
- External genital, vaginal, or cervical ulcerations, erythema, or pigment changes
- Diffuse or focal vulvar erythema especially around the orifices of the Bartholin, Skene, periurethral, or vestibular glands
- Abnormal vaginal discharge suggestive of infection or inflammation
- Tenderness of the minor vestibule with the "Q-tip test"
- Trigger or tender points of the vaginal or pelvic musculature

Most Important Diagnostic Studies

- Vaginal cultures
- Urine cultures
- Vaginal wet preps
- Vaginal pH
- Testing for sexually transmitted diseases
- Biopsies of the vulva if vulvar dystrophy is suspected

Treatments

- Specific reeducation regarding the couple's sexual attitudes and practices
- Education about sexual anatomy, physiology, and behavior
- Kegel exercises
- Graduated vaginal dilators
- Use of water-soluble lubricants
- Systemic or vaginal estrogen replacement
- Treatment of the vulvar dystrophies with topical corticosteroids
- Specific treatment of chronic or recurrent vulvovaginitis
- Avoidance of perfumed soaps, douches, vaginal sprays, or scented tampons
- Wearing of cotton underwear and loose-fitting clothing
- Treatment of vestibulitis with:
  Calcium citrate and avoidance of dietary oxalate
  Tricyclic antidepressants
  Topical treatment with acyclovir ointment, corticosteroids, 5% lidocaine, 5-flurouracil, or capsaicin

Injection of triamcinolone or alpha-interferon

- Individual or couple treatment with a therapist who specializes in sexual dysfunction
- Surgical treatment specific to diseases that may be the cause of deep dyspareunia
- Perineoplasty (for introital stricture)
- Excision of one or both Bartholin glands (for tumor, obstruction, inflammation)
- Surgical excision of part or all of the hymenal ring (for scarring and pain of hymenal remnant)
- Vestibulectomy (for vulvar vestibulitis)

REFERENCES

1. Steege JF, Ling FW. Dyspareunia. *Obstet Gynecol Clin North Am* 1993;20:779–793.
2. Bornstein J, Shapiro S, Rahat M, et al. Polymerase chain reaction search for viral etiology of vulvar vestibulitis syndrome. *Am J Obstet Gynecol* 1996;175:139–144.
3. Bazin S, Bouchard C, Brisson J, et al. Vulvar vestibulitis syndrome: an exploratory case-control study. *Obstet Gynecol* 1994;83:47–50.
4. Plouffe L. Screening for sexual problems through a simple questionnaire. *Am J Obstet Gynecol* 1985;151:166–169.
5. Bachmann GA, Leibleum SR, Grill J. Brief sexual inquiry in gynecology practice. *Obstet Gynecol* 1989;73:425–427.
6. Beard RW, Reginald PW, Wadsworth J. Clinical features of women with chronic lower abdominal pain and pelvic congestion. *Br J Obstet Gynaecol* 1988;95:153–161.
7. Lamont J. Vaginismus. *Am J Obstet Gynecol* 1978;131:632–636.
8. Robinson C, Reich L, Piar G, et al. The office management of sexual problems: brief therapy approaches. *J Reprod Med* 1975;15:127–144.
9. Scholl GM. Prognostic variables in treating vaginismus. *Obstet Gynecol* 1988;72:231–235.
10. Cattaneo A, Carli P, DeMarco A, et al. Testosterone maintenance therapy. Effects on vulvar lichen sclerosus treated with clobetasol propionate. *J Reprod Med* 1996;41:99–102.
11. Sideri M, Origoni M, Spinaci L, et al. Topical testosterone in the treatment of vulvar lichen sclerosus. *Int J Gynaecol Obstet* 1994;46:53–56.
12. Bracco GL, Carli P, Sonni L, et al. Clinical and histologic effects of topical treatments of vulval lichen sclerosus. A critical evaluation. *J Reprod Med* 1993;38:37–40.
13. Marinoff SC, Turner MLC. Vulvar vestibulitis syndrome: an overview. *Am J Obstet Gynecol* 1991;165:1228–1233.
14. Solomons CC, Melmed MH, Heitler SM. Calcium citrate for vulvar vestibulitis: a case report. *J Reprod Med* 1991;36:879–882.
15. Massey LK, Roman-Smith H, Sutton RAL. Effect of dietary oxalate and calcium on urinary oxalate and risk of formation of calcium oxalate kidney stones. *J Am Diet Assoc* 1993;93:901–906.
16. Baggish MS, Sze EHM, Johnson R. Urinary oxalate excretion and its role in vulvar pain syndrome. *Am J Obstet Gynecol* 1997;177:507–511. Baggish MS, Sze EHM, Johnson R. Urinary oxalate excretion and its role in vulvar pain syndrome. *Am J Obstet Gynecol* 1997;177:507–511.
17. Friedrich EG Jr. Therapeutic studies on vulvar vestibulitis. *J Reprod Med* 1988;33:514–518.
18. Sarrel PM, Steege JF, Maltzer M, et al. Pain during sex response due to occlusion of the Bartholin gland duct. *Obstet Gynecol* 1983;62:261–264.
19. Mindsager NT, Young TW. Pain during sexual response due to bilateral Bartholin's gland adenomas. A case report. *J Reprod Med* 1992;37:983–985.
20. Grillo L, Grillo D. Management of dyspareunia secondary to hymenal remnants. *Obstet Gynecol* 1979;56:510–514.
21. Woodruff JD, Parmley TH. Infection of the minor vestibular gland. *Obstet Gynecol* 1983;62:609–612.
22. Bornstein J, Goldik Z, Alter Z, et al. Persistent vulvar vestibulitis: the continuing challenge. *Obstet Gynecol Surv* 1997;53:39–44.
23. Bornstein J, Goldik Z, Stolar Z, et al. Predicting the outcome of surgical treatment of vulvar vestibulitis. *Obstet Gynecol* 1997;89:695–698.
24. Mann MS, Kaufman RH, Brown D, et al. Vulvar vestibulitis: significant clinical variables and treatment outcome. *Obstet Gynecol* 1992;79:122–125.
25. Baggish MS, Miklos JR. Vulvar pain syndrome: a review. *Obstet Gynecol Surv* 1995;50:618–627.
26. Bornstein J, Abramovici H. Combination of subtotal perineoplasty and interferon for the treatment of vulvar vestibulitis. *Gynecol Obstet Invest* 1997;44:53–56.
27. Bornstein J, Goldik Z, Alter Z, et al. Persistent vulvar vestibulitis: the continuing challenge. *Obstet Gynecol Surv* 1997;53:39–44.

13

ENDOCERVICAL AND ENDOMETRIAL POLYPS

JAMES E. CARTER

KEY TERMS AND DEFINITIONS

Endocervical polyps: Pedunculated tumorous formations at the surface of the cervix which are a hyperplastic phenomenon of the epithelium and stroma rather than a true neoplasm.

Endometrial polyps: Pedunculated tumorous formations of the endometrium which are a hyperplastic phenomenon of the epithelium and stroma rather than a true neoplasm.

INTRODUCTION

Cervical polyps are hyperplastic tumor-like formations of the cervix formed of epithelium and stroma. They are not true neoplasms. They are pedunculated, roughly pear-shaped, soft, smooth, and red or purple, and they vary from a few millimeters to 3 cm long. The pedicle almost always rises from the cervical canal but occasionally may arise from the external surface of the cervix (1). In most cases cervical polyps project beyond the external os.

Cervical polyps are found in about 4% of all routine gynecologic exams (2). In a study of age distribution, 2% occurred in patients less than 30 years of age, 18%, age 31 to 40; 34%, age 41 to 50; 28%, age 51 to 60; 10%, age 61 to 70; and 8%, age 70 to 81 (3).

Endometrial polyps are found in up to 27% of patients who have a cervical polyp (4). This is notably higher than the 7% prevalence of endometrial polyps in women without a cervical polyp. In menopausal patients endometrial polyps are found in 57% of patients who have an apparent cervical polyp. All cervical polyps present during tamoxifen treatment have been found to be associated with endometrial polyps (5). Premenopausal patients taking combined oral contraceptives are the least likely to have coexistent endometrial polyps (5). Cervical polyps are a strong independent risk factor for endometrial polyps (2).

ETIOLOGY

The etiology of cervical polyps is not known, but the fact that they are more frequent in multigravidas speaks in favor of traumatic or inflammatory irritation of the endocervical mucosa leading to their growth (6). Abnormal local responsiveness to hormonal stimulation or a localized vascular congestion of cervical blood vessels could also be a cause of focal hyperplasia of the glandular epithelium. Because cervical polyps are often associated with endometrial hyperplasia, this adds further support to the theory that high levels of estrogen may have a significant etiologic role (7).

PATHOLOGY

Polyps consist of stroma and endocervical glands and are covered by columnar mucus-secreting epithelium that may be replaced by metaplastic squamous epithelium. The histologic picture varies depending on the amount and type of the stroma and the glands. Inflammation and superficial ulceration are common features of endocervical polyps (6). Microscopically, polyps are found to be a hyperplastic condition of the endocervical epithelium. They usually have a large number of blood vessels, especially near the surface. They are frequently edematous and inflamed (1). The development of dysplasia and *in situ* or invasive carcinoma in a polyp occurs in less than 1% of cases (5).

SYMPTOMS OR HISTORY

In 60% of women with cervical polyps the finding is incidental and is made during a routine examination. About 40% of women with cervical polyps are symptomatic. Menometrorrhagia occurs in 40%, postmenopausal bleeding in 30%, postcoital bleeding in 12%, and abnormal vaginal discharge in 18% of patients. Eleven percent of patients have had a previous dilatation and curettage for the same indication in the past (3). Cervical polyp is one of the most common causes of intermenstrual vaginal bleeding (3). Occasionally, women with endocervical polyps present with dysmenorrhea or with intermittent cramping pelvic pain.

PHYSICAL EXAMINATION

The examination of a woman with endocervical or endometrial polyps is generally normal other than the presence of a polyp at the cervical os. The polyp is often felt during bimanual examination, but in some patients it may not be evident until speculum examination is performed (1). Sometimes mucus or blood obscures the polyp, so the cervix should be completely cleared after cytology and culture specimens are obtained. Rarely, the polyp or the cervix is tender to palpation, and less often the uterus may be tender.

DIAGNOSTIC STUDIES

All menopausal patients with a cervical polyp would benefit from a diagnostic hysteroscopy (5). Sonohysterography is very effective in distinguishing endometrial thickening from endometrial polyps (8) and, in the presence of a cervical polyp, will usually demonstrate the presence of an associated endometrial polyp. Conventional transvaginal sonography will sometimes miss an endometrial polyp (9). If polypectomy alone is performed in asymptomatic patients, endometrial polyps may be missed in up to about one-third of premenopausal patients (4). This is even more significant in postmenopausal patients in whom hyperplasia of the polyp or the endometrium is often associated with cervical and endometrial polyps. In patients with cervical polyps who are asymptomatic, malignant endometrial pathology has not been discovered, so the safest and least destructive evaluation using cervical polypectomy and endometrial biopsy is recommended (4). In patients with cervical polyps who are symptomatic, significant endometrial pathology has been found in about 8%. This includes endometrial adenocarcinoma as well as endometrial polyps with atypical hyperplasia. Therefore in patients who are symptomatic with cervical polyps, hysteroscopy, curettage, and cervical polypectomy are all appropriate (4). Vaginal sonography, two-dimensional hysterosonography, and three-dimensional hysterosonography are also appropriate when combined with endometrial sampling (8–10).

Menorrhagia and leukorrhea are the chief symptoms of cervical polyps, but they are often asymptomatic.

DIAGNOSES

The final diagnosis depends on the histology of the polyp after its removal. In one series of 127 cases of asymptomatic cervical polyps, 90% were benign, and in 223 symptomatic patients with polyps, 82% were benign (4).

Other diagnoses thought to be cervical polyps are blood clots, leiomyomas, endometrial carcinoma, and endometrial polyps (3). Müllerian adenosarcoma also has presented as a benign cervical polyp (11).

MANAGEMENT OR TREATMENT

The treatment of polyps is usually simple. If the polyp is large, a clamp can be applied approximately 0.5 cm above the origin of the pedicle. A surgical ligature should be tied between the clamp and the cervix, and then the clamp can be removed. The polyp can be excised by cutting along the line of the crush. All tissue removed should be sent for pathologic review, because a malignancy can arise in these benign-appearing structures in up to 2% of cases (3). The cervical canal can be dilated after removal of the body of the polyp to allow destruction of the base of the polyp by electrocautery or laser vaporization (1). Excessive bleeding requiring hospitalization occurs in 3% of patients at the time of removal of cervical polyps (3).

Removal of cervical polyps as an outpatient procedure is recommended for the asymptomatic patient. Polypectomy and endometrial sampling are recommended for the symptomatic patient. Endometrial polyps found by sonography, hysterosonography, or hysteroscopy should be removed in symptomatic patients.

KEY POINTS
Differential Diagnosis

- Müllerian adenosarcoma
- Endometrial polyp
- Blood clots
- Leiomyoma

Most Important Questions to Ask

- Has the patient had a previous polypectomy?
- Is the patient experiencing bleeding or discharge?

Most Important Physical Examination Findings

- Visualization of the polyp

Most Important Diagnostic Studies

- Histologic evaluation of the polyp
- Endometrial biopsy
- Sonography

- Hysterosonography
- Hysteroscopy

Treatments

- Removal

REFERENCES

1. DiSaia PJ. Disorders of the uterine cervix. In: Scott JR, DiSaia PJ, Hammond CB, et al., eds. *Danforth Obstetrics and Gynecology.* Philadelphia: JP Lippincott, 1994:892–924.
2. Vilodre LF, Bertat R, Petters R, et al. Cervical polyp as risk factor for hysteroscopically diagnosed endometrial polyps. *Gynecol Obstet Invest* 1997;44:191–195.
3. Golan A, Ber A, Wolman I, et al. Cervical polyp: evaluation of current treatment. *Gynecol Obstet Invest* 1994;37:56–58.
4. Coeman D, Van Belle Y, Vanderick G, et al. Hysteroscopic findings in patients with a cervical polyp. *Am J Obstet Gynecol* 1993; 169:1563–1565.
5. Aaro LH, Jacobson LJ, Soule EH. Endocervical polyps. *Obstet Gynecol* 1963;21:659–665.
6. Bychkov V, Isaacs JH. *Pathology in the practice of gynecology.* St Louis: Mosby, 1995:133.
7. Pradhan S, Chenoy R, O'Brien PMS. Dilatation and curettage in patients with cervical polyps: a retrospective analysis. *Br J Obstet Gynecol* 1995;102:415–417.
8. Cohen JR, Luxman D, Sagi J, et al. Sonohysterography for distinguishing endometrial thickening from endometrial polyps in postmenopausal bleeding. *Ultrasound Obstet Gynecol* 1994;4: 227–230.
9. Bonilla-Musoles F, Raga F, Osborne NG, et al. Three-dimensional hysterosonography for the study of endometrial tumors: comparison with conventional transvaginal sonography, hysterosalpingo-sonography, and hysteroscopy. *Gynecol Oncol* 1997; 65:245–252.
10. Van Den Bosch T, Vandendael A, Van Schoubroeck DV, et al. Combing vaginal ultrasonography and office endometrial sampling in the diagnosis of endometrial disease in postmenopausal women. *Obstet Gynecol* 1995;85(3):349–352.
11. Kerner H, Lichtig C. Mullerian adenosarcoma presenting as cervical polyps: a report of seven cases and a review of the literature. *Obstet Gynecol* 1993;81:655–659.

14

ENDOMETRIOSIS AND ENDOSALPINGIOSIS

FRED M. HOWARD

KEY TERMS AND DEFINTIONS

Atypical endometriosis: Usually red or clear papular lesions, which are generally superficial new lesions that produce prostanglandins and which are exposed to peritoneal fluid and can cause functional pain symptoms, like dysmenorrhea.

Endometriosis: The presence of ectopic endometrial glands and stroma.

Endosalpingiosis: The presence of ectopic tubal epithelium.

Metaplasia of coelomic epithelium: Induced change (metaplasia) of any areas of coelomic epithelium, the type of epithelium from which the müllerian duct is derived, that can result in conversion to endometriosis.

Sampson's theory: That endometriosis is due to retrograde flow of menstrual effluent through the fallopian tubes into the peritoneal cavity.

Typical endometriosis: The black-brown, black, or puckered black stellate scar lesions that are classically recognized as endometriosis and probably cause pain by the formation of cystic nodules, scar tissue, and fibrotic infiltration, which generate nociceptor stimulation by mechanical pressure or by stretching tissue.

INTRODUCTION

Endometriosis is the presence of ectopic endometrial glands and stroma—that is, endometrium located outside of the endometrial cavity. It has been found in numerous locations (Table 14.1). The name "endometriosis" was first applied to ectopic endometrium by Sampson in 1921 (1–3). Although a monumental amount has been written about endometriosis since Sampson's landmark papers, there is still a great deal about it that is unclear and controversial, and it remains an enigmatic disorder in that the etiology, the natural history, and the precise mechanisms by which it causes pain are not completely understood (4). In some patients it

behaves almost like a malignancy, yet in others it is a seemingly irrelevant and insignificant finding; in some it is associated with incapacitating symptoms, but in others it is just an incidental histologic diagnosis; and in some cases it recurs "like dandelions in the grass," while in others excision results in its total and permanent elimination. It is truly a disease of contrasting characteristics (Table 14.2).

The prevalence of endometriosis in the general population is believed to be 1% to 7% (5,6). Because it is accurately diagnosed only by surgical biopsy with histologic confirmation, the true prevalence and incidence of endometriosis have been difficult to determine. In many women with patent fallopian tubes, it may be a normal consequence of menses, rather than a "disease" (7). Yet in some of these women it becomes a progressive process that results in symptoms and is rightly considered a disease. Currently, there are no prospective criteria to identify which women are at risk for progression (8).

In women who undergo a laparoscopy to evaluate chronic pelvic pain (CPP), the prevalence of endometriosis is about 33% (Table 5.5) (9). In patients undergoing laparoscopy for infertility, the prevalence is about 40%. These high prevalences, when compared to the baseline

TABLE 14.1. POSSIBLE SITES OF ENDOMETRIOSIS

Common Sites	Less Common or Rare Sites
Ovaries	Umbilicus
Round ligaments	Laparotomy scars
Broad ligaments	Hernial sacs
Uterosacral ligaments	Small intestine
Rectovaginal septum	Rectum
Appendix	Sigmoid
Pelvic peritoneum	Ureters
Bladder	Vulva
Pelvic lymph nodes	Extremities
Cervix	Pleural cavity
Vagina	Lung
Fallopian tubes	Nasal mucosa

TABLE 14.2. ENDOMETRIOSIS AS A DISEASE OF CLINICAL CONTRASTS

Characteristic	Contrasting Characteristic
Benign disease	Locally invasive
Benign disease	Widespread disseminated foci
Benign disease	Proliferates in pelvic lymph nodes
Minimal disease	Severe pain
Many large endometriomas	Asymptomatic
Cyclic hormones cause growth	Continuous hormones reverse the growth pattern

prevalence in the general population, suggest an association of endometriosis with CPP. Additionally, it appears that about 70% of women with endometriosis have some type of pelvic pain symptoms (10). The association of endometriosis and CPP is further supported by the significant improvement in CPP that is observed with treatment of endometriosis. However, deeper delving into the research on the association of CPP and endometriosis is a truly bewildering experience. Although the data on the incidence of endometriosis suggest an association with pelvic pain and it is widely believed that endometriosis is a cause of pelvic pain (and infertility), it is difficult to prove with these data that endometriosis actually causes pelvic pain. In fact, it has been recently suggested that asymptomatic endometriosis occurs much more frequently than previously reported and that the 1% to 7% incidence determined in laparoscopic studies of asymptomatic, fertile women over the last decade may be erroneously low. For example, Rawson (7) has recently documented endometriosis in 45% of 86 women undergoing laparoscopy without a history of pelvic pain or infertility (72% were stage I). Even before the advent of laparoscopy, the association of pelvic pain and endometriosis was not clear. Certainly, it has long been accepted and taught that endometriosis can cause dysmenorrhea, dyspareunia, and other pelvic pain. It has been generally stated that 70% to 75% of women with endometriosis have some type of pelvic pain, with 25% to 30% pain-free. Inexplicably, it has been observed that the severity of pain frequently does not correlate with the severity of endometriosis (11). A critical examination of these observations led Vercellini et al. (12) to suggest that "the association between CPP and endometriosis is based on unverified clinical tenets and anecdotal reports." One can question whether the current data even justifies the conclusion that endometriosis, per se, is a cause of pelvic pain. In fact, Slocumb (13) has stated that the evidence could be interpreted as suggesting that endometriosis is actually a manifestation rather than a cause of chronic pelvic pain, because "many women not only have the pain long before the finding of endometriosis, but also may have the same pain after treatment or total pelvic clean-out."

ETIOLOGY

There are several general theories of etiology of endometriosis (Table 14.3). None of these theories alone explains the protean manifestations of endometriosis, or the predilection of some women, but not others, to symptomatic endometriosis. *Sampson's theory* is that endometriosis is due to retrograde flow of menstrual effluent through the fallopian tubes into the peritoneal cavity. This theory is supported observationally by the increased incidence of endometriosis in adolescents with obstructive reproductive tract anomalies (14), in adult women with cervical stenosis (15), and experimentally by evidence that monkeys develop endometriosis if their cervix is sutured closed. However, it has been shown laparoscopically and in dialysis patients that most women experience some degree of retrograde menstruation, so there must be more to the development of endometriosis than just retrograde flow. *Metaplasia of coelomic epithelium,* the epithelium from which the müllerian duct is derived, can result in endometrium. The decidual reaction of peritoneum during pregnancy is an example of this process. Metaplasia needs an induction phenomenon or factor, which might be menstrual debris, estrogen, or progesterone. Metaplasia may best explain endometriosis in the umbilicus or deep in the rectovaginal septum. The theory of *lymphatic and vascular metastases* is invoked to explain the occurrence of endometriosis in remote locations such as the pleura, nose, and spinal column. It has been reported that endometriosis is present in pelvic lymph nodes in 30% of women with pelvic endometriosis, which supports this theory. A *defect of the immunologic system* is supported by a good deal of research, and it helps to explain why not all women develop endometriosis secondary to retrograde menstruation. This remains an area of active research. It also ties into the theory of *genetic predisposition,* because any immunologic disorder may well be inherited. Familial predisposition was noted by Sampson in his early studies. He found a sevenfold increase of endometriosis in relatives of women with the disease. Finally, recent research has focused on the endometrial cells that are present in endometriosis and found a number of abnormalities that may contribute either to initiation or development of endometriosis. For example, endometriosis cells have been found to have abnormal production of aromatase cytochrome P_{450}, an enzyme that is not present in normal endometrium and is

TABLE 14.3. THEORIES OF ETIOLOGY OF ENDOMETRIOSIS

Retrograde menstruation (Sampson's theory)
Metaplasia
Lymphatic and vascular metastases
Immunologic defect
Genetic predisposition
Abnormal endometrium in endometriosis

integral to the conversion of androstenedione and testosterone to estrogen. This ability to produce estrogen locally may directly stimulate the growth of endometrial cells of endometriotic lesions. Endometriosis cells have also been observed to have increased amounts of vascular endothelial growth factor and interleukin-6. The true importance of these abnormalities is not yet clear.

It is worthwhile to especially note the role of estrogen, because there are several clinical observations that suggest that the development and persistence of endometriosis are estrogen dependent. First, endometriosis is rare before puberty or after menopause unless the woman is on estrogen replacement therapy (5). Second, bilateral oophorectomy typically results in regression of endometriotic lesions. Third, decreased levels of estradiol via gonadotropin-releasing hormone (GnRH) agonist treatment results in regression of endometriosis. Estradiol levels of 10 to 20 pg/mL usually result in atrophy of endometriotic lesions (levels greater than 60 pg/mL usually are associated with growth of endometriotic lesions) (16). Fourth, endometriosis can develop in the prostatic utricle of a male with DES treatment for prostatic cancer. Finally, immunohistochemical studies show that virtually all endometriosis lesions contain estrogen receptors.

In addition to estrogen, there are several other risk factors for the development of endometriosis that are worth noting. Short menstrual cycles with frequent menses and long menstrual duration increase the risk of endometriosis. Risk is decreased by 40% in women with cycles of greater than 35 days in length (relative risk of 0.6), while those with shorter cycles of less than 27 days have about twice the risk of developing endometriosis (relative risk of 2.1) when compared to women with a 28- to 34-day cycle. Duration of menses of greater than 8 days increases the risk of endometriosis by twofold to threefold over that of women with menstrual flow of 7 or less days per cycle. Exercise also influences the risk of endometriosis. Women who exercise an average of 7 or more hours per week have an 80% decrease in risk of developing endometriosis (relative risk of 0.2) compared to women who do not exercise (5). Intercourse during menses may also be a risk factor. Women giving a history of coitus during menses are found to have an incidence of endometriosis of 18%, compared to an incidence of 11% in women giving a history of avoiding intercourse during menses (17).

Even if the etiology of endometriosis were well-understood, it would still be necessary to explain the etiology of symptoms associated with its presence in some women, but not in others. It has been hypothesized that minimal or microscopic endometriosis is a natural occurrence in menstruating women with patent fallopian tubes; this is based on the demonstration by some researchers of asymptomatic endometriosis in 20% to 45% of women (7,18), as well as on the finding that endometriosis can be histologically documented in 13% of biopsies of normal peritoneum in women with known endometriosis and in 6% of biopsies of normal peritoneum in women without visible endometriosis (19). Experimentally, this is also supported by an interesting study of baboons in captivity. It was shown that 10 of 24 baboons that had proven fertility in the wild developed endometriosis during observation over 12 to 22 months with no interventions except laparoscopies. Nine had subtle or atypical lesions, and four had typical or classical lesions. In this study, life-table analysis showed cumulative incidences of 40% at 12 months and 70% at 32 months. That nearly all endometriotic lesions (94%) that developed in baboons during observation were subtle lesions supports the concept that subtle lesions are "young" implants (20). Other observations that suggest that minimal endometriosis is a common asymptomatic condition in menstruating primates are (a) a 31% prevalence of spontaneous minimal endometriosis in baboons with greater than 2 years in captivity (21) and (b) a 20% to 40% prevalence of minimal to mild endometriosis in women of proven fertility having laparoscopic tubal ligations (22,23). Pelvic pain is thought to occur when these minimal implants are able to grow and invade deeply into pelvic tissue. One theory, as mentioned previously, is that there is an immunologic defect that allows aggressive growth of the endometrial cells and the development of symptomatic disease (24). This aggressive endometriosis might produce symptoms due to swelling of the tissue with hormonal stimulation, plus extravasation of blood and menstrual debris into surrounding tissues, with production of prostaglandins as possible chemical mediators of pain and inflammation (which could also lead to scarring and adhesions). It is also hypothesized that atypical lesions (i.e., red or clear papular lesions), which are more superficial and are fresh or new lesions and are less likely to cause symptoms by the above mechanism, are exposed to peritoneal fluid, produce prostanglandins, and cause functional pain symptoms, like dysmenorrhea, via direct production of prostanglandins, rather than secondary to inflammation. There are data supporting this explanation. Vernon et al. (25) have shown that atypical lesions produce much more prostaglandin F than lesions that are black or "powder-burn" in appearance. Characteristics that correlated with increased prostaglandin F synthetic activity were (a) red, vascular appearance, (b) presence of endometrial glands and stroma, and (c) low or no hemosiderin content. Atypical lesions, which are usually superficial and relatively small, may cause pain (26), and these findings suggest at least one possible mechanism by which that might occur. These atypical lesions are exposed to peritoneal fluid and through this exposure may cause functional pain symptoms like dysmenorrhea that are related to prostaglandin levels, in contrast to typical lesions that may cause organic pain due to mechanical pressure and from stimulation of pain fibers by scars and stretching of areas of fibrotic infiltration. Prostaglandin synthetic activity has been shown to be greater in moderate and mild disease than in severe or extensive disease (25). This may be at least a partial explanation for the seeming paradox of significant pain in the face of minimal disease, because atypical lesions may be easily overlooked, missed, or ignored.

It has been suggested that typical lesions cause pain by the formation of cystic nodules, scar tissue, and fibrotic infiltration, which generate nociceptor stimulation by mechanical pressure or by stretching tissue. Such a mechanism would predict that larger lesions and more deeply infiltrating lesions would cause more frequent or more severe pain. Consistent with this, Koninckx and co-workers (4,27) have published evidence showing that the presence and severity of pelvic pain in patients with endometriosis correlated with the depth of infiltration of the implants. However, their data did not show a correlation between total pelvic area of endometriosis and pelvic pain. Although the correlation of infiltration depth and pain was statistically significant, it was not absolute. For example, 43% of patients with pelvic pain had lesions that infiltrated to a depth of 2 mm or more, and 24% of patients with pain had lesions that infiltrated to 6 mm or more. In comparison, in patients with infertility, but no pain, 24% had lesions that infiltrated to 2 mm or more, and 9% had lesions that infiltrated to 6 mm or more. All patients with implants that infiltrated 10 mm or more had severe pelvic pain. An earlier study by the same group showed that 17% of women with superficial infiltration (<2 mm) had pain, while 53% with intermediate infiltration (2 to 6 mm), and 37% with deep infiltration (>6 mm) had pelvic pain (27). Koninckx and co-workers believe that their data support the theory that deep infiltrating endometriosis is the main cause of pelvic pain due to endometriosis. Obviously, although depth of infiltration appears to be related to pelvic pain, it does not seem to be the only possible mechanism by which pain occurs with endometriosis.

No correlation has been found between the Revised AFS classification of endometriosis and the depth of infiltration of lesions. For example, in one study, stage I disease had a 3% frequency of deeply infiltrating lesions (>6 mm); stage II, 34%; stage III, 15%; and stage IV, 22% (4). This finding led Koninckx and co-workers to propose yet another classification scheme for endometriosis, one which includes depth of infiltration (Table 14.4). Ripps and Martin (28) evaluated depth of infiltration in a small series of 59 endometriosis patients and found that the average depth of infiltration of lesions in patients with focal tenderness was 5.4 mm, while in patients without focal tenderness the average depth was 3.4 mm. While not statistically significant, this small sample is suggestive; and further prospective evaluations of CPP, focal pelvic tenderness, and depth of endometriosis infiltration, possibly using Koninckx's classification, may be a fruitful endeavor.

Innately, it would seem that if endometriosis is indeed a cause of CPP, there should also be some correlation between the presence or the severity of pain and the amount of

TABLE 14.4. STAGING SYSTEM FOR ENDOMETRIOSIS BASED ON THE DEPTH OF INFILTRATION OF THE DEEPEST LESION AND THE PRESENCE OR ABSENCE OF ENDOMETRIOMAS

Condition	Superficial Infiltration (≤6 mm)	Deep Infiltration (>6 mm)
No endometrioma		
Pelvic area involved <3 cm²	Is	Id
Pelvic area involved >3 cm²	IIs	IId
Endometrioma present		
Endometrioma <2 cm³	IIIs	IIId
Endometrioma >2 cm³ or bilateral or dense adhesions also present and >5 cm²	IVs	IVd

endometriosis present. However, that has not been the anecdotal experience of clinicians, nor have attempts to correlate either the presence or severity of pain with various methods of staging of endometriosis been fruitful. For example, recent laparoscopic studies (29,30) have found no correlation between careful staging according to the Revised AFS classification and the presence or the severity of pain. Koninckx et al. (4) have also evaluated the total pelvic area of endometriosis, as well as the total volume of endometriomas, and found that neither correlated with pelvic pain. Thus, studies of the amount of endometriosis have not supported the belief that endometriosis is a cause of CPP.

Fidele et al. (29), by studying the location of endometriosis implants compared to the localization of pain symptoms in 160 women, evaluated the hypothesis that if endometriosis were a cause of pain, then it should cause pain at its site(s) of implantation. They found no correlation between the location of endometriosis and of pelvic pain. However, Ripps and Martin (28) in a prospective study of 82 women with either pelvic pain or infertility, 59 of whom had endometriosis, found that 76% of the patients with endometriosis had localized tenderness that correlated with an area of endometriosis. However, it should be noted that more than one-half (58%) of these patients also had areas of endometriosis that were not tender. Ripps and Martin also attempted to evaluate the types of endometriotic lesion to see if any correlation existed with focal tenderness and found no specific correlation with either typical or atypical lesions. As an aside, in patients with focal tenderness, endometriosis was the most frequent diagnosis (45 of 68 diagnoses or 66%). Although these data can be used to suggest that if a woman with endometriosis has focal tenderness on examination, then most likely endometriosis will be found in that area (as well as other areas), it is still not very strong evidence for the assertion that endometriosis is a cause of CPP.

The attribution of CPP to endometriosis in women with minimal disease is particularly problematic. Small endometriotic lesions are found with sufficient frequency in normal-appearing peritoneum of pain-free women and in women without pain having gynecologic surgery that it is difficult not to believe that minimal disease is an incidental finding, rather than cause of or contributor to pain. For example, Rawson (7) found that about 40% of women undergoing laparoscopically assisted hysterectomy visually had endometriosis, greater than 90% of whom had stage I or II disease.

PATHOLOGY

All of the following descriptive terms have been aptly applied to describe the many possible gross appearances of endometriosis: red raspberries, purple raspberries, blueberries, blebs, peritoneal pockets, whitish scar tissue, stellate scar tissue, strawberry-colored lesions, red vesicles, white vesicles, clear vesicles, powder burns, peritoneal windows, yellow-brown patches, brown-black patches, adhesions, clear polypoid lesions, red polypoid lesions, red flame-like lesions, black puckered spots, white plaques with black puckers, and chocolate cysts (31–34). Based on the gross appearance, lesions are often categorized into atypical and typical lesions. Atypical lesions are often nonpigmented and difficult to see. Atypical lesions tend to be superficial with 2 mm of infiltration or less. In contrast, typical lesions tend to be deeply infiltrating. Yet, as previously discussed, the atypical lesions can be symptomatic and may actually be the most metabolically active endometriosis. The presence of pelvic pain does not correlate specifically with either typical or atypical lesions. It may correlate with pigmentation, however. For example, Jansen and Russell noted that women with both pigmented and nonpigmented lesions were more likely to have dyspareunia or significant dysmenorrhea than women with only nonpigmented lesions (26).

Left untreated, nonpigmented atypical lesions have been observed to progress to pigmented typical endometriosis within 6 to 24 months. This supports the hypothesis that the nonpigmented lesions are early endometriosis, while the pigmented, dark lesions are a late consequence of the cyclic growth and regression of lesions, with hormonal change and tissue bleeding resulting in discoloration by blood pigment. Also, both Redwine (25) and Koninckx et al. (4) have published observational data suggesting a progression over time from nonpigmented to pigmented lesions; atypical lesions were found to decrease in incidence with increasing patient age, while typical black lesions increased in incidence with increasing patient age. The observations that atypical lesions inversely correlate with the age of the patients and typical lesions increase with patient age suggest that endometriosis is a progressive disease. This is further supported by the observations that the total volume of disease increases with increasing patient age and that the depth of infiltration of lesions increases with increasing age.

TABLE 14.5. CORRELATION OF GROSS APPEARANCE OF LESIONS WITH THE HISTOLOGIC CONFIRMATION OF ENDOMETRIOSIS

Type of Lesion	Number with Lesion	Number with Confirmed Endometriosis	Percentage with Confirmed Endometriosis
Scarred black	35	33	94
Scarred brown	45	36	80
Scarred white	20	16	80
Red polypoid	12	9	75
Red flat	12	4	33
Red raised	6	2	33
Black vesicles	5	4	80
Brown vesicles	18	13	72
Clear vesicles	23	15	65
White vesicles	19	11	58
Peritoneal pockets	36	14	39
Yellow	9	5	56
Yellow-brown	18	4	22
Grain-like	10	2	20
Carbon	6	1	17

Gross appearance is insufficient to make a diagnosis, because endometriosis is a pathologic diagnosis (Table 14.5). To definitively diagnose endometriosis, one must see histologically both endometrial glands and stroma (36,37). Hemosiderin-filled macrophages are also often seen, but are not essential to the diagnosis. Occasionally, "powder burn" lesions show only hemosiderin-laden macrophages and no endometrial glands and stroma. Although it is sometimes stated that this represents "burned-out" endometriosis, there is no evidence to support this conclusion. It is not justified to histologically make a diagnosis of endometriosis unless glands and stroma are identified.

Interestingly, deep endometriotic lesions are more likely to correlate with the endometrium in histologic phase of the menstrual cycle than are superficial or intermediate depth lesions (27). Deep lesions correlate about 75% of the time, while superficial lesions correlate about 60% of the time and intermediate lesions correlate about 40% of the time.

SYMPTOMS OR HISTORY

Endometriosis is a disease of women of reproductive age, so most women with endometriosis-associated pain are 20 to 45 years of age. However, it has been reported in girls as young as 10 years, and it may be a more common cause of pain in teenagers than is generally recognized. It may also occur in postmenopausal women, particularly if they are on estrogen replacement. About 70% of women with endometriosis and CPP are nulligravid. There may be a history of prior miscarriages, because there is a twofold to threefold increase in the risk of abortion with endometriosis.

Classically, the woman with endometriosis presents with one or more of the following triad: an adnexal mass (endometrioma), infertility, or pelvic pain (38). Estimates are that 5% to 40% of women with endometriosis have CPP. Pelvic pain most often starts as dysmenorrhea and about 75% of women with endometriosis-associated pelvic pain have dysmenorrhea as a component of their pain symptoms. Classically, the dysmenorrhea pain of endometriosis is worst during the first several days of menses, but also may be significant for several days prior to menses. Dyspareunia with deep penetration is also a frequent component of endometriosis-associated pain, occurring in 8% to 33% of cases. It may also continue postcoitally for several hours. Sometimes there is point tenderness with intercourse. When this occurs, women may describe pain when a specific area is hit during coitus. When dyspareunia is referred to the rectum or lower sacrococcygeal area, it may suggest rectovaginal septum or uterosacral ligament involvement. Up to 50% of women with endometriosis-associated pain have more than one of these pain symptoms. Although CPP, dyspareunia, and dysmenorrhea are significantly more common in women with endometriosis than in women with a normal pelvis, these pain symptoms are not as specific nor diagnostic for endometriosis as is commonly thought, and by themselves do not justify a diagnosis of endometriosis. Also, neither the presence nor the severity of pain allows an estimate of the extent of endometriosis. Neither of these correlates with the stage or extent of endometriosis. However, patients with both pain and infertility are more likely to have higher-stage disease. Forty percent to 50% of patients with either pain or infertility have stage I disease, whereas only 20% with both pain and infertility have stage I disease. Additionally, often the location of pain symptoms does not correlate with the location of lesions, although patients with deeply invasive lesions are more likely to have pain at the area of the implants.

Pain symptoms may or may not be associated with a pelvic mass or endometrioma: It is not unusual for a woman with a large endometrioma to be asymptomatic. When symptoms are present with endometriomas, generally about one-third have dysmenorrhea, one-third have dyspareunia, two-thirds have CPP, and about one-third have all three symptoms.

Abnormal uterine bleeding, particularly intermenstrual bleeding, may occur in women with endometriosis. There is no increase of menorrhagia, however.

Intestinal involvement occurs in 12% to 37% of women with endometriosis. Again, severity of symptoms does not correlate with the extent of involvement. Also, symptoms related to the gastrointestinal tract may not fluctuate with menses. Symptoms that may occur with intestinal involvement are abdominal pain, dyspareunia, tenesmus, dyschezia, constipation, diarrhea, low back pain, and, rarely, hematochezia or symptoms of bowel obstruction. The rectosigmoid and anterior rectum are the portions of the intestinal tract most often involved. The appendix or cecum may also be involved, and when involved they occasionally cause acute symptoms.

Urinary tract involvement occurs in 10% to 20% of women with endometriosis, most often at the bladder peritoneum and anterior cul-de-sac. Involvement of the distal one-third of the ureter is possible and may lead in rare cases to obstruction. Often there are no symptoms secondary to bladder involvement, but frequency, pressure, dysuria, or hematuria occasionally are present.

Endometriosis may rarely cause significant pulmonary symptoms with lung involvement, such as dyspnea on exertion, pleural effusion, and lung collapse. Catamenial hemothorax has been reported. A cyclically bleeding or a cyclically tender mass in an incisional scar may also occur with endometriosis.

SIGNS OR EXAMINATION

In many women with endometriosis-associated pelvic pain the physical examination is completely normal. In others there is tenderness only during menses. For this reason it is sometimes helpful to do the examination during the first day or two of menstrual flow in women with suspected endometriosis. This may also increase the likelihood of finding tender endometriotic nodules in the pelvis or rectovaginal septum. Some women with endometriosis have persistent areas of tenderness in the pelvis consistent with sites of endometriosis, whether or not they are menstruating. In particular, a fixed retroverted uterus with tenderness posterior to it may be found and is suggestive of endometriosis. Tender nodularity of the uterosacral ligaments and cul-de-sac on rectovaginal examination is a classically described finding with endometriosis, but is not that frequently present. Narrowing of the posterior vaginal fornix may rarely be present. Asymmetrically enlarged, tender ovaries that are fixed to the broad ligaments or pelvic sidewalls are sometimes found. In patients with endometriomas a tender adnexal mass may be noted.

Focal tenderness may be noted in women with endometriosis. Ripps and Martin (28) found that 76% of women with endometriosis had focal tenderness at the site of one or more of their endometriosis lesions. Of the remaining patients with endometriosis, 20% had no tenderness and 4% had tenderness, but not at the site of endometriosis. Consistent with the previous discussion of correlation of pelvic pain and the depth of infiltration of lesions, in those women with focal tenderness the average depth of infiltration of endometriosis was 5.4 mm compared to 3.4 mm in those without focal tenderness. Fibrotic lesions were the most likely to be tender, while red lesions were the least likely to be tender.

DIAGNOSTIC STUDIES

The symptoms and signs that might lead to a clinical diagnosis of endometriosis are not reliable enough to justify diagnosis and treatment, as the clinical diagnosis is confirmed at the time of surgical evaluation only about half of the time (39). At the present time an accurate diagnosis can only be made by surgical and histologic confirmation (41). Before the introduction of diagnostic laparoscopy, this required an exploratory laparotomy, which obviously was not done without considerable and serious symptoms (41). Laparoscopy is a much less invasive procedure than laparotomy and is currently the recommended diagnostic procedure for any patient suspected of having endometriosis (42). Most authorities believe that confirmation by laparoscopy or laparotomy is mandatory before a patient is diagnosed with or treated for endometriosis.

There are a number of advantages of laparoscopy over laparotomy for the diagnosis of endometriosis. Small lesions of 180 to 400 μm may be seen with near-contact laparoscopy, which gives a four- to eight-power magnification. The angle of the view with laparoscopy allows a better visualization of the cul-de-sac, the areas under the ovaries, and the upper abdomen. The incisions are smaller, cosmetically more appealing, and less painful. There are lower rates of wound infections and other wound complications. Laparoscopy allows an outpatient surgical procedure and shorter recovery time. These advantages are especially important when the diagnosis of endometriosis is *not* confirmed. CPP is the reason for 40% of laparoscopies, and endometriosis is diagnosed in about 40% of these procedures (43).

Many gynecological surgeons believe it appropriate to exclude or diagnose endometriosis solely on the basis of visual findings (14,44,45). However, recent studies have clearly shown that endometriosis presents with a variety of appearances (Table 14.6), which may make laparoscopic visual diagnosis inaccurate in some cases (Table 14.5) (26,39). As has already been discussed, these varied appearances have been categorized into "atypical" or "subtle" lesions versus "typical" or "classic" lesions. Atypical generally means the red, yellow, white, or clear lesions, whereas typical refers to the black-brown, black, or puckered black stellate scar lesions. Typical lesions are the appearances classically recognized as endometriosis, while atypical or subtle lesions have often been overlooked or gone unnoticed (47). This oversight can lead to significant underdiagnosis, because it has been reported that up to one-third of patients with endometriosis have only lesions of the atypical type and up to 15% have only nonpigmented lesions. Missing the diagnosis and underestimating the extent of disease may occur in 7% and 50% of cases, respectively, especially with atypical lesions (39).

Thus laparoscopic evaluation for possible endometriosis must be thorough and complete. The common sites in the pelvis and abdomen that must be closely inspected include the ovaries (all surfaces) and ovarian fossae, pelvic peritoneum (particularly the cul-de-sac, periureteral, and bladder peritoneum), uterine ligaments, sigmoid colon, appendix, fallopian tubes, and rectovaginal septum. In a study of 716 women with endometriosis, Koninckx et al. (18) found the following anatomic distributions: cul-de-sac and uterosacrals, 69%; ovaries, 45%; fossa ovarica, 33%; and vesicouterine fold, 24%. Unfortunately, they did not give data from any of the less common pelvic sites. Perez (48) found that endometriosis involved the appendix in 1 of 25 patients with pelvic endometriosis. If one wishes to adequately evaluate all of these anatomic sites, as well as the variety of abnormalities that can be noted during inspection of these areas, it is usually necessary to use at least a double-puncture technique. "Near-contact" laparoscopy, which results in up to an eightfold magnification, may be helpful in searching for atypical, nonpigmented endometriosis as well as for peritoneal lesions as small as 400 μm. Redwine (48) has suggested that "painting" the peritoneal surfaces with blood may also be helpful for visualizing nonpigmented lesions. The laparoscopic appearance of endometriotic lesions does not significantly change during the menstrual cycle, and the accuracy and frequency of diagnosis do not change with menstrual phase, so timing of diagnostic laparoscopy during a particular phase of the cycle is not crucial if the evaluation is being done for CPP (4). Martin et al. (39) found that with increased awareness of atypical lesions and liberal use of biopsies, the frequency of diagnosis of endometriosis at laparoscopy markedly increased (from 42% in 1982 to 72% in 1988). Such observations may also justify repeat laparoscopy in women with a history of a negative laparoscopy, but with persistent symptoms consistent with endometriosis. For example, Jansen and Russell (26) found that six women with only nonpigmented, endometriotic lesions at the time of initial laparoscopic biopsies, who were not otherwise treated, had classic pigmented lesions at the time of a second-look laparoscopy 6 to 24 months later. Missed diagnoses are also likely if the traditional pattern of seeking only black lesions is followed. One study of 137 consecutive women with endometriosis

TABLE 14.6. CLASSIFICATION OF POSSIBLE APPEARANCES OF ENDOMETRIOTIC LESIONS INTO 20 TYPES

Fibrotic white	Yellow-brown
Fibrotic brown	Yellow
Fibrotic black	Carbon
Clear vesicles	Psammoma bodies
White vesicles	Peritoneal pockets
Brown vesicles	Adhesions
Black vesicles	Ovarian adhesions
Flat red	Typical
Raised red	Subtle
Polypoid red	Other

showed that 60% had black lesions, 66% had nonblack lesions, 35% had only black lesions, and 40% had no black lesions (36).

Conversely, solely visual diagnosis can lead to overdiagnosis, because by appearance the following lesions have been confused with both typical and atypical endometriosis: hemangiomas, old suture, ovarian carcinoma, residual carbon deposits from prior surgery, ectopic pregnancy, adrenal cortical rest, Walthard rest, breast carcinoma, epithelial inclusions, reaction to oil-based hysterosalpingogram medium, inflammatory cystic inclusions, inflammation with or without Psammoma bodies, splenosis, endosalpingiosis, submesothelial microbleeding, and normal peritoneum. Table 14.5 shows the correlation between visual and biopsy diagnoses with some of the varied appearances possible with endometriosis (39). Obviously, the wide variation of appearances can prove deceptive. In a retrospective review of 132 cases of endometriosis diagnosed laparoscopically by 54 gynecologists, biopsies were sent in only 15 cases (11%), and in all 15 the diagnoses were not confirmed by histology (49). Furthermore, when all cases surgically diagnosed as endometriosis were evaluated, including those diagnosed by laparotomy or hysterectomy, histologic confirmations of endometriosis were obtained in only 143 of 212 cases (67%). In another study, 142 patients were diagnosed with endometriosis by laparoscopic appearance, 110 (77%) had biopsies taken, and in only 84 (59%) did the biopsies confirm the diagnosis (27). Clearly the potential for overdiagnosis and for underdiagnosis is high enough that it is best to consider almost any abnormality potentially as endometriosis and to biopsy it. Furthermore, with the underlying uncertainty about the role of endometriosis in CPP, histologic confirmation of a visual diagnosis should always be obtained before CPP is attributed to endometriosis. It is worth repeating that Sampson originally defined endometriosis in 1921 as "the presence of ectopic tissue which possesses the histological structure and function of the uterine mucosa," a definition that is still valid (50–52) and a definition that clearly requires histologic confirmation before the diagnosis can be made.

Adhesions are common in association with endometriosis. They may contain endometriosis in up to one-half of cases, so it may be wise also to histologically evaluate adhesions in patients with CPP.

Peritoneal defects represent one of many categories of appearance of endometriosis (Table 14.6) and are a particularly interesting finding at the time of laparoscopy (Fig. 14.1). These defects should be excisionally biopsied, including the surrounding ridge of tissue. They have been noted in 4% to 17% of patients with CPP, and about two-thirds of the time they are endometriotic lesions (33,34). About 20% of patients with endometriosis have peritoneal pockets. Locations of peritoneal defects, in decreasing order of frequency, are the posterior cul-de-sac, right broad ligament, left broad ligament, left uterosacral ligament, right uterosacral ligament, and anterior cul-de-sac.

Documentation of laparoscopic findings is important to treatment and follow-up of women with endometriosis. For this reason, various staging systems have been proposed. The revised American Fertility Society (AFS) staging system is the most widely used system at the present time (Fig. 14.2). This system, and most others, were developed for infertility evaluations, not for pelvic pain, and they give more value or weight to disease involving the ovaries and fallopian tubes. Recently, AFS (now the Society of Reproductive Medicine) suggested a new staging system for patients with pain (Fig. 2.3). It has not been used enough to know if it is helpful in predicting prognosis or response to treatment.

A preoperative ultrasound seems prudent before a laparoscopic evaluation for CPP, in case endometriosis and ovarian enlargement are found at the time of laparoscopy.

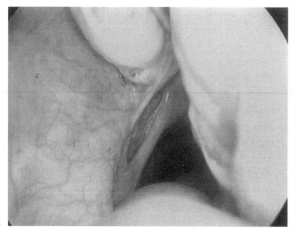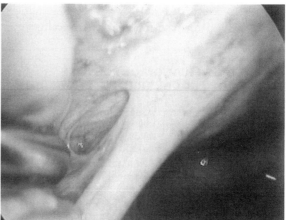

A

B

FIGURE 14.1. A,B: Appearance of peritoneal pocket. Such pockets are endometriosis about two-thirds of the time and should be excisionally biopsied, including the surrounding ridge of tissue.

Patient's Name _____ Date_____

Stage I   (Minimal) - 1-5
Stage II (Mild)   - 6-15
Stage III (Moderate) - 16-40
Stage IV (Severe)   - >40
Total_____

Laparoscopy_____ Laparotomy_____ Photography_____
Recommended Treatment_____
_____
Prognosis_____

PERITONEUM	**ENDOMETRIOSIS**	<1cm	1-3cm	>3cm
	Superficial	1	2	4
	Deep	2	4	6
OVARY	R Superficial	1	2	4
	Deep	4	16	20
	L Superficial	1	2	4
	Deep	4	16	20

	POSTERIOR CULDESAC OBLITERATION	Partial	Complete
		4	40

	ADHESIONS	<1/3 Enclosure	1/3-2/3 Enclosure	>2/3 Enclosure
OVARY	R Filmy	1	2	4
	Dense	4	8	16
	L Filmy	1	2	4
	Dense	4	8	16
TUBE	R Filmy	1	2	4
	Dense	4*	8*	16
	L Filmy	1	2	4
	Dense	4*	8*	16

*If the fimbriated end of the fallopian tube is completely enclosed, change the point assignment to 16.

Additional Endometriosis: _____   Associated Pathology: _____
_____   _____
_____   _____
_____   _____

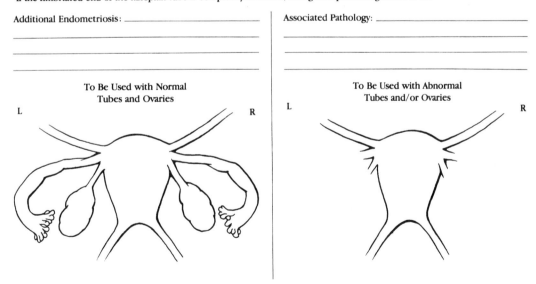

To Be Used with Normal   To Be Used with Abnormal
Tubes and Ovaries   Tubes and/or Ovaries
L   R   L   R

FIGURE 14.2. The revised American Fertility Society (AFS) staging system for endometriosis.

About 15% to 20% of women with endometriosis have endometriomas, generally ranging in size from 3 to 8 cm, so they are not always palpable on examination. When an ultrasound is done preoperatively and shows a cyst in a patient with endometriosis, needle puncture of the ovary has been suggested to detect occult endometriomas and properly stage endometriosis. In one reported series of patients with endometriosis, all of the endometriomas in the patients with "positive" ovarian punctures were visualized by preoperative sonography (53). When endometriosis is not visualized anywhere else in the pelvis and a preoperative ultrasound shows normal ovaries, there is no proven

TABLE 14.7. THE RELIABILITY OF CA-125 LEVELS IN THE DIAGNOSIS OF PELVIC ENDOMETRIOSIS

	All Stages	Stages III and IV
Sensitivity	53	85
Specificity	86	86
Positive predictive value	89	87
Negative predictive value	46	67

TABLE 14.8. GENERAL TREATMENT OPTIONS FOR WOMEN WITH ENDOMETRIOSIS-ASSOCIATED PELVIC PAIN

Observation with palliative treatment
Conservative surgery
Hormonal suppression
Combined medical and surgical treatments
Definitive extirpative surgery

role for ovarian needle puncture in the laparoscopic evaluation of patients with CPP. Circumspection is important because not all chocolate cysts are endometriomas. For example, Martin and Berry (36) have reported that 60% are endometriomas, 27% are corpora lutea or albicans, and 12% are nondiagnostic.

Ca-125 levels have been evaluated as aids to diagnosis and follow-up. However, as a diagnostic test Ca-125 has a low sensitivity and specificity, although it is more reliable for advanced-stage disease (Table 14.7) (54). One concern is that Ca-125 levels are also elevated with cancers of the ovary, endometrium, gastrointestinal tract, fallopian tube, and breast. They are also increased with pelvic inflammatory disease, pregnancy, menses, and leiomyomata (55). Although Ca-125 levels have been shown to decrease with medical treatment, the decreases did not correlate with clinical response to therapy.

Adolescents with endometriosis should be evaluated for obstructive anomalies, because about 10% will have such an anomaly. Hysterography and magnetic resonance imaging may be helpful in such an evaluation.

In patients in whom intestinal endometriosis is suspected, evaluation of the intestinal tract is usually normal, because most patients have involvement of the serosa or muscularis, not the mucosa. Sigmoidoscopy may show a bluish submucosal mass in some of these cases. Mucosal lesions may be diagnosed by sigmoidoscopy, colonoscopy, or barium enema studies, but these evaluations are certainly not necessary on a routine basis (57).

In patients with suspected urinary tract involvement, cystoscopy and intravenous pyelography or computerized tomography of the kidney, ureters, and bladder may be indicated.

MANAGEMENT OR TREATMENT

Because there are many different medical and surgical treatments for endometriosis-associated pelvic pain (Table 14.8), none of which can be considered ideal for all patients (and the efficacies of which are not completely clear) (57,58) many factors must be considered in planning treatment. The patient needs to be informed about her disease and the options for treatment, and she should be actively involved in the decisions. The patient's understanding of

the disease will influence decisions about treatment. It is important to use common sense, but it is especially critical to consider the patient's unique needs and problems. It is necessary to incorporate into planning the location and extent of endometriosis, as well as severity of symptoms; and any other pelvic pathology that may be important. The patient's age, reproductive plans, duration of infertility, and attitude toward surgery or toward hormonal medications may be vital components of the patient's needs or concerns. The patient's motivation and her emotional state may influence options and choices. Plans may need to be modified based on the tolerance of drug therapies or persistence or worsening of symptoms.

Ideally, the efficacy of any therapy is substantiated by data from randomized clinical trials. Fortunately, such studies are available for medical and surgical treatment of endometriosis-associated pelvic pain. These data will be used as the basis for this discussion of treatment. Unfortunately, most of the published studies on treatment of endometriosis do not specifically address CPP. Instead, they provide general evaluations of efficacy for the combination of pelvic pain, dysmenorrhea, and dyspareunia, and sometimes also pelvic tenderness and induration. By using a combined scoring system, those treatments that induce amenorrhea, by definition, relieve dysmenorrhea; and if the data are reported as combined scores with equal weighting of pelvic pain, dyspareunia, and dysmenorrhea (and this is in fact what most of the studies report), then a decrease of up to one-third occurs in the score *a priori*. In many studies this may result in a statistically significant decrease of pain, but this does not automatically translate into clinically significant decrease of pain.

MEDICAL TREATMENT

Some of the options for medical treatment of endometriosis are listed in Table 14.9.

Danazol

Danazol, a 17-ethinyl-testosterone derivative, is one of the most commonly used medical treatments and has been used as the "gold standard" or control treatment for the evaluation of most other medical treatments. It was first reported

TABLE 14.9. MEDICAL TREATMENTS FOR ENDOMETRIOSIS

Methyltestosterone, 5–10 mg/day
Oral contraceptives
  Enovid (high dose pill originally popularized by Kistner as "pseudopregnancy")
  Low-dose pills, start on day 3 of cycle continuously; double dose for 5 days if breakthrough bleeding occurs
  Low-dose pills, taken cyclically
Medroxyprogesterone acetate, 100 mg/day
Danazol, 200–400 mg b.i.d.
Gonadotropin-releasing hormone analogues (GnRH analogues)
  Nafarelin, 200–400 μg b.i.d.
  Leuprolide, 3.75–7.5 mg q28 days
  Goserelin, 3.6 mg q28 days
  Triptorelin, 3.75 mg q28 days

for treatment of endometriosis in 1971 by Greenblatt et al. (59) Food and Drug Administration (FDA) approval for this indication occurred in 1976. Danazol is contraindicated in patients with abnormal uterine bleeding, pregnancy, breastfeeding, or impaired renal, cardiac, or hepatic function. It is mildly androgenic and anabolic, activities that account for many of its side effects. It does not significantly affect luteinizing hormone (LH) and follicle-stimulating hormone (FSH) levels in premenopausal women, but it lowers estrogen levels by directly inhibiting steroidogenesis at the ovarian and adrenal levels. It induces atrophic changes in the endometrium and endometriosis by its effect on estrogen levels. Its half-life is about 4 to 5 hours, so it must be dosed at least twice a day. Side effects are acne, edema, weight gain, hirsutism, voice changes, hot flushes, abnormal uterine bleeding, decreased breast size, decreased libido, vaginal dryness, nausea, weakness, and muscle cramps. From a placebo-controlled study, the absolute risk of side effects that were statistically greater than those in the placebo group were: acne, 57%; edema, 41%; muscle cramps, 32%; and irregular spotting, 63% (60). Weight gain averaged 2.6 kg in the danazol-treated patients, versus no weight gain in placebo-treated patients. Exercise may decrease the number of side effects reported by patients receiving danazol by as much as one-half. However, it has no effect on relief of pain or time to recurrence over that obtained with danazol only without an exercise program (61).

In early uncontrolled studies, about 75% of patients had relief of either pelvic pain or dysmenorrhea, and about 60% had relief of dyspareunia (62). There is only one placebo-controlled, double-blind randomized clinical trial of danazol for the treatment of endometriosis-associated pelvic pain. This was reported by Telimaa et al. (63) and evaluated both danazol and medroxyprogesterone acetate. They enrolled 20 patients with laparoscopically confirmed endometriosis, stage I or II, into the danazol group and 19 patients into the placebo group. Eighteen and 17 patients completed the trial, respectively. Danazol was given at a dose of 600 mg per day for 6 months. Unfortunately, this study had several significant flaws. The method of randomization was not specified, the method of assessment of pelvic pain was inadequate, and the power was insufficient. Also, one-fourth of the patients in each group had electrocoagulation of endometriosis implants at the time their diagnostic laparoscopies, and four patients (of the total of 59 in the study) who experienced side effects that led to discontinuation of medication were simply dropped from the study and excluded from analysis. If these inadequacies are ignored, then this trial shows a decrease of mean pain scores of 80%, with a confidence interval of 59% to 102%, at the end of 6 months of medical treatment with danazol (Table 14.10). At 12 months, 6 months after discontinuation of medication, the average decrease of pain scores was 65%. From the data reported, it appeared that of evaluable patients, 3 (17%) of 18 had severe painful symptoms (included pelvic pain, low back pain, diarrhea, dysuria, and dyspareunia) at the end of 6 months of treatment with danazol, compared to 12 (75%) of 16 in the placebo group

TABLE 14.10. EFFICACY BASED ON CHANGES IN PAIN SEVERITY SCORES, OF MEDICAL TREATMENTS OF ENDOMETRIOSIS-ASSOCIATED PELVIC PAIN

	MPA[a]	Danazol[b]	Leuprolide[c]
Decrease at 3 months in the mean pelvic pain scores	2.8 (2.5–3.3)[d]	3.5 (2.2–4.8)[d]	3.3
Percentage decrease at 3 months in the mean pelvic pain scores	49% (29–69%)	49% (28–71%)	—
Decrease at 6 months in the mean pelvic pain scores	4.2 (3.1–5.3)	5.3 (4.1–6.6)	3.0
Percentage decrease at 6 months s in the mean pelvic pain score	71% (50–92%)	80% (59–102%)	—

[a]MPA (medroxyprogesterone acetate), 100 mg/day × 6 months.
[b]Danazol, 600 mg/day × 6 months.
[c]Depo-leuprolide, 3.75 mg q4 weeks × 6 doses.
[d]Numbers in parentheses are 95% confidence intervals.

(63). This means that there is about a 58% decrease in the number of patients with severe pain symptoms due to danazol treatment, or that about two patients need to be treated with danazol to eliminate severe pain in one patient.

Progestagens

Medroxyprogesterone acetate (MPA) has been a recommended treatment for many years. Breakthrough bleeding is a significant problem with MPA treatment, and sometimes estrogen treatment is necessary to stop the bleeding. Also, prolonged amenorrhea and anovulation may occur after discontinuation of depot MPA treatment. Mood changes, depression, and irritability may also occur. In a placebo-controlled trial of MPA at 100 mg per day the risk of side effects due to MPA were: acne, 33%; edema, 61%; muscle cramps, 17%; and irregular spotting, 56%. Weight gain with 6 months of treatment was 2.2 kg (61). Bone mineral density is decreased in women who use depot MPA, even in the lower doses used for contraception (150 mg every 3 months). The amount of bone density loss in general correlates with the duration of use of depot MPA, with a spinal bone density Z score of -0.48 after less than 15 years of use versus -0.91 after greater than 15 years of use (64).

Some of the suggested doses of MPA have been 10 mg three times a day orally or intramuscularly 100 mg every 2 weeks for 3 months, then 200 mg per month for 4 months. However, the only placebo-controlled, randomized, double-blind trial showing efficacy was with 100 mg per day orally for 6 months. As previously noted, this study had several flaws. Also, only 20 patients were enrolled in the MPA group and there was follow-up on just 16 of them. The efficacy of MPA at this high dosage was not statistically different from that of danazol. At completion of treatment at 6 months there was a 71% (confidence interval, 50% to 92%) decrease of pelvic pain scores, and a 47% decrease 6 months after discontinuation of treatment (Table 14.10). The number needed to treat for MPA for severe pain symptoms was two, the same as that for danazol.

Gestrinone, a 19-nortestosterone derivative with mostly progestagenic and low androgenic activity, has been studied in at least two randomized clinical trials comparing it to danazol (65) and leuprolide acetate (66). The study against danazol was of 269 women with all stages of endometriosis, 144 of whom had pelvic pain, randomized to oral gestrinone, 2.5 mg twice weekly, or oral danazol, 200 mg twice daily, for 6 months. Pain was relieved in 70% to 75% of patients in this study, with no significant difference between treatments. Side effects were similar with the two treatments, although more patients experienced hirsutism with gestrinone (about 40% versus 10%) and leg cramps with danazol (about 25% versus 15%). The randomized study of gestrinone versus leuprolide compared oral gestrinone 2.5 mg twice per week to intramuscular leuprolide acetate 3.75

mg every 4 weeks for 6 months in 55 women with pelvic pain. Nonmenstrual pelvic pain was evaluated with VAS scores and was not different between the gestrinone and leuprolide groups pretreatment (4.1 and 4.7, respectively) or at the end of 6 months of treatment (1.2 and 1.6, respectively). However, 6 months after completion of treatment there was a lower pain level in the gestrinone group (1.1 versus 3.4, respectively). Bone density evaluations in this study showed that there was a decrease of 3.0% ± 4.8% at the end of treatment with leuprolide compared to a slight increase of 0.9% ± 2.1% with gestrinone. The leuprolide group only recovered to a decrease of 1.1% ± 3.3% by the time of the 6-month follow-up. Gestrinone lowered high-density lipoprotein (HDL) levels by about 35%, whereas leuprolide caused no significant change.

Gonadotropin-Releasing Hormone Analogues

Gonadotropin-releasing hormone (GnRH) agonists are analogues of naturally occurring GnRH. The GnRH agonists currently available for use in the United States are nafarelin, leuprolide, and goserelin. They all work at the hypothalamic–pituitary level to shut down LH and FSH production and release, although their initial effect is stimulation of activity. This "down-regulation" leads to a dramatic decline in estradiol levels. It has been suggested that rarely GnRH agonist therapy may fail to decrease pain due to a failure to sufficiently suppress serum estradiol levels (67). Because it has been shown that inadequate suppression of estradiol correlates with failure to relieve dysmenorrhea, it may be appropriate to check estradiol levels in women with endometriosis-associated pelvic pain who do not improve with GnRH agonist treatment. GnRH agonists may also have efficacy related to their effect on the immune system. For example, GnRH agonists have been shown to increase natural killer cell numbers and T-cell mitogenic activity (68).

Nafarelin is administered intranasally at a dose of 200 to 400 µg twice a day. Leuprolide is most often given intramuscularly in a depot form at a dose or 3.75 mg or 7.5 mg every 28 days. There is also a 3-month depot form. Goserelin is administered as a depot subcutaneous insertion or implant, 3.6 mg every 28 days. GnRH analogue treatment is usually continued for 6 months. Side effects of the GnRH agonists are loss of bone density, hot flashes, vaginal dryness, decreased libido, headaches, emotional lability, acne, and reduced breast size. Nafarelin may cause nasal irritation. In a placebo-controlled trial of leuprolide, the absolute risk of side effects were hot flashes in 59% and headaches in 24%. Bone density loss was 11.8% after 6 months (69).

Only two GnRH agonists, depot leuprolide acetate and triptorelin, have been evaluated in randomized, placebo-controlled clinical trials (69,70). Dlugi et al. (69) enrolled 63 women, 48 of whom had pelvic pain, with laparoscopically diagnosed stages I, II, III, or IV endometriosis into a prospective, randomized, double-blind, multicenter, placebo-controlled study of leuprolide acetate given every 4 weeks for a total of six 3.75-mg injections. A major flaw in this study was that blinding was broken at 3 months if significant pain persisted, and this led to 70% of the placebo group being switched to leuprolide treatment after 3 months. This left only six patients in the placebo group for analysis, making it impossible to analyze the data by intention-to-treat analysis criteria and to evaluate efficacy at 6 months. At 3 months there was a mean decrease of pelvic pain scores of 1.2 (on a 0 to 3 scale) compared to a 0.3 decrease in the placebo group, which was statistically significant (Table 14.10).

In the triptorelin trial, 49 women with endometriosis-associated pelvic pain were randomized to receive 3.75 mg of depot triptorelin or placebo injections every 28 days. There was a mean decrease in visual analog scale pain scores of 4.9 (84%) in the treated group (24 patients) and 2.1 (34%) in the placebo group (25 patients) at the end of treatment at 6 months. Thus the mean decrease in pain scores attributable to treatment was 50%. All but one patient in this study had mild to moderate stage disease. Dysmenorrhea was totally relieved, because all women receiving triptorelin were amenorrheic during treatment. Dyspareunia was relieved in 10 (77%) of 13 triptorelin-treated women and 9 (45%) of 20 placebo-treated women. This gives an absolute risk reduction of 32% and a number needed to treat of 3 for dyspareunia.

There are a number of randomized clinical trials comparing the GnRH agonists leuprolide (71), goserelin (72,73), and nafarelin (74–76) to danazol. They show that there is no significant difference in efficacy of treatment of pelvic pain, dysmenorrhea, and dyspareunia between the GnRH agonists and danazol, with relief of symptoms in 50–70% of patients with either treatment. One of the

larger trials of two different doses of nafarelin allowed a separate evaluation of these three pain symptoms (Table 14.11), and the results suggest that about one-half of treated patients have significant pain relief with either treatment at the end of 6 months of treatment and 6 months after treatment (77). With either GnRH analogue or danazol treatment, pain symptoms begin to return within the first year after discontinuation of treatment. For example, the trial of leuprolide versus danazol by Wheeler et al. (72) showed return of pelvic pain within 1 year in 30% to 60% and of dysmenorrhea in 65% to 75% of patients. As an aside, this study also looked at analgesic usage and did not show any change in the use of analgesics during treatment with either leuprolide or danazol.

Differences in side effects of GnRH analogues and danazol can be evaluated from these trials. Hot flashes, headaches, vaginal dryness, and decreased libido are generally more frequent with GnRH agonists, although they also occur with danazol. Weight gain and adverse effects on lipid profiles are significant with danazol and generally do not occur with GnRH analogues. Patients receiving treatment with GnRH analogues are about one-third less likely to discontinue treatment than those taking danazol, and most of this difference is attributed to side effects (64).

Several important points should be considered in basing treatment decisions on these randomized clinical trials of danazol versus GnRH analogues. First, these studies included patients with all stages of endometriosis, not just mild to moderate stages as in the placebo-controlled trials. However, the groups were still heavily weighted toward patients with stage I and II disease. Second, there are no placebo groups in these studies, so it is difficult to know how large the placebo effects were in each trial, and thus no conclusions can be drawn regarding absolute efficacies from these trials. Third, almost all of the trials included few, if any, patients with severe pelvic pain; most patients with

TABLE 14.11. RESULTS OF TREATMENT OF PAIN SYMPTOMS FROM A DOUBLE-BLIND, RANDOMIZED CLINICAL TRIAL COMPARING NAFARELIN TO DANAZOL IN THE TREATMENT OF ENDOMETRIOSIS

Pain Symptom	Nafarelin		Danazol	
	Number with Symptom	Percentage with Symptom	Number with Symptom	Percentage with Symptom
Pelvic pain, pretreatment	77	100	28	100
Pelvic pain, posttreatment	30	39	10	36
Pelvic pain, 6 months posttreatment	41	53	14	50
Dysmenorrhea, pretreatment	90	100	34	100
Dysmenorrhea, posttreatment	1	1	2	6
Dysmenorrhea, 6 mos. posttreatment	59	66	17	50
Dyspareunia, pretreatment	57	100	23	100
Dyspareunia, posttreatment	18	32	4	17
Dyspareunia, 6 months posttreatment	18	32	7	30

nonmenstrual pain had mild to moderate pain only. For example, in the large European trial of nafarelin with 315 enrolled patients, of the patients they were able to follow for 1 year after treatment only 67 had pelvic pain, and of these 67, 18 had moderate pelvic pain and only 1 had severe pelvic pain (76). Fourth, not all patients respond to GnRH agonist therapy (or danazol). Second-look laparoscopy studies show that with both GnRH analogue and danazol treatments, the stage or amount of endometriosis shows no change or worsening in 15% to 20% of cases, whereas improvement occurs in 60% to 70%, and complete resolution in only 15% to 20% (77). Endometriomas 1 cm or more in size appear to not respond to medical treatment. Clinically even more significant is that no more than one-half of patients are *pain-free* after 6 months of medical treatment (78). Fifth, after discontinuation of treatment symptoms tend to recur in many patients. For example, in one longer-term study, after 6 months of GnRH agonist therapy, 45% of patients who improved during initial therapy had recurrence of pain attributed to endometriosis during several years of follow-up (79). The mean time to recurrence of symptoms severe enough to warrant retreatment appears to be between 8 and 11 months. Recurrence after danazol appears to be similar, with recurrences from 6 to 24 months after initially successful treatment.

When patients have a recurrence of pain within 1 year of treatment, retreatment with GnRH analogues appears to be fairly effective, with about two-thirds of patients showing a significant reduction of pain levels during retreatment (80). However, retreatment with GnRH analogues within 1 year of completing a course of treatment results in further loss of bone density that is additive. For example, mean bone density loss with 3 to 6 months of nafarelin treatment at 400 μg per day was 1.4 ± 0.4%, loss with retreatment within 1 year was 0.6 ± 0.4%, and total loss of bone density with treatment and retreatment was 1.9 ± 0.8%.

Because of concerns about loss of bone density, studies have been done looking at less than 6 months of treatment and at add-back treatment with estrogen or progestagen. For example, Hornstein et al. (81) compared 3 months of nafarelin (plus 3 months of placebo) to 6 months of nafarelin in a double-blind, randomized clinical trial of 179 women with pelvic pain. They found similar decreases in combined pain levels (dysmenorrhea, dyspareunia, pelvic pain, pelvic tenderness, and pelvic induration) at the end of treatment in both groups and reported that about 74% of women had at least some improvement in both groups. Only 82 patients completed the full 18 months of the study, but of those completing the study there were no significant differences in pain levels at any of the evaluations during the 18 months (although pain levels steadily increased during the 12 months of follow-up after discontinuation of treatment). Twenty-four women (29%) in the 3-month group and 23 (28%) in the 6-month group dropped out of the study due to inadequate pain relief. An interesting aside from this study was that the degree of suppression of estradiol levels correlated with relief of dysmenorrhea, but did not correlate with or predict relief of dyspareunia or pelvic pain (Table 14.12).

An example of a study of add-back therapy is that by the Lupron Add-Back Group (82). They randomized 201 patients with endometriosis-associated pelvic pain to four different treatment groups for 1 year each: (a) leuprolide, 3.75 mg every 28 days, and oral placebo daily; (b) leuprolide, 3.75 mg every 28 days, and oral norethindrone acetate, 5 mg daily; (c) leuprolide, 3.75 mg every 28 days, and norethindrone acetate, 5 mg daily, plus conjugated equine estrogen, 0.625 mg daily; or (d) leuprolide, 3.75 mg every 28 days, and norethindrone acetate, 5 mg daily, plus conjugated equine estrogen, 1.25 mg daily. There were significant differences in loss of bone density between the groups. Those who received only leuprolide lost 6.3% ± 2.3% in their mean bone density over the 52 weeks of the trial. In contrast, the mean bone density losses in the lower and higher estrogen add-back groups

TABLE 14.12. CORRELATION OF RELIEF OF PAIN SYMPTOMS WITH SUPPRESSION OF ESTRADIOL LEVELS DURING NAFARELIN TREATMENT OF ENDOMETRIOSIS

Symptoms Evaluated	Estradiol Levels			*p* Values
	<19 pg/mL	20–39 pg/mL	>40 pg/mL	
Dysmenorrhea improved with treatment	84 (99%)	33 (100%)	17 (81%)	<0.01
Pelvic pain improved with treatment	58 (72%)	25 (81%)	15 (75%)	0.19
Dyspareunia improved with treatment	47 (85%)	33 (100%)	6 (75%)	0.54
Pelvic tenderness improved with treatment	54 (83%)	22 (92%)	15 (79%)	0.30

were 0.2% ± 3.3% and 0.7% ± 4.1%, respectively. Mean bone density loss in the group that received only norethindrone acetate add-back was 1.0% ± 2.4%. Similarly, hot flashes were significantly decreased by about 50% in all three add-back groups. Suppression of menses also differed between the groups, with 100% suppression in both the leuprolide only group and the norethindrone acetate only add-back group, compared to 70% and 40% suppression in the lower and higher estrogen add-back groups, respectively. Suppression of menses correlated with suppression of mean estradiol levels (15 pg/mL versus 9 pg/mL versus 17 pg/mL versus 28 pg/mL, respectively). Differences in efficacy of treatment of dysmenorrhea, pelvic pain, and pelvic tenderness did not reach statistical significance. However, the higher estrogen add-back group approached significance for less effectiveness in efficacy for dysmenorrhea and pelvic pain. Also, this group had more patients who dropped out of the trial prior to the completion of 1 year due to lack of improvement of symptoms than the other groups. Seventeen percent of the 1.25-mg/day estrogen add-back group dropped out of the study due to pain compared to 2% in the leuprolide-only group, 5% in the norethindrone acetate add-back group, and 6% in the 0.625-mg/day estrogen add-back group. This study supports add-back therapy with 5 mg per day of norethindrone acetate, with or without 0.625 conjugated equine estrogen, for GnRH analogue treatment of endometriosis-associated pelvic pain without any significant effect on efficacy, but with notable improvement of safety for up to 1 year of treatment.

Oral Contraceptives

Oral contraceptive (OC) treatment was popularized by Kistner (84). He used high-dose pills such as Enovid and induced "pseudopregnancy" with the high levels of estrogen and progesterone. It is more common now to use low-dose pills in a cyclical manner to decrease dysmenorrhea or in a continuous method to induce amenorrhea. If breakthrough bleeding occurs with the continuous method, then the dose is doubled for 5 days to stop the bleeding, and then decreased back to one per day for 6 to 9 months. No more than three or four pills per day should be used in trying to maintain amenorrhea. Anecdotally, it has been reported that endometriomas can enlarge and rupture during the first 6 weeks of OC treatment. Side effects are weight gain, breast tenderness, nausea, chloasma, abnormal uterine bleeding, enlargement of myomas, thrombophlebitis and thromboembolism, increased apetite, irritability, depression, edema, hypertension, and increased vaginal discharge. They are contraindicated in women with a history of or high risk of thrombosis or a history of breast cancer and are relatively contraindicated with diabetes, collagen vascular disease, or hypertension.

There is surprisingly little literature about the treatment of endometriosis with OCs, despite their apparent widespread use in clinical practice. There appears to be only one randomized clinical study of OCs used for endometriosis-associated pain (84). This was a study of 57 patients with laparoscopic biopsy-confirmed diagnoses of endometriosis randomized to 6 months' treatment with either low-dose contraceptive pills (0.02 mg ethinyl estradiol with 0.15 mg desogestrel daily taken cyclically) or monthly subcutaneous injections of goserelin 3.6 mg. The dose of ethinyl estradiol was increased to 0.03 mg if breakthrough bleeding occurred in the contraceptive group. Although goserelin was more effective at relieving dysmenorrhea and possibly dyspareunia during treatment, there was no difference in relief of nonmenstrual pelvic pain. Six months after discontinuation of treatment, there were no differences between the two treatments, with OCs decreasing the severity of symptoms as effectively as goserelin. However, symptoms had recurred in all patients. Hot flashes, insomnia, and vaginal dryness were significantly more common in the goserelin group. Headache and weight gain tended to be more common in the OC group; one patient in the OC group withdrew because of severe headaches.

Based on this randomized clinical trial, OCs offer reasonable efficacy in the treatment of endometriosis-associated pelvic pain. Compared to other hormonal treatments, all of which have limited durations of therapy, OCs have the advantage that they can be given indefinitely. This is a significant advantage considering that it is well known that symptoms frequently recur when medications are stopped. If other studies are done that show OCs to be at least as effective as the other existing well-recognized hormonal therapies, OCs would offer a wider choice of treatment options and offer long-term symptom control. Obviously, other larger studies are needed.

Androgens

Androgen therapy with *methyltestosterone* is rarely used anymore and has not been evaluated in randomized clinical trials. Doses over 300 mg per month carry a significant risk of virilization. Other side effects include hirsutism, oily skin, acne, hepatocellular jaundice, and virilization of the female fetus if inadvertently given during pregnancy. Unless studies are done in the future showing significant efficacy, methyltestosterone should not be used to treat endometriosis-associated pelvic pain.

Anti-progesterones

Preliminary results with mifepristone suggest that it induces amenorrhea and improves endometriosis-associated pelvic pain when given at doses of 50 to 100 mg daily. It may be possible to achieve similar results with lower doses, but this remains to be adequately studied (85).

SURGICAL TREATMENT

In the woman with CPP and endometriosis, conservative management (i.e., without extirpation of the uterus, tubes, and ovaries) is indicated when preservation of reproductive potential is important or when the patient wishes to retain her reproductive organs for personal, social, or psychologic reasons. Medical treatment is a good option in such patients and, as has been discussed already, GnRH analogues, danazol, and high-dose MPA result in an 80% to 90% decrease in pain levels and complete relief of pain in up to 50% of patients during treatment (86,87). However, pain has generally recurred after discontinuation of the medication (88–91). Because all of these medications except OC have significant side effects and significant cost that preclude their long-term use, the fact that pain recurs after cessation of therapy is a serious limitation of their usefulness for the treatment of CPP. Also, it should be pointed out that even though AFS scores decrease by 30% to 55%, up to 10% of patients actually have laparoscopically documented progression of endometriosis during medical treatment. Such ruminations can be used to argue for surgical treatment of endometriosis in CPP patients.

Not surprisingly, it has been suggested that symptomatic endometriosis be surgically treated at the time of laparoscopic diagnosis (92). The technical objectives of surgery are to restore normal pelvic anatomy and to resect, coagulate, or vaporize all endometriosis implants (31). The clinical objective is to relieve pelvic pain. The technical objectives can be accomplished with a number of different surgical techniques, but pain relief does not always follow. There are a number of surgical procedures that have been performed to treat endometriosis and endometriosis-associated pelvic pain (Table 14.13).

Surgery for endometriosis can be challenging, tedious, and frustrating, rivaling that for invasive carcinoma. The surgeon must be well-versed in pelvic surgery, especially retroperitoneal dissection. Tissue planes are often obliterated, and lesions may involve vital viscera. Injuries to bowel, bladder, or ureter may be necessary components of the surgery in some patients. Inadvertent injuries to these

TABLE 14.13. CONSERVATIVE SURGICAL PROCEDURES THAT ARE PERFORMED LAPAROSCOPICALLY IN THE TREATMENT OF ENDOMETRIOSIS-ASSOCIATED PELVIC PAIN

Coagulation of endometriotic lesions
Vaporization of endometriotic lesions
Resection of endometriotic lesions
Adhesiolysis
Ovarian cystectomy
Oophorectomy
Salpingectomy
Uterosacral neurectomy (uterosacral ligament transection)
Presacral neurectomy

organs, especially without recognition, are complications that obviously must be guarded against vigorously. The components of conservative surgery for endometriosis are (a) fine suture when suturing is necessary, (b) reperitonealization or use of adhesion barriers, (c) microsurgical techniques, (d) meticulous hemostasis, and (e) complete resection of lesions and adhesions.

The core of surgical treatment is the removal or destruction of all endometriotic lesions. This may be done with mechanical, thermal, electrical, or laser energy, and there are no objective data that one is better than the other. Coagulation of lesions occurs with temperatures of less than 100°C. Vaporization occurs at temperatures over 100°C. Enzymes denature at 40°C to 65°C and DNA denatures at over 80°C. These temperatures can be generated by application of heat, electricity, or laser energies. The surgeon's knowledge, familiarity, and competence with the energy sources are far more important than any differences between them. It seems important for best results to ensure complete, full-depth resection or destruction of all implants, including atypical lesions (93). Usually the border between normal tissue and endometriosis is fairly obvious during resection, coagulation, or vaporization, but it can be difficult at times with deep lesions. Excision or destruction of deeply infiltrating endometriosis, which is found predominantly in the rectovaginal septum, uterosacral ligaments, and uterovesical folds, can be especially challenging. Recognition of the depth of infiltration can also be problematic, because many deeply infiltrating lesions appear as isolated black puckered spots or as larger white plaques with a black puckered spot within the plaque. Without full exposure and excision, these may be treated as only superficial lesions. Any peritoneal lesion 5 mm or more in size should be excisionally biopsied, rather than coagulated, to aid in ensuring complete removal of larger and deeper disease, as well as giving histologic confirmation of the diagnosis.

There is, however, only one placebo-controlled, double-blind, randomized clinical trial of surgical treatment, which was published by Sutton et al. (94) in 1994 and used laser energy to destroy the lesions. They enrolled 74 women with stage I, II, or III endometriosis into a prospective comparison of surgical treatment via operative laparoscopy to expectant management after diagnostic laparoscopy. Operative laparoscopy consisted of laser ablation of endometriosis, lysis of any adhesions, and bilateral uterine nerve transection. Sixty-three women completed the study: 32 in the laser laparoscopy group and 31 in the diagnostic laparoscopy group. The loss of 15% of their subjects (2 pregnancies, 5 hormonal contraceptive treatments, 1 psychotic depression, and 3 lost) represents the only significant weakness of this study. A "worst-case scenario" reanalysis with inclusion of the excluded patients significantly changes the outcome results, so this loss must be considered excessive. Blinding is difficult in surgical

TABLE 14.14. EFFICACY AT 3 AND 6 MONTHS OF SURGICAL TREATMENT OF PELVIC PAIN BASED ON CHANGES IN PAIN SEVERITY SCORES

	Three Months	Six Months
Median decrease in VAS pain scores in control group	1.2	−0.2
Percentage decrease in VAS pain scores in control group	16%	−2.0%
Median decrease in VAS pain scores in treated group	2.6	3.8
Percentage decrease in VAS pain scores in treated group	30%	45%
Median decrease in VAS pain scores attributable to surgical treatment	1.4	4.0
Percentage decrease in VAS pain scores attributable to surgical treatment	14%	47%

studies, but this was accomplished in Sutton's study. A three-puncture technique was used in all procedures and patients were not told if they had laser ablation or simply diagnostic laparoscopy. Follow-up data were collected by a study nurse also blinded to treatment group. Blinding was not broken until 6 months postoperatively. The 3-month and 6-month results of treatment are summarized in Table 14.14. At 3 months there is a significant placebo effect and there is no statistical difference between the placebo or control group [15 (48%) of 31 improved] and the treated or experimental group [18 (56%) of 32 improved]. At 6 months the placebo effect was greatly decreased [only 7 (23%) of 31 improved]. The percentage change in median pain scores at 6 months that can be attributed to surgical treatment is 47%. In clinical terms this means that an average decrease of pain of about 50% can be expected 6 months after laser laparoscopy due solely to the effect of treatment in a population of women with endometriosis-associated pelvic pain.

A clinically more useful analysis of the outcomes of laser laparoscopy for endometriosis-associated pelvic pain, based on evidence-based medicine terminology (95), is presented in Table 14.15. Forty percent of women had alleviation of pain 6 months after laser laparoscopy due to the treatment, which is called the absolute benefit increase

(ABI). From this it is possible to calculate a number needed to treat (NNT) of 2.5. This means that to obtain pain relief at 6 months in one woman it was necessary to surgically treat two to three women. Another useful analysis (not shown in the table) is of the need for a repeat laparoscopy due to persistent significant pelvic pain in the 6 to 12 months after the initial laparoscopy. Of the laser laparoscopy patients, 5 (16%) had another laparoscopy for continued significant pelvic pain, versus 16 (52%) of the patients with diagnostic laparoscopy and expectant care. This gives an absolute risk reduction (ARR) of 36% and an NNT of 2.8. In other words, laser laparoscopic treatment of three women with endometriosis-associated pelvic pain is necessary to prevent one repeat laparoscopy within 12 months due to persistent CPP (when compared to diagnostic laparoscopy only).

Sutton et al. (96) have continued to follow the patients in this study in an unblinded manner; two of the patients with symptom relief at 6 months had recurrent pain, while one without pain relief at 6 months was symptom free at 12 months without any other treatment, giving a 59% (19 of 32) response at 12 months. Of the other 11 patients without pain relief at 6 months after laser laparoscopic surgical treatment, one responded to treatment for irritable bowel syndrome, two had repeat laparoscopy and

TABLE 14.15. EVIDENCE-BASED MEDICINE ANALYSIS OF THE OUTCOME OF LASER LAPAROSCOPIC TREATMENT OF ENDOMETRIOSIS FOR THE ALLEVIATION OF PELVIC PAIN

	At 3 Months	At 6 Months	At 12 Months
Rate of improvement with laser laparoscopic treatment (EER)	56% (39–73%)[a]	63% (46–79%)[a]	59% (42–76%)[a]
Rate of improvement with diagnostic laparoscopy only (CER)	48% (30–66%)	23% (8–37%)	—
Relative benefit increase (EER − CER)/CER	17%	174%	—
Relative benefit EER/CER	1.2	2.7	—
Absolute benefit increase (ABI) (EER − CER)	8% (−17–33%)	40% (18–62%)	—
Number needed to treat (1/ABI)	12.5	2.5 (1.6–5.7)	—

[a]Numbers in parentheses are 95% confidence intervals.

treatment of endometriosis with pain relief, five continued to have symptoms without further treatment, one was pregnant, and one was lost to follow-up. In the expectant or control group, all 24 with continued symptoms underwent a second laparoscopy and had laser treatment. Fifteen (63%) were relieved of symptoms at subsequent six months follow-up, 7 (29%) had still not improved, and two (8%) were lost to follow-up. Evaluation of this follow-up data from the aspect of repeat laparoscopy is also worthwhile. Overall, 26 patients underwent a second laparoscopy due to continued CPP, two in the laser laparoscopy group and 24 in the expectant group. Seventeen (65%) had relief of pain symptoms at 6 months' follow-up, a proportion almost identical to the response rate at the time of the initial laparoscopies. Although there is no way to know, as this follow-up was only observational, it seems reasonable to assume that the placebo response would again have been about 20% to 25% and that the NNT would also have again been 2.5.

It is important to note that this study, the only published, placebo-controlled, double-blind, randomized clinical trial of surgical treatment, excluded women with stage IV endometriosis. Although there seems to be no reason *a priori* to assume that similar results would not occur in women with stage IV disease, it must be stated that there is no similar evidence regarding the efficacy of conservative, laparoscopic surgical treatment of endometriosis-associated pelvic pain in women with stage IV disease.

Other studies of surgical treatment are observational in design or compare different surgical treatments to one another. The number of such studies is overwhelming, so the remainder of the discussion of surgical treatment in this chapter will necessarily be incomplete and will reflect only a selection of available data.

Adhesiolysis is a frequent component of surgery for endometriosis as adhesions are common in association with endometriosis. The possible role of adhesions in CPP, and their treatment, has been discussed elsewhere in this text (Chapter 8). In women with endometriosis, adhesions may contain endometriosis in up to one-half of cases, especially periovarian adhesions, so it may be wise also to histologically evaluate adhesions in patients with CPP. Thus it is important to not simply lyse adhesions in patients with endometriosis, but rather to try to excise, ablate, or remove the entire adhesive band.

Ovarian endometriomas may be treated by *cystectomy* or *salpingoophorectomy*. Endometriomas can be removed laparoscopically as long as care is taken to exclude malignancy (97,98). Even when the appearance suggests a benign cyst, the cyst wall should be biopsied to adequately evaluate the ovary for any possibility of cancer and for histologic confirmation of the diagnosis. At this point, the further management of endometriomas becomes unclear and controversial. The approaches usually recommended are (a) cystectomy by wedge resection, (b) cystectomy by

stripping of the lining, (c) laser or electrical coagulation of the cyst lining, or (d) wide incision and drainage. Simply puncturing and aspirating an endometrioma through the laparoscope is inadequate surgery because of the possibility of missing a malignancy and an unacceptably high recurrence rate (99,100). Fayez and Vogel (101) have published one of the larger series on laparoscopic treatments of patients with endometriomas, in which they compared four different surgical techniques. They concluded that wide incision with drainage and irrigation was the best treatment because wedge excision resulted in severe adhesions and removal or ablation of the cyst lining resulted in the same recurrence rates as with wide incision and drainage (about 28%). They histologically evaluated 66 of 159 endometriomas and did not find endometrial glands or stroma in *any* of them. They concluded that endometriomas' "walls do not have endometriotic tissue" and, thus it is unnecessary to remove the cyst walls. It may be more appropriate to wonder how one makes a diagnosis of ovarian endometriosis without any endometriosis in the ovary. However, in spite of not finding endometriosis in the endometriomas, their recurrence rate 8 weeks after incision and drainage, ablation, or stripping was 28%, while it was 0% with wedge excision. A subsequent randomized clinical trial reported by Beretta et al. (103) showed different results from those of Fayez and Vogel. Sixty-four patients with endometriomas 3 cm or more in diameter were randomized to either cystectomy (Group 1) or drainage and bipolar coagulation of the lining (Group 2). Group 1 had lower cumulative recurrence rates of dysmenorrhea, deep dyspareunia, and nonmenstrual pelvic pain than Group 2. For example, over 24 months, 10% of Group 1 had recurrent pelvic pain versus 53% of Group 2. Median time to recurrence of pain was also longer in Group 1 than in Group 2, 19 months versus 10 months. In this study, 89% of the endometriomas had endometrial glands and stroma in their linings. This trial strongly supports cystectomy as the preferred approach over incision and coagulation of the lining. Evidence presented by Martin and Berry (103) is pertinent to this dilemma. They have stressed that not all "chocolate cysts" are endometriomas, even when clinically thought to be so. In a histologic study of 41 chocolate cysts, 36 of which were the thought clinically to be endometriomas, only 25 were histologically confirmed by the presence of endometrial glands and stroma, with 11 of the 41 definitely corpora lutea or albicans and 5 nondiagnostic. Although it is not absolutely resolved, it seems most appropriate at this time to perform ovarian cystectomy, with histologic confirmation, when an endometrioma is suspected and conservative treatment is desired.

Both presacral neurectomy (104–108) and uterosacral neurectomy (uterine nerve resection or transection of the uterosacral ligament) (108–110) have been recommended for relief of CPP associated with endometriosis. For both

TABLE 14.16. RESULTS OF A RANDOMIZED CLINICAL TRIAL OF TREATMENT OF PELVIC PAIN (NOT DYSMENORRHEA OR DYSPAREUNIA) IN PATIENTS WITH STAGE III OR IV ENDOMETRIOSIS WITH CONSERVATIVE LAPAROTOMY SURGERY WITH VERSUS WITHOUT PRESACRAL NEURECTOMY (PSN)[a]

Severity of Pelvic Pain	Preoperatively No PSN (n = 15)	Postoperatively No PSN (n = 15)	Preoperatively PSN (n = 17)	Postoperatively PSN (n = 17)
None	—	10 (67%)	—	14 (82%)
Mild	4 (27%)	2 (13%)	3 (18%)	0 (0%)
Moderate	6 (40%)	2 (13%)	8 (47%)	1 (6%)
Severe	5 (33%)	1 (7%)	6 (35%)	2 (12%)

[a]Of 71 patients randomized in this study, 32 had pelvic pain.

procedures the evidence for efficacy is mostly from observational studies of case series, although *presacral neurectomy* (PSN) has been evaluated in at least two randomized clinical trials. In the first, only eight patients with dysmenorrhea, four with PSN and four without PSN, were randomized (111). However, due to results in 18 nonrandomized patients combined with the results in the eight randomized cases, the monitoring committee stopped the study because of the marked difference in relief of dysmenorrhea between the groups. All patients had moderate to severe dysmenorrhea and stage III–IV endometriosis. Of the 17 patients undergoing presacral neurectomy, only 2 had a recurrence of pain, compared to 0 out of 9 with relief in the group without presacral neurectomy. There were no difference in relief of lateral pain, back pain, or dyspareunia between the groups. In a larger randomized trial, Candiani et al. (112) found that only midline dysmenorrhea was affected by adding PSN to conservative surgery for endometriosis. Randomization was of 71 patients with moderate or severe endometriosis and midline dysmenorrhea to conservative surgery alone or conservative surgery and presacral neurectomy. Presacral neurectomy markedly reduced the midline component of menstrual pain, but no statistically significant differences were observed between the two groups in the frequency and severity of dysmenorrhea, pelvic pain, or dyspareunia (Tables 14.16 to 14.18). The ability to detect a difference may have been limited by the study's sample size though. After presacral neurectomy, constipation developed or worsened in 13 patients and urinary urgency occurred in three. Taken together, these trials suggest that presacral neurectomy has a role in conservative surgery for endometriosis, but is most effective for the treatment specifically of midline dysmenorrhea. There appears to be a small effect, if any, on nonmenstrual pelvic pain or dyspareunia. In women with failure or recurrent pain after PSN, it is unwise to repeat the PSN due to retroperitoneal fibrosis and distorted anatomy.

Uterosacral neurectomy (USN), also called laparoscopic uterosacral nerve ablation (LUNA), has not been subjected to a randomized clinical trial in the treatment of endometriosis-associated pelvic pain. The only published randomized trial was of central dysmenorrhea in women without endometriosis (113). This study of 21 women showed no improvement in any patient in the control group and relief in 5 (45%) of 11 in the USN group at 1 year of follow-up. Sutton et al. included USN as part of their surgical procedure in their randomized trial of surgical treatment of endometriosis. Subsequently, they have undertaken a trial to evaluate the role of USN combined

TABLE 14.17. RESULTS OF A RANDOMIZED CLINICAL TRIAL OF TREATMENT OF DYSMENORRHEA IN PATIENTS WITH STAGE III OR IV ENDOMETRIOSIS WITH CONSERVATIVE LAPAROTOMY SURGERY WITH VERSUS WITHOUT PRESACRAL NEURECTOMY

Severity of Dysmenorrhea	Preoperatively No PSN (n = 36)	Postoperatively No PSN (n = 36)	Preoperatively PSN (n = 35)	Postoperatively PSN (n = 35)
None	0 (0%)	21 (58%)	0 (0%)	23 (66%)
Mild	0 (0%)	6 (17%)	0 (0%)	5 (14%)
Moderate	8 (22%)	4 (11%)	6 (17%)	4 (11%)
Severe	28 (78%)	5 (14%)	29 (83%)	2 (6%)

TABLE 14.18. RESULTS OF A RANDOMIZED CLINICAL TRIAL OF TREATMENT OF PATIENTS WITH STAGE III OR IV ENDOMETRIOSIS AND DYSPAREUNIA WITH CONSERVATIVE LAPAROTOMY SURGERY WITH VERSUS WITHOUT PRESACRAL NEURECTOMY

Severity of Dyspareunia	Preoperatively No PSN (*n* = 18)	Postoperatively No PSN (*n* = 18)	Preoperatively PSN (*n* = 19)	Postoperatively PSN (*n* = 19)
Absent	—	11 (61%)	—	15 (79%)
Mild	5 (28%)	3 (17%)	4 (21%)	0 (0%)
Moderate	7 (39%)	1 (6%)	6 (32%)	2 (11%)
Severe	6 (33%)	3 (17%)	9 (47%)	2 (11%)

with resection or ablation of endometriotic lesions and preliminary, unpublished results suggest that it adds little, if any, benefit to the surgery (personal communication). This is not too surprising as endometriosis-associated pelvic pain is rarely only midline pain or dysmenorrhea.

In women who have recurrent pain after a conservative procedure, there is some benefit in trying another conservative procedure. For example, Candiani et al. (114) found that only about 20% of their patients had recurrent pain and about 15% required a third surgery for endometriosis-associated pain over 2 to 10 years of follow-up after a second conservative procedure. All of them had stage III or IV disease.

Finally, it should be noted that although the number of patients studied are limited, the data from all of the placebo-controlled trials suggest that about one woman out of every two or three treated (NNT = 2 or 3), whether by surgery or medical treatment, will obtain a clinically significant decrease in her pain level. The data do not allow a conclusion as to whether medical or surgical treatment is more effective in the treatment of endometriosis associated pelvic pain (Table 14.19).

COMBINED MEDICAL AND SURGICAL TREATMENT

There is no consensus on the role of combined medical and surgical treatment of endometriosis in CPP patients. Some authors suggest preoperative medical treatment (115) in cases of known endometriosis, and some suggest postoperative medical treatment if there is extensive disease (116). Theoretically, potential advantages of preoperative medical therapy include (a) suppression of ovulatory activity so functional cysts are not confused with endometriosis, (b) decreased inflammation at the areas of endometriosis, (c) decreased general pelvic vascularity, and (d) decreased size of endometriosis implants. However, there are also some potential disadvantages of preoperative medical therapy: (a) appearance of endometriosis may be more difficult to diagnosis; (b) medication is costly and has numerous side effects; and (c) if the patient is interested in conception, medical therapy requires a significant time delay. There are no clinical trials of preoperative medical treatment on which to base a decision.

There are, however, at least three randomized, placebo-controlled clinical trials of postoperative medical treatment

TABLE 14.19. EFFICACY OF TREATMENT OF PELVIC PAIN, BASED ON CHANGES IN PAIN SEVERITY SCORES, AT THE END OF 6 MONTHS OF MEDICAL TREATMENT WITH MEDROXYPROGESTERONE ACETATE, DANAZOL, OR TRIPTORELIN COMPARED TO EFFICACY 6 MONTHS AFTER LASER LAPAROSCOPIC SURGICAL TREATMENT

	MPA After 6 Months of Treatment[a]	DAN After 6 Months of Treatment[b]	TRP After 6 Months of Treatment[c]	Six Months After Surgery
Absolute decrease in pain scores attributable to treatment	2.8 (1.7–4.0)[d]	4.8 (3.6–6.2)[d]	3.1	4.0
Relative decrease in pain scores attributable to treatment	50% (30–71%)	74% (54–95%)	53%	47%

[a]MPA (medroxyprogesterone acetate), 100 mg/day for 6 months.
[b]DAN (danazol), 600 mg/day for 6 months.
[c]TRP (triptorelin), 3.75 mg/month for 6 months.
[d]Numbers in parentheses are 95% confidence intervals.

(117–119). In the study of Telimaa et al., 60 patients with surgical debulking via laparotomy of stages I–IV endometriosis were randomized to treatment for 6 months with danazol (600 mg per day), medroxyprogesterone acetate (100 mg per day), or placebo. Second-look laparoscopies were done at 6 months, at the completion of medical treatment. Fifty-one patients completed the entire 12 months of follow-up of the study. The results showed that medroxyprogesterone acetate decreased average pain levels by 54% and that danazol decreased pain levels by 32% relative to placebo. However, a very worrisome finding in this study was that the 12-month pain levels in the control group were back to pretreatment levels. (The authors did not respond to requests for clarification.) This level of pain suggests that there was no therapeutic effect from surgical treatment, and this is not consistent with the results of the other two studies of postoperative treatment or the previously discussed study by Sutton et al. of surgical treatment only.

The second study, reported by Parazzini et al. (118), was limited to 75 women with stage III or IV endometriosis debulked via laparotomy. They were randomized to 3 months of nafarelin (400 µg per day) or placebo nasal spray. A combined visual analog score of pelvic pain and dysmenorrhea was then evaluated at 12 months in the 61 women who did not conceive. At 12 months postoperatively, nafarelin treatment resulted in no difference in pain levels. Unfortunately, the authors did not report data at 6 months.

The third study, done by Hornstein et al. (119), enrolled 109 women with stages I–IV endometriosis who underwent "reductive" laparoscopic surgery via laser or electrosurgery. Surgery was followed by 180 days of medical therapy with nafarelin, 200 µg b.i.d., or placebo nasal spray b.i.d. The goal was to follow all patients for 18 months after completion of medical therapy, but follow-up data on only 93 (85%) of the women were reported. Also, only 56 (51%) of the women had moderate or severe pelvic pain preoperatively, and the publication does not break down the pelvic pain data, but rather reports a pain score based on combined zero to three ratings of pelvic pain, dysmenorrhea, and dyspareunia (dysmenorrhea–dyspareunia–pelvic pain (DDP) pain scores). In women who were not sexually active, a dyspareunia score was still assigned by multiplying the sum of the pelvic pain and dysmenorrhea scores by 1.5. In the study, 16 patients who were randomized were excluded from analysis: 9 of 53 in the placebo group and 7 of 56 in the nafarelin group. A worst-case scenario reanalysis significantly changes the major outcome results of this study. Also, 16 patients were dropped from the study due to early discontinuation of therapy or noncompliance. Although at 6 months postoperatively, at the termination of medical treatment, the nafarelin treated group had slightly lower DDP scores,

this difference may have been due only to the absence of dysmenorrhea attributable to the amenorrhea induced by nafarelin. At 12 months (6 months after discontinuation of nafarelin) there was no statistically or clinically significant difference in pain scores between the nafarelin and placebo treated groups. The other major outcome studied by Hornstein et al. (120) was the need for alternative or other therapies postoperatively. Overall, during the course of the study, 25 (57%) of 44 placebo-treated patients required other treatment and 15 (31%) of 49 nafarelin-treated patients required other treatment. This difference gives an absolute risk reduction of 26% and a number needed to treat of 3.8 (95% confidence interval of 2.2 to 14.3).

It is not possible from the three available trials to clearly conclude whether medical treatment after surgical treatment is efficacious. At this time the evidence appears to suggest that 6 months of treatment with either nafarelin at 400 µg per day, danazol at 600 mg per day, or MPA at 100 mg per day lowers pain levels at 6 months postoperatively, but possibly does not affect pain levels at 12 months postoperatively. Three months of nafarelin therapy after surgical debulking of endometriosis does not appear to offer any improvement of response of endometriosis-associated CPP (Table 14.20). A reasonable way to interpret and apply these data is to initiate medical treatment after conservative surgical debulking therapy if patients have persistent or recurrent pain, rather than treat all patients postoperatively.

In summary, gynecologists must recognize that the finding of endometriosis in women with CPP does not ensure that medical or surgical treatment of endometriosis will result in effective relief of pain. To the contrary, although treatment of endometriosis in women with pelvic pain is clearly indicated based on randomized, placebo-controlled, double-blind clinical trials, pain relief of 6 or more months' duration due to treatment can be expected in only about 40% to 70% of women with endometriosis-associated CPP.

If fertility is not desired, then hysterectomy, with or without bilateral salpingo-oophorectomy, is often recommended for endometriosis-associated pelvic pain. There is no consensus as to the advisability of removal of both ovaries if one or both are not directly involved by endometriosis. In one study evaluating this dilemma, recurrence of pain when one or both ovaries are preserved has been reported to occur in 62% of cases compared to 10% when both ovaries are removed, giving a relative risk for pain recurrence of 6.1 (confidence interval 2.5 to 14.6) (120). Reoperation for pain was also more likely with ovarian preservation, with 31% requiring reoperation compared to 4% if both ovaries were removed at the time of hysterectomy for endometriosis. Although uncommon, endometriosis has been reported to recur after hysterectomy and bilateral salpingo-oophorectomy, with and without estrogen replacement therapy (121–123).

TABLE 14.20. EFFICACY OF MEDICAL TREATMENT OF ENDOMETRIOSIS-ASSOCIATED PELVIC PAIN AFTER SURGICAL DEBULKING OF ENDOMETRIOSIS

	MPA × 6 Months, Pain Relief at 6 Months[a]	DAN × 6 Months, Pain Relief at 6 Months[b]	NAF × 6 Months, Pain Relief at 6 Months[c,d]	MPA × 6 Months, Pain Relief at 12 Months	DAN × 6 Months, Pain Relief at 12 Months	NAF × 3 Months, Pain Relief at 12 Months	NAF × 6 Months, Pain Relief at 12 Months[d]
Surgery plus placebo: Mean decrease in pain scores	0.1[e]	0.1[e]	1.0	0.0[e]	0.0[e]	6.9	1.0
Surgery plus medical treatment: Mean decrease in pain scores	4.0	6.0	3.2	3.0 (1.7–4.4)	1.9 (0.6–3.2)	7.0	1.4
Decrease in mean pain scores attributable to medical treatment	3.8	4.3	2.2 (1.4–3.0)	3.1 (1.8–4.4)	1.9 (0.6–3.3)	0.1	0.4 (–0.4–1.2)
Percentage decrease in mean pain scores attributable to medical treatment	66%	71%	44% (28–61%)	54% (30–88%)	32% (8–57%)	—	8% (–8–24%)

[a]MPA (medroxyprogesterone acetate), 100 mg/day for 6 months.
[b]DAN (danazol), 600 mg/day for 6 months.
[c]NAF (nafarelin), 400 μg/day for 3 months.
Numbers in parentheses are 95% confidence intervals.
[d]In this study, pain relief was based on the aggregate decrease of dysmenorrhea, dyspareunia, and pelvic pain, in contrast to the other studies in which the data in this table represent only relief of nonmenstrual pelvic pain.
[e]These results, which are all from one study, are disconcerting and hard to explain because they suggest that surgery has no effect on pain postoperatively. See the text for further descriptions of the three studies summarized in this table.

ENDOSALPINGIOSIS

Endosalpingiosis is the presence of ectopic oviduct epithelium. The term endosalpingiosis, like endometriosis, is attributed to Sampson. Typical locations of endosalpingiosis are similar to those of endometriosis: pelvic peritoneum, uterus, fallopian tubes, ovaries, cul-de-sac, omentum, bladder serosa, bowel serosa, periaortic area, and skin (124). It is probably underreported, because much of the surgery for endometriosis consists of ablation of all recognized peritoneal abnormalities without histologic evaluation. In one series of 51 cases of laparoscopy for CPP, with histologic confirmation of endometriosis or endosalpingiosis in 23 cases (45%), two patients (4%) had only endosalpingiosis and 4 (8%) had both endosalpingiosis and endometriosis. In this series, women with endosalpingiosis represented 26% of CPP cases with a histologic diagnosis (125).

Endosalpingiosis is thought to be commonly associated with previous tubal surgery such as tubal ligation or salpingectomy, as well as with "chronic salpingitis." Theories of origin are similar to those for endometriosis, because it is thought to be spread locally from the endosalpinx via retrograde menstrual flow, to occur due to *in situ* coelomic metaplasia, or to occur due to lymphatic or hematagenous spread.

Grossly, endosalpingiosis usually appears as punctate, 1 to 2 mm, white to yellow, opaque or translucent, fluid-filled, cystic lesions that give a granular appearance to the involved peritoneum. Histologically, endosalpingiossis is diagnosed by the presence of benign ciliated and nonciliated columnar cells along with peg cells in abnormal locations. Psammoma body formation is associated with symptomatic endosalpingiosis. Hemorrhagic response to hormonal stimuli does not occur with endosalpingiosis like it does with endometriosis.

There has been one report of a patient with pain thought due to endosalpingiosis whose pain improved with danazol treatment (124). Two patients have been reported with response to GnRH analogue treatment (125).

KEY POINTS

Most Important Questions to Ask

- Did pain start initially as menstrual cramps (dysmenorrhea)?
- Does your pain worsen with menses or just before menses?
- Do you have pain with deep penetration during intercourse? If so, does it continue afterwards?

- Do you have rectal pain, especially with bowel movements?
- Have you had problems conceiveing?
- Do you have irregular uterine bleeding, particularly intermenstrual bleeding?
- Do you have urinary frequency, pressure, dysuria (pain with urination), or hematuria (blood in your urine)?

Most Important Physical Examination Findings

- Pelvic tenderness or nodularity only during menses
- Localized tender areas in the pelvis
- A fixed retroverted uterus with tenderness posterior to it
- Tender nodularity of the uterosacral ligaments and cul-de-sac on rectovaginal examination
- Narrowing of the posterior vaginal fornix
- Asymmetric, enlarged, tender ovaries that are fixed to the broad ligaments or pelvic sidewalls
- A tender adnexal mass

Most Important Diagnostic Studies

- Diagnostic laparoscopy
- Preoperative ultrasound
- Needle puncture of the ovary
- Ca-125 levels
- Hysterography and magnetic resonance imaging (adolescents with endometriosis)
- Sigmoidoscopy
- Colonoscopy
- Barium enema
- Cytoscopy
- Intravenous pyelography or computerized tomography

Treatments

- Observation with palliative treatment
- Conservative surgery
- Coagulation of endometriotic lesions
- Vaporization of endometriotic lesions
- Resection of endometriotic lesions
- Adhesiolysis
- Ovarian cystectomy
- Oophorectomy
- Salpingectomy
- Uterosacral neurectomy (uterosacral ligament transection)
- Presacral neurectomy
- Hormonal suppression
- Methyltestosterone, 5 to 10 mg per day
- Oral contraceptives
- Enovid (high-dose pill originally popularized by Kistner as "pseudopregnancy")
- Low-dose pills, start on day 3 of cycle continuously; double dose for 5 days if breakthrough bleeding occurs
- Low-dose pills, taken cyclically
- Medroxyprogesterone acetate, 100 mg per day
- Danazol, 200 to 400 mg b.i.d.
- Gonadotropin-releasing hormone analogues (GnRH analogues)
- Nafarelin, 200 to 400 μg b.i.d.
- Leuprolide, 3.75 to 7.5 mg q28 days
- Goserelin, 3.6 mg q28 days
- Triptorelin, 3.75 mg q28 days
- Combined medical and surgical treatments
- Definitive extripative surgery

REFERENCES

1. Sampson JA. Peritoneal endometriosis due to dissemination of endometrial tissue into the peritoneal cavity. *Am J Obstet Gynecol* 1927;14:422.
2. Sampson JA. Benign and malignant endometrial implants in the peritoneal cavity and their relationship to certain ovarian tumors. *Surg Gynecol Obstet* 1924;38:287.
3. Sampson JA. Perforating hemorrhagic (chocolate) cysts of the ovary. *Arch Surg* 1921;3:245.
4. Koninckx PR, Lesaffre E, Meuleman C, et al. Suggestive evidence that pelvic endometriosis is a progressive disease, whereas deeply infiltrating endometriosis is associated with pelvic pain. *Fertil Steril* 1991;55:759–765.
5. Barbieri RL. Etiology and epidemiology of endometriosis. *Am J Obstet Gynecol* 1990;162:565.
6. Mahmood TA, Templeton AA, Thomson L, et al. Menstrual symptoms in women with pelvic endometriosis. *Br J Obstet Gynaecol* 1991;98:558–563.
7. Rawson JMR. Prevalence of endometriosis in asymptomatic women. *J Reprod Med* 1991;36:513–515.
8. Martin DC. Letter to the editor. *Fertil Steril* 1991;56:792.
9. Howard FM. The role of laparoscopy in chronic pelvic pain: promise and pitfalls. *Obstet Gynecol Surv* 1993;48:357–387.
10. Kistner RW. *Gynecology: principle and practice.* Chicago: Year Book Medical Publishers, 1979:447–448.
11. Kistner RW. *Gynecology: principles and practice.* Chicago: Year Book Medical Publishers, 1979:447.
12. Vercellini P, Bocciolone L, Vendola N, et al. Peritoneal endometriosis: morphologic appearance in women with chronic pelvic pain. *J Reprod Med* 1991;36:533–536.
13. Slocumb JC. Chronic somatic, myofascial, and neurogenic abdominal pelvic pain. *Clin Obstet Gynecol* 1990;33:145.
14. Goldstein DP, DeCholnoky C, Emans SJ, et al. Laparoscopy in the diagnosis and management of pelvic pain in adolescents. *J Reprod Med* 1980;24:251.
15. Barbieri RL. Stenosis of the external cervical os: an association with endometriosis in women with chronic pelvic pain. *Fertil Steril* 1998;70:571–573.
16. Barbieri RL. Hormone treatment of endometriosis: the estrogen threshold hypothesis. *Am J Obstet Gynecol* 1992;166:740–745.
17. Filer RB, Wu CH. Coitus during menses: its effect on endometriosis and pelvic inflammatory disease. *J Reprod Med* 1989;34:887.
18. Koninckx PR, D'Hooghe TD, Oosterlynck D. Response to letter to the editor. *Fertil Steril* 1991;56:590–591.
19. Nisolle M, Paindaveine B, Bourdon A, et al. Histologic study of

peritoneal endometriosis in infertile women. *Fertil Steril* 1990;53:984–988.

20. D'Hooghe TM, Bambra CS, Raeymaekers BM, et al. Development of spontaneous endometriosis in baboons. *Obstet Gynecol* 1996;88:462–466.

21. D'Hooghe TM, Bambra CS, DeJonge I, et al. The prevalence of sponaneous endometriosis in the baboon increases with the time spent in captivity. *Acta Obstet Gynecol Scand* 1996;75: 98–101.

22. Liu DTY, Hitchcock A. Endometriosis: its association with retrograde menstruation, dysmenorrhea and tubal pathology. *Br J Obstet Gynaecol* 1986;93:859–862.

23. Moen MH, Muus KM. Endometriosis in pregnant and non-pregnant women at tubal sterilization. *Hum Reprod* 1991;6: 699–702.

24. Dmowski WP. Visual assessment of peritoneal implants for staging endometriosis: do number and cumulative size of lesions reflect the severity of a systemic disease? *Fertil Steril* 1987;47: 382–384.

25. Vernon MW, Beard JS, Graves K, et al. Classification of endometriotic implants by morphological appearance and capacity to synthesize prostaglandin F. *Fertil Steril* 1985;46: 801–806.

26. Jansen RP, Russell P. Nonpigmented endometriosis: clinical, laparoscopic, and pathologic definition. *Am J Obstet Gynecol* 1986;155:1154–1159.

27. Cornillie FJ, Oosterlynck D, Lauweryns JM, et al. Deeply infiltrating pelvic endometriosis: histology and clinical significance. *Fertil Steril* 1990;53:978–983.

28. Ripps BA, Martin DC. Focal pelvic tenderness, pelvic pain, and dysmenorrhea in endometriosis. *J Reprod Med* 1991;36:470–472.

29. Fedele L, Parazzini F, Bianchi S, et al. Stage and localization of pelvic endometriosis and pain. *Fertil Steril* 1990;53:155–158.

30. Nezhat N, Winer W, Nezhat F, et al. Laparoscopic treatment of endometriosis with laser and videocamera augmentation (videolaseroscopy). *J Gynecol Surg* 1989;5:163–168.

31. Cook AS, Rock JA. The role of laparoscopy in the treatment of endometriosis. *Fertil Steril* 1991;55:663–680.

32. Vercellini P, Bocciolone L, Vendola N, et al. Peritoneal endometriosis: morphologic appearance in women with chronic pelvic pain. *J Reprod Med* 1991;36:533–536.

33. Chatman DL. Pelvic peritoneal defects and endometriosis: Allen–Masters syndrome revisited. *Fertil Steril* 1981;36:751–756.

34. Chatman DL, Zbella EA. Pelvic peritoneal defects and endometriosis: further observations. *Fertil Steril* 1986;46:711–712.

35. Redwine DB. Age-related evolution in color appearance of endometriosis. *Fertil Steril* 1987;48:1062–1063.

36. Martin DC, Berry JD. Histology of chocolate cysts. *J Gynecol Surg* 1990;6:43.

37. Jansen RP, Russell P. Nonpigmented endometriosis: clinical, laparoscopic, and pathologic definition. *Am J Obstet Gynecol* 1986;155:1154–1159.

38. Adamson GD. Diagnosis and clinical presentation of endometriosis. *Am J Obstet Gynecol* 1990;162:568–569.

39. Martin DC, Hubert GD, Vander Zwaag R, et al. Laparoscopic appearances of peritoneal endometriosis. *Fertil Steril* 1989;51:63.

40. Sutton C, Hill D. Laser laparoscopy in the treatment of endometriosis: a 5-year study. *Br J Obstet Gynaecol* 1990; 97:181.

41. Muse K. Clininical manifestations and classification of endometriosis. *Clin Obstet Gynecol* 1988;31:813–822.

42. Israel R. Endometriosis: diagnostic evaluation. In: Mishell DR,

43. Brenner PL, eds. *Common problems in ob/gyn.* NJ: Medical Economics, 1988:589.

43. Howard FM. The role of laparoscopy in chronic pelvic pain: promise and pitfalls. *Obstet Gynecol Surv* 1993;48:357–387.

44. Fayez JA, Vogel MF. Comparison of different treatment methods of endometriomas by laparoscopy. *Obstet Gynecol* 1991;78: 660–665.

45. Chatman DL, Zbella EA. Biopsy in laparoscopically diagnosed endometriosis. *J Reprod Med* 1987;32:855–857.

46. Stripling MC, Martin DC, Chatman DL, et al. Subtle appearance of pelvic endometriosis. *Fertil Steril* 1988;49:427–431.

47. Perez JJ. Laparoscopic presacral neurectomy: results of the first 25 cases. *J Reprod Med* 1990;35:625–630.

48. Redwine DB. Peritoneal blood painting: an aid in the diagnosis of endometriosis. *Am J Obstet Gynecol* 1989;161:865–866.

49. Martin DC, Ahmic R, El-Zeky FA, et al. Increased histologic confirmation of endometriosis. *J Gynecol Surg* 1990;6:275.

50. Nunley WC. Medical management of endometriosis: a review. *Hosp Formul* 1985;20:704.

51. Droegemueller W, Herbst AL, Mishell DR, et al. *Comprehensive gynecology.* St Louis: Mosby, 1987:493.

52. Barbieri RL. Etiology and epidemiology of endometriosis. *Am J Obstet Gynecol* 1990;162:565–567.

53. Candiani GB, Vercellini P, Fedele L. Laparoscopic ovarian puncture for correct staging of endometriosis. *Fertil Steril* 1990; 53:994–998.

54. Lanzone A, Marane R, Muscatello R, et al. Serum Ca-125 levels in the diagnosis and management of endometriosis. *J Reprod Med* 1991;36:603.

55. Adamson GD. Diagnosis and clinical presentation of endometriosis. *Am J Obstet Gynecol* 1990;162:568–569.

56. Rapkin AJ, Mayer EA. Gastroenterologic causes of chronic pelvic pain. *Obstet Gynecol Clin North Am* 1993;20:663–683.

57. Adamson GD, Nelson HP. Surgical treatment of endometriosis. *Obstet Gynecol Clin North Am* 1997;24:375–409.

58. Kettel LM, Hummel WP. Modern medical management of endometriosis. *Obstet Gynecol Clin North Am* 1997;24:361–73.

59. Greenblatt RB, Dmowski WP, Mahesh VB, et al. Clinical studies with an antigonadotropin-danazol. *Fertil Steril* 1971;22: 102–112.

60. Telimaa S, Puolakka J, Ronnberg L, et al. Placebo-controlled comparison of danazol and high-dose medroxyprogesterone acetate in the treatment of endometriosis. *Gynecol Endocrinol* 1987;1:13.

61. Carpenter SE, Tjaden B, Rock JA, et al. The effect of regular exercise on women receiving danazol for treatment of endometriosis. *Int J Gynecol Obstet* 1995;49:299–304.

62. Barbieri RL, Evans S, Kistner RW. Danazol in the treatment of endometriosis: analysis of 100 cases with 4-year follow-up. *Fertil Steril* 1982;37:737–746.

63. Farquhar C, Sutton C. The evidence for the management of endometriosis. *Curr Opin Obstet Gynecol* 1998;10:321–332.

64. Cundy T, Cornish J, Roberts H, et al. Spinal bone density in women using depot medroxyprogesterone acetate contraception. *Obstet Gynecol* 1998;92:569–573.

65. Bromham DR, Booker MW, Rose GL, et al. Updating the clinical experience in endometriosis—the European perspective. *Br J Obstet Gynaecol* 1995;102(Suppl 12):12–16.

66. The Gestrinone Italian Study Group. Gestrinone versus a gonadotropin-releasing hormone agonist for the treatment of pelvic pain associated with endometriosis: a multicenter, randomized, double-blind study. *Fertil Steril* 1996;66:911–919.

67. Tamaya T, Misao R, Nakanishi Y. The failed suppression of serum estradiol level by gonadotropin-releasing hormone agonist in a case of pelvic endometriosis. *Am J Obstet Gynecol* 1998;179:828–829.

68. Hsu CC, Lin YS, Wang ST, et al. Immunomodulation in women with endometriosis receiving GnTH agonist. *Obstet Gynecol* 1997;89:993–998.

69. Dlugi AM, Miller JD, Knittle J. Lupron depot (leuprolide acetate for depot suspension) in the treatment of endometriosis: a randomized, placebo-controlled, double-blind study. *Fertil Steril* 1990;54:419–427.

70. Bergqvist A, Bergh T, Hogstrom L, et al. Effects of triptorelin versus placebo on the symptoms of endometriosis. *Fertil Steril* 1998;69:702–708.

71. Wheeler JM, Knittle JD, Miller JD. Depot leuprolide versus danazol in treatment of women with symptomatic endometriosis. I. Efficacy results. *Am J Obstet Gynecol* 1992;167:1367–1371.

72. Rock JA, Truglia JA, Caplan RJ, and the Zoladex Endometriosis Study Group. Zoladex (goserelin acetate implant) in the treatment of endometriosis: a randomized comparison with danazol. *Obstet Gynecol* 1993;82:198–205.

73. ANZ Zoladex Group. Goserelin depot versus danazol in the treatment of endometriosis. The Australian/New Zealand experience. *Fertil Steril* 1995;63:504–507.

74. Henzyl MR, Corson SL, Moghissi K, et al. Administration of nasal nafarelin as compared with oral danazol for endometriosis. A multicenter double-blind clinical trial. *N Engl J Med* 1988;318:485–489.

75. Kennedy SH, Williams IA, Brodribb J, et al. A comparison of nafarelin acetate and danazol in the treatment of endometriosis. *Fertil Steril* 1990;53:998–1003.

76. Nafarelin European Endometriosis Trial Group. Nafarelin for endometriosis: a large-scale, danazol-controlled trial of efficacy and safety, with 1-year follow-up. *Fertil Steril* 1992;57:514–522.

77. Adamson GD, Kwei L, Edgren RA. Pain of endometriosis: effects of nafarelin and danazol therapy. *Int J Fertil* 1994;39:215–217.

78. Henzyl MR, Kwei L. Efficacy and safety of nafarelin in the treatment of endometriosis. *Am J Obstet Gynecol* 1990;162:570.

79. Waller KG, Shaw RW. Gonadotropin-releasing hormone analogues for the treatment of endometriosis: long-term follow-up. *Fertil Steril* 1993;59:511–515.

80. Hornstein MD, Yuzpe AA, Burry K, et al. Retreatment with nafarelin for recurrent endometriosis symptoms: efficacy, safety, and bone mineral density. *Fertil Steril* 1997;67:1013–1018.

81. Hornstein MD, Yuzpe AA, Burry KA, et al. Prospective randomized double-blind trial of 3 versus 6 months of nafarelin therapy for endometriosis associated pelvic pain. *Fertil Steril* 1995;63:955–962.

82. Hornstein MD, Surrey ES, Weisberg GW, et al., for the Lupron Add-Back Study Group. Leuprolide acetate depot and hormonal add-back in endometriosis: a 12-month study. *Obstet Gynecol* 1998;91:16–24.

83. Kistner RW. Treatment of endometriosis by inducing pseudopregnancy with ovarian hormones. *Fertil Steril* 1959;10:539–554.

84. Vercellini P, Trespidi L, Colombo A, et al. A gonadotrophin-releasing hormone agonist versus a low-dose oral contraceptive for pelvic pain associated with endometriosis. *Fertil Steril* 1993;60(1):75–79.

85. Kettel LM, Murphy AA, Morales AJ, et al. Preliminary report on the treatment of endometriosis with low-dose mifepristone (RU-486). *Am J Obstet Gynecol* 1998;178:1151–1156.

86. Shaw RW. Nafarelin in the treatment of pelvic pain caused by endometriosis. *Am J Obstet Gynecol* 1990;162:574–576.

87. Rolland R, van der Heijden PFM. Nafarelin versus danazol in the treatment of endometriosis. *Am J Obstet Gynecol* 1990;162:586–588.

88. Henzyl MR. Role of nafarelin in the management of endometriosis. *J Reprod Med* 1989;34:1021–1024.

89. Fedele L, Arcaini L, Bianchi S, et al. Comparison between cyproterone acetate and danazol in the treatment of pelvic pain associated with endometriosis. *Obstet Gynecol* 1988;73:1000–1004.

90. Henzl MR, Kwei L. Efficacy and safety of nafarelin in the treatment of endometriosis. *Am J Obstet Gynecol* 1990;162:570–574.

91. Betts JW, Buttram VC Jr. A plan for managing endometriosis. *Contemp Ob/Gyn* 1980;15:121.

92. Howard FM. Laparoscopic evaluation and treatment of women with chronic pelvic pain. *J Am Assoc Gynecol Laparosc* 1994;1:325–331.

93. Davis GD, Brooks RA. Excision of pelvic endometriosis with the carbon dioxide laser laparoscope. *Obstet Gynecol* 1988;72:816–819.

94. Sutton CJG, Ewen SP, Whitelaw N, et al. Prospective, randomized, double-blind trial of laser laparoscopy in the treatment of pelvic pain associated with minimal, mild, and moderate endometriosis. *Fertil Steril* 1994;62:696–700.

95. Sackett DL, Haynes RB. Summarising the effects of therapy: a new table and some more terms. *Evidence-Based Med* 1997;2:103–104.

96. Sutton CJG, Pooley AS, Ewen SP, et al. Follow-up report on a randomized controlled trial of laser laparoscopy in the treatment of pelvic pain associated with minimal to moderate endometriosis. *Fertil Steril* 1997;68:1070–1074.

97. Daniell JF, Kurtz BR, Gurley LD. Laser laparoscopic management of large endometriomas. *Fertil Steril* 1991;55:692–695.

98. Reich H, McGlynn F. Treatment of ovarian endometriomas using laparoscopic surgical techniques. *J Reprod Med* 1986;31:577–584.

99. Frangenhein H. The range and limits of operative laparoscopy in the diagnosis of sterility. In: Phillips JM, ed. *Endoscopy in gynecology.* Downey, CA: American Association of Gynecologic Laparoscopist, 1978:276.

100. Nezhat C, Winer WK, Nezhat F. A comparison of the CO_2, argon, and KTP/532 lasers in the videolaseroscopic treatment of endometriosis. *Colposc Gynecol Laser Surg* 1988;4:41.

101. Fayez JA, Vogel MF. Comparison of different treatment methods of endometriomas by laparoscopy. *Obstet Gynecol* 1991;78:660–665.

102. Beretta P, Franchi M, Ghezzi F, et al. Randomized clinical trial of two laparoscopic treatments of endometriomas: cystectomy versus drainage and coagulation. *Fertil Steril* 1998;70:1176–1180.

103. Martin DC, Berry JD. Histology of chocolate cysts. *J Gynecol Surg* 1990;6:43–46.

104. Polan ML, DeCherney A. Presacral neurectomy for pelvic pain in infertility. *Fertil Steril* 1980;34:557–560.

105. Lee RB, Stone K, Magelssen D, et al. Presacral neurectomy for chronic pelvic pain. *Obstet Gynecol* 1986;68:517–521.

106. Tjaden B, Schlaff WD, Kimball A, et al. The efficacy of presacral neurectomy for the relief of midline dysmenorrhea. *Obstet Gynecol* 1990;76:89–91.

107. Black WT. Use of presacral sympathectomy in the treatment of dysmenorrhea. A second look after twenty-five years. *Am J Obstet Gynecol* 1964;89:16.

108. Doyle JB, Des Rosiers JJ. Paracervical uterine denervation for relief of pelvic pain. *Clin Obstet Gynecol* 1963;6:742.

109. Lichten E. Three years experience with LUNA. *Am J Gynecol Health* 1989;5:9.

110. Lichten EM, Bombard J. Surgical treatment of primary dysmenorrhea with laparoscopic uterine nerve ablation. *J Reprod Med* 1987;32:37–41.

111. Tjaden B, Schlaff WD, Kimball A, et al. The efficacy of pre-

sacral neurectomy for the relief of midline dysmenorrhea. *Obstet Gynecol* 1990;76:89–91.

112. Candiani GB, Fedele L, Vercellini P, et al. Presacral neurectomy for the treatment of pelvic pain associated with endometriosis: a controlled study. *Am J Obstet Gynecol* 1992;167:100–103.

113. Lichten EM, Bombard J. Surgical treatment of primary dysmenorrhea with laparoscopic uterine nerve ablation. *J Reprod Med* 1987;32:37–41.

114. Candiani GB, Fedele L, Vercellini P, et al. Repetitive conservative surgery for recurrence of endometriosis. *Obstet Gynecol* 1991;77:421–424.

115. Marrs RP. The use of potassium-titanyl-phosphate laser for laparoscopic removal of ovarian endometriomas. *Am J Obstet Gynecol* 1991;164:1622–1626.

116. Martin DC. CO_2 laser laparoscopy for endometriosis associated with infertility. *J Reprod Med* 1986;31:1089–1094.

117. Telimaa S, Ronnberg L, Kauppila A. Placebo-controlled comparison of danazol and high-dose medroxyprogesterone acetate in the treatment of endometriosis after conservative surgery. *Gynecol Endocrinol* 1987;1:363–371.

118. Parazzini F, Fedele L, Busacca M, et al. Postsurgical medical treatment of advanced endometriosis: results of a randomized clinical trial. *Am J Obstet Gynecol* 1994;171:1205–1207.

119. Hornstein MD, et al. Use of nafarelin versus placebo after reductive laparoscopic surgery for endometriosis. *Fertil Steril* 1997;68:860–864.

120. Namnoum AB, Hickman TN, Goodman SB, et al. Incidence of symptom recurrence after hysterectomy for endometriosis. *Fertil Steril* 1995;64:898–902.

121. Metzger DA, Lessey BA, Soper JT, et al. Hormone-resistant endometriosis following total abdominal hysterectomy and bilateral salpingo-oophorectomy: correlation with histology and steroid receptor content. *Obstet Gynecol* 1991;78:946–950.

122. Redwine DB. Endometriosis persisting after castration: clinical characteristics and results of surgical management. *Obstet Gynecol* 1994;83:405–413.

123. Dmowski WP, Radwanska E, Rana N. Recurrent endometriosis following hysterectomy and oophorectomy: the role of residual ovarian fragments. *Int J Gynecol Obstet* 1988;26:93–103.

124. Davies SA, Maclin VM. Endosalpingiosis as a cause of chronic pelvic pain. *Am J Obstet Gynecol* 1991;164:495–496.

125. Keltz MD, Kliman HJ, Arici AM, et al. Endosalpintiosis found at laparoscopy for chronic pelvic pain. *Fertil Steril* 1995;64:482–485.

15

UTERINE LEIOMYOMAS

C. PAUL PERRY

KEY TERMS AND DEFINITIONS

Intramural leiomyoma: A myoma located in the myometrium.

Leiomyoma: A benign tumor derived from smooth muscle; other names are fibroid, fibromyoma, or myoma.

Menorrhagia: Excessive and prolonged bleeding occurring at the regular intervals of menstruation.

Parasitic leiomyoma: An unusual variant of leiomyoma that is pedunculated originally, but develops alternate blood supply from omentum or other pelvic structures and detaches from the uterus.

Pedunculated myoma: A myoma that is attached to the uterus only by a pedicle.

Submucosal leiomyoma: A myoma that is located immediately below the endometrium.

Subserosal myoma: A myoma located just beneath the uterine serosa.

INTRODUCTION

Uterine leiomyomas are benign tumors of uterine smooth muscle. They are also referred to as myomas, fibroids, and fibromyomas. Uterine leiomyomas are the most common tumors of the female pelvis occurring in one in every four to five women, with the highest incidence in the fifth decade (1). About 175,000 hysterectomies are performed annually for this condition at an expense of over $1 billion.

ETIOLOGY

Myomas may be solitary tumors, but most often there are multiple leiomyomas. Each myoma is of single muscle cell origin. They may result from a chromosomal abnormality, most commonly number 12.

The size of myomas depends on differences in vascular supply, proximity to adjacent tumors, degenerative changes, and hormonal growth factors (2). Estrogen and growth hormone are known to sometimes stimulate the growth of fibroids, whereas androgens and progesterone may some-

times inhibit their growth. Intracellular estrogen is increased when fibroids are compared with nonneoplastic myometrial cells. The reduction in size after menopause is thought to be owing to this regulatory mechanism. Peak levels of growth hormone in response to insulin-induced hypoglycemia is twice as high in women with myomas than in a control group. However, this "Estrogen-Growth Hormone Hypothesis" cannot explain all the variations of growth. Genetically determined tendencies or blood supply may play a major role (1).

PATHOLOGY

Most often these tumors are submucosal (submucous), intramural, subserosal, or pedunculated. Submucosal myomas are located immediately below the endometrium. Intramural leiomyomas are located in the myometrium. Subserosal myomas are located just beneath the uterine serosa. Pedunculated myomas are attached to the uterus by a pedicle. Parasitic leiomyomas, an unusual variant, are pedunculated originally, but develop alternate blood supply from omentum or other pelvic structures and detach from the uterus. Myomas of the round ligament, broad ligament, cervix, and fallopian tube are also occasionally found.

Ascites has been reported with these fibroids (3). Also, benign metastasizing leiomyoma, disseminated peritoneal leiomyomatosis, and intravenous leiomyomatosis have been reported (4). Polycythemia and leiomyosarcoma are rare complications of these tumors. It is not clear if leiomyomas truly degenerate into malignant sarcomas or whether sarcomas arise spontaneously as separate neoplasms. Clearly, the concern that a suspected myoma might be a sarcoma is a clinical conundrum, but the reality is that uterine leiomyosarcomas are rare and leiomyomas are common.

SYMPTOMS

Although most fibroids are asymptomatic, 10% to 40% may produce abnormal uterine bleeding, infertility, or pain. Menorrhagia is often associated with the presence of uterine fibroids, especially submucosal myomas. Patients may have experienced this for so long that they consider it normal. To ask if their menstruation is such that "they will bleed through their protection" is a useful screen. Stress urinary incontinence is seen in some patients who have external pressure on the bladder from the fibroid. With increased abdominal pressure, the tumor acts as a plunger and urine leakage occurs.

Chronic pain symptoms with myomas are generally dysmenorrhea or pressure. Although one of three women with myomas experiences pain, this pain is most often dysmenorrhea. Pressure-type pain from the myoma's size (if large) or from growth or enlargement may occasionally present as chronic pelvic pain (CPP), but CPP is attributed to uterine fibroids far more frequently than justified. There is evidence that most of the time CPP is produced by associated pathology (e.g., endometriosis or adhesions) rather than the uterine fibroid (1). In addition to pressure-type pain, impingement of leiomyomata on surrounding structures can cause a variety of symptoms depending on their size and location. The onset of pain is usually gradual. Collision dyspareunia, rectal pressure, and pelvic discomfort are likely with a fixed retroverted fibroid that may fill the cul-de-sac. Ureteral compression from very large myomas can produce hydronephrosis and back pain, but complete obstruction has not been described. Recurrent, sharp pelvic pain in the patient with a pedunculated leiomyoma could be caused by intermittent torsion. Acute pelvic pain may also occur with myomas in specific conditions such as acute red degeneration during pregnancy and transcervical prolapse of a submucous fibroid ("aborting fibroid").

It is germane to again state that chronic pelvic pain from uterine leiomyomas is atypical. Other conditions such as adenomyosis, endometriosis, irritable bowel syndrome, and interstitial cystitis should be suspected when pain is the presenting symptom (5).

PHYSICAL EXAMINATION

Diagnosis of uterine fibroids is accomplished with great accuracy by physical examination. Pelvic examination reveals an enlarged, firm, irregularly shaped uterus. With degeneration, the consistency of the myomas may become softer, or even cystic, to palpation. Rarely, the uterus may be tender. By clinical examination, though it is sometimes difficult to differentiate the uterine tumors from an adnexal tumor. Whether the tumor moves as part of the uterus or independently may help with this distinction, but is not a completely reliable finding because ovarian cancer may fix the ovary to the uterus. Pregnancy may also account for an enlarged uterus.

Smaller submucosal myomas may be symptomatic but not palpable. Prolapse of a pedunculated submucosal

myoma can often be diagnosed visually by the presence of the myoma at the cervical os.

DIAGNOSTIC STUDIES

Ultrasonography has been valuable to document the number of fibroids, their location, degree of calcification, and rate of growth. Other imaging techniques such as computerized tomography (CT) and magnetic resonance imaging (MRI) are too expensive to be routinely used, but may sometimes be helpful in distinguishing ovarian from uterine masses. Hysterosalpingography may yield important information regarding conservative management of the infertile patient. Hysteroscopy is often helpful in diagnosing (and treating) patients with submucosal myomas. Laparoscopy is helpful to discover associated pathology in CPP patients.

DIAGNOSIS

Ultimately, the diagnosis of leiomyomas requires histological confirmation. However, clinical evaluation is usually sufficiently accurate that biopsy or excision can be avoided except in unclear or extenuating circumstances.

Differential diagnoses of pelvic masses thought to be myomas include pregnancy, ovarian masses, and colorectal neoplasia. In women thought to have CPP associated with myomas, other common causes of CPP are more likely the etiology and should be considered prior to attributing CPP to leiomyomas.

TREATMENT
Medical Treatment

Size, location, growth rate, and symptoms make individualization of management of patients with uterine leiomyomas one of the great arts of gynecology. Treatment of CPP from uterine fibroids includes expectant management, and medical and surgical therapy. Some older criteria for treatment, such as greater than a 12-week-size pregnancy or inability to evaluate the adnexa, no longer apply (5). If symptoms are not severe and the patient is approaching menopause, repeat examinations can be performed every 6 months to assure there is no rapid growth. Nonsteroidal antiinflammatory drugs (NSAIDs) can be used to treat dysmenorrhea and iron therapy may be necessary to treat anemia. Oral contraceptives and progesterone may be of limited benefit in treatment of dysmenorrhea or menorrhagia associated with myomas. Gestrinone (an androgen) and RU486 (an antiprogesterone) are currently under investigation for hormonal treatment of leiomyoma.

Gonadotrophin releasing hormone agonists (GnRH-a) have been most effective in reducing the size and symptoms of leiomyoma. By creating a hypoestrogenic environment, the smooth muscle cellular component is reduced up to 50% in volume. Response to GnRH-a therapy is directly related to the cellularity and inversely related to the amount of collagen present before treatment. Maximum reduction in size occurs after 3 months of therapy, but long-term control can be produced by prolonging the hormonal suppression. Unfortunately, regrowth to pretreatment size will occur within 12 weeks after cessation of the GnRH-a. Risk and cost benefits do not favor this medical approach to painful myomas. However, short-term therapy has been useful to reduce blood loss and to convert an abdominal to a vaginal hysterectomy. Preoperative GnRH-a with oral iron supplement may be useful in patients with menorrhagia to treat iron deficiency anemia.

Surgical Treatment

Surgical treatment of painful leiomyomas includes hysterectomy, transcervical resection, myomectomy, embolization, and myolysis. Hysterectomy is considered the gold standard for successful treatment with complete resolution of symptoms and an acceptable morbidity rate. The vaginal route is preferred, either after GnRH-a, or by morcellation in skilled surgical hands. Laparoscopic hysterectomy or laparoscopically assisted vaginal hysterectomy may be performed with some of the advantages of a transvaginal hysterectomy. Laparoscopic supracervical hysterectomy is also an option in those patients with good pelvic support who wish to avoid a laparotomy.

Myomectomy is an option for those patients wishing to retain their reproductive potential. Myomectomy is sometimes discouraged because of a belief of an inordinate risk of blood loss and adhesion formation. There is no evidence that complications are increased with myomectomy versus hysterectomy. Use of dilute vasopressin, limited uterine incisions and careful hemostasis assure reasonable blood losses and reduce postoperative adhesions. Laparoscopic myomectomy can now be performed with little blood loss and decreased recovery (7). However, uterine incision closure can be difficult and requires a surgeon skilled in laparoscopic suturing. Because of this, in many cases the size of the fibroid should be limited to below 5 cm if the laparoscopic approach is to give good results. Powered morcellators have greatly facilitated the extraction of large myomas laparoscopically. Further refinements in technique may make this the procedure of choice in the future.

Hysteroscopic transcervical resection of submucous myomas is becoming more common in the surgical approach to infertility and abnormal uterine bleeding, but little is known regarding its benefit in those patients with pain. Other nonmedical therapies, including myolysis by electrodesiccation or cryotherapy, are under investigation. Arterial embolization has been demonstrated to decrease the size of fibroids, but long-term results are lacking (8).

The treatment of CPP should be tailored to each patient with leiomyomata. A rush to judgment regarding the palpable fibroid being etiologic may lead to improper diagnosis and treatment. Many more options are now available to our patients and the physician must educate the patient in risks and benefits of the appropriate alternatives.

KEY POINTS

Differential Diagnosis

- Pregnancy
- Extrauterine masses, especially ovarian
- Other common causes of pelvic pain

Most Important Questions to Ask

- Rapid or slow onset of pain
- Pain experienced during pregnancy
- Recent onset of stress urinary incontinence
- Collision dyspareunia
- Pelvic pressure
- Bleeds through protection during menstruation

Most Important Physical Examination Sign

- Enlarged, firm, irregularly shaped uterus
- Pelvic mass

Most Important Diagnostic Study

- Pelvic ultrasound

Treatments

- Expectant
- Nonsteroidal antiinflammatory drugs
- GnRH agonist
- Myomectomy: hysteroscopy, laparotomy, or laparoscopy
- Hysterectomy
- Embolization

REFERENCES

1. Buttram VC, Reiter RC. Uterine leiomyomata: etiology, symptomalology, and management. *Fertil Steril* 1981;36:433–445.
2. ACOG Technical Bulletin. Uterine leiomyomata. 1994;No. 192.
3. Prayson RA, Hart WR. Pathologic considerations of uterine smooth muscle tumors. *Obstet Gynecol Clin NA* 1995;22: 637–657.

4. Brand AH, Scurry JP, Planner RS, et al. Grapelike leiomyoma of the uterus. *Am J Obstet Gynecol* 1995;173:959–961.

5. Hutchins FL. Uterine fibroids. *Obstet Gynecol Clin NA* 1995;22:659–665.

6. Kawamura N, Shibata S, Ito F, et al. Correlation between shrinkage of uterine leiomyoma treated with buserelin acetate and histopathologic findings of biopsy specimen before treatment. *Fertil Steril* 1997;68:632–636.

7. Reich H. Laparoscopic myomectomy. *Obstet Gynecol Clin NA* 1995;22:757–759.

8. Ravina JH, Herbreteau D, Ciraru-Vigneron N, et al. Arterial embolisation to treat uterine myomata. *Lancet* 1995;346:671–672.

16

OVARIAN RETENTION SYNDROME

AHMED M. EL-MINAWI
FRED M. HOWARD

KEY TERMS AND DEFINITIONS

Ovarian remnant syndrome: The persistence of functional ovarian tissue after intended extirpation of both ovaries with or without hysterectomy.

Ovarian retention syndrome (residual ovary syndrome): The presence of persistent pelvic pain, dyspareunia, or a pelvic mass after intended conservation of one or both ovaries at the time of hysterectomy.

INTRODUCTION

The majority of physicians when discussing the sequelae of retained ovaries following hysterectomy tend to speak in terms of *residual ovary syndrome,* a term popularized by Grogan, Christ, and Lotze, rather than *ovarian retention syndrome* (1,2). Both of these terms are readily confused by gynecologists with the *ovarian remnant syndrome,* a disorder occurring after oophorectomy in which inadvertent incomplete removal of all ovarian tissue has occurred (3). Ovarian retention syndrome is, in our opinion, the preferable name for an ovarian mass or ovarian pain occurring after hysterectomy, because *retention* is defined as the act of retaining or the state of being retained (i.e., to keep in possession of or hold intact) (4). On the other hand, *residual* refers to the remainder left after a portion or part is separated or taken and that remains effective for some time. By definition a *remnant* is a small part or trace remaining of a larger entity and thus *residual* and *remnant* mean basically the same thing (4). When applied to the presence of ovarian tissue, they both are most appropriately used when describing a piece of ovary that is inadvertently left after oophorectomy. Neither of these two terms is correct if applied to the deliberate retention of one or more ovaries at the time of hysterectomy, in which instance the term *retention* is more appropriate. We propose that ovarian retention syndrome be used for the syndrome characterized by the presence of persistent pelvic pain, dyspareunia, or a pelvic mass after conservation of one or both ovaries at the time of hysterec-

tomy. The distinction between ovarian retention syndrome and ovarian remnant syndrome is dependent on the surgical history and pain symptoms of the patient.

There is not a great deal published regarding ovarian retention syndrome. Even determining its frequency is difficult because of the relatively few series published and the retrospective manner in which they are reported. A major stumbling block is that cases may be listed that were not originally performed by the reporting gynecologist; thus, no accurate denominator of the total number of hysterectomies can be given. The lowest incidence is the 0.9% reported by Ranney and Abu-Ghazaleh, which represents 14 patients out of a total of 1,557 hysterectomies with ovarian conservation done exclusively by the two authors (5). The highest incidence is reported by Grogan and Duncan who had 19 patients (4.9%) in a series of 390 cases of hysterectomy with retained ovaries (6). Estimates of the incidence of ovarian retention syndrome from published series are listed in Table 16.1 (7–9).

ETIOLOGY

A possible major etiological factor in the occurrence of ovarian retention syndrome is pelvic adhesion formation from either the hysterectomy or previous surgery. Grogan proposed that pain with ovarian retention syndrome "may reflect ovarian dysfunction secondary to pelvic adhesions and perioophoritis (10)." These adhesions, in his opinion, interfere with ovarian function and ovulation, leading to a pelvic mass composed of multiple cystic, atretic, or hemorrhagic follicles that produce pelvic pain. Similarly, Christ and Lotze surmise that pelvic adhesions somehow interfere with ovarian function and ovulation and give rise to persistent follicular and corpus luteum cysts (2). Sidall-Allum et al. are of the opinion that the pain from the ovary arises from its inability to cyclically expand because of its encapsulation in dense adhesions (11). The presence of functioning ovarian tissue is a requirement for pain in these theories. Dekel et al. have attempted to explain the increase in cyst

TABLE 16.1. REPORTED INCIDENCE OF THE OVARIAN RETENTION SYNDROME IN THE LITERATURE

Investigator(s)	Hysterectomies with conservation	Retention syndrome patients	Incidence in series (%)	Hysterectomy done at same institute (%)
Ranney and Abu-Ghazaleh	1,557	14	0.9	100
Funt et al.	922	13	1.4	100
Bukovsky et al.	329	6	1.8	100
Gevaerts	303	6	1.9	100
Hwu et al.	1,520	35	2.3	—
Dekel et al.	2,561	73	2.8	99
Christ and Lotze	6,188	202	3.1	22
Mackenzie	252	9	3.5	100
De Neef and Hollenbeck	161	7	4.3	100
Grogan and Duncan	390	19	4.9	—
Grogan, 1958	—	30	—	80
Grogan, 1967	—	92	—	45
El-Minawi and Howard	—	29	—	24
Carey and Slack	—	8	—	—
Siddall-Allum et al.	—	7	—	0

occurrence as ovarian dysfunction caused by disturbance of the ovarian blood supply during hysterectomy, part of which is derived from the uterine arteries (12). It is well established that ovaries in posthysterectomy patients maintain ovarian function and hormonal production for extended periods (13).

Data from clinical reports support a possible role of pelvic adhesions (Table 16.2). Christ and Lotze reported that 85% of their cases had extensive adhesions involving the ovaries at the time of surgery in addition to 57% having cystic ovaries (2). Hwu et al. report that extensive pelvic adhesions was the "typical" operative finding (14). Bukovsky and Sidall-Allum both report adhesions in 100% of their cases, which is the same figure found in our series of 29 patients who underwent surgery for ovarian retention syndrome (11,15,16). On the other hand, Ranney and Abu-Ghazaleh report operating on only two patients with pelvic adhesions (17%) as a primary finding, but do not report on adhesions possibly found in other patients (5) Carey and Slack reported finding dense adhesions in only two (25%) of their patients on repeat surgery (17).

It also appears that the etiology of ovarian retention syndrome is in some way related to the patient's past history. A history of pelvic surgery prior to hysterectomy may be a contributing factor and is present in 35% to 79% of cases (Table 16.3) (10,16). One possible explanation is that the preexisting adhesions make the hysterectomy more difficult and lead to even more severe adhesive disease. Also, in some cases there may be nociceptive signals arising from the adhesions, causing pelvic pain that continues or recurs with adhesions of the retained ovaries (18).

The previous symptoms or the indication for hysterectomy may also have a bearing on the occurrence of ovarian retention syndrome. Many patients in the reported series have documented histories of pelvic pain prior to hysterectomy. Whether this has a direct bearing on the subsequent condition (as in case of pain arising from pelvic adhesions from prior surgery) needs further investigation. If the pain was caused by some other process, such as pelvic congestion syndrome, then pain would definitely recur on the side of a retained ovary. This was discussed by Sidall-Allum et al., who recommended bilateral oophorectomy in patients undergoing surgical treatment for pelvic

TABLE 16.2. FREQUENCY OF PELVIC ADHESIONS IN PATIENTS WITH OVARIAN RETENTION SYNDROME

Investigators	Retention syndrome	Percent with pelvic adhesions
Carey and Slack	8	25
Funt et al.	13	69
Gevaerts	6	83
Christ and Lotze	202	85
Bukovsky et al.	6	100
Sidall-Allum et al.	7	100
El-Minawi and Howard	29	100

TABLE 16.3. FREQUENCY OF PRIOR SURGERY AMONG OVARIAN RETENTION SYNDROME PATIENTS

Investigator(s)	Retention syndrome patients	Percent with history of prior abdominopelvic surgery
Grogan	122	35
Christ and Lotze	202	40
Bukovsky	6	50
El-Minawi and Howard	29	79

TABLE 16.4. COMMON PREOPERATIVE INDICATIONS FOR HYSTERECTOMY IN OVARIAN RETENTION SYNDROME PATIENTS

Authors	Cases	Pelvic Pain (%)	Leiomyoma (%)	Bleeding (%)	Endometriosis (%)
Christ and Lotze	202	10	23	20	10
Grogan	92	20	24	21	—
Grogan	30	27	13	37	—
Funt et al.	13	15	77	15	8
Bukovsky et al.	6	0	83	67	33
El-Minawi and Howard	29	34	7	34	28

congestion syndrome so as to prevent recurrent pain (11). In their series of seven cases, five had pain symptoms prior to their hysterectomies. Myomas and bleeding are also common primary preoperative diagnoses (Table 16.4). Endometriosis is another prehysterectomy diagnosis that may lead in many cases to dense adhesions that may recur following hysterectomy. In our series of 29 patients, chronic pelvic pain and bleeding were equally represented (34%) as causes for hysterectomy, where leiomyomas contributed to the indication for hysterectomy in only two patients (16).

The age of the patient may also be a factor in development of the syndrome. It should be more common in younger women with greater ovarian activity, based on the belief that ovarian retention syndrome stems from ovarian dysfunction. The majority of women with ovarian retention syndrome had their hysterectomies in their third or fourth decade and the average age at time of diagnosis of ovarian retention syndrome is in their fourth and fifth decades (Table 16.5). This is a period when there is still vigorous ovarian function.

It is also possible that the route of hysterectomy has a role in the etiology of ovarian retention syndrome (12,15). There appears to be a significantly higher incidence of ovarian retention syndrome following the abdominal route as compared to the vaginal route. After abdominal hysterectomy the incidence of ovarian retention syndrome is 4% to 5% and after vaginal hysterectomy it is 0.4% to 0.5%. This difference may reflect only the previously alluded to role of pelvic adhesions (which are greater in abdominal cases) as a major factor in the etiology of ovarian retention syndrome.

Dekel et al. have examined the role or unilateral versus bilateral ovarian preservation in the subsequent development of ovarian retention syndrome (12). They found no statistically significant difference between the two groups.

PATHOLOGY

A variety of different histological patterns may be found with ovarian retention syndrome. Table 16.6 summarizes the most commonly encountered benign pathology in the published studies. The large series of Christ and Lotze reported atretic or hemorrhagic follicular cysts in 30% of cases, corpora lutea in 42%, endometriosis in 14%, and benign neoplasms in 23% (2). Grogan's series showed corpora lutea in 33% of cases, follicular or hemorrhagic or atretic cysts in 47%, endometriosis in 10%, and benign neoplasia in 14%. Our series showed the highest incidence of endometriosis at 34%, with other findings of functional ovarian cysts in 59% and benign neoplasia in 24%.

TABLE 16.5. AGE AT THE TIME OF HYSTERECTOMY AND AT THE TIME OF DIAGNOSIS OF OVARIAN RETENTION SYNDROME

Series	Number of Cases	Age Range at Hysterectomy	Mean Age at Hysterectomy	Age Range at Diagnosis	Mean Age at Diagnosis
Bukovsky et al.	6	28–39	35	33–43	39
Sidall-Allum et al.	7	29–44	37	36–46	42
Carey and Slack	8	—	—	29–49	39
Finan et al.	27	23–43	31	26–68	40
Funt et al.	13	27–40	34	27–44	37
El-Minawi and Howard	29	20–40	31	28–50	37
Grogan	30	20–39	—	30–39	—

TABLE 16.6. SOME OF THE TYPES OF PATHOLOGY FOUND IN PATIENTS WITH OVARIAN RETENTION SYNDROME

Commonly found pathology
  Corpus luteum cysts
  Follicular cysts
  Hemorrhagic cysts
  Atretic cysts
Less commonly found
  Endometriosis
  Benign neoplasms
  Paraovarian cysts
Least commonly found
  Malignant neoplasms

Malignancies have also been reported, although less frequently. Interpretation of the results of studies as regards malignant potential of the retained ovary depends on how the statistics were compiled (2,12). Most of the studies done can be criticized for the absence of a denominator that provides the total number of patients who had undergone hysterectomy with ovarian conservation. Follow-up of all hysterectomy patients with preserved ovaries is the most reliable method of determining the incidence of malignancy in retained ovaries. With this method Christ and Lotze found ovarian cancer in six (0.1%) of 6,188 patients and Dekel et al. found cancer in nine (0.35%) of 2,561 patients with ovarian conservation (2,12). In Ranney and Abu-Ghazaleh's series the incidence of cancer of the ovary was 0.2% (four of 1,557 patients with one or more preserved ovaries) (5). On the other end of the spectrum, employing the no-denominator method, Grogan's cumulative series of 122 cases showed an incredibly high 8.2% malignancy rate (10). Although acknowledging the high rate in his study, Grogan notes that other investigators have reported high (3.6% to 6.7%) malignancy rates also in conserved ovaries (19–21). These rates, a result of not knowing the total number of hysterectomies with ovarian conservation, falsely suggest a high risk for malignant transformation in the retained ovary.

SYMPTOMS

Chronic lower abdominal or pelvic pain is the main symptom in at least two-thirds of patients with ovarian retention syndrome (Table 16.7). Prospectively recording pain on a calendar is helpful in determining any pattern of the pain. The intensity and cyclicity of pain may vary, with some patients complaining of cyclic pain while others suffer continuously (10). A cyclic pattern of pain may be more likely to occur if the ovary is encapsulated in dense adhesions (18). The quality of pain also differs and can range from a bothersome ache to recurrent colicky pain and incapacitating cramps. Pelvic pain is often referred to the site of the retained ovary (1,11). The pain can also radiate to the lower back and down into the legs.

Deep dyspareunia occurs in at least one-fifth of patients with ovarian retention syndrome (Table 16.7). It is usually not a solitary complaint, but when it is the only symptom it usually is located directly at the site of the retained ovary (10). This may be more common when the vaginal cuff closure incorporates the utero-ovarian ligament (2,3). Other pain symptoms of ovarian retention syndrome include dysuria, recurrent renal colic, and recurrent urinary tract infections (15). Other less commonly reported symptoms include malaise, fever, weakness, nausea, and vomiting.

PHYSICAL EXAMINATION

Physical examination is an important part of the diagnostic evaluation. Vaginal examination in particular is revealing because, as shown in Table 16.7, many of these patients present with tender pelvic masses at the vaginal vault that may vary in size from 4 to 18 cm in size, with the majority in the range of 5 to 10 cm (1,2,12,15,17). In some cases there is

TABLE 16.7. VARIOUS PRESENTING SYMPTOMS AND SIGNS AND THEIR INCIDENCE

Author(s)	Cases	Pelvic Pain	Dyspareunia	Asymptomatic Mass	Pain and Mass	Other Symptoms
Bukovsky et al.	6	6 (100%)	5 (83%)	0	1 (17%)	6 (100%)
Sidall-Allum et al.	7	6 (86%)	4 (57%)	0	1 (14%)	3 (43%)
Carey and Slack	8	7 (87%)	2 (25%)	1 (12%)	1 (12%)	0
Funt et al.	13	7 (54%)	0	5 (38%)	8 (62%)	1 (8%)
Finan et al.	27	9 (30%)	—	17 (63%)	—	—
El-Minawi and Howard	29	28 (96%)	18 (62%)	1 (3%)	8 (28%)	—
Grogan	30	15 (50%)	5 (17%)	8 (27%)	—	—
Dekel et al.	73	52 (71%)	—	18 (25%)	—	3 (4%)
Grogan	92	44 (48%)	4 (4%)	24 (26%)	20 (22%)	—
Christ and Lotze	202	156 (77%)	59 (29%)	29 (14%)	113 (56%)	10 (5%)
Total	487	330 (68%)	97 (20%)	103 (21%)	152 (31%)	22 (4%)

just thickening at the vaginal cuff with exquisite tenderness to palpation (2). Bimanual examination may also reproduce the pain of dyspareunia at the retained ovary or ovaries. Steege suggests that in thin patients, bimanual examination usually outlines the anatomy sufficiently to provide a diagnosis (18).

DIAGNOSTIC STUDIES

Diagnosis of ovarian retention syndrome is helped by the use of abdominal or vaginal ultrasound (11,15,17). Computerized tomography and magnetic resonance imaging are rarely used, but may help characterize a pelvic mass in cases of ovarian retention syndrome (22). Intravenous pyelograms may be used to identify any effect the previous operations or the current condition has had on the ureters and their locations. This is of importance because of the frequency of dense pelvic adhesions encountered in these cases that may distort the anatomy and make the ureters difficult to identify during surgery (23).

A diagnostic approach using GnRH agonists has been suggested based on the theory that because functional ovarian are an integral part of ovarian retention syndrome, suppressing their function should produce an amelioration of symptoms (17). GnRH agonists may cause symptom relief by (a) suppression of ovarian follicle formation, (b) suppression of cellular activity and stromal proliferation, (c) reduction in ovarian blood flow, and (d) alteration of inflammatory mediator activity. Of eight patients treated with goserelin, 3.6 mg subcutaneously every 28 days, only one did not have pain relief. Six of the patients who reported marked improvement underwent oophorectomy. Obviously more cases of ovarian retention syndrome must be evaluated before it is clear whether GnRH analogue suppression is a useful diagnostic test.

Laparoscopy may also be used as a diagnostic test and has the advantage of being diagnostically and therapeutically beneficial. At laparoscopy the surgeon is able to identify any pathology of the retained ovary. Steege advocates the use of microlaparoscopy and conscious pain mapping in cases where the diagnosis is not clear-cut (24).

DIAGNOSIS

The diagnosis of ovarian retention syndrome can be challenging. Christ and Lotze state that the correct diagnosis based on clinical grounds is made in only 30% of cases (2). It should be suspected in a hysterectomized patient with conserved ovary(ies) having pelvic pain or a tender pelvic mass in the vicinity of the vaginal cuff. Many patients with ovarian retention syndrome are not seen by the surgeons who performed their hysterectomies. This is owing in part to the relatively long intervals between the hysterectomy

TABLE 16.8. TIME INTERVAL BETWEEN HYSTERECTOMY AND ONSET OF SYMPTOMS OR SURGERY FOR OVARIAN RETENTION SYNDROME

Investigators	Number of Cases	Mean Time Interval (yr)	Range of Time Interval (yr)
Bukovsky et al.	6	—	1½–4
Sidall-Allum et al.	7	—	1–18
Christ and Lotze	202	—	0–5 = 53%
			5–10 = 24%
			>10 = 23%
Grogan	30	—	0–5 = 60%
			5–10 = 30%
			>10 = 10%
Grogan	92	—	>5 = 65%
Dekel et al.	73	—	≤5 = 47%
			>5 = 53%
Hwu et al.	35	—	≤5 = 60%
			>5 = 40%
El-Minawi and Howard	29	6.4	1–18
Funt et al.	13	3.0	1/2–8
Ranney and Abu-Ghazaleh	14	7.8	4–22

and the beginning of symptoms in most patients. The time of onset of symptoms and presentation following hysterectomy is quite varied, ranging from less than 6 months to more than 20 years (Table 16.8) (5,25).

TREATMENT

Medical Treatment

Medical and conservative treatment, rather than difficult surgery, have been suggested, but published results of such treatment are scarce. Grogan considered a conservative approach to be best, reserving surgery only when these measures failed to produce relief. He stated that "reassurance rather than operative intervention" worked best in patients whose discomfort was associated with other menstrual molimina, such as breast engorgement. He suggested the use of hormonal replacement therapy, but did not provide data on outcomes. Steege says that hormonal suppression, using either oral contraceptives, GnRh agonists, or continuous medroxyprogesterone, may be sufficient in treating the condition (18). He also advocates analgesics and watchful waiting, with surgical treatment only if medical therapy fails. Although these may in fact be helpful, no data are available to validate them. Certainly, Carey and Slack's innovative use of GnRH agonists in a small series of cases as a diagnostic tool supports the possibility of medical therapy, because most of their patients had amelioration of symptoms while receiving GnRH analog. Further evaluation is needed because this was only a preliminary study.

Surgical Treatment

Surgery remains the most common treatment for ovarian retention syndrome. Oophorectomy is the best way to treat symptomatic ovarian retention syndrome, provided the ovaries are the actual cause of the pain. Obviously, if the symptoms are not caused by ovarian retention syndrome, then cure by oophorectomy is unlikely.

The actual surgery differs from case to case but mainly involves salpingo-oophorectomy and extensive adhesiolysis, and in some cases excision or destruction of endometriosis. Almost all reported series have employed an abdominal laparotomy as the surgical approach (1,2,5,6,10–12,15,17, 25). Our series is the only one exclusively using operative laparoscopy in treatment of ovarian retention syndrome (16). Steege states that the majority of cases can be accomplished by an experienced operative laparoscopist, a statement with which we totally agree (18). In our series the mean blood loss for the 25 cases completed laparoscopically was only 70 mL, compared to the average of 325 mL of the four cases converted to laparotomy. The hospital stay in our laparoscopically treated series was also low, with 70% of the cases staying 23 hours or less in the hospital.

The surgery is technically demanding because of the preponderance of adhesions found at surgery. Division of these adhesions can be time-consuming and risky. Bowel preparation is import, because in some cases bowel resection may be needed and bowel injury is not uncommon. The ovaries are often densely adherent to the pelvic sidewall, vaginal cuff, sigmoid and mesocolon, small bladder, omentum, and bladder. Identification of the ureters is crucial because of the adhesions to the pelvic sidewalls. Extensive retroperitoneal dissection of the ureters is often necessary to free the ovaries and can be difficult and painstaking. Placement of ureteral stents may be helpful in cases where distortion of the anatomy prevents easy visualization of the ureters, especially for laparoscopic procedures (18).

Because of the extensive adhesiolysis and the location of the pathology in these patients, complications can and do occur. Bowel injury during dissection has been reported by several authors (16,25,26). Ureteric injuries have also been reported (2,11). It is vital that such injuries be recognized and repaired at the time of the surgery.

The usual definitive procedure is ophorectomy or salpingo-oophorectomy. There was one report where ovariopexy was performed in a young patient (15). At times, surgeons have elected to remove only one ovary, assuming it was the cause of pain and sparing the other. Christ and Lotze reported leaving one ovary in 12 of their patients, but they did not comment on follow-up (2). In our series, six patients with ovarian retention syndrome were also left with one ovary, but three of these were reoperated on at a later date for recurrent ovarian retention syndrome. In light of this high rate of recurrence we recommend that any ovarian retention syndrome patient with both ovaries have bilateral oophorectomy if undergoing surgery for the condition.

Results of surgical treatment of ovarian retention syndrome have been encouraging. All of the six patients reported by Bukovsky et al. were pain free at $1\frac{1}{2}$ to 3 years after surgery (15). Five of these were treated by salpingo-oophorectomies and one by ovariopexy. Sidall-Allum et al. report that six of their seven patients were pain free 12 months after salpingo-oophorectomy (11). The one failed patient was thought to have an ovarian remnant. Carey and Slack reported that five of their patients (who had all received GnRH for diagnosis) were pain free 12 months after surgery (17). One patient continued to have persistent pain 1 year later. In our series, nine of 29 patients had recurrent or persistent pain after surgery. As mentioned previously, three of these were ovarian retention syndrome occurring in the ovary left at first surgery. Other diagnoses believed to be responsible for recurrent pain were ovarian remnant syndrome (1), nerve entrapment (1), vulvar vestibulitis (1), inguinal hernia (1), chronic appendicitis (1) and chronic pelvic pain of undetermined etiology (1).

KEY POINTS

Most Important Questions to Ask

- Is there chronic lower abdominal or pelvic pain?
- Does the intensity and cyclicity of pain may vary?
- Is the pain consistently in one location?
- Does the pain radiate to the lower back and down into the legs?
- Is there deep dyspareunia?

Most Important Physical Examination Findings

- A tender pelvic mass at the vaginal vault

Most Important Diagnostic Studies

- Abdominal and vaginal ultrasound
- Computerized tomography
- Magnetic resonance imaging (rarely)
- Intravenous pyelogram
- GnRH agonists suppression of ovarian function

Treatments

- Hormonal suppression with estrogen and/or progestin
- GnRH analogue suppression
- Salingo-oophorectomy
- Ovariopexy

REFERENCES

1. Grogan RH. Residual ovaries. *Obstet Gynecol* 1958;12(3):329–332.
2. Christ JE, Lotze EC. The residual ovary syndrome. *Obstet Gynecol* 1975;46(5):551–556.
3. Steege JF. Ovarian remnant syndrome. *Obstet Gynecol* 1987;70(1):64–67.
4. *Webster's new collegiate dictionary.* Springfield, MA: Merriam Co., 1979.
5. Ranney B, Abu-Ghazaleh S. The future function and fortune of ovarian tissue which is retained in vivo during hysterectomy. *Am J Obstet Gynecol* 1977;128(6):626–634.
6. Grogan RH, Duncan CJ. Ovarian salvage in routine abdominal hysterectomy. *Am J Obstet Gynecol* 1955;70:1277–1283.
7. De Neef JC, Hollenbeck ZJR. The fate of ovaries preserved at the time of hysterectomy. *Am J Obstet Gynecol* 1966;96(8):1088–1097.
8. Gevaerts POH. Abdominale totale uterus extirpatie of supravaginale uterus amputatie. Thesis, Leiden, Holland, 1963. Quoted in De Neef JC, Hollenbeck ZJR. The fate of ovaries preserved at the time of hysterectomy. *Am J Obstet Gynecol* 1966;96(8):1088–1097.
9. Mckenzie LL. On discussion of the frequency of oophorectomy at the time of hysterectomy. *Am J Obstet Gynecol* 1968;100:724–725.
10. Grogan RH. Reappraisal of residual ovaries. *Am J Obstet Gynecol* 1967;97(1):124–129.
11. Sidall-Allum J, Rae T, Rogers V, et al. Chronic pelvic pain caused by residual ovaries and ovarian remnants. *Br J Obstet Gynaecol* 1994;101:979–985.
12. Dekel A, Efrat Z, Orvieto R, et al. The residual ovary syndrome: a 20-year experience. *Eur J Obstet Gynecol Reprod Biol* 1996;68:159–164.
13. Backstrom CT, Boyle H. Persistence of premenstrual symptoms in hysterectomized women. *Br J Obstet Gynecol* 1981;88:530–535.
14. Hwu YM, Wu CH, Yang YC, et al. The residual ovary syndrome. *Chin Med J* 1989;43(5):335–340.
15. Bukovsky I, Liftshitz Y, Langer R, et al. Ovarian residual syndrome. *Surg Gynecol Obstet* 1988;167(8):132–134.
16. El-Minawi AM, Howard FM. Operative laparoscopic treatment of ovarian retention syndrome. Presented at the second annual meeting of the International Pelvic Pain Society, October 21–22, 1997.
17. Carey MP, Slack MC. GnRH analogue in assessing chronic pelvic pain in women with residual ovaries. *Br J Obstet Gynecol* 1996;103:150–153.
18. Steege JF. Pain after hysterectomy. In: Steege JF, Metzger DA, Levy BS, eds. *Chronic pelvic pain. An integrated approach.* Philadelphia: W.B. Saunders, 1998:135–144.
19. Thorp D. Ovarian carcinoma susequent to hysterectomy. *West J Surg* 1951;59:440–447.
20. Pemberton FA. Carcinoma of ovary. *Am J Obstet Gynecol* 1940;40:751–763.
21. Counseller VS, Hunt W, Haisler FR Jr. Carcinoma of the ovary following hysterectomy. *Am J Obstet Gynecol* 1955;69:628–638.
22. Price FV, Edwards R, Buchsbaum HJ. Ovarian remnant syndrome: difficulties in diagnosis and management. *Obste Gynecol Suury* 1990;45(3):151–156.
23. Berek JS, Darney PD, Lopkin C, et al. Avoiding ureteral damage in pelvic surgery for ovarian remnant syndrome. *Am J Obstet Gynecol* 1979;133:221–222.
24. Steege JF. Microlaparoscopy. In: Steege JF, Metzger DA, Levy BS, eds. *Chronic pelvic pain. An integrated approach.* Philadelphia: W.B. Saunders, 1998;337–346.
25. Funt MA, Benigno BB, Thompson JD. The residual adnexa–asset or liability? *Am J Obstet Gynecol* 1977;129(3):251–254.
26. Finan MA, Kwark JA, Joseph GF, et al. Surgical resection of endometriosis after prior hysterectomy. *J La State Med Soc* 1997;149:32–35.

17

OVARIAN REMNANT SYNDROME

AHMED M. EL-MINAWI
FRED M. HOWARD

KEY TERMS AND DEFINITIONS

Ovarian remnant syndrome: The persistence of functional ovarian tissue inadvertently not removed at the time of intended extirpation of one or both ovaries, with or without hysterectomy.

Ovarian retention syndrome: The presence of persistent pelvic pain, dyspareunia, and/or a pelvic mass after intended conservation of one or both ovaries at the time of hysterectomy; also called *residual ovary syndrome*.

INTRODUCTION

Ovarian remnant syndrome is one of the least considered and least recognized conditions in the patient with pelvic pain who has had an oophorectomy (1,2). The condition arises from the persistence of ovarian fragments unintentionally left *in situ* during oophorectomy. It may occur after ooophorectomy performed by either laparotomy or laparoscopy. The syndrome has classically and most commonly been described in patients presenting with pelvic pain or a pelvic mass after a previous bilateral salpingo-oophorectomy and hysterectomy. It is important to note that it is not synonymous with the ovarian retention syndrome (Chapter 16), supernumerary ovary, or accessory ovary (Chapter 6), all of which are different in their etiologies, although sometimes sharing similar symptoms (3). Supernumerary ovary refers to the presence of one or more extra ovaries entirely separate from normally placed ovaries, and is rare. Accessary ovary is also rare and refers to excess ovarian tissue situated near the normally placed ovary that may be connected with it and have developed from it.

Although ovarian remnant syndrome is also a rare condition, it occurs more commonly than generally thought. The prevalence and incidence are difficult to establish with any reliability because most cases are not reported and those that have been reported are usually sporadic case reports rather than prospective cohorts (Table 17.1). Steege suggested that the condition is more common than implied by the fact that there had been only 50 previously published cases when he reported his cases (4). This opinion is particularly supported by the reports of Symmonds and Petite and of Petite and Lee (5,6). Both series were from the Mayo Clinic. In the first series, Symmonds and Petit reported 20 surgically confirmed cases over a 28-year period from 1950 to 1978. Then from the same institution Petit and Lee reported 31 cases of ovarian remnant during the 5-year interval from 1980 to 1985, representing almost a tenfold increase in prevalence. This increase in published cases most likely represents an increased awareness among physicians, coupled with more sensitive diagnostic techniques. Price et al. in a 1990 review found 93 reported cases (3).

TABLE 17.1. REPORTED SERIES OF OVARIAN REMNANT SYNDROME FROM THE PERSPECTIVE OF THE NUMBER OF CASES PER YEAR

	No. of Cases	Dates	Time in Years	Mean/Year
Symmonds and Petit	20	1950–1978	28	0.7
Shemwell and Weed	12	1960–1970(?)	10	1.2
Steege	13	1981–1985	4	3.2
Price et al.	31	1980–1985	5	6.2
Webb	27	1981–1988(?)	7	3.8
Nezhat and Nezhat	13	1989–1990	0.83	15
Elkins et al.	20	1988–1991	3.4	5.9

ETIOLOGY

Shemwell and Weed formally described the ovarian remnant syndrome in 1970 (7). They stated that, "when removing ovaries for chronic tubo-ovarian abscesses or ovarian endometriosis, it is virtually impossible to remove all ovarian tissue" and this "residual ovarian tissue sometimes becomes functional (and) ... becomes painful." In an elegant animal experiment, Minke et al. showed that devascularized ovarian tissue could re-implant and function (8). Revascularization of ovarian tissue occurred in 75% of the experimental cases, with 43% of the viable ovaries showing follicle formation. Estrogen effects were displayed in 37% of the rats. These data clearly show the potential for growth and function of incompletely excised ovarian cortical tissue that is adherent to peritoneal surfaces at the time of initial surgery, and underscore the necessity for meticulousness during oophorectomy.

The ovarian remnant syndrome most often represents a complication of a difficult oophorectomy. Predisposing factors include pelvic inflammatory disease, adhesive disease from prior surgery, and endometriosis. The studies of Mattingly and Frederick and of Symmonds and Pettit suggest three major factors that may complicate the initial surgery and increase the possibility of leaving an ovarian remnant: (a) difficulty in hemostasis owing to increased pelvic vascularity, (b) dense adhesions causing distortion of the anatomy and difficult dissection, and (c) alteration of the anatomy by a neoplasm (5,9). Vascular changes in the soft tissue of the pelvis as a result of endometriosis, neoplasms or inflammatory diseases may have a pathogenetic role, because the increased vascularity may allow ovarian remnants to thrive and function in ectopic locations (10). Adhesions, whether from prior abdominopelvic surgery or diseases that cause adhesions, appear to be a quite important etiological factor. The adhesive disease makes the oophorectomy more difficult, increasing risk of incomplete removal and leading to a more severe adhesive process. Often the surgeon will use blunt dissection rather than remove the adherent peritoneum along with the ovary.

Preexisting conditions appear to play a significant role. Endometriosis and pelvic inflammatory disease (PID) are preexisting conditions that are important risk factors (Table 17.2). Both conditions predispose to extensive adhesions that make resection of the ovaries difficult, increasing the risk of incomplete ovarian resection. Inflammatory bowel disease and adnexal tumors are additional risk factors (5). The technique used in treating previous conditions, particularly "pelvic cysts," may play a role in subsequent evolution of this syndrome. Often these "cysts" are removed by simply clamping the ovarian vessels very close to the ovary, with the associated risk of retaining a portion of ovarian tissue attached to the vessels on the proximal side of the clamp (1).

It has also been suggested that the increasing use of laparoscopic surgery for complex procedures, particularly with the presence of dense adhesions, will lead to an increase in the frequency of ovarian remnant syndrome owing to the lack of tactile sensation, and the possibility of leaving behind small parts of the specimen when attempting to remove it through the trocars (8,11). Nezhat and Nezhat reported two patients with ovarian remnant syndrome following laparoscopic salpingo-oophorectomy using endoloop ligatures (12). They were of the opinion that these cases signaled a possible long-term complication of the endoloop technique of oophorectomy. In addition to surgical technique that ensures complete excision of ovarian tissue, the use of laparoscopic tissue retrieval bags and good irrigation may also reduce the incidence of this complication by preventing peritoneal seeding of ovarian tissue.

Rarely are cases of ovarian remnant preceded by a single pelvic operation. A history of two or three prior procedures

TABLE 17.2. DIAGNOSES PRIOR TO THE DEVELOPMENT OF OVARIAN REMNANT SYNDROME

	Endometriosis	PID	Inflam. Bowel	Ovarian Tumor	Uterine Tumor	Adhesive Disease	Unknown	No. of Cases
Steege	6	2	1	2	1	?	3	13
Berek et al.	—	2	—	—	—	?		2
Petit and Lee	15	14	13	—	1	?	1	31
Symmonds and Petit	2	1	—	—	—	2	—	2
Price et al.	2	—	—	—	—	1	—	3
Elkins et al.	3	—	—	1	5	6	—	10
Symmonds and Petit	10	4	1	3	4	?	3	20
Scott et al.	2	—	—	—	—	3	—	3
Lafferty et al.	1	1	2	3	—	?	—	8
Shemwell and Weed	6	2	—	—	—	—	2	10
Total	47	26	17	9	11	12	9	102

The operative diagnoses at the time of previous hysterectomies and/or oophorectomies.

TABLE 17.3. MEAN AGE AT INITIAL OOPHORECTOMY AND AT DIAGNOSIS OF OVARIAN REMNANT SYNDROME

Investigators	Patient ages at oophorectomy	Mean age at oophorectomy	Patient ages at diagnosis of ORS	Mean age at Dx of ORS
Shemwell and Weed, 1970	14–40 yrs	33.1 ± 7.9 yrs	26–57 yrs	39.5 ± 7.9 yrs
Lafferty et al., 1996	21–41	34.1 ± 6.9	24–44	37.0 ± 6.7
Webb, 1989	NA	20 yrs	29–54	36.0 ± ??
Pettit and Lee, 1988	NA	NA	23–56 (28 < 40)	NA
Steege, 1987	NA	NA	25–46	36.3 ± 5.1
Nezhat and Nezhat, 1992	24–42	35.6 ± 4.5	25–43	36.9 ± 4.9
Sidall-Allum et al., 1994	21–47	36.0 ± 8.9	33–50	42.6 ± 5.7
Kaminski et al., 1995	NA	NA	32–42	36.3 ± 4.6

is far more common. Webb reported a mean of 4.3 previous pelvic procedures with a range of one to nine (1). Lafferty et al. reported eight patients who had a total of 45 prior procedures, with a range of two to eight per patient (13). Steege's series of 13 patients had a mean of 3.2 previous pelvic surgeries (4). Additionally, previous surgery for ovarian remnant syndrome is a significant risk factor. Many of the patients with multiple previous procedures have had at least one prior attempt at excising the remnant(s) and the recurrence rate ranges from 8% to 10% (14).

Ovarian remnant syndrome is a disorder that usually occurs in the reproductive years. Women with this disorder often have had oophorectomies at a relatively young age, giving ample time for regrowth of the remnants. Table 17.3 shows the data from a number of investigators as to the age at which the oophorectomy was performed and the age at which a surgical diagnosis of ovarian remnant syndrome was made, and shows that the majority of patients are less than 35 years old at the time of oophorectomy and are 35 to 40 years of age at the time of diagnosis. The only study in which there was a slightly higher mean age was the prospective study of Sidall-Allum et al. (15).

The actual cause of pain in ovarian remnant syndrome remains poorly understood. The best explanation at present is that pain results from continued function of ovarian tissue that is covered by extensive pelvic adhesions and scar tissues, and this combination of dense pelvic adhesions and functioning ovarian tissue results in symptomatic painful cysts. Histologic findings in ovarian remnants confirm that ovarian function continues. Algesic chemicals released from the ovarian remnant into this confined area could also contribute to pain production. Additionally, the patient may have nociceptive signals arising from the scarring that may have developed into a pain syndrome, and thereby add to the ovarian pain (16). How frequently ovarian remnants exist without causing pain, or any other signs or symptoms, is not known. Of the 20 histologically confirmed cases reported by Symmonds and Petit, one had no symptoms or signs, but was incidentally diagnosed at the time of unrelated surgery.

PATHOLOGY

The pathology of ovarian remnants varies, ranging from mostly fibrovascular tissue to malignancy (Table 17.4)

TABLE 17.4. HISTOLOGICAL DIAGNOSES IN OVARIAN TISSUE IN CASES OF OVARIAN REMNANT SYNDROME

	Corpora Lutea of Follicular Cysts	Normal Ovarian Tissue	Benign Neoplasias	Carcinoma	Endometriosis	Total
Symmonds and Petit	2	—	—	—	—	2
Webb	25	—	2	—	—	27
Symmonds and Petit	16	—	3	—	1	20
Petit and Lee	16	10	2	—	3	—
Nezhat and Nezhat	5	3	—	—	4	12
Steege	6	—	2	—	—	8
Shemwell and Weed	6 (?)	2 (?)	—	1	1	10
Total	76	15	9	1	9	110

(7,28). The majority of cases show normal ovarian tissue, often with small follicular cysts. Corpora lutei, corpora albicans, and hemorrhagic cysts are common findings. Endometriosis is occasionally present and may involve the ovary, adhesions, and other areas in the pelvis. It is of interest that even though endometriosis accounts for about 50% of the original oophorectomies in women who later develop ovarian remnant syndrome (Table 17.2), less than 10% of cases of ovarian remnants show residual or recurrent endometriosis (Table 17.4). Rarer findings include ovarian fibromas, mucinous cystadenomas, and dermoid cysts (1,6).

Malignancy has been reported in ovarian remnants and is a particular concern. Fortunately, it does not appear to be a common occurrence. There have been, however, at least five reported cases of adenocarcinoma or low malignant potential tumors of ovarian remnants; therefore, it is vital that this possibility be considered whenever a pelvic mass is found after oophorectomy (7,17–19,26).

SYMPTOMS AND HISTORY

The syndrome occurs in women who have a history of bilateral or unilateral oophorectomy, with or without hysterectomy. It usually presents as chronic pain of varying quality and severity in the abdominopelvic area, with or without a palpable pelvic mass. Patients with an ovarian remnant often suffer for years before a diagnosis is made. Because most of these patients have undergone multiple surgeries, including a hysterectomy and bilateral salpingo-oophorectomy, the possibility of a gynecological cause is usually not recognized. Typically, the woman has seen many physicians before a suspicion of ovarian remnant as a potential cause of her pain arises.

Most of the patients, as previously mentioned, are in their mid- to late thirties and almost all are less than 50 years of age. In fact, of 111 published cases that we reviewed with patients' ages available, only two women were over 50 years of age. The majority have histories of appendectomies or ovarian cystectomies in their youth, later followed by complaints of pain. Often there is a history of a diagnosis of endometriosis, for which one or more surgical procedures have been performed. All of these patients' surgical histories reveal either bilateral or (less commonly) unilateral oophorectomy, with or without hysterectomy. Some of them may even have histories of prior surgery for treatment of a remnant, which should point the physician in the direction of ovarian remnant syndrome, not away from it. Typically, the patient with ovarian remnant syndrome presents anywhere from a few months to 5 years or more after the oophorectomy (Table 17.3). This may be highly variable and affected by the number of previous surgical procedures and the resultant adhesive process within the pelvis. An interval of 3 to 5 years appears to be the most common before onset of the symptoms.

The common presenting symptoms are (a) pelvic pain, (b) dyspareunia, (c) bowel symptoms, and (d) urinary symptoms (Table 17.5). Symptoms are variable, but abdominopelvic pain is most common and is present in more than 65% of patients. The pain may be dull, diffuse, nonradiating, or localized, consistent with the vague nature of visceral pain. Chronic pelvic pain is most common, but some patients experience periodic exacerbations and others have pain that is intermittent or cyclic (1,4–7). The chronicity or cyclicity is most probably dependent on whether or not the ovarian remnant has functional cystic activity. Acute exacerbations are sometimes severe enough to cause patients to seek emergency care.

The location of the pain is most often in the lower abdomen or pelvis and ipsilateral to the remnant, although occasionally it is variable. Patients may also complain of flank pain, groin pain, and dyspareunia (1,7,13,15,20,21). In addition, in those who still have a uterus there may be significant lateral pelvic and lower back pain accompanying dysmenorrhea (11).

The absence of hot flushes in a woman not receiving hormonal replacement following bilateral oophorectomy should be heralded as a signal to investigate carefully for ovarian remnant. Of reported cases, 70% to 100% have had no history of postmenopausal vasomotor symptoms in spite of not receiving hormonal replacement therapy (7,21). In the rare woman with a history of bilateral oophorectomy

TABLE 17.5. PRESENTING SIGNS AND SYMPTOMS WITH OVARIAN REMNANT SYNDROME

	Pelvic Pain	Pelvic Mass	Dyspareunia	Pain with Defecation	Dysuria	Other
Petit and Lee	30/31	27/31	—	—	—	—
Symmonds and Petit	13/20	13/20	—	—	—	5/20
Price et al.	3/3	2/3	2/3	—	—	—
Steege	13/13	8/13	—	—	—	—
Nezhat and Nezhat	13/13	10/13	—	—	—	—
Webb	27/27	23/27	14/27	8/27	5/27	–4/27
Shemwell and Weed	10/10	10/10	10/10	—	—	—
Total	109/117 (93%)	93/117 (79%)	26/40 (65%)	8/27 (30%)	5/27 (19%)	9/27 (33%)

without a hysterectomy, cyclic vaginal bleeding is also very suggestive of endogenous ovarian estrogen production by an ovarian remnant (22).

Deep dyspareunia is present in 40% to 50% of patients. Most often it is during deep thrusting and of a "collision" type owing to pressure against the vagina apex, adhesions, and the remnant. Postcoital ache, similar to that with pelvic congestion syndrome, may also occur in up to 40% of cases (15).

Constipation is sometimes present and is probably most commonly secondary to adhesions, but may also be the result of small bowel and large bowel compression by remnants (10,13,23). The constipation is usually chronic and can be worsened by use of bulking agents because of the obstructive etiology. There are published reports of at least one case of small bowel obstruction and several of large bowel compression by ovarian remnants (3).

Flank pain may occur and when present is particularly worrisome because it may suggest ureteral involvement and obstruction. There are at least 15 published reports of unilateral ureteral obstruction (3). In Webb's series of 27 patients, 15% presented with unilateral ureteral obstruction (1). Ureteral obstruction may occur even in cases of unilateral oophorectomy and subsequent ipsilateral ovarian remnant syndrome. Flank pain with ovarian remnant is most often unilateral, particularly when associated with ureteral obstruction (20,24,25). Urinary tract involvement may be accompanied by additional symptoms such as urgency, frequency, or bladder pressure (13). In cases with significant acute ureteral obstruction there may be associated nausea and vomiting (24). These urinary tract symptoms are of particular concern in cases of recurrent ovarian remnant syndrome, because they can be the result of retroperitoneal fibrosis. When present, retroperitoneal fibrosis may be a slowly progressive process that results in stricture and obstruction, and may require ureteral diversion or reimplantation to resolve (26).

SIGNS AND PHYSICAL EXAMINATION

The abdominal examination is usually not remarkable other than the finding of multiple surgical scars consistent with a history of prior surgical procedures. Ovarian remnants are usually too small to be palpated abdominally. Tenderness to deep palpation may be present and if present is usually on the same side as the remnant (3). Abdominal tenderness may be marked in cases with urinary complications, and there can also be costovertebral angle tenderness and signs of peritoneal irritation (20,24). Constipation occurring as result of adhesions and ovarian remnant may lead to increased abdominal girth and rarely decreased bowel sounds on auscultation.

At pelvic examination, inspection of the external genitalia and vagina usually reveals signs of estrogen effect, with normal-sized labia and moist, well-cornified vaginal mucosa (7). Pelvic palpation may reveal tenderness in one or both fornices. Bimanual pelvic examination may reveal a palpable mass, although its absence does not preclude the diagnosis. Pettit and Lee reported a mass or thickening in 65% of their cases, and overall it appears that in more than one-half of cases a mass is palpable by pelvic examination (6). It is usually tender, small (less than 5 cm), and located on the pelvic sidewall (close to the ureters) or at the lateral vaginal apex, lateral to the vaginal fornices (4). The mass may be soft and smooth, or be felt as a dense thickening (2,6).

DIAGNOSTIC STUDIES

The history, symptoms, and signs are frequently not enough to allow a diagnosis of ovarian remnant syndrome (1,6,22). Often the diagnosis has been made at surgery, after investigating vague chronic pelvic pain for which no preoperative diagnosis was reached. With increased awareness of the condition, physicians have begun to suspect and diagnose it without resort to surgery except for treatment. Some of the criteria for nonsurgical diagnosis follow:

1. History of previous bilateral (or, rarely, unilateral) oophorectomy
2. Pelvic mass by palpation, ultrasound, or computerized tomography
3. Evidence of continuing ovarian activity as defined by premenopausal follicle-stimulating hormone (FSH) (less than 40 mIU/mL) or estradiol levels (more than 30 pg/mL), provided there is no exogenous hormonal replacement
4. Cyclic vaginal bleeding in the absence of exogenous hormonal replacement
5. Positive clomiphene citrate stimulation of remnants as identified by ovarian follicle formation by ultrasound
6. A significant rise in estradiol levels within the first 7 days after depot-leuprolide injection, in the absence of exogenous hormonal replacement

Vaginal ultrasound shows a pelvic mass in 50% to 85% of cases (6,12). The mass is usually cystic or multiseptated with a well-defined solid tissue ring surrounding it (13,20). The diagnostic accuracy of ultrasound may be improved by pretreatment with clomiphene citrate (26,27). A 5- to 10-day course of clomiphene citrate, 100 mg daily, appears to stimulate follicular formation in up to 90% of cases; this may permit easier sonographic visualization. Not all ovarian remnants have functional follicles; therefore, this technique is not consistently helpful (15).

Computerized tomography has also been used as a diagnostic imaging technique, but is considerably more expensive than ultrasound. It is possibly more useful when the remnant is extremely small or is surrounded by dense adhesions and is not cystic. Theoretically magnetic resonance imaging should be very accurate in detecting an ovarian remnant, but there have not been published reports to allow an evaluation of its utility. Overall, more than 80% of patients with ovarian remnant syndrome present with a pelvic mass that is detectable by palpation or by imaging studies.

Measurement of FSH levels can be useful in cases of suspected ovarian remnant syndrome (2,4,6,12,13,15,22,26, 27). If the woman is not on hormonal replacement, or it is withheld for 3 weeks or more, premenopausal FSH levels lower than 40 mIU/mL are present in about 50% to 75% of women with an ovarian remnant (4,25). However, it is not clear how long hormonal replacement must be withheld prior to measuring FSH and it may be necessary to abstain from hormonal treatment for as much as 8 to 12 weeks to improve the diagnostic reliability. A postmenopausal level of FSH is not absolute proof of the absence of an ovarian remnant because the remnant may be of low metabolic activity and simply fail to produce estrogen levels sufficient to suppress FSH. Steege found two of eight women with ovarian remnant syndrome had FSH levels over 40 mIU/mL (88 and 98 mIU/mL, respectively), and Price et al. reported a case with an FSH of 295 mIU/mL (3,4). As an interesting aside to the use of FSH levels to diagnose ovarian remnant, Elkins et al. reported that two of 10 cases with an adnexal mass and FSH levels less than 40 mIU/mL had no histologically confirmed ovarian tissue at the time of surgery (26).

Another method for diagnosing ovarian remnant syndrome is the gonadotropin releasing hormone agonist (GnRH-a) stimulation test (21). GnRH agonists initially stimulate gonadotropin production and, therefore, ovarian estrogen production. This observation is used in the GnRH-a stimulation test, in which a baseline level of estradiol is measured and GnRH agonist (depot-leuprolide, 3.75 mg intramuscularly once, or leuprolide, 1 mg a day for 3 days subcutaneously) is administered, followed by repeat a measurement of estradiol 4 to 7 days later. If hormonally responsive ovarian tissue is present, then a significant rise in estradiol occurs. This test may not be reliable if exogenous hormones are being taken. The advantages of this test include the ease with which the marker can be detected, its widespread availability, and its ability to produce a response even when the remnant is extremely small.

Additional diagnostic techniques include intravenous pyelography or computerized tomography with contrast to investigate the urinary tract. Involvement of the ureter, sometimes with obstruction, is not unusual with an ovarian remnant, and even when not necessary for diagnosis, these evaluations can be crucial prior to attempted surgical treatment (20,28). Serum urea nitrogen and levels should be obtained if there is evidence of ureteral dilation, hydronephrosis, or ureteral deviation.

Barium enema radiography to evaluate the lower gastrointestinal tract may be advisable if there is any suspicion of involvement or stricture of the colon as a cause of pelvic pain.

In some cases the diagnosis of ovarian remnant can only be made at the time of surgery; even then it can be difficult. Laparoscopy is an inconsistent diagnostic tool, as dense adhesions frequently hide an ovarian remnant (1,6). Petit and Lee reported that of 31 patients with ovarian remnant syndrome, 17 had undergone a prior laparoscopy without the diagnosis being made (6). They attributed this to the presence of dense adhesions obscuring the remnants. If diagnostic laparoscopy is used in the evaluation of a patient with suspected ovarian remnant, the surgeon must be prepared to perform extensive and potentially complicated adhesiolysis. The same is true if exploratory laparotomy is performed. Typically a tedious and time-consuming procedure involving exhaustive lysis of adhesions is necessary prior to locating the remnant, which commonly is embedded in dense scar tissue (4,12,27). The most common locations are along the pelvic sidewall, with a predilection to ureteral involvement (1,12,13,22,24,27,28). Remnants are also found attached to the colon, vaginal cuff, and presacral areas (1,6). Other pelvic structures are often attached to the remnant by dense adhesions. The ovarian remnants usually are 3 to 5 cm in diameter, although they can be large and cystic and measure up to 10 cm (4,12). Sometimes they can only be distinguished from the surrounding fibrous and adhesive tissue by histological evaluation. Further complicating the operative diagnosis is the fact that ovarian remnants may be bilateral and there may be multiple remnants unilaterally (1,5).

DIAGNOSIS

The diagnosis of ovarian remnant syndrome should be considered in any woman with lower abdominal pain or an ipsilateral pelvic mass several months or more after an oophorectomy. This is especially true in those with prior hysterectomy and bilateral salpingo-oophorectomy. Too often it is assumed to be impossible for these women to have a gynecologic disease and therefore no evaluation for such pathology is undertaken. This is unfortunate because 30% to 60% of such women with chronic pelvic pain may have ovarian remnant syndrome (29).

Two categories of diagnosis of ovarian remnant syndrome are necessary: "definitive" and "probable" (4). *Definitive diagnosis* is restricted to cases with histologic documentation of ovarian tissue in a patient in whom the ovary was previously surgically removed, with the remnant usually found ipsilateral to the previous oophorectomy. *Probable diagnosis* can be made with (a) a history of prior bilateral oophorectomy, (b) premenopausal levels of follicle-stimulating hormone or estradiol in the absence of estrogen or progestin replacement therapy, and (c) a pelvic mass by palpation or by visualization on ultrasound or CT scan. A probable diagnosis category is necessary because not all patients with ovarian remnant syndrome are evaluated or treated surgically.

In women with pelvic pain or a pelvic mass after hysterectomy and bilateral salpingo-oophorectomy, ovarian remnant syndrome is probably more common than is generally recognized. Some of the other possible diagnoses that must be considered include interstitial cystitis, postoperative peritoneal cysts, fallopian tubal remnant syndrome, ovarian carcinoma, primary peritoneal carcinoma, irritable bowel syndrome, retroperitoneal fibrosis, intermittent bowel obstruction, inflammatory bowel disease, gastrointestinal neoplasia, abdominopelvic adhesive disease, and vaginal apex neuroma. The diagnostic studies suggested in this chapter and in the respective chapters covering each of these diagnoses will often allow a nonsurgical, probable diagnosis. However, in some cases there will be too much uncertainty and surgical evaluation will still be necessary to establish a satisfactory diagnosis.

TREATMENT OR MANAGEMENT

Ovarian remnant syndrome is not only difficult to diagnose, it is also difficult to treat. Thus, as with most illnesses, the ideal treatment of ovarian remnant syndrome is prevention. At the time of difficult oophorectomy the surgeon should not be timid. Wide dissection and stripping of the adherent peritoneum along with the ovary should be done. Exposure of the ureter, sometimes with the use of ureteral stents, is essential to assure complete removal of the ovary in most difficult cases. When attempting laparoscopic oophorectomy, proper exposure and lysis of adhesions is also crucial for proper excision (30,31). Theoretically, the use of bags to remove the specimen followed by copious irrigation may help to prevent ovarian remnant caused by spillage during laparoscopic specimen retrieval. In spite of these aggressive efforts, ovarian remnant syndrome still seems to occur or reoccur in some women.

Properly performed surgical excision appears to be the optimum treatment for the woman with chronic pelvic pain who has an ovarian remnant (4–6). Having said this, there is a postoperative recurrence rate of 8% to 15%, and multiple surgeries for remnants are not uncommon (4,14). The alternatives include medical treatment and radioablative therapy. Sonographically directed aspiration of cysts has also been suggested (32).

Medical Treatment

Medical therapy usually consists of hormonal suppression of the function of the ovarian tissue. Depot-medroxyprogesterone acetate (150 mg intramuscularly each month), danazol (600 mg per day orally), depot-leuprolide acetate (3.75 mg intramuscularly each month), and combined estrogen-progestagen therapy have all been used in small case series with mixed results, and there are limited data on their successful use (2,4,28). For example, of the 13 patients reported by Steege, 10 were unsuccessfully treated with hormonal regimens: two with danocrine, five with conjugated estrogen, two with medroxyprogesterone acetate, and one with both conjugated estrogen and

progestogen. All of these patients underwent subsequent surgery. Three patients that did not have surgery were also treated medically, two of whom continued to have mild to moderate pelvic pain. In the surgical series reported by Nezhat and Nezhat, 8 of 13 had undergone unsuccessful hormonal treatment (12). Of the 31 patients in the series from Petit and Lee, 24 had received prior hormonal treatments without improvement: danazol in 11, medroxyprogesterone acetate in four, conjugated estrogens in four, and combination of medroxyprogesterone acetate and conjugated estrogens in five (6). However, Steege (personal communication) has used, and we (unpublished data) have also used, GnRH agonist treatment with estrogen add-back therapy for the long-term treatment of ovarian remnant syndrome with good pain control and minimal side effects without any significant loss of bone density in a small number of cases (33).

Radioablation of the ovarian remnant has been successfully used in a limited number of cases. Success may be age-related, with better responses in women over 45 years of age (34). One concern with this therapy is illustrated by the series of eight patients reported by Shemwell and Weed who were treated with radiation only or a combination of radiation and surgery (7). Although five of their patients did reasonably well, one of the patients initially treated with only radiation was subsequently found to have adenocarcinoma in the endometriotic ovarian remnant. If radioablation is selected to treat a patient with ovarian remnant syndrome, clearly it is important that all laboratory (e.g., Ca-125) and imaging studies (e.g., ultrasound or CT scan) suggest a benign process. Overall, results with radiation therapy have been mixed (6). It may be a particularly reasonable option in cases of failed surgical treatment for ovarian remnant syndrome (34). Treatment with 1,000 to 2,000 rads seems to be a sufficient dose to sterilize the ovarian remnant while minimizing the risk of radiation-associated complications.

A minimally invasive approach to treatment using sonographically directed needle aspiration of symptomatic remnants has been reported (32). Three of 10 cases were successfully treated this way with relief of pain and no recurrence, but the follow-up was short.

Surgical Treatment

Surgical treatment remains the mainstay of management of ovarian remnant syndrome (Table 17.6). Although surgery may be done via laparoscopy or laparotomy, laparotomy has been used far more often (4–6,13). Advocates of laparotomy cite the dense adhesions and the marked difficulty of surgery in most cases as reasons that make laparoscopy inappropriate. Additionally, there is significant risk of ureteral or bowel injuries, plus in some cases it is not possible to excise the remnant without resection of bowel, bladder, or ureter. There is legitimate concern that a laparoscopic approach might predispose to less than optimal

TABLE 17.6. RESULTS OF SURGICAL TREATMENT OF OVARIAN REMNANT SYNDROME

Author	No. of Patients	Cured or Improved	Not Cured or Improved	Mean follow-up (years)	Re-operated
Petit	31	26	5	? (0.8–5)	2
Webb	27	24	3	3.8 (1–6)	1
Symmonds	20	15	(5 lost)	?	0
Steege	10	8	2	1.5	2
Price	3	3	0	0.5 (3–8 mos)	0
Nezhat	13	9	4	?	3
Howard	5	3	2	3–8	2
Total	109	88	16 (plus 5 lost)	—	10

resection. Despite this there have been reports of successful laparoscopic treatment of the condition (11,12,30,31).

Regardless of the surgical approach, there are some preoperative actions that can be helpful. In cases with small nonpalpable remnants the use of clomiphene citrate to stimulate ovarian growth can facilitate identification at the time of surgery (27). Preoperative urinary tract pyelography, computerized tomography, or sonography can help identify those at risk for intraoperative ureteral injury. Full bowel preparation is also important because bowel damage or resection may be necessary.

A retroperitoneal approach to excision of an ovarian remnant is probably best in almost all cases (31). Often lengthy and tedious adhesiolysis is required before the retroperitoneal dissection can even be started. The technique that usually allows the best access involves complete dissection of the pelvic course of the ureter starting at the pelvic brim, with coagulation or ligation of any vascular supply to the remnant that is identified during the dissection. Dissection along the course of the ureter usually leads to the mass, which in many cases lies on the pelvic sidewall peritoneum near the angle of the vaginal vault. Dissection of the bladder off the vaginal vault often may be needed. In addition, resection of a portion of the vagina, bladder, colon, or ureter is sometimes unavoidable if the mass is adherent to any of these structures (13,26). Ureteral stents may be helpful in avoiding ureteral injury, although there is controversy over their usefulness (1). Anecdotally we have found them particularly useful if laparoscopic excision is being attempted. The placement of radiopaque vascular clips in the area of the removed remnant may be reasonable because this may help direct radioablative treatment or reoperation in the event of a recurrence (26). With up to a 15% recurrence rate, an aggressive approach is mandatory and affords the best opportunity to excise adherent peritoneum and ensure complete resection of the remnant.

Another potential complication of surgery for ovarian remnant is retroperitoneal fibrosis. This may be a slowly progressive process that results in stricture and obstruction of the ureter, and may require ureteral diversion or reimplantation to resolve (35).

KEY POINTS

Differential Diagnosis

- Postoperative peritoneal cysts
- Fallopian tubal remnant syndrome
- Ovarian carcinoma
- Primary peritoneal carcinoma
- Irritable bowel syndrome
- Interstitial cystitis
- Retroperitoneal fibrosis
- Intermittent bowel obstruction
- Abdominopelvic adhesive disease
- Vaginal apex neuroma

Most Important Questions to Ask

- Have you had previous surgical removal of one or both ovaries?
- How many surgical procedures have you had? What were they and what were they for?
- Were previous surgeries difficult?
- Where is your pain located?
- Do you have pain with intercourse with deep penetration or aching pain after intercourse?
- Do you have pain with bowel movements?
- Do you have urgency, frequency, bladder pressure, or pain with urination?
- Do you have pain in the flank area?
- Did you have hot flushes after removal of both ovaries or do you have hot flushes if you do not take your hormonal replacement?
- Do you have problems with constipation?

Most Important Physical Examination Findings

- Abdominal surgical scars
- Abdominal tenderness to deep palpation
- Costovertebral angle tenderness
- Normal signs of estrogen effect, with moist, well-cornified vaginal mucosa

- Tenderness in one or both vaginal fornices
- A tender, palpable mass on pelvic examination

Most Important Diagnostic Studies

- Ultrasonography, with or without clomiphene stimulation
- Computerized tomography
- Estradiol levels while not on hormonal replacement
- GnRH agonist stimulation test
- Magnetic resonance imaging
- FSH levels while not on hormonal replacement
- Intravenous pyelography or computerized tomography with contrast
- Barium enema radiography
- Laparoscopy

Treatment

- Meticulous dissection and exposure during oophorectomy can help reduce its occurrence.
- Surgical excision
- Radioablative therapy
- Sonographically directed aspiration of cysts
- Hormonal suppression
    Depot-medroxyprogesterone acetate
    Danazol
    GnRH agonist
- Combined estrogen-progestagen therapy

REFERENCES

1. Webb MJ. Ovarian remnant syndrome. *Aust NZ J Obstet Gynecol* 1989;29(4):433–435.
2. Nelson DC, Avant GR. Ovarian remnant syndrome. *S Med J* 1982;75(6):757–758.
3. Price FV, Edwards R, Buchsbaum HJ. Ovarian remnant syndrome: difficulties in diagnosis and management. *Obstet Gynecol Surv* 1990;45:151–156.
4. Steege JF. Ovarian remnant syndrome. *Obstet Gynecol* 1987;70(1):64–67.
5. Symmonds RE, Petit PDM. Ovarian remnant syndrome. *Obstet Gynecol* 1979;54(2):174–177.
6. Pettit PD, Lee RA. Ovarian remnant syndrome: diagnostic dilemma and surgical challenge. *Obstet Gynecol* 1988;71(4):580–583.
7. Shemwell RW, Weed JC. Ovarian remnant syndrome. *Obstet Gynecol* 1970;36:299–303.
8. Minke T, DePond W, Winkelmann T, et al. Ovarian remnant syndrome: study in laboratory rats. *Am J Obstet Gynecol* 1994;171(6):1440–1445.
9. Mattingly RF, Frederick EG. Difficult hysterectomy. *Clin Obstet Gynecol* 1972;15:877–801.
10. Payan HM, Gilbert EF. Mesenteric cyst-ovarian implant syndrome. *Arch Pathol Lab Med* 1987;111:282–283.
11. Rana N, Rotman C, Hasson HM, et al. Ovarian remnant syndrome after laparoscopic hysterectomy and bilateral salpingo-oophorectomy for severe pelvic endometriosis. *JAAGL* 1996;3(3):423–426.
12. Nezhat F, Nezhat C. Operative laparoscopy for the treatment of ovarian remnant syndrome. *Fertil Steril* 1992;57(5):1003–1007.
13. Lafferty HW, Angioli R, Rudolph J, et al. Ovarian remnant syndrome: experience at Jackson Memorial Hospital, University of Miami, 1985 through 1993. *Am J Obstet Gynecol* 1996;174(2):641–645.
14. Riva JM, Mikuta JJ. Ovarian remnant syndrome. *Postgrad Obstet Gynecol* 1984;4:1–2.
15. Sidall-Allum J, Rae T, Rogers V, et al. Chronic pelvic pain caused by residual ovaries and ovarian remnants. *Br J Obstet Gynaecol* 1994;101:979–985.
16. Steege JF. Pain after hysterectomy. In: Steege JF, Metzger DA, Levy BS, eds. *Chronic pelvic pain. An integrated approach.* Philadelphia: W.B. Saunders, 1998:135–144.
17. Bruhwiler H, Luscher KP. Ovarialkarzinom bei ovarian remnant syndrome. *Geburtshilfe Frauenheilkd* 1991;51:299–303.
18. Glaser D, Burrig KF, Mast H. [Ovarian cancer in ovarian remnant syndrome]? *Geburtshilfe Frauenheilkd* 1992;52(7):436–437.
19. Kazadi Buanga J, Laparte Escorza MC, Lopez Garcia G. [Ovarian remnant syndrome. A case report of a malignancy.] *J Gynecol Obstet Biol Reprod (Paris)* 1992;21(7):769–772.
20. Phillips HE, McGahan JP. Ovarian remnant syndrome. *Radiology* 1982;142(2):487–488.
21. Scott RT Maj, Beatse SN Lt Col, Illions EH Lt Col, et al. Use of the GnRH agonist stimulation test in the diagnosis of ovarian remnant syndrome. A report of three cases. *J Reprod Med* 1995;40(2):143–146.
22. Kaminski PF, Meilstrup JW, Shackelford DP, et al. Ovarian remnant syndrome, a reappraisal: the usefulness of clomiphene citrate in stimulating and pelvic ultrasound in locating remnant ovarian tissue. *J Gynecol Surg* 1995;11(1):33–39.
23. Wilder JR, Barnes WA. Obstruction of the small intestine by corpus luteum cyst: report of a case. *JAMA* 1953;151:730–731.
24. Berek JS, Darney PD, Lopkin C, et al. Avoiding ureteral damage in pelvic surgery for ovarian remnant syndrome. *Am J Obstet Gynecol* 1979;133:221–222.
25. Major FJ. Retained ovarian remnant causing ureteral obstruction. *Obstet Gynecol* 1968;32:748–749.
26. Elkins TE, Stocker RJ, Key D, et al. Surgery for ovarian remnant syndrome. Lessons learned from difficult cases. *J Reprod Med* 1994;39(6):446–448.
27. Kaminski PF, Sorosky JI, Mandell MJ, et al. Clomiphene citrate as an adjunct in locating ovarian tissue in ovarian remnant syndrome. *Obstet Gynecol* 1990;76(5 Part 2):924–926.
28. Koch MO, Coussens D, Burnett L. The ovarian remnant syndrome and ureteral obstruction: medical management. *J Urol* 1994;152:158–160.
29. Howard FM. Laparoscopic evaluation and treatment of women with chronic pelvic pain. *JAAGL* 1994;1:325–331.
30. Howard FM. Laparoscopic treatment of ovarian remnant and ovarian retention syndrome. *JAAGL* 1995;2(Suppl):S20.
31. Kamprath S, Possover M, Schneider A. Description of a laparoscopic technique for treating patients with ovarian remnant syndrome. *Fertil Steril* 1997;68(4):663–667.
32. Fleischer AC, Tait D, Mayo J, et al. Sonographic features of ovarian remnants. *J Ultrasound Med* 1998;17(9):551–555.
33. Hornstein MD, Surrey ES, Weisberg GW, et al. Leuprolide acetate depot and hormonal add-back in endometriosis: a 12-month study. *Obstet Gynecol* 1998;91:16–24.
34. Thomas WW, Hughes LL, Rock J. Palliation of recurrent endometriosis with radiotherapeutic ablation of ovarian remnants. *Fertil Steril* 1997;68:938–940.
35. Elkins TE, Stocker RJ, Key D, et al. Surgery for ovarian remnant syndrome. Lessons learned from difficult cases. *J Reprod Med* 1994;39(6):446–448.

18

PELVIC VARICOSITIES AND PELVIC CONGESTION SYNDROME

AHMED M. EL-MINAWI

KEY TERMS AND DEFINITIONS

Allen-Masters syndrome: A syndrome characterized particularly by dyspareunia believed to be secondary to a hypermobile uterus with tears or windows in the posterior broad ligament.

Deep dyspareunia: Pain with intercourse that occurs with deep penile penetration into the vagina, as opposed to entry dyspareunia that occurs with initial entry of the penis.

Pelipathia vegetativa: An early term applied to the syndrome that is now generally referred to as pelvic congestion syndrome.

Pelvic congestion syndrome (PCS): Syndrome characterized by pelvic pain and dyspareunia, and associated with pelvic varicosities and congestion (slow drainage of dilated pelvic veins with resultant stasis).

Pelvic varicosities: Pelvic veins that are consistently dilated more than is normal, generally 5 or 6 mm or more.

Posttubal ligation syndrome: Syndrome characterized by pelvic pain and/or dyspareunia that has its onset after performance of a tubal sterilization procedure.

INTRODUCTION

Chronic pelvic pain (CPP) is gynecology's archetypal rebel without a cause or, more accurately, a rebel for whom gynecologists are constantly *seeking* a cause. Among the causes that have slowly gained legitimacy is the often-disputed pelvic congestion syndrome. The association of pelvic varicosities and pelvic pain was first alluded to in the nineteenth century and later confirmed in the twentieth century (1–5). Pelvic congestion, or varicocele, was first described by Richet in 1857, who used the term *hématocele péri-utérine* to describe the huge varicosities he encountered (1). Although this condition is characterized by dilated, incompetent ovarian veins, the pelvic congestion syndrome (PCS) is best defined as pelvic varicosities accompanied by chronic pelvic pain (6,7).

The widely variable symptomatology and the highly prevalent emotional and psychological disturbances encountered in these patients caused few physicians to accept pelvic congestion as a legitimate diagnosis. The term *pelipathia vegetativa*, as reported by Gauss, was derived from terminology used in earlier works he reviewed, which suggested the uniqueness of the syndrome and also denoted their authors' impression of a psychomotor-autonomic dysfunction (8). It was owing to Howard Taylor that physicians finally began to listen to these unfortunate women. His thought-provoking landmark paper, entitled "Vascular Congestion and Hyperemia," presented to the American Gynecological Society in 1948, piqued the interest of many physicians (9). It was presented at a time when the pathophysiology of the disorder was not understood and afflicted women were thought to be neurotic. Hysterectomy was being resorted to as a solution despite the apparent absence of pelvic pathology. Although Taylor attempted to caution overzealous surgeons by stating, in 1957, that, "premature resort to surgery is the characteristic error in the present-day management" of CPP patients, his own early results hardly supported his statements (10). This was pointed out to him during his 1948 presentation, by a physician named Schumann, who noted that, "in Dr. Taylor's whole series of patients but one was classified as completely cured and that was by hysterectomy (9)." Even so, Taylor's subsequent publications had a great influence on gynecologists' perceptions of pelvic congestion as a psychosomatic disease (10–12). Although his and Duncan's joint hypothesis that "chronic vascular congestion is a psychosomatic complaint" was unsupported by hard evidence, it was a milestone in the long road toward understanding the syndrome (11).

During the late 1960s interest surged briefly in pelvic congestion because of a suggested association with the so-called posttubal ligation syndrome, but no in-depth investigation of the pelvic pain-pelvic congestion connection was done until the late 1970s (13). It was then that investigators began to carefully study pelvic varicosities and their relation to CPP, menstrual dysfunction, and tubal sterilization procedures (14–17). The greater part of present-day understanding of this controversial syndrome is owing to the efforts of Beard and his colleagues in London, who have practically monopolized recent publications on pelvic congestion (5,14,18–20).

ANATOMY

Anatomists have shown that the elaborate pelvic venous system consists of a visceral and a parietal system that interconnect via numerous anastamoses. The parietal system encompasses the anterior, posterior presacral, and lateral pelvic plexuses that all are tributaries of the internal iliac veins. The internal iliac vein receives blood from the exterior of the pelvis via the inferior and superior gluteal, internal pudendal, sciatic, and the obturator veins. The radichial plexuses and the inferior vena cava drain the parietal system posteriorly.

The visceral venous tributaries of the internal iliac encompass several plexuses, most important of which are the uterine veins and plexuses. The visceral venous system also includes the ovarian veins, which terminate into the inferior vena cava on the right and left renal vein on the left. The ovarian venous system forms a plexus near the ovary and within the broad ligament, which communicates with the uterine plexus. Additionally, the visceral venous system includes the vesical and rectal veins and their plexuses, which have numerous anastamotic connections to the vaginal (and therefore uterine) plexuses (21,22).

Veins function as both collectors and reservoirs. The latter is a function of their internal valves, which play an important role in maintaining normal circulation (23). Anatomists and investigators have relentlessly studied the valvular structures of the limb veins because of the well-known complications of their incompetence but have rarely investigated the pelvic venous valvular system. The majority of present-day information on the internal iliac veins and its tributaries comes from the work of LePage et al., who dissected 82 iliac venous systems in 42 human cadavers (22). Despite older texts having been vague about the presence of valves within the internal iliac, LePage et al. found that 10% had valves (22). This low figure led him to consider that the occurrence of vascular congestion and varicosities was probably not just a function of valvular incompetence, but also a result of genetic anomalies or disturbances in the venous wall collagen structure.

ETIOLOGY

The syndrome of pelvic congestion raises etiopathogenic problems that remain only partly solved (24). Over the years various hypotheses have been put forward to explain the congestive state in affected women and, although each of these theories appears to have merit when viewed in its

TABLE 18.1. CLASSIFICATION OF PCS

Etiopathological Classification of Pelvic Congestion Syndrome
Anatomic dysfunction
Orgasmic dysfunction
Psychosomatic dysfunction
Hormonal dysfunction
Iatrogenically induced dysfunction

original context, each is deficient under different circumstances. In attempting to present and review these hypotheses, I propose classifying the condition according to the possible variations in etiopathology. Table 18.1 lists the classification, which seems to encompass the various theories presented over the years.

Anatomic Dysfunction

Given the complexity of the pelvic venous system it was only natural for investigators to attempt to solve the question of PCS by implicating this system as a primary cause of dysfunction.

Venous Overload and Valvular Incompetence

As first suggested by Dudley in 1888, LeFevre in 1964, and Beard et al. in 1984, pelvic varicocele is considered to be an etiologic factor (2,5,25). Pelvic varicosities are thought to occur in a mechanism similar to that of varicose veins, via the effect of gravity on an incompetent venous valvular system. The resultant venous stasis produces congestion and the pain typical of the syndrome (26). This was demonstrated by Reginald et al. by using the selective venoconstrictor dihydroergotamine (DHE) to reduce both venous congestion and pelvic pain in women with PCS (27). Their results suggested that the cause of the pain was the dilated pelvic veins, but could not differentiate whether it was owing to the congestive state or the venous distension.

Investigators have also approached the venous overload/incompetence mechanism from a different viewpoint; that is, that of a *pregnancy-induced state*. Dudley speculated that pregnancy resulted in postpartum varicosities (2). Taylor's early work had suggested that PCS is a disease of the reproductive years, a finding confirmed by Steege's review and by the data of Beard and colleagues, in which the mean age was 32.4 years (4,18,28). Hodgkinson indicated that during pregnancy a potential increase in the capacity of the ovarian veins of up to 60 times could occur and last for up to 6 months postpartum (29). Hughes and Curtis found that dilated veins were more frequently present with increasing parity and noted that pregnancy might be a risk factor for PCS (30). Giacchetto et al., utilizing a combination of ultrasound and retrograde phlebography, showed that parity was significantly higher in women with proven pelvic varices (31). A previous study by the same group showed that venous flow increases greatly during pregnancy, dilating veins and potentially damaging valves in an already compromised system, a view also shared by LePage and associates (22,32). These findings, when combined with the venous kinking caused by a malpositioned gravid uterus, likely lead to venous stagnation, flow reversal, and ensuing varicosities (33).

A pregnancy-induced anatomical dysfunction was also at the heart of Allen and Master's controversial "fascial defect" mechanism of pelvic congestion and pelvic pain. The defects in the broad ligament, they argued, were related to traumatic delivery and these defects led to uterine malpositioning and pelvic congestion (34). In a later commentary, Allen noted that patients seen with this syndrome were parous and speculated whether a normal delivery accompanied by a minor fetal malpresentation, as a mildly deflexed OP, would be enough to induce the syndrome (9).

Uterine malposition, in the absence of Allen-Master's fascial defects, was also considered a possible etiology of PCS by some. Interestingly, the association of uterine malposition, or "displacement," with pelvic pain and "pelvic congestion" or "varicocele" was recognized as far back as 1888 (2). A similar association was reported by Lydston in 1895 while attempting to counter adverse comparisons of the then-new fad of bicycling with use of sewing machines among women. He explained that the symptoms caused by the latter were owing to the sewing posture which caused the woman's "corset-steel" to dig into her abdomen (35). (Strangely enough, the seamstress-PCS connection is mentioned 94 years later by Menkiszak, who noted that "hypokinesis and piece-work claiming far advanced precision as well as monotony of the performed activity lead, in consequence, to congestion of organs in the small pelvis." (36) In 1973, Truc and Masset reviewed the literature and concluded there is a close association of retroversion of the uterus, pelvic pain, and dilated pelvic veins (37). The mechanism suggested was kinking of the veins in a manner similar to that proposed by Capasso (33).

Orgasmic Dysfunction

Orgasmic dysfunction was suggested as a possible pathophysiologic mechanism for occurrence of PCS based on the work of Masters and Johnson, who carefully described the physiologic responses to sexual stimulation (38,39). Visceral vasocongestion and cul-de-sac transudate were shown to occur during the primary phase of stimulation. When a woman is stimulated up to, but not reaching, orgasm (the plateau phase), some pain caused by the vasocongestion may be felt in the pelvic area. That such events can produce pelvic discomfort and psychic irritation is very clear, but whether this can produce permanent pathologic changes in the pelvic organs is debatable (38).

Psychosomatic Dysfunction

Taylor wrote that, "Psychiatric disturbances, usually of an emotional character, are a common accompaniment of pelvic congestion...." This was recognized by late nineteenth century physicians and, as a result, their patients' main complaint of pelvic pain was looked on as a psychogenic state (*pelipathia vegetativa*) by some or as "hysteria" by others (4,8). The phenomenon of psychological disturbances in these patients begs us to address the chicken-or-egg question of what occurs first: the chronic pain or psychopathology? It is clear now that chronic pain is a complex psychophysiological behavior pattern that cannot be broken down into distinct components (40). Modern concepts of pain have replaced the overly simplistic dichotomous view of pain, in which symptoms are either somatogenic or psychogenic. The modern biopsychosocial model of pain is a multidimensional one. In attempting to answer the chicken-and-egg dilemma, investigators in chronic pain have made inroads toward solving it both directly and indirectly. The latter method is much more feasible and utilizes either retrospective or cross-sectional studies. Such studies have dominated research into PCS since Taylor reviewed his first series of 105 patients in 1948. It was Taylor's opinion that an important factor in the etiology of PCS was "the effect of a primary state of emotional tension on the smooth muscle and secretory cells in the pelvis in producing 'psychosomatic' effects (4)." His belief that the psyche played a role led him to further investigation and, in 1952, he and Duncan voiced their opinion that stress actually led to chronic vascular congestion and subsequent PCS (11). Their study, which involved thermography of the vaginal vault, showed that increased nervous tension led to excessive pelvic visceral blood flow. In retrospect, this study was flawed in two ways: First, their finding was later proven to occur in all women under tension, and second, and more importantly, they could not rule out pelvic pathology, because present-day investigative techniques, such as laparoscopy, were not available (18,41). Partial support to Duncan and Taylor's theories was provided by well-designed studies by Beard and colleagues that confirmed that women with pelvic pain of apparently no cause were psychologically different from women without pain. According to Beard these patients "tend to be more neurotic ... and ... form less rewarding relationships." Beard et al.'s work supported the hypothesis that some pelvic pain could have a psychosomatic origin (14,19).

Investigators in other fields have also attempted to provide insight in the cause-and-effect relation between chronic pain and psychological disturbances. For example, Blanchard et al. performed a series of statistical analyses of cross-sectional data on a large number of headache patients of various ages and at various points in their lifetime course of headaches (42). Their results support the hypothesis that preexisting psychopathology may be a significant factor in "causing" chronic headache. Whether such studies can be applied to PCS and its accompanying psychosocial disturbances remains to be seen, but they are probably applicable to an extent. The shortcoming of the retrospective and cross-sectional methodologies lies in their inability to identify factors that predispose individuals to the development of chronic pain, because the characteristics of chronic pain patients may be consequences of their pain. The chicken-and-egg once more! A later prospective study by Beard et al. attempted to resolve this controversy (20). In following a group of PCS patients with psychosocial disturbances who had undergone total abdominal hysterectomy and bilateral salpingo-oophorectomy (TAH-BSO) as treatment, they noted that 35 of the 36 women reported absence of pain and return to normal lifestyles. Their tentative conclusion was that the patients' overt preoperative behavioral disturbances were caused by the pain.

Realistically, the only way to identify the causal antecedents of chronic pain is by conducting a prospective study *before* the patients develop pain and observing them while their chronic pain syndromes unfold. Although this seems impractical, several prospective studies have actually been attempted (43–45). According to Grzesiak their results "have suggested that various psychosocial factors—especially symptoms of depression—may be risk factors for later development of pain (46)."

Hormonal Dysfunction

A possible hormonally induced etiology was touched upon by Beard et al. in 1984, who mentioned that the varicosities seen with PCS could be "a result of relaxation of the smooth muscle in the walls of the pelvic veins caused by some vasoactive substance as yet unidentified (5)." Based on evidence from previous studies showing that PCS occurred exclusively in the reproductive years and fortified by observations by their own group, Reginald et al. speculated that PCS could be caused by ovarian hormones, possibly estrogen (4,5,14,15,18,19,47,48). Their study entailed suppressing ovarian function in 22 women with PCS using medroxyprogesterone acetate (MPA). There was a venographically demonstrated reduction in pelvic congestion in 17 of the patients, of whom 16 had become amenorrheic. This significant association between MPA-induced ovarian suppression and decreased pelvic congestion implicated the ovarian hormones, particularly estrogen, in playing a central role in the pathogenesis of the condition (49,50). Partial support for this theory comes from a randomized controlled trial of MPA and psychotherapy by Farquhar et al., showing a statistically significant reduction in pain after 4 months of treatment with MPA alone; but it must be added, less than the reduction with MPA combined with psychotherapy (51). In addition, Adams et al. reported a 56% incidence of polycystic ovaries (PCO) in a group of 55

patients with venographically proven PCS (49). The women were also found to have significantly larger uteri and thicker endometrium as compared with a control group of normal women, all of which led them to consider a role for estrogen in causing both the pelvic congestion and the associated uterine changes.

Iatrogenically Induced Dysfunction

Even more controversial than PCS, the so-called *posttubal ligation syndrome* may also lead to a PCS-like condition, usually accompanied by menstrual disturbances. An association of chronic pelvic pain following tubal ligation has been suspected since the 1920s, when Sampson speculated that it might be owing to a form of localized endometriosis (52). Interruption of the utero-ovarian circulation with consequent functional and anatomical changes, including the formation of pelvic varicosities, has been suggested as the cause of the syndrome (17,53–57). El-Minawi et al. have shown that these pelvic vascular abnormalities tend to occur especially after more destructive midsegment tubal sterilization procedures. They reported that 23 (58%) of 40 posttubal ligation patients presented with pelvic pain and in 70% of these pelvic varicosities were found by vaginal ultrasound (58). A more recent unpublished study by El-Minawi and El-Minawi showed that 83 (8.5%) of 978 patients undergoing laparoscopy for chronic pelvic pain had pelvic varicosities, subsequently documented either by venography or ultrasound, and of these 60% had a history of tubal ligation (59). Stock reported that 13 of 75 women with a history of prior tubal ligation had varicosities at the time of hysterectomy (60). Of these, five (39%) had symptoms consistent with pelvic congestion syndrome, whereas the remaining patients had pain localized only to the side where the varicosities were prominent. Lu and Chun, in a follow-up of 1,055 cases of postpartum tubal ligation, reported the incidence of pelvic discomfort as 16% in those cases with varicosities (53). From the wide disparity in figures it can be surmised that tubal ligation has an association with pelvic varicosities and that its association with PCS, although probable, is less clear.

Investigators have also found another link between pelvic pain, varicosities, and previous tubal sterilization. Ruifang et al. studied the peritoneal fluid in 18 women with history of tubal sterilization and complaints of pain consistent with pelvic congestion (61). On comparing the findings with those in ten controls with a history of tubal ligation but no pain and ten normal healthy controls, they found marked differences. The levels of 6 keto-prostaglandin F1 alpha (6-keto-PGF1α) were significantly increased in the 18 pain patients. Likewise, the volume of peritoneal fluid was markedly increased in these same women as compared to the controls. They suggested that tubal ligation led to an increase in 6-keto-PGF1α levels, which played an important role in the causation of pelvic pain in association with the pelvic varicosities.

Another possible iatrogenic cause of pelvic congestion and associated pain was reported on by Osman and colleagues (62). They laparoscopically and venographically assessed 39 Lippes loop C users (1 to 12 years duration of use) complaining of chronic pelvic pain and in whom myometrial overactivity had been excluded. They found the incidence of demonstrable pelvic varicosities to be 95% venographically and 52% laparoscopically in these women, in addition to good correlation between the site of maximum pain and the sites of maximum varicosities. They could not explain the connection between the IUD and the varicosities.

SYMPTOMS

One of the problems in establishing PCS as a legitimate diagnosis is the wide range of presenting symptoms, which in Taylor's words, "form a considerable part of office gynecologic practice (4)." Both Taylor's and Beard's work have provided insight as to the clinical characteristics and presentations of women with PCS. The syndrome almost always afflicts women in their reproductive years, typically multiparous patients in their third or fourth decades (4,18). The following symptoms may occur separately or, more commonly, as combinations.

Pain

Dull, aching pain in the pelvic area is the most common type of pain, similar in character to that produced by varicose veins in the legs. It is usually not constant and may be brought on by simple acts, such as walking or changing posture. Evidence suggests that it is directly related to the congestive state of the tissues. Although most often unilateral it can occur on both sides simultaneously. It is usually localized to the lateral lower abdominal quadrant. It is also most severe premenstrually (2,4,14,18). Occasional *acute exacerbations of sharp pain* may occur, at times severe enough to result in emergency evaluation and lead to mistaken diagnoses such as acute appendicitis or pelvic inflammatory disease (4,18). Additionally, Taylor noted that a distinguishing feature is the disproportionate degree of agitation and reaction to the pain, which he speculated might be caused by the sudden engorgement and stretching of the ovarian capsule (4). *Low backache*, apparently a result of the generalized congestion and increased uterine size, has also been frequently reported (4,8,18,34,37). Backache is characteristically sacral in position and made worse by standing. Sacrodynia and hypogastric pain have been reported in women working in nonergonomic positions (36).

Sexually related pain is very common, so much so that one earlier investigator made it the central feature of PCS

(63). Notably, *deep dyspareunia* is one of the most consistent symptoms of PCS, with an incidence ranging from 71% to 78% in Beard's and Taylor's studies, respectively, despite their being almost 40 years apart (4,18). Postcoital ache, lasting in some cases up to 24 hours, was reported in 65% of Beard and colleagues' cases and also seems to be a common complaint (19).

Menstrually related pain also seems to be a consistent symptom, with *congestive dysmenorrhea* being the most common type of pain (4,54,60). It was reported by 89% of Beard and colleagues' cases with pelvic congestion (18). In addition to these common types of pain, researchers have also reported instances of burning urination, vague burning vulvar pain, and rectal pain (4).

Menstrual Disorders and Genital Symptomatology

In addition to the previously mentioned premenstrual pain, changes in menstrual frequency, duration, or amount may occur. Dysfunctional uterine bleeding occurs in 54% of women with PCS (18). In cases with previous tubal ligation procedures, menorrhagia and menometrorrhagia may also be present (54,58,60). Taylor reported intermenstrual spotting in 25% of cases and attributed it to minute hemorrhages from an excessively congested endometrium or endocervix (4). Vaginal discharges are also a common symptom, most often being clear mucoid in nature (4,18).

Gastric and Intestinal Disturbances

Nausea, flatulence, and epigastric distress have been noted. Likewise, vague abdominal cramping and changes in bowel habits have been mentioned, although the changes are not as consistent as in patients with irritable bowel syndrome (4,18).

Urinary Tract Symptoms

Frequency and urgency have been reported, in addition to the previously mentioned burning micturition. Cystoscopy may reveal congestion and edema of the trigone. Urine cultures typically are negative (4,18). Interestingly, Bochorishvili and colleagues commented on 78 patients complaining of vague pelvic pain and urinary tract disturbances that could not be reliably attributed to either urologic or gynecologic disorders (64). These patients underwent simultaneous excretory urography and transuterine pelvic phlebography revealing the lower part of the ureters to be entangled in the vaginouterine veins. Patients with urodynamic disorders on one side were found to have more varicosities on that same side, leading them to believe that the varicosities compressed the ureter and led to the patient's symptoms.

Symptoms of Nervous System Disturbance

Various symptoms have been described, but headache, fatigue, and insomnia are the most common and consistent (4,11,18). Headache is characteristically a migraine-type headache. Fatigue occurs as loss of energy and exhaustion in the absence of physical exertion.

Psychiatric and Emotional Disturbances

These disturbances have been associated with PCS since it was first recognized. Patients may show a wide range of emotional disorders ranging from simple anxiety to depression with attempted suicide. Some show signs of emotional immaturity and strong dependency needs, whereas others lapse into states of depression (4,8,11,18). Psychological evaluation and counseling are useful when dealing with the PCS patient. Properly done they lead to relevant information on the patient's mood state, past and current experience with pain and illness, and provide insight as to the patient's beliefs about the nature of her pain. They can provide the physician, at times, with evidence that the symptoms stem from an emotional disturbance, thus providing a gateway to possible successful nonsurgical treatment (14). Psychometric instruments can help in pointing the physician toward a proper diagnosis, and also prepare the patient in dealing with her condition, whatever treatment path is chosen (65).

SIGNS

On inspection of the external genitalia, superficial vulvar and paravulvar varices have often been described (4,6,7,66). These may only involve the immediate medial aspect of the thigh or, in more severe cases, extend into the posteromedial thigh and buttock and spread down over the posterior aspect of the legs.

Abdominal palpation usually reveals tenderness at the *ovarian point*, which lies at the junction of the upper and middle thirds of a line drawn from the anterior superior iliac spine to the pubic symphysis (18,19). Deep abdominal pressure at this point reproduces the pelvic pain complained of by the patient. This is believed to be owing to ovarian vein compression, leading to back-pressure on the plexus of veins at the ovarian hilum. Beard and colleagues found that one of the most discriminating combinations of signs and symptoms was ovarian point tenderness on abdominal palpation and postcoital ache (18). This combination is 94% sensitive and 77% specific for pelvic congestion as confirmed by pelvic venography.

Vaginal examination and bimanual palpation of the cervix, uterus, and ovaries are of great value. Inspection of the cervix often reveals an excessive clear mucoid discharge, whereas the cervix itself is often blue because of engorgement (4,67). Bimanual examination of the cervix elicits pain and tenderness on movement. Some investigators have noted that tenderness of the uterosacral ligaments and the parametrium are the most characteristic sign of PCS, whereas others have noted that ovarian and adnexal tenderness on bimanual examination to be the most distinguishing sign (4,15). Beard et al. have found that ovarian pain elicited by gentle compression on vaginal examination when combined with postcoital ache is 97% sensitive and 64% specific in diagnosing PCS (18).

Although some investigators have pointed out an increased size in uterine volume with PCS in their cases, it has not been found to be a reliable, reproducible sign (49).

DIAGNOSTIC STUDIES

Diagnostic Laparoscopy

Pelvic pain is the most common indication for diagnostic laparoscopy but in 60% of cases no diagnosis is made (68). Many gynecologists use this technique as a screening method prior to other diagnostic procedures when PCS is suspected, and it is still the only reliable method of excluding endometriosis. Priou reported limited success in diagnosing varicosities by laparoscopy (69). Metzger states that

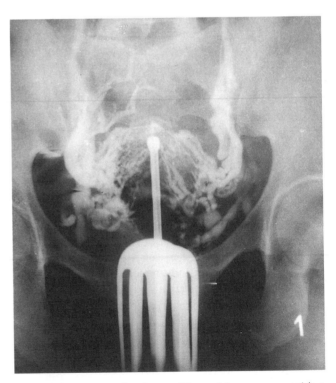

FIGURE 18.1. Example of a positive pelvic venogram with a transuterine Rocket needle technique.

laparoscopy is not a definitive method of diagnosing pelvic varicosities because the patient's intrabdominal pressure is high and Trendelenburg positioning leads to venous drainage, thereby decreasing venous distention and increasing false negative diagnoses (28). Although agreeing with her statement, in our experience it is possible to visualize these varicosities by decreasing the intraabdominal pressure and gradually placing the patient in a reverse Trendelenburg position. This technique was recently reported by El-Minawi and El-Minawi in a study of 83 patients with suspected varicosities at laparoscopy that were later confirmed by venography or ultrasound (59). Osman et al. used this technique to diagnose pelvic varicosities in 52% of their patients with venographically proven varicosities (62). It should also be noted that some investigators have shown that in women with CPP and negative laparoscopies, up to 91% had dilated veins and pelvic congestion on venography (5).

Pelvic Venography

Pelvic venography has proved to be an invaluable tool in the diagnosis of pelvic varicosities (18). Although invasive, the advantages lie in its ability to provide a detailed picture of the pelvic venous anatomy, the exact locations of any varicosities and grading of their severity. A variety of techniques have been used, the two most common being selective retrograde ovarian venography and transuterine venography.

Transuterine venography has been the most commonly employed method owing to its relative ease and low cost (18,70,71). Water soluble contrast medium is introduced into the uterine venous system via injection into the myometrium of the uterine fundus with a special single-lumen needle (Rocket Needle, Rocket Co., London, England). The needle is passed through the cervix via a special concentric metal sheath that covers all but the final 0.5 cm tip of the needle. With the patient on her back, 20 to 30 mL of the contrast medium are injected, with or without abdominal compression. The first image is taken immediately at the end of injection, followed by a second image 20 sec later (or after release of compression, if used) and a third image at 60 sec (Fig. 18.1). Some authors recommend the injection of 3 to 10 mL of hyaluronidase immediately prior to the contrast medium, whereas others do not, believing it could produce an artificial intramural uterine venous network (18,27,72). Although this method is advantageous in that it provides information on the uterine and broad ligamentary vascular systems as well as the ovarian veins, it also has several drawbacks. Giaccheto regards this method as being hemodynamically incorrect, considering it an anterograde venography that fails to take into account the pathological retrograde reflux resulting from gravity in an incompetent vascular system (31). In addition Metzger notes that even with compression the ovarian veins may not always be

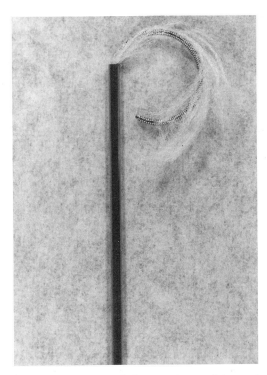

FIGURE 18.2. Gianturco coil that can be used for embolization of ovarian veins. When completely extruded from the cannula the coil rolls into a circle.

filled and that discomfort that may require heavy sedation of the patient (28). Because of concerns about excessive pain, we used heavy sedation or general anesthesia in some of our cases (59).

Beard and colleagues have described a venogram scoring system based on the maximum diameter of the ovarian veins, time of disappearance of contrast, and the degree of congestion of the ovarian plexus (Table 18.2) (5). The score can range from 3 to 9, with 3 or 4 being normal and 5 to 9 suggesting increasingly severe pelvic congestion. This scor-

TABLE 18.2. SCORING SYSTEM FOR ASSESSING PELVIC VENOGRAPHY

	SCORE		
	1	2	3
Maximal diameter of ovarian veins (mm)	1–4	5–8	>8
Time to disappearance of end of contrast medium after injection (seconds)	0	20	40
Ovarian plexus congestion	Normal	Moderate	Extensive

From Beard RW, Highman JH, Pearce S, et al. Diagnosis of pelvic varicosities in women with chronic pelvic pain. *Lancet* 1984;ii:946–949, with permission.

ing system is not influenced by the parity or stage of menstrual cycle of the patient. Using a score of 5 or more as diagnostic of PCS, Beard et al. reported a sensitivity of 91% and a specificity of 89% in a study of 18 women without and 45 women with PCS. This gives a likelihood ratio of 8.3 for a positive test and a likelihood ratio 0.1 for a negative test.

Selective ovarian venography can either be performed via a jugular venous approach or via the much more commonly used transfemoral approach (7,32,33,73). The technique is performed under local anesthesia and involves puncturing the common femoral vein and placing a small-diameter introducer sheath. Special teflon catheters are passed under fluoroscopic guidance into the ovarian veins and nonionic water-soluble contrast medium injected. Because the right ovarian vein drains directly into the inferior vena cava, it is more difficult to cannulate and usually involves using a different type or size catheter than the left side (33). Some consider this invasive technique to be the method of choice for diagnosis of pelvic varicosities. The following criteria, described by Kennedy and Hemmingway, are suggestive of venous congestion: maximal ovarian vein diameter of 10 mm, congestion of the ovarian venous plexus, filling of veins across the midline, or filling of vulvar and thigh varicosities (74).

Another much less commonly used technique of venography is vulvar phlebography, as described by Craig and Hobbs, whereby injection of contrast medium is done via vulvar vein injection (75). Likewise, selective ovarian venography via vulvar vein puncture has also been used (76).

Ultrasound and Doppler

The advantages of ultrasound in diagnosing pelvic congestion were reported by Montanari in 1975 almost a decade before investigators in the mid-1980s reported its use in documenting pelvic varicosities (4,77,78). Taylor et al. in 1985 introduced Doppler to measure pelvic blood flow and this was followed later by the use of transvaginal ultrasound in documenting and measuring pelvic varicosities (31,58,79). The use of color Doppler, although appealing, has not yet reached the stage where it can be applied in the diagnosis of PCS. It has been mentioned by some, but mainly for identification of arterial flow disturbances associated with the condition and not actual measurement of venous flow patterns (80,81).

The fact that ultrasound is noninvasive allows it to be used in all patients suspected of having pelvic congestion. Utilizing transvaginal ultrasound, Giacchetto et al. reported the presence of linear or circular anechogenic structures of a diameter greater than 5 mm, and lateral to the uterus and cervix, that increased by Valsalva or by standing suggested pelvic varices (31). By means of pulsed Doppler duplex transvaginal scanning, El-Minawi et al. noted a significant

increase in the resistance index (RI) of uterine artery blood flow in women with posttubal ligation venous congestion as compared to normal control patients (0.8 ± 0.05 versus 0.7 ± 0.04, $p < 0.001$). This was directly proportional to the size of the varices (58). Doppler duplex sonography has also been used in the follow-up of PCS patients treated by ovarian vein embolization. Capasso et al. reported good concordance of clinical findings with follow-up Doppler studies in 11 patients who experienced complete symptomatic relief following embolization (33). Of these, 72% showed excellent correlation (i.e., complete symptomatic relief and variceal thrombosis), whereas 18% had incomplete variceal thrombosis.

Radioisotopes and Magnetic Resonance Imaging

Over two decades ago, Clavero Nunez and colleagues attempted to diagnose pelvic varicosities utilizing intravenous 13 mIn and a Gamma camera detector (82). Their findings, although interesting, were not specific enough to be useful. In the 1980s, Xenon 133 clearance was used in diagnosing pelvic congestion in a group of patients with pelvic pain undergoing surgery (83). Although it showed that blood flow was slower in those with proven pelvic congestion at laparotomy than in those without, the predictive value was not high enough to merit continued study by investigators.

Gupta and McCarthy, using conventional MRI, have commented on the appearance of pelvic varices (84). Researchers in Japan have developed new techniques utilizing MRI that show promise and could possibly be applied to aid in the diagnosis of PCS. Joja and colleagues have reported the use of MRI and magnetic resonance angiography (MRA) in diagnosis of a uterine cirsoid aneurysm in a 51-year-old patient (85). Conventional T1- and T2-weighted images showed multiple fluid voids, whereas MRA gave images equal to pelvic angiography. Kamoi used three dimensional magnetic resonance venography (3D-MRV) to investigate the role of the internal pudendal vein in the etiology of pelvic varicosities in 27 males (86). 3D-MRV enabled him to detect a significant interruption in flow in the ascending portion of the vein, in the vicinity of Alcock's canal.

It remains to be seen whether these new technologies, with further refinement, can replace the current gold standards for diagnosing pelvic varicosities.

TREATMENT

At this point, it should be clear that a physician presented with a patient with suspected PCS must be open-minded in the extreme. She or he must be open to many approaches to treatment, even Fothergill's observation that, "A change of employment often works like a charm" (3). As has been reviewed, the etiology may be multifactorial.

Because of the chronicity of the condition and because of the biosychosocial origins, it is my opinion that part of proper management, even after an evidence-based diagnosis has been reached, is to continue psychological counseling. On one hand it may actually be part of proper psychotherapy if the patient's profile and diagnostic results point to a significant psychogenic component, whereas on the other hand, it will be beneficial in that patients can be brought to understand that chronic conditions are not always amenable to a 100% cure, even if surgical treatment is justified. The benefits of integrating psychotherapy with standard treatment regimens are stressed by Smith and Reginald, and supported by the work of Farquhar et al., whose results showed that combined treatment with medroxyprogesterone acetate (MPA) and psychotherapy was significantly more effective than MPA or psychotherapy alone (50,51).

SURGICAL TREATMENT

Hysterectomy

Historically, most physicians have treated women with PCS with hysterectomy (4). Although this treatment should now have little if any role in therapy, it is interesting to note the various attitudes and opinions dealing with it.

One view is that in women with emotional disturbances and insecure family relations, physical suffering is an escape from mental and social conflicts. In such patients hysterectomy as a therapy is believed to be the worst route to take. Duncan and Taylor argued that taking away the physical pain might leave these patients in such intense psychic pain that acute psychosis or even suicide might result (11).

Another perspective on the relative inadequacy of hysterectomy comes from a retrospective study by Stovall et al., who evaluated the long-term outcome of hysterectomy in 99 women who underwent surgery for pelvic pain of at least 6 months' duration (87). Although there was no evidence these women had PCS, all had symptoms and physical examination findings suggestive of disease confined to the uterus. Patients were excluded if there was previously documented extrauterine pelvic disease, extrauterine pelvic disease at the time of surgery, or uterine weight exceeding 200 g. Patients were followed after hysterectomy for an average of 22 months. Nearly a quarter of the patients (22%) had persistent pelvic pain after hysterectomy.

On the other hand, Beard et al. performed hysterectomy plus bilateral salpingo-oophorectomy on 36 women with PCS documented by venography, 33 of whom had failed to obtain relief with long-term medical therapy (20). Their results showed a dramatic improvement in pain scores, a return to normal lifestyles, and a significant increase in frequency of intercourse. Smith and Reginald commented on

these observations and argued that failure to remove the ovaries may have led to recurrent pain, as in Stovall's series (50). Accordingly, they recommended bilateral oophorectomy be performed if hysterectomy is contemplated. Because the majority of these women are in their reproductive years, the benefits of such surgery must be carefully weighed against the drawbacks of loss of fertility and the necessity of long-term use of hormone replacement therapies.

Ovarian Vein Ligation

One of the first treatments for this condition, ovarian vein ligation, has been practiced since the early 1900s (3). The transperitoneal route was the first to be employed, followed later by the retroperitoneal approach (6). Drawbacks to these methods are the large incisions, the relatively long hospital stay and convalescence period, and the inability to properly assess the pelvic cavity directly. Mathis et al. and Grabham and Barrie have reported a laparoscopic transperitoneal technique of ovarian vein ligation using titanium clips, providing a solution to the drawbacks of the open methods (66,76). A similar laparoscopic method involving suture ligation has been used, but minimal data on results are published. Metzger reviewed a number of studies dealing with ovarian vein ligation and observed that only 52% of patients were cured, 17% showed improvement and the remainder had no change in symptoms (28). She likewise made three points that, in her opinion, could improve the outcome of the procedures. These included ligation of both the distal and proximal vessels to prevent thrombosis, ligation of the vessels of both ovaries to prevent recurrence on the opposite side, and ligation only if the congestion is directly caused by the ovarian veins.

MEDICAL THERAPY

Hormonal Therapy

The previously mentioned studies of Reginald et al. and Farquhar et al. imply ovarian hormones are important in the etiology of PCS (48,51). Their use of medroxyprogesterone acetate (MPA) reduced the diameter of the pelvic varices and ameliorated the patients' symptoms to some extent. In addition, Adam and colleagues' data showing increases in the incidence of PCO and increases in uterine size in women with PCS imply a hormonal origin (49). Reginald and colleagues' study involved suppression of ovarian function using 30 mg of MPA daily for 6 months in 22 women with lower abdominal pain caused by pelvic congestion (48). In 17 of 22 women (77%) there was a venographically demonstrable reduction in pelvic congestion. There was also a statistically significant reduction in these 17 women's pain scores as compared to the other five women with no change in venographic scoring. The idea for Farquhar et al.'s study arose from Reginald et al.'s findings (51). This study was a double-blind, randomized, controlled trial of treatment with MPA or psychotherapy (51). The results showed that MPA therapy alone significantly reduced pain, but also suggested that results should not be expected for at least 2 months, because the efficacy of MPA increases over time (50). Although MPA is well tolerated and safe, breakthrough bleeding occurs in a significant number of patients. In addition, pain returns when treatment is stopped (48).

The overall opinion of the British researchers is that ovarian suppression alone is not enough, as revealed by the failure of oral contraceptives to relieve pelvic congestion and by the insignificant pain relief shown in Gangar and colleagues' study using a combination of GnRH agonists, estradiol valerate, and MPA (9,88). Hormonal treatment is not generally a feasible long-term treatment, particularly in the younger woman. It may be beneficial for short-terms treatment until a more permanent solution to the patients' symptoms is found.

Radiologic Transcatheter Embolization of the Ovarian Veins

Edwards et al. first reported the use or transcatheter ovarian vein embolization to treat pelvic pain patients in 1993 (89). There have been five other published reports, in addition to an unpublished series by Machan mentioned by Metzger (7,28,33,73,90,91). Together these reports have involved a total of 53 patients, with no serious complications reported (Table 18.3). Likewise, no case of postembolization has yet to be reported. The procedure is similar to transfemoral selective venography, previously described, with the additional step of injecting the embolizing agent(s). Most experts do not recommend the use of liquid sclerosing agents, to avoid inadvertent systemic dissemination and prefer to use either enbucrilate (Histoacryl L Transparent, B. Braun, Melsungen, Germany) or small 5- to 15-mm diameter stainless-steel coils (Gianturco Coils, Cook Inc., Bloomington, IN) (Fig.

18.2) or a combination of the two (33,89). The reported follow-up of these cases ranged from 6 months to 4 years (73,89). Various degrees of relief have been noted by investigators following this procedure. Capasso et al. note that 11 (58%) of their 19 patients had complete relief of symptoms, three (16%) had only partial relief, and five (26%) had persistent pain (33). This level of relief is not far from the 73% attributed to Machlan et al. by Metzger. The 100% cure rates reported by some investigators are misleading because they are either case reports or involve very small numbers. Ovarian vein embolization is a promising treatment option with the advantages of being an outpatient procedure, involving no prolonged convalescence, and being less costly than surgical treatments. The disadvantages are the relatively high dose of radiation to which the patient is exposed during flouroscopy and the lack of longer follow-up data. More prospective studies are needed to determine its eventual role in the management of PCS.

KEY POINTS

Differential Diagnoses

Endometriosis
- Adenomyosis
- Adhesions
- Psychological disorders

Most Important Questions to Ask

- Where is your pain located? Is on only one side or both sides? Do you have low back pain or backache?
- What is the nature or quality of your pain? Is it dull and aching? Is it acute and sharp?
- Is your pain brought on by walking or changing posture?
- Is your pain most severe premenstrually?
- Do you have pain with intercourse or pain after intercourse?

TABLE 18.3. OVARIAN VEIN EMBOLIZATION CASES, TECHNIQUES, AND COMPLICATIONS IN THE LITERATURE

Investigators	Cases	Technique used	Cured	Complications
Edwards et al. (89)	1	Stainless steel coils	100%	None reported
Florio et al. (90)	1	Sclerosing agent	100%	None reported
Abbas et al. (91)	1	Stainless steel coils	100%	None reported
Sichlau et al. (7)	3	Stainless steel coils	2 of 3	None reported
Machan et al.[a]	22	[b]	16 of 22	[b]
Capasso et al. (33)	19	Enbucrilate (80%) Stainless steel coils	11 of 19	Two ovarian vein perforations by guidewire
Tarazov et al. (73)	6	Stainless steel coils	6 of 6	One mild hematoma at puncture site Two patients had low grade fever >24 hrs

[a]Unpublished but quoted by Metzger.
[b]Not mentioned.

- Do you have irregular or heavy menstrual bleeding, or bleeding in between your periods?
- Do you have headaches, fatigue, or insomnia?

Most Important Physical Examination Findings

- Superficial vulvar and paravulvar varices
- Abdominal tenderness at the ovarian point
- Excessive clear mucoid cervical discharge
- Blue-appearing cervix
- Tenderness on bimanual examination of the cervix
- Tenderness on bimanual examination of the adnexae

Most Important Diagnostic Studies

- Diagnostic laparoscopy in a reverse Trendelenburg position with decreased intraabdominal pressure
- Transuterine pelvic venography
- Selective retrograde ovarian venography
- Transvaginal ultrasound with or without Doppler
- MRI

Treatments

- Hormonal ovarian suppression
- Psychotherapy
- Oophorectomy
- Ligation of ovarian veins
- Embolization of ovarian veins

REFERENCES

1. Richet MA. *Traité pratique d'anatomie medico-chirurgicale.* Paris: E. Chamerot Libraire Editeur, 1857.
2. Dudley AP. Varicocele in the female: what is its influence upon the ovary? *NY Med J* 1888;48:147–149.
3. Fothergill WE. Varicocele in the female. *BMJ* 1921;2:925–926.
4. Taylor HC. Vascular congestion and hyperemia, their effect on structure and function in the female reproductive organs. Part II. The clinical aspects of the congestion-fibrosis syndrome. *Am J Obstet Gynecol* 1949;57:637–653.
5. Beard RW, Highman JH, Pearce S, et al. Diagnosis of pelvic varicosities in women with chronic pelvic pain. *Lancet* 1984;ii:946–949.
6. Hobbs JT. The pelvic congestion syndrome. *Practitioner* 1976;216:529–540.
7. Sichlau MJ, Yao JST, Vogelzang RL. Transcatheter embolotherapy for the treatment of pelvic congestion syndrome. *Obstet Gynecol* 1994;83(5 Part 2):892–896.
8. Gauss CJ. Eine haufig vorkommende, mehrfach beschriebene, meist verkannte und oft operativ umsont angegangene Erkrankung: die Pelipathia vegetativa. *Deutsch Med Wchnschr* 1949;74:1288–1290.
9. Allen WA. Chronic pelvic congestion and pelvic pain. *Am J Obstet Gynecol* 1971;109:198–202.
10. Taylor HC. The problem of pelvic pain. In: Meigs JV, Somers HS, eds. *Progress in gynecology.* New York: Grune & Stratton, 1957:191–207.
11. Duncan CH, Taylor HC. A psychosomatic study of pelvic congestion. *Am J Obstet Gynecol* 1952;64:1–12.
12. Taylor HC. Pelvic pain based on a vascular and autonomic nervous disorder. *Am J Obstet Gynecol* 1954;67:1177–1196.
13. Ringrose CAD. Post tubal ligation menorrhagia and pelvic pain. *Int J Fertil* 1974;19:168.
14. Beard RW, Belsey EM, Lieberman BA, et al. Pelvic pain in women. *Am J Obstet Gynecol* 1977;128:566–570.
15. Renaer M, Nijs P, van Assche A, et al. Chronic pelvic pain without obvious pathology. Personal observations and a review of the problem. *Eur J Obstet Gynaecol Reprod Biol* 1980;10:415–463.
16. Renaer M. Chronic pelvic pain without obvious pathology. In: *Chronic pelvic pain in women.* New York: Springer-Verlag, 1981:162–175.
17. El-Minawi MF, Mashhor N, Reda MS. Pelvic venous changes after tubal sterilization. *J Reprod Med* 1983;28(10):641–648.
18. Beard RW, Reginald PW, Wadsworth J. Clinical features of women with chronic lower abdominal pain and pelvic congestion. *Br J Obstet Gynaecol* 1988;95:153–161.
19. Beard RW, Reginald PW, Pearce S. Psychological and somatic factors in women with pain due to pelvic congestion. *Adv Exp Biol Med* 1988;245:413–421.
20. Beard RW, Kennedy RG, Gangar KF, et al. Bilateral oophorectomy and hysterectomy in the treatment of intractable pelvic pain associated with pelvic congestion. *Br J Obstet Gynaecol* 1991;98:988–992.
21. Gray H. The blood-vascular system. In: Pick TP, Howden R, eds. *Gray's Anatomy,* 15th ed. New York: Bounty Books, 1977:616–618.
22. LePage PA, Villaviciencio JL, Gomez ER, et al. The valvular anatomy of the iliac venous system and its clinical implications. *J Vasc Surg* 1991;14:678–683.
23. Thibodeau GA, ed. *Anatomy and physiology.* St. Louis: Times Mirror/Mosby College Publishing, 1987:455.
24. Charles G. Congestive pelvic syndromes. *Revue Francaise de Gynecologie et d'Obstetrique* 1995;90(2):84–90.
25. LeFevre H. Broad ligament varicocele. *Acta Obstet Gynecol Scand* 1964;43(Suppl 7):122–123.
26. Pelvic congestion (Editorial). *Lancet* 1991;337:398–400.
27. Reginald PW, Beard RW, Kooner JS, et al. Intravenous dihydroergotamine to relieve pelvic congestion with pain in young women. *Lancet* 1987;ii:351–353.
28. Steege JF. Chronic pelvic pain: clinical perspectives. In: Dinnerstein, Burrows, eds. *Handbook of psychosomatic obstetrics and gynaecology.* Amsterdam: Elsevier Biomedical Press, 1983:401–412.
29. Hodgkinson CP. Physiology of the ovarian veins during pregnancy. *Obstet Gynecol* 1953;1:26–37.
30. Hughes RR, Curtis DD. Uterine phlebography: correlation of clinical diagnoses with dye retention. *Am J Obstet Gynecol* 1962;83:156–164.
31. Giacchetto C, Cotroneo GB, Marincolo F, et al. Ovarian varicocele: ultrasonic and phlebographic evaluation. *J Clin Ultrasound* 1990;18:551–555.
32. Giacchetto C, Catizone F, Cotroneo GB, et al. Radiologic anatomy of the genital venous system in female patients with varicocele. *Surg Gynecol Obstet* 1989;169:403–407.
33. Capasso P, Simons C, Trotteur G, et al. Treatment of symptomatic pelvic varices by ovarian vein embolization. *Cardiovasc Intervent Radiol* 1997;20:107–111.
34. Allen WM, Masters WH. Traumatic laceration of uterine support. *Am J Obstet Gynecol* 1955;70:500–513.
35. Lydston FL (1895). Quoted In: Martensen RL. Of a bicycle built for two [... in perspective]. *JAMA* 1995;274:1321.
36. Menkiszak J. Pain in the lumbosacral region in pelvic congestion syndrome in women working under conditions of limited motor activity. *Annales Academiae Medicae Stetinensis* 1989;35:167–178.

37. Truc JB, Musset R. Pathologie de tissue cellulaire pelvien et grossesse. In: De Brux J, ed. *Le tissue cellulaire pelvien.* Paris: Masson, 1973.

38. Daly MJ. Evaluation and preferred management of premenstrual tension-pelvic congestive syndrome and allied states. In: Reid DE, Christian CD. *Controversy in obstetrics and gynecology II.* Philadelphia: W.B. Saunders, 1974:776–779.

39. Masters WH, Johnson VE. *Human sexual response.* Boston: Little, Brown, 1966.

40. Gatchel RJ. Psychological disorders and chronic pain. Cause-and-effect relationships. In: Gatchel RJ, Turk DC, eds. *Psychological approaches to pain management. A practitioner's handbook.* New York: Guilford Press, 1996:33–52.

41. Osofsky HJ, Fisher S. Pelvic congestion: some further considerations. *Obstet Gynecol* 1968;31:406–410.

42. Blanchard EB, Kirsch CA, Applebaum KA, et al. Role of psychopathology in chronic headache: cause or effect? *Headache* 1989;29:295–301.

43. Leino P, Magni G. Depressive and distress symptoms as predictors of low back pain, neck-shoulder pain, and other musculoskeletal morbidity: A 10 year follow-up of metal industry employees. *Pain* 1993;54:89–94.

44. Von Korff M, Le Resche L, Dworkin SF. First onset of common pain symptoms: a prospective study of depression as a risk factor. *Pain* 1993;55:251–258.

45. Pietri-Taleb F, Riihimaki H, Viikari-Juntura E, et al. Longitudinal study on the role of personality characteristics and psychological distress in neck trouble among working men. *Pain* 1994; 58:261–267.

46. Grzesiak R, Ury GM, Dworkin RH. Psychodynamic psychotherapy with chronic pain patients. In: Gatchel RJ, Turk DC, eds. *Psychological approaches to pain management. A practitioner's handbook.* New York: Guilford Press, 1996:148–178.

47. Adams J, Beard RW, Franjs S, et al. Pelvic ultrasound findings in women with chronic pelvic pain: correlation with laparoscopy and venography. Quoted In: Reginald PW, Adams J, Franks S, et al. Medroxyprogesterone acetate in the treatment of pelvic pain due to venous congestion. *Br J Obstet Gynaecol* 1989;96:1148–1152.

48. Reginald PW, Adams J, Franks S, et al. Medroxyprogesterone acetate in the treatment of pelvic pain due to venous congestion. *Br J Obstet Gynaecol* 1989;96:1148–1152.

49. Adams J, Reginald PW, Franks S, et al. Uterine size and endometrial thickness and the significance of cystic ovaries in women with pelvic pain due to congestion. *Br J Obstet Gynaecol* 1990;97: 583–587.

50. Smith KM, Reginald PW. Treatment options in women with unexplained chronic pelvic pain. In: Studd J, ed. *The Yearbook of the Royal College of Obstetricians and Gynaecologists.* London: RCOG Press, 1996:193–204.

51. Farquhar CM, Rogers V, Franks S, et al. A randomized controlled trial of medroxyprogesterone acetate and psychotherapy for the treatment of pelvic congestion. *Br J Obstet Gynaecol* 1989;96: 1153–1162.

52. Sampson J. Endometriosis following salpingectomy. *Am J Obstet Gynecol* 1928;16:461–463.

53. Lu T, Chun D. A long-term follow-up study of 1,055 cases of post partum tubal ligation. *Obstet Gynaecol Br Commonw* 1967; 74:875–880.

54. Ringrose CA. Post tubal ligation menorrhagia and pelvic pain. *Int J Fertil* 1974;19(3):168–170.

55. Neil JR, Noble AD, Hammond GT, et al. Late complications of sterilization by laparoscopy and tubal ligation. *Lancet* 1975; 2(7937):699–700.

56. Uchida H. Uchida tubal sterilization. *Am J Obstet Gynecol* 1975;121(2):153–158.

57. Hefnawi F, Kandil O, El-Sheikha Z. Study of sequelae of various surgical methods of female sterilization. Proceedings of the 2nd International Conference on Voluntary Sterilization. Alexandria, VA: Moharemm Press, 1975:151.

58. El-Minawi MF, Derbala S, Ahmed MM, et al. Transvaginal Doppler sonographic study in patients with post tubal ligation syndrome. *Med J Cairo Univ* 1991;59(4):1003–1010.

59. El-Minawi MF, El-Minawi AM. Laparoscopy in chronic pelvic pain: 25 years experience. Presented at the International Congress of Gynecologic Endoscopy, AAGL 26th Annual Meeting. Seattle, Washington, Sept. 23–28, 1997.

60. Stock RJ. Sequelae of tubal ligation: an analysis of 75 consecutive hysterectomies. *S Med J* 1984;77(10):1255–1260.

61. Ruifang W, Zhenhai W, Lichang L, et al. Relationship between prostaglandin in peritoneal fluid and pelvic venous congestion after sterilization. *Prostaglandins* 1996;51(2):161–167.

62. Osman MI, Din Shafeek MA, Abdalla MI, et al. Chronic pelvic pain in Lippes IUD users. Laparoscopic and venographic evaluation. *Contracept Deliv Syst* 1981;2:41–51.

63. Kehrer E. Munchen. med. Wchnschr. 1922. Quoted In: Taylor HC. Vascular congestion and hyperemia, their effect on structure and function in the female reproductive organs. Part II. The clinical aspects of the congestion-fibrosis syndrome. *Am J Obstet Gynecol* 1949;57:637–653.

64. Bochorishvili GG, Siterman SL, Meparishvili ASH. The diagnostic value of simultaneous ecretory urography and transuterine phlebography in a urodynamic study of the upper urinary tract. *Urolgiia I Nefrologiia* 1990;2:38–41.

65. DeGood DE, Dane JR. The psychologist as a pain consultant in outpatient, inpatient and workplace settings. In: Gatchel RJ, Turk DC, eds. *Psychological approaches to pain management. A practitioner's handbook.* New York: Guilford Press, 1996:33–52.

66. Mathis BV, Miller JS, Lukens ML, et al. Pelvic congestion syndrome: a new approach to an unusual problem. *Am Surg* 1995; 61:1016–1018.

67. Beard RW, Reginald PW, Pearce S. Pelvic pain in women. *BMJ* 1986;293:1160–1162.

68. Howard FM. The role of laparoscopy in chronic pelvic pain: promises and pitfalls. *Obstet Gynecol Surv* 1993;48:357–387.

69. Priou G, Arvis P, Rind A. Etude de l'apport diagnostique de la coelioscope dans le bilan des algies pelviennes chroniques. A propos de 184 cas. *J Gynecol Obstet Biol Repr* 1984;13(4):395–402.

70. Hammen R. The technique of pelvic phlebography. *Acta Obstet Gynecol Scand* 1965;44:370–374.

71. Bellina JH, Dougherty C, Michal A. Transmyometrial pelvic venography. *Obstet Gynecol* 1969;34(2):194–199.

72. Murray E, Comparato MR. Uterine phlebography. *Am J Obstet Gynecol* 1968;102(8):1088–1093.

73. Tarazov PG, Prozorovskij KV, Ryzhkov VK. Pelvic pain syndrome caused by ovarian varices. Treatment by transcatheter embolization. *Acta Radiologica* 1997;38:1023–1025.

74. Kennedy A, Hemmingway A. Radiology of ovarian varices. *Br J Hosp Med* 1990;44:38–43.

75. Craig O, Hobbs JT. Vulval phlebography in the pelvic congestion syndrome. *Clin Radiol* 1974;25:517–525.

76. Grabham JA, Barrie WW. Laparoscopic approach to pelvic congestion syndrome. *Br J Surg* 1997;84:1264–1266.

77. Montanari GD, Alfieri G, Grella P, et al. Ultrasonic tomography in the diagnosis of pelvic congestion. *Minerva Ginecologica* 1975; 27(3):219–223.

78. Frede TE. Ultrasonic visualization of varicosities in the female genital tract. *J Ultrasound Med* 1984;3(8):365–369.

79. Taylor KJW, Burms PN, Woodcock JP. Blood flow in deep abdominal and pelvic vessels: ultrasonic and pulsed Doppler analysis. *Radiology* 1985;154:487–493.

80. Fleischer AC, Kepple DM. Transvaginal color duplex sonography: clinical potentials and limitations. *Semin Ultrasound, CT, MR* 1992;13(1):69–80.

81. Smith MR. Pulsatile pelvic masses: options for evaluation and management of pelvic arteriovenous malformations. *Am J Obstet Gynecol* 1995;172(6):1857–1863.

82. Clavero Nunez JA, Ortiz Quintana L, Becerro de Bengoa Callua C. A new method for the diagnosis of pelvic pathology by gammagraphy. Part I: description of the method and normal results. *Acta Europaea Fertilitatis* 1975;6(2):167–171.

83. Pellegri PP, Montanari GD. The preoperative diagnosis of pelvic congestion by means of 133 Xenon injected into the cervical myometrium. *Acta Obstet Gynecol Scand* 1981;60(5):447–449.

84. Gupta A, McCarthy S. Pelvic varices as a cause for pelvic pain, MRI appearance. *MRI* 1994;12(4):679–681.

85. Joja I, Asakawa M, Motoyama K, et al. Uterine cirsoid aneurysm: MRI and MRA. *J Assisted Tomogr* 1996;20(2):290–294.

86. Kamoi K. Pathologic significance of the internal pudendal vein in the development of intrapelvic venous congestion syndrome. *Japan J Urol* 1996;87:1214–1220.

87. Stovall TG, Ling FW, Crawford DA. Hysterectomy for chronic pelvic pain of presumed uterine etiology. *Obstet Gynecol* 1990; 75:676–679.

88. Gangar KF, Stones RW, Saunders C, et al. An alternative to hysterectomy? GnRH analogue combined with hormone replacement therapy. *Br J Obstet Gynaecol* 1993;100:360–364.

89. Edwards RD, Robertson IR, MacLean AB, et al. Case report: pelvic pain syndrome–successful treatment of a case by ovarian vein embolization. *Clin Radiol* 1993;47:429–431.

90. Florio F, Balzano S, Nardella M, et al. Varicocele ovarico trattato con scleroembolizzazione percutanea. Descrizione di un caso. *Radiol Med* 1993;85:295–297.

91. Abbas FM, Currie JL, Mitchell S. Selective vascular embolization in benign gynecologic conditions. *J Reprod Med* 1994;39:492–496.

19

PELVIC INFLAMMATORY DISEASE

JAMES E. CARTER
FRED M. HOWARD

KEY TERMS AND DEFINITIONS

Bacterial vaginosis: A complex synergistic vaginal infection associated with *G. vaginalis, bacteroides* species, *Peptostreptococcus,* the mobile curved anaerobic rod *Mobiluncus, alpha hemolytic streptococci,* and *M. hominis.*

Pelvic inflammatory disease: Comprises a spectrum of inflammatory disorders of the upper female genital tract, including any combination of endometritis, salpingitis, tuboovarian abscess, and pelvic peritonitis.

Post-pelvic inflammation disease chronic pelvic pain: Chronic abdominopelvic pain as a sequela or pelvic inflammatory disease.

INTRODUCTION

Pelvic infections can be separated into three basic categories: (a) infections that occur postpartum and postabortion involving intrauterine trauma, (b) postoperative infections usually developing from organisms that are introduced into the operative site from the skin or vagina, or less frequently the gastrointestinal tract, during surgery, and (c) pelvic inflammatory disease (PID), a bacterial infection that usually occurs in the nonpregnant patient without preceding surgical entry of the abdominal or endometrial cavity (1). PID comprises a spectrum of inflammatory disorders of the upper female genital tract, including any combination of endometritis, salpingitis, tuboovarian abscess, and pelvic peritonitis (2).

PID can occur as an acute episode, recurrent episodes, or as a chronic condition. The etiology, pathology, pathogenesis, symptoms, history, risk factors, examination, differential diagnosis and therapies for acute, recurrent, and chronic PID are very similar. These conditions are a continuum within a patient who may begin with an episode of PID that is not recognized or is undertreated in its acute phase and then develops a chronic inflammatory condition. These patients are difficult to distinguish from patients who have recurrent infections because the examination and etiologies are so similar.

PID is an important consideration in caring for women with chronic pelvic pain (CPP), as CPP is a frequent sequela of PID. As sequelae of PID, CPP is very highly correlated with fallopian tubal damage and adhesions (14).

EPIDEMIOLOGY

In the United States there are an estimated 1.2 million visits for PID per year to physicians' offices, of which approximately 420,000 are initial visits for PID. Additionally, about 280,000 women per year are hospitalized for PID; of these, approximately 65% of cases are attributed to acute PID and 35% to chronic PID (3–6). In addition, an estimated 150,000 surgical procedures are performed annually for complications of salpingitis (2,4,7). For 1990 it is estimated there were 200,000 hospitalized cases of PID with an additional 1,277,000 outpatient cases (8). The estimated incidence of PID is 14.2 per 100 women and among women 15 to 44 years, the hospitalization rate is 2.2 per 1,000 women (7). The rate of hospitalization for PID is inversely related to age (2).

Long-term sequelae, including infertility, ectopic pregnancy, and CPP, develop in approximately 25% of women with PID (9). In addition, recurrent PID is a frequent occurrence. Involuntary infertility occurs in approximately 20% and ectopic pregnancies are increased six to tenfold (9–11).

CPP, dyspareunia, hydrosalpinx, tubo-ovarian abscess, pelvic adhesions, and inflammatory residua, often leading to surgical interventions, are estimated to occur in 15 to 20% of cases (2). CPP as a sequelae of PID is a fairly common outcome. Seventeen percent of women who are treated for PID develop CPP and 18% of laparoscopy-confined cases of PID report chronic pelvic pain lasting more than 6 months (9,12). In women who are hospitalized for treatment of PID, 24% develop CPP (13). The incidence of CPP rises to 67% of women with three or more episodes of PID (9). At a second look laparoscopy 88% of post-PID women with CPP had morphologic changes of the fallopian tubes or ovaries and the CPP was highly correlated with the extensiveness of post-PID adhesions (Table 19.1) (14).

TABLE 19.1. PERITUBAL ADHESIONS AND DISTAL TUBAL PATHOLOGY AMONG PID PATIENTS WITH CHRONIC PAIN

		Women with chronic pain	
	Total women	Number	Rate %
Adhesions			
None	57	5	9
Slight	23	3	13
Moderate	40	25	63
Extensive	32	29	91
Fimbriated ends			
Normal	74	23	31
Phimotic	18	8	44
Clubbed	41	23	56

From Westrom L. Chronic pain after acute PID. In: Belfort P, Piatti JA, Eskes TKAB, eds. *Advances in gynecology and obstetrics.* Proceedings of the XIIth World Congress Gynecol Obstet, Rio de Janiero, October 1988, with permission.

ETIOLOGY

The exact etiology of CPP after PID is not known, but most often it is believed secondary to adhesive and tuboovarian disease. A discussion of the relationship of CPP to adhesions is found in Chapter 8. In some cases, CPP may be related to chronic inflammation owing to host immunologic responses or recurrent infections caused by repeated infectious exposures and weakened host defenses secondary to previous infectious damage.

The etiology of PID is a polymicrobial infection (3,15). Microorganisms that have been recovered from the upper genital tracts include *N. gonorrhoeae, C. trachomatis,* mycoplasmas, anaerobic and aerobic bacteria from the endogenous vaginal floor such as *bacteroides, Peptostreptococcus, Gardnerella vaginalis, Escherichia coli, haemophilus influenza,* and *aerobic streptocci* (3). In the hospitalized cases of PID a sexually transmitted organism was present in 65% of cases; *N. gonorrhea* and *C. trachomatis* were recovered from 55% and 22%, respectively (16). However, in one study, although nearly 50% of patients had *N. gonorrhoeae* recovered from the endocervix, it was isolated from the fallopian tube in only 23%. In 30% of cases, only anaerobic or facultative bacteria were isolated. Anaerobic or facultative organisms were frequently (nearly 50%) recovered from the upper genital tract in patients with STD organism (3,16). In a separate study, 25% to 50% of PID cases do not have detectable Chlamydial or gonococcal infection, but rather other anaerobic or facultative bacteria have been isolated from the upper genital tract (17).

It has been postulated that gonococcus or chlamydia initiates PID and produces tissue damage and changes in the local environment, which in turn allows access to the upper genital tract for anaerobic and aerobic organisms from the vaginal and cervical flora (18–20). It has also been proposed that PID initially has a polymicrobial etiology (21–23).

It has been suggested that bacterial vaginosis, an overgrowth of anaerobic and aerobic flora of the vagina, may predispose or facilitate the ascent of gonorrhea or chlamydia into the upper genital tract (24). Many of the microorganisms found in PID have been implicated in bacterial vaginosis. Bacterial vaginosis is a complex synergistic vaginal infection associated with *G. vaginalis, bacteroides species, Peptostreptococcus,* the mobile curved anaerobic rod *Mobiluncus, alphahemolytic streptococci,* and *M. hominis* (3). An association between bacterial vaginosis and PID has been demonstrated (24–27). Bacterial vaginosis is present in 30% to 60% of women with laparoscopically confirmed PID (24).

Anaerobic bacteria are usually the most frequent fallopian tube isolates in patients with salpingitis. Isolates obtained from the endometrial cavity more closely mirror those in the fallopian tube than those obtained via culdocentesis (3).

PATHOGENESIS

Most PID results from intracanalicular spread of microorganisms from the endocervix and vagina to the endometrium and fallopian tubes (3). *N. gonorrhoeas, C. trachomatis,* and bacterial vaginosis all result in ascending infection of the endometrial cavity documented by the presence of histological endometritis (3).

Four factors may contribute to the ascent of bacteria from the endocervix and vagina: (a) uterine instrumentation facilities upward spread of vaginal and cervical microorganisms, (b) hormonal changes during menses and menstruation lead to cervical changes resulting in loss of the mechanical barrier that helps prevent ascent, (c) retrograde menstruation favors the bacterial ascent from the endometrium to the fallopian tubes and the peritoneal cavity, and (d) individual microorganisms with potential virulent factors (3). Bacterial vaginosis may facilitate ascent of STD and other aerobic and anaerobic bacteria through enzymatic degradation by proteolytic enzymes associated with bacterial vaginosis bacteria (24).

Unlike most bacterial infections in which tissue damage results from the direct effect of bacterial replication, the damage and scarring associated with *C. trachomatis* is a result of the host immune response to the infection (28,29). Repeated infection produces extensive tubal scarring, distal tubal obstruction and peritubular adhesions (29). These changes are believed to be the major pathogenesis of CPP after chlamydial PID. The scarring of the fallopian tube also leads to tubal infertility or ectopic pregnancy (3,17).

Nongonococcal, nonchlamydial (NG, NC) PID is likely to occur when a critical number of organisms overwhelms local defense mechanisms in the cervix allowing an infection to ascend to the upper genital tract (30). It seems likely there is a continuum from bacterial vaginosis, which is associated with significantly increased and very high colony counts of anaerobic bacteria and gardnerella vaginalis, and occurrence of NG, NC salpingitis (3).

SYMPTOMS OR HISTORY

Post-Pelvic Inflammatory Disease Chronic Pelvic Pain

As previously discussed, it is most commonly believed that CPP after PID is associated with adhesive and tubal damage. These adhesions are generally believed to cause pelvic pain that is exacerbated by sudden movements, intercourse, and certain physical activities. Often the pain is consistent in its location, although over time the area of involvement may expand. Pain as a sequela of PID is usually not related to the menstrual cycle, but in some patients it worsens premenstrually or at the time of menses. A history of repeated episodes of PID makes the diagnosis of CPP as a sequela of PID more likely. However, a history of prior pelvic inflammatory is not always easy to obtain.

Acute Pelvic Inflammatory Disease

Because aggressive treatment of PID may lessen the chance of subsequent CPP, it is worthwhile to review the symptoms of acute PID. PID is difficult to diagnose because of the wide variation in the symptoms and signs. Many women with PID have subtle or mild symptoms that do not readily indicate PID. Consequently, delay in diagnosis and effective treatment probably contributes to inflammatory sequelae in the upper reproductive tract. A diagnosis of PID usually is based on clinical findings. However, the clinical diagnosis of PID is imprecise. A clinical diagnosis of symptomatic PID has a positive predictive value of 65% to 90% (2). Many episodes of PID go unrecognized. Some cases are asymptomatic and others are unrecognized because the patient or the health care provider fails to recognize the implications of mild or nonspecific symptoms or signs (e.g., abnormal bleeding, dyspareunia, or vaginal discharge). Because of the difficulty of diagnosis and the potential for damage to the reproductive health of women even by apparently mild or atypical PID, health care providers should maintain a low threshold for the diagnosis of PID (2).

Even though PID is an infectious disease, 30% to 50% of patients are afebrile at presentation. Nausea and vomiting are present in less than one-half of patients. Pain is usually of less than 2 weeks duration. Gonococcal PID often presents within 1 to 2 weeks of menses.

There is a strong correlation between exposure to sexually transmitted organisms and PID. Up to 75% of PID in women under the age of 25 was associated with culture or serologic evidence of infection with *N. Gonorrhoeae*, *C. trachomatis*, or *Mycoplasma hominis* (31). Several aspects of

sexual behavior have been proposed to be associated with an increased risk of PID. These include having more than one sex partner in the previous 30 days, intercourse during menses, and lack of contraception at time of intercourse (3,32–34). Barrier methods (mechanical and chemical) when properly used, decrease the risk of STD, PID, and sequelae of PID (35). Condom use decreases the risk of developing PID (36). Vaginal douching is a potential risk factor for PID and PID-associated sequelae. Women with PID are more likely to have a history of douching than are women who do not douche, with an adjusted relative risk of 1.7 if douching occurred in the previous 2 months (37,38). Although women who use oral contraceptives may be at increased risk for cervical chlamydial infections, the incidence of PID and its clinical and laparoscopic severity are reduced in patients using oral contraceptives (39–41). Oral contraceptives may mask the signs and symptoms of ascending infection leading to an increase of subclinical cases that are associated with tubal infertility, ectopic pregnancy, and chronic pelvic pain (17).

Patients who give a history of lower abdominal pain, irregular menses, fevers or chills, sexual contact with known carriers of sexually transmitted diseases, urinary symptoms, gastrointestinal symptoms, in the proper age group and marital status for risk of PID may not have PID and these symptoms have been found to have a very low sensitivity for prediction of this condition (41).

SIGNS AND EXAMINATION

Post-Pelvic Inflammatory Disease Pelvic Pain

As noted in the preceding, CPP associated with prior PID is generally owing to adhesions or tubal disease. There are no specific findings on examination that allow a diagnosis of adhesions. Occasionally with dense uterine adhesions the uterus is found in a fixed, immobile retroverted position. Also tenderness on examination may correlate with the location of adhesions. With hydrosalpinges or tuboovarian complexes, a tender adnexal mass may be palpable.

Acute Pelvic Inflammatory Disease

Minimum criteria for a clinical diagnosis of pelvic pain owing to PID, if no other causes for the pain can be identified, are bilateral lower abdominal tenderness, bilateral adnexal tenderness, and cervical motion tenderness. Additional criteria which may be used to enhance the specificity of the minimum criteria include the flowing: oral temperature greater than 101°F (greater 39.3°C), abnormal cervical or vaginal discharge, elevated erythrocyte sedimentation rate, elevated C-reactive protein, and laboratory documentation of cervical infection with *N. gonorrhoeae* or *C. trachomatis* (2).

A speculum examination may show cervical or vaginal discharge. It is best first to assess the parts of the abdomen away from the area of tenderness. In the presence of abdominal guarding, it is helpful to have the patient voluntarily contract and relax the abdominal muscles before the examination. Tenderness over the liver may be related to perihepatitis (Fits-Hugh-Curtis syndrome) (42). This is a clinical syndrome characterized by right upper quadrant pain and tenderness in association with PID. It is estimated to occur in 1% to 10% of patients with PID (43,44).

Laparoscopic studies have shown that the clinical diagnosis of PID is often inaccurate. PID is frequently found in patients undergoing laparoscopy for other causes of acute pelvic pain (3).

DIAGNOSTIC STUDIES

Laparoscopy is the current gold standard diagnostic study for both acute PID and for CPP secondary to prior PID. Laparoscopic conscious pain mapping (Chapter 5) may be the best option for CPP, but it is limited by procedural pain in women with acute PID and probably not advisable. Logistically and economically routine laparoscopy is impractical for all patients suspected of having acute PID (3).

Other useful studies for diagnosing acute PID include histopathological evidence of endometritis on endometrial biopsy, transvaginal sonography or other imaging techniques showing thickened fluid-filled tubes with or without pelvic fluid or tuboovarian complex, elevated erythrocyte sedimentation rate (ESR), elevated C-reactive protein, and laboratory documentation of cervical infection with pathogenic organisms. However, other than laparoscopy, there is no diagnostic test specific for PID (45). C-reactive protein levels are elevated in PID, but have a sensitivity as low as 74% and a specificity as low as 50% (3). Similarly, an elevated ESR has a sensitivity as low as 64% and a specificity as low as 43% (3). Endometrial biopsy demonstrating endometrial inflammation is more reliable, with a 90% correlation with laparoscopically confirmed salpingitis (25,46). Histologic features of endometritis associated with salpingitis include plasma cells in the endometrial stroma, polymorphonuclear leukocytes in the endometrial surface epithelium, intraluminal polymorphonuclear leukocytes, dense subepithelial stromal lymphocytic infiltration, and germinal centers containing transformed lymphocytes (46).

Transvaginal sonography can facilitate and improve the ultrasound diagnosis of PID. A sonogram suggestive of PID would include thickened fluid-filled tubes with or without free pelvic fluid. Transvaginal ultrasound may also be useful in CPP after PID by revealing a fluid-filled hydrosalpinx or complex mass consistent with a tuboovarian complex.

On MRI inflammatory exudates exhibit a signal intensity equal or greater than that of simple fluid on both T1- and T2-weighted images (48). On T1-weighted images, changes in the fat planes, indistinct borders of pelvic organs, and accentuated fascial lines can be observed. The ovary will be swollen, with multiple cystic structures, indicating an early stage of abscess formation or prominent edema. If the lesion is untreated or incompletely treated in the early inflammatory phase, an overt tuboovarian abscess can be formed, which may persist for a long period after the lesion has subsided into a subacute or chronic stage. Tuboovarian abscesses are frequently ill-defined. The fluid content commonly has a signal intensity identical to or slightly greater than that of simple fluid on both T1- and T2-weighted images, but signal characteristics similar to that of blood may be observed. The inner layer of the cyst wall occasionally exhibits a faint hyperintensity on T1-weighted images, possibly indicating a blood element. It is occasionally difficult to distinguish these subacute or chronic inflammatory masses from adnexal neoplasms on the basis of either the imaging characteristics or the clinical course. Extensive changes of the fat plane and a serratus appearance of the uterus and bowel loops despite the small size of the mass may be the clue permitting diagnosis (48).

In patients in whom hysterectomy was performed for persistent irregular vaginal bleeding and pain, samples for both aerobic and anaerobic bacteria and STDs were taken after hysterectomy (49). Nearly one-fourth of all patients harbored one or more microorganisms in the uterus, mostly *Gardnerella vaginalis*, *Enterobacter*, and *streptococcus agalactiae*. In symptomatic patients the uterine cavity is frequently colonized with potentially pathogenic organisms that may play a causative role in endometritis. In patients with persistent irregular vaginal bleeding, hysteroscopic examination for inflammation of the uterine cavity could be conducted prior to hysterectomy being undertaken (49). However, the danger of spreading infection from the lower genital tract to the peritoneal cavity by way of the fallopian tubes or the systemic circulation has led some to recommend avoidance of hysteroscopy if infection is suspected (50).

TREATMENT
Medical Therapy

PID treatment regimens must provide empiric, broad-spectrum coverage of likely pathogens. Antimicrobial coverage should include *N. gonorrhoeae*, *C. trachomatis*, anaerobes, Gram-negative faculative bacteria, and *streptococci*. Anaerobic bacteria have been isolated from the upper reproductive tract of women who have PID and data from *in vitro* studies have revealed that anaerobics such as *Bacteroides fragilis* can cause tubal and epithelial destruction. In addition bacterial vaginosis is also diagnosed in many women who have PID. The recommended regimen should have anaerobic coverage.

Hospitalization should occur if the diagnosis is uncertain and the patient seems ill, the patient is pregnant, the patient does not respond clinically to oral antimicrobial therapy, the patient is unable to follow or tolerate an outpatient oral regimen, the patient has severe illness, nausea and vomiting, or high fever, the patient has a tuboovarian abscess, or the patient is immunodeficient.

Oral treatment can be given with the following regimens.

Regimen A: Ofloxacin 400 mg orally twice a day for 14 days, plus Metronidazole 500 mg orally twice a day for 14 days.

Regimen B: Ceftriaxone 250 mg IM once or Cefoxitin 2 g IM, plus Probenecid 1 g orally in a single dose concurrently, or other parenteral third generation cephalosporin (e.g., Ceftizoxime or Cefotaxime).

Doxycycline: 100 mg orally twice a day for 14 days is to be given with Regimen B (2).

Oral Ofloxacin was investigated as a single agent in clinical studies and was found to be effective against *N. gonorrhoeae* and *C. trachomatis,* but its lack of anaerobic coverage was a concern (2).

Empiric oral therapy is often tried in women with CPP in whom prior, chronic, or recurrent PID is suspected. There are no studies supporting efficacy for this approach in the treatment of CPP.

There are no efficacy data comparing parental with oral regimens. Most trials have used parenteral treatment for at least 48 hours after the patient demonstrates substantial clinical improvement, although this is an arbitrary designation. The recommended parenteral regimen is Cefotetan 2 g IV every 12 hours or Cefoxitin 2 g IV every 6 hours, plus Doxycycline 100 mg IV or orally every 12 hours. Doxycycline should be administered orally when possible, even when the patient is hospitalized because of the pain associated with infusion. An alternate regimen is Clindamycin 900 mg IV every 8 hours, plus Gentamicin loading dose IV or IM (2 mg/kg of body weight), followed by a maintenance dose (1.5 mg/kg) every 8 hours. Parenteral therapy may be discontinued 24 hours after a patient improves clinically, and continuing oral therapy should consist of Doxycycline 100 mg orally twice a day or Clindamycin 450 mg orally four times a day to complete a total of 14 days of therapy. When tuboovarian abscess is present, Clindamycin provided more effective anaerobic coverage for treatment.

Surgical Treatment

Hydrosalpinges, tuboovarian abscesses and pyosalpinges can be treated by ultrasonographic guided transvaginal aspiration (51). In addition, ultrasonographically guided transvaginal aspiration with placement of drainage catheter can also be utilized for resolution of tuboovarian abscesses (52). If these techniques fail then therapy via laparoscopy or laparotomy would become necessary.

The surgical treatment for PID requires drainage of all abscesses and may require removal of diseased tissue, even including hysterectomy and bilateral salpingo-oophorectomy. The surgical treatment for the sequelae of PID is primarily the treatment of the adhesions that form as a result of this condition. This requires a laparoscopic approach for the pelvic adhesions (Chapter 8), as well as for the treatment of the perihepatitis of the Fitz-Hugh-Curtis syndrome (3). Hysterectomy with bilateral salpingo-oophorectomy is commonly performed for sequelae of PID, although there is not much published information documenting efficacy for CPP.

KEY POINTS
Most Important Questions to Ask

- How many sexual partners do you have and have you had in the past?
- What form of birth control are you using?
- Any past history of sexually transmitted diseases or PID?

Most Important Physical Examination Findings

- Lower abdominal tenderness, cervical tenderness, adnexal or uterine

Most Important Diagnostic Studies

- Laparoscopy
- Ultrasonography
- Endometrial biopsy

REFERENCES

1. Eschenbach DA, Holmes KK. Acute inflammatory disease: current concepts of pathogenesis, etiology, and management. *Clin Obstet Gynecol* 1975;18:35–56.
2. Centers for Disease Control. 1998 guidelines for treatment of sexually transmitted diseases. *MMWR* 1998;47:79–86.
3. Sweet RL, Gibbs RS, eds. Pelvic inflammatory disease. In: Sweet and Gibbs, eds. *Infectious diseases of the female genital tract.* Baltimore: Williams & Wilkins, 1995:379–428.
4. Curran JW. Economic consequences of pelvic inflammatory disease in the United States. *Am J Obstet Gynecol* 1980;138:848–851.
5. Jones OG, Saida AA, St John RK. Frequency and distribution of salpingitis and pelvic inflammatory disease in short stay in hospitals in the United States. *Am J Obstet Gynecol* 1980;138:905–908.
6. Centers for Disease Control. Pelvic inflammatory disease, guidelines for prevention and management. *MMWR* 1991;40:1–25.
7. Washington AE, Cates W, Sadi AA. Hospitalizations for pelvic inflammatory disease. Epidemiology and trends in the United States, 1975 and 1981. *JAMA* 1984;251:2529–2533.
8. Rolfs RT, Galaid E, Zaidi AA. Epidemiology of pelvic inflammatory disease: trends in hospitalization and office visits, 1979–1988. Joint Meeting of the Centers for Disease Control and National Institutes of Health about pelvic inflammatory disease prevention, management and research in the 1990's. Bethesda MD, September 4–5, 1990.

9. Westrom LV, Berger GS, eds. *Consequences of pelvic inflammatory disease.* New York: Raven Press, 1992:101–114.

10. Westrom L. Incidence, prevalence and trends of acute pelvic inflammatory disease and its consequences in industrialized countries. *Am J Obstet Gynecol* 1980;138:880–892.

11. Westrom L. Effect of acute pelvic inflammatory disease on fertility. *Am J Obstet Gynecol* 1975;121:707–713.

12. Falk V. Treatment of nontuberculous salpingitis with antibiotics alone and in combination with glucocorticoids. *Acta Obstet Gynecol Scand* 1965;44(Suppl 6):3–118.

13. Safrin S, Schachter J, Dahrouge D, et al. Long-term sequelae of acute PID. *Am J Obstet Gynecol* 1992;166:1300–1305.

14. Westrom L. Chronic pain after acute PID. In: Belfort P, Piatti JA, Eskes TKAB, eds. *Advances in gynecology and obstetrics* Proceedings of the XIIth World Congress Gynecol Obstet Rio de Janeiro, October 1988.

15. Eschenbach DA, Buchanan T, Pollock HM, et al. Polymicrobial etiology of acute pelvic inflammatory disease. *N Engl J Med* 1975;293:166–171.

16. Jossens MOR, Eskenazi B, Schacter J, Sweet RL. Risk factors associated with pelvic inflammatory disease of differing microbial etiologies. *Sexually Trans Dis* 1996;23:239–247.

17. Rice PA, Schachter J. Pathogenesis of pelvic inflammatory disease. *JAMA* 1991;266:2587–2593.

18. Cunningham FG, Hauth JC, Gilstrap LC, et al. The bacterial pathogenesis of acute pelvic inflammatory disease. *Obstet Gynecol* 1978;52:161–164.

19. Chow AW, Maikasian KL, Marshall J Jr, et al. The bacteriology of acute pelvic inflammatory disease. *Obstet Gynecol* 1975;122:876–879.

20. Monif GRG, Welkos SL, Baer H, et al. Cul-de-sac isolates from patients with endometritis, salpingitis, peritonitis and gonococcal endocervicitis. *Am J Obstet Gynecol* 1976;126:158–161.

21. McCormack WM, Nowroozi K, Alpert S. Acute pelvic inflammatory disease: characteristics of patients with gonococcal infection and evaluation of their response to treatment with aqueous procaine penicillin G and spectromycin hydrochloride. *Sex Transm Dis* 1977;4:125–131.

22. Eschenbach DA. Epidemiology and diagnosis of acute pelvic inflammatory disease. *Obstet Gynecol* 1980;55:1425–1535.

23. Sweet DL, Draper DL, Schachter J, et al. Microbiology and pathogenesis of acute salpingitis as determined by laparoscopy: what is the appropriate site to sample? *Am J Obstet Gynecol* 1980;138:985–989.

24. Soper DE, Brockwell NJ, Dalton HP, et al. Observations concerning the microbial etiology of acute salpingitis. *Am J Obstet Gycecol* 1994;170:1008–1017.

25. Paavonen J, Tersala K, Heinonen PK, et al. Microbiological and histopathological findings in acute pelvic inflammatory disease. *Br J Obstet Gynecol* 1987;94:454–460.

26. Eschenbach DA, Hiller S, Critchlow C, et al. Diagnosis and clinical manifestations of bacterial vaginosis. *Am J Obstet Gynecol* 1988;158:819–828.

27. Miller SL, Kiviat NB, Critchlow C, et al. Bacterial vaginosis-associated bacteria as etiologic agents of pelvic inflammatory disease (abstract). Proceedings of the annual meeting Infections Disease Society of Obstetrics and Gynecology, San Diego CA, August 6, 1992.

28. Patton DL, Halbert SA, Kuo CC, et al. Host response to Chlamydia trachomatis infection of the fallopian tube in pig-tailed monkeys. *Fertil Steril* 1983;40:829–840.

29. Patton DL, Kuo CC, Wong SP, et al. Distal obstruction induced by repeated Chlamydia trachomatis salpingeal infection in pig-tailed macaques. *J Infec Dis* 1987;155:1292–1299.

30. Eschenbach DA, Holmes KK. Acute PID: current concepts of pathogenesis, etiology and management. *Clin Obstet Gynecol* 1975;18:35–36.

31. Mardh PA, Lind I, Svensson L, et al. Antibodies to *Chlamydia trachomatis, Mycoplasma hominis* and *Neisseria gonorrhoeae* in serum from patients with acute salpingititis. *Br J Vener Dis* 1981; 57:125–129.

32. Eschenbach DA, Stevens C, Critchow C, et al. Epidemiology of acute PID. Presented at the International Society of STD Research 9th International Meeting. October 6–9, 1991, Banff, Alberta, Canada.

33. Wolner-Hanssen P, Eschenbach DA, Paavonen J, et al. Decreased risk of symptomatic chlamydial PID associated with oral contraceptive use. *JAMA* 1990;264:54–59.

34. Marchbanks PA, Lee NC, Peterson HB. Cigarette smoking as a risk for PID. *Am J Obstet Gynecol* 1990;162:639–644.

35. Kani J, Adler MW. Epidemiology of PID. In: Berger GS, Westrom LS, eds. *PID.* New York: Raven Press, 1992:7–22.

36. Austin H, Louv WC, Alexander WJ. A case-control study of spermacides and gonorrhea. *JAMA* 1984;251:2822–2824.

37. Wolner-Hanssen P, Eschenbach DA, Paavonen J, et al. Association between vaginal douching and acute PID. *JAMA* 1990; 263:1936–1941.

38. Zhang J, Thomas AG, Leybovich E. Vaginal douching and adverse health effects: a meta analysis. *Am J Pub Health* 1997; 87:1207–1210.

39. Washington AE, Goves S, Schachter J, et al. Oral contraceptives. *Chlamydia trachomatis* infection and PID. *JAMA* 1985; 124:2246–2250.

40. Washington AE, Aral SO, Wolner-Hanssen P, et al. Assessing risk for PID and its sequelae. *JAMA* 1991;266:2481–2586.

41. Kahn JG, Walker CK, Washington AE, et al. Diagnosing PID. A comprehensive analysis and considerations for developing a new model. *JAMA* 1991;266:2596–2604.

42. Duleba AJ, Keltz MD, Olive DL. Evaluation and management of chronic pelvic pain. *Jrnl AAGL* 1996;3:205–227.

43. Fitz-Hugh T. Acute gonococcal peritonitis in the right upper quadrant in women. *JAMA* 1934;102:2091–2096.

44. Stanley MM. Gonococcal peritonitis of the upper abdomen in young women. *Arch Intern Med* 1946;78:1–13.

45. Paavonen J, Westrom LV. Diagnosis of acute PID. In: Berger GS, Westrom LV, eds. *PID.* New York: Raven Press, 1992:49–78.

46. Paavonen J, Aine R, Teisala K, et al. Comparison of endometrial biopsy and peritoneal fluid cytology with laparoscopy in the diagnosis of acute PID. *Am J Obstet Gynecol* 1985;151:645–650.

47. Cacciatore B, Leminen A, Ingman-Friberg S, et al. Transvaginal sonographic findings in ambulatory patients with suspected PID. *Obstet Gynecol* 1992;80:912–916.

48. Togashi K. *MRI of the female pelvis.* Tokyo: Igaku-Shoin, 1993: 282(1–325).

49. Moller BR, Krostiansen FV, Thorsen P, et al. Sterility of the uterine cavity. *Acta Obstet Gynecol Scand* 1995;74:216–219.

50. Baggish MS, Barbot J, Valle RF. *Diagnostic and operative hysteroscopy: a text and atlas.* Chicago: Yearbook Medical Publishers, 1989;97:1–234.

51. Aboulghar MA, Mansour RT, Serour G. Ultrasonographically guided transvaginal aspiration of tuboovarian abscesses and pyosalpinges: an optional treatment for acute PID. Egyptian IVF-ET Center 85, Mosby Year-Book, 1995.

52. Feld R, Eschelman DJ, Sagerman JE, et al. Treatment of pelvic abscesses and other fluid collections: efficacy of transvaginal sonographically guided aspiration and drainage. *AJR* 1994;163: 1141–1145.

20

PELVIC FLOOR RELAXATION DISORDERS

JAMES E. CARTER

KEY TERMS AND DEFINITIONS

Arcus tendineus pelvic fascia (white line): The tendineus aponeurosis of the obturator internus muscle anteriorly and of the levator ani complex posteriorly into which the vaginal pubocervical fascia is attached.

Cystocele: Defective support of the upper portion of the vagina above the urethrovesical crease that allows the bladder to prolapse toward or through the vaginal introitus.

Cystourethrocele: Loss of support of entire anterior wall.

Enterocele: Intestine herniates through a defect between pubocervical and rectovaginal fascia. Peritoneum is in contact with vaginal mucosa.

Iliococcygeus muscle: Arises from a fibrous band on the pelvic wall (arcus tendineus levator ani) and forms a relatively horizontal sheet that spans the opening within the pelvis and forms a shelf on which the organs may rest.

Levator ani muscles: Formed by two portions, the pubovisceral muscle and the iliococcygeus muscle.

Occult uterovaginal prolapse: Prolapse of the uterine cervix and upper vagina that is detected only with traction applied to the cervix by a tenaculum or ring forceps.

Paracolpium: The viscero-fascial layer that attaches to the upper two-thirds of the vagina.

Parametrium: The viscero-fascial layer that attaches to the uterus and forms the cardinal and uterosacral ligaments.

Paravaginal defect: Defect as a result of detachment of the pubocervical fascia from its lateral attachment to the fascia of the obturator internal muscle at the level of the arcus tendineus fascia of the pelvis (white line).

Pelvic floor: The muscular and fascial layers that prevent the abdominal and pelvic organs from falling through the opening within the bony pelvis.

Pelvic floor dysfunction: This phrase usually refers to genital prolapse, abnormal continence and evacuation, and can also encompass problems such as dyspareunia or obstructive labor.

Pseudorectocele: A defect in the perineal body in which the posterior wall appears to, but does not bulge into the vagina.

Pubococcygeus muscle: Is the most cephalic portion of the levator ani and passes from the pubic bones to insert on the inner surface of the coccyx.

Puborectalis muscle: Portion of the pubovisceral levator ani muscle that passes beside the vagina, where the lateral vaginal walls are attached to it, and continues dorsally where some fibers penetrate the rectum between the internal and external sphincter, whereas others pass behind the anorectal junction.

Pubovisceral muscle: The thick U-shaped muscle that arises from the pubic bones on either side of the midline and passes behind the rectum forming a slinglike arrangement; includes both the pubococcygeus and puborectalis portions of the levator ani.

Rectocele: Defect present when the anterior rectal wall and overlying vagina prolapse toward or through the vaginal introitus and hymenal ring.

Rectovaginal septum (Denonvilliers or rectovaginal fascia): A distinct layer of fibromuscular tissue lying immediately beneath the vaginal mucosa that separates the dorsal rectal compartment from the ventral urogenital compartment, with attachments to the cul-de-sac peritoneum, the fascia covering the levator ani muscles, the base of the cardinal and uterosacral ligaments, the posterior cervix, and the perineal body.

Urethrocele: Descent of the lower anterior vaginal wall to the level of the hymenal ring during straining; owing to loss of urethral support.

Urogenital hiatus of levator ani: The opening in the levator ani muscle through which the urethra, vagina, and rectum pass and through which prolapse occurs. The borders of the hiatus are: anteriorly, the pubic bones; laterally, the levator ani muscles; and posteriorly, the perineal body and external anal sphincter.

Uterosacral ligaments: Visible and palpable medial margin of the cardinal-uterosacral (parametrial) ligament complex.

Uterovaginal prolapse: Prolapse of the uterine cervix and upper vagina toward or through the vaginal introitus.

Vaginal prolapse: Term usually applied posthysterectomy to a defect of pelvic support that allows the vaginal apex to prolapse toward or through the vaginal introitus.

Viscero-fascial layer: The layer of the pelvic floor created by the endopelvic fascia that attaches the pelvic organs to the pelvic walls, thereby suspending the pelvic organs; a combination of the pelvic viscera and endopelvic fascial wall.

INTRODUCTION

The pelvic floor is the supportive layer that prevents the abdominal and pelvic organs from falling through the opening of the bony pelvis (1,2). It depends on the coordinated action of the striated muscles of the levator ani and the smooth muscles of the pelvic organs. With damage or loss of strength of the fascia and muscle of the pelvic floor, relaxation or support defects may occur. Pelvic support disorders are common and account for almost 400,000 surgical procedures annually for women in the United States (3). Most of these surgical procedures are for correction of function, not for the relief of pelvic pain. However, relaxation disorders of the pelvic floor cause pelvic and back pain, and should be considered as possible causes or contributors during the evaluation of the woman with chronic pelvic pain (CPP). As the diagnosis is usually apparent from the physical examination and pain is most often mild in intensity, it is common to neglect the potential role of pelvic floor support defects in CPP.

ETIOLOGY

The normal resting tone of the pubovisceral muscle closes the rectum, vagina, and urethra by compressing them against the pubic bone. Lateral to this the flat sheetlike iliococcygeus muscle forms a horizontal shelf on which the upper pelvic organs rest. As long as the pelvic musculature functions normally, the pelvic floor is closed and the ligaments and fascia are under no tension. They simply act to stabilize the organs in their position above the levator ani muscles. When the pelvic floor muscles relax or are damaged, the pelvic floor opens and the vagina lies between the high intraabdominal pressure and low atmospheric pressure where it must be held in place by the ligaments. Although the ligaments can sustain these loads for short periods of time, if the pelvic muscles do not close the pelvic floor, then the connective tissue will become damaged and eventually fail to hold the vagina in place (Fig. 20.1). (2).

DeLancy has proposed anatomic levels of pelvic support that help to understand both normal anatomy and relaxed or damaged support anatomy. DeLancey Level I refers to the upper one-fourth of the vagina, which is suspended by the cardinal/uterosacral ligament complex. DeLancey Level II refers to the middle one-half of the vagina that is maintained by its lateral attachments. DeLancey Level III refers to the lower one-fourth of vagina that is maintained in it anatomic position by fusion of the lower vagina to the urogenital diaphragm and perineal body.

The function of the levator ani muscle can be compromised either by direct injury to the muscle or by damage to the nerve supply of the muscles. The neuromuscular injury occurs as a result of small nerves being torn away from their muscle fibers resulting in a diminished ability of the muscle to contract and a loss of normal function (1).

The pelvic connective tissue is more likely to be damaged by rupture than by stretching. Generalized stretching or attenuation is the exception (4). However, once the vagina or uterus descends below its normal position, the constant load placed on them by the weight of the abdominal contents probably causes the same type of connective tissue elongation associated with stretching of any ligament or tendon. The failure of ligaments under this strain results not only from acute damage, but also from an inability of the connective tissue to repair itself (1).

The factors involved in pelvic organ prolapse include: (a) the inborn strength of the connective tissue and muscle; the loss of connective tissue strength which can occur because

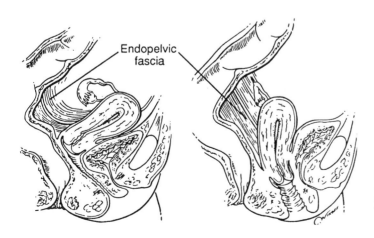

FIGURE 20.1. The cardinal-uterosacral ligament complex is able to sustain significant stretch when the levator ani muscles are open, but if the pelvic muscles do not close the pelvic floor, then the connective tissue will become damaged and eventually fail to hold the vagina in place.

of damage at childbirth, deterioration with age, and poor collagen repair, (b) the loss of levator function that can occur because of neuromuscular damage during childbirth or metabolic diseases that affect muscle function, (c) increased loads on the supportive system including prolonged lifting or chronic coughing from chronic pulmonary disease, and (d) disturbance of the balance of the structural parts such as alteration of the vaginal axis by urethral suspension or failure to reach the cardinal ligaments at hysterectomy (2).

The changes that vaginal birth causes in the pelvic floor deserve special examination. Damage to the levator ani muscles and their innervation is common during vaginal birth. Loss of the muscle's ability to support the pelvic organs and unload the ligaments may be partially responsible for the breakage and elongation of the ligaments later in life. Some damage to the connective tissue of the parametrium and paracolpium occurs during childbirth and can also contribute to subsequent prolapse. The paracolpium is responsible for suspending the apex of the vagina. It attaches to the upper two-thirds of the vagina.

Childbirth is found to be associated with a variety of muscular and neuromuscular injuries to the pelvic floor that are linked to the development of pelvic organ prolapse. Risk factors for pelvic floor injury include forceps delivery, episiotomy, prolonged second stage of labor, and increased fetal size. Cesarean delivery appears to be protective, especially if the patient does not labor before delivery. Obstetricians may be able to reduce pelvic floor injuries by minimizing forceps deliveries and episiotomies, by allowing passive descent in the second stage, and by selectively recommending elective cesarean section (5).

The levator ani and the sphincter muscles of the pelvic floor are innervated by the anterior sacral nerve roots S2–S4. Direct motor branches of these nerve roots travel over the cranial surface of the pelvic floor, where they are vulnerable to stretching and compression during parturition. During childbirth the pelvic floor is exposed to direct compression from the fetal presenting part, as well as downward pressure from maternal expulsive efforts. These forces stretch and distend the pelvic floor, resulting in functional and anatomic alterations in the muscles, nerves, and connective tissue of the pelvic floor. Obstetricians are most familiar with muscular injuries such as lacerations to the perineum and external anal sphincter. Little is known about damage to the levator ani muscles during childbirth because these muscles are not usually visible at delivery.

Childbirth can affect the pelvic floor by damaging the peripheral nerves that innervate the levator ani and sphincter muscles. Childbirth causes stretching or compression of the pelvic nerves as they traverse the pelvic floor. The resultant injury causes partial denervation of the pelvic floor musculature. Recovery may occur as the denervated muscles are reinnervated by surrounding intact nerves (5). Denervation injuries of the pubococcygeus and external anal sphincter muscles have been demonstrated after 42% to 80% of vaginal deliveries (6,7). Denervation has not been seen after elective cesarean delivery, although it has been associated with cesarean deliveries performed during labor.

Many women demonstrate evidence of pelvic floor neuropathy in the immediate postpartum period, but most will subsequently recover neuromuscular function and only a minority experience long-term sequelae (5). Denervation injury may be cumulative with increasing parity (7).

The fascia and connective tissues of the pelvic floor may also be injured during labor and delivery. The mechanisms of connective tissue injury and repair in the pelvis are poorly understood (3). The endopelvic fascia is probably torn or ruptured (rather than stretched) during childbirth. Isolated breaks in the endopelvic fascia have been implicated in the genesis of cystoceles, vaginal support defects, and genuine stress incontinence (4). After an acute injury to connective tissue, new collagen is formed. Because the new collagen is never as strong as the original connective tissue, the endopelvic fascia may be weaker after childbirth (3).

The normal position of the uterus is not over the urogenital hiatus, as was believed previously, but rather over the levator plate. The active basal tone of the levator ani muscles helps to maintain this relationship by keeping the urogenital hiatus closed. The role of the endopelvic fascia may be to fix the pelvic organs in an appropriate position over the levator plate via attachments to the pelvic sidewall. If levator tone deteriorates the pelvic organs become suspended over a widened urogenital hiatus by their ligaments and connective tissue supports. Under these circumstances, the endopelvic fascia will gradually stretch and weaken as a result of chronic tension. Thus decreased levator function may be the first step in a process that ultimately causes failure of the connective tissue support of the pelvic organs. In addition, an inherent weakness of the endopelvic fascia may contribute to the problem. For example, fibroblasts from women with pelvic organ prolapse produce weaker types of collagen than women with normal pelvic organ support (5).

Genital organ prolapse is a direct consequence of weakening of the pelvic floor. The pelvic floor is weaker after vaginal delivery (6,8). Childbirth is a potential cause of genital organ prolapse. Pelvic floor neuropathy associated with childbirth may also play a role in the genesis of pelvic organ prolapse. Fifty percent of women with symptomatic pelvic organ prolapse have evidence of levator ani muscle denervation. Parous women with prolapse have more pronounced histologic and electromyographic evidence of levator denervation (5). Other factors, such as inherent variations in connective tissue quality and isolated breaks in the fascial attachments of the pelvic organs also undoubtedly play roles.

SYMPTOMS OR HISTORY

There are several symptoms that all types of prolapse have in common. Once the vagina prolapses below the introitus, it becomes a structural layer between the high pressures in the intraabdominal space and the relatively low atmospheric pressure. The downward force this pressure differential creates puts tension on the fascia and ligaments that support the vagina and uterus. This results in a painful, dragging sensation where the tissues connect to the pelvic wall, usually identified by the patient as occurring in the groin and pelvis, and sacral backache caused by traction on the uterosacral ligaments. The symptoms may subside when the patient is lying down, owing to reduced downward pressure, and seem minimal in the morning, but increase progressively the longer she is erect and active (9). She may feel or see tissue prolapsing to or through the vaginal introitus. In addition, exposure of the moist vaginal wall leads to a sensation of perineal wetness that may be confused with urinary incontinence, and it may also give rise to ulceration of the vaginal wall. Most patients also have an underlying sense of heaviness, fullness, or insecurity that it is difficult for them to describe and is often expressed as a feeling that "something is just not right." Although this is difficult for patients to put into words, it causes significant distress and should not be ignored.

Patients with pelvic floor relaxation disorders may be unable to initiate a stream, may be unable to void easily and may not be able to empty their bladders completely. Manual replacement of the bladder back inside the vaginal canal may be required before initiation of voiding can occur. Recurrent urinary tract infections may occur.

There may be pain during sexual intercourse or penetration may be obstructed because of tissue protruding outside the introitus. The frequency of intercourse may be diminished because of anxiety on the part of the partner.

Symptoms of Anterior Wall Prolapse: Cystourethrocele

Loss of urethral support and support of the lower vaginal wall is associated with stress urinary incontinence. It is helpful to get a detailed history about urinary incontinence in such women. A diary or uroflow chart is a good way to obtain this history. For a period of 7 days the patient records the time and volume of each episode of micturition (voluntary or involuntary), incontinence, fluid intake, and episodes of urgency. In patients with detrusor instability the frequency of micturition is significantly increased and the mean volume voided and largest single void in the day are significantly reduced. Women with genuine stress incontinence have increased total daily urine output, frequency of micturition, and the largest single void in the daytime. Normal total voided volume is 1,350 mL per 24 hours. Frequency of micturition per 24 hours is 5.5, mean voided volume is 240 mL. Largest single voided volume is 450 mL (11).

Loss of support of the upper anterior vaginal wall and bladder base can cause difficulty in emptying the bladder. This is believed to be a possible cause of recurrent or persistent urinary tract infection (Chapter 31).

If a woman voids by Valsalva, a cystocele simply gets bigger and no impulse is provided for urine to flow through the urethra. Many patients also complain of urinary urgency and frequency that comes from stretching of the bladder base that accompanies its prolapse through the vaginal introitus.

Symptoms Associated With Prolapse of the Uterus, Vaginal Apex, or Enterocele

These patients usually complain of the generalized symptoms of prolapse mentioned above. Some have urgency and frequency.

Symptoms of Rectocele

The cardinal symptom of a rectocele is difficulty emptying the rectum. As a woman bears down to evacuate, stool is pushed into the rectocele and the harder she strains, the bigger the rectocele becomes. This results in a vicious cycle, with the rectocele causing constipation, which in turn causes worsening of the rectocele, and so on. Many women find that pressing between the vagina and rectum helps with defecation.

PHYSICAL EXAMINATION

If present, pelvic floor relaxation defects can almost always be found by physical examination. At times the exact organ prolapsing is difficult to identify and imaging studies may be needed for exact identification. Also, sometimes if the examination is done early in the day in only the lithotomy position, some or all defects are missed. Whenever symptoms suggest pelvic floor relaxation and it is not found at the time of pelvic examination, it is important to repeat the examination in the standing position, and possibly late in the day after the patient has been erect for several hours.

At the time of examination it is important to identify and describe the severity, anatomic location, and organ or organs prolapsing as accurately as possible.

Describing Severity of Prolapse

A reliable and universally understandable system of describing how big a prolapse is involves the distance each element of the prolapse descends below or rises above the hymenal ring when the prolapse is at its largest. For example, there is little ambiguity in saying that the uterine cervix is 4 cm below the hymen during straining and that an accompanying rectocele is 2 cm below this landmark. In addition, the diameter of the prolapse may be mentioned and assist in describing the severity of the lesion present. The component elements of the prolapse should be listed separately.

Describing the Anatomic Defect

Anterior Vagina

The anterior vaginal wall should be above the hymenal ring. Descent of the anterior vaginal wall to the hymenal ring during straining is characteristic of a urethrocele.

The anterior vaginal wall above the urethrovesical crease usually lies in a plane at about 45-degree angle from the horizontal plane of the perineum. Descent below the level of the hymenal ring is significant and can be caused by one of three things:

1. Separation of the paravaginal attachment of the pubocervical fascia from the white line
2. Loss of the vagina's attachment to the cervix
3. Tearing in the pubocervical fascia that results in herniation of the bladder through this layer

These may lead to defects involving the anterior vaginal wall in the midline, laterally or paravaginally, superiorly, or any combination of these sites (4,10) (Fig. 20.2). Defects may be identified clinically by evaluating each individual area. Using curved sponge forceps with the curve pointed posteriorly toward the ischial spines, the lateral aspects of the anterior vagina and pubocervical fascia can be returned to their normal point of attachment along the arcus tendineus fasciae pelvis. The forceps then are placed laterally, and the patient is asked to strain maximally. If she strains and there are no evident anterior defects, she has lateral or paravaginal loss of support. If, when she strains, there is some improvement in anterior support, but she continues to have a midline bulge through the open arms of the forceps, she also has a midline defect in the pubocervi-

cal fascia. The forceps may be closed and used to support the base of the bladder centrally. When the patient strains and she has no midline descent, the support defect is midline or central (9).

Superior loss of support is characterized by several clinical clues. When the patient strains, if the anterior vaginal epithelium appears thin and shiny, with loss of rugae from the vaginal cuff along the base of the bladder, and the anterior vaginal wall is longer than the posterior vagina, the patient is likely to have superior loss of support of her pubocervical fascia. Superior defects frequently are associated with midline defects.

Anterior enteroceles, where intestine herniates into a defect in the pubocervical fascia can occur. This can be difficult to distinguish from a high cystocele. Often the base of bladder can be drawn into the top of the defect (11).

Cervix or Vaginal Cuff

The location of the cervix is customarily used to gauge the severity of uterine prolapse. Its position relative to the hymenal ring should be noted while the prolapse is at its largest. If the cervix is not visible because of the presence of a cystocele or rectocele, then its location may be palpated while having the patient strain. When the cervix descends to within 1 cm of the hymenal ring, there is significant loss of support. In instances where the uterus is not necessarily going to be removed, the normality of uterine support should be tested before assuming that the uterus is well supported. This can be done by grasping the cervix with a tenaculum or ring forceps and applying traction until it stops descending (12). Occult prolapse in which the cervix comes below the hymenal ring can be detected in this way.

The cervix or cuff depends on DeLancey Level I support, the cardinal uterosacral ligament complex. With inadequate cardinal uterosacral ligament support, the cervix may descend from its normal position, halfway to the hymen, to

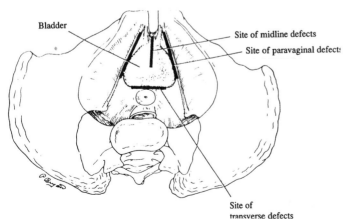

FIGURE 20.2. Illustration of the location of midline, paravaginal, and transverse defects of vaginal support.

the hymen, halfway outside the hymen, or fully outside the hymen, as in the woman who has uterine procidentia. In the woman who has a normally supported vaginal cuff, dimples can be seen at the 3 and 9 o'clock areas signifying the location of the cardinal uterosacral ligament attachment. The scar where the cuff was closed after hysterectomy also serves to identify the location of the vaginal apex. As the cuff descends from its normal position, it usually is possible to continue to see dimples at the 3 and 9 o'clock positions. Dimples serve as an objective reference point allowing discrimination between loss of support for the bladder anteriorly and loss of support for the cul-de-sac and cuff posteriorly (9).

The apical enterocele occurs when intestine herniates into the defect created by the separation of the pubocervical from the rectovaginal fascia in a posthysterectomy patient. It is usually associated with loss of apical, uterosacral and cardinal ligament support and vault descent (11).

Posterior Vagina

Rectoceles and posterior enteroceles involve some defects in the rectovaginal fascia (11). The posterior vaginal wall is the site of both rectoceles and enteroceles. A rectocele is present when the anterior rectal wall and overlying vagina protrude below the hymenal ring. Posterior enterocele exists when the cul-de-sac becomes distended with the intestine and bulges the posterior vaginal wall outward. There are also occasions in which the posterior wall appears to bulge into the vagina, not because the rectal wall is poorly supported but because of a deficiency in the perineal body. This has been referred to as a pseudorectocele and can be easily differentiated from a true rectocele because the anterior wall contour is normal on rectal examination (13).

Discrimination between enterocele and a rectocele however may be clinically difficult. The "double bubble," the discreet appearance of a hernia sac on the anterior surface of a rectocele, is clinically indicative of an enterocele but generally not present. Examination of the patient in the standing position may allow the discrimination between an enterocele and a rectocele. The index finger is placed in the anterior rectal ampulla and the thumb in the vaginal vault, palpating the rectovaginal septum for evidence of small bowel between the rectum and the vagina (9).

Anatomically posterior enterocele extends from the apex of the vagina downward, whereas a rectocele typically begins in the lower portion of the vagina. The hallmark of a typical rectocele is the formation of a pocket that allows the anterior rectal wall to balloon down through the introitus. When a rectal examination is performed with the prolapse fully developed, a rectocele exists if there is an extension of the rectal lumen below the axis of the anus. This not only provides the diagnosis but also illustrates the mechanism by which rectoceles create symptoms. As long as the anterior rectal wall has a smooth contour and no sacculation, even though it may be more mobile than normal, stool will pass out through the anus. However, when a pocket develops as the patient strains, stool becomes trapped and difficulty with evacuation can occur (2).

The rectovaginal fascia extends from the cul-de-sac superiorly to the perineal body distally and laterally to the levator fascia (Fig. 20.3). Defects in this fascial support structure occur most commonly in the midline but may occur laterally or transversely near the perineum or the vaginal cuff. As with the anterior segment, the rectum normally does not cross the midvaginal axis on straining. The curved ringed forceps may be placed posteriorly and laterally in an effort to reduce the posterior defect. If there continues to be a bulge between the open arms of the forceps, the defect is midline. The forceps may be closed and used to support the midline. If there is no loss of support when the patient strains, the defect is in the midline. Loss of support at the cul-de-sac or at the perineal body is best identified intraoperatively (9).

Patients who have prolapse after hysterectomy are assessed as to whether prolapse of the vaginal apex is present. Examination of the patient who has previously had a hysterectomy should include a specific effort to determine the location of the vaginal apex when the prolapse is at its largest. The apex is identified by the scar that exists where the cervix was removed. Vaginal prolapse is present when the vaginal apex lies below the level of the hymenal ring. If the apex descends to within the lower one-third of the vagina with straining, a significant deficit in support of the apex is present and the vagina should be resuspended during repair (2).

Assessment of Pelvic Floor Muscularity

The next portion of the pelvic floor evaluation is to determine the ability to produce voluntary pelvic floor muscle

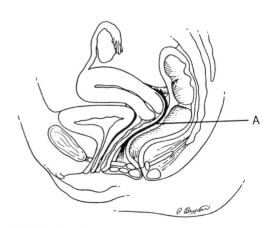

FIGURE 20.3. Illustration of the rectovaginal septum.

contractions and the ability to keep the pelvic floor muscle contracted during stress situations. The levator muscles are evaluated for symmetry and defects (such as muscle hernias, scarring, and the volume of the muscles) (14), and for trigger points (a focus of hyperirritability in a tissue that, when compressed, is locally tender and, if sufficiently hypersensitive, gives rise to referred pain and tenderness and sometimes to referred autonomic phenomena and distortion of proprioception) (15,16). Types of trigger points include myofascial, cutaneous, ligamentous, and periosteal trigger points. Palpable taut bands or nodules are sought by flat palpation, which is examination by finger pressure that proceeds across the muscle fibers at a right angle to their length, while compressing them against a firm underlying structure, such as bone. These are groups of taut muscle fibers that are associated with a myofascial trigger point and are identifiable by tactile examination. Contraction of the fibers in this band produces the local twitch response (15,16).

Examination of contractility is the next important step in evaluation of pelvic floor function. The pelvic floor is evaluated for voluntary contractions and the symmetry of the contractions is determined. The bladder neck is palpated to determine if contraction leads to a dislocation and the vaginal wall is palpated during coughing to determine if contractions occur with abdominal stress situations. Contractility can easily be assessed by vaginal or rectal examination (14).

The clinical evaluation of pelvic floor function is determined by evaluating the state of the muscles at rest and during a maximum voluntary contraction (Table 20.1). This involves inspection, palpation, and testing of the muscles. The patient should be positioned in good light with knees bent apart. Using disposable gloves and water soluble lubricating jelly, the labia are parted and the area carefully examined and the genitoanal area are inspected to evaluate the skin condition, muscle tone, and presence of prolapse (17). To observe during a pelvic floor contraction the patient is told to "squeeze and lift" the pelvic floor muscles as if preventing the escape of flatus and urine.

During the evaluation of the pelvic floor it is also important to observe for extraneous muscle activity. When the patient is asked to perform a pelvic floor muscle contraction it is not uncommon to observe the patient holding her

TABLE 20.1. SOME OF THE IMPORTANT COMPONENTS OF THE PHYSICAL EXAMINATION OF THE PELVIC FLOOR (17)

Observation at rest	The presence of urethrocele, cystocele, uterine prolapse, and rectocele
Excoriation	Suggests almost continuous state of wetness and may give an indication of the severity of incontinence
Dry erythematous tissue	Vaginitis Urethritis May cause frequency, urgency, and dysuria
Observation during a pelvic floor contraction Strong levators and contraction	Voluntary strength of the levator ani Puckering and indrawing of the vaginal introitus, anal sphincter, and perineal body
Weak levators and contraction	Slight puckering or inability to produce any movement of the perineum
Observations during a cough Healthy, strong pelvic floor	Produces little or no movement; either at the vaginal introitus or the perineum as a whole
Weak pelvic floor	Perineal descent Vaginal introitus will bulge and gape Caudal movement of any prolapse Short spurt of urine may be observed Repeat the cough contracting the pelvic floor muscles, to test whether she can minimize the perineal descent
Observation standing	At rest, during a pelvic floor muscle contraction and on coughing
Weak muscles Strong muscles	Prolapse is more likely to be provoked No difference from lithotomy examination

From Laycock J. Clinical evaluation of the pelvic floor. In: Schussler B, Laycock J, Norton P, et al., eds. *Pelvic floor re-education principles and practices*. London: Springer-Verlag, 1994:42–48, with permission.

breath and contracting the abdominal, gluteal, and adductor muscles in an effort to produce a maximum contraction. These extraneous muscles are generally recruited when the pelvic muscles are tiring. Observation and palpation of these auxiliary muscles will determine the extent of their involvement and the examiner should make the patient aware of these unwanted muscle contractions. Contraction of the abdominal muscles produces an increase in intraabdominal and intravesical pressures, which may produce incontinence. To avoid breath holding, women should be initially taught to contract their pelvic floor muscles while breathing out. Although this involves some abdominal muscle activity, it prevents Valsalva and bearing down, which some patients erroneously perceive as the correct contraction technique (17).

Palpation of the pelvic floor muscle can be performed per vagina or per rectum. Palpation permits an evaluation of muscle bulk, resting tone, contractile strength, and reflex response to cough. In addition, reduced sensation and pain should be identified. Transvaginal palpation is performed with a gloved, lubricated index finger introduced 3 to 4 cm into the vagina and rotated through 360 degrees (Fig. 20.4). The strong levator ani of a young woman will be felt as a thick (approximately 1 to 2 cm), firm band of muscle, compared with the weak levator ani of an elderly woman, which will feel thin and may have lack of tone that renders it indistinguishable from the surrounding tissues. Areas of atrophy can be detected as zones of reduced muscle bulk. An active voluntary contraction is felt as a tightening, lifting, and squeezing action under the examining finger. Active voluntary contraction during palpation should also be performed in a standing position. The contractility of the muscles during a maximum voluntary contraction is assessed by introducing two fingers (index and middle) in both the anterior-posterior and side to side planes (17).

Transrectal palpation enables examination of the puborectalis and external anal sphincter at rest and during maximum voluntary contraction. This is best carried out with the patient in the left lateral position with the examiner using a gloved lubricated index finger. The index finger is introduced 3 to 4 cm transrectally and the puborectalis muscle palpated with the distal pad of the index finger. The effect of a pelvic floor muscle contraction is felt as tension on the examining finger as the slinglike puborectalis pulls the rectum anteriorly. A contraction of the external anal sphincter is detected on withdrawing the finger to a position 1 to 2 cm inside the anal canal (17). The assessment of muscle strength involves introducing the index and middle fingers into the distal 3 cm of the vagina for parous women (using one finger only for those women with a small diameter vagina) and assessing the Power (P), Endurance (E), number of Repetitions (R), and number of Fast (F) (1 second) contractions; furthermore, Every (E) Contraction (C) is Timed (T). This mnemonic (PERFECT) provides a simple reminder of

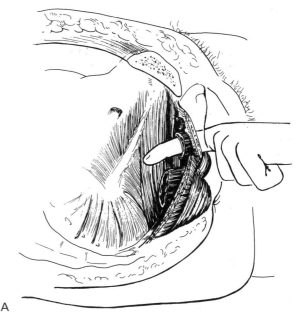

A

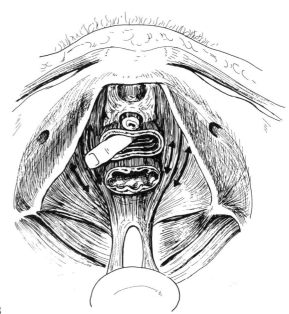

B

FIGURE 20.4. A,B: Transvaginal palpation of the pelvic floor muscles may be performed with a gloved, lubricated index finger introduced 3 to 4 cm into the vagina and rotated through 360 degrees.

pelvic floor muscle assessment and also provides data regarding the fast and slow twitch muscle fibers.

Q-Tip Testing

At the time of the physical examination, hypermobility of the urethroversical junction during stress situations and coughing can be demonstrated and roughly quantified by the so-called Q-tip test (18). A Q-tip is inserted into the proximal part of the urethra. During coughing or straining the bare end of the Q-tip is displaced upward. The extent of change of the angle during this displacement roughly reflects the degree of mobility. Because of its lack of sensitivity and specificity, use of this method for the *diagnosis* of stress urinary incontinence should be abandoned. For pelvic floor reeducation, however, it is quite useful (18).

During voluntary contraction of the pelvic floor muscle, the mobile urethra moves toward the symphysis, thereby causing the Q-tip stem to move gradually downward. The increase in the angle is dependent on the extent to which the stem is moved and therefore dependent on the extent of the pelvic floor muscle contraction.

A patient who is unable to contract the pelvic floor voluntarily will not be able to move the Q-tip. Therefore, they will require electrostimulation of the pelvic floor muscles as a first step prior to pelvic floor reeducation. The use of the Q-tip test allows quantification of improvement in the pelvic floor and possible contractility during the course of treatment. The test can be of great help in biofeedback control especially in those patients who are not able to voluntarily contract the pelvic floor at the beginning of the reeducation program.

DIAGNOSTIC STUDIES

Ultrasound

Ultrasound imaging is regarded as the most conclusive investigation for evaluation of pelvic floor muscle function. Movements of the urethrovesical junction and bladder base with contractions of the pelvic floor muscles are seen to be more cranial than ventral when the medial urethral attachment to the puborectalis sling is intact. Opposite movements are seen with straining. Coughing results in fast, caudally oriented movement of the bladder and the urethra. The extent of movement increases with insufficiency of the urethrovesical attachments. Ultrasound imaging, a relatively noninvasive technique, is of practicable value (Table 20.2). Vaginal sonography, perineal ultrasound, introital sonography, and rectosonography can all be used. Perineal and introital applications of linear array and mechanical sector scanners have been found to be most suitable for patients with lower urinary tract disorders.

Application of imaging techniques to demonstrate the urethrovesical anatomy in patients with genuine stress incontinence relates to one of the aims of pelvic floor reeducation, to demonstrate effective elevation of the urethrovesical unit by voluntary or reflex contraction of the pelvic floor muscles. Sonographic techniques can act as biofeedback and also can be of help in learning the correct contractions and activation of pelvic floor muscles by demonstrating movement of the urethrovesical unit in an anterior and upward direction and thus elevating the bladder neck toward the symphysis region which causes mechanical closure of the urethra (19).

TABLE 20.2. USES OF ULTRASOUND IN THE EVALUATION OF THE PELVIC FLOOR IN WOMEN

Identification of static and dynamic disturbances of pelvic floor muscle function
Dynamic examination of the bladder and urethra
Objective comparison of changes owing to pelvic floor muscle reeducation
Easy visualization of bladder neck movement during pelvic floor muscle contractions
Measurement of muscle thickness

Perineal ultrasound is a reliable technique that allows reproducible static and dynamic evaluation. Lateral chain urethrocystography is superior to perineal ultrasound only if bladder neck funneling is the aim of the evaluation. It is inferior if bladder neck mobility during maximal Valsalva is being investigated (20).

Colporectocystourethrography

Colporectocystourethrography (CRCU) is a radiological technique that allows visualization of the urethra and bladder neck, vagina, rectum, and anal canal by radiopacity (21). CRCU enables visualization of the dynamic changes not only of the urethrovesical junction, but of all pelvic organs caused by pelvic floor muscle activity. As long as MRI produces only static pictures, CRCU is the only method for obtaining dynamic images of pelvic floor muscle activity. Using this technique it is possible to demonstrate that patients cured using pelvic floor reeducation for the treatment of urinary stress incontinence show a higher decrease of anorectal and urethrovesical inclination and a greater uplift of the bladder base and posterior walls of the rectum with pelvic floor muscle activity. However, CRCU requires a significant radiation dose and significant effort and preparation. Therefore, it is not a method that is useful in routine clinical evaluation (21).

Cystograms, Viscerograms, Colpocystograms, and Defecography

Cystourethrograms allow analysis of the posterior urethrovesical angle. Dynamic pelvic viscerograms with injection of the levator muscles with contrast solution (levator myography) demonstrate that in the erect posture the vagina assumes a horizontal position at rest and during straining. They show that during increases in abdominal pressure, the vagina and rectum are forced downward toward the sacrum over the levator plate. They also demonstrate that patients with support defects have an enlarged levator hiatus (22). A colpocystogram adds opacification with contrast medium of the bladder, urethra, rectum and vagina and allows a dynamic study of pelvic support and function. For example, a colpocystogram can demonstrate how a large rectocele can conceal urinary incontinence by buttressing the bladder neck and explain how urinary leakage, funneling, and bladder neck descent can occur after a repair of a large rectocele. Defecography or dynamic proctography is particularly helpful in evaluating rectoceles and provides information regarding pelvic floor descent and rectocele formation. Although the identification of a rectocele by physical examination is not enhanced by dynamic defecography, it is more sensitive than physical examination in identifying enteroceles and also can identify sigmoidoceles preoperatively so they can be properly corrected during surgery (22).

Dynamic Fluoroscopic Evaluation of the Pelvic Floor

Dynamic fluoroscopic evaluation of the pelvic floor involves making the urinary, genital, and gastrointestinal tracts opaque. Once the small bowel is opacified, the vaginal canal is opacified with a dilute barium sulfate suspension paste. Two hundred milliliters of water soluble contrast is placed into the bladder with a small urethral catheter. The rectum is then made opaque. The patient is seated on a radiologic commode and resting images are obtained during squeezing and straining. The contraction of the puborectalis may be observed during the squeezing frame. Indentation of the posterior rectum is noted. The dynamic portion of the examination follows as the patient empties her rectum completely. This form of study has excellent clinical value and is the best study and most practical technique for radiographic evaluation of women with prolapse (22).

Magnetic Resonance Imaging

The unique feature of magnetic resonance imaging (MRI) is its ability to provide soft tissue contrast resolution. This technique can distinguish the various fascial and muscular layers of pelvic support. However, the supine position that is required is not a gravity dependent position and therefore is not the best position for the evaluation of a prolapse. It is also not the proper physiological position for urination or defecation. With advancing technology, this imaging technique may be valuable for the evaluation of patients with pelvic support defects. During dynamic imaging significant differences in the amount of descent with straining are noted on fast MRI. Studies indicate that dynamic MRI may play a clinical role in the evaluation and treatment of patients with recurrent prolapse, incontinence, suspected enterocele, and multicompartment prolapse, as well as patients with equivocal findings on physical examination. Dynamic MRI may also be helpful in clarifying anorectal defects (22).

MRI can currently demonstrate asymmetry between the two sides of the pelvic floor muscles, recognize defects

within the pelvic floor muscles themselves, and determine muscle volume. With respect to pelvic floor exercise, it may be possible to use MRI to measure pelvic floor muscle volumes as an objective parameter of the training effect (23). Defects in the paracolpium at vaginal support DeLancey levels I, II, and III can be found by magnetic resonance imaging scans prior to surgery in patients with symptomatic pelvic relaxation. Postoperative scans after paravaginal repair demonstrate disappearance of these defects (24).

Urodynamics

The use of urodynamic investigation accurately diagnoses genuine stress incontinence and allows selection of patients with this problem who are most likely to respond to pelvic floor reeducation. Resting urethral pressure may increase following successful treatment, although it seems more likely that pelvic floor reeducation is effective by improving the transmission of increases in intraabdominal pressure to the urethra, as a result of improved efficiency of voluntary and reflex contraction of the pelvic floor muscle. More specific urodynamic variables predictive of success of pelvic floor reeducation have not been fruitful to date (25).

Electrophysiology

In order to understand how electrophysiological information is obtained two basic procedures need to be understood—recording and stimulation. One can record the ongoing spontaneous bioelectrical activity for muscle and nerves but often an artificially evoked activity is diagnostically more informative. For this, stimulation is needed. Both recording and electrical stimulation are achieved through the use of electrodes. These are usually either "needle" or "surface" electrodes. Surface electrodes have comparatively large active surfaces and are thus nonselective. If used for recording, they take up bioelectrical activity from the source in an integrated fashion. Most patients do not find pelvic floor electromyography (EMG) uncomfortable (26).

The EMG can measure the bioelectrical activity of a muscle that is the most practical indicator of its contractility (Kinesiological EMG). It can also demonstrate whether a muscle is normal, myopathic or denervated or reinnervated (motor unit EMG).

For rehabilitation a kinesiological EMG measures the bioelectrical activity providing a qualitative and quantitative description of its activity over time. A meaningful EMG can only be performed on an innervated muscle. Motor unit EMGs of pelvic floor muscles are used in neurophysiological laboratories interested in neurogenic sacral dysfunctions (conus and cauda equina lesions, myelodysplasia, postoperative or postirradiation injuries, differential diagnosis between multiple system atrophy and idiopathic Parkinson's disease). There are also patients with sacral dysfunctions (urinary or fecal incontinence) that are not associated with signs of neurologic injury or disease. For example, women with stress incontinence have partially denervated pelvic floor muscles. Concentric needle EMG is a worthwhile investigation for women with urinary retention as it can reveal isolated abnormality of the urethral sphincter. Peripheral motor pathways such as the pudendal nerve can be evaluated by electrical stimulation using surface type electrodes. The demonstration of a preserved response is the most important finding. Central motor pathways can also be assessed. Significant prolongation of central motor conduction time has been demonstrated in patients with multiple sclerosis and sphincter disturbance (26).

Somatosensory evoked potentials (SEPs) can be obtained by stimulating somatosensory system in the periphery. A pudendal SEP study is obtained by placing EEG ear clip electrodes over the labia and over the clitoris. The absence of the pudendal SEP is abnormal. Latencies are sensitive to demyelination, being prolonged in multiple sclerosis (26).

Sacral reflexes include the bulbocavernosus and the anal reflex. The bulbocavernosus reflex is elicited by squeezing the clitoris and the anal reflex by pricking the perianal skin. Bulbocavernosus reflex latencies above 45 msec are abnormal. Prolonged latencies in the bulbocavernosus reflex have been found in patients with stress incontinence supporting the neurogenic hypothesis of this disorder. Although it seems intrinsically worthwhile to make as refined a diagnosis as possible regarding a neurogenic pelvic floor muscle lesion, the clinical relevance of detailed assessment is as yet not clarified (26).

DIFFERENTIAL DIAGNOSIS

The differential diagnosis of pelvic floor relaxation disorders is divided into two sections. First, the specific relaxation disorder itself; second, the etiology of the specific disorder.

The specific disorders of the pelvic floor that must be differentiated have been listed and include differentiation between cystocele and cystourethrocele with differentiation between support defects in the midline, laterally or paravaginally, superiorly or in combination of these sites. In addition, the rectocele must be differentiated from the pseudorectocele and the enterocele. Also, it is helpful to realize that defects in the support level of DeLancey levels III and II result in cystocele and rectocele, whereas loss of upper suspensory fibers (DeLancey level I) is responsible for the development of vaginal uterine prolapse. Especially important with the rectocele is to recognize that breaks in the rectovaginal septum have occurred for a rectocele to be present (27). All rectoceles are not alike; the specific defect in the rectovaginal septum must be recognized prior to any repair.

With regard to etiology it is important to recognize that after vaginal delivery the mechanism of pelvic floor muscle activity is impaired. The relaxed pelvic floor is not able to actively counterbalance intraabdominal pressure in order to prevent further damage. The only mechanism that may be able to overcome pelvic floor relaxation related problems during situations of physical stress is active pelvic floor muscle contraction. However, this is not ready for use as it is not a normal physiological mechanism but is the result of training (28).

Other causes of pelvic floor relaxation must be considered such as multiple sclerosis, Parkinson's disorder, senile atrophy, and connective tissue disorders. However, these conditions account for only a small proportion of pelvic floor relaxation disorders.

MANAGEMENT OF PELVIC FLOOR RELAXATION DISORDERS

Medical Therapy

Current therapy of pelvic floor relaxation involves physiotherapy to recover some muscle function or surgery to compensate and in some cases or correct anatomic defects. None of these treatments is able to restore the pelvic floor to its original structure and function. Prevention of pelvic floor insufficiency is a major goal of pelvic floor reeducation. Widening of the levator hiatus is an etiology of genital prolapse. The hiatus is determined by the levator ani sling and ligaments and fascial planes that connect these muscles to their bony pelvic anchors. Pelvic floor reeducation has a role in prevention of pelvic relaxation owing to muscular weakness. Pelvic floor reeducation acts by (a) increasing muscular strength and endurance of the pelvic floor, (b) increasing the reflex action of these muscles through fast twitch recruitment, and (c) increasing awareness of these muscles (29).

EMG studies performed in patients with a significant history of long-term moderate to severe chronic introital dyspareunia and tenderness of the vulvar vestibule demonstrate increased resting tension levels of the pelvic floor muscles. After 4 months of daily at-home, biofeedback-assisted pelvic floor rehabilitation exercises, pelvic floor muscle contractions increased 95%, resting tension levels decreased 68%, and the instability of the muscle at rest decreased by 62%. Subjective reports of pain decreased an average of 83%. Seventy-five percent of the patients were able to resume intercourse by the end of the treatment. Pelvic floor muscle instability was found to be a critical factor in pain associated with vulvar vestibulitis syndrome. A biofeedback-assisted exercise program that stabilized the pelvic floor muscles significantly reduced and in some cases eliminated symptoms of vulvar vestibulitis syndrome (30,31).

Pelvic floor reeducation is also helpful for the treatment of painful intercourse caused by abnormal tone of the superficial muscles of the perineum (vaginal hypertonia). This is not to be confused with vaginismus, which is an impenetrable spasm reflecting an involuntary act of defense against vaginal penetration. For treatment of vaginal hypertonia sessions of relaxation therapy, which can include perineal massage to mobilize the musculature, combined with biofeedback techniques are helpful (32).

Techniques for Pelvic Floor Reeducation

Biofeedback is a giving of immediate information to a subject about bodily processes that are usually unconscious. These processes can then be subject to operant conditioning. Because many women with pelvic floor relaxation syndrome are not aware of the pelvic floor muscles and are unable to produce a voluntary contraction, biofeedback is a useful method of pelvic floor muscle reeducation.

Techniques that can be used for biofeedback include: (a) digital biofeedback where the pelvic floor muscles are stressed during digital palpation, which enhances sensory awareness and may trigger a contraction (stretch reflex), (b) use of a perineometer, which demonstrates pressure changes registered on a monitor (care must be taken to insure that an increase in intravaginal pressures is owing to a pelvic floor muscle contraction and not a manifestation of concomitant abdominal muscle activity), and (c) electromyography, which uses vaginal electrodes to monitor the action potentials in the paravaginal muscles and an abdominal muscle electrode to ensure the abdominal muscles are not activated at the same time. Using biofeedback, an individual training program can be designed for the specific patient. A generally applicable program involves pelvic floor muscle evaluation, followed by 15-minute sessions of pelvic floor strengthening exercises using the biofeedback system. Three to six months are now considered necessary to bring about a change in pelvic floor muscle strength (33). The introduction of neuromuscular electrical stimulation modalities, which provide greater cortical awareness and enhanced pelvic floor muscle contraction, may shorten the length of time required for improvement in pelvic floor muscle strength (34).

The aim of neuromuscular electrical stimulation (NMES) is to excite motor and sensory fibers of the pudendal nerves, produce a pelvic floor muscle (PFM) contraction and thus increase the strength of those muscles. The electrical stimuli produce a contraction of the PFM's and simultaneously reflex inhibition of the detrusor muscle. NMES is a suitable therapy for pelvic floor relaxation syndromes, as well as detrusor instability and sphincter incompetence. At the beginning of any treatment program it helps the patient to establish an adequate awareness of those muscles relevant to maintain continence and to improve her ability to contract them correctly. NMES is combined with muscular pelvic floor training; thus, it is difficult to assess particular effects of electrical stimulation alone (35).

Stimulation technique utilizes a frequency individualized to the patient's comfort between 10 and 25 Hz with pelvic floor contractions occurring for 10 seconds in every 30 seconds with a session lasting for 10 to 15 minutes in one protocol (36). NMES is applied in two main categories: acute maximum and chronic low intensity stimulation. There are important stimulation parameters that include frequency pattern of stimuli, pulse width, and frequency and duration of treatment. Acute maximum stimulation is used to strengthen muscle; this is done through maximum (up to 120 mA) tolerated current applied for 10 to 30 minutes, one to three times per week for several weeks. A wide range of pulse widths and frequencies can be used; however, pulse widths in the range of 200 to 400 microseconds appear to be best suited. Chronic low intensity stimulation is a low frequency (10 Hz) stimulation applied for up to several hours per day for several months. NMES using maximum stimulation increases muscle strength in a similar manner to voluntary exercise by repeatedly overloading the pelvic floor muscles by repeated maximum contractions. In addition, electrically elicited contractions targeting fast twitch muscle fibers train these fibers more effectively than volitional exercise. Improved reflex responses are a sequel to maximum NMES. Low frequency, low intensity chronic stimulation modifies the physiological and metabolic characteristics of muscle atrophy by disuse. The chronically stimulated muscle assumes the properties of slow muscle units increasing endurance (37).

A current with a frequency in the range of 10 to 40 Hz with duration of approximately 250 microseconds will activate fast and slow motoneurons. A current with a frequency of 35 to 40 Hz will optimally elicit a comfortable tetanic contraction with minimal fatigue. The duty cycle is the ratio between the time the stimulator is on and the time it is off. A 5/15 (5 S on and 15 S off) may be selected for very weak muscles, progressing to 5/10 and later 5/5 as the muscles become stronger. Treatment time should be increased as muscles become stronger, increasing treatment time from 10 to 30 minutes for maximal stimulation. Maximal stimulation at 35 Hz, 250 to 350 microseconds and appropriate duty cycle can be applied until a patient can produce a moderate contraction with a small degree of lift, lasting 4 seconds. Treatment then continues with pelvic floor exercises, biofeedback and/or cones together with NMES (38).

Interferential therapy stems from the concept of two medium frequency currents (range 2,000 to 5,000 Hz) producing an amplitude modulated interference current with a frequency equal to the difference between the two applied currents. A low frequency 35 Hz effect can be produced in deep muscles by the interaction of two medium frequency currents such as 4,000 and 4,035 Hz. Interferential therapy reduces the discomfort perceived by the patient because of the intensity of the low frequency current required to activate deep seated muscles. This occurs because the main resistance to low frequency currents is encountered at the electrode–skin interface, and when the skin resistance is high, a larger voltage has to be applied in order to achieve an adequate current flow. By increasing the frequency, the resistance is decreased and less voltage is required to drive the current to the underlying muscles. Neuromuscular tissue responds to current intensity, frequency, and pulse width, and interferential therapy simply produces bursts of short duration current of selected frequency just like other forms of NMES (34).

Vaginal Cones

Vaginal cones were designed to compensate for major deficiencies of various methods of pelvic floor muscle exercises. Once the correct performance of voluntary contractions of the pelvic floor muscles is taught by utilizing biofeedback techniques and neuromuscular electrical stimulation or digital intravaginal palpation, vaginal cones can be utilized as a biofeedback method for exercising the pelvic floor muscles. When a cone of the appropriate weight is inserted into the vagina it tends to slip out. The feeling of losing the cone provides a sensory feedback that makes the pelvic floor contract around the cone retaining it. This principle is used to teach a pelvic floor muscle contraction and to test the strength of the pelvic floor muscle and to exercise the pelvic floor muscle correctly. The heaviest cone that can be actively retained for 1 minute by contracting the pelvic floor muscles is a standardized measure of the pelvic floor muscle strength. The patient should begin exercise with the heaviest weight she can retain for 1 minute. She should aim to increase the time she is able to retain the cone without losing it, up to a maximum of 15 minutes and to repeat this twice a day. She should increase the amount of movement by walking around, stair climbing, running, coughing, and hand washing, up to a period of 15 minutes. Vaginal cones allow for the correct and reliable identification testing and exercising of pelvic floor muscles and distinguishing their contraction from contraction of the abdominal muscles. The cone will be pulled up by proper contraction of the pelvic floor muscles; if it is pushed out the patient has contracted abdominal muscles (38).

Surgical Therapy

Surgical therapy for pelvic floor relaxation addresses specific defects in the fascial layer that have been disrupted. The appropriate surgical reapproximation of this fascial layer depends on the accurate diagnosis of the fascial layer involved. Details of surgical repair are not discussed in this text, because such reconstructive surgery constitutes a major component of gynecological surgical education and training, and is discussed in depth in many surgical texts and in many of the references cited in this chapter.

Because surgical repair addresses only the fascial layer, pelvic floor muscle dysfunction must be addressed to optimize the opportunity for success of the surgical therapy. Also, dyspareunia can follow the repair of a rectocele or enterocele if this is not addressed.

The laparoscopic approach to pelvic floor defects has been described for the apical enterocele (pubocervical fascia separated from rectovaginal fascia) and for vaginal/uterine prolapse (break in cardinal/uterosacral suspensory ligaments) (39,40,41,42) as well as for paravaginal defects (43) and for posterior compartment defects (rectocele) (42,44). All support defects present as a bulge into the vagina. A bulge indicates a break in the tube itself or the tube has lost its apical suspension, lateral attachment or distal fusion. The integrity of the tube must be restored and it must be re-suspended, reattached laterally, and re-fused distally (11).

Prevention of Pelvic Floor Relaxation Disorders

A careful examination and a directed history may identify women with early signs of pelvic floor dysfunction. In these cases pelvic floor exercises may be beneficial. Because pelvic floor exercise can strengthen the levator ani muscle, it follows that improved muscle strength may prevent or ameliorate pelvic organ prolapse. Women with early signs of pelvic floor dysfunction may also benefit from education regarding correct lifting techniques, weight reduction, prevention of constipation, and avoidance of cigarette smoking (12).

KEY POINTS
Differential Diagnosis

- The specific relaxation disorder itself
- The etiology of the specific disorder

Most Important Questions to Ask

- What do you see or feel when you are standing up for a long time?
- What is your most severe symptom—loss of urine with cough, constipation, pressure, pain, urgency, feeling of heaviness?
- Did you have a vaginal delivery, what was the length of time of the second stage, what was the size of the baby, and were there any episiotomies or tears?
- Do you have pain or lack of feeling with intercourse?

Most Important Physical Examination Findings

- Protrusion of portion of the pelvic floor below the hymenal ring

- Hypertonicity or hypotonicity of the vaginal muscles
- Palpable weakness or tenderness of the levator ani muscles

Most Important Diagnostic Studies

- Physical examination
- Ultrasound
- Surface EMG studies

Treatments

- Pelvic floor reeducation using biofeedback controlled EMG together with neuromuscular stimulation
- Surgical repair of the specific defects in the fascial wall

REFERENCES

1. DeLancey JOL. Anatomy and biomechanics of genital prolapse. *Clin Obstet Gynecol* 1993;36:897–909.
2. DeLancey JOL. Pelvic organ prolapse. In: Scott JR, DiSaia PJ, Hammond CP, et al, eds. *Danforth's obstetrics and gynecology,* 7th ed. Philadelphia: JB Lippincott, 1994:803–825.
3. Norton PA. Pelvic floor disorders: the role of fascia and ligaments. *Clin Obstet Gynecol* 1996;36:926–938.
4. Richardson AC, Lyon JB, Williams NL. New look at pelvic relaxation. *Am J Obstet Gynecol* 1976;126:568–573.
5. Handa VL, Harris TA, Ostergard DR. Protecting the pelvic floor: obstetric management to prevent incontinence and pelvic organ prolapse. *Obstet Gynecol* 1996;88:470–478.
6. Allen RE, Hosker GL, Smith ATB, et al. Pelvic floor damage and childbirth: a neurophysiological study. *Br J Obstet Gynaecol* 1990; 97:770–779.
7. Snooks SJ, Swash M, Setchell M, et al. Injury to innervation of pelvic floor sphincter musculature in childbirth. *Lancet* 1984; ii:546–550.
8. Rockner G, Jonasson A, Olung A. The effect of mediolateral episiotomy at delivery on pelvic floor muscle strength evaluated with vaginal cones. *Acta Obstet Gynecol Scand* 1991;70:51–54.
9. Shull BL. Clinical evaluation of women with pelvic support defects. *Clin Obstet Gynecol* 1993;36:939–951.
10. Youngblood JP. Paravaginal repair for cystourethrocele. *Clin Obstet Gynecol* 1993;36:960–966.
11. Richardson AC. The anatomic defects in rectocele and enterocele. *J Pelv Sur* 1995;1:214–221.
12. Bartscht KD, DeLancey JOL. A technique to study the passive supports of the uterus. *Obstet Gynecol* 1988;72:940–943.
13. Nichols DH, Randall CL. *Vaginal surgery,* 3rd ed. Baltimore: Williams & Wilkins, 1989:403–412.
14. Schussler B. Aims of pelvic floor evaluation. In: Schussler B, Laycock J, Norton P, et al., eds. *Pelvic floor re-education principles and practice.* London: Springer-Verlag, 1994:39–41.
15. Slocumb JC. Chronic somatic, myofascial, and neurogenic abdominal pelvic pain. *J Clin Obstet Gynecol* 1990;33:145–153.
16. Simons D, Travell JG, Simons LS. *Myofascial pain and dysfunction: the trigger point manual.* Baltimore: Williams & Wilkins, 1999;1:1–140.
17. Laycock J. Clinical evaluation of the pelvic floor. In: Schussler B, Laycock J, Norton P, et al., eds. *Pelvic floor re-education principles and practices.* London: Springer-Verlag, 1994:42–48.
18. Schussler B, Hesse U. Q-tip testing. In: Schussler B, Laycock J, Norton P, et al., eds. *Pelvic floor re-education principles and practices.* London: Springer-Verlag, 1994:49–50.
19. Kolbl H. Ultrasound. In: Schussler B, Laycock J, Norton P, et al., eds. *Pelvic floor re-education principles and practices.* London: Springer-Verlag, 1994:64–74.
20. Schaer GN, Koechli OR, Schussler B, Haller U. Perineal ultrasound for evaluating the bladder neck and urinary stress incontinence. *Obstet Gynecol* 1995;85:220–224.
21. Schussler B. Radiological evaluation of the pelvic floor invscera. In: Schussler B, Laycock J, Norton P, et al., eds. *Pelvic floor re-education principles and practices.* London: Springer-Verlag, 1994:75–77.
22. Brubaker L, Heit MH. Radiology of the pelvic floor. *Clin Obstet Gynecol* 1993;36:952–959.
23. Debus-Thide G. Magnetic resonance imaging (MRI) of the pelvic floor. In: Schussler B, Laycock J, Norton P, et al., eds. *Pelvic floor re-education principles and practices.* London: Springer-Verlag, 1994:78–82.
24. Huddleston HT, Dunnihoo DR, Huddleston PM, et al. Magnetic resonance imaging of defects in DeLancey vaginal support levels I, II, and III. *Am J Obstet Gynecol* 1995;172:1778–1784.
25. Hilton P. The role of urodynamics in pelvic floor re-education. In: Schussler B, Laycock J, Norton P, et al., eds. *Pelvic floor re-education principles and practices.* London: Springer-Verlag, 1994:51–63.
26. Vodusek D. Electrophysiology. In: Schussler B, Laycock J, Norton P, et al., eds. *Pelvic floor re-education principles and practices.* London: Springer-Verlag, 1994:83–97.
27. Richardson AC. The rectovaginal septum revisited: its relationship to rectocele and its importance in rectocele repair. *Clin Obstet Gynecol* 1993;36:976–983.
28. Schussler B, Anthuber C, Warrell D. The pelvic floor before and after delivery. In: Schussler B, Laycock J, Norton P, et al., eds. *Pelvic floor re-education principles and practices.* London: Springer-Verlag, 1994:105–110.
29. Norton P. Treatment of stress urinary incontinence. In: Schussler B, Laycock J, Norton P, et al., eds. *Pelvic floor re-education principles and practices.* London: Springer-Verlag, 1994:123–126.
30. Glazer HI, Rodke G, Swencionis C, et al. Treatment of vulvar vestibulitis syndrome with electromyographic biofeedback of pelvic floor musculature. *J Reprod Med* 1995;40:283–290.
31. Simons D, Travell JG, Simons LS. *Myofascial pain and dysfunction: the trigger point manual.* Baltimore: Williams & Wilkins, 1999;1:1–1038.
32. Pigne A, Oudin G. Treatment of sexual dysfunction. In: Schussler B, Laycock J, Norton P, et al., eds. *Pelvic floor re-education principles and practices.* London: Springer-Verlag, 1994:126–129.
33. Laycock J. Biofeedback control. In: Schussler B, Laycock J, Norton P, et al., eds. *Pelvic floor re-education principles and practices.* London: Springer-Verlag, 1994:154–156.
34. Laycock J. Interferential therapy. In: Schussler B, Laycock J, Norton P, et al., eds. *Pelvic floor re-education principles and practices.* London: Springer-Verlag, 1994:168–169.
35. Anthuber C, Pigne A. Neuromuscular electrical stimulation. In: Schussler B, Laycock J, Norton P, et al., eds. *Pelvic floor re-education principles and practices.* London: Springer-Verlag, 1994:163–167.
36. Schussler B, Prince S. Concept of an individualized combined pelvic floor reeducation program. In: Schussler B, Laycock J, Norton P, et al., eds. *Pelvic floor re-education principles and practices.* London: Springer-Verlag, 1994:169–176.
37. Laycock J, Plevnik S, Senn E. Electrical stimulation. In: Schussler B, Laycock J, Norton P, et al., eds. *Pelvic floor re-education principles and practices.* London: Springer-Verlag, 1994:143–153.
38. Plevnik S. Vaginal cones. In: Schussler B, Laycock J, Norton P, et al., eds. *Pelvic floor re-education principles and practices.* London: Springer-Verlag, 1994:139–142.

21

VULVODYNIA

C. PAUL PERRY

KEY TERMS AND DEFINITIONS

Allodynia: Pain resulting from a nonnoxious stimulus to the skin.

Neuralgia: Paroxysmal pain, which extends along the course of one or more nerves.

Neuroma: An unorganized bulbous or nodular mass of nerve fibers produced by accidental or purposeful sectioning of a nerve.

Nociceptor: A nerve receptor for pain.

Vestibulitis: Pain in the space between the labia minora into which opens the urethra and vagina.

Vulvodynia: Pain in the female external genitalia.

Vaginismus: Painful involuntary spasm of the vaginal musculature usually so intense as to prevent intercourse; pelvic floor myalgia.

INTRODUCTION

Vulvodynia, as defined by the International Society for the Study of Vulvar Disease, is a "chronic vulvar discomfort, especially that characterized by the patient's complaint of burning, stinging, irritation, or rawness" (1). This symptom complex may be subdivided into four categories by etiology: (a) periorificial dermatitis (cyclic vulvovaginitis, steroid rebound dermatitis, lichen sclerosus); (b) vulvar vestibulitis; (c) dysesthetic vulvodynia or pudendal neuralgia; and (d) vulvar neuroma formation (2). A fifth category of vulvodynia, vestibular papillomatosis, was dropped after initial evidence that the human papillomavirus (HPV) might be etiologic was unsubstantiated.

Each of these four categories of vulvodynia is characterized by distinctive symptoms. Vulvar burning or dyspareunia with skin changes suggests periorificial dermatitis, which involves cyclic vulvovaginitis, steroid rebound dermatitis, and lichen sclerosus. Dyspareunia without skin changes characterizes vulvar vestibulitis. Vulvar burning without skin changes is consistent with dysesthetic vulvodynia or pudendal neuralgia. Focal or localized vulvodynia without skin changes or dyspareunia suggests vulvar neu-

roma. Although they overlap somewhat, these divisions help clinicians make an accurate diagnosis and treat with the best possibility of success (2).

It is estimated that over 200,000 women in the United States have significant vulvar pain. The personal nature of the problem makes it difficult to obtain accurate figures, and many patients have been embarrassed into silence by being told that their problem was "all in their head." Patients with vulvodynia appear normal to the outside world. No one else can appreciate their pain—not family, not spouse, and frequently not even physicians (3).

PERIORIFICIAL DERMATITIS
Etiology

Periorificial dermatitis is characterized by vulvar burning or dyspareunia with skin changes. Causes of periorificial dermatitis include cyclic vulvovaginitis, steroid dermatitis, and lichen sclerosus. Each of these conditions will be considered individually.

Cyclic Vulvovaginitis

Symptoms of Cyclic Vulvovaginitis
Cyclic vulvovaginitis is characterized by recurrent itching and burning often related to menses. The symptoms may initially respond to anticandidal agents, but the recrudescence is often interpreted by the patient as an incorrect diagnosis. Topical drugs may irritate the inflamed tissue and become ineffective. Perspiration, semen, vaginal discharge and soaps can exacerbate the symptoms. The irritation can be labial and vaginal. Usually erythema and edema are noted. Fissures may occur with intercourse and periodic scaling or pustules may be present. The typical patient is premenopausal, with a history of frequent yeast infections or recurrent bacterial infections (e.g., chronic sinusitis, cystitis, or bronchitis) requiring antibiotics.

Diagnosis of Cyclic Vulvovaginitis
Diagnostically, wet preps and cultures confirming *Candida* are most helpful. Biopsies are usually not helpful.

Treatment of Cyclic Vulvovaginitis

Treatment of chronic vulvodynia produced by cyclic vulvovaginitis requires long-term systemic suppression. Ketoconazole in doses of 200 mg twice a day for 10 days, followed by 100 mg every day for 30 days may be required. If the infection has been poorly controlled for years, some patients may need 50 mg every other day for 3 months. Due to potential liver toxicity, this regimen may be supplanted by Fluconazole 150 mg every week for 4 weeks and every other week for 8 weeks or longer (4).

Rebound Dermatitis

Symptoms of Steroid Rebound Dermatitis

A second type of burning with skin changes can be seen in women who have used topical steroids for prolonged periods, producing a rebound steroid dermatitis. The symptoms are usually described as an irritation that may be ameliorated by topical corticosteroids, but a rebound in pain and discomfort occurs upon discontinuation of the medication. These patients often have a history of recurrent *Candida* with the use of full-strength fluorinated topical steroids. Intercourse usually produces swelling and pain.

Diagnosis of Steroid Rebound Dermatitis

The vulva may be erythematous with telangiectasis. There may also be hyperplasia of the sebaceous glands and a papular rash on the labia majora (4).

Treatment of Steroid Rebound Dermatitis

Treatment consists of an oral anticandidal regimen prophylactically used while tapering off the topical steroids. Avoidance of all other topical medication is preferable.

Lichen Sclerosus

Symptoms of Lichen Sclerosus

The third skin condition producing burning or dyspareunia with visible skin changes is lichen sclerosus. The etiology of this condition is uncertain. The degree of itching and burning is variable. Dyspareunia is present if the skin becomes friable. Patients may describe a tearing and even bleeding at the introitus with penetration.

Diagnosis of Lichen Sclerosus

Examination of the vulva may reveal depigmentation, tissue friability, petechiae, introital narrowing, and resorption of the labia minora (5). This condition is easily diagnosed by an experienced clinician in its advanced forms, but should always be confirmed by biopsy. The thickest area of affected skin should be selected for biopsy.

Treatment of Lichen Sclerosus

Testosterone in petrolatum is no longer the treatment of choice. Greater relief with more rapid reversal of the skin changes is provided by clobetasol 0.05%. This should be applied twice a day for 1 month, once a day for 1 month, and then as needed (4,6).

VULVAR VESTIBULITIS

There are two common conditions that produce dyspareunia with little or no skin changes: vestibulitis and vaginismus. They often occur in the same patient. They remain undiagnosed unless Q-tip palpation of the vestibule and digital palpation of the pelvic floor muscles is compulsively performed in all patients with dyspareunia. Vulvodynia produced by these two conditions remains one of the greatest sources of misery for patients suffering with chronic pelvic pain. This etiology of dyspareunia is very often misdiagnosed, to the misfortune of many patients.

Etiology of Vestibulitis

The etiology of vulvar vestibulitis is probably multifactorial, but it may have a final common pathway. Among the agents thought to cause this condition are (a) infections, (b) irritants, (c) psychologic stress, and (d) neuropathic changes. This neuropathic mechanism could be the result of various traumas including chronic visceral pain. We now have evidence to support this change in the innervation of the minor vestibular glands. This neurogenic mechanism could be the thread that leads to a better understanding of this condition and vaginismus.

Recurrent candidal infections were once thought to predispose patients to vestibulitis. Probably this was related to the fact that most of these patients feel as if they have recurrent yeast infections with burning and painful intercourse. These presumed infections are reported as fact to their physicians. However, no relationship to positive wet preps or cultures can be established. Even attempts to desensitize patients to *Candida albicans* antigen were shown to have no effect (7). Bacterial and viral agents have been suggested, but no clear link has been established. The prevalence of herpes simplex and cytomegalovirus was nil. There was a flurry of interest in the greater than 50% association of HPV and vestibulitis (8,9). While the presence of HPV DNA in patients was common, there has been no correlation in treatment response rates and the virus is no longer thought to play an etiologic role (10).

The most commonly mentioned irritant in association with vestibulitis is calcium oxalate crystals. In 1991, Solomons et al. (11) reported a single patient who seemed to have exacerbations of vestibulitis corresponding to measured increases in urinary oxalate levels. It is a testimony to the desperation of these patients that from this one case report a cottage industry rapidly developed around the measurement of urinary oxalate and the prescription of timed administration of calcium citrate. We are indebted to this report for highlighting the paucity of scientific study. It also fueled the establishment of the "Vulvar Pain Foundation," a lay organization that has pressured the medical community to devote more attention to the diagnosis and treatment of vulvodynia. While calcium citrate and diet will reduce urinary oxalate absorption and excretion, Baggish demonstrated that a 3-month course of this regimen did not alter the symptoms of patients with the highest oxalate levels (12,13). The theory of sharp oxalate crystals causing severe burning on contact with the vestibule cannot be scientifically verified despite numerous patient testimonials. This is true of most of the treatments now employed for this condition.

There is no doubt that patients with vulvodynia from vestibulitis experience psychosexual dysfunction due to their severe dyspareunia. History of previous sexual abuse is thought to be higher in patients with chronic pelvic pain in general, but this has recently been questioned specifically for vestibulitis (14). The psychological stress of these patients was underscored by Jantos in a study that found depression in 89% (severe in 49%) and suicidal ideation in 57% of patients with chronic vestibulitis (15). This is likely more secondary than primary.

There is mounting evidence in support of vestibulitis as a neuropathic syndrome, with multiple initiators and neuropathy as the final common pathway. It may start with physiologic visceral or somatic pain and progress to hyperalgesia and allodynia. Sensitization of nerve endings may be peripheral or central. Nerve endings become increasingly responsive to both painful and innocuous stimuli (15). Noxious input can reflexly induce sympathetic activity that in turn activates somatic peripheral nerves. Several theories have been put forth to explain this phenomenon (16). It is known that prostaglandins, mediated through the nitric oxide system of neurotransmitters, are involved in production of this allodynia (17). Understanding these mechanisms will permit a more rational approach to treatment of this difficult condition and offers hope of moving away from empiricism.

Symptoms of Vestibulitis

Vestibulitis was first described by Skene as "focal vulvitis" over 100 years ago. In 1928, Howard Kelly noted the presence of "tender red spots on the vestibule making intercourse intolerable" (18). Friedrich (19) designated vulvar vestibulitis syndrome a subset of vulvodynia in 1987. He described the constellation of symptoms: (a) severe pain on vestibular touch or attempted vaginal entry, (b) tenderness to pressure localized to the vulvar vestibule, and (c) physical findings confined to various degrees of vestibular erythema. Skene had noted the same syndrome: "Pruritus was absent and external manifestations of disease lacking, but when the examining finger comes in contact with the hyperesthetic part, the patient complains of pain which is sometimes so great as to cause her to cry out" (19).

Onset of vestibulitis is usually abrupt and has been diagnosed as early as 14 years and as late as 65 years of age. The most typical patient is between the ages of 20 and 45 years (15). Patients may have great difficulty in describing their symptoms. Terms such as soreness, burning, dryness, rawness, deep irritation, and pressure might be used. Patients may say that they can't seem to clear up a yeast infection because other women or physicians suggested this possibility. Rarely will she describe itching. The discomfort almost never awakens her from sleep. Intercourse and speculum exams are always painful. Tight clothing, exercise, and prolonged sitting or walking may exacerbate her symptoms (15,20). Symptoms might vary with time of day, level of stress, or course of the menstrual cycle. Duration of symptoms vary from 6 months to more than 5 years (21).

Diagnosis of Vestibulitis

Patients are usually Caucasian and nulligravida. They may have other types of pelvic pain such as severe dysmenorrhea (with or without endometriosis), interstitial cystitis, vaginismus, abdominal wall trigger points, or painful adhesions. This lends credence to the neuropathic etiology of vestibulitis with central nervous system sensitization of peripheral nerve endings. In this case, segmental hyperesthesia of the pudendal nerve (S_{2-4}), which is the main innervation of the vestibule, may be produced by the other chronic pelvic pain.

The sine qua non of diagnosing vestibulitis by physical examination is the Q-tip test (Fig. 12.2). The importance of performing this simple maneuver on all patients with dyspareunia, chronic pelvic pain, or vague pelvic complaints cannot be overemphasized. While applying gentle tactile stimulation to specific areas of the vestibule, the patient can rate her discomfort. The vestibule is bounded superiorly by the clitoris and inferiorly by the posterior fourchette and fossa navicularis. It extends inward to the hymen, which delineates its border with the vagina, and laterally it extends from the hymenal ring to a line of more keratinized skin on the labia minora called Hart's line (22). Starting at 12 o'clock (just below the clitoris and above the urethra) and proceeding clockwise, the most tender areas may be at 4 and 8 o'clock at the opening of the Bartholin glands. Tender lesions should be mapped for each patient on a scale of 0 to 4 (a 4 will cause the patient to involuntarily move—"positive jump sign"). This system has been shown to be remarkably reproducible (21). Erythematous foci may or may not be present. This could be a result of localized prostaglandin release producing vasodilation. Biopsy of these lesions are not helpful and cause these patients unnecessary emotional and physical trauma. No pathognomonic histologic lesions are yet known.

Treatment of Vestibulitis

Approximately one-half of patients with vestibulitis will experience spontaneous remission of symptoms within the first 6 months of onset. However, as in most chronic pain, the rate of spontaneous remissions has an inverse relationship to duration (21). Due to the likelihood of spontaneous remission and lack of controlled studies, as well as the neuropathic nature of vestibulitis pain being affected by pain levels elsewhere in the pelvis, present treatment is largely anecdotal.

Treatments may be divided into oral, topical, injectable, and surgical. Treatment protocols should proceed from least to most invasive, making surgery the treatment of last resort.

Our treatment protocol begins with low-dose tricyclic antidepressants. Amitriptyline doses as low as 10 mg per day may be sufficient to give good relief. Doses up to 100 mg per day may be used, but patients may not tolerate the dry mouth, constipation, drowsiness, and weight gain of these higher doses. Most patients with vestibulitis are depressed. As in all neuropathic pain, it is extremely important to treat this aggressively. This can be accomplished by adding a selective serotonin reuptake inhibitor in the morning to the bedtime doses of amitriptyline.

Topically, we begin with acyclovir ointment massaged into the tender vestibular areas by the patient twice a day for a month. If pain mapping indicates improvement, then acyclovir is continued with frequent evaluations until cure or failure is apparent. Second-line topical treatment is with 5-flurouracil. One tablespoonful is left on the vestibule for 2 hours twice a week. Patients are instructed to wash thoroughly after the 2-hour application and to skip doses if soap and water begin to burn. They are cautioned to set a timer so as not to exceed 2 hours. Follow-up is the same as for acyclovir. The next line of therapy is a compounded gel of ketoprofen, carbamazepine, 5% lidocaine, and amitriptyline, used 4 to 6 times a day.

If topical therapy proves ineffective, intralesional injection of triamcinolone 20 mg (0.5 mL of triamcinolone solution mixed with 0.5 mL of 0.5% bupivicane) is begun. Before all vestibular injections, benzocaine ointment is applied for 15 minutes to decrease the pain of injections as much as possible. Patients are asked to return in 2 weeks to evaluate response. If improvement is noted, injections may be repeated up to three times every 2 weeks for maximum resolution. The next line of therapy in our treatment armamentarium is alpha-interferon. We inject at 1, 3, 4, 8, 9, and 11 o'clock a total of 2.5 million units (1 mL) in divided doses twice a week for 4 weeks. Remapping of the allodynia is done before benzocaine is applied for the eighth injection. If improvement is noted, repeat the treatment once a week for 4 weeks. Allow 2 weeks off before final evaluations to resolve tenderness from injections. This course of treatment is cost-effective before resorting to surgery (23). It has been our experience that approximately 20% response rate can be expected for each of these treatment modalities, so we proceed from least to most costly and invasive. Surgery is usually not required for relief of symptoms.

For surgical treatment, the vestibule is excised and the vaginal tissue is advanced to cover the defect (Fig. 12.4) (22,24,25). Success rates as high as 95% have been reported for vestibulectomy; but with long-term follow-up, success rates are lower. Baggish and Miklos (22) suggest removal of the Bartholin glands at the time of vestibulectomy (22). They also mention the use of the CO_2 laser for excision, but our experience with pudendal neuralgia after laser application to the vulva causes concern. Bornstein and co-workers (24,25) suggest either removal of the vestibular tissue above the urethra or injecting this area with alpha-interferon to decrease long-term failures. It is clear that vestibulectomy is effective, but is a treatment of last resort. If the patient is so unfortunate as to fail vestibulectomy, few options remain. Neuroma formation is a feared complication of this procedure and remains one of our most difficult challenges.

VAGINISMUS

Etiology of Vaginismus

Vaginismus is the other common condition that produces dyspareunia with little or no skin changes. It is produced by involuntary spasm of the pelvic floor musculature. It is also commonly referred to as pelvic myalgia. Fields (16) explains how impulses originating from distant structures (vestibulitis, endometriosis, interstitial cystitis, etc.) may cause the reflex activation of motoneurons, which produces muscle contraction and activation of muscle nociceptors. This spasm can also arise as a result of direct injury (vaginal delivery, surgery of pelvic floor, traumatic intercourse, etc.). Muscles most commonly involved are the pubococcygeus, piriformis, and obturator internus (Chapter 45).

Symptoms of Vaginismus

The most consistent complaint is penetration dyspareunia—that is, pain with vaginal entry. Pelvic aching after intercourse is common in patients with vaginismus. Sitting for long periods will aggravate this aching. If the piriformis is involved, pain will radiate into buttocks and down the posterior thigh, especially when walking up inclines or stairs.

Diagnosis of Vaginismus

Direct digital palpation of the muscle will illicit pain if spasm is present. Care must be taken to isolate each muscle on each side and to grade the spasm on a 1 to 4 scale depending on patient response.

Treatment of Vaginismus

The treatment of pelvic floor myalgia is twofold. First find and treat any persistent tissue injury that may be triggering the spasm (for example, endometriosis or interstitial cystitis). Second, begin muscle retraining with physical therapy. Patients can be instructed to perform pubococcygeus and piriformis stretching. Biofeedback can be useful in alleviating painful vestibulitis and vaginismus. Heat, exercise, and trigger point injections are also helpful adjuncts to full recovery (26,27).

PUDENDAL NEURALGIA

Dysesthetic vulvodynia, essential vulvodynia, and pudendal neuralgia are diagnostic terms applied when complaints are of constant burning of the vulva and the perineum is without skin changes. This affected area is bound laterally by the labiocrural fold, anteriorly by the mons pubis, and posteriorly by the anus and coccyx. This corresponds to the innervation of the cutaneous division of the pudendal nerve (S_{2-4}).

Etiology of Pudendal Neuralgia

The etiology of pudendal neuralgia may be divided into metabolic, traumatic, and idiopathic. The determinative factor is that the signaling mechanism of this motor and sensory nerve of the pelvic floor becomes abnormal or neuropathic. Diabetic neuropathy can produce this condition as well as multiple sclerosis and leprosy. Trauma from vaginal delivery, sacrospinous vaginal vault suspension, or aggressive colporrhaphy may produce injury. This can occur from suture ligature or scar entrapment. The etiology of many neuralgias remain obscure.

Symptoms of Pudendal Neuralgia

Constant burning pain is the typical complaint of patients with pudendal neuralgia. Characteristically, there is no dyspareunia with dysesthetic vulvodynia.

Diagnosis of Pudendal Neuralgia

Usually the patient has seen a number of physicians for this condition. Often she has been diagnosed with intractable yeast infections or told that the problem was "all in her head." This is due to the total absence of positive physical findings. These patients are more likely to be postmenopausal. They may have a history of a previous painful surgical procedure such as CO_2 laser vaporization of the vulva. On physical exam, there are no skin changes. The Q-tip test is negative. There may be a difference in tactile sensation between the right and left side. This could be hypoesthesia or hyperesthesia. Occasionally, patients report that perspiration exacerbates symptoms. Tight clothing may increase discomfort. Vaginismus is absent.

Treatment of Pudendal Neuralgia

Oral medications for neuropathic pain may be effective. The first drug of choice is amitriptyline. Starting at low doses, the medication is slowly pushed to tolerance or maximum benefit. If amitriptyline is not helpful, diphenylhydantoin, carbamazepine, gabapentin, divalproex sodium, tarazadone, pamelor, and sinequan should be tried separately. Care should be taken to observe all drug precautions and avoid harmful interactions in these sometimes elderly patients.

VULVAR NEUROMA

Vulvar neuroma is the most common cause of localized vulvodynia without skin changes or dyspareunia. A neuroma may be formed any time a nerve is interrupted distal to its cell body. The terminus of this nerve can be exquisitely sensitive and generate spontaneous action potentials, which are interpreted as pain.

Etiology of Vulvar Neuroma

Neuromas are caused by traumatic or iatrogenic transection of peripheral nerve fibers. Classic examples are straddle injuries in young girls and in the excisional scar of a patient undergoing vestibulectomy.

Symptoms of Vulvar Neuroma

Patients can be in all age groups. If there is no history of vulvar surgery, careful questioning may bring to mind an injury suffered long before the symptoms occurred. The patient will usually describe a deep pain of gradual onset becoming more intense with time. The pain is unilateral without dyspareunia. Exercise or prolonged sitting aggravates the pain. Tight clothing is uncomfortable due to the development of hyperalgesia.

Diagnosis of Vulvar Neuroma

The sine qua non of a neuroma is point tenderness that duplicates the pain. Frequently, a tiny nodule is palpable in the soft tissue, and most often patients can put their finger right on this area.

Treatment of Vulvar Neuroma

Currently, there is no reliable efficacious treatment that will ensure no recurrence. Cryotherapy, chemical ablation, surgical resection, and radiofrequency ablation have been tried with mixed results.

KEY POINTS

Differential Diagnosis

- Recurrent Candidiasis
- Skin disorder: steroid rebound, lichen sclerosus, irritant or contact allergy
- Neuropathic: vestibulitis, vaginismus, pudendal neuralgia

Most Important Questions

- Is there itching?
- Is there burning pain?
- Is the pain deep?
- Is penetration of the vagina painful? Is there pain with initial entry?
- Is pain aggravated by perspiration, semen, tight clothing, or sitting?
- Is there pelvic aching after intercourse?
- Is there a history of bacterial infections requiring antibiotics?
- Is there diabetes mellitus?
- Is there a history of previous vulvar surgery or trauma?

Most Important Physical Examination Findings

- Vulvar erythema, edema, fissuring, sebaceous hyperplasia, telangiectasis, papular rash, scaling, or pustules
- Whitening of the skin with loss of vulvar architecture
- Focal erythema of minor vestibular gland
- Q-tip test
- Pelvic floor muscle palpation
- Small tender nodule in the soft tissue, palpation of which duplicates the patient's pain

Most Important Diagnostic Studies

- Wet preps and cultures
- Biopsy of possible lichen sclerosus
- Grading vestibular and muscle tenderness on a scale of 0 to 4

Treatments

- Candidiasis: long-term suppression with oral agents
- Steroid rebound dermatitis: gradual withdrawal of topical steroids while maintaining oral anticandidal therapy
- Lichen sclerosus: Clobetasol
- Vestibulitis: topicals, injectables, biofeedback, and surgery

- Vaginismus: physical therapy, trigger point injections, and biofeedback
- Vulvar neuroma: neuropathic medications, cryotherapy, chemical ablation, radiofrequency ablation, and surgical resection

REFERENCES

1. Burning vulva syndrome: report of the ISSVD task force. *J Reprod Med* 1984;29:457.
2. McKay M. Vulvodynia: diagnostic patterns. *Dermatol Clin* 1992; 10:423–433.
3. Jones KD, Lehr ST. Vulvodynia: diagnostic techniques and treatment modalities. *Nurse Pract* 1994;4:34–46.
4. McKay M. Vulvodynia. In: Steege JF, Metzger DA, Levy B, eds. *Chronic pelvic pain: An integrated approach,* 1st ed. Philadelphia: WB Saunders, 1998:188–196.
5. McKay M. Vulvodynia versus pruritus vulvae. *Clinical Obstet Gynecol* 1985;28:123–133.
6. Bornstein J, Heifetz S, Kellner Y, et al. Clobetasol dipropionate 0.05% versus testosterone propionate 2% topical application for severe vulvar lichen sclerosus. *Am J Obstet Gynecol* 1998;178:80–84.
7. Marinoff SC, Turner MLC. Hypersensitivity to vaginal candidiasis of treatment vehicles in the pathogenesis of minor vestibular gland syndrome. *J Reprod Med* 1986;31:796–799.
8. Turner MLC, Marinoff SC. Association of human papillomavirus with vulvodynia and the vulvar vestibulitis syndrome. *J Reprod Med* 1988;33:533–537.
9. Bornstein J, Shapiro S, Rahat M, et al. Polymerase chain reaction search for viral etiology of vulvar vestibulitis syndrome. *Am J Obstet Gynecol* 1996;175:139–144.
10. Bornstein J, Shapiro S, Goldshmid N, et al. Severe vulvar vestibulitis: relation to HPV infection. *J Reprod Med* 1997;42: 514–518.
11. Solomons CC, Melmed MH, Heitler SM. Calcium citrate for vulvar vestibulitis: a case report. *J Reprod Med* 1991;36:879–882.
12. Massey LK, Roman-Smith H, Sutton RAL. Effect of dietary oxalate and calcium on urinary oxalate and risk of formation of calcium oxalate kidney stones. *J Am Diet Assoc* 1993;93: 901–906.
13. Baggish MS, Sze EHM, Johnson R. Urinary oxalate excretion and its role in vulvar pain syndrome. *Am J Obstet Gynecol* 1997; 177:507–511.
14. Edwards L, Mason M, Phillips M, et al. Childhood sexual and physical abuse: incidence in patients with vulvodynia. *J Reprod Med* 1997;42:135–139.
15. Jantos M, White G. The vestibulitis syndrome: medical and psychosexual assessment of a cohort of patients. *J Reprod Med* 1997;42:145–152.
16. Fields HL. *Pain,* 1st ed. New York: McGraw-Hill, 1987:82–95.
17. Minami T, Nishihara I, Seiji I, et al. Nitric oxide mediates allodynia induced by intrathecal administration of prostaglandin E_2 or prostaglandin F_2 in conscious mice. *Pain* 1995;61:285–290.
18. Marinoff SC, Turner MLC. Vulvar vestibulitis syndrome: an overview. *Am J Obstet Gynecol* 1991;165:1228–1233.
19. Friedrich EG. Vulvar vestibulitis syndrome. *J Reprod Med* 1987; 32:110–114.
20. Lynch PJ. Vulvodynia: a syndrome of unexplained vulvar pain, psychologic disability and sexual dysfunction: the 1985 ISSVD presidential address. *J Reprod Med* 1986;31:773–780.
21. Peckham BM, Maki DG, Patterson JJ, et al. Focal vulvitis: a characteristic syndrome and cause of dyspareunia: features, natural history, and management. *Am J Obstet Gynecol* 1986;154:855–864.

22. Baggish MS, Miklos JR. Vulvar pain syndrome: a review. *Obstet Gynecol Surv* 1995;50:618–627.

23. Marinoff SC, Turner ML, Hirsch RP, et al. Intralesional alpha interferon: cost-effective therapy for vulvar vestibulitis. *J Reprod Med* 1993;38:19–24.

24. Bornstein J, Goldik Z, Alter Z, et al. Persistent vulvar vestibulitis: the continuing challenge. *Obstet Gynecol Surv* 1997;53:39–44.

25. Bornstein J, Abramovici H. Combination of subtotal perineoplasty and interferon for the treatment of vulvar vestibulitis. *Gynecol Obstet Invest* 1997;44:53–56.

26. White G, Jantos M, Glazer H. Establishing the diagnosis of vulvar vestibulitis. *J Reprod Med* 1997;42:157–160.

27. Costello K. Myofascial syndromes. In: Steege JF, Metzger DA, Levy BS, eds. *Chronic pelvic pain: an integrated approach,* 1st ed. Philadelphia: WB Saunders, 1998:251–266.

22

CARCINOMA OF THE COLON

JAMES E. CARTER

KEY TERMS AND DEFINITIONS

Colorectal carcinoma: Cancer of the large intestine or rectum; the second most common cause of cancer deaths in the United States.

Colorectal polyp: A grossly visible protrusion from the mucosal surface that may be classified pathologically as a nonneoplastic hamartoma (juvenile polyp), a hyperplastic mucosal proliferation (hyperplastic polyp), or an adenomatous polyp; only adenomas are clearly premalignant.

INTRODUCTION

Cancer of the colon or rectum can cause chronic lower abdominal pain in women, although it is not a common diagnosis in women with chronic pelvic pain (CPP) (1). For example, Demco found one case in 100 patients undergoing laparoscopic evaluation for CPP (2). Most series of CPP patients report no cases. Because of this it is not often considered in the differential diagnosis of women with CPP, an oversight that is occasionally quite detrimental to the unfortunate woman with colorectal carcinoma.

Cancer of the large bowel is second only to lung cancer as a cause of cancer deaths in the United States. Colorectal cancers display regional differences within the United States, with the highest incidence in the Northeast. The incidence of this disease varies from 3.5 per 100,000 in India to 32.3 per 100,000 in Connecticut (3). The occurrence of colorectal cancer starts to rise sharply after the age of 40 years and is most common in individuals 50 years of age or older (4). However, it can also occur in the third or fourth decade.

ETIOLOGY AND PATHOLOGY

Most colorectal cancers are believed to arise from adenomatous polyps. A polyp is a grossly visible protrusion from the mucosal surface and may be classified pathologically as a

nonneoplastic hamartoma (juvenile polyp), a hyperplastic mucosal proliferation (hyperplastic polyp), or an adenomatous polyp. Only adenomas are clearly premalignant, and only a minority of these lesions ever develop into cancer. Adenomatous polyps are found in the colons of about 30% of middle-aged or elderly people. Fewer than 1% of polyps ever become malignant. Most polyps produce no symptoms and remain clinically undetected. Occult blood in the stool may be found in fewer than 5% of patients with such lesions.

The risk factors for the development of colorectal cancer include diet, especially diets very high in animal fat and low in fiber; hereditary syndromes (autosomal dominant inheritance) such as polyposis coli, and nonpolyposis syndrome; inflammatory bowel disease; *Streptococcus bovis* bacteremia; and possibly tobacco use. The available data strongly associate a high intake of animal fat with the development of large bowel cancer.

Therefore, both inherited predisposition and environmental factors seem to be implicated in carcinogenesis in the colon and rectum. In countries with a high incidence of colon cancer, the average fat content in the diet is about 40% of total calories, in contrast to the dietary fat content of 15% to 20% or less of total calories in countries with a low cancer incidence. Fat in the colon increases biliary sterol excretion, leading to increase colonic epithelial proliferation, modification of cell membranes, and stimulation of the synthesis of prostaglandins that induce cellular proliferation. Dietary fiber appears to reduce colonic carcinogenesis by diluting and binding carcinogens in the lumen, by modifying colonic bacterial flora, and by acidifying the colonic lumen by short-chain fatty acids. Anticarcinogens found in fruits and vegetables (indoles, thioethers, dithiothiones, retinoids) may play a factor in protecting against carcinoma of the colon.

The vast majority of colorectal cancers are adenocarcinomas. The tumors exhibit varying degrees of glandular differentiation and produce variable amounts of mucin. Grossly, they may be divided into two major groups: polypoid and annular constricting lesions. The polypoid lesion is most commonly found on the right side, and the annular constricting lesion is more common on the left side of the colon. Adenocarcinomas of the rectum may be sessile or polypoid. Seventy-five percent of colorectal cancers occur in the descending colon, rectosigmoid, and rectum. The cecum and ascending colon are involved in 15%, and the transverse colon is involved in 10%. Carcinoma of the colon spreads by direct extension through the wall of the bowel and into the pericolic fat and mesentery, by invasion of surrounding organs, by way of lymphatic to the regional lymph nodes, and via the portal vein to the liver. Additionally, the tumor may spread throughout the peritoneal cavity and to the lungs and bones.

SYMPTOMS

The major symptoms of colorectal cancer are rectal bleeding, pain, and change in bowel habits. Of patients with colorectal carcinoma, 74% were with a change in bowel habits, 65% with abdominal pain, and 51% with rectal bleeding (1). Pain with left-sided cancers is usually colicky and increased after meals. Those on the right side are often asymptomatic or present with vague symptoms, and bleeding may be occult. Tumors of the cecum and ascending colon rarely obstruct early. Changes in bowel habit (with reduction in stool caliber or progressive constipation) and hematochezia are more common with left-sided lesions. Constipation alternating with increased frequency of stools may also occur, which occasionally leads to an initial erroneous diagnosis of irritable bowel syndrome. Adenocarcinomas of the colon may present with a localized perforation and with signs of peritonitis. An abdominal mass or symptoms and signs of liver metastasis may be the earliest clinical manifestations of the underlying colorectal cancer.

Colorectal cancer must be suspected when patients present with rectal bleeding, a change in bowel habits, a decrease in stool caliber, iron deficiency anemia, or unexplained abdominopelvic pain. Such symptoms are especially worrisome if there is also a history of prior removal of an adenoma or a cancer, previous or present inflammatory bowel disease, or a family history of one of the inherited colorectal cancer syndromes.

SIGNS

Adenocarcinomas of the colon may present with signs of peritonitis due to perforation. An abdominal mass or hepatomegaly due to liver metastasis may be one of the earliest clinical manifestations of an underlying colorectal cancer. A digital rectal examination is essential in determining the presence of a distal rectal cancer or of a perineal or pelvic spread. Stool is often positive for blood by guiaic or hemoccult testing.

DIAGNOSTIC STUDIES

Laboratory tests may reveal iron deficiency anemia or an abnormality of liver enzymes. Radiologic studies should include a chest x-ray or computerized tomography (CT) scan of the abdomen and pelvis. The digital rectal exam is followed by colonoscopy or double-contrast barium enema following sigmoidoscopy.

DIAGNOSIS

The major differential diagnoses include hemorrhoids, angiodysplasia, diverticulosis, and other benign and malignant gastrointestinal tumors. Although imaging and endoscopic studies may be very suggestive, histologic confirmation with colonoscopic biopsies clearly establishes the diagnosis of colorectal cancer.

MANAGEMENT OR TREATMENT

The most important goal of treatment for primary malignancies of the colon and rectum is complete removal. Surgical resection of the affected segment, including omentum and lymph nodes, is performed. Radiation therapy plays an important role in the postoperative management of rectal cancer. The combination of radiation and chemotherapy, 5-fluorouracil, is standard therapy and reduces local recurrence and distant metastasis (3,4).

Aspirin and other nonsteroidal antiinflammatory drugs, which are thought to suppress cell proliferation by inhibiting prostaglandin synthesis, reduce the risk of colonic adenomas and carcinomas as well as death from large bowel cancer. Diets rich in fruits and vegetables are associated with lower rates of colorectal cancer. Estrogen replacement therapy has been associated in prospective cohort studies with the reduction in the risk of colorectal cancer in women, conceivably by an effect on bioacid synthesis and composition (4).

KEY POINTS
Differential Diagnosis

- Hemorrhoids
- Angiodysplasia
- Diverticulosis
- Other benign and malignant tumors

Most Important Question to Ask

- Has there been a change in bowel habits, abdominal or pelvic pain, and/or rectal bleeding?

Most Important Physical Examination Finding

■ Digital examination and test of stool for occult blood

Most Important Diagnostic Study

■ Colonoscopy

Treatments

■ Surgical resection, radiation, and 5-flourouracil

REFERENCES

1. McSherry CK, Cornell GN, Glenn F. Carcinoma of the colon and rectum. *Ann Surg* 1969;169:502–509.
2. Demco LA. Effect on negative laparoscopy rate in chronic pelvic pain patients using patient assisted laparoscopy. *J Soc Laparoendosc Surg* 1997;1:319–321.
3. Levin B. Neoplasms of the large and small intestines. In: Bennett JC, Plum F, eds. *Cecil textbook of medicine,* vol 1. Philadelphia: WB Saunders, 1996:721–728.
4. Mayer RJ. Gastrointestinal tract cancer. In: Fauci AS, Braunwald E, Isselbacher KJ, et al, eds. *Harrison's principles of internal medicine,* vol 1. New York: McGraw-Hill, 1998:568–578.

23

CHRONIC INTERMITTENT BOWEL OBSTRUCTION

C. PAUL PERRY

KEY TERMS AND DEFINITIONS

Dysmotility: Abnormal peristalsis and evacuation of the bowel.

Ileus: Obstruction of the intestines from lack of motility (adynamic) or occlusion (dynamic).

Obstipation: Intractable lack of bowel evacuation.

Pseudoobstruction: A disorder of intestinal contents propulsion due to a disturbance in the small bowel and colonic myoelectric activity.

INTRODUCTION

Chronic pelvic pain may be produced by a number of conditions affecting bowel motility. With normal motility a cyclic pattern occurs every 2 hours. It begins in the stomach and migrates in an orderly fashion along the entire small intestine. This is called the interdigestive migrating complex. Feeding interrupts this cycle and establishes a postprandial pattern of intermittent contractions that depends upon the nutrient and caloric content of the meal (1). Any pathology disturbing this pattern may produce ileus and pain. To produce chronic pelvic pain, this condition must be recurrent, be perceived low in the abdomen or pelvis, and be limited to incomplete disruption of bowel function. Intermittent bowel obstruction, dynamic or adynamic, is this sort of condition.

ETIOLOGY

Intermittent bowel obstruction may be produced by extrinsic or intrinsic pathology. Extrinsic factors, in order of decreasing frequency, include adhesions, inflammatory lesions, herniation, and neoplasms (2). Intrinsic pathology includes dysmotility with irritable bowel syndrome and chronic intestinal pseudoobstruction.

Extrinsic Pathology

Most commonly a patient with pain due to intermittent bowel obstruction has a luminal compromise from an adhesive band. The bowel becoming entrapped by fibrosis from previous surgery usually produces this. A congenital abnormality such as a persistent omphalomesenteric ligament may rarely produce intermittent obstruction (3). The distinction between partial and complete small bowel obstruction is based upon established clinical criteria. Implied in the clinical diagnosis of partial obstruction is the expectation that there may be resolution without emergent surgical intervention (4).

Inflammatory lesions such as Crohn's disease and diverticulitis are well known to present as chronic pelvic pain in women. Especially in the early stages of Crohn's disease, before bloody diarrhea has become a prominent symptom, intermittent cramping may be attributable to the reproductive tract. Diverticulitis may produce sufficient inflammation to partially obstruct the bowel. Left-lower-quadrant chronic pelvic pain is frequently the presenting complaint in older women with diverticulitis.

Herniation of the bowel with intermittent obstruction may be an uncommon cause of chronic pelvic pain. Indirect and direct inguinal hernias and femoral hernias have all been implicated. Spigelian hernias of the anterior abdominal wall may occur at the lateral edge of the rectus muscle in the transversalis fascia. Pain produced from intermittent bowel entrapment is often diffuse and poorly localized (5). The referred component of this visceral pain is to the same dermatomes as referred pain from the reproductive tract, making the diagnosis difficult at times.

Neoplasms are responsible for some episodes of intermittent obstruction. Leiomyomata of the small bowel may present with intermittent pain and obstruction. Occasionally, the tumor may drop into the pelvis and present as a pelvic mass. Neoplastic lesions such as colon, ovarian, and bladder cancer can produce partial intermittent obstruction of the small or large bowel (6). Nausea, vomiting, and pain are present at varying degrees depending upon what portion of the bowel is involved (7).

The ileum is an area of bowel that seems especially vulnerable to partial obstruction when advanced endometriosis is present. Bowel involvement by endometriosis is thought to occur in 12% to 37% of cases. Small bowel is less likely to be obstructed (7%) than colon. The terminal ileum is the major locus for this cyclic luminal narrowing which produces right-lower-quadrant pain and sometimes nausea and vomiting. Patients have difficulty distinguishing this pain from menstrual cramping (8).

Intrinsic Pathology

Symptoms of intermittent bowel obstruction can originate with intrinsic abnormalities of bowel motility (dysmotility). The most common condition of this type is irritable bowel syndrome. Although it is thought to be a pathologic disturbance of the large bowel, the small bowel function may also be abnormal. This condition affects women of all ages, but is especially common in the younger women experiencing school or career stresses. It may often be a component of complex pelvic pain syndromes such as endometriosis, vestibulitis, and pelvic floor myalgia. There are two distinct patterns: constipation-dominant and diarrhea-dominant. The small bowel dysmotility is most often seen in the patient complaining of multiple loose stools per day (diarrhea-dominant) (9). These patients will have intermittent sharp abdominal and pelvic pain with bloating (Chapter 28).

A less common and more difficult to diagnose abnormality of small bowel motility is chronic intestinal pseudoobstruction (CIP). This is a disorder of the propulsion of intestinal contents caused by a disturbance in the intestinal or colonic myoelectric activity (10). CIP is actually a spectrum of dysmotilities, which give rise to symptoms mimicking bowel obstruction. Obstipation may result from colonic involvement. Two types of CIP have been described: a myogenic and a neurogenic form. Decreased frequency and intensity of intestinal contractions distinguish the myogenic type. The neurogenic type has normal amplitude and frequency, but the contractions are disorganized and nonperistaltic. These patients experience recurrent bouts of abdominal swelling, pain, nausea, and vomiting. The painful episodes are not related to eating and are usually severe. The dysmotility will often promote bacterial overgrowth; when this occurs, symptoms may begin to follow meals (11).

SYMPTOMS

Sharp, intermittent, unilateral or bilateral, lower abdominopelvic pain, nausea, and abdominal bloating are the most common symptoms of intermittent bowel obstruction. The patient may describe sudden pain that "almost brings me to my knees." The dysmotility class of patients experience a more gradual onset sometimes rising to a crescendo of cramp. A positive relationship between pain sequence and meals is important to elicit. A history of constipation, as defined as a decrease in the usual frequency of bowel movements, will help delineate the constipation dominant type of irritable bowel.

A history of cyclic pain related to menses is strongly suggestive of some hormonal exacerbation. Endometriosis is highly likely to be an associated condition, especially if premenstrual dysmenorrhea is present.

EXAMINATION

Peritoneal signs are usually absent in the early phases. If the symptoms are sufficiently sporadic, abdominal and pelvic examinations will be normal. Tenderness over the cecum and rectosigmoid is a suspicious sign for bowel etiology. Bowel sounds may vary from hyperactive to hypoactive, depending on the pathology. In the partial mechanically obstructed patient, pain is accompanied by audible high-pitched bowel sounds.

DIAGNOSIS

Chronic intermittent bowel obstruction may be difficult to diagnose between attacks. Gastrointestinal endoscopy and laparoscopy may serve a limited role. They are mainly reserved to rule in or out other associated pathology. Flat plate x-ray of the abdomen with upright view can distinguish complete, versus partial, bowel obstructions by the presence of dilated loops of small bowel and the absence or presence of gas in the colon. Contrast studies such as barium enema and small bowel follow-through x-rays are often diagnostic of inflammatory bowel diseases. When pelvic masses are palpable, ultrasound exams can be diagnostic for extrinsic obstruction etiologies. Computerized axial tomography (CAT) scan or magnetic resonance imaging (MRI) may augment the workup when necessary.

Dysmotility disorders are diagnosed by exclusion. The history and lack of positive findings on the above studies suggest their presence as etiologies for the chronic pelvic pain. Motility studies can be used to confirm this diagnosis. A therapeutic trial for irritable bowel syndrome may be helpful.

TREATMENT

Although episodes of acute intermittent partial bowel obstruction should be treated conservatively, prevention of recurrence requires the location and amelioration of the intestinal narrowing. Adhesion formation from previous surgery is the most common surgical finding. Patients with previous laparotomies should be approached laparoscopically only after a thorough decompression of the bowel. A preoperative mechanical bowel preparation is necessary to decrease the risk of postoperative complications. A left-upper-quadrant approach may be the best to prevent entry injuries.

Laparotomy is sometimes required to adequately run the bowel. Strictures may be subtle, and tactile confirmation cannot be underestimated. Hernias can sometimes be diagnosed and repaired laparoscopically, but transperitoneal laparotomy remains the gold standard. Medical treatment for intermittent bowel obstruction by endometriosis is at best temporizing, and a resection of the affected intestine will be necessary. Neoplastic extrinsic obstruction is relieved by tumor resection and bowel diversion as necessary.

Functional dysmotility is treated with an irritable bowel regimen (Chapter 28). Medications required will depend on whether the constipation-dominant or diarrhea-dominant type is present. CIP may require parenteral nutrition or small bowel transplant (10).

KEY POINTS

Differential Diagnosis

- Discriminate between partial and complete obstruction.
- Discriminate between mechanical and dysmotility obstruction.
- Discriminate between extrinsic and intrinsic mechanical obstruction.
- Discriminate between congenital and acquired mechanical obstruction.

Most Important Questions to Ask

- Is the pain constant or intermittent?
- Are the symptoms related to the menstrual cycle?
- Is the location constant?
- Are the pains sharp or dull?
- Are the pains more frequent after meals?
- Is there associated nausea or vomiting?
- Is there associated painful premenstrual dysmenorrhea?
- Is diarrhea or constipation present?

Most Important Physical Examination Findings

- Presence of pelvic mass
- Right-lower-quadrant or left-lower-quadrant tenderness

- Positive blood in the stool
- Hyperactive bowel sounds in association with painful episode
- Hard palpable stool in the colon

Most Important Diagnostic Studies

- Flat and upright x-rays of the abdomen
- Barium enema or small bowel follow-through
- Pelvic ultrasound for mass
- Lower bowel endoscopy
- CAT scan or MRI of abdomen and pelvis
- Bowel motility studies
- Laparoscopy

Treatments

- Surgical alleviation of bowel compromise
- Medical treatment of dysmotility

REFERENCES

1. Cullen JJ, Caropreso DK, Hemann LL, et al. Pathophysiology of adynamic ileus. *Dig Dis Sci* 1997;42:731–737.
2. Raf LE. Causes of small intestinal obstruction. *Acta Chir Scand* 1969;135:67–72.
3. Perry CP. Recognition and treatment of persistent omphalomesenteric ligament: a report of two cases. *J Reprod Med* 1990;35:636–638.
4. Brolin RE. Partial small bowel obstruction. *Surgery* 1984;95:145–149.
5. Daoud I. General surgical aspects. In: Steege JF, Metzger DA, Levy B, eds. *Chronic pelvic pain: an integrated approach* 1st ed. Philadelphia: WB Saunders, 1998:329–336.
6. Krebs HB, Goplerud DR. Mechanical intestinal obstruction in patients with gynecologic disease: a review of 368 patients. *Am J Obstet Gynecol* 1987;157:577–583.
7. Martorell RA. Jejunal obstructions. *Am Surg* 1960;126:481–484.
8. Rubio MG, Fernandez R, De Cuenca B, et al. *Am J Gastroenterol* 1997;92:525–526.
9. Kellow JE, Phillips SF, Miller LJ, et al. Dysmotility of the small intestine in irritable bowel syndrome. *Gut* 1988;29:1236–1243.
10. Papadatou B, Ferretti F, Gambarara M, et al. Clinical heterogeneity of chronic intestinal pseudo-obstruction. *Transplant Proc* 1997;29:1872–1873.
11. Whitehead WE. Gastrointestinal disorders. In: Steege JF, Metzger DA, Levy B, eds. *Chronic pelvic pain: an integrated approach*. Philadelphia: WB Saunders, 1998:205–206.

24

COLITIS

JAMES E. CARTER

KEY TERMS AND DEFINITIONS

Infectious enterocolitis: Intestinal infection that causes pain and diarrhea due to either the infectious organism or a released toxin or both.

Pseudomembranous colitis: A toxin induced inflammatory process due to *Clostridium difficile*, characterized by exudative plaques or pseudomembranes attached to the surface of the inflamed colonic mucosa.

Ulcerative colitis: An inflammatory disease of the mucosa of the colon or rectum that is of unknown etiology.

INTRODUCTION

Ulcerative colitis is an inflammatory disease of the mucosa of the colon that is of unknown etiology. It generally presents with acute pain and diarrhea, but can go undiagnosed for years and thus present as chronic pelvic pain (CPP). Ulcerative colitis is discussed in detail in Chapter 27.

Infectious enterocolitis also presents most commonly as acute abdominopelvic pain and diarrhea; but as with ulcerative colitis, if it is neglected the infected woman may present with CPP and chronic diarrhea. Infectious enterocolitis may occur at all ages. Pseudomembranous colitis due to *Clostridium difficile* is a particularly virulent type of colitis found in hospitalized patients or in those on antibiotic therapy.

ETIOLOGY AND PATHOLOGY

The etiologic agent of pseudomembranous colitis, *Clostridium difficile*, may be detected in the colonic flora of 3% to 5% of healthy adults and it is widely distributed in our environment, including soil and water. It is especially common in hospitals and nursing homes, where as many as 20% to 30% of patients who have received antibiotics may be asymptomatic carriers and where spread of the organism from people who have colitis to others treated with antibiotics is likely to occur (1).

Growth of the organism is promoted by poorly understood antibody-induced alterations in the normal intestinal flora (2). The disease is caused by the elaboration of two or more toxins during growth of *C. difficile*. The inflammatory and secretory effects of toxin A of *C. difficile* involve intrinsic neural pathways. Through these pathways, toxin A leads to mast-cell degranulation and the secretion of multiple inflammatory mediators (3,4).

Enterocolitis is commonly caused by *Vibrio cholerae* or enteropathic *Escherichia coli*. However, both of these organisms lead to explosive diarrhea with massive loss of intestinal fluid, so they are rarely, if ever, a source of CPP. Other organisms, such as salmonella, shigella, *E. coli,* and *Campylobacter*, may produce crampy lower abdominal pain and mucoid stools. Thus in some women they may occasionally be a source of CPP. Tuberculosis of the intestinal tract is uncommon in the United States. However, with the recent resurgence of tuberculosis, it may become a more common problem and cause of CPP in women.

SYMPTOMS AND HISTORY

Most patients with infectious entercolitis present with crampy abdominopelvic pain and watery or multiple mucoid stools. Rectal burning is also common. About 33% have bloody stools, and up to 40% may have fever.

Pseudomembranous colitis may begin as early as 1 day after initiation of antibiotic therapy or as late as 6 weeks after it has been discontinued. The most frequent symptoms are profuse watery diarrhea and cramping abdominal pain. The patients may also have a fever and leukocytosis (5).

Gastrointestinal tuberculosis usually presents with nonspecific chronic abdominopelvic pain and diarrhea that is intermittent. History of a fever is uncommon (6).

SIGNS AND PHYSICAL EXAMINATION

With tuberculosis of the gastrointestinal tract a right lower quadrant mass may be palpable. Mild to moderate tenderness is usually present with all types of infectious enterocolitis. With psedomembranous colitis, however, lower abdominal tenderness is sometimes quite marked. Rebound tenderness is not characteristic, but may occasionally be noted, particularly with pseudomembranous colitis (5). Bowel sounds are generally hyperactive.

DIAGNOSTIC STUDIES

With infectous entercolitides, microscopic examination of stool samples reveals multiple polymorponuclear leukocytes and red blood cells. Stool cultures may be used to identify the etiologic organism. Tuberculosis may be more difficult to isolate, and endoscopic biopsies may be needed to confirm the diagnosis. A chest x-ray showing active disease is also presumptive supportive evidence (6).

With pseudomembranous colitis, testing for fecal leukocytes has a sensitivity of 30% to 50%, and a positive test rules out benign or simple antibiotic diarrhea. A stool culture for *C. difficile* is not diagnostic because 10% to 25% of patients in hospitals may carry the organism and only 75% of isolates produce toxins. The gold standard is to test for the presence of fecal toxins such as the cytopathic effect of toxin B in tissue cultures. This is time-consuming, expensive, and not widely available. The test for toxin A by enzyme-linked immunosorbent assay (ELISA) is rapid, widely available, and relatively inexpensive. The sensitivity varies, however, and may only be fair. False positives may be a problem. The latex agglutination test for *C. difficile* is rapid and inexpensive, but also has many false positives and false negatives. Radiologic studies such as plain film of the abdomen, barium enema, and computerized tomography shows primarily nonspecific findings (2). Flexible sigmoidoscopy is the most rapid way to make the diagnosis, but is expensive and misses about 10% of cases. Biopsy of minor or nonspecific lesions increases the yield. Colonoscopy is a rapid and most sensitive way to make the diagnosis, but again it is expensive and may be hazardous. *C. difficile* toxin-induced colitis can mimic the endoscopic appearance of ulcerative colitis or Crohn's disease.

Rarely, a patient with tuberculosis may have stenosis or fistula formation. Abdominal computerized tomography with radiographic contrast material will generally demonstrate these findings if they are present.

DIAGNOSIS

Colitis is usually distinguished from other potential causes of CPP by the presence of diarrhea. In an occasional patient it may be confused with irritable bowel syndrome. Conversely, many patients with irritable bowel syndrome present with a history of having been diagnosed as having chronic colitis. Positive cultures, fecal leukocytes and red blood cells, and positive tests for toxins generally establish the diagnosis. Tuberculosis is diagnosed by positive skin testing, abnormal chest or abdominal x-ray findings, positive stool cultures, and biopsies confirming the presence of tuberculous bacilli.

The differential diagnosis for pseudomembranous colitis includes acute and chronic diarrhea caused by other enteric pathogens, an adverse reaction to medications other than antibiotics, idiopathic inflammatory bowel diseases, and intraabdominal sepsis.

MANAGEMENT OR TREATMENT

For the rare patient with CPP associated with infectious enterocolitis, antibiotic sensitivity testing of the cultured organism allows specific, definitive antibiotic therapy.

For pseudomembranous colitis, discontinuing all antimicrobial agents is desirable. Replacing fluid and electrolyte losses may resolve symptoms without further specific therapy. Antiperistaltic drugs are best avoided because they may cause worsening of the illness. Therapy with metronidazole or vancomycin is usually given for about 7 to 10 days, using antibiotics orally to prevent the organism from growing and producing toxins. Metronidazole 250 or 500 mg four times a day is usually successful in the treatment, but occasional isolates of *C. difficile* are resistant to this treatment. For seriously ill patients, vancomycin 125 to 500 mg orally four times a day for 7 to 14 days is active against virtually all isolates of *C. difficile*.

KEY POINTS
Differential Diagnosis

- Infectious enterocolitis
- Tuberculosis
- Pseudomembanous colitis
- Adverse reaction to medications other than antibiotics
- Inflammatory bowel diseases
- Irritable bowel syndrome

Most Important Questions to Ask

- Do you have diarrhea or frequent loose or mucoid stools?
- Have you been on antibiotic therapy recently?

Most Important Physical Examination Findings

- Tender lower abdomen

- Hyperactive bowel sounds
- Right-lower-quadrant mass

Most Important Diagnostic Studies

- Stools for leukocytes and red blood cells
- Stools for culture, ova, parasites, and toxins
- Sigmoidoscopy or colonoscopy

Treatment

- Appropriate antibiotics

REFERENCES

1. Waler KJ, Gilliland SS, Vance-Bryan K. *Clostridium difficile* colonization in residents of long term care facilities: prevalence in risk factors. *J Am Geriatr Soc* 1993;41:9–40.
2. Fekety R. Pseudomembranous colitis. In: Bennett JC, Plum F, eds. *Cecil textbook of medicine,* vol 2. Philadelphia: WB Saunders, 1996:1633–1635.
3. Vanner S, Jiang MM, Suprenant A. Mucosal stimulation evokes vasodilatation in submucosal arterioles by neuronal and non-neuronal mechanisms. *Am J Physiol* 1993;264:G202–G212.
4. Goyal RK, Hirano I. The enteric nervous system. *N Engl J Med* 1996;334:1106–1115.
5. Kelly CP, Pothoulakis C, Lamont JT. *Clostridium difficile* colitis. *N Engl J Med* 1994;330:257–262.
6. Rapkin AJ, Mayer EA. Gastroenterologic causes of chronic pelvic pain. *Obstet Gynecol Clinics North Am* 1993;20:663–683.

25

CONSTIPATION

AHMED M. EL-MINAWI

KEY TERMS AND DEFINITIONS

Chagas' disease: An infection caused by Trypanosoma cruzi, and endemic in South America, that may cause constipation via destruction of the myenteric plexus of the distal colon and rectum.

Colonis dysmotility or inertia: A functional cause of constipation due to slow colonic transit times found predominantly in young to middle-aged women presenting with abdominal distention, cramping, heavy straining, and infrequent defecation.

Congenital aganglionosis or Hirschsprung's disease: First described in 1888 by Hirschprung, this is an absence of myenteric neurons in the segment of colon just proximal to the anal sphincter, leading to a segment of contracted bowel that causes obstruction and proximal dilatation. It may affect various lengths of the colon, sometimes extending beyond the sigmoid colon and rarely (and fatally) to the entire intestine.

Constipation: There are three commonly cited definitions of constipation: (a) frequency of less than three stool passages per week, (b) decreased stool bulk and caliber, and (c) straining with stool passage.

Megarectum: An acquired anatomic cause of constipation, which is distinguished by a volumetric increase in the capacity of the rectum with significant alteration of rectal compliance; can be either primary and idiopathic, or secondary to rectal or anal obstruction (as in Hirschsprung's), or secondary to a myenteric plexus injury as in Chagas' disease.

Paradoxical puborectalis contraction: Obstructive constipation due to failure of normal relaxation of the puborectalis to allow straightening of the anorectal angle during defecation; also known as *anismus, spastic pelvic floor syndrome*, and *nonrelaxing puborectalis syndrome*.

INTRODUCTION

Constipation can be thought of as a great equalizer. It transcends social, economical, racial, and national boundaries.

Yet constipation is only a symptom and not a disease. It has been with us for millennia, with countless ancient treatments and concoctions having been passed down over the centuries without notable success. The ancient Egyptians discovered the enema by observing storks inject themselves with sea water. In the Middle Ages, Arabs introduced senna tea and rhubarb to Europe. The obsession of people with some of these remedies reached a pinnacle in seventeenth-century Europe when constipation was thought to be the source of all viles, and enemas were all the rage (1). Even today this inclination continues as asserted by the numerous "colonic lavage" clinics in trendy Venice Beach in California and across the border in Mexican "alternative therapy" clinics.

Despite its prominent history, there is no consensus as to a precise definition of constipation. Because it is a symptom, it may be influenced by multiple factors and thus a combination of objective and subjective criteria may be used to define it. There are three commonly cited definitions of constipation: (a) less than three stool passages per week (2), (b) decreased stool bulk and caliber, and (c) straining with stool passage (3). The first definition is the least subjective, but not necessarily accurate in all patients. The second and third definitions are very dependent on identifying what is "normal" in each individual patient and greatly broaden the spectrum of people who fall under the definition of constipation. Whatever the definition, it remains certain that constipation, which is more common in women (4), plays a role in the etiology or severity of chronic pelvic pain in some women.

EPIDEMIOLOGY

Constipation is an important symptom that leads to approximately 2.5 million visits to physicians per year in the United States alone (5). This does not take into account the far greater numbers who do not seek professional treatment and symptomatically treat themselves with over-the-counter drugs. The prevalence of the disorder actually varies somewhat depending on country, socioeconomic status, gender, and age. In the United States the general population prevalence is 2%, increasing to 4.5% in the 65- to 74-year age group and greater than 10% in the over-75-year age group (4). Likewise, studies have shown a higher prevalence of constipation among African-Americans (17%) than among Caucasians (12%) (6). Other countries have not had surveys as widespread as those in the United States, so the figures may not be reliable, but in general the figures in other developed countries are similar to the U.S. figures (3). That constipation is related to diet is evident by the much lower incidence in Third World countries with high-fiber, low-animal-fat diets (7).

Gender has a significant role, with females twice as likely to have constipation as men (8). The reasons for this are still unclear, but it is known that idiopathic slow colonic transit times occur most often in young women (9), and some have suggested that alterations in hormonal levels affect bowel motility (10). This notion seems reasonable because it is known that high progesterone levels in pregnancy lead to smooth muscle relaxation and slower colonic transit times.

ETIOLOGY

Current beliefs are that constipation is a multifaceted disorder with many possible etiologies (Table 25.1) (11). Con-stipation may be colonic or extracolonic in origin. Colonic origin may be congenital or acquired, while extracolonic causes may be neurogenic or endocrine. *Congenital agan-glionosis* or *Hirschsprung's disease* is characterized by an absence of myenteric neurons in the segment of colon just proximal to the anal sphincter, leading to a segment of con-tracted bowel that causes obstruction and proximal dilata-tion. The disease may affect various lengths of the colon, sometimes extending beyond the sigmoid colon (12) and rarely (and fatally) with total intestinal involvement (13). The exact reasons for this disorder, first described in 1888 by Hirschsprung (14), remain unclear. The disease probably has a genetic component, with the incidence of familial occurrence averaging about 4% (15). The absence of the ganglionic cells has been thought to be due to either (a) fail-ure of migration of neural crest cells during embryogenesis (16), (b) failure of development of neural crest cells after migration (17), or (c) pathologic destruction of the cells after migration (18). There is a variant of the disease that presents during adulthood.

A large proportion of cases of constipation are due to acquired colorectal disease, either anatomic or functional. Among the former are strictures of the colorectum or anus induced by a variety of disorders. *Endometriotic lesions* may lead to strictures either directly due to extensive sigmoid lesions or indirectly through massive adhesions induced by advanced disease in the pelvis (19). *Adhesions* secondary to

TABLE 25.1. CAUSES OF CONSTIPATION

Mechanical	Pharmacologic	Metabolic and Endocrine	Neurogenic	Idiopathic
Obstructive	Analgesics	Amyloidosis	*Peripheral*	*Colonic*
Neoplastic	Anesthetics	Diabetes	Hirschsprung	Inertia
Postsurgical	Anticholinergics	Hypercalcemia	Autonomic neuropathy	Megabowel
Hernia	Anticonvulsants	Hyperparathyroidism	Chagas' disease	Intussusception
Volvulus	Antidepressants	Hypokalemia	Ganglioneuromatosis	*Pelvic*
Endometriosis	Antiparkinsonian agents	Hypopituitarism	Multiple endocrine neoplasia (IIb)	Paradoxical puborectalis contraction
Diverticulitis	Antacids	Hypothyroidism	*Spinal*	Rectocele
Ischemic colitis	Barium sulfate	Pheochromocytemia	Cauda equina tumor	Descending perineum
Functional	Diuretics	Porphyria	Iatrogenic	
Irritable bowel syndrome	Ganglionic blockers	Pregnancy	Meningocele	
Proctitis	Hematinics	Scleroderma	Multiple sclerosis	
Diverticular disease	Hypotensives	Uremia	Paraplegia	
Inadequate dietary fiber	Laxative abuse		Resection of nervi erigentes	
Inadequate water intake	Metallic intoxication		Shy–Drager syndrome	
	Monoamine oxidase inhibitors		Tabes dorsalis	
	Opiates		Trauma	
	Paralytic agents		*Central*	
	Parasympatholytic		Parkinson's disease	
	Phenothiazines		Stroke	
	Psychotherapeutics		Tumors	

pelvic inflammatory disease (20) or pelvic surgery can also lead to strictures and resulting constipation. *Inflammatory bowel diseases*, such as Crohn's disease, ulcerative colitis, diverticulitis, or ischemic colitis, often are stricture-inducing disorders (11). Other causes include an obstructing *colonic neoplasm* or *intussusception*. *Sigmoid volvulus*, usually a disorder of the elderly, can present as chronic intermittent constipation.

Rectocele, which is protrusion of the anterior rectal wall into the vaginal vault, is sometimes a cause of dysfunctional defecation. Weakening of the pelvic floor muscles and rectovaginal septum lead to difficult evacuation. The result is straining, which either causes or enlarges any defect or weakness in the rectovaginal septum, leading to the belief that constipation may cause, and may also increase the size of, a rectocele. Once present, a rectocele causes constipation or obstipation through ballooning of the defect during bearing down, with diversion of the fecal pathway. Up to 75% of women with rectocele have constipation as a presenting symptom (21).

Another acquired anatomic cause is *megarectum*, which is distinguished by a volumetric increase in the capacity of the rectum with significant alteration of rectal compliance (22). The constipation results from dysmotility or flaccidity. Usually the rectal wall is not hypertrophic or thickened. Megarectum can be either primary idiopathic or secondary to rectal or anal obstruction (as in Hirschsprung's), or secondary to a myenteric plexus injury as in Chagas' disease. Idiopathic megarectum is usually not associated with aganglionosis, although there may be a variety of ganglionic pathology that can range from normal to complete absence (23).

Chagas' disease is an infectious cause of constipation. Caused by the *Trypanosoma cruzi*, it is endemic in South America. The organisms multiply within the subcutaneous tissue, and they migrate in their leishmanial form to the muscle coat of the gut. The myenteric plexus is destroyed and replaced by histoplasmocytic infiltrate and fibrosis, along with hypertrophy of the longitudinal and circular muscles (24). There is a debate over whether the destruction is due to neurotoxin liberation or direct invasion by the organisms (25). The destroyed segment (most commonly the distal colon and rectum) becomes dyskinetic and dilates, leading to functional obstruction and constipation.

Colonic dysmotility or inertia is a functional cause of constipation due to slow colonic transit times. This disorder is predominantly seen in young to middle-aged women presenting with abdominal distention, cramping, heavy straining, and infrequent defecation. Several theories have been suggested to explain this etiologically obscure condition. One is that it is secondary to a primary sigmoid motility disorder. Another relates the condition to abnormalities in intestinal hormone levels, the most specific being a decrease in vasoactive inhibitory peptide in the muscularis of the colon (26). One group of investigators attempted to explain colonic inertia as a manifestation of systemic smooth muscle motility disease resulting in motility disorders of all hol-

low viscera. Interestingly, 15% of their female patients had associated galactorrhea (27).

Another cause of constipation that is more common in women than men is *paradoxical puborectalis contraction* (PPC), also known as *anismus, spastic pelvic floor syndrome*, and *nonrelaxing puborectalis syndrome*. Women with pelvic floor pain syndrome often have this problem also (Chapter 45). During defecation the puborectalis muscle normally relaxes, straightening the anorectal angle and opening the anal canal. Failure of this mechanism due to puborectalis contraction leads to obstructed rectal emptying. Studies suggest that the underlying pathophysiology is more complex than this, because anismus can occur in normal people also (28,29). Anorectal sensitivity in these patients is decreased and may play a role. Others believe it to be an adult-onset focal dystonic syndrome as a result of prolonged efforts to empty the rectum (30).

Among the extracolonic causes are the metabolic abnormalities that may be associated with constipation. As many as 20% of *diabetic neuropathy* patients may have constipation, which is due to alterations in smooth muscle contractile patterns (31). *Hypothyroidism* is often accompanied by constipation and is likewise due to increased transit times. *Porphyrias* can lead to disturbed gastrointestinal motility, with both spasmodic and dilated areas of the gut, leading to constipation. A rare cause is *pheochromocytoma*. *Pregnancy*, although a normal condition, causes an increase in progesterone levels. Transit time is increased, as is colonic water absorption. Thirty-five percent to 40% of women suffer from constipation during their pregnancies (32).

Neurologic causes of constipation include *peripheral nerve injuries* such as stretch of parasympathetic nerve branches during prolonged labor. This can lead to disordered colonic motility and constipation. High and low *traumatic cord transection* patients have constipation. *Multiple sclerosis* has many effects, many of which contribute to the occurrence of constipation.

A variety of *medications* can lead to constipation. These include those with anticholinergic properties, such as antidepressants, antipsychotics, and narcotic analgesics. The chronic use of laxative drugs may lead to local injury to the colonic innervation and subsequent dysmotility and constipation (33). Nonsteroidal antiinflammatory drugs are at times the cause of serious constipation, albeit in a very small percentage of users (34).

Surgical interventions may lead to constipation as previously mentioned. Although in most cases it is a result of decreased intestinal mobility due to adhesions, it can also result from nerve dysfunction brought upon by the surgery. There is evidence that gynecologic pelvic surgery directly increases the incidence of constipation. In a retrospective cohort study, patients who had a presacral neurectomy appeared to have the highest incidence of constipation (32%), but women who had a hysterectomy also had significant rates of persistent constipation (28%). In the control group, with no history of gynecologic surgery, only 10% of women had constipation (35).

HISTORY

Patients with chronic pelvic pain and constipation, a not uncommon combination, are a diagnostic (and therapeutic) dilemma. The constipation may be a result or cause of the pain symptoms. Thus a detailed history is of great significance in evaluating constipation. Because it is a symptom and is highly subjective, the physician must endeavor to define the "normal" state of the individual patient to accurately evaluate the condition. Moreover, it is important to obtain detailed information regarding the patient's current typical bowel habits, including frequency, consistency, timing, and duration of straining. Sometimes patients have detailed logs of their bowel movements; but if not, having patients do a prospective stool diary, combined with objective evaluations, can be particularly useful (36). All aspects of the bowel movements should be broached in the hope of finding some clue as to the cause. Colonic inertia patients may report abdominal bloating and discomfort between meals. The need for enemas or suppositories can be important points. Eliciting a history of digital manipulation to enable defecation is also important, particularly in cases of rectocele and nonrelaxing puborectalis syndrome. Complaints of a sensation of bearing down or pressure in the perineum point to a rectocele, perineal descent syndrome, or instussception, as does a sensation of incomplete rectal emptying.

Socially acceptable defecation and bowel habits are learned and under conscious control, so it is not surprising that constipation may have a psychologic component (37). This is particularly true for the woman with chronic pelvic pain and constipation. Many have a history of suffering from emotional disturbances, especially depression, which may be risk factors for later development of pain and/or constipation (38). The patient's mannerisms and the nonverbal communication or body language used by the patient may lead the practitioner to delve further into the psychologic background of the individual. In particular, past history of childhood sexual abuse has been found to greatly increase the occurrence of constipation in later years (39). Aspects of the patient's adult life should be taken into consideration, including workplace and social stresses. Sexual history can be important. Vaginismus has been found to be linked with a decreased amplitude of the recto-anal inhibitory reflex (40). Additionally, patients with irritable bowel syndrome often have pain during or after intercourse (41). Because chronic pelvic pain is the main complaint of the patient, special emphasis must be placed upon gathering as much information regarding the type, quality, duration, and severity of the pelvic pain symptoms. The relation of the pain to activities other than defecation should be explored, because pelvic pain, like constipation, can be

multifactorial. History of physical activities such as bicycling or horseback riding may be important in some instances, because they may be the cause of a pudendal neuropathy that may manifest in both chronic pain and constipation. In these cases, in addition to the constipation and deep pelvic pain, there will be history of burning pain in the vulvar and inner thigh area.

One of the more important aspects in the history is age of onset. Onset as an infant points to possible congenital etiology, whereas later onset suggests an acquired condition. Although constipation is thought of as a symptom of middle age, changes in colonic motility with age have not been adequately assessed. Constipation in elderly individuals may be due to other factors besides age and should be investigated accordingly.

Another aspect that should be probed is that of nutritional and medicinal intake. Lack of adequate fiber intake as well or adequate intake with poor liquid consumption may induce constipation. The excessive ingestion of high-protein "junk food" such as hamburgers may lead to constipation, because the high protein and low fiber content leads to formation of small compacted stools. Likewise, excessive intake of iron-rich vitamin supplements may lead to constipation. History of chronic laxative use is also important because, as previously mentioned, these lead to dysfunctional intestinal motility. In chronic users, a syndrome of sorts occurs, usually heralded by violent colicky pain that usually follows meals. These painful contractions fail to expel fecal matter and may involve the whole abdomen and grow closer together. Patients may become depressed as a result of hypersecretion brought on by the laxatives leads to potassium depletion with resulting fatigue and tetany in severe cases (1).

Additionally a detailed medical history is of importance to identify any pre-existing conditions that are associated with constipation (Table 25.1). History of prior pelvic surgical interventions should be sought as well.

PHYSICAL EXAMINATION

A properly done examination is of utmost importance. Since constipation is a multifaceted disorder, care must be taken to not overlook any possible systemic disease. The practitioner should start by exclusion of the most commonly associated systemic diseases, especially any signs suggestive of diabetes or hypothyroidism.

Particular attention should then be directed to the abdominal and anorectal examinations. Inspection of the contour of the abdomen may reveal distention as a result of collected stool or gas. Percussion should differentiate this from ascites or intraabdominal tumors. Auscultation of intestinal borborygmi and their locations can differentiate the condition from intestinal obstruction or paralytic ileus. Both superficial and deep palpation should be done. Large obstructive lesions may be felt in slim patients, as will hard stool impaction. Tenderness may point to an inflammatory process such as pelvic inflammatory disease or diverticulitis. An examination of the possible hernial orifices should be done, because they may be a cause of constipation. Special attention should be paid to the detection of femoral hernias because they are commonly overlooked (33).

The anorectal examination is an important aspect of evaluation of constipation. The gynecologic pelvic examination is usually done in a lithotomy position, but the anorectal exam is best performed in Sims' position. Initial visual examination may reveal the presence of soiling of the undergarments or perineal area and may point to incontinence secondary to fecal impaction. Careful inspection should be done for fissures or stenosis, which cause pain and may cause functional constipation because of the patient's fear of defecation. Ectopic anus should also be looked for. Signs of sexual abuse include abrasions or multiple fissures of the anal orifice. The next step is an assessment of the resting anal tone. The patient should be asked to bear down for assessment of the function of the internal and external sphincters (42). Anismus can be suspected if the anal sphincters contract in response to the normal anorectal reflex. The digital examination can also reveal the presence and consistency of stool within the rectum. Likewise, this will reveal the presence of strictures or obstructing tumors in the lower end of the rectum. Levator spasm can also be detected. Nerve dysfunction is suspected with loss of reflex to light stroking of the anal skin. In patients where a possible pudendal neuropathy is suspected, the anorectal examination is important.

A complete and thorough pelvic exam should be done to rule out gynecologic causes. Deep bimanual palpation is done to elicit any tenderness that might point to endometriosis. Levator spasm or trigger points within the muscle should be checked for. Rectocele and prolapse should be looked for. Rectal examination will reveal areas of weakness in the anterior rectal wall as bulges into the vagina. The patient should strain, and the extent of perineal descent should be noted, if any, and graded. Because the loss of support is a fascial defect that may be either superior, lateral, or midline, this should be assessed in the normal manner by insertion of the examiner's finger along the posterior vaginal wall and asking the patient to bear down. Additionally, examination of the patient in a standing position is important for the diagnosis of enterocele.

LABORATORY AND IMAGING STUDIES

In most cases a thorough history and examination are usually sufficient to reach a preliminary diagnosis and begin treatment. But at times these are not enough and further studies are needed. One basic complementary investigation is colonic contrast radiography using barium enemas. This excludes anatomic abnormalities or obstructing lesions of the rectum or colon. Its usefulness is limited by the fact that some conditions, such as megacolon, have been described in normal individuals.

Other studies to uncover anatomic abnormalities are anoscopy, flexible sigmoidoscopy, and colonoscopy. Mucosal changes such as dark pigmentation (melanosis coli) due to excessive laxative use may be observed, in addition to anatomic disorders such as ulcers, hemorrhoids, neoplasms, or strictures.

When anatomic abnormalities are not revealed by the above methods, functional abnormalities should be looked for. Defecography and/or colonic transit times are usually the next steps. Defecography, or evacuation proctography as it is sometimes called, is a radiographic study that provides dynamic assessment of defecation and allows selection of patients who may require surgery. It is valuable when one suspects rectocele, enterocele, sigmoidocele, rectal prolapse, occult prolapse, or idiopathic incontinence. The technique is relatively painless and easy to perform. No bowel preparation is needed. The rectum is filled with a radiopaque paste using a special applicator and the patient is seated on a radiolucent toilet seat. Evacuation should be done as quickly and completely as possible (43). When this is done as specific evaluation of prolapse, rectocele, or cystocele, complete pelvic visceral opacification is needed. The so-called "four-contrast defecography" technique (44) may be used. The vagina is filled with barium paste while the bladder is filled with a water-soluble contrast. The patient ingests barium 2 hours prior to the procedure while the rectum is filled with barium paste. Additionally, radiopaque markers are placed on specific areas on the perineum. These permit assessment of structures in relation to the perineal body. This technique is probably a better method of objectively evaluating rectoceles and enteroceles, along with their clinical significance in constipation, because pelvic examination is not always effective in detecting them, particularly enteroceles (45). Nonrelaxing puborectalis syndrome can be evaluated with this technique, also (46).

Colonic transit time studies are helpful when a diagnosis of chronic idiopathic constipation is made. They can assist in determining the severity of constipation as well as neuropathic and myopathic small bowel dysmotility. There are a number of methods available, such as radiopaque markers, scintigraphy, breath hydrogen concentration, and liquid transit (47). The technique most commonly utilized is radiopaque marker ingestion. An abnormal transit time is usually more than 72 hours.

Some patients have specific abnormalities of the sphincter that may lead to constipation. These patients may have loss of the recto-anal inhibitory reflex, as in Hirschsprung's disease or in intestinal neuronal dysplasia. Recto-anal balloon manometry is one method of detection of this disorder, using a manometer attached to a balloon placed through the anus and into the rectum. Patients with poor rectal sensation may need more than the usual volume of 60 mL of air to initiate a reflex, those with Hirschsprung's will have absence of inhibition, and patients with sphincter hypertonia will have excessively high pressures coupled with inhibition (48).

Anal electromyography (EMG) and measurement of pudendal nerve terminal latency (PNTML) are of value in assessing the electrical activity of the pelvic floor. Anal EMG is particularly useful in diagnosing paradoxical puborectalis contraction and in revealing neuromuscular damage related to chronic straining. The technique uses an anal plug electrode to measure electrical activity of the anal sphincter apparatus. EMG recording of the external anal sphincter muscle shows a paradoxical increase in activity during evacuation efforts in cases of paradoxical puborectalis contraction or anismus (49). The technique of measuring PNTML is of use in assessing pudendal nerve injury and discovering intrinsic neurologic injury to the striated sphincter muscles of the pelvic floor. It involves a glove-mounted nerve stimulating and recording device that is introduced through the rectum and brought into contact with the ischial spine on each side. A reading is taken three times from each pudendal nerve. A PNTML value greater than 2.2 msec is considered abnormal. Thus in patients with chronic pelvic pain, injury to the pudendal nerve may be the cause of both their pain and the accompanying constipation. Additional diagnostic procedures include the balloon expulsion test and scintigraphic defecography.

In patients with chronic pelvic pain and constipation whose histories and physical examinations point towards possible pelvic and intestinal endometriosis, laparoscopy is an extremely beneficial diagnostic and therapeutic modality (50). Garcha et al. (19) reported on laparoscopic diagnosis and removal of sigmoid colon endometriosis causing constipation.

None of the above will be effective in evaluating the patient if a concomitant metabolic disorder exists that may be exacerbating the condition. Thus simple lab tests to evaluate anemia, glucose levels, renal function, and thyroid function, at a minimum, may need to be a part of the evaluation if there is any suggestion of these conditions (33).

TREATMENT

Due to the multifactorial etiology of constipation, there is no single specific treatment plan. Rather, treatment must be tailored to the individuals history and specific pathophysiology (51). After the history and physical examination the physician should have a good idea of whether he or she is dealing with a "temporary" constipation brought on by various transient causes or a chronic constipation of pathologic cause(s). Examples of temporary constipation include that following abdominopelvic surgery or extensive travel with time changes, an altered schedule, and dietary irregularity. Temporary constipation may flare or exacerbate the pain of patients with chronic pelvic pain, but usually respond to

reassurance and common sense interventions with hydration, increased dietary bulk, natural bowel stimulants, and, occasionally, transient use of laxatives. Chronic constipation is a more serious and difficult problem.

Medical conditions that may cause constipation, such as diabetes or hypothyroidism, should be appropriately treated. In such cases, patients can usually be reassured that their constipation will gradually improve. Additional help in the form of dietary supplements may be offered, in accordance with the guidelines to be discussed below.

Patients with a history of chronic laxative use should, in general be weaned from them. There may be exceptions to this recommendation—for example, those with adult-type Hirschsprung disease. Weaning can be particularly difficult in the elderly chronic user for whom the concept of not having a bowel movement every day is frustrating. Reassurance and reeducation are the keys to treatment in these patients. The patient should understand that assessment of their bowel function, without laxative interference, is of great importance.

Patient education is an extremely important part of the therapy (1), both for idiopathic and nonidiopathic constipation. The first thing is to explain what the normal expectations for bowel movements should be. Often patients have preformed misconceptions that modifies their behavior and worsens the condition. Attempting to plan bowel movements is another part of education. Because movements are stimulated by food ingestion, the patient should be taught to attempt evacuation a short while after meals. The importance of liquid intake in large quantities is to be emphasized. Three quarts a day should be the target. Physical exercise and proper muscle usage should be taught, because exercise is a crucial component of normal bowel function. Sedentary lifestyles are constipating, so patients with constipation have much to gain from daily exercise. The associated increased flexibility can also be helpful in attaining a proper position during defecation. Flexion of the thighs and pelvis bring the body close to the most efficient position, which is squatting. Increasing the tone of the abdominal muscles is also important in helping defecation by increasing intraabdominal pressure. Teaching the patient to do isometric abdominal muscle contractions is effective, particularly in connection with breathing exercises to strengthen the diaphragm.

Following these initial attempts at behavioral modification, dietary modification should be the next step. Dietary fiber intake should be greatly increased, with 25 to 30 g per day the goal. Bran, cereals, raw vegetables, and fruits are all effective agents with the added benefit of providing needed minerals and vitamins.

Failure of these simple measures may lead to trial use of laxatives. Laxatives are many types: (a) bulk-forming agents, (b) lubricant, (c) emollients, (d) stimulants, and (e) osmotic laxatives. *Bulk laxatives* include plantago seed (psyllium), guar, malt soup extract, and methylcellulose. These are effective, provided that water intake of 2 of 4 L per day is achieved. Otherwise, constipation may be worsened by these agents.

This treatment is useful in patients with anal fissure, pregnancy, diverticular disease, or irritable bowel syndrome (52). While largely safe and well-tolerated, there are some precautions to be taken. Patients with obstruction or megacolon may become worse (33). *Lubricants* are usually a form of mineral oil. Mineral oil is contraindicated in elderly patients with history of stroke due to the risk of pulmonary aspiration. Other forms of commercial lubricants should be used cautiously since they often contain stimulants. *Stimulant laxatives* should generally not be used for treatment of chronic constipation. Their only role is in amelioration of acute attacks. *Hyperosmolar agents* are useful when other measures fail. Sorbitol is a hyperosmolar agent that is very effective and low in cost, but should not be used as a long-term laxative.

Prokinetic agents such as cisapride have been shown to increase stool frequency and decrease stomach emptying time (53). Studies have proven it effective in chronic constipation in paraplegics (54) and in children with idiopathic constipation.

Patients with constipation and psychiatric symptoms or disorders will usually be one of three types: (a) symptomatizing as a result of constipation, (b) having symptoms contributing to constipation, or (c) having unrelated symptoms needing treatment (55). The majority are a mixture of the first and second types. Psychiatric treatment should be sought if it is felt that psychiatric factors are a major instigator. Judicious use of antidepressants is often effective in alleviating depression symptoms and motivating the patient.

While many patients will benefit from the above-mentioned treatments, there are some that will not. Some of these patients will be found to have anatomic or functional abnormalities. Treatment of these patients should be geared to correct the suspected pathophysiology. Others will have chronic idiopathic constipation with no identifiable cause. The results of their colonic transit tests are helpful in managing them. Patients with idiopathic constipation and normal transit times, who did not get relief with dietary or behavioral modification, are candidates for further investigations including psychologic evaluation. Patients with long transit times will have usually undergone further testing. Patients with slow transit constipation often become worse on bulking agents because they increase the severity of their symptoms (56). These patients have bowel frequencies between once a week and once a month. When pelvic floor dysfunction is not present and the symptoms are causing severe decrease in quality of life, then surgery may be called for. The most commonly done procedure is colectomy. Subtotal colectomy and ileorectal anastomosis are usually effective in improving quality of life in these patients. Duthie et al. (57) reported that 67% of their patients were satisfied in the long term; bowel frequency improved, but abdominal bloating was still a problem. Surgery should only be resorted to in these patients as a last measure, after all other methods fail.

In the same vein, patients with slow transit and a documented pelvic outlet obstruction should not undergo colonic resection surgery unless absolutely necessary. Surgery will not correct the obstructive defect unless it happens to be a colonic tumor. The main disorder seen in the slow transit–pelvic obstruction patients is paradoxical puborectalis contraction (anismus). As previously discussed, this can usually be diagnosed using anal probe EMG and cinedefecography. Investigators have attempted surgical division of the puborectalis to prevent its action on the sphincter, but this is a procedure with notable morbidity (58). Biofeedback has proven a popular alternative to surgery due to its success in ameliorating the condition and its relatively low cost and lack of morbidity. Several types of biofeedback are available, but EMG-based biofeedback is most commonly employed. It is relatively simple to set up, gives a tangible visual result for the patient, and is relatively economical. Results from various studies have shown good short-term results (up to 70% success), (33) but long-term data are lacking.

Pelvic floor weakness, as with a rectocele, should only be treated surgically after clear evidence of its involvement in constipation. The previously mentioned investigative procedures can provide evidence of the role of a rectocele. Too often surgeons operate on mild rectoceles that have not been thoroughly investigated, with detrimental effects on the patient's psyche after failure of the procedure to ameliorate the constipation. Surgical techniques differ depending on the surgical training background. Gynecologists usually repair rectoceles transvaginally, while colorectal surgeons prefer a transanal approach through the rectal wall. Rectal or mucosal prolapses are indications for surgical treatment because they may be sources of pain leading to voluntary constipation. In cases in which reproductive tract diseases such as endometriosis are suspected, laparoscopic surgery is an excellent approach.

KEY POINTS

Most Important Question to Ask

- What do you believe is normal bowel function?
- How often do you usually have a bowel movement?
- What time of the day do you usually have a bowel movement?
- What are your bowel movements usually like? Hard? Formed? Loose or runny? Small caliber? Pellet-like?
- Do you usually have to strain to have a bowel movement?
- Do you have abdominal bloating and discomfort? When does this usually occur?
- Do you regularly use laxatives, enemas, or suppositories to have a bowel movement?
- Do you put your finger in the vagina or rectum to aid in bowel movements?
- Do you feel like you empty your bowel completely when you have a bowel movement?
- Do you have pain with intercourse?
- Is there any history of sexual or physical abuse?

- Were deliveries of children difficult? What were the weights of the babies?
- Do you perform physical activities such as bicycling or horseback riding regularly?
- At what age did you start having problems with constipation?
- Do you take any medications, vitamins, or iron?
- What are the sources of fiber in your diet?
- How much water or other liquids do you drink each day?
- Have you ever had any pelvic or abdominal surgery?

Most Important Physical Examination Findings

- Any signs of systemic disease
- Abdominal distention
- Abdominal or pelvic mass
- Abdominal or pelvic tenderness
- Abdominal or inguinal hernias
- Soiling of the undergarments or perineal area
- Anal fissures or stenosis
- Ectopic anus
- Assessment of the resting anal tone
- Abnormal anal tone, fecal impaction, or anorectal mass at digital rectal examination
- Levator ani spasm or trigger points
- Loss of anal reflex
- Rectocele, enterocele, or rectal prolapse

Most Important Diagnostic Studies

- Air contrast barium enemas
- Anoscopy, flexible sigmoidoscopy, and colonoscopy
- Defecography
- Colonic transit times
- Recto-anal balloon manometry
- Anal electromyography
- Pudendal nerve terminal latency
- Laparoscopy
- Hematocrit
- Thyroid stimulating hormone
- Fasting and 2-hour glucose levels
- Serum creatinine

Treatments

- Treatment is tailored to the patient dependent on the suspected etiology
- Psychiatric evaluation and treatment may be important
- Treat any medical conditions, such as diabetes or hypothyroidism
- Patients with a history of chronic laxative use, in general, should be weaned from them
- Patient education
- Normal expectations for bowel movements
- Plan bowel movements a short while after meals
- Large quantities of liquid intake (3 quarts a day)
- Physical exercise and proper muscle usage, including isometric abdominal muscle contractions and breathing exercises
- Increase dietary fiber intake to 25 to 30 g per day
- Trial use of laxatives in some cases
- Prokinetic agents such as cisapride in some cases
- Subtotal colectomy and ileorectal anastomosis, rarely
- Biofeedback
- Surgical treatment of rectocele, other prolapses, or other pelvic diseases if there is clear evidence of involvement in constipation

REFERENCES

1. Thiroloix J. *La constipation et ses consequences.* Paris: Editions Robert Laffont. 1974:ix–x.
2. Martelli H, Devroede G, Ahran P. Some parameters of large bowel motility in normal man. *Gastroenterology* 1978;75:612–618.
3. Ehrenpreis ED. Definitions and epidemiology of constipation. In: Wexner SD, Bartolo DCC, eds. *Constipation. Etiology, evaluation and management.* Oxford: Butterworth-Heinemann, 1995:3–7.
4. Sonnenburg A, Koch TR. Epidemiology of constipation in the United States. *Dis Colon Rectum* 1989;32:1–8.
5. Sonnenburg A, Koch TR. Physician visits in the United States for constipation. *Dig Dis Sci* 1989;34:606–611.
6. Sandler RS, Jordon MC, Skelton BJ. Demographic and dietary determinants of constipation. *Am J Publ Health* 1990;80(2):185–189.
7. Langman MS, Logan RFA. The epidemiology of human colonic diseases. In: Kirsner JB, Shorter RG, eds. *Diseases of the colon, rectum and anal canal.* Baltimore: Williams and Wilkins, 1988:179–180.
8. Everhart JE, Go VL, Johannnes RS. A longitudinal survey of self-reported bowel habits in the United States. *Dig Dis Sci* 1989;34(8):1153–1162.
9. MacDonald A, Shearer M, Paterson PJ, et al. Relationship between outlet obstruction constipation and obstructed urinary flow. *Br J Surg* 1991;78:613–615.
10. Hinds JP, Stoney B, Wald A. Does gender or the menstrual cycle affect colonic transit? *Am J Gastroenterol* 1989;84(2):123–126.
11. Wexner SD, Jagelman DG. Chronic constipation. *Postgrad Adv Colorect Surg* 1989;1(12):1–22.
12. Kleinhaus S, Boley SJ, Sheran M. Hirschsprung's disease. A survey of the members of the American Academy of Pediatrics. *J Pediatr Surg* 1979;14:588–597.
13. DiLorenzo M, Yazbeck S, Brochu P. Aganglionosis of the entire bowel: four new cases and review of the literature. *Br J Surg* 1985;72:657–658.
14. Hirschsprung H. Stuhltragheit Neugeborener infolge Dilatation und Hypertrophy des Colons. *Jahresbericht Kinderheilk* 1888;27:1.
15. Oakley JR, Lavery IC. Etiology of congenital colorectal disease. In: Wexner SD, Bartolo DCC, eds. *Constipation. Etiology, evaluation and management.* Oxford: Butterworth-Heinemann, 1995:9–11.
16. Okamoto E, Ueda T. Embryogenesis of intramural ganglia of the gut and its relation to Hirschsprung's disease. *J Pediatr Surg* 1967;2:437–443.
17. Fujimoto T, Hata J, Yokayama S. A study of the extracellular matrix protein as the migration pathway of neural crest cells in

the gut: analysis in human embryos with specific reference to the pathogenesis of Hirschsprung's disease. *J Pediatr Surg* 1989; 24:550–556.

18. Earlam RJ. A vascular cause for Hirschsprung's disease? *Gastroenterology* 1985;88:1274–1279.

19. Garcha IS, Perloie M, Strawn EY, et al. Laparoscopic resection of sigmoid endometrioma. *Am Surg* 1996;62(4):274–275.

20. Girardot C, Legmann Pand Le Goff JY. Rectal stenosis. A rare complication of chronic salpingitis caused by an intrauterine device. *J Radiol* 1990;71(1):23–26.

21. Capps WF. Rectoplasty and perineoplasty for the symtomatic rectocele: a report of fifty cases. *Dis Colon Rectum* 1975;18:237–244.

22. Verduron A, Devroede G, Bouchoucha M. Mega rectum. *Dig Dis Sci* 1988;33:1164–1174.

23. Gemlo BT, Wong WD. Etiology of acquired colorectal disease. In: Wexner SD, Bartolo DCC, eds. *Constipation. Etiology, evaluation and management.* Oxford: Butterworth-Heinemann, 1995:19–20.

24. Cutait DE, Cutait R. Surgery of chagasic megacolon. *World J Surg* 1991;15:188–197.

25. Okumura M, Franca LCM, Correa Neto A. Comentarios sobre a patogenia da molestia de chagas; especial referencia a infeccao eperimental em camundongos. *Rev Hosp Clin* 1963;18:161.

26. Koch TR, Carney JA, Go L, et al. Idiopathic chronic constipation is associated with decreased colonic vasoactive intestinal peptide. *Gastroenterology* 1988;94:300–310.

27. Watier A, Devroede G, Duranceau A. Constipation with colonic inertia: a manifestation of systemic disease? *Dig Dis Sci* 1983;28: 1025–1033.

28. Kuijpers HC, Bleijenberg G. The spastic pelvic floor syndrome: a cause of constipation. *Dis Colon Rectum* 1985;28:669–672.

29. Read NW, Timms JM, Barfield LJ. Impairment of defecation in young women with severe constipation. *Gastroenterology* 1986; 90:53–60.

30. Mathers SE, Kempster PA, Swash M, et al. Constipation and paradoxical puborectalis contraction in anismus and Parkinson's disease: a dystonic phenomenon? *J Neurol Neurosurg Psych* 1988; 51:1503–1507.

31. Battle WM, Cohen JD, Snape WJ. Disorders of colonic motility in patients with diabetes mellitus. *Yale J Biol Med* 1983;56:277–283.

32. Anderson AS. Constipation during pregnancy: incidence and methods used in its treatment in a group of Cambridgeshire women. *Health Vis* 1984;12:363–364.

33. Barrett M, Rauh SM. Constipation. In: Leppert PC, Howard FM, eds. *Primary care for women.* Philadelphia: Lippincott-Raven, 1997:467–477.

34. Tremaine WJ. Chronic constipation: causes and management. *Hosp Pract* 1990;April 30:89–100.

35. Perry CP. Relationship of gynecologic surgery to constipation. *J Am Assoc Gynecol Laparosc* 1999;6(1):75–78.

36. Ashraf W, Park F, Lof J, et al. An examination of the reliability of reported stool frequency in the diagnosis of idiopathic constipation. *Am J Gastroenterol* 1996;91:26–32.

37. Devroede G, Bouchoucha M, Girard G. Constipation, anxiety and personality: what comes first? In: Bueno L, Collins S, Junior JL, eds. *Stress and digestive motility.* London: John Libbey, 1989:55–60.

38. Grzesiak R, Ury GM, Dworkin RH. Psychodynamic psychotherapy with chronic pain patients. In: Gatchel RJ, Turk DC, eds. *Psychological approaches to pain management. A practitioner's handbook.* New York: The Guilford Press. 1996:148–178.

39. Talley NJ, Helgeson S, Zinmeister AR. Are sexual and physical abuse linked to functional gastrointestinal disorders? *Gastroenterology* 1992;89:A523.

40. Weber J, Ducrotte P, Touchais JY, et al. Biofeedback training for constipation in adults and children. *Dis Colon Rectum* 1987;30: 844–846.

41. Guthrie E, Creed FH, Whorwell PJ. Severe sexual dysfunction in women with the irritable bowel syndrome: comparison with inflammatory bowel disease and doudenal ulceration. *Br Med J Clin Res* 1987;295(6598):577–578.

42. Beck DE. Initial evaluation of constipation. In: Wexner SD, Bartolo DCC, eds. *Constipation. Etiology, evaluation and management.* Oxford: Butterworth-Heinemann, 1995:31–35.

43. Kuijpers HC. Defaecography. In: Wexner SD, Bartolo DCC, eds. *Constipation. Etiology, evaluation and management.* Oxford: Butterworth-Heinemann, 1995:75–77.

44. Altringer WE, Saclarides TJ, Dominguez JM, et al. Four-contrast defecography: pelvic "floor-oscopy." *Dis Colon Rectum* 1995; 38(7):695–699.

45. Kelvin FM, Maglinte D, Hornback JA, et al. Pelvic prolapse: assessment with evacuation proctography (defecography). *Radiology* 1992;184:547–551.

46. Blatchford GJ, Cali RL, Christensen MA. Surgical treatment of rectocele. In: Wexner SD, Bartolo DCC, eds. *Constipation. Etiology, evaluation and management.* Oxford: Butterworth-Heinemann, 1995:199–209.

47. von der Ohe M, Camilleri M. Measurement of small bowel and colonic transit: indications and methods. *Mayo Clin Proc* 1992; 67:1169–1179.

48. Stein BL, Roberts PL. Manometry and the rectoanal inhibitory reflex. In: Wexner SD, Bartolo DCC, eds. *Constipation. Etiology, evaluation and management.* Oxford: Butterworth-Heinemann, 1995:63–76.

49. Preston DM, Lennard-Jones JE. Anismus in chronic constipation. *Dig Dis Sci* 1985;30:413–418.

50. Howard FM. The role of laparoscopy in chronic pelvic pain: promise and pitfalls. *Obstet Gynecol Surv* 1993;48:357–387.

51. Orr WC, Johnson P, Yates C. Chronic constipation: a clinical conundrum. *JAGS* 1997;45:652–653.

52. Tedesco FJ. Laxative use in constipation. *Am J Gastroenterol* 1985;80(4):303–309.

53. Muller-Lissner SA. Bavarian constipation study. Treatment of chronic constipation with cisapride and placebo. *Gut* 1987; 28:1033–1038.

54. Binnie NR, Creasy GH, Edmond P. The action of cisapride on chronic idiopathic constipation of paraplegia. *Paraplegia* 1988; 26:151–158.

55. Strickland MC, Heymen. Psychiatric treatment of constipation. In: Wexner SD, Bartolo DCC, eds. *Constipation. Etiology, evaluation and management.* Oxford: Butterworth-Heinemann, 1995: 251–261.

56. Yoshioka K, Keighley MRB. Clinical results of colectomy for chronic constipation. *Br J Surg* 1989;76:600–604.

57. Duthie GS, Bartolo DCC, Miller R, et al. Anismus does not adversely affect the outcome of colectomy and ileorectal anastomosis for slow transit constipation. *Gut* 1989;30:A735 (abstract).

58. Kamm MA, Hawley PR, Lennard-Jones JE. Lateral division of the puborectalis muscle in the management of severe constipation. *Br J Surg* 1988;75:661–663.

26

DIVERTICULAR DISEASE

C. PAUL PERRY

KEY TERMS AND DEFINITIONS

Diverticular disease: The spectrum of problems that may be caused by the presence of diverticula.

Diverticulitis: The presence of peridiverticular infection and inflammation.

Diverticulosis: The presence of diverticula within the colon without inflammation.

Diverticulum: A saccular outpouching of all layers of the colonic wall.

Dyschezia: Painful evacuation of feces from the colon.

False diverticulum: Herniation of only the mucosal layer of the colon.

Phlegmon: A mass produced by the inflammatory reaction of diverticulitis. It is often composed of thickened bowel wall, mesocolon, and adjacent structures such as bladder, uterus, small bowel, and omentum.

INTRODUCTION

Diverticular disease may present as chronic pelvic pain. More commonly, patients are diagnosed and treated during an initial attack and do not become an uncertain chronic pain problem. Diverticulosis is rare in females less than 30 years of age and uncommon in patients less than 40, but thereafter the incidence increases linearly. It occurs in one-third of the population over 45 and two-thirds of the population over 85 years of age. Five percent of all autopsies in the United States, United Kingdom, and Australia reveal the presence of diverticulosis. Of those requiring surgery, 16% are operated on within the first month and 50% are operated on within the first year. Men predominate in patients under 50 years of age, but women predominate in the older group (1).

Because the lower ileum, colon, and sigmorectum share the same innervation as the cervix, uterus, and adnexa, it may be difficult to determine if lower abdominal–pelvic pain is gynecologic or enterocolic in origin. The pain is usually diffuse and poorly localized. Visceral afferent nerves supplying the distal ileum, cecum, and transverse colon are carried by the sympathetic splanchnic nerves traversing the inferior mesenteric plexus. These enter the spinal cord at the T_{10}–L_2 level. The remaining portions of the colon, from the splenic flexure to the rectum, are supplied by afferent nerves traveling with the parasympathetic nerves of the nervi eregentes and enter the spinal cord at the S_{2-4} level. Thus, pain from diverticulitis is perceived to originate below the umbilicus and thereby often thought gynecologic in origin.

Because of viscerosomatic convergence (Chapter 55), there are two types of pain that may be experienced with diverticulitis: true visceral pain and referred pain. Visceral pain, in contrast to somatic pain, is usually perceived to be deep and difficult to localize. It is often accompanied by autonomic reflexes such as nausea, vomiting, diaphoresis, and restlessness (2). Somatic referred pain may be manifested by abdominal wall trigger points or muscle spasm.

ETIOLOGY

Diverticular disease is mainly a disease of Western civilization. It is much less common in the East and is virtually unheard of in Africa (1). The rectosigmoid is the most common site of diverticula. Eighty percent of diverticula are found in the sigmoid, 10% in the transverse colon, 4% in the rectum, 4% in the ascending colon, and 2% in the cecum (3).

A right-sided, or cecal, diverticulum is congenital. A left-sided, or rectosigmoid, diverticulum is acquired. Cecal diverticulosis is rare except in certain population groups such as Japanese, Hawaiians, Chinese, and Samoans (4). Eighty-four percent of all diverticula are left-sided (3). The etiology of acquired diverticula is thought to be a function of abnormal motility. These so-called "pulsion diverticula" may be caused from abnormally high intraluminal pressures created by diets low in fiber. Evidence supporting this etiology comes from both clinical and laboratory observations. The rectosigmoid usually develops waves of pressure in the 10-mmHg range, but when diverticular disease is present, pressures of up to 90 mmHg have been measured. Laboratory rats consuming a diet relatively low in fiber develop diverticula at a rate similar to that of humans in Western population. Raised intracolonic pressures found in patients with diverticular disease may be lowered by adding fiber to their diets (1).

PATHOLOGY

Diverticula are saccular outpouchings of the colon (Fig. 26.1). In the sigmoid colon, diverticula are formed by a herniation of mucosa and muscularis mucosae. These are called false or pseudodiverticula. More proximal in the colon, true diverticula are found containing all layers of the bowel wall. In the uninflamed condition, diverticula freely communicate with the colonic lumen. Their ostia vary from 0.5 cm to 1 cm and project through arcs of circular muscle at the point where blood vessels supplying the mucous membrane normally penetrate. Thus, an artery and vein are usually closely associated with each diverticulum. This anatomic relationship accounts for the bleeding seen with some cases of diverticulitis.

Normally, feces freely communicate between the diverticulum and the bowel lumen. When inflammation is present, it usually begins at the apex and spreads to the peri-

colic and mesenteric fat. This produces swelling and entrapment of inspissated feces, abrasion of the diverticular mucosa and possible ulceration or rupture of the sac. Localized peritonitis may spread to involve more diverticula in this fashion (1).

SYMPTOMS

There is some potential for diverticulosis to cause mild chronic pain, but there is no evidence that this is a common problem. Generally, diverticulosis produces no symptoms until inflammation occurs. The most common complaint of patients suffering with diverticulitis is lower abdominal pain. Usually, the pain is constant and localized to the left lower quadrant. It may start in the periumbilical area or right lower quadrant. This depends on the site of the diverticulum and the degree of peritonitis present. The pain is usually aggravated by eating and decreased with bowel movements or the passage of flatus. The patient may also manifest crampy diarrhea, constipation, flatulence, or dyspepsia. Varying degrees of nausea and vomiting may be present. Anorexia is common. Low-grade fever may be present. Urinary frequency and dysuria has been noted in up to 20% of patients with diverticulitis. This is due to the close proximity of the urinary

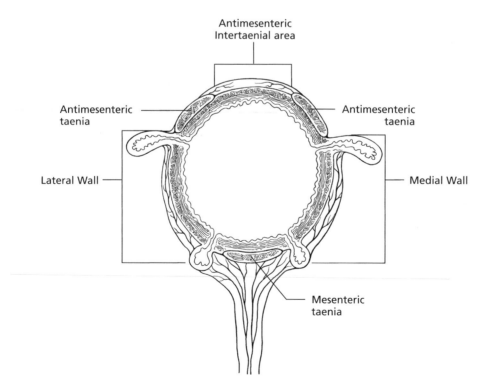

FIGURE 26.1. Cross-sectional drawing of colon, showing principal points of diverticular formation between the mesenteric and antimesenteric teniae. (From Goligher JC. *Surgery of the anus, rectum, and colon,* 5th ed. London: Bailliére Tyndall, 1984, with permission.)

bladder. Complications of diverticulitis include perforation, bleeding, abscess, and fistula formation. Death may result from sepsis, exsanguination, or surgical complications (1,2).

EXAMINATION

The abdominal examination usually reveals tenderness in the left lower quadrant. A firm, tender, cylindrical sigmoid can be rolled under the fingertips. Abdominal wall trigger points may be elicited. These will be found in the iliohypogastric, ilioinguinal, and genitofemoral nerve distribution. A palpable mass may be noted on the bimanual pelvic exam. Fever and tachycardia are seen with advanced inflammation. Hypoactive bowel sounds, rebound tenderness, and abdominal rigidity are found in those patients with colonic perforation (1,2).

DIAGNOSTIC STUDIES

Leukocytosis and an elevated sedimentation rate are helpful initial laboratory findings. Gross or occult blood may be found in the stool. Barium enemas and sigmoidoscopy should be performed with caution in the acutely ill patient for fear of causing perforation. When peritoneal signs are present, meglumine diatrizoate (Gastrografin) should be used in the event that the patient has unrecognized perforation. This could cause some fluid shift into the peritoneal cavity, but will avoid the potentially disastrous consequences of barium peritonitis. In evaluation of chronic pain, this contrast study can be diagnostic. Certain radiologic signs are characteristic of diverticular disease: abscess, deformed diverticula, fistula formation, narrowed segments, obstruction, pericolic mass, sinus tracts, spasms, stricture, and thickened colonic wall.

A computerized tomography (CT) scan may be more helpful and relatively noninvasive. Magnetic resonance imaging (MRI) is no more diagnostic, but more expensive. These studies can identify pericolic abscesses and may reveal small bowel distention if the ileum or jejunum form part of the wall of the phlegmon. Radionuclide scanning with labeled red blood cells is safe if bleeding is suspected. If positive, the scan may be followed by selective inferior or superior mesenteric angiography (1).

DIAGNOSIS

The location of the diverticulum will determine how easily the diagnosis is made. Not surprisingly, left-lower-quadrant pain and tenderness are most common. Diverticulitis especially should be considered in the older female patient with chronic pelvic pain. A past history of diverticulosis should raise the level of suspicion. Varying degrees of gastrointesti-

nal symptoms may be elicited. A mass can sometimes be palpated, but may be mistaken for a tuboovarian complex in many cases. Differential diagnosis for these findings must also include: ischemic colitis, pelvic inflammatory disease, pyelonephritis, colon cancer, colonic polyps, ulcerative colitis, and torsion of the left adnexum (1).

Right-sided diverticulitis is uncommon. It usually presents as an acute process, is more difficult to diagnose, and occurs at a younger age. The incidence does not increase with age. Patients presenting with cecal diverticulitis are clinically indistinguishable from those with appendicitis. Crohn's disease, Meckel's diverticulitis, pelvic inflammatory disease, torsion of the right adnexum, cholecystitis, ischemic bowel syndrome, and pyelonephritis can have similar presentations.

TREATMENT

Medical Treatment

When a diagnosis of chronic pelvic pain due to recurrent bouts of diverticulitis is made, medical therapy should be immediately instituted. Initially, bowel rest and oral antibiotics are started. Minocycline hydrochloride or sulfamethoxazole—trimethoprim with metronidazole have been effective treatments. After symptoms improve, high-fiber diet and fiber supplements with increased water intake become part of the secondary preventive maintenance regimen (1).

Surgical Treatment

Colonic resection is reserved for those patients with recurrent diverticulitis poorly controlled with medical therapy. Certain complications such as intractable bleeding, fistula formation, obstruction, and abscess formation will require surgery. Younger patients are more likely to have persistent pain and recurrence. Therefore, patients less than 55 years of age with one or more episodes of diverticulitis associated with complications are considered surgical candidates. Patients more than 55 years of age should experience at least two episodes before surgery is recommended. Factors to be considered in surgical judgment include: general health, persistent pain or leukocytosis, obstructive symptoms, inability to distinguish lesion from carcinoma, urinary tract symptoms, perforation, and fistula formation (1).

Simple diverticulectomy and oversewing of the diverticulum have been reported, but are rarely performed. Resection of the involved segment of colon with primary anastomosis is done most frequently after bowel prep in the absence of abscess. When anastomotic breakdown is feared, a two- or three-stage operation is preferred. Resection with colostomy followed by reanastomosis is performed in two steps. Colostomy with mucous fistula followed by resection, followed by reanastomosis, is performed in a three-stage procedure (1).

KEY POINTS

Differential Diagnosis

- Left-lower-quadrant pain: ischemic colitis, pelvic inflammatory disease, carcinoma, pyelonephritis, ulcerative colitis, and torsion of left adnexum.
- Right-lower-quadrant pain: appendicitis, ischemic colitis, Crohn's disease, Meckel's diverticulum, cholecystitis, carcinoma, pyelonephritis, and torsion of right adnexum.

Most Important Questions to Ask

- Any history of diverticulosis?
- Gastrointestinal symptoms: anorexia, nausea, vomiting, diarrhea, constipation?
- Any blood in the stool?
- Is the pain constant or cramping?
- Any fever?
- Are bowel movements painful?
- Is there any relief with the passage of stool or flatus?
- Is the pain aggravated by eating?
- Is there any urinary frequency or painful urination?

Most Important Physical Examination Findings

- Palpable, tender lower abdominal–pelvic mass
- Fever
- Tachycardia

- Hypoactive bowel sounds
- Rebound tenderness

Most Important Diagnostic Studies

- Complete blood count with sedimentation rate
- Stool for occult blood
- CT scan
- Barium enema or colonoscopy in the nonacute patient
- Gastrografin enema
- Radionuclide scan and angiography

Treatments

- Medical: broad-spectrum antibiotics, bowel rest
- Preventive maintenance: high-fiber diet, fiber supplements, and increased water intake
- Surgical: colon resection with reanastomosis in one, two, or three stages

REFERENCES

1. Veidenheimer MC, Roberts PL. *Colonic diverticular disease.* Boston: Blackwell Scientific Publications, 1991,1–155.
2. Rapkin AJ, Mayer EA. Gastroenterologic causes of chronic pelvic pain. *Obstet Gynecol Clin North Am* 1993;20:663–683.
3. Sardi A, Gokli A, Singer JA. Diverticular disease of the cecum and ascending colon: a review of 881 cases. *Am Surg* 1987;53:41–45.
4. Al-Hilaly MA, Razzaq HA, El-Salfiti JI, et al. Solitary caecal diverticulitis. *Acta Chir Scand* 1989;155:475–478.

27

INFLAMMATORY BOWEL DISEASE

JAMES E. CARTER

KEY TERMS AND DEFINITIONS

Crohn's disease: An inflammatory bowel disease that is characterized by focal, asymmetric, transmural inflammation affecting any portion of the gastrointestinal tract from the mouth to the anus; the symptoms and signs are determined by the sites and extent of inflammation.

Inflammatory bowel disease: Idiopathic, chronic inflammatory bowel diseases, including Crohn's disease and ulcerative colitis.

Ulcerative colitis: An inflammatory bowel disease characterized by abdominopelvic pain, rectal bleeding, tenesmus, and the passage of mucopus with a spectrum of diffuse, continuous, superficial inflammation of the colon, which begins within the rectum and extends to involve a variable, contiguous, proximal segment of colonic mucosa.

INTRODUCTION

Ulcerative colitis and Crohn's disease occur among all age groups, but have a peak incidence in the second and third decades. The incidence of Crohn's disease has risen over the past 20 years, and it now shares incidence and prevalence rates with ulcerative colitis of 5 per 100,000 and 50 per 100,000, respectively. The combined prevalence of the diseases is approximately 100 per 100,000 population. These disorders are seen most commonly in Northern Europe and North America. They are rare in Central America, South America, Africa, the Middle East, and Asia. Approximately 20% of individuals with inflammatory bowel disease have a relative with ulcerative colitis or Crohn's disease. Cigarette smoking appears to protect against ulcerative colitis and is associated with Crohn's disease. More than 80% of patient's with ulcerative colitis are nonsmokers, whereas 80% of patients with Crohn's disease smoke cigarettes [1].

Chronic abdominopelvic pain and discomfort are reported by patients with inflammatory bowel disease [2], so they must be considered in women with chronic pelvic pain. However, gastrointestinal symptoms are significant with all but the earliest manifestations of inflammatory bowel disease, which usually limits the initial differential diagnosis to gastrointestinal diseases.

ETIOLOGY

The causes of ulcerative colitis and Crohn's disease are not known. Although genetic, biochemical, and immunologic patterns are recognized, a definitive etiopathogenesis remains elusive. The absence of an appropriate animal model for chronic inflammatory bowel disease has hampered progress in determining pathogenesis. No infectious agent has been related to ulcerative colitis or to Crohn's disease, although it is speculated that exposure to a common bacterial antigen stimulates an autoimmune reaction against a shared host antigen via molecular mimicry [1].

A popular view is that a defect exists in the down-regulation of immune events allowing persistent amplification of tissue damaging processes. The inflammatory reaction in inflammatory bowel disease mimics infectious enterocolitis with the exception of the failure to halt progressive tissue destruction. There are subtle differences between the immunologic findings of ulcerative colitis and Crohn's disease, and misclassification is recognized as the clinical pathologic process evolves over time. When the diagnosis changes, it is almost always from ulcerative colitis to Crohn's disease and virtually never the reverse [1].

Potential initiating events in inflammatory bowel disease include increased intestinal permeability, aberrant epithelial processing of antigen, improper epithelial utilization of short-chain fatty acids, and molecular mimicry between a luminal antigen and components of intestinal mucosa [1].

Nonsteroidal inflammatory drugs damage the proximal and distal intestinal epithelium, increase intestinal permeability, and tend to exacerbate inflammatory bowel disease. Once initiated, many of the pathophysiologic events in inflammatory bowel disease are related to amplification of the inflammatory process [1].

The release of inflammatory mediators, including prostaglandins and leukotrienes, histamine from mast cells, and neuropeptides such as substance P or vasoactive intestinal peptide, alters epithelial function and contributes to the intestinal secretory process, including diarrhea. The enteric nervous system helps to regulate the local and systemic immune system, linking the association of stress and psychologic factors with disease flare ups. It is thought that one or more antigens, which have yet to be identified, activate macrophages and T cells beneath the superficial epithelial cells; these epithelial cells then secrete cytokines and chemotactic agents that can induce differentiation of B cells to immunoglobulin-secreting plasma cells. Consequently, increased concentration of cytokines (such as the interleukins) and of the immunoglobulins act directly to destroy the epithelial cells (2).

Patients with inflammatory bowel disease report chronic symptoms of abdominal pain (3). The effect of recurring intestinal tissue irritation on lumbosacral visceral afferent pathways was determined. Chronic ileal inflammation, such as that found in Crohn's disease, was associated with increased thresholds for discomfort and greatly diminished systemic autonomic reflex responses. In contrast, patients with irritable bowel syndrome showed lower thresholds for discomfort associated with increased autonomic responses. The findings in Crohn's patients may result from descending bulbospinal inhibition of sacral dorsal horn neurons in response to chronic intestinal tissue irritation (2).

One might expect that inflammation of the small intestine in Crohn's disease would result in hyperalgesia of splanchnic afferent pathways projecting to the thoracolumbar spinal cord. However, contraregulatory mechanisms activated by persistent tissue irritation may explain the absence of hyperalgesia in chronic inflammatory conditions of the gut.

Several lines of evidence support a possible role for the enteric nervous system in the pathogenesis of inflammatory bowel disease. Psychologic stress may exacerbate inflammatory bowel disease, suggesting important interactions among the brain, enteric nervous system, and gastrointestinal tract. In both Crohn's disease and ulcerative colitis, the immunoreactivity of substance P is increased and the binding sites for the substance P receptor are expressed more widely (4).

PATHOLOGY

Ulcerative colitis encompasses a spectrum of diffuse, continuous, superficial inflammation of the colon, which begins within the rectum and extends to involve a variable, contiguous, proximal segment of colonic mucosa. In 25% of patients the disease is limited to the rectum (proctitis); in another 25% to 50% the rectum and sigmoid (proctosigmoiditis) or the descending colon (left-sided colitis) is involved. In 33% of patients, the inflammation extends proximal to the splenic flucture (extensive colitis) or involves the entire colon (pancolitis). The gross or endoscopic appearance of the colonic mucosa in ulcerative colitis ranges from normal-appearing mucosa to complete denudation. Mild inflammatory changes include absence of the mucosal vascular pattern, fine granularity of the mucosa, pinpoint hemorrhage to mucosal swabbing, and exudation of mucopus. The inflammatory features are constant within the involved segment of the colon; and, once established, the upward margin of inflammation usually remains constant in the same individual (1).

Patients with inflammation throughout the colon may develop distal terminal ileitis. The inflammation extends beneath the lamina propria only in severe cases, when submucosal involvement produces a thinning of the circular and longitudinal muscles leading to colonic distention (toxic megacolon). Ulcerative colitis is primarily a mucosal process, and removal of the entire mucosa is curative (1). In the active phase of inflammation, acute inflammatory cells, primarily polymorphonuclear leukocytes, accumulate near the epithelium, invade the crypts, and are concentrated within the crypt lumen (crypt abscess). Progressive changes include degeneration or necrosis of the crypt epithelium with coalescence of crypt abscesses to produce shallow ulceration extending to the lamina propria. Epithelial dysplasia may occur in long-standing ulcerative colitis and is highly associated with the presence of colonic malignancy as a long-term complication (1).

Crohn's disease is characterized by focal, asymmetric, transmural inflammation affecting any portion of the gastrointestinal tract from the mouth to the anus. The ileum and right colon are most often involved, but any segment of the gastrointestinal tract can be inflamed (1). Microscopic changes often are identified distant from the sites of macroscopic disease. These focal changes and the tendency of Crohn's disease to recur after segmental resection suggest that subtle changes of Crohn's disease exist throughout the alimentary tract. Most commonly, the distal ileum and right colon are macroscopically inflamed. The colon is involved in about 20% of patients; approximately 15% to 20% have gross disease limited to the small bowel. The stomach or duodenum is involved in less that 10% of patients. Diseases of the anal canal, including deep fissures, fistulas, and prominent hemorrhoidal skin tags, are common (1).

The mucosa in Crohn's disease is involved in a focal discontinuous manner, both microscopically and macroscopically. The focal, transmural inflammation and the potential for proximal gastrointestinal tract involvement distinguishes Crohn's disease from ulcerative colitis. The earliest macroscopic lesion of Crohn's disease is by minute aphthoid ulcer invariably occurring over a lymphoid aggregate. These ulcerations can extend deep throughout the layers of the bowel wall, producing a fissure that can become a fistula into the mesentery or a contiguous organ. Inflammatory changes in Crohn's disease are typically transmural, accounting for the thickening of the bowel wall and narrowing of the lumen. As Crohn's disease heals, fibrotic changes replace acute inflammation, creating permanent focal strictures. In gross specimens, changes include thickened, sausage-shaped bowel with serosal hyperemia along the antimessenteric border and thickening and lymphoid hyperplasia of the adjacent mesentery. Lymphoid aggregates are common throughout all layers of the mucosa, submucosa, and serosa with characteristic aggregates of histiocytes forming noncaseating granulomas in up to 50% of resected specimens. The presence of noncaseating granuloma also distinguishes Crohn's disease from ulcerative colitis but is not necessary for the diagnosis. Microscopic changes are present throughout the gastrointestinal tract, distant from grossly involved segments of intestines (1).

HISTORY AND PHYSICAL EXAMINATION

Ulcerative Colitis

Patient's with proctitis have rectal bleeding, tenesmus, and the passage of mucopus. The consistency of stools is variable, and many patients with ulcerative proctitis are constipated. The greater the extent of colon involved, the more likely the patient is to suffer from diarrhea. Rectal urgency reflects reduced compliance of the inflamed rectum. Abdominal cramping is common, but abdominal pain or tenderness, reflecting transmural disease and stimulation of serosal or peritoneal pain receptors, is not typical of the superficial (mucosal) nature of ulcerative colitis. As the severity of the inflammation increases, the patient is more likely to suffer from systemic symptoms. Low-grade fever, malaise, occasional nausea and vomiting associated with defecation, night sweats, and arthralgias are frequent complaints. With severe ulcerative colitis, patients present with fever, dehydration, tachycardia, and symptoms of abdominal tenderness, reflecting progressive inflammation into deeper layers of the colon (1).

Crohn's Disease

The symptoms and signs of Crohn's disease are determined by the sites and extent of inflammation. Gastroduodenal Crohn's disease mimics peptic ulcer disease, with nausea, vomiting, and epigastric pain. Patients with small intestinal involvement have abdominal cramping, diarrhea, and abdominal tenderness. The pain and tenderness of Crohn's disease are due to transmural inflammation. Transmural inflammation leads to fibrosis and narrowing of the intestinal lumen, which produce symptoms of obstruction: nausea, vomiting, waves of abdominal pain, and a reduced output of stool. On physical exam, an abdominal mass may be found if the mesentery is involved. Patients with colonic Crohn's disease present with abdominopelvic pain, cramping, or localized pain, rectal bleeding, and diarrhea. Weight loss occurs in Crohn's disease because of small-bowel-related malabsorption. Systemic symptoms, including fever, night sweats, malaise, and arthralgias, are common (1).

Symptoms of rectal bleeding, tenesmus associated with the passage of pus, nocturnal pain and diarrhea, fever, night sweats, weight loss, or extra intestinal symptoms or signs generally exclude an uncomplicated irritable bowel syndrome. On physical examination, evidence of significant weight loss or extraintestinal signs, a palpable abdominal mass or tenderness, or significant perianal disease suggests inflammatory bowel disease (1).

DIAGNOSTIC STUDIES

Ulcerative Colitis

Laboratory studies reflect the severity of colitis. Iron deficiency anemia secondary to chronic blood loss is common. A low serum ferritin confirms the presence of iron deficiency anemia. Elevated erythrocyte sedimentation rate and other acute-phase reactants are inconstant features in ulcerative colitis. A low serum albumin occurs with extensive colitis as a manifestation of protein exudation from the inflamed colon. Serum alkaline phosphatase and GGTP may be modestly elevated in patients with pericholangitis; greater changes in bilirubin or hepatocellular enzymes suggest sclerosing cholangitis or chronic hepatitis (1).

Crohn's Disease

Laboratory features reflect blood loss, malabsorption, protein-losing enteropathy, and elevation of acute-phase reactions. Anemia may be due to a deficiency in iron (blood loss) or malabsorption of folic acid or vitamin B_{12}. Serum albumin and total protein are reduced with either malnutrition or protein losing enteropathy. Electrolyte abnormalities reflect the severity of diarrhea, and lowered serum calcium may reflect reduced serum albumin, calcium malabsorption, or vitamin D deficiency. Patients with ileal disease malabsorb fat-soluble vitamins, which can produce clinically significant symptoms (1).

There are no pathognomonic clinical endoscopic or histologic features of the idiopathic inflammatory bowel diseases. A cardinal feature is the exudation of inflammatory cells into the lumen, manifested by fecal leukocytes or red blood cells on stool examination. The presence of anemia, electrolyte disorders, hypoalbuminemia, an elevated erythrocyte sedimentation rate, and/or C-reactive protein is sufficient but not necessary to suggest inflammatory bowel disease. When suspicion of the diagnosis warrants, endoscopic and radiographic studies, in conjunction with histologic interpretation of biopsy specimens, confirm the diagnosis. The degree of illness at presentation should determine the aggressiveness of the diagnostic workup (1).

Patients presenting with colitis symptoms of rectal bleeding, cramping, tenesmus, mucopus, or watery diarrhea in conjunction with fecal leukocytes warrant a colonic examination. A proctoscopic examination or flexible sigmoidoscopy reveals the presence and pattern of distal colonic inflammation. Diffuse continuous mucosal changes with a distinct upper boundary to adjacent normal-appearing mucosa are typical of ulcerative proctitis or proctosigmoiditis. Focal inflammation with aphthoid ulcers, linear or stellate ulcers with normal mucosa, or inflammatory changes beginning above the rectum in previously untreated patients suggests Crohn's disease. Findings can be correlated with mucosal biopsy studies and radiographic evaluation (1).

Radiographically, a supine and upright view of the abdomen is performed. In colitis, a plain view of the abdomen often demonstrates a tubular, ahaustral segment of colon in the presence of distal ulcerative colitis. Air contrast barium studies of the colon reveal diffuse, contiguous granularity, superficial ulceration, and absent haustration in active ulcerative colitis. Pseudopolyps or a tubular-appearing colon may be found in chronic ulcerative colitis. Focal, asymmetric ulcerations with linear or fissuring ulcers, the presence of fistulas, rectal sparing, or diseased terminal ileum with reflux of the barium define the radiographic extent and severity of colonic Crohn's disease. A small bowel follow-up demonstrates the extent of small intestinal involvement in Crohn's disease (1).

DIAGNOSIS

Inflammatory bowel disease is distinguished from those diseases of the bowel of established origin such as viral, bacterial, and parasitic infections, diverticulitis, radiation enteritis or colitis, drug- or toxin-induced enterocolitis, and vasculitis of the intestinal tract. The differential diagnosis for inflammatory bowel disease includes irritable bowel syndrome, enteric infections, parasitic infections, mesenteric adenitis, ischemic bowel disease, recurrent diverticultis, intestinal lymphomas, radiation enteritis, eosinophlilic gastroenteritis, celiac sprue, and drug-related enterocolitis colonic carcinoma (1).

Patients with irritable bowel syndrome rarely present with inflammatory features. Most enteric infections are self-limited. Viral gastroenteritis lasts 1 to 4 days without rectal bleeding or fecal leukocytes. Bacterial pathogens produce self-limited disease lasting less than 7 to 14 days. *Campylobacter jejuni* produces protracted symptoms, and *clostridium C. difficile* toxin-induced colitis can mimic the symptoms, signs, and endoscopic appearance of ulcerative colitis or Crohn's disease. Stool cultures for enteric pathogens and studies for *C. difficile* toxin should be obtained to rule out infections. Studies can be performed for *Yersinia enterocoliticia*, tuberculosis, and actinomycocis. Parasitic infections such as amebiasis may cause diarrhea, rectal bleeding, and sigmoidoscopic appearance similar to that of inflammatory bowel disease. Fresh stool specimens are examined repeatedly for amebic cysts or trophozoites. Persistent rectal bleeding should not be attributed to hemorrhoids unless a flexible sigmoidoscopy has excluded inflammatory bowel disease. Radiation enteritis is limited to a patient with a history of radiation therapy. Eosinophilic gastroenteritis presents with diarrhea, malabsorption, and protein-losing enteropathy, but the associated peripheral blood eosinophilia and biopsies are distinguishing. The diffuse, proximal malabsorptive pattern of celiac sprue, associated with diffuse villous atrophy, is distinct from the focal, distal small bowel changes of Crohn's disease (1).

MANAGEMENT OR TREATMENT

Surgical Treatment

A proctocolectomy cures ulcerative colitis. Ulcerative colitis can be cured by colectomy, which alleviates the symptoms, lessens medication requirements, and can prevent potential long-term complications of colitis (cancer). Indications for surgery include toxic megacolon, perforation, intractable hemorrhage, complications in medical therapy, failure to improve with medical therapy, and evidence of confirmed dysplasia or cancer.

Surgery does not cure Crohn's disease. Surgery for Crohn's disease is limited to treatment of complications. Surgery is indicated for recurrent intestinal obstruction, complicated fistulas, intractable hemorrhage, disease refractory to medical therapy or complicated by inability to withdraw corticosteroids, growth retardation that does not respond to medical or nutritional intervention in children, and cancer (1).

Medical Treatment

Aminosalicylates

Sulfalazine combines sulfapyridine with a salicylate (5-amniosalicylic acid) for delivery into the connective tissue of the colon. Sulfalazine is effective in a dose-dependent manner for treating acute ulcerative colitis and for maintaining remission of quiescent ulcerative colitis. Sulfalazine has also been effective for mild to moderate Crohn's disease when the colon is involved (1).

Corticosteroids

Corticosteroids are indicated to induce remission in either ulcerative colitis or Crohn's disease. Oral prednisone is indicated for moderate to severe ulcerative colitis at doses of 400 mg daily initially followed by gradual tapering according to the clinical course (1).

Immunosuppressives

6-Mercaptopurine is effective in the long-term therapy of ulcerative colitis and Crohn's disease at doses that are not immunosuppressive, but probably have antiinflammatory activity (1).

Mild ulcerative proctitis can be treated with topical corticosteroids or topical mesalamine provided as enemas or foam. Proctosigmoiditis responds to hydrocortisone or mesalamine enemas in combination with oral amniosalicylates (1).

Unlike in ulcerative colitis, nutritional therapies have a more prominent role in treatment of Crohn's disease and prevention of complications. Supplemental nutrition is required in patients with Crohn's disease who have enhanced requirements for iron, protein, calcium, magnesium, folic acid, and water-soluble vitamins. In addition, patients with ileo-Crohn's disease require therapy for malabsorption of fat-soluble vitamins and vitamin B_{12}. No maintenance therapy has proved effective in Crohn's disease clinical trials. Corticosteroids should not be continued once clinical benefit has been obtained because of their severe long-term sequelae and their lack of benefit in preventing relapse. Many patients who respond to sulfalazine will worsen on withdrawal. Metronidazole results in long-term toxicity (neuropathy) (1).

The glucocorticoid drug budesonide provides antiinflammatory relief to the lower intestine and upper colon with fewer side effects than seen in studies of other steroid drugs. It was more effective with fewer side effects than mesalamine. Sixty-two percent of patients who took budesonide had remission after 16 weeks (5).

A new approach comes with the understanding that people with Crohn's disease produce cytokines in an abnormal fashion. Drugs are being engineered to attack specific abnormalities central to the disease process. These drugs will block the cytokines that are being produced by patients with Crohn's disease. The administration of monoclonal antibodies to the proinflammatory cytokine tumor necrosis factor alpha (TNF-α) has provided the most promising results. Recently, cA II (infliximab), a chimeric monoclonal antibody to TNF-α, was tested in patients with Crohn's disease. A single intravenous dose of cA II resulted in improvement of 65% of patients as compared with a response of 17% among patients given placebo (6).

KEY POINTS

Differential Diagnosis

- Irritable bowel syndrome
- Enteric infections
- Parasitic infections
- Mesenteric adenitis
- Ischemic bowel disease
- Recurrent diverticulitis
- Intestinal lymphomas
- Radiation enteritis
- Eosinophilic gastroenteritis
- Celiac sprue
- Drug-related enterocolitis
- Colon carcinoma

Most Important Question to Ask

- Are you experiencing symptoms of rectal bleeding, rectal spasms, passage of pus, abdominal cramping, diarrhea, or abdominal tenderness?

Most Important Physical Examination Finding

- Presence of abdominal pain or tenderness

Most Important Diagnostic Studies

- Exudation or inflammation into the bowel lumen manifested by fecal leukocytes or red blood cells on stool examination
- Sigmoidoscopy or colonoscopy findings of characteristic lesions

Treatments

- Aminosalicylates
- Corticosteroids
- Immunosuppressives
- Monoclonal antibodies
- Surgical therapy for unresponsive ulcerative colitis

REFERENCES

1. Hanauer SB. Inflammatory bowel disease. In: Bennett JC, Plum F, eds. *Cecil textbook of medicine,* vol 1. Philadelphia: WB Saunders, 1996:707–715.
2. Bernstein CN, Niazi N, Robert M, et al. Rectal afferent function in patients with inflammatory and functional intestinal disorders. *Pain* 1996;66:151–161.
3. Gray GM. Inflammatory bowel disease. In: Dale DC, Federman DD, eds. *Scientific American medicine,* vol 4. New York: Scientific American Inc. 1995:1–18.
4. Mazundar S, Das KM. Immunocytochemical localization of vasoactive intestinal peptide of substance P in the colon from normal subjects and patients with inflammatory bowel disease. *Am J Gastroenterol* 1992;87:176–181.
5. Thomsen OO, Cortot A, Jewell D, et al. A comparison of budesonide and mesalamine for active Crohn's disease. *N Engl J Med* 1998;339:370–374.
6. Bickston SJ, Cominelli F. Treatment of Crohn's disease at the turn of the century [Editorial]. *N Engl J Med* 1998;339:401–402.

28

IRRITABLE BOWEL DISEASE

FRED M. HOWARD

KEY TERMS AND DEFINITIONS

Basal myoelectrical cyclic rhythm of the colon: Also referred to as the slow-wave frequency; dominant (90% of the time) myoelectric frequency of six cycles per minute present in the colon of normal healthy individuals; the colon contracts when spiked potentials are superimposed on this basal myoelectrical rhythm.

Discreet clustered contractions: Continuous irregular bursts of contractions during phase 2 of small bowel motility that are believed to be propulsive and occur more commonly in IBS patients.

Enteric nervous system: A collection of neurons in the gastrointestinal tract that can function independently of the central nervous system and controls motility, exocrine and endocrine secretions, and microcirculation of the gastrointestinal tract.

Irritable bowel syndrome: A common functional bowel disorder of uncertain etiology characterized by a chronic, relapsing pattern of abdominopelvic pain and bowel dysfunction with constipation and/or diarrhea.

Migrating motor complex: Motor activity or motility of the normal small bowel in the fasting state that is characterized by a cycle every 60 to 120 minutes that may be divided in four phases: quiescence, irregular intermittent contractions, uninterrupted rhythmic contractions (propagation or "housekeeper" phase), and transition.

Rapidly propagating contractions: Prolonged, large-amplitude, rapidly propagating contractions that occur during phase 2 of small bowel motility, last more than 12 seconds, and are propulsive; occur more commonly in IBS patients.

INTRODUCTION

Irritable bowel syndrome (IBS) is one of the most common disorders associated with chronic pelvic pain (CPP) in women. Symptoms suggestive of IBS are present in 50% to 80% of women with CPP (1,2). It is an intriguing syndrome that has confounded clinicians and distressed patients for over a century. The term *irritable bowel syndrome* is applied to a hodgepodge of gastrointestinal disorders and is known by many other names, an unfortunate fact that confuses patients (and clinicians). Some of the other names include spastic colitis, neurogenic mucous colitis, mucous colitis, membranous enteritis, membranous colitis, and nervous colitis. In particular the use of the term *colitis* is inappropriate. There is no inflammation of the colon either grossly or microscopically in patients with IBS. Nor is IBS confined to the colon; it also involves the small intestine. These alternative names should be discarded in favor of irritable bowel syndrome.

In the evaluation of pelvic pain, IBS needs to be ruled out. Of women with IBS, 21% aged 18 to 40 years have undergone hysterectomies. This is significantly higher than the national average of about 6% (3). IBS is common. It affects 15% of Western and Chinese populations. It accounts for 3 million visits a year to primary care providers, leading to 2 million medical prescriptions. IBS is the second most common reason for absenteeism from work, after the common cold. Approximately 25% to 50% of all referrals to gastroenterologists are related to this diagnosis. However, only 20% to 25% of patients with IBS consult a physician. In most Western countries, IBS is three times more common in women than in men. IBS is more common in the white population by a 5:1 margin. Jewish people also tend to have a higher incidence compared with the non-Jewish population. In half of those affected, symptoms begin before 35 years of age. Forty percent of patients with IBS are 35 to 50 years of age (4).

As a syndrome, IBS is defined by the presence of a combination of symptoms and signs. In 1978, Manning et al. (5) published the following criteria for IBS: (a) abdominal pain relieved by a bowel movement; (b) more frequent stools with onset of pain; (c) looser stools with onset of pain; and/or (d) abdominal distention evident by tighter clothing or by visible distention. The more criteria present, the more likely the patient has IBS. These criteria have continued to be used, but their sensitivity has been found to be as low as 42%. In the early 1990s, the International Congress of Gastroenterology published more specific criteria to define IBS (6). These criteria, known as the *Rome criteria*, are listed in Table 28.1.

TABLE 28.1. THE "ROME" DIAGNOSTIC CRITERIA FOR IRRITABLE BOWEL SYNDROME

At least 3 months of continuous or recurrent symptoms of:
1. abdominal pain or discomfort that is:
   a. relieved with defecation,
   b. and/or associated with a change in frequency of stool,
   c. and/or associated with a change in consistency of stool;
   and
2. two or more of the following, at least one-quarter of occasions or days:
   a. altered stool frequency,[a]
   b. altered stool form (lumpy/hard or loose/watery stool),
   c. altered stool passage (straining, urgency, or feeling of incomplete evacuation),
   d. passage of mucus,
   e. bloating or feeling of abdominal distention.

[a]For research purposes "altered" may be defined as more than three bowel movements per day or less than three bowel movements per week.

Patients with IBS often are difficult to manage. However, much has been learned recently about IBS, due to improved techniques in evaluating the small and large intestines, and treatment modalities are continually improving.

ETIOLOGY

IBS is a functional disorder, which means that by definition no structural or biochemical abnormalities are present that explain the symptoms. It is one of several functional digestive disorders. Others affect the esophagus, stomach, and biliary system. Categorization as a functional disorder does not imply that IBS is a psychiatric disorder, although initially it was thought of as primarily a psychiatric disease. Symptoms can be influenced by psychologic factors and stressful situations.

The pathophysiologic mechanisms that cause IBS are not completely understood and likely are multifactorial. The physiologic makeup of the bowel is a complicated subject. Multiple control mechanisms are at work, including the central nervous system, autonomic nervous system, enteric nervous system, and hormonal input.

Similarly to women with CPP generally, approximately 70% to 80% of patients with IBS have abnormal psychologic profiles, with increased somatization, hypochondriasis, and depression. It has been found that 50% of patients report onset of symptoms during a stressful period of their life and report exacerbations of these symptoms with stressful events. However, data suggest that the symptoms of psychologic stress have nothing to do with the development of IBS. They do influence the decision to consult a physician. This has been termed the "self-selection" hypothesis. Patients with IBS who do not seek medical treatment do not have profiles that are different from those of a control population without IBS. Thus it is not

clear if these psychologic changes are etiologic or secondary, and they do not seem sufficient to explain the syndrome. Therefore, other mechanisms to explain the etiology of IBS must be sought.

One potential explanation relates to the basal myoelectrical cyclic rhythm of the colon. This rhythm also is referred to as the *slow-wave frequency*. The colon contracts when spiked potentials are superimposed on this basal myoelectrical rhythm. Normal healthy individuals typically have a dominant frequency of six cycles per minute 90% of the time. Patients with IBS more commonly have a slow-wave frequency of three cycles per minute. However, this slower rhythm does not seem to be specific for IBS. Psychoneurosis is another diagnosis that seems to have a similar rhythm. Patients with IBS also seem to have slower changes in motor activity in response to anger, pain, psychologic stress, hormonal stimulation, and balloon distention.

Small bowel motility is also altered in IBS patients. Normal motility of the small bowel in a fasting healthy subject is characterized by a migrating motor complex that occurs cyclically every 60 to 120 minutes in four phases. Phase 1 is quiescence. Phase 2 consists of irregular intermittent contractions that increase in frequency and amplitude over a 30-minute period. Phase 3 consists of a sequence of uninterrupted rhythmic contractions that last 5 to 15 minutes. The phase 3 propagation of contractions allows food to be swept out of the stomach and is commonly referred to as the "housekeeper" phase. Phase 4 is the short time between the phase 3 activity and phase 1 inactivity. In the nonfasting or fed state, the pattern of small bowel motility consists of continuous irregular contractions.

In IBS patients there are two specific motor patterns that are seen more commonly than in non-IBS controls. Both patterns occur during phase 2. One of these patterns consists of continuous irregular bursts of contractions called discreet clustered contractions (DCCs). DCCs are believed to be propulsive. The other pattern is characterized by prolonged, large-amplitude, rapidly propagating contractions (RPCs) that last more than 12 seconds. RPCs are propulsive. Normal women also can have DCCs and RPCs, but women with IBS appear to have increased pain and sensitivity to them. Kellow et al. (7) found that 61% of intermittent RPCs were associated with pain in IBS patients compared to only 17% in control subjects. Small bowel motor activity also seems to be increased in IBS patients in response to fatty meals and hormonal stimulation.

Unfortunately, it has been difficult to consistently show a direct association between the symptoms of IBS and specific changes in colon and small bowel motility. Although clearly there are abnormalities of motility with IBS, more needs to be known.

Another alteration that may account for some symptoms of IBS is increased visceral sensitivity. Patients with IBS have abnormal pain levels with intestinal distention. This may explain the common complaint of excessive bloating and gas, because it has been suggested that patients with IBS may not actually have elevated amounts of intestinal gas. Rather, they may have abnormal pain at a given volume of gas. This has been demonstrated by studies in which inflated balloons in the rectums of patients with IBS and controls showed that IBS patients exhibited pain at a much lower interstitial wall tension than normal patients (8). This increased anorectal sensitivity may explain the pain before bowel movements and the sense of incomplete evacuations often complained of by IBS patients. IBS patients do not have a generally increased sensitivity to painful stimuli. For example, response to hand immersion in ice water is the same in IBS patients as in normal subjects.

Colonic fermentation in patients with IBS appears to be abnormal, and this might also have a role in the production of symptoms (9). In a crossover controlled trial in six female IBS patients and six female controls of a standard diet and an exclusion diet matched for macronutrients, the maximum rate of gas excretion, total gas production, and hydrogen production were greater in patients than in controls. In patients, the exclusion diet reduced symptoms and produced a fall in maximum gas excretion. After a lactulose challenge, breath hydrogen was greater on the standard than on the exclusion diet. Such data suggest that colonic gas production, particularly of hydrogen, is greater in patients with IBS than in controls and that fermentation may be an factor in the pathogenesis of IBS.

Investigations continue on the possible roles of peptides that are found in the gut and brain, such as vasoactive interstinal polypeptide, substance P, cholecystokinin, and enkephalins, and seem to have integrative activities, but their roles in IBS are as yet unclear.

HISTORY AND SYMPTOMS

The characteristic symptoms of IBS are abdominal pain, bloating, belching, excessive flatus, diarrhea, constipation, painful defecation, and the sensation of incomplete evacuation. A complete history also includes questions about anorexia, early satiety, nausea, vomiting, number of bowel movements per day, number of bowel movements per week, urgency to defecate, prolonged evacuation attempts, straining to defecate, stool color, weight loss without dieting, and increase of symptoms with sex or menses. Symptoms generally start in late adolescence or early adulthood. Onset in later life is less common.

Abdominal pain is most often in the left lower quadrant, but may be located in the middle and/or lower abdominal area as well. Many patients have two or more sites of pain. Less often, abdominal pain is poorly localized. The pain typically does not radiate. Pain may be described as cramping, burning, dull, sharp, steady, bloating, or knife-like. Eating commonly precipitates pain, and defecation often relieves it.

Either diarrhea or constipation, or alternating episodes of both, may be present. It is helpful to ask the patient to describe her bowel movements precisely. In particular, many individuals complain of constipation if they do not have a bowel movement daily, and they do not realize that normal stool frequency is anywhere from three times a day to every 3 days. In patients with IBS and diarrhea the volume of diarrhea is small, less than 200 mL per day. Diarrheic stool volumes greater than 200 mL per day suggest the diagnosis is not IBS.

Characteristically, both pain and diarrhea resolve during sleep. Diarrhea associated with IBS also characteristically resolves during a 24-hour fast. Awakening and noting pain is not the same as being awakened by pain, and it is important to try to have the patient make this distinction if possible. Depression, not uncommon in women with IBS, may be the cause of nighttime wakening, and this should not lead the physician away from considering IBS as a possible diagnosis. Similarly, awakening and then noting the urge to defecate should be distinguished from being wakened by the need to evacuate. The latter suggests a a true secretory cause for diarrhea, not IBS. Also, if diarrhea continues during a 24-hour fast, it suggests a secretory etiology, not IBS. As an aside, it is usually very difficult to have a patient maintain a true 24-hour fast, so this symptom characteristic is not particularly useful as a diagnostic intervention.

Typically in patients with diarrhea-dominant IBS, with an episode or exacerbation the initial stool is formed, then subsequent stools are increasingly loose and eventually are liquid. Patients with constipation-dominant IBS typically have small, "pellet-like" stools. Occasionally, patients with IBS may give a history of pencil-thin stools. This has been attributed to rectal and sigmoid spasm.

Patients with IBS are more likely to have gastrointestinal reflux with heartburn, dysphagia, globus sensation, and noncardiac chest pain than those without IBS. They also have more urologic dysfunction, fatigue, and reproductive tract problems (10).

IBS symptoms often exacerbate during menses, so direct questions should be asked about a cyclic pattern corresponding with menses; this correlation should not be assumed to mean that the pain is of gynecologic origin (11). Even in women without IBS, there is an increased occurrence of diarrhea, constipation, and increased gas at menses. These changes may be related to prostaglandin levels. Some preliminary research suggests that suppression of the menstrual cycle with gonatropin-releasing hormone agonists is efficacious in IBS. The role of prostaglandin antagonists has not been well-studied. Women with IBS also have a higher frequency of dyspareunia than do women without IBS.

A detailed dietary history should be taken. It is helpful to have the patient keep at least a 7-day diary of the quality and quantity of food and drink consumed during symptomatic periods. Particular note should be taken of whether the patient is a binge eater. Because lactose intolerance can mimic IBS and can contribute to the symptoms of IBS, the dietary history should also include detailed information about lactose consumption. About 40% of patients with IBS also have lactose intolerance. Lactose intolerance affects 90% of Asians and Africans and up to 50% of southern Europeans. Lactose is present in a wide variety of foods, therefore, it is important that the patient learn to read labels to provide information about lactose consumption and, if lactose is found to be a contributor to symptoms, to eliminate it from her diet.

Sorbitol, which is a common sweetening agent used in "sugar-free" and other dietetic foods, may also contribute to symptoms, so the history should include information on its consumption. Normally, at least 90% of ingested sorbitol is absorbed in the small intestine by passive diffusion. Ingestion of more than 30 g of sorbitol is known to cause osmotic diarrhea, but some individuals tolerate much less and may react with consumption of only 10 g. Ten grams of sorbitol can be present in four to five sugar-free mints. Severe sorbitol intolerance is found in about 30% of blacks and 4% of whites.

Fructose, a major sugar component of fruit, also can cause significant abdominal distress. Fructose is added to a variety of processed foods. Symptoms seem to be related to its fermentation by colonic bacteria and malabsorbed carbohydrates. The combination of sorbitol and fructose can contribute to the patient's diarrhea; therefore, should be eliminated from the diet, at least on a trial basis, if the history reveals their consumption.

Caffeinated products (including coffee, tea, and cola), carbonated products, and gas-producing foods may contribute to bloating. Common gas-producing foods include broccoli, cabbage, brussel sprouts, asparagus, cauliflower, and beans. Smoking and chewing gum lead to more swallowed air and may increase gas and bloating. Excessive alcohol consumption may lead to increased rectal urgency.

A detailed medication history, including all current and past medications, both prescribed and over-the-counter, is necessary. Many medications alter bowel motility and may exacerbate symptoms of IBS. In particular, many patients take laxatives and do not realize that laxatives contribute to their symptoms. Antacids containing magnesium or aluminum can cause diarrhea or constipation, respectively.

A history of any abdominal surgery can be important. Postoperative adhesions may cause symptoms that mimic IBS.

A complete social history including questions related to sexual and physical abuse is pertinent. Drossman and colleagues found that 44% of patients with functional gastrointestinal disorders have a history of sexual or physical abuse in childhood or later in life (12). All but one of the physically abused patients had been sexually abused also. Patients are unlikely to volunteer this information unless specifically asked.

Travel history, particularly overseas, is often important in the differential diagnostic evaluation of symptoms suggesting IBS. Family history of gastrointestinal diseases, especially inflammatory bowel disease, colon cancer, or malabsorption states such as sprue, is important in differential diagnostic evaluation, also.

A history of rectal bleeding suggests a diagnosis other than IBS unless the bleeding is related to hemorrhoids or a fissure from straining. Similarly, a history of weight loss suggests that the diagnosis is not IBS. Weight loss is unusual in a patient with IBS unless there is concomitant depression.

The symptoms of IBS are chronic, although variable in severity. Pain and bowel symptoms that are of a steadily progressive nature suggest a diagnosis other than IBS. Also, as a chronic disorder, IBS usually has an onset of symptoms that is gradual and vague, and it is unusual for the patient to be able to relate an exact date of onset of symptoms. If so, it is likely that she does not have IBS.

SIGNS AND PHYSICAL EXAMINATION

On general appearance patients with IBS often seem anxious and tense. They may have tachycardia and hypertension. In contrast, however, they are sometimes depressed in their affect and behavior. Otherwise, the general physical examination is usually normal.

On abdominal examination, inspection may reveal mild to moderate distention. Surgical scars are important to note and correlate with the history. On palpation, tenderness may be elicited. It is most often in the left lower quadrant, if present, but may be generalized. Rebound tenderness occasionally may be elicited, but is not a common finding. Rectal and pelvic examinations are important to assess for masses or anal disease, such as hemorrhoids or fissures, that could explain some of the symptoms.

Signs suggesting an acute abdomen, with generalized tenderness or board-like rigidity, rebound tenderness, tympanitic bowel sounds, and a fever, are not consistent with IBS, and they should lead the physician to evaluate expeditiously for a serious intraabdominal process. Such findings are not consistent with the diagnosis of IBS.

DIAGNOSTIC STUDIES

In the patient with suspected IBS a complete blood cell count with differential, chemistry profile and sedimentation rate are suggested. The complete blood cell count helps rule out anemia and inflammation or infection. The sedimentation rate similarly helps rule out an inflammatory process. The white blood cell differential is useful in evaluating parasitic infection (which often causes eosinophilia), tuberculosis (which causes monocytosis), and inflammation (which may cause toxic granulation). With IBS the chemistry profile should be normal, whereas in inflammatory bowel disease electrolyte abnormalities are more likely. To rule out infection with *Giardi*, amoeba, and other parasites, three stool specimens should be sent for ova-and-parasite (O&P) testing.

Stool also should be checked for occult blood; results should be negative in IBS patients. Similarly, methylene blue stain of stool to look for white blood cells should be negative with IBS, because the presence of large numbers of white blood cells is diagnostic of inflammation. A Sudan stain for fat can be performed by adding 2 drops of acetic acid, 2 drops of Sudan III, and 95% alcohol to a slide with a stool specimen. The slide is then gently heated to boiling. Normally, only a few small red-staining fat globules are seen. In severe steatorrhea, many large fat globules are seen. Stools should be checked for *Clostridium difficile* toxin if there has been antibiotic exposure within the last 6 weeks.

In women less than 40 years of age, proctosigmoidoscopy with biopsy should be performed. Although the mucosa may appear grossly normal, biopsy may reveal microscopic or collagenous colitis. With patients older than 40 years, a barium enema and flexible sigmoidoscopy or a full colonoscopy may be indicated to rule out neoplasia. The insufflation during an air-contrast barium enema or colonoscopy often reproduces the patient's IBS symptoms.

The possibility of lactose intolerance can be formally tested with a hydrogen breath test if there is any question. The breath test is much more sensitive than the blood test.

Irritable bowel syndrome is a diagnosis of exclusion. Unfortunately, there is no one simple physical finding, blood test, or x-ray that unquestionably confirms the diagnosis. The difficulty of diagnosis is further confounded by the fact that IBS may coexist with other bowel problems.

TREATMENT OR MANAGEMENT
Medical Treatment

Because IBS is a syndrome of uncertain etiology, treatment is not specific to the disease, but rather is directed to relief of symptoms. For the purpose of treatment, patients may be sorted into one of three major subclassifications, depending on which symptom(s) is dominant. The three symptom subclassification are (a) abdominal pain, gas, and bloating, (b) constipation predominant, and (c) diarrhea predominant. Unfortunately, many patients do not fall clearly into one of these three groups, but have overlapping symptoms. The severity of the symptoms also influences the choice of treatment.

In patients with predominately abdominal pain, gas, and bloating symptoms, if there is clearly no evidence of small bowel obstruction, then a trial of an antispasmodic is suggested. The commonly used antispasmodics are dicyclomine (Bentyl), hyoscyamine (Levsin), Donnatal, and Librax. None of these has been shown to be consistently efficacious. Treatment with any of these drugs is started at a low dose

and increased gradually. Unfortunately, sometimes efficacy is obtained only at a level at which side effects are troublesome. Potential side effects of antispasmodic, anticholinergic medications include urinary retention, xerostomia, and mydriasis. It is helpful to discuss these side effects with the patient before initiating treatment. Because many patients have these symptoms postprandially, the timing of the dosing is crucial. Generally, it is best to give each of these medications 30 minutes before meals. However, if a sublingual preparation is prescribed, then it an be given at the time that the discomfort begins. In patients with predominately gas and bloating symptoms, Beano (a D-galactosidase) or a simethicone preparation (Gas X, Phazyme) also can be tried.

If the patient's symptomatology is predominately constipation, then a trial of increased roughage and psyllium is prescribed. Many patients have increased gas with increased fiber, and about 15% cannot tolerate fiber therapy. It is recommended, therefore, that fiber be increased gradually and be taken with a meal (usually breakfast). Sometimes tap water enemas during the initiation of fiber supplements are helpful. If necessary, a stool softener or osmotic laxative also can be used temporarily. An insufficient dose of fiber is a frequent cause of failure. Chronic use of stimulant laxatives should be discouraged. If constipation persists, then further investigation with a colonic transit test is indicated. This is done by ingestion of 20 radiopaque markers, followed by x-rays taken on days 4 and 7 after ingestion. Anorectal manometry, tests of rectal sensation and expulsion, and assessment of the pelvic floor for descent are sometimes necessary also.

There may be a role for prokinetic agents in constipation (13,14). Cisapride (Propulsid), which seems to work by facilitating acetylcholine release from the myenteric plexus, has been shown to increase small bowel transit and may be helpful. However, in a randomized, placebo-controlled trial in 96 patients with constipation-predominant IBS, cisapride 5 mg three times daily for 12 weeks did not change symptoms any more than placebo (abdominal pain, 31% versus 31% improvement, respectively; constipation, 56% versus 58%, respectively; and abdominal bloating; 27% versus 27%, respectively) (15). Only the difficulty of stool passage showed a significantly higher improvement with cisapride. In a different randomized, double-blind, placebo-controlled study of cisapride, 5 mg three times daily for 12 weeks, the reduction in severity and frequency scores for abdominal pain was significantly greater in the cisapride group (60% and 61%) than in the placebo group (40% and 32%) (16). Abdominal distention and flatulence were also significantly improved. In 71% of cisapride-treated versus 39% of placebo-treated patients the overall rating of response to treatment was good or excellent. More evidence is needed to clearly demonstrate whether cisapride is efficacious in the treatment of IBS.

Metoclopramide (Reglan) is not recommended because, although it is a prokinetic agent, it does not act on the large intestine. Tricyclic antidepressants should be avoided in these patients because they may aggravate constipation because of their anticholinergic side effects.

In IBS patients with diarrhea-predominant symptomatology, loperamide (Imodium) is the most commonly used agent (17). It is available over the counter. The dose is 2 to 4 mg four times a day up to a maximum dose of 16 mg per day. Loperamide decreases intestinal transit time, enhances intestinal water absorption, and strengthens rectal sphincter tone. In a double-blind placebo-controlled trial of loperamide in patients with diarrhea-predominant IBS, loperamide was found to significantly improve stool consistency, pain, and urgency (18). Loperamide does not cross the blood–brain barrier, but other antidiarrheal agents, such as Lomotil and codeine, do cross the blood–brain barrier. Patients with IBS often are especially sensitive to antidiarrheal agents. Sometimes a single dose causes constipation, so caution must be exercised in prescribing antidiarrheals. It is prudent to try a soluble dietary fiber (psyllium, pectin, or oat bran) before using loperamide or other antidiarrheals. A low-fat diet and smaller meals also may help. Tricyclic antidepressants, due to their anticholinergic properties, may alleviate diarrhea and associated pain in some patients.

Idiopathic bile acid catharsis, a disorder in which bile acid entering the colon irritates the large bowel, can be a cause of functional diarrhea. A trial of cholestyramine (up to 4 g every 6 hours) is warranted in women with diarrhea-predominant symptoms. There is a high false-negative rate (up to 25%) and an appreciable false-positive rate with cholestyramine use. In specialized centers, bile acid malabsorption can be assessed by the ^{75}Se HCAT test.

Ondansetron, a serotonin receptor antagonist (5HT3), slows colonic transit time and may be useful in the treatment of diarrhea-predominant IBS (19). In a double-blind, placebo-controlled crossover study of ondansetron in 50 patients with irritable bowel syndrome, it reduced bowel frequency and improved stool consistency in diarrhea-predominant patients and did not cause a deterioration of bowel habits in constipation-predominant subjects (20). No statistically significant improvement was seen for abdominal pain or distention, although those patients who did respond were approximately twice as likely to be taking ondansetron than placebo. In another randomized double-blind parallel group trial it has been shown that a potent and selective 5-HT3 antagonist (Alosetron) increases the compliance of the colon to distention and modulates visceral sensitivity in a dose-dependent manner (21). These changes could contribute to changes in perception of colonic distention and improvement in the symptoms of IBS. However, the 5-HT3 antagonists are not approved by the Food and Drug Administration for this indication.

Peppermint oil is the major constituent of several over-the-counter remedies for IBS. Because this represents a safe and inexpensive treatment, there is a ready market for such products. In a prospective, randomized, double-blind, placebo-controlled clinical study of 110 patients with symptoms of IBS, peppermint oil in an enteric-coated formulation (Colpermin), taken three to four times daily, 15 to 30 minutes before meals, for 1 month, decreased abdominal pain in 79% of patients compared to 43% in the placebo group (absolute benefit increase of 36% and number needed to treat of 2.8) (22). Peppermint oil also decreased abdominal distention in 83% of patients compared to 29% with placebo (absolute benefit increase of 54% and number needed to treat of 1.9), reduced stool frequency in 83% compared to 32% with placebo (absolute benefit increase of 51% and number needed to treat of 2.0), decreased borborygmi in 73% versus 31% with placebo (absolute benefit increase of 42% and number needed to treat of 2.4), and reduced flatulence in 79% compared to 22% with placebo (absolute benefit increase of 57% and number needed to treat of 1.8). Thus, in this trial, Colpermin was effective and well tolerated. A recent review of eight randomized, controlled trials suggests that peppermint oil could be efficacious for symptom relief in IBS, but methodological flaws preclude a definitive judgment about efficacy (23).

The use of anxiolytic medications is controversial, but their use in combination with other agents may be beneficial. One study of diazepam combined with octylonium bromide showed that combination therapy, compared to monotherapy, reduced abdominal pain intensity and gas distention (24).

Pharmacologic therapy is not necessary in all individuals and, at times, may be counterproductive due to side effects. The foundation of treatment involves confidence in the diagnosis and a strong physician–patient relationship (25). IBS is a chronic disorder, so management is best accomplished with a strong therapeutic relationship and good communication. Ensuring that the patient understands her disorder is very important. She should know that IBS is a real disorder in which the intestine is abnormally sensitive to stimuli, even normal stimuli. She should understand that her active participation in treatment is essential to achieve improvement. Some patients believe that they may have cancer, so it may be necessary to clearly state that IBS is the diagnosis and that IBS does not lead to cancer, require surgery, or shorten life expectancy. Psychotherapy with cognitive-behavioral therapy (including stress management), dynamic psychotherapy, hypnosis, and relaxation therapy may be helpful. If family dysfunction exacerbates symptoms, then family counseling can be useful also. Combining psychologic treatment with medical therapies improves the clinical response over that with the medical treatment only (26,27). Factors that predict a good response to psychotherapy include predominately diarrhea and pain, the association of overt psychiatric symptoms, intermittent pain exacerbated by stress, short durations of bowel complaints, and few sites of abdominal pain (28). Patients with constant abdominal pain do poorly with psychotherapy or hypnotherapy. A recent review of controlled trials of psychologic treatments for irritable bowel syndrome found that

8 out of 14 studies reported that psychologic therapy was significantly superior to control treatment in reducing the primary symptoms of IBS (29). Five studies failed to detect a significant effect, although three of these did report that symptoms were significantly reduced after psychologic treatment compared with baseline measures. However, only one study (a hypnotherapy trial) had acceptable methodologic quality, and this study was poorly generalizable due to sample selection.

Complementary medical therapies are frequently used by patients with IBS. In particular, relaxation response training, hypnosis, and biofeedback appear to be helpful. However, complementary treatments must be subjected to the same scientific scrutiny as traditional treatments. For example, a randomized clinical trial of 18 weeks of two phytotherapeutic agents, Extr. *Fumaria officinalis* or Extr. *Curcuma xanthorrhiza*, failed to show any differences in pain, bloating, or quality of life over that of placebo (the placebo response in this trial was 65%) (30).

SURGICAL TREATMENT

Women with IBS have a disproportionately high predisposition to undergo hysterectomy (31). Clearly, it is important that accurate diagnosis and comprehensive treatment modalities be tried before hysterectomy is performed in women with pelvic pain and symptoms suggestive of IBS. Whether hysterectomy is capable of causing or worsening IBS symptoms is not clear.

Adhesiolysis may have a limited role in the treatment of IBS, if adhesions are thought responsible for some or all of the symptoms. There are no methodologically valid trials that allow an evaluation of this approach to treatment, so it seems best reserved for isolated unusual cases or for experimental trials.

KEY POINTS

Differential Diagnoses

- Neoplasia
- Inflammatory bowel disease
- Vascular insufficiency
- Chronic constipation
- Complications of constipation
- Chronic diarrhea
- Intestinal parasites
- Lactase deficiency
- Gynecologic disorders
- Psychologic disorders

Most Important Questions to Ask

- Have you had continuous or recurrent abdominopelvic pain for at least 3 months?
- Is your abdominal pain relieved with passing a bowel movement?
- Is your pain associated with a change in frequency of stool?
- Is your pain associated with a change in consistency of stool?
- Do you have, at least one-fourth of the time, more than three bowel movements per day or less than three bowel movements per week?
- Do you have, at least one-fourth of the time, lumpy and hard or loose and watery stools?
- Do you have, at least one-fourth of the time, straining or urgency with stool passage or a feeling of incomplete evacuation?
- Do you have, at least one-fourth of the time, passage of mucus with bowel movements?
- Do you have, at least one-fourth of the time, bloating or a feeling of abdominal distention?
- Have you had any significant weight loss without dieting?
- Does your pain or diarrhea occur during the night while you are sleeping?
- Do any of your symptoms worsen just before or during your menses?
- Do a dietary recall.
- Do you take any medications or laxatives?
- Do you have a history of any abdominal or pelvic surgery?
- Have you ever been sexually or physically abused?

Most Important Physical Examination Findings

- Patient may seem anxious and tense or depressed
- Mild to moderate abdominal distention examination
- Surgical scars
- Abdominal tenderness may be elicited
- Rectal and pelvic examinations to assess for masses or anal disease

Most Important Diagnostic Studies

- Complete blood cell count with differential
- Chemistry profile
- Sedimentation rate
- Three stool specimens for ova-and-parasite testing
- Stool for occult blood
- Methylene blue stain of stool for white blood cells
- Sudan stain of stool for fat
- Stools for *Clostridium difficile* toxin
- In women less than 40 years of age, proctosigmoidoscopy with biopsy
- In patients older than 40 years, a barium enema and flexible sigmoidoscopy or a full colonoscopy
- Hydrogen breath test for lactose intolerance
- Anal manometry

Treatments

- Pain-predominant syndrome

- Belladonna, 5 to 10 drops orally t.i.d. before meals
- Dicyclomine, 10 to 20 mg t.i.d.–q.i.d.
- Cimetropium bromide, 50 mg t.i.d.
- Amitriptylline, 10 to 75 mg q.h.s.
- Desipramine, 25 to 75 mg q.h.s.
- Hyoscyamine (Levsin), 0.125 to 0.25 mg t.i.d.–q.i.d.
- Donnatal, 1 to 2 tablets t.i.d.–q.i.d.
- Librax, 1 to 2 capsules t.i.d.–q.i.d.
- Beano (a D-galactosidase)
- A simethicone preparation (Gas X, Phazyme)
- Peppermint oil
- Constipation-predominant syndrome
  - Wheat bran, 10 to 30 g per day
  - Psyllium, ¹/₂ to 1 tbsp per day
  - Ispaghula, 20 g per day
  - Polycarbophil or methylcellulose, 1 to 2 tbsp per day
  - Cisapride, 5 to 10 mg t.i.d.
- Diarrhea-predominant syndrome
  - Loperamide (Imodium), 2 to 4 mg q.i.d.
  - Wheat bran, 10 to 30 g per day
  - Psyllium, ¹/₂ to 1 tbsp per day
  - Polycarbophil or methylcellulose, 1 to 2 tbsp per day
  - Amitriptylline, 25 to 75 mg q.h.s.
  - Desipramine, 10 to 75 mg q.h.s.
  - Ondansetron, 16 mg t.i.d.
  - Peppermint oil
  - Psychotherapy
  - Adhesiolysis

REFERENCES

1. Walker EA, Katon WJ, Jemelka R, et al. The prevalence of chronic pelvic pain and irritable bowel syndrome in two university clinics. *J Psychosom Obstet Gynecol* 1991;12(Suppl):65.
2. Longstreth GF, Preskill DB, Youkeles L. Irritable bowel syndrome in women having diagnostic laparoscopy or hysteroscopy. Relation to gynecologic features and outcome. *Dig Dis Sci* 1990;35:1285–1290.
3. Prior A, Whorwell PJ. Gynaecological consultation in patients with the irritable bowel syndrome. *Gut* 1989;30:996.
4. Talley NJ, Zinsmeister AR, VanDyke C, et al. Epidemiology of colonic symptoms and the irritable bowel syndrome. *Gastroenterology* 1991;101:927–934.
5. Manning AP, Thompson WG, Heaton KW, et al. Towards positive diagnosis of the irritable bowel. *Br Med J* 1978;2:653–654.
6. Thompson WG. Functional bowel disease and functional abdominal pain. *Gut* 1999;45(Suppl 2):1143–1147.
7. Kellow JE, Gill RC, Wingate DL. Prolonged ambulant recordings of bowel motility demonstrate abnormalities in the irritable bowel syndrome. *Gastroenterology* 1990;98:1208–1218.
8. Slater BJ, Plusa SM, Smith AN, et al. Rectal hypersensitivity in the irritable bowel syndrome. *Int J Colorectal Dis* 1997;12:29–32.
9. King T, Elia M, Hunter JO. Abnormal colonic fermentation in irritable bowel syndrome. *Lancet* 1998;352:1187–1189.
10. Lynn RB, Friedman LS. Irritable bowel syndrome. *N Engl J Med* 1993;329:1940–1945.
11. Whitehead WE, Cheskin Lj, Heller BR, et al. Evidence for exacerbation of irritable bowel syndrome during menses. *Gastroenterology* 1990;98:1485.
12. Drossman DA, Leserman J, Nachman G, et al. Sexual and physical abuse in women with functional or organic gastrointestinal disorders. *Ann Intern Med* 1990;113:828–833.
13. Schutze K, Brandstatter G, Dragosics B, et al. Double-blind study of the effect of cisapride on constipation and abdominal discomfort as components of the irritable bowel syndrome. *Aliment Pharmacol Ther* 1997;11:387–394.
14. Noor N, Small PK, Loudon MA, et al. Effects of cisapride on symptoms and postcibal small-bowel motor function in patients with irritable bowel syndrome. *Scand J Gastroenterol* 1998;33:605–611.
15. Schutze K, Brandstatter G, Dragosics B, et al. Double-blind study of the effect of cisapride on constipation and abdominal discomfort as components of the irritable bowel syndrome. *Aliment Pharmacol Ther* 1997;11:387–394.
16. VanOutryve M, Milo R, Toussaint J, et al. "Prokinetic" treatment of constipation-predominant irritable bowel syndrome: a placebo-controlled study of cisapride. *J Clin Gastroenterol* 1991;13:49–57.
17. Efskind PS, Bernklev T, Vatn MH. A double-blind placebo-controlled trial with loperamide in irritable bowel syndrome. *Scand J Gastroenterol* 1996;3:463–468.
18. Lavo B, Stenstam M, Nielsen AL. Loperamide in treatment of irritable bowel syndrome—a double-blind placebo controlled study. *Scand J Gastroenterol (Suppl)* 1987;130:77–80.
19. Goldberg PA, Kamm MA, Setti-Carraro P, et al. Modification of visceral sensitivity and pain in irritable bowel syndrome by 5-HT3 antagonism (ondansetron). *Digestion* 1996;57:478–483.
20. Maxton DG, Morris J, Whorwell PJ. Selective 5-hydroxytryptamine antagonism: a role in irritable bowel syndrome and functional dyspepsia? *Aliment Pharmacol Ther* 1996;10:595–599.
21. Delvaux M, Louvel D, Mamet JP, et al. Effect of alosetron on responses to colonic distension in patients with irritable bowel syndrome. *Aliment Pharmacol Ther* 1998;12:849–855.
22. Liu JH, Chen GH, Yeh HZ, et al. Enteric-coated peppermint-oil capsules in the treatment of irritable bowel syndrome: a prospective, randomized trial. *J Gastroenterol* 1997;32:765–768.
23. Pittler MH, Ernst E. Peppermint oil for irritable bowel syndrome: a critical review and metaanalysis. *Am J Gastroenterol* 1998;93:1131–1135.
24. Capurso L, Del SF, Tarquini M, et al. Octylonium bromide plus diazepam versus diazepam or octylonium bromide alone in the treatment of irritable bowel syndrome. An open controlled clinical trial. *Curr Ther Res Clin Exp* 1992;52:368–377.
25. Drossman DA, Thompson WG. The irritable bowel syndrome: review and a graduated multicomponent treatment approach. *Ann Intern Med* 1992;116:1009–1016.
26. Guthrie E, Creed F, Dawson D, et al. A controlled trial of psychological treatment for the irritable bowel syndrome. *Gastroenterology* 1991;100:450–457.
27. Svedlund J, Ottosson JO, Sjodin I, et al. Controlled study of psychotherapy in irritable bowel syndrome. *Lancet* 1983;2:589–591.
28. Guthrie E, Creed F, Dawson D, et al. A controlled trial of psychological treatment for the irritable bowel syndrome. *Gastroenterology* 1991;100:450–457.
29. Talley NJ, Owen BK, Boyce P, et al. Psychological treatments for irritable bowel syndrome: a critique of controlled treatment trials. *Am J Gastroenterol* 1996;91:277–286.
30. Brinkhaus B, Hentschel C, Lindner M, et al. Phytotherapy in irritable bowel syndrome: a randomised double blind, placebo-controlled clinical trial (presented at the 5th Annual Symposium on Complementary Healthcare, 10–12 December 1998, Exeter). *FACT: Focus on Alternative and Complementary Therapies* 1998;3:182–183.
31. Longstreth GF, Wolde-Tsadik G. Irritable bowel-type symptoms in HMO examinees. Prevalence, demographics, and clinical correlates. *Dig Dis Sci* 1993;38:1581–1589.

29

PERITONEAL CYSTS

FRED M. HOWARD

KEY TERMS AND DEFINITIONS

Multicystic mesothelioma: A rare lesion consisting of multiple mesothelial-lined cysts that affect various parts of the abdominopelvic peritoneal surface; also called cystic mesothelioma, cystic mesothelial hyperplasia, or benign mesothelial cyst.

Peritoneal inclusion cysts: Benign adnexal masses that occur secondary to fluid trapped among adhesions surrounding an ovary.

Postoperative peritoneal cyst: A rare postoperative complication resulting in an abdominal or pelvic cyst that is lined by mesothelial cells and is associated with adhesions and most often pain.

INTRODUCTION

Peritoneal mesothelial cysts are rare. When present, they are frequently associated with chronic pelvic pain (CPP). The proper nomenclature for these cysts is not clear, nor is it clear if the diverse cases reported with varied names represent the same process. Although Ross et al. (1) believe that all of the various terms, such as *cystic peritoneal mesothelioma, multicystic peritoneal mesothelioma, inflammatory cysts of the peritoneum, postoperative peritoneal cysts, benign papillary peritoneal cystosis*, and *infiltrating adenomatoid tumor* are the same, my bias is that of the multicystic masses that are associated with CPP, at least two distinct types exist. One is related to surgical adhesive disease and is probably best termed *postoperative peritoneal cyst* or *peritoneal inclusion cyst*. The other is a reactive mesothelial proliferation and may or may not be related to surgery and adhesive disease. It is probably best termed *benign cystic mesothelioma* or *multicystic peritoneal mesothelioma*. Neither are neoplasms, and neither are premalignant.

The formation of postoperative peritoneal cysts (POPCs) is an infrequent postoperative complication (2). They may occur months to years after surgery and occur after a variety of operative procedures. They have been reported only in women. Almost all women with these cysts present with abdominopelvic pain and a palpable pelvic mass (3). The mean age at presentation in a series of seven cases was 38 years, with a range of 24 to 46 years (4).

Benign cystic mesotheliomas (BCMs) have also been referred to as multicystic peritoneal mesotheliomas, multilocular peritoneal cysts, and infiltrating adenomatoid tumors (5). They are also relatively rare lesions, but have been reported more frequently than postoperative peritoneal cysts. Some confusion may arise because the mesothelial cell is often not included in the differential considerations in the gynecologic pathology of a cystic mass (6). Benign mesothelial cysts have been reported in men, but are much more common in women. Of 37 cases reported by Weis and Tavassoli (7), 31 were in women. All five cases reported by Katsube et al. (8) were in women. Although benign mesothelial cysts may occur anywhere in the peritoneum, they are most commonly found in the pelvis. In the series of Weiss and Tavassoli, 19 of 37 cases occurred in the pelvis, where they typically involved the uterus, cul-de-sac, bladder, or rectum. Mean ages of the women in the two largest reported series of cases were 38 years (31 cases) (7) and 33 years (25 cases) (1).

ETIOLOGY

Neither of these types of cysts are neoplasms. Postoperative peritoneal cysts are loculated areas between adherent viscera in which fluid accumulates. Although they have been reported after removal of both ovaries, they appear to be more common if one or both ovaries remain. This may be due to the fact that ovaries are the main producers of peritoneal fluid (9). Thus in patients with ovaries they may produce postoperative peritoneal cysts if they are surrounded by adhesions. Of course this causes the sonographic appearance of a complex adnexal mass. Postoperative or pelvic infection may also have an etiologic role. In one series of four cases, all had a history of postoperative fever or pelvic inflammatory disease.

Benign cystic mesothelioma is thought to be due to nonneoplastic reactive mesothelial proliferation. Many, but not all, patients have a history of endometriosis, pelvic inflammatory disease, or prior abdominal surgery. For example, in the cases of multicystic mesothelioma reported by Weiss and Tavassoli, (7) of the 17 cases with a known history, only 9 had prior surgical procedures. The patient with a 23-cm benign cystic mesothelioma reported by Birch et al. (5) had a history of only a prior laparoscopic tubal ligation. Although asbestos has been linked to malignant mesothelioma, no link to benign cystic mesothelioma has been shown (10).

PATHOLOGY

The walls of both types of cysts are mesothelial in origin and do not contain smooth muscle. Cyst walls are lined by cuboidal or flat mesothelial cells, with minimal inflammation or lymphocytic infiltration. This helps to differentiate them from lymphangiomas. Often the lining reveals reactive mesothelial cells and some lymphocyte infiltration. However, there is no microbiologic evidence of acute infection. Gram stains and cultures are negative.

Benign multicystic mesotheliomas appear grossly as multiple, translucent, membranous cysts that usually group together to form a confluent mass or line the surface of the peritoneum in a discontinuous fashion. Rarely, they are free-floating in the abdomen or pelvis. Weiss and Tavassoli (2) found that 6 cases of multicystic mesothelioma were actually solitary lesions, 15 were localized but multifocal, and 16 were diffuse. Reported sizes range from 4 cm to 23 cm for cystic mesotheliomas (5,6).

TABLE 29.1. CLASSIFICATION OF PERITONEAL MESOTHELIOMAS

I. Benign
   Fibrous mesothelioma
   Adenomatoid tumor
   Benign papillary mesothelioma
   Benign cystic mesothelioma

II. Malignant
   Fibrosarcomatous mesothelioma
   Epithelial mesothelioma
   Mixed forms

Endometriosis is the most common concurrent disease found with benign multicystic mesotheliomas. For example, in one series it was present in 8 of 25 cases (1). Evidence of prior salpingitis is also sometimes present; Ross et al. (1) found this in 3 of 25 cases.

Table 29.1 summarizes one possible pathologic classification of peritoneal mesotheliomas.

SYMPTOMS OR HISTORY

Most patients with either POPC or BCM present with abdominopelvic pain. Combining the results of 100 cases from eight published reports shows that 81 of the patients presented with pain (1–3,7,8). In almost all of the cases the pain was chronic or recurrent. Acute pelvic pain, although occasionally the presenting symptom, was much less common. Pain often starts as a gradual development of lower abdominal fullness and distention. There may be associated dysuria and constipation. Patients may present with abdominal bloating, particularly with a benign cystic mesothelioma (11). Most of the reported cases without pain have presented with asymptomatic abdominopelvic masses.

As implied by the name, almost all patients with POPCs have a history of prior surgery. Only one case of a cyst consistent with POPC has been described in a patient without a history of prior surgery (12). Most patients have had multiple operations before the development of POPCs. In a series of seven cases, the 11 prior surgeries were: hysterectomy (2); hysterectomy and oophorectomy (1); appendectomy with abscess (1); colectomy for Crohn's and left oophorectomy (1); ileal resection and colectomy for Crohn's (1); and cholecystectomy and ovarian abscess (1). In another series of four cases, the previous operative procedures were: cesarean section times three, tubal ligation, and abdominal hysterectomy (1); myomectomy and ovarian wedge resection and right salpino-oophorectomy and myomectomy (1); cystectomy with ilioconduit, cholecystectomy, adhesiolysis, and abdominal hysterectomy and bilateral salpingo-oophorectomy (1); and right salpingostomy, right salpingectomy, and abdominal hysterectomy with adhesiolysis (1) (2). The time from prior surgery to presentation with a postoperative peritoneal cyst varies from as little as 6 months to as much as 21 years (Table 29.2).

TABLE 29.2. BASELINE HISTORIES IN REPORTED CASES OF POSTOPERATIVE PERITONEAL CYSTS

Study	Number of Cases	Mean Age	Mean Number of Prior Operations	Mean Interval From Last Operation
Falk and Bunkin (18)	6	43.7 (38–48)	1.3 (1–2)	8.1 yrs (3–13)
Monafo and Goldfarb (19)	4	26.2 (17–46)	2.5 (1–4)	7.8 yrs (3.5–12)
Lees et al. (12)	3	25.3 (17–32)	1.7 (0–4)	3–8 yrs
Gussman et al. (2)	4	36 (31–40)	3 (2–4)	6.6 mos (1.5–8)
Lipitz et al. (3)	6 (recurrent)	45.3 (32–56)	2.5 (1–4)	N/A

In patients with benign cystic mesotheliomas the history of prior surgery is less absolute. The patient with a 23-cm benign cystic mesothelioma reported by Birch et al. (5) had a history of only a prior laparoscopic tubal ligation. In the cases of multicystic mesothelioma reported by Weiss and Tavassoli (7), of the 17 cases with a known history, 9 had prior surgical procedures. In two cases reported by Nirodi et al. (10) both had prior surgery: one a tubal ligation and the other an appendectomy and right salpingectomy. Ross et al. (1) reported that 15 of 23 with a known history had prior surgery.

SIGNS OR PHYSICAL EXAMINATION

Tenderness in the area of a POPC or PCM is usually present, although a cyst is not always palpable. Only two of seven cases of POPC that presented with pelvic pain had a palpable adnexal mass (4). In the four cases of cystic mesothelioma reported by Schneider et al. (6), three had tenderness on pelvic examination and two had a palpable pelvic mass. When present, the mass is generally soft, cystic, and tender (2). Sizes of palpable cysts have ranged from 4 to 24 cm (1,2). Most of the masses are pelvic in location. In the series of 25 cases reported by Ross et al. (1), all of the primary lesions involved the pelvis and 12 were totally confined to it.

DIAGNOSTIC STUDIES

Ultrasonography almost always reveals POPCs and PCMs as large, complex, cystic masses with thin walls and septations. In patients with ovaries, the ovarian fluid may produce cysts around the ovaries if adhesions are present. Of course this causes the sonographic appearance of a complex adnexal mass. By transvaginal ultrasound it may be distinguished from a malignancy by the appearance of an intact ovary amid septations and fluid (2,4). Location of the mass is variable. For example in one series of seven cases it was right-sided in five cases, left-sided in one, and midline in one (4). As noted previously, most of the cysts are pelvic in location.

If intravenous pyelogram and barium enema are performed, they generally show only the compressive effects of a large mass (2). Computerized tomography shows findings similar to those of ultrasonography.

Laboratory studies, including complete blood counts, serum chemistries, and enzymes, are normal (2,5). Cultures and gram stains of the cyst fluid are negative (2,5).

DIAGNOSIS

In the acute postoperative period, one must consider the possibility of hematomas, abscesses, seromas, and lympho-cysts. More remotely from surgery, hydrosalpinges, ovarian cysts, matted adherent organs, retroperitoneal cysts, omental cysts, and ovarian cancer must be included in the differential diagnosis. Others possible diagnoses are lymphangioma, endosalpingiosis, cystic mesonephric remnants, and epithelial inclusion cysts.

MANAGEMENT OR TREATMENT

Medical Treatment

Observation is an option if symptoms are controlled and there is no evidence of malignancy (4).

Tamoxifen, 20 mg per day, has been used to treat one case of benign cystic mesothelioma in a 19-year-old woman. After 4 weeks of treatment there was a decrease of volume of the cystic mass to about one-half of its initial volume. It stabilized at that size during 18 months of therapy (13).

Depot leuprolide, 3.75 mg per month, was used to treat another patient with recurrent benign cystic mesothelioma because the cystic mass had been steadily increasing in size and had become symptomatic (14). It had a pretreatment volume of 3969 cm^3. There was an initial marked increase in volume, followed after 4 weeks by a decrease to about the pretreatment volume. There was no change in volume in the subsequent 6 months of treatment, until add-back therapy with conjugated estrogen, 0.625 mg per day, and medroxyprogesterone acetate, 2.5 mg per day, was started. With add-back the volume increased rapidly and the patient became symptomatic with pain again after 8 weeks. All medications were then discontinued. The patient refused surgical therapy and after 3 months had a mass with a volume of 29,273 cm^3. Depot leuprolide was started again with a decrease of the cystic mass to 23,118 cm^3, at which time surgery was performed.

Surgical Treatment

Surgical treatment may be excision or simply adhesiolysis if the POPC is a pseudocyst (4). POPCs are invariably adherent to adjacent structures, and tissue planes are poorly defined. Most often the surgery is difficult and complicated. It is usually not feasible to perform the surgery laparoscopically. Laparoscopic excision has been reported for benign cystic mesotheliomas (15). BCMs are generally retroperitoneal (5). With POPCs and BCMs the risk of recurrence is 30% to 50% after surgical resection (4). In the Mayo Clinic series, six of eight cases had recurrences after surgical treatment (16). It is important to distinguish peritoneal cysts from cystic tumors of the ovary, because the former do not require removal of the ovary and carry no risk of malignant potential.

Transvaginal or percutaneous aspiration with ultrasound guidance is also a treatment option (2,4). Aspiration is not always successful, especially with large masses, and about 50% of cases recur (5). In cases that recur after drainage, drainage followed by ethanol instillation may be an option. This has been done in six patients transvaginally using a 17-gauge needle to instill 20 to 30 mL of 95% ethanol after drainage of the cyst fluid. Patients have significant discomfort with this procedure and may require analgesia for 2 to 3 hours afterwards. One patient had a recurrence of a 15-cm cyst and underwent repeat treatment with ethanol. All the others had no recurrence over 9 to 22 months of follow-up (3). Cystic mesothelioma has also been successfully treated in one patient with recurrence by using tetracycline, 25 mL of 1.3% solution, as a sclerosing agent (17).

KEY POINTS

Differential Diagnoses

- Hematoma
- Abscess
- Seroma
- Lymphocyst
- Hydrosalpinges
- Ovarian cysts
- Matted adherent organs
- Retroperitoneal cyst
- Omental cyst
- Ovarian cancer
- Lymphangioma
- Endosalpingiosis
- Cystic mesonephric remnants
- Epithelial inclusion cysts

Most Important Questions to Ask

- Do you have pain in the same location all the time?
- Have you had prior surgery or pelvic infection?

Most Important Physical Examination Finding

- Tender cystic mass

Most Important Diagnostic Studies

- Ultrasound
- Computerized tomography
- Intravenous pyelography
- Barium enema

Treatments

- Observation
- Tamoxifen
- Depot leuprolide acetate
- Aspiration
- Sclerosis
- Surgical excision

REFERENCES

1. Ross JM, Welch WR, Scully RE. Multilocular peritoneal inclusion cysts (so-called cystic mesotheliomas). *Cancer* 1989;64:1336–1346.
2. Gussman D, Thickman D, Wheeler JE. Postoperative peritoneal cysts. *Obstet Gynecol* 1986;68:53S–55S.
3. Lipitz S, Seidman DS, Schiff E, et al. Treatment of pelvic peritoneal cysts by drainage and ethanol instillation. *Obstet Gynecol* 1995;86:297–299.
4. Sohaey R, Gardner TL, Woodward PJ, et al. Sonographic diagnosis of peritoneal inclusion cysts. *J Ultrasound Med* 1995;14:913–917.
5. Birch DW, Park A, Chen V. Laparoscopic resection of an intra-abdominal cystic mass: a cystic mesothelioma. *Can J Surg* 1998;41:161–164.
6. Schneider V, Partridge JR, Gutierrez F, et al. Benign cystic mesothelioma involving the female genital tract: report of four cases. *Am J Obstet Gynecol* 1983;145:355–359.
7. Weiss SW, Tavassoli FA. Multicystic mesothelioma: an analysis of pathologic findings and biologic behavior in 37 cases. *Am J Surg Pathol* 1988;12:737–746.
8. Katsube Y, Mukai K, Silverberg SG. Cystic mesothelioma of the peritoneum: a report of five cases and review of the literature. *Cancer* 1982;50:1615–1622.
9. Koninckx PR, Renaer M, Brosens IA. Origin of peritoneal fluid in women: an ovarian exudation product. *Br J Obstet Gynaecol* 1980;87:177–183.
10. Nirodi NS, Lowry DS, Wallace RJ. Cystic mesothelioma of the pelvic peritoneum. Two case reports. *Br J Obstet Gynaecol* 1984;91:201–204.
11. Birch DW, Park A, Chen V. Laparoscopic resection of an intra-abdominal cystic mass: a cystic mesothelioma. *Can J Surg* 1998;41:161–164.
12. Lees RF, Feldman PS, Brenbridge ANAG, et al. Inflammatory cysts of the pelvic peritoneum. *Am J Roentgenol* 1978;131:633–636.
13. Letterie GS, Yon JL. The antiestrogen tamoxifen in the treatment of recurrent benign cystic mesothelioma. *Gynecol Oncol* 1998;70:131–133.
14. Letterie GS, Yon JL. Use of a long-acting GnRH agonist for benign cystic mesothelioma. *Obstet Gynecol* 1995;85:901–903.
15. Navarra G, Occhionorelli S, Santini M, et al. Peritoneal cystic mesothelioma treated with minimally invasive approach. *Surg Endosc* 1996;10:60–61.
16. Carpenter HA, Lancaster RJ, Lee RA. Multilocular cysts of the peritoneum. *Mayo Clin Proc* 1982;57:634–638.
17. Benson RC, Williams TH. Peritoneal cystic mesothelioma: successful treatment of a difficult disease. *J Urol* 1990;143:347–348.
18. Falk HC, Bunkin IA. Intraperitoneal cysts simulating ovarian cysts. *Obstet Gynecol* 1953;1:183–187.
19. Monafo W, Goldfarwb W. Postoperative peritoneal cyst. *Surgery* 1963;53:470–473.

30

BLADDER CANCER

CHARLES W. BUTRICK

KEY TERMS AND DEFINITIONS

Hematuria: Significant if gross hematuria is seen in two out of three clean voided specimens that demonstrate greater than three red blood cells per high-power field.

Bladder washing: Simple office technique to obtain a specimen for cytologic examination.

Tumor markers: Substances that can be measured in voided urine to help identify patients with bladder cancer.

Intravesical therapy: Placement of therapeutic agents directly into the bladder that treat bladder cancer or attempt to prevent its recurrence after primary therapy.

Continent urinary diversion: Any surgical technique used after a radical cystectomy that involves the construction of a urinary reservoir with a stoma that is brought through the abdominal wall.

Orthotropic bladder replacement: Surgical technique used after cystectomy where the reconstructed urinary reservoir is attached to the urethra, thus alleviating the need for catheterizing and abdominal wall stoma (see above).

INTRODUCTION

Bladder cancer is the fourth most common cancer and the twelfth leading cause of death in the United States. The American Cancer Society estimates that 54,200 new cases of bladder cancer will occur in the United States in 1999. Women are one-third less likely to be affected than men. It is the eighth most common type of cancer in women, with most cases occurring after the age of 60 (1). Cigarette smoking is associated with a dose-dependent twofold to fivefold increase in the risk of bladder cancer. Occupational exposure to certain aromatic amines, such as beta-naphthyl amines, xenylamine, 4-nitrobiphenyl, and benzidine, is also a well-established risk factor with a latency period of 5 to 50 years between exposure to these substances and the development of bladder cancer (2).

These aromatic amines are typically used in the textile, leather, rubber, dye, paint, hairdressing, or organic chemi-

cal industries. Other potential factors that are causally linked to bladder cancer include excessive caffeine intake, analgesic abuse, artificial sweeteners (including saccharine and cyclamate), chronic cystitis, the presence of chronic indwelling catheters (2% to 10% of paraplegics with chronic indwelling catheters will develop bladder cancer), prior pelvic radiation, prior cyclophosphamide use (ninefold increase risk), and the rare familial tendency toward bladder cancer.

The incidence of bladder cancer has been shown to be increasing over the last several years despite the general population's reduction in smoking. The cause of this is unknown, but increasing exposure to chemicals in our environment is thought to be the cause. The incidence of diagnosed bladder cancer is approximately 16.5 per 100,000 persons per year, and this incidence has increased approximately 50% in the last 3 years (3). Most bladder cancers present as superficial disease, and these lesions are likely to recur in 50% to 75% of cases. Thus, the ongoing prevalence of bladder cancer far exceeds its primary incidence (4).

CLINICAL FEATURES

Pelvic pain is not a prominent symptom of bladder cancer. However, 20% of patients complain of irritative lower urinary tract symptoms such as frequency, urgency, or dysuria. Evaluation of patients sent to a tertiary center for these same irritative symptoms demonstrates that approximately 2% will be found to have bladder cancer as the cause of these symptoms. There is a high prevalence of multifocal carcinoma *in situ* or poorly differentiated advanced disease in patients with irritative symptoms. These irritative symptoms and pain with voiding are similar to those of interstitial cystitis and urethral syndrome. During the evaluation of a patient with pelvic pain and irritable bladder symptoms, it is crucial that the clinician exclude bladder cancer as a diagnosis.

Gross or microscopic hematuria is the most frequent presenting sign of bladder cancer, occurring in 80% of patients with bladder cancer. Hematuria is typically intermittent, which makes it a commonly ignored sign that therefore delays evaluation and diagnosis. Significant hematuria is defined as greater than three red blood cells per high-power field, especially when seen on at least two out of three voided specimens (5). Anytime gross hematuria is found, a single sample is all that is necessary. If a culture positive urinary tract infection (UTI) is identified, treatment of that UTI should be followed by urinalysis to verify resolution of the hematuria. Persistent hematuria demands evaluation of both the lower and the upper urinary tracts.

INITIAL EVALUATION

During the workup of pelvic pain, all patients with significant hematuria in the absence of a UTI need further evaluation. The lower urinary tract should be evaluated with cystourethroscopy; if no lesion is found, then a sample for bladder cytology should be collected. Additionally, the upper tracts should be evaluated by intravenous urography [renal ultrasound or renal computerized axial tomography (CAT) scan can be used, but an intravenous pyelogram (IVP) is the standard approach]. Urine cytology can result in inaccuracies and, therefore, certainly cannot be relied upon to rule out disease. The accuracy of bladder washings, however, can be markedly improved by not collecting simply a voided sample, but instead having a catheter inserted to drain the bladder of all urine, then filling the bladder with at least 50 mL of saline and then draining the saline and thus providing a true accurate sample without the artifacts that can be caused by a simple voided sample. False-negative urine cytologies are frequently seen with a well-differentiated tumor. Yet even in high-grade tumors, the false-negative rate can be as high as 20%. Despite its inaccuracies, urine cytology can identify a high-grade lesion in the upper tract or carcinoma *in situ* of the bladder in those patients with very little, if any, cystoscopic abnormalities. For initial evaluation of hematuria, see Figure 30.1.

Recent reports have proposed that the presence of "markers" in voided urine may help in the detection of transitional cell carcinoma. Tumor markers under investigation include bladder tumor antigen (BTA), nuclear matrix protein (NMP) 22, and pelomerase, to name a few. The hope is that these tumor markers will help in identifying early bladder lesions and decrease the need for invasive procedures such as intravenous pyelography and cystoscopy. Additionally, these markers may decrease the need for surveillance cystoscopy in patients after initial treatment for superficial bladder cancer. At this point, NMP22 appears to be the most promising tumor marker due to its greater sensitivity relative to BTA or cytology (70% versus 50% versus 30% to 40%) (6).

The goals of cystoscopy are to diagnosis the presence of a papillary or solid transitional cell cancer involving the bladder, to establish whether more than one focus of disease is present, to identify the location of the lesion, and to visualize any additional abnormal mucosal areas (7). Visible bladder lesions should be biopsied, preferably under a general or regional anesthetic. Office biopsies are certainly safe and very well tolerated, with a relatively low incidence of bleeding complications. However, transurethral resection done under general anesthesia not only allows for a more careful bimanual examination to determine the potential for extravesical spread of cancer, but also allows for a deep resection to assess the depth of invasion. Additional random biopsies should be undertaken, as well as biopsies along the lateral margins of the site of resection. These biopsies are important steps in determining the stage and the prognosis. The presence of diffuse or multifocal carcinoma *in situ* of course demands a different therapeutic approach than those with a single isolated lesion and no evidence of multifocal disease. Patients with a high-grade and/or deeply invasive lesion also require evaluation of possible pelvic extension of the cancer. The most common approaches include computerized tomography (CT) scan, magnetic resonance imaging (MRI), and/or lymph angiography for tumors not invading the detrusor muscle.

STAGING OF BLADDER CANCER

Endoscopic and pathologic findings at the time of initial evaluation form the basis for clinical staging. About 75% of patients are diagnosed as having superficial bladder cancer. Superficial cancers are papillary tumors that are confined to the mucosa, whereas carcinoma *in situ* may replace or undermine the normal mucosa and can involve either focal or diffuse areas of the uroepithelium. Invasive cancers are generally nodular tumors that infiltrate the muscularis and/or the serosa with associated increased likelihood of the development of metastatic disease.

DIFFERENTIAL DIAGNOSIS

Most women with bladder cancer do not present with pain or irritable bladder symptoms. Eighty percent present with painless hematuria. Thus, the differential diagnosis generally revolves around evaluation of hematuria. A thorough evaluation of hematuria typically involves a history, physical examination, urine culture, urine cytology, cystourethroscopy, and IVP. If the urine culture is positive, treatment should be initiated and then urine reevaluated to determine if the hematuria is persistent.

As many as 10% to 18% percent of women with hematuria are found not to have an identifiable cause for the hematuria; but if followed for 2 years and reevaluated, 16% of these patients will be found to have a detectable lesion. Exercise-induced trauma typically results in hematuria that will resolve within 24 to 48 hours. Nonsteroidal antiin-

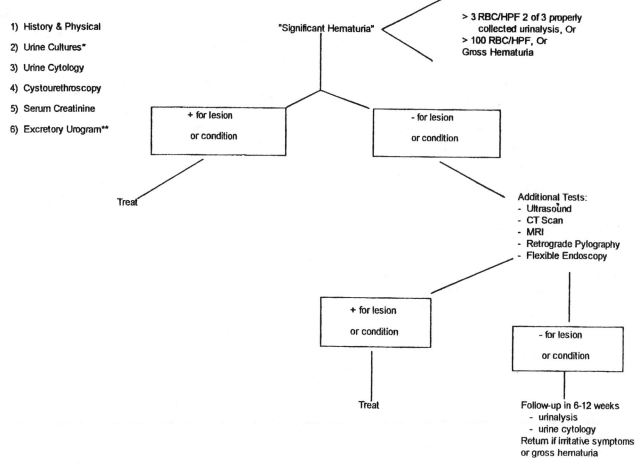

1) History & Physical

2) Urine Cultures*

3) Urine Cytology

4) Cystourethroscopy

5) Serum Creatinine

6) Excretory Urogram**

"Significant Hematuria"

> 3 RBC/HPF 2 of 3 properly
collected urinalysis, Or
> 100 RBC/HPF, Or
Gross Hematuria

+ for lesion
or condition

- for lesion
or condition

Treat

Additional Tests:
- Ultrasound
- CT Scan
- MRI
- Retrograde Pylography
- Flexible Endoscopy

+ for lesion
or condition

- for lesion
or condition

Treat

Follow-up in 6-12 weeks
- urinalysis
- urine cytology
Return if irritative symptoms
or gross hematuria

FIGURE 30.1. Clinical evaluation based on endoscopic and pathologic findings at the time of initial presentation with hematuria.

flammatory drugs (NSAIDs) and anticoagulants may induce hematuria, yet it is not rare that these drugs can actually unmask an asymptomatic lesion. The association with NSAIDs is of particular relevance to women with pelvic pain. Therefore, a full evaluation is still indicated despite the use of these drugs.

Hematuria due to renal stones is usually associated with renal colic, yet silent hematuria can certainly occur. Acute glomerular disease (nephritis) is associated with hematuria with classic clinical findings of nephritis and typical findings of protein casts in the urinary sediment.

Except for bladder cancer, extrarenal sources of hematuria typically are associated with irritative symptoms such as urgency, frequency, and dysuria. The most common etiology of hematuria in women is bacterial cystitis. Noninfectious causes of hematuria involving the lower urinary tract includes inflammatory or hypersensitive syndromes such as interstitial cystitis, trigonitis, and urethritis. In women with significant secondary dysmenorrhea and dyspareunia, consideration of endometriosis involving the bladder and/or ureter is appropriate. Classically, however, endometriosis of the bladder causes cyclic hematuria that has a close temporal relationship with the patient's menstrual cycle.

TREATMENT OF SUPERFICIAL BLADDER CANCER

The prognosis and treatment of bladder cancer changes significantly once muscle invasion occurs. Approximately 76% of bladder cancers found are superficial in a nonscreened population (8). The primary treatment for papillary bladder tumors that do not invade the detrusor muscles is transurethral resection. Small, low-grade, noninvasive tumors can be fulgurated or lasered, but this is less than ideal because with these techniques no specimen is made available for pathologic evaluation.

Despite complete tumor resection, two-thirds of patients develop a tumor recurrence within 5 years; and by 15 years, 88% of patients develop a recurrence. With close surveillance, only 10% of those recurrences will actually progress to a lesion that invades the detrusor muscle. It is because of this high incidence of recurrence that management must involve not only complete resection with careful evaluation for other mucosal lesions, but also close long-term follow-up and therapy to minimize these recurrences.

SURVEILLANCE IN PATIENTS WITH SUPERFICIAL BLADDER CANCER

Because recurrence is so frequently seen, diagnosis of early recurrence is the primary goal of any surveillance program. The second goal is to rule out upper tract disease that occurs in 2% to 5% of patients with superficial bladder cancer. Traditional surveillance includes serial cystoscopy occurring every 3 months for 2 years, then every 6 months for 2 years, and then yearly. In addition, urine cytology should be done immediately post resection to ensure complete resection. The use of cytology as a screening tool to monitor for recurrence is not a substitute for serial cystoscopies as outlined above. However, cytology may be helpful to identify the presence of unsuspected upper tract disease. An IVP is still considered the gold standard in evaluating the upper urinary tract. Approximately 2% to 5% of low-risk patients with superficial bladder cancer, and up to 21% of high-risk patients with superficial bladder cancer, will go on to develop upper urinary tract disease (9). The average interval between the initial diagnosis of superficial bladder cancer and the development of upper urinary tract tumors is approximately 70 months.

Patients at risk for recurrent bladder cancer after treatment for superficial bladder cancer include those with multiple primary tumors, Grade III lesions, submucosal lesions, positive postresection cytology, or dysplasia/carcinoma *in situ* on random biopsies done at the time of original surgical resection. Patients with any of these risks factors should undergo postresection intravesical therapy in order to limit the likelihood of recurrence and hopefully to improve their long-term prognosis.

INTRAVESICAL THERAPY

Intravesical chemotherapy became popular in the early 1960s, when thiotepa was demonstrated by many investigators to reduce tumor recurrence and eradicate papillary tumors (10). While intravesical chemotherapy does seem to show a reduction in tumor recurrence in short-term follow-up studies (2 years), long-term follow-up has not shown this same reduction in tumor recurrence or in progression of disease (11). Intravesical bacille Calmette Guérin (BCG) is now recognized to be the treatment of choice for carcinoma *in situ* of the bladder. It is also considered to be the best prophylactic therapy for patients with high-risk superficial bladder cancer for the prevention of recurrent disease and for decreased incidence of disease progression. With BCG maintenance

therapy (three weekly treatments which are repeated at 6-month intervals), follow-up studies demonstrate a 50% to 83% reduction in recurrent tumors (12).

Adjunctive therapies to prevent recurrence of superficial bladder cancer also include intravesical interferon-alpha-2B and interleukin-2, both of which have shown promise with complete response rate of 47% in patients with carcinoma *in situ*. However, the response was maintained in only half of the patients who seemed to respond initially when followed long term. Intravesical photodynamic therapy using intravenous photofrin II as a photosensitizer has also been considered in patients at risk for recurrent bladder cancer. While photodynamic therapy demonstrates a high response rate, posttherapy symptoms and bladder contractures are quite common (13). Additional therapies that have shown some promise include oral *Lactobacillus casei* and high-dose therapies, including vitamin A, B_6, C, and E.

TREATMENT OF INVASIVE BLADDER CANCER

Once bladder cancer has spread into the detrusor muscle, treatment changes radically. At that stage, treatment must be aggressive because 5-year survival rate drops to as low as 50%. Even in patients with superficial muscle invasion (stage T2), 5-year survival averages only 50% to 60% (14).

Patients with invasive bladder cancer must have an individualized approach to their therapy. Therapeutic options are determined only after a careful evaluation of the extent of cancer, the grade of the tumor, and the general medical condition of the patient. Options include surgery (with or without bladder preservation), external beam radiation, chemotherapy, or any combination thereof.

While radiotherapy alone allows bladder preservation, the 5-year survival rates with this treatment for patients with T2, T3, and T4 tumors are only 40%, 20%, and 10%, respectively (15). Chemotherapy alone yields a complete response in only 20% of patients with invasive bladder cancer. Recently, the combination of radiation after systemic chemotherapy (which sensitizes the cancer to radiation) has provided a more acceptable response rate with a 4-year survival rate of approximately 58% (16).

TABLE 30.1. INVASIVE BLADDER CANCER FIVE-YEAR SURVIVAL RATES

Type of therapy	Five-Year Survival Rate (%)
Transurethral resection	57–70
Partial cystectomy	40–60
Simple cystectomy	54–62
Radiation therapy	19–57
Neoadjunctive therapy plus cystectomy	45–92

SURGICAL OPTIONS FOR INVASIVE BLADDER CANCER

For disease confined to the bladder (stages T1 through T3A), surgical treatment alone provides the best chance of achieving a disease free state and the best overall survival rate. There are many surgical options. The best approach is chosen based upon depth of invasion, location of the tumor, and the surgeon's own expertise.

Traditionally, transurethral resection alone is not sufficient therapy even in patients with small lesions if muscle invasion is found. If the patient is not medically fit to tolerate a more radical approach, one can expect a 40% 5-year survival rate with a solitary superficial muscle invasive lesion.

In women, the standard surgical approach for invasive bladder cancer is an anterior pelvic exenteration with wide excision of the bladder, urethra, uterus, fallopian tubes, ovaries, anterior vaginal wall, and pelvic lymph nodes. It is important to remove the urethra and anterior vaginal wall because they are involved in 36% of women with invasive bladder cancer (as compared to men, where recurrent bladder cancer in the urethra is found in less than 5% when their treatment includes urethral conservation). Additionally, evaluation of the distal ureter by frozen section (to ensure there is no residual cancer) is an important part of any radical surgical approach for the treatment of bladder cancer.

In the past, urinary diversion with external collective devices has been the result of such radical cystectomies. Now, continent urinary diversion allows patients to avoid external collection devices and therefore maintain a more positive body image. The most common continent diversion is the Indiana pouch. An Indiana pouch uses detubularized right colon and 10cm of the terminal ileum. From this pouch a small stoma is brought to the lower abdomen. The patient then performs intermittent catheterization from this small stoma to empty the pouch.

Orthotropic bladder replacement (neobladder) is an attempt to avoid even the need for intermittent catheterization. Here, the neobladder is constructed again of either colon and/or terminal ileum and then is attached to the urethra. This is quite practical in men but is used less frequently in women because of the high incidence of urethral involvement with bladder cancer. However, this is an option in selected female patients whose lesion is not involving the urethra. Under these circumstances, it offers ideal reconstruction in the patient undergoing radical surgical treatment of bladder cancer. Voiding is accomplished by intermittent catheterization and/or valsalva voiding techniques. Continence control is also a problem in women with this type of reconstruction. Because the urethral sphincter mechanism is often located at, or proximal to, the line of resection, very careful patient selection is required in this regard as well.

ADJUNCTIVE CHEMOTHERAPY

One of the most controversial issues in treating locally invasive bladder cancer is the timing and use of systemic chemotherapy. Most patients with invasive cancer who have tumor recurrence ultimately succumb to distant metastases. Therefore, adjunctive chemotherapy is used in an attempt to eradicate lymph node and occult distant metastases at the time of initial therapy. Potential benefits also include that cisplatin may act as a radiation sensitizer and that systemic chemotherapy prior to radiation therapy may eliminate the problem of reduced drug access to the tumor that result from radiation-induced vascular sclerosis. The most promising regime is a four-drug combination, including methyltrexate, vinblastin, adriamycin, and cisplatin. This regime is called M-VAC.

Encouraging results have also been reported with a variety of bladder-sparing approaches. An example of this approach involves (a) transurethral resection of the primary tumor and (b) the combination of cisplatin, methotrexate, and vinblastin administered for two cycles and then followed with 4,000-Gy radiation and concomitant cisplatin. The approach has resulted in a 53% complete response rate; and when cystoscopy, cytology, and a cancer workup for persistent or metastatic disease are all negative, an additional 2,480-Gy radiation and cisplatin are readministered. Results are only preliminary, but the response rate seems quite high.

MANAGEMENT OF METASTATIC DISEASE

At least 30% of patients with invasive transitional cell carcinoma will have metastases at some time during their therapy. Half of them will present with local or distant spread at the time of initial treatment. The other half will relapse after the initial treatment is completed. Distant metastasis are spread hematogenously to the liver, lungs, and bone. Once this is seen, death often follows quickly (2-year surgical rate less than 5%).

Salvage in these patients with metastatic disease is typically attempted with systemic chemotherapy. Single-agent chemotherapy does not produce a prolonged response, and rarely is it curative. Therefore, multiagent chemotherapy is the treatment of choice. M-VAC is believed to be the most effective regime currently available (17). M-VAC therapy demonstrates a 57% to 70% initial response rate, yet only a 25% complete response rate. In those patients with a complete response, two-thirds will relapse within 2 years. Therefore, only 17% of patients treated with M-VAC will be found to be tumor free at 3-year follow-up. This low success rate is achieved at a relatively high cost of significant toxicity, including 3% of patients expiring from the consequences of myelosuppression (3).

SUMMARY

Although bladder cancer is uncommon in women with pelvic pain, all clinicians should maintain a high index of suspicion when hematuria is found. Early diagnosis and treatment are the keys to management of any cancer, and this is certainly the case when caring for patients with bladder cancer. Superficial bladder cancer is unique in that recurrence is almost to be expected. Therefore, close surveillance after initial therapy is very important so that recurrences can quickly be identified and eradicated. Additionally, early diagnosis of recurrence will minimize the patient's chance of progression into a more advanced form of invasive bladder cancer.

KEY POINTS

- Bladder cancer is not rare in women; in fact the incidence is increasing. Therefore, evaluation of significant hematuria is always indicated and should not be delayed.
- Cystourethroscopy, IVP, and cytology are important diagnostic tests in the evaluation of any patients with hematuria.
- While most cases of bladder cancer are found to be superficial at the time of diagnosis, recurrence is very common. Therefore, posttherapy surveillance is mandatory.
- Adjunctive prophylactic therapy in patients with superficial bladder cancer should be considered in patients with high-risk lesions.
- Continent urinary diversion and orthotopic bladder replacement are two new adjunctive surgical approaches to help patients maintain a positive body image.

REFERENCES

1. Landis SH, Murray T, Bolden S. Cancer statistics, 1998, *CA Cancer J Clin* 1998;48:6.
2. Lamm DL, Torti FM. Bladder cancer, 1996. *Cancer* 1996;46(2) 93–112.
3. Catalona WJ. Urothelial tumors of the urinary tract. *Campbell's urology.* Ch.28, 1995, 1094–1158.
4. Heney NM, Ahmed F, Flanagan MJ, et al. Superficial bladder cancer: progression and recurrence. *J Urol* 1983;130:1083.
5. Fantl JA. Hematuria. *Primary Care Update: Ob/Gyn* 1994;1(6): 257–259.
6. Soloway MS, Briggman V, Carpinito GA, et al. Use of a new tumor marker, urinary NMP 22 in the detection of transitional cell carcinoma of the bladder. *J Urol* 1998;159:394–398.
7. Droller MJ. Bladder cancer: state of the art care. *CA Cancer J Clin* 1998;48:269–284.
8. Messing EM. Comparison of bladder cancer outcome in men undergoing hematuria home screening versus those with standard clinical presentation. *Urology* 1995;45:387–396.
9. Cookson MS, Herr HW, Zhang ZF, et al. The treated natural history of high risk superficial bladder cancer: 15-year outcome. *J Urol* 1997;158:62–67.
10. Bateman JC, Lamm DL, Griffith JG. Intravesical therapy: does it affect the natural history of superficial bladder cancer? *Semin Urol* 1992;10:39–44.
11. Lamm DL. Apparent failure of current intravesical chemotherapy prophylaxis to influence the long term course of superficial transitional cell cancer of the bladder. *J Urol* 1995;153:1444–1450.
12. Herr HW. BCG therapy for superficial bladder cancer: a ten year follow-up. *J Urol* 1992;147:1020–1023.
13. Harty JI. Complication of whole bladder dehematoprophyrine-ther photodynamic therapy. *J Urol* 1989;141:1341–1346.
14. Whitmore WF. Selection of treatment for muscle infiltrating transitional cell bladder cancer. *Arch ESP Urol* 1990;43:219–222.
15. Wesson MF. Radiation therapy in regionally advanced bladder cancer. *Urol Clin North Am* 1992;19(4):725–734.
16. Kaufman DJ. Selective bladder preservation by combination treatment of invasive bladder cancer. *N Engl J Med* 1993;329 (19):1377–1382.
17. Sternberg, et al. Preliminary results of M-VAC for transitional cell carcinoma of the urothelium. *J Urol* 1985;133:403.

31

CHRONIC AND RECURRENT URINARY TRACT INFECTIONS

C. PAUL PERRY

KEY TERMS AND DEFINITIONS

Asymptomatic urinary tract infection: Microbial colonization of the urine without tissue inflammation.

Glycocalyx: The glycoprotein and polysaccharide covering of certain bacteria that allows their adherence to tissue surfaces.

Lower urinary tract syndrome: Suprapubic pain, dysuria, frequency and urgency.

Stranguria: The slow and painful discharge of urine.

Urinary tract infection: Microbial colonization of the urine and inflammation of the tissues concerned with production, storage, and excretion of urine.

Uropathogens: Microbes that are inherently more virulent than others.

INTRODUCTION

The urinary tract is a contiguous epithelial surface from the kidneys to the urethral meatus. In the absence of infection, these tissues are bathed in a constant flow of sterile urine. Any of these structures are at risk for injury when pathogens invade the common urinary stream. If the pathogens are eliminated before tissue injury, an asymptomatic or silent infection occurs. Pathogens can be bacterial, viral, or fungal. Infections are usually ascending. That is, they arise from the microorganisms gaining access by way of the distal urethral meatus. Infections may also be descending or hematogenous (1).

Infection of the urinary tract is usually manifested by acute symptoms of pain requiring immediate attention. However, if the infection becomes chronic or recurrent, sensitization and chronic pelvic pain may result. Chronic inflammation from infection may cause a decreased threshold in nociceptive receptors. They then can become activated by even normal stimuli (e.g., bladder filling). Visceral nerve hypersensitivity produces pelvic muscle spasm, soft tissue trigger points, and skin hyperesthesia through the convergence–projection phenomenon. These changes may persist long after the initial insult. This mechanism is responsible for chronic and recurrent urinary tract infections becoming a generator of chronic pelvic pain. Some investigators feel that interstitial cystitis (Chapter 32)is an end stage of this process, but no microorganisms have been discovered to cause interstitial cystitis despite rigorous attempts to do so.

Urinary tract infections are one of the most common conditions encountered in clinical practice. In 1990, in the United States, about 5.7 million office visits were for one of the following complaints: painful urination, frequency and urgency, or urinary tract infection. Women account for 75% of all patients seen with urinary tract infections. The incidence of urinary tract infection increases with increasing age. The prevalence of asymptomatic bacteriuria rises about 1% per decade and may be as high as 10% in elderly women. The risk is independent of socioeconomic status and is not increased in diabetes (1).

ETIOLOGY

The most common uropathogens are gram-negative bacteria belonging to the family of Enterbacteriacea. This includes *Escherichia coli, Klebsiella, Enterobacter, Proteus, Salmonella,* and *Shigella.* The most common yeast is *Candida albicans.* Commensal organisms that colonize the urethra, such as *Lactobacilli* and *Gardnerella,* are considered urethral or vaginal contaminants. They grow poorly in urine (1).

Invasive infection occurs when uropathogens gain access by way of the urethra. They then attach to and penetrate the urothelial lining. Ascent is generally thought to be by Brownian motion, but may be augmented by motile flagella and, in some cases, by the spread of extracellular glycocalyx. Gram-negative organisms release endotoxins and induce interleukins.

The increased susceptibility of the female to this process is thought to be due to three factors: (a) the comparatively short urethra, (b) the ability of uropathogens to colonize the periurethral zone, and (c) the presence of specific receptors to the adhesive strains of bacteria on urothelial cells. The roles of sexual activity, feminine hygiene, and fluid intake continue to be debated. Two groups seem especially vulnerable to recurrent infections. One is the elderly female, while the other is the genetically predisposed female. In the older female, bacteria more easily colonize the atrophic menopausal genitourinary tract. Also, there is an increased receptivity of their uroepithelium to the attachment of these pathogens (2). Vaginal administration of estriol has been shown to reverse this trend (3). There is another group of women with an increased risk of infections throughout life. They are of B or AB blood types. They allow certain bacteria to colonize the gut, attach to the urothelium, and invade the urinary tract of an otherwise healthy host (1).

Urethral obstruction and urethral stasis from stenosis or a urethral diverticulum have also been implicated as predisposing to this condition. Success in relieving some patients' symptoms by urethral dilation and surgical urethroplasty is offered as proof for this belief.

SYMPTOMS

Lower urinary tract hypersensitivity is a term used for such conditions as urethral syndrome, chronic trigonitis, and chronic nonbacterial cystitis. Many patients experience an insidious onset of their symptoms; some relate onset to an acute severe bacterial cystitis. These severe infections are accompanied by intense dysuria and often hematuria. While initial symptoms resolve with antibiotics, they may return at another time despite sterile urine (4). Although initiated by infection, there may be no persistent infection after the cascade of events is set in motion. An overly sensitive bladder leads to uncoordinated, low-volume urination. Voiding dysfunction and pain before, during, and after emptying may be present. Postmicturition dribbling may occur if retained urine is present in a urethral diverticulum.

Neuropathic pain and myofascial pain are hallmarks of this lower urinary tract hypersensitivity. Women who describe their pain as "burning" or "electric shock-like" should be considered to have neuropathic pain. Musculoskeletal pain is probably the most frequently misdiagnosed component of these chronic pelvic pain syndromes. This symptom is usually a dull, poorly localized pain. Patients will describe postcoital ache or throbbing that lasts up to 48 hours. They may also complain of fullness in the vagina.

Nocturia and frequency are functions of bladder sensitivity. Over time, this creates a smaller bladder capacity, which potentiates the abnormal voiding pattern. Dehydration often produces increased symptoms. Dietary factors such as caffeine, carbonated beverages, acidic or spicy foods can aggravate the sensitized bladder. Some patients report more pain with sugar or aspartame. Sitting or standing for long periods can aggravate the musculoskeletal components. Anxiety, depression, and fatigue are also exacerbating

factors. Intercourse can cause exacerbations. Premenstrual times are often more uncomfortable (4).

EXAMINATION

Abdominal wall, suprapubic, and sacral trigger points should be sought. Bladder and distal ureteral pain are generally referred to the lower abdomen and suprapubic area (Fig. 3.17) and may result in trigger points in this area. It is important to rule out an acute process by being certain that diffuse abdominal tenderness, guarding, and rebound are absent.

Q-tip palpation of the vulva should always be done to rule out vulvar vestibulitis (Chapter 21). It is not infrequently an associated finding with lower urinary tract hypersensitivity. Careful palpation of the pubococcygeus, piriformis, and obturator muscles is made for spasm and trigger points. A one-finger exam is started at the urethra to determine tenderness. The examination proceeds proximally, attempting to reproduce the patient's pain. The trigone and each ureteral insertion should be palpated separately. Milking the urethra may reveal pus or urine, indicative of a suburethral diverticulum.

DIAGNOSTIC STUDIES

The diagnosis of chronic pelvic pain originating from a hypersensitive lower urinary tract depends on the above history and physical examinations with repeatedly negative urine cultures. A voiding diary and urinalysis is central. If no pyuria is found, lower urinary tract syndrome is present. If interstitial cystitis is suspected, hydrodistention and cystoscopy can be performed under anesthesia. Usually, cystoscopy and radiologic studies are normal and not helpful. One exception is urethrography with a double-balloon catheter to demonstrate a suspected urethral diverticulum.

Urodynamics may reveal uninhibited bladder contractions. Uroflowmetry when the patient experiences stranguria demonstrates the erratic prolonged flow characteristic of vesical–sphincter dyssynergia (5). Pelvic floor electromyography and pressure studies can also objectively document muscle spasm and inability to relax during voiding.

DIAGNOSIS

Recurrent urinary infections are diagnosed by urine cultures. The hypersensitive disorders of the urinary tract are defined by excluding other clinical entities, such as true infection and interstitial cystitis. This may seem imprecise when compared with more definite diagnostic techniques available for other diseases. However, the definition of any sensory disorder is made largely by exclusion, with negative rather than positive features (4).

TREATMENT

Medical Treatment

The treatment of chronic pelvic pain due to recurrent infection starts with prevention of prolonged visceral nerve stimulation. Asymptomatic bacteriuria and all episodes of cystitis should be promptly treated with appropriate antimicrobials. Relief of dysuria should be quickly obtained with phenazopyridine hydrochloride. Long-term and prophylactic courses may be required. Patients with chronic frequency, urgency, and dyspareunia should be checked for a tender trigone of the bladder. Long-term trimethoprim of 100 mg twice a day for 10 days followed by 100 mg at bedtime for 30 days will often alleviate these symptoms even in the absence of a positive culture. The patient should be monitored for resolution of symptoms and resolution of trigonal tenderness.

Some patients may notice consistent exacerbations with intercourse. In these, postcoital prophylaxis with nitrofurantoin is usually effective to stop this recurrent pain. Other measures such as voiding after intercourse and increased water intake should also be discussed. Atrophic changes may be reversed by estrogen vaginal cream. One-gram application at the top of the vagina at bedtime two to three times per week will accomplish this.

When nocturia is present more than twice a night, tricyclic antidepressants such as imipramine pamoate, 100 mg at bedtime, are helpful to break this habit. This therapy is most helpful when the nocturia occurs early after retiring; but if it occurs throughout the night, the bladder capacity may be restricted. In this case, frequency during the day will be present and bladder training will be necessary. Keeping a voiding diary will allow the patient to consciously increase the time between voiding and thereby increase the bladder capacity. Oxybutynin chloride 5 mg or tolterodine 2 mg may be administered twice a day to help decrease frequency.

If stranguria or hesitancy is present and vesical–sphincter dyssynergia is documented by uroflowmetry, diazepam 2.5 to 10 mg every 6 hours may be helpful. Terazosin may also be successful starting at 1 mg at bedtime.

If a constant burning pain is a primary complaint, neuropathic treatments should be used. Gabapentin is effective in a dose range of 100 to 400 mg three times per day. Electric shock-like pain can often be controlled with carbamazepine 200 mg twice per day. Other medications helpful for neuropathic pain include topiramate, mexiletine hydrochloride, and lamotrigine.

SURGICAL TREATMENT

Surgical therapy for chronic lower urinary tract syndrome is controversial. Repeated urethral dilation has been effective to relieve symptoms of terminal dysuria in some patients. External urethroplasty has been employed for the treatment of frequency, nocturia, and "slow stream" (6). Transurethral cauterization of the trigone is advocated by some as treatment for chronic trigonitis. Neuroablative procedures such as presacral neurectomy or uterovaginal ganglion excision have been inconsistent in relieving symptoms of the hypersensitive bladder (7).

KEY POINTS

Differential Diagnosis

- Recurrent bacterial infection
- Hypersensitive lower urinary tract syndrome
- Vestibulitis
- Vesical–sphincter dyssynergia
- Atrophic vaginitis and urethritis
- Interstitial cystitis

Most Important Questions to Ask

- What are the location, frequency, and quality of the pain?
- Is the pain burning or electric and shock-like?
- Does intercourse affect the occurrence?
- Is there painful penetration or deep thrust pain?
- Is there aching or vaginal fullness long after intercourse?
- Does prolonged sitting increase the pain?
- Is there a stopping and starting of the urinary stream?
- Is there dryness or burning with intercourse?
- How often and when during the night does nocturia occur?
- Does post voiding dribbling of urine occur after standing?

Most Important Physical Examination Findings

- Presence of abdominal wall, suprapubic, or dorsal wall trigger points
- Q-tip test
- Urethral tenderness
- Milking of the urethra
- Trigonal tenderness
- Reproduction of symptoms by one-finger palpation
- Presence of pelvic floor myalgia
- Presence of atrophic vaginal changes

Most Important Diagnostic Studies

- Urinalysis
- Urine culture
- Urodynamics

- Uroflowmetry
- Pelvic floor electromyography
- Cystoscopy with hydrodistention
- Urethrography with double-balloon catheter

Treatments

- Active infection: sensitivity-specific antimicrobial
- Urinary tract prophylactic antisepsis: trimethoprim, nitrofurantoin
- Dysuria: phenazopyridine hydrochloride
- Frequency: oxybutynin chloride, imipramine pamoate, bladder training
- Pelvic floor myalgia: physical therapy
- Vesical–sphincter dyssynergia: diazepam, tolterodine
- Neuropathic pain: gabapentin, carbamazepine, mexiletine, lamotrigine

REFERENCES

1. Kunin CM. *Urinary tract infections: detection, prevention, and management*, 5th ed. Baltimore: Williams and Wilkins, 1997, 2–188.
2. Reid G, Zorzitto ML, Bruce AW, et al. Pathogenesis of urinary tract infection in the elderly: the role of bacterial adherence to uroepithelial cells. *Curr Microbiol* 1984;11:67–72.
3. Raz R, Stamm WE. A controlled trial of intravaginal estriol in postmenopausal women with recurrent urinary tract infections. *N Engl J Med* 1993;329:753–756.
4. George NJR. Gosling JA, eds. *Sensory disorders of the bladder and urethra*. New York: Springer-Verlag, 1986, 2–121.
5. Kaplan WE, Firlit CF, Schoenberg HW. The female urethral syndrome: external sphincter spasm as etiology. *J Urol* 1980;124:48–49.
6. Richardson FH. External urethroplasty in women: technique and clinical evaluation. *J Urol* 1969;101:719–723.
7. Perry CP. Laparoscopic uterine nerve ablation, presacral neurectomy, and uterovaginal ganglion excision. In: *Practical Manual of Operative Laparoscopy and Hysteroscopy*, 2nd ed. Azziz RA, Murphy AA, eds. New York: Springer, 1992:173–180.

32

INTERSTITIAL CYSTITIS

FRED M. HOWARD

KEY TERMS AND DEFINITIONS

Glomerulations: Characteristic petechial, submucosal hemorrhages of the bladder mucosa that occur after distention of the bladder.

Glycosaminoglycans: The extremely hydrophilic polysaccharides of the bladder surface that help form a layer of micelles of water on the bladder epithelium. This micellar layer acts as a barrier between the transitional epithelial cells and urine.

Hunners ulcer: A linear cracking or ulcer of the bladder mucosa that is thought to be pathognomonic of interstitial cystitis, but is not a consistent finding. Named for Hunner, who first described interstitial cystitis in 1914.

Interstitial cystitis: A chronic inflammatory condition of the bladder characterized by frequency and urgency of urination, nocturia, and sometimes chronic pelvic pain and dyspareunia. The diagnostic criteria are controversial, but most commonly it is diagnosed if there is absence of objective evidence of another disease that could cause the symptoms and there are characteristic cystoscopic glomerulations or Hunners ulcer of the bladder.

Irritable bladder syndrome: Symptoms of frequency, urgency, nocturia, and bladder or pelvic pressure, with or without pelvic pain or dysuria, suggestive of interstitial cystitis but without the characteristic cystoscopic and histologic findings of interstitial cystitis.

INTRODUCTION

Interstitial cystitis (IC) is a chronic inflammatory condition of the bladder that may cause chronic pelvic pain (CPP). The definition and diagnostic criteria of IC are controversial and unclear, but most commonly it is defined clinically by the following triad: (a) irritative voiding symptoms, (b) absence of objective evidence of another disease that could cause the symptoms, and (c) a characteristic cystoscopic appearance of the bladder (1–4).

IC tends to occur predominantly in women at 30 to 59 years of age (1). Up to 85% of cases have been reported at 40 to 45 years of age (2,5). The disease appears to be unrelated to menopausal status, occurring both premenopausally and postmenopausally. The incidence is not known, but has been estimated as 36 cases per 100,000 women in the United States and 18 cases per 100,000 women in Finland (2). Pelvic pain is an inconsistent finding, with diurnal and nocturnal frequency usually the most distressing symptoms for the patient. However, pelvic pain is reported by up to 70% of women with IC, and occasionally it is the presenting symptom or chief complaint (2). In a series of 57 women with CPP and negative laparoscopies reported by Reiter and Gambone (6), only one was found to have IC. In a consecutive series of 197 women that I have cared for with CPP as a presenting complaint, four were diagnosed with IC. Although IC is an uncommon diagnosis in CPP patients, physicians caring for women with CPP must still be familiar with it. In many cases the diagnosis has not been made until the patient has undergone numerous operative procedures such as laparoscopies, neurolytic procedures, hysterectomy, and salpingo-oophorectomy.

ETIOLOGY

The etiology of IC is unknown. It is possible that more than one etiology and more than one disease are encompassed in the syndrome. Current thinking suggests that patients with IC have defects in the glycosaminoglycan layer of the bladder wall, although there is no evidence that the glycosaminoglycan is intrinsically defective or abnormal. The glycosaminoglycans of the bladder surface are extremely hydrophilic polysaccharides that form a layer of micelles of water on the bladder epithelium. This micellar layer acts as a barrier between the transitional epithelial cells and urine (3). In IC, it is hypothesized that a defect in this layer allows "leaking" of the epithelium, resulting in a dysfunctional epithelium with excessive permeability and exposure of the transitional epithelium and muscularis to noxious substances in the urine (1). Such leaking of urinary constituents into the bladder wall might explain the nonspecific inflammatory reaction characteristically found in the submucosa and muscularis of bladder biopsies of patients with IC. This explanation, however, is only partial, possibly explaining the end-effect mechanism of IC. It does not address the mechanism by which the permeability or leakiness of the glycosaminoglycan layer occurs.

An autoimmune cause of this leakiness seems possible. Several researchers have demonstrated an increased number of mast cells in the bladder wall of patients with IC, potentially consistent with an autoimmune process (1). Detection of antinuclear antibodies and increased excretion of eosinophilic cationic protein in the urine also support an autoimmune mechanism. Other proposed mechanisms include viral infection(s), toxin(s) exposure, or other inflammatory mediators (5). However, the failure to culture an organism and the failure of antibiotic therapy to alleviate symptoms argues against a bacterial infectious etiology (7).

The physiologic causes of pain with interstitial cystitis are also not clear. The inflammatory reaction of the bladder wall may, via algesic substances released by this reaction, cause niociceptor stimulation of visceral neural pathways. This inflammation results in a contracted bladder of limited capacity in some patients that may cause pain as well as urgency and frequency. Such chronic visceral pain may result in spasm of the pelvic floor muscles (levator ani syndrome) with resultant pelvic pain.

One-third to one-half of patients with IC have increased numbers of mast cells in the bladder wall. Mast cell degranulation releases histamine, prostaglandins, and leukotrienes that may affect bladder muscle and nerve endings. The increase of pain seen in some women with IC at the time of menses may result from mast cell degranulation due to changes in hormonal levels.

SYMPTOMS OR HISTORY

Unremitting frequency and urgency of urination are the characteristic symptoms of IC. Dysuria is not a characteristic symptom, but the urgency and frequency experienced is so severe that these women commonly give histories of recurrent treatment for urinary tract infections. Typically, there is a history of 3 to 7 years of symptoms before the diagnosis is established. Nocturia, with voiding three or more times per night, is also a characteristic and troublesome symptom. Incontinence does not generally occur.

Pelvic pain, although not as universal a symptom of IC as urgency, frequency, and nocturia, occurs in 50% to 70% of women with IC. Typically, the pain is suprapubic, and it may radiate to the low back or groin. Most of the women with chronic pelvic pain associated with IC also have dyspareunia. Pain associated with IC is thought to be secondary to inflammation of the bladder wall and pelvic floor muscle spasm. In many patients, pain increases with bladder filling and decreases after voiding. Pain with void-

ing (dysuria), although occasionally present, is not a characteristic symptom of IC.

The symptoms of IC generally worsen over the first several years after onset, eventually reaching a relatively stable level of intensity. However, it is not unusual for the intensity of symptoms to fluctuate and vary. About 10% of women with IC have spontaneous resolution of symptoms.

Obviously, it is vital that a thorough clinical history relating to the urinary tract be taken from women with CPP and urologic symptoms. Such a history is crucial for planning an efficient and accurate diagnostic evaluation. It may also be useful in subsequent therapeutic interventions. For patients whose symptoms suggest IC, the history should include specific questions about the number of times the patient voids during the day at her best and at her worst. It should also include the number of voidings during the night, both at best and worst. The patient should also be asked to estimate the volume voided at urination, both daytime and nighttime. Finally, the patient should be asked to recall her voiding habits prior to the onset of irritative bladder symptoms. A voiding diary is often helpful.

SIGNS OR EXAMINATION

The physical examination in women with IC is usually normal. Some may have anterior vaginal wall tenderness under the trigone and suprapubic pelvic tenderness, but this is variable. Many women with IC also may have significant tenderness of the pelvic floor muscles; especially during episodes of acute exacerbation of pain, levator ani or piriformis muscle tenderness may be present. At the time of the examination it is important to try to exclude findings consistent with urethral diverticula, adnexal pathology, endometriosis, and uterine abnormalities.

DIAGNOSTIC STUDIES

The symptoms of frequency and urgency are consistent with urinary tract infection, necessitating urinalysis and urine culture. A history of recurrent urinary tract infections, and improvement with antibiotic therapy (usually without culture positive documentation), does not negate the need for urinalysis and urine culture. Empiric antibiotic therapy should not be done in these patients because it only delays the diagnosis and further confuses the patient. A patient without infection, but with such a history, may respond to antibiotic treatment due to (a) the natural history of the disease, (b) the placebo effect, and (c) the increase in fluid intake usually recommended along with the antibiotics (dilute urine is less irritating to the bladder). After antibiotics are completed, fluid intake usually returns to its low, pretreatment level with recurrence of full-blown symptoms.

In patients with IC without infection, a urinalysis is generally normal. About 20% of patients have 5 to 10 white blood cells per high-power microscopic field, and less than 10% have greater than 10 white blood cells per high-power field (4). Less than 10% of women with IC have greater than 5 red blood cells per high-power field in a urinalysis. In the occasional patient with hematuria, urine cytology is essential. Some have suggested that urine cytologies are advisable in all patients prior to the diagnosis of IC. If the patient has a history of smoking, there is little debate—urine cytology should be done. Of course, cytologies should be negative in patients with IC.

Because several other diseases, especially urinary tract infections and urethral syndrome, may cause similar symptoms, and because a finding of characteristic petechial, submucosal hemorrhages (termed "glomerulations") is one of the essential criteria for diagnosis, cystoscopy is a mandatory diagnostic test in patients suspected of having IC. It addition to the glomerulations (Figs. 5.1A,B) that show up on a second filling of the bladder, linear cracking and Hunners ulcer, named for Hunner who first described IC in 1914, may also be noted, but are not a consistent finding. Because significant bladder distention is needed and this is very painful in women with IC, general or spinal anesthesia is usually necessary. Cystoscopy for the diagnosis of IC is performed in a somewhat standardized manner for the best diagnostic results without confusing artifactual findings. After urethroscopy is completed the bladder is not allowed to collapse around the cystoscope, as this may traumatize the bladder mucosa and cause iatrogenic artifacts. The bladder is passively distended to 60 to 80 cm of water pressure for 2 to 3 minutes. This may require compression of the urethra by upward digital compression of the anterior vaginal wall against the urethroscope to prevent leakage. Although the risk is low, it is possible to rupture the bladder in IC patients during this distention (2). Findings during this first filling are usually normal, although occasionally increased trabeculation may be noted. As soon as maximal capacity is reached, the volume is noted and the irrigant is drained. If videocystoscopy is performed and the bladder is visualized during this emptying phase, diffuse bleeding from the mucosa is noted that causes the terminal portion of drained irrigant to be blood-tinged (see Fig. 5.1). Mean cystoscopic bladder capacity in IC patients is 545 mL (under anesthesia at 70 to 80 cm water pressure) with a range of 150 to 950 mL (5). The bladder is refilled and examination reveals splotchy, submucosal hemorrhages throughout the bladder of the patient with IC. These hemorrhages are called glomerulations. Glomerulations do not occur in a normal bladder, but may rarely occur in other bladder disorders. A Hunners ulcer may rarely be seen; when noted, it is diagnostic. Patients with markedly decreased bladder capacity are more likely to show Hunners ulcer. Bladder biopsies are useful, but not essential unless other abnormalities are seen. In such cases, biopsies must be

done to rule out carcinoma *in situ* or cancer. Up to 1% of women diagnosed with IC may actually have carcinoma *in situ* (8). If biopsies are performed at the time of cystoscopic diagnosis, the histologic finding of increased mast cells (special fixation and staining required) has been reported to be useful for confirmation of IC. Histologic findings of non-specific inflammation in the bladder submucosa and muscularis, as well as vasodilation and edema in the submucosa, are characteristic but not pathognomonic of IC. It is important that any infection has been cleared for several weeks before cystoscopy, not only because of infection concerns, but also because current or recent infection may cause cystoscopic findings similar to those of IC. Postprocedure pain may be decreased by instillation of a dilute solution of local anesthetic after completing cystoscopy (for example, 30 mL of 0.25% bupivicaine).

Cystometrics reveal decreased bladder capacities in almost all women with IC. In fact, this decrease in bladder capacity is sometimes used as a diagnostic criteria (9). Bladder compliance is also decreased. If bladder capacity is measured without general or spinal anesthesia, it is less than 600 mL. Significant pain and urgency occur with such volumes. In fact, if a patient tolerates bladder volumes of 600 to 700 mL without severe pain and urgency (some suggest 350 mL as the upper limit), then the diagnosis of IC is quite unlikely (4).

The potassium challenge or Parsons test has also been shown to be a useful diagnostic test for IC. The patient is asked to rate their baseline pain level, and then the bladder is infused with 40 mL of sterile water and she is again asked to rate her pain level, as well as any sensation of urgency, after the water is retained for 3 to 5 minutes. Patients with IC generally do not have a change of pain level with this volume of sterile water. The water is then drained and 40 mL of a 400 mEq/L solution of potassium chloride is infused into the bladder (this solution is easily made by mixing 40 mEq of potassium chloride with sterile water and bringing the volume to 100 mL), and the patient is again asked to rate her symptoms. The grading system and questions used by Parsons are shown in Fig. 32.1(10). A positive test is when the patient does not have a change with the water solution and has a change of two or more on the pain or urgency scale with the potassium chloride solution. The potassium challenge test is negative in 96% of normal controls and is positive in 70% of patients with IC (11). Patients with radiation cystitis also have positive responses to the potassium challenge test. The sensitivity of the potassium challenge is diminished if the patient has had recent therapy for IC, especially DMSO or anesthetic instillations.

Radiographic studies are mostly useful to rule out other conditions, but not to specifically confirm the diagnosis of IC. Thus, in selected patients, intravenous pyelography, voiding or static cystography, skeletal and pelvic x-rays, sonography, or computerized tomography may be indicated. Again, any of these studies should be normal if the diagnosis is IC.

Grading Scale:

Pain   None   Mild   Moderate   Severe

              0   1   2   3   4   5

Urgency   None   Mild   Moderate   Severe

              0   1   2   3   4   5

Questions:

1. Which solution is worse?

    ___Solution 1   ___Solution 2   ___Neither

2. Is the difference between solutions:

    ___None   ___Mild   ___Moderate   ___Severe

FIGURE 32.1. Grading scale and questions used for the potassium challenge or Parsons test.

Ongoing research has suggested potential usefulness of other tests, such as antinuclear antibodies, eosinophil cationic protein, histamine metabolites, epidermal growth factor, and glycosaminoglycan layer component assays, but there is not sufficient evidence to warrant routine clinical use of any of these determinations, as yet.

DIAGNOSIS

The major symptoms of IC—urgency, frequency, nocturia, and pelvic pain—may be associated with several other diagnoses. Acute, recurrent, or chronic infections of the urinary tract must be especially considered. A urine culture showing 100,000 or more bacterial colonies of one organism confirms a bladder infection (cystitis). Infections of the urethra (urethritis) may show similar culture results, but more commonly show either lower colony counts with bacterial urethritis or negative bacterial cultures with chlamydial urethritis. A positive chlamydial antigen or polymerase chain reaction (PCR) screening test from the urethra, Skenes glands, urine, or cervix suggests chlamydial urethritis (nongonococcal urethritis or NGU in older references). Gonococcal urethritis must also be considered, and appropriate cultures for *Nisseria gonorrhoeae* must be performed from the urethra, Skenes, and cervix. Tuberculous cystitis is also a possibility, particularly with aseptic pyuria. A positive tuberculin skin test and chest x-ray findings of tubercular disease support this diagnosis. However, urine cultures and stains for acid-fast bacilli, as well as histologic findings on bladder biopsy consistent with tubercular cystitis, are needed to confirm the diagnosis.

Bladder tumors, including carcinoma *in situ*, may also present with symptoms similar to those of IC. The presence of microscopic hematuria may suggest this possibility. Because of the possibility of bladder tumors in the differential, urine cytologies and cystoscopically directed bladder biopsies should generally be performed as part of the diagnostic workup.

Chronic urethral syndrome is a possible diagnosis in women with CPP that may be similar to IC in presentation. Cultures will similarly be negative, but with urethral syndrome there is usually marked tenderness to palpation of the anterior vaginal wall under the urethra and to passage of a catheter or cytourethroscope. Neither of these occur with IC.

Another syndrome, probably best termed irritable bladder, has the same symptoms and findings as IC, except that cystoscopy and bladder histology are normal (12). The etiology (or etiologies) of irritable bladder is also not known, but probably results from some source of bladder irritation that causes increased pelvic muscle activity. This muscle activity causes pelvic pressure with a strong desire to void when there is little urine in the bladder. Subsequent urination is dysfunctional because the bladder volume is insufficient to trigger normal reflex, coordinated micturition via detrusor contraction with simultaneous outlet relaxation. Urination is accomplished by straining, producing pain, hesitancy, and an intermittent stream. This may cause further bladder irritation, producing a "vicious cycle" of urgency, frequency, and pain. The original cause of bladder irritation is undoubtedly varied, including such things as acute cystitis, coital trauma, or sexual abuse, but this usually cannot be discerned at the time of clinical presentation. Treatment for irritable bladder is similar to the behavior modification and autodilation methods for IC that will be discussed later. Additionally, water consumption should be increased and dietary bladder irritants should be avoided (coffee, tea, carbonated beverages, citrus, cranberry juice, tomato juice and sauces, and alcohol). Treatment with warm baths and local heat, relaxation training, biofeedback, or physical therapy may be helpful. Symptomatic, medical therapy for irritable bladder syndrome is sometimes indicated. Antispasmodics, smooth and skeletal muscle relaxants, and analgesic or nonspecific medications such as those listed in Table 32.1 may be empirically tried. It is best to avoid narcotic medications in the treatment of irritable bladder. Again, cystoscopic findings distinguish irritable bladder from IC.

Other conditions may mimic the cystoscopic "glomerulations." These include infections (particularly tubercular or fungal), certain toxins (e.g., cyclophosphamide or formalin), radiation cystitis, neoplasms (especially carcinoma *in situ*), and overdistention of a defunctionalized bladder (4). These diagnoses may be distinguished from IC by history or by histologic findings. Most are not causes of CPP.

In summary, the differential diagnosis of IC is not always easy. In a sense, it is a diagnosis of exclusion, being a disease of variable symptoms, of unknown etiology, of possibly heterogeneous causation, and with no specific marker (except possibly Hunners ulcer, a finding generally not present). More specific diagnostic criteria for IC have been proposed by the National Institutes of Health, but these have not been widely accepted for clinical use (13).

MANAGEMENT OR TREATMENT

Treatment of IC can be a frustrating experience for both the patient and her physician(s), because none of the currently available therapies are curative. Significant biopsychosocial consequences are not surprising, considering that the patient is being told she has a disease of unknown cause with no known cure and with potentially incapacitating but not fatal consequences. Such consequences may be compounded by the triviality sometimes accorded her urinary symptoms and pain by family, physicians, and friends. Because of such issues, it is crucial that the physician educate and involve the patient fully in her diagnostic evaluation and treatment. When possible or appropriate, education of family members may also be helpful. IC tends to be a relapsing disease, even after seemingly successful treatment. It is important to educate the women about this characteristic of the disease both before treatment is instituted and after successful treatment is finished. Subsequent acceptance of the need for possible retreatment may be made easier by such education (5). However, this need not be presented in such a negative way that only hopelessness is conveyed. The real possibility of long periods of remission after successful treatment, especially with active patient participation in behavioral modification, can be optimistically presented without any deceit on the physician's part. Some of the self-help measures can be initiated even prior to cystoscopic diagnosis. Table 32.2 is an example of a handout of some self-interventions that the patient can initiate either before or after diagnosis (12).

MEDICAL TREATMENT

A useful treatment, as long as the patient does not have severe pain, is autodilation. This is a behavioral modification modality whereby the patient gradually increases her bladder capacity through gradually increasing the intervals between voidings (1). With this technique it is useful if the patient keeps a diary of times and volumes of urination and of fluid intake, of pain intensity (VAS rating), and of any suspected factors that might affect symptoms (for example, menses, sexual activity, or stress) (12). The patient and physician review the initial diary to establish baseline severity of symptoms and set concrete treatment goals. It is important that very specific goals be set and followed. The goals must be slow, gradual progression; if the patient attempts to progress too rapidly, failure is

TABLE 32.1. MEDICATIONS FOR IRRITABLE BLADDER SYNDROME

Medication	Dose
Anticholinergics/Antispasmodics	
Flavoxate hydrochloride	100–200 mg q6–8h
Hyoscyamine sulfate	0.125–0.30 mg q6–8h
Oxybutynin chloride	5 mg q6–12h
Smooth-Muscle Relaxants	
Phenoxybenzamine hydrochloride	10–20 mg q8–12h
Prazosin hydrochloride	1–5 mg q8–12h
Terazosin hydrochloride	1–5 mg q.d.
Skeletal-Muscle Relaxants	
Carisoprodol	350 mg q6–8h
Cyclobenzeprine	10 mg q8–12h
Methocarbamol	500–1,000 mg q6–8h
Diazepam	2–10 mg q6–12h
Analgesics/Others	
Phenazopyridine	200 mg q8h
Ketorulac tromethamine	10 mg q6h
Naproxen sodium	275–550 mg q6–12h
Ibuprofen	200–800 mg q6–8h
Amitryptilline	25–75 mg q.d.

TABLE 32.2. SELF-HELP FOR IRRITABLE BLADDER SYMPTOMS

There are things you can do that may help relieve irritative bladder symptoms of frequency, urgency, or pain on urination. These symptoms may have several different causes, including bacterial infection, substances in the urine causing irritation, or intrinsic bladder problems such as interstitial cystitis or tumors. Antibiotics are only indicated for bacterial infections, so a urine culture should be taken before starting any antibiotic, unless your physician specifically advises you otherwise.

At the first signs of discomfort or urgency, increase your intake of fluids. Some have found that starting with 16 oz. of water mixed with one teaspoon of baking soda helps relieve symptoms. You should continue drinking 8 oz. of plain water every 20 minutes over the next several hours. This dilution of urine or "flushing out" the bladder occasionally relieves symptoms completely. If not, it is okay to use acetaminophen or ibuprofen for pain relief. Bladder analgesics such as pyridium may also help and will not alter the results of a subsequent urine culture. If the increased fluid intake does not relieve symptoms completely, it is important to call your physician to arrange to have a urine culture done. This may be obtained via a midstream voided specimen or may require a catheterization for accurate culture results.

Some patients with chronic or recurrent irritative bladder problems find that specific foods or beverages flare or contribute to their symptoms. Some of the more common dietary irritants are listed below. You can try to discover if any of these foods contribute to your symptoms by following an elimination diet with add-back of one food or beverage at a time. In other words, you eliminate all of the foods and beverages listed, or only the ones you suspect may flare your symptoms, for at least 10 days. This may bring marked relief of symptoms in some cases. Then you begin to add back to your diet the eliminated foods, only one at a time, every 10 to 14 days. If symptoms return, this suggests that the specific food or beverage is an irritant for you and is best avoided. You may find that foods or beverages other than those listed contribute to your symptoms.

Alcoholic beverages	Cranberries and cranberry	Rye bread or rye products
Apples and apple juice	juice	Shortening
Artificial sweeteners	Fava jeans	Smoked or barbecued foods
Avocado	Fried foods	Sour cream
Brewer's yeast	Grapes	Soy sauce or tamari
Cantaloupe	Guava	Spicy (hot) foods
Carbonated drinks	Lima beans	Strawberries
Cheese (especially aged)	Margarine	Sugar
Chili and similar spicy foods	Mayonnaise	Tap water
Citrus fruit	Onions	Tea
Chicken liver	Peaches	Tomatoes and tomato juice
Chocolate	Pickled herring	Vitamin B complex
Coffee	Pineapple	Vinegar and vinegar products
Corned beef	Plums	Yogurt

inevitable. An initial increase of voiding intervals of no more than 15 minutes should be attempted. After about a month of successfully increasing the minimum voiding interval by 15 minutes, the minimum interval should be increased again. Generally, it is reasonable to try to increase the voiding interval by 15 minutes each month until a minimum interval of 3 to 4 hours is attained. The patient should continue to keep her diary throughout this treatment. This assists with compliance, adherence, motivation, and monitoring of her progress. Monthly physician visits are also helpful for the same reasons. Remission rates of 80% to 85% have been obtained with this treatment (Table 32.3). However, relapse of symptoms is likely if the patient is not vigilant with the training. Success with autodilation is limited to those patients with mild or controllable pain.

TABLE 32.3. THERAPY OF INTERSTITIAL CYSTITIS

Method	Success Rate (%)
Hydrodistention of bladder	50 (6–10 months)
Autodilation	80–85 (selected patients)
Dimethylsulfoxide, 50%, intravesical	40–50
Heparin, intravesical	40–50
Heparin, subcutaneous	30–35
Pentosanpolysulfate, oral	40–50
Nonsteroidal antiinflammatory drugs	—
Oxychlorosene, 0.4%, intravesical	—
Chromaline sodium	—
Transcutaneous electrical nerve stimulation (TENS) unit	—
Nd:YAG laser	—
Cystectomy and diversion	—

Urinary alkalization has been suggested by clinical experience to decrease symptoms of IC. In addition to an acid-restricted diet (see Table 32.2), urine can be made more alkaline by taking potassium citrate, 30 mL three times a day.

Dimethylsulfoxide (DMSO, Rimso-50) was the first drug with an FDA-approved indication for IC. DMSO is a product of the wood pulp industry, a derivative of lignin. It is a superb solvent, being miscible with water, lipids, and organic agents. DMSO has a number of pharmacologic properties that led to interest in its use for IC: (a) membrane penetration without membrane damage; (b) enhancement of drug absorption (e.g., steroids); (c) antiinflammatory activity; (d) topical analgesic activity via interruption of conduction in peripheral nerves; (e) promotion of collagen breakdown or dissolution via weakening of cross-linking; (f) muscle relaxation; (g) bacteriostasis; (h) vasodilation; and (i) enhancement of mast cell histamine release. All but the last of these pharmacologic properties are potential mechanisms by which DMSO might decrease symptoms in IC. In contrast, the DMSO effect on mast cells could account for the initial transient worsening of symptoms in some IC patients with DMSO treatment.

DMSO has very low systemic toxicity. It is primarily excreted via the renal system as unchanged DMSO and as dimethylsulfone ($DMSO_2$). A small percentage is excreted via the respiratory system as dimethylsulfide (DMS). DMS accounts for the garlic-like taste and breath odor after DMSO treatment. Some early animal studies raised concerns of lenticular opacities, but this has never been reported with therapeutic doses or human use. DMSO has

been reported to be teratogenic in animal studies, so its use in pregnancy is contraindicated.

Initial attempts to use DMSO for IC were transdermal, and results were mediocre. This led to trials of intravesical administration, which gave more promising results and led to FDA approval. Intravesical treatment with DMSO can be readily done as an office procedure. It is best to perform a urinalysis prior to treatment to exclude bacteriuria. Additionally, DMSO treatment should not be done until at least 3 to 4 weeks after bladder biopsies to avoid excessive absorption via the unhealed biopsy sites. The urethra may be anesthetized with 2% lidocaine topically. Sometimes the treatment is painful, so analgesics prior to treatment may be beneficial. Some have also suggested vesical nerve block via subvesical injection of 10 to 20 mL of 1% lidocaine (Fig. 32.2), but definitive evidence has not been presented that this improves comfort during the procedure or enhances the therapeutic response. A small urethral catheter (8–12 French) is inserted and the bladder emptied. A 50-mL volume of 50% DMSO (Rimso-50) is instilled and the catheter removed. The patient waits 15 to 30 minutes before voiding. Treatments are usually repeated four to eight times at 1- to 2-week intervals. As mentioned above, some patients find this treatment painful, so in these patients a pretreatment dose of ibuprofen, naproxen sodium, or ketorulac tromethamine might be considered. Some patients complain of significant irritation and burning of the urethra with DMSO treatment. This can be diminished by leaving the catheter in and clamped for the 15 to 30 minutes of treatment, then emptying the DMSO via the catheter before removal. Painful bladder spasms occur in about 10% of

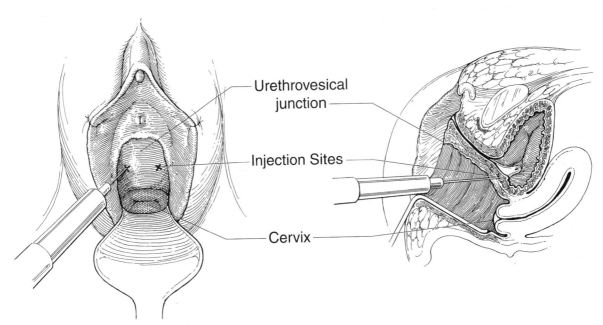

Urethrovesical junction

Injection Sites

Cervix

FIGURE 32.2. Vesical neural block for DMSO treatment of interstitial cystitis.

patients, and these may be treated with anticholinergics or belladonna and opium suppositories. All patients note a garlic-like odor of breath and taste in the mouth for 24 to 48 hours after DMSO treatment. This can be personally and socially unpleasant for the patient, so it is important that each patient be counseled about this side effect. Not uncommonly, symptoms worsen transiently after the first treatment, so success cannot be determined until more than two treatments are done. In addition to subjective evidence of decreased symptoms, objective evidence of significantly increased bladder capacity (greater than 100-mL increase) has also been demonstrated (2,14). Unfortunately, DMSO treatments result only in remission of disease, not cure. At least 30% to 60% of patients relapse within the first year after successful treatment. Compounding this, retreatment with DMSO after relapse of symptoms is less effective, and many patients ultimately become resistant to DMSO treatment (5). A suggestion has been made that the addition of 100 mg of hydrocortisone to the 50-mL dose of 50% DMSO might improve the response in patients without improvement after initial or retreatment courses of DMSO (14). However, no outcome results have been published for this regimen.

Other intravesical therapies for IC have been less extensively studied than DMSO. Additionally, none of the intravesical drug therapies other than DMSO have FDA approval for treatment of IC. Although this does not preclude their use, it does mean that patients should be appropriately counseled as to the "investigational" nature of the treatment.

Heparin has been used both subcutaneously and intravesically for IC. Both of these modalities have the advantage that the patient can be taught self-administration. Given subcutaneously, the usual dose is 2,500 to 5,000 units three times per week. Although anticoagulation is unlikely with this dose, it is still advisable to check several partial thromboplastin times over the first 3 weeks of treatment. Response rates with subcutaneous heparin are no higher than one in three (Table 32.3). In patients with a clinical response, this treatment should not generally be continued more than 8 to 10 weeks, because chronic heparin use may cause osteoporosis and hair loss. In a patient with a good response, but with recurrence after a full course of therapy, retreatment may be tried if the patient has been off heparin for at least 3 months.

Intravesical heparin has been slightly more effective than subcutaneous heparin, with about 40% to 50% of patients responding (Table 32.3). Three to five times per week, 10,000 units of heparin in 10 mL of sterile water are instilled into the bladder via a small urethral catheter (8–12 French). The patient can be taught to do this herself. She retains the heparin without voiding for at least 1 hour. Heparin is not significantly absorbed into the circulation from the bladder, so partial thromboplastin time assays are not needed. A prophylactic antibiotic dose with each treatment is recommended.

Patients not responsive to these modalities can be treated with intravesical oxychlorosene sodium (Clorpactin) (15). This treatment is painful, so general or regional anesthesia is necessary and the perineum must be protected during use to avoid contact from spillage.

Another intravesical therapy that has been suggested is capsaicin. A randomized clinical trial of treatment of 36 patients with 10 μg of capsaicin versus placebo showed significant improvements in frequency and nocturia, but no improvement in pain levels compared to the control group (16).

Peters et al. (17) found that intravesical bacillus Calmette-Guérin (BCG) is efficacious in the treatment of pelvic pain and urinary frequency associated with interstitial cystitis. In a prospective, double-blind, placebo-controlled trial they showed that BCG resulted in a response rate of 60%, compared to a response rate of 27% in the placebo group. In responders, the mean decrease of pelvic pain was 81%. The absolute benefit increase of BCG is 33% and the number needed to treat is 3. If this response rate can be confirmed by others, BCG may represent a useful addition to the armamentarium for the treatment of interstitial cystitis.

Sodium pentosan polysulfate (PPS) is a polyanionic analogue of heparin that has been used to treat IC. It may be administered orally (1). Reported results of its effectiveness have been mixed, but at least one placebo-controlled, double-blinded study showed a 50% response rate, compared to the placebo response of 23% (3). Decreased pelvic pain, in particular, occurred in 45% of patients, compared to 18% with placebo. PPS dosage in this study was 100 mg orally three times a day. PPS is the only FDA-approved oral medication for IC and is sold under the brand name Elmiron.

The exact modes of action of heparin and PPS are not known. However, both are complex sulfated polysaccharides and are extremely hydrophilic. Because of this, when bound to the surface epithelium, they are capable of forming or enhancing the layer of micelles of water over the epithelium. Thus, at least theoretically, they may improve the barrier and antiadherance activity of the endogenous glycosaminoglycan layer of the bladder epithelium. However, in spite of this possible mechanism, there is no evidence of any intrinsic abnormalities of the glycosaminoglycan of patients with IC.

Other nonsurgical treatments for IC have been reported, but evidence of their effectiveness is scant. *Cyclosporine*, an immunosuppressive drug, in an uncontrolled, nonblinded study resulted in improvement in 10 of 11 patients (18). Doses were 2.5 to 5 mg/kg daily for 3 to 6 months, followed by maintenance doses of 1.5 to 3 mg/kg daily. Doses had to be lowered in two patients due to hypertension. Symptoms recurred in these patients when cyclosporine was discontinued. Oral *L*-arginine, 1.5 g daily for 6 months, resulted in improvement in urinary frequency and pain in an uncontrolled, nonblinded study of 10 women with IC (19). The mode of action is thought to be related to increasing nitric oxide levels, because L-arginine is the substrate for nitric oxide synthase. *Nifedipine*, in an open trial of 10 women with IC, resulted in improvement in eight, with complete resolution of symptoms in three, but there are no controlled studies of its use (20). It is advisable to do a nifedipine titration test before instituting treatment. This is done by measuring a baseline blood pressure, giving 10 mg nifedipine orally, and repeating blood pressure measurements every 15 minutes. If by 1 hour there is not significant decrease of blood pressure (less than 20 mmHg drop of systolic and no change in diastolic), then a second 10-mg dose is given and the process repeated. Patients who tolerated this titration test can be started on 30 mg of slow-release nifedipine per day for 2 weeks, then increased to a maintenance dose of 60 mg of slow-release nifedipine per day. Patients with significant decreases of blood pressure during the titration will only tolerate 30 mg of nifedipine per day. *Antihistamines*, such as hydroxyzine, have also been used with some success. *Hydroxyzine* is started at 25 mg at bedtime and gradually increased to 50 mg at bedtime and 25 mg during the day. In an uncontrolled, nonblinded study of hydroxyzine, 37 of 40 women had improvement in symptoms, by an average of about 35% decrease of frequency and pain scores (21). *Tricyclic antidepressants*, particularly *amitriptyline*, have been frequently used to treat IC, yet little is published regarding efficacy. Uncontrolled, nonblinded studies have suggested improvement in 65% to 90% of

those able to tolerate amitriptyline at doses of 25 to 75 mg daily at bedtime (22,23). Evidence of usefulness of tricyclic antidepressants with other chronic pain syndromes would imply at least some effectiveness for pain symptoms in IC.

Transcutaneous electrical nerve stimulation (TENS) therapy has been used for the treatment of IC with variable results, with 20% to 80% of patients showing at least some degree of improvement. TENS frequency settings used for IC range from 2 to 50 Hz. Patients usually start treatment with high-frequency stimulation and switch to low frequency if there is no response after 1 month. The placement of electrodes is 10 to 15 cm apart and just superior to the pubic symphysis (Fig. 32.3).

SURGICAL TREATMENT

The mainstay of urologic treatment of IC for more than 50 years has been hydrodistention of the bladder. This procedure can be performed at the time of diagnostic cystoscopy if general or spinal anesthesia is used. If the patient has IC, it is too painful to be done without anesthesia. After diagnostic evaluation is completed, the bladder is filled to maximal capacity at 80 to 100 cm water pressure for 2 minutes. There is some risk of bladder rupture with this procedure, estimated at less than 15% (2). Patients complain of increased pain immediately postoperatively, and it is generally several weeks until they note a remission of symptoms. About 50% of patients have a successful response to hydrodistention (Table 32.3). Remission generally lasts for six to ten months, with a gradual recurrence of symptoms in almost all patients. Retreatment with hydrodistention has a greatly diminished success rate. The mechanism of action of hydrodistention is not know. Speculation is that one or both of the following mechanisms may apply: (a) The dysfunctional epithelium is damaged and regeneration of normal epithelium is stimulated or (b) there is significant nerve damage with resultant denervation. The latter mechanism is not totally consistent with the observed increased symptoms postoperatively. Regardless of the actual mechanism, hydrodistention is a reasonable initial therapy. It has a good, albeit temporary, response rate, it is fairly easy and safe to perform, and it can be done at the same time as the diagnostic cystoscopy.

Neurolytic surgery via laser destruction of the vesicoureteric plexus has been reported with some degree of success (24), but these have been uncontrolled studies with limited follow-up and require further confirmation before this procedure is widely used. Presacral neurectomy has a limited, if any, role in surgical treatment. Up to one-third of patients have improvement with presacral neurectomy, but in those with relief it appears to be temporary (25).

Approximately 5% of patients have unresponsive, intractable, incapacitating symptoms that justify surgical

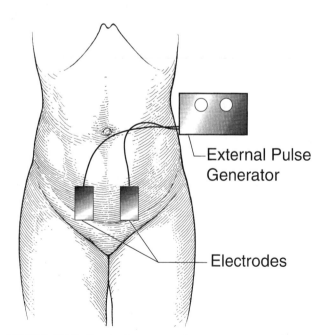

External Pulse Generator

Electrodes

FIGURE 32.3. Usual placement of transcutaneous electrical nerve stimulation (TENS) electrodes for the treatment of interstitial cystitis. Electrodes are 10 to 15 cm apart and just superior to the pubic symphysis.

treatment. Such patients usually have small-capacity bladders (<400 mL), void 18 to 20 times per day, and have severe, uncontrolled pain. Augmentation cystoplasty and cystectomy–urethrectomy–continent diversion with a Kock or Indiana pouch have been the most successful and acceptable aggressive or radical surgical treatments. However, in one series of such patients, 2 of 15 developed subsequent pouch pain.

A less aggressive surgical approach, with some degree of success, is Nd:YAG laser ablation of the bladder lining (26). Of 39 patients (33 women) treated with the Nd:YAG laser, 30 had an initial response. More than 50% had subsequent recurrence of symptoms and required re-treatment. Additionally, two of the patients had small bowel perforations due to unrecognized laser injury, both presenting with the complications several days after laser irradiation. Obviously, Nd:YAG laser treatment must be considered experimental at this time and should be done under study or protocol conditions by surgeons experienced with use of the Nd:YAG laser.

In summary, the mainstays of current treatment for IC are hydrodistention, autodilation, and DMSO. Individually, these treatments generally achieve 40% to 60% remission rates. The effectiveness of combining these modalities has not been well-studied. A great deal more research on treatment effectiveness for IC is needed, but is difficult to perform. Because the major clinical characteristics of IC are subjective symptoms, it is crucial that objectivized measurements such as VAS pain ratings, voiding intervals, voided volumes, and VAS ratings of urgency be used. Also, placebo-controlled studies are needed, because currently available studies show placebo responses of 10% to 25% in IC patients.

KEY POINTS

Differential Diagnoses

- Acute urinary tract infection
- Bladder tumors, especially carcinoma *in situ*
- Chlamydial urethritis or cystitis
- Chronic infection of the urinary tract
- Chronic urethral syndrome
- Endometriosis
- Gonococcal urethritis
- Irritable bladder syndrome
- Recurrent urinary tract infection
- Tuberculous

Most Important Questions to Ask

- How often do you usually urinate during the daytime?
- How often do you usually get up at nighttime to urinate?
- Do you have pain during urination? If so, what kind of pain is it?

- Do you have pain when your bladder is full, or is your pain made worse when your bladder is full?
- Does emptying your bladder make this pain better or worse?
- Is your pain worse immediately after emptying your bladder?
- Do you ever lose urine?
- Do you have a childhood history of infections, incontinence, or bedwetting?
- If so, were any procedures such as urethral dilation or cutting of the urethral opening performed to correct these problems?
- Did the onset of bladder symptoms correspond with any of the following:
    Becoming sexually active?
    A new sexual partner?
    A change of birth control?
    A change of jobs?
    Increased stress at home, work, or school?
    Changes in menses?
    Pelvic surgery or other pelvic procedures?
- Are your symptoms the same 24 hours a day, 7 days a week?
- If not, how do they vary?
- Do they vary with your menstrual cycle?

Most Important Physical Examination Findings

- Tenderness of the anterior vagina under the trigone and bladder
- Pelvic floor muscle tenderness

Most Important Diagnostic Studies

- Cystourethroscopy, with fill–refill technique
- Potassium challenge or Parsons test
- Urinalysis
- Urine culture
- Urine cytologies, especially if a history of smoking
- Bladder biopsies
- Computerized tomography
- Intravenous pyelography
- Skeletal and pelvic x-rays
- Sonography
- Urodynamic studies
- Voiding or static cystography

Treatments

- Antihistamines, such as hydroxyzine
- Augmentation cystoplasty
- Autodilation
- Capsaicin, intravesically
- Cyclosporine, orally

- Cystectomy–urethrectomy–continent diversion with a Kock or Indiana pouch
- Dietary modification and restriction
- Dimethylsulfoxide (DMSO), intravesically
- Education
- Heparin, intravesically or subcutaneously
- Hydrodistention of the bladder
- L-arginine, orally
- Nd:YAG laser ablation of the bladder lining
- Nifedipine, orally
- Oxychlorosene (Clorpactin), intravesically
- Sodium pentosan polysulfate (Elmiron)
- Transcutaneous electrical nerve stimulation (TENS) therapy
- Tricyclic antidepressants, particularly amitriptyline
- Urinary alkalization with potassium citrate
- Neurolytic surgery via laser destruction of the vesicoureteric plexus or presacral neurectomy

REFERENCES

1. Summit RL Jr. Urogynecologic causes of chronic pelvic pain. *Obstet Gynecol Clin North Am* 1993;20:685–698.
2. Ramahi AJ, Richardson DA. A practical approach to the painful bladder syndrome. *J Reprod Med* 1990;35:805–809.
3. Parsens CL. Sodium pentosanpolysulfate treatment of intersitial cystitis: an update. *Urology (Suppl)* 1987;29:14–16.
4. Messing EM. The diagnosis of intersitial cystitis. *Urology (Suppl)* 1989;29:4–21.
5. Parsons CL. Interstitial cystitis: what options? *Contemp Obstet Gynecol* 1992;August:23–28.
6. Reiter RC, Gambone JC. Nongynecologic somatic pathology in women with chronic pelvic pain and negative laparoscopy. *J Reprod Med* 1991;36:253–259.
7. Ratliff TL, Klutke CG, McDougall EM. The etiology of interstitial cystitis. *Urol Clin North Am* 1994;21:21–30.
8. Utz DC, Zincke H. The masquerade of bladder cancer *in situ* as interstitial cystitis. *J Urol* 1974;111:160–161.
9. Parsons LH, Stoval TG. Surgical management of chronic pelvic pain. *Obstet Gynecol North Am* 1993;20:765–778.
10. Parsons CL. Potassium sensitivity test. *Tech Urol* 1996;2:171–173.
11. Parsons CL, Stein PC, Bidair M, et al. Abnormal sensitivity to intravesical potassium in interstitial cystitis and radiation cystitis. *Neurourol Urodyn* 1994;13:515–520.
12. Bavendam TG. Irritable bladder—a commonsense approach. *Contemp Obstet Gynecol* 1993;April:70–77.
13. Gillenwater JY, Wein AJ. Summary of the National Institute of Arthritis, Diabetes, Digestive and Kidney Diseases workshop on intersititial cystitis, National Institutes of Health, Bethesda, Maryland, August 28–29, 1987. *J Urol* 1988;140:203–206.
14. Sant GR. Intravesical 50% dimethyl sulfoxide (RIMSO-50) in treatment of intersitial cystitis. *Urology (Suppl)* 1987;29:17–21.
15. Sant GR, LaRock DR. Standard intravesical therapies for interstitial cystitis. *Urol Clin North Am* 1994;21:73–83.
16. Lazzeri M, Beneforti P, Benaim G, et al. Intravesical capsaicin for treatment of severe bladder pain: a randmized placebo controlled study. *J Urol* 1996;156:947–952.
17. Peters KM, Diokno AC, Steinart BW, et al. The efficacy of intravesical bacillus Calmette-Guérin in the treatment of interstitial cystitis: long-term followup. *J Urol* 1998;159:1483–1486.
18. Forsell T, Fuutu M, Isoniemi H, et al. Cyclosporine in severe interstitial cystitis. *J Urol* 1996;155:1591–1593.
19. Smith SD, Wheeler MA, Foster HE Jr, et al. Improvement I interstitial cystitis symptom scores during treatment with L-arginine. *J Urol* 1997;158:703–708.
20. Fleischmann JD, Huntley HN, Shingleton WB, et al. Clinical and immunological response to nifedipine for treatment of interstitial cystitis. *J Urol* 1991;146:1235–1239.
21. Theoharides TC. Hydroxyzine in the treatment of interstitial cystitis. *Urol Clin North Am* 1994;21:113–119.
22. Hanno PM, Wein AJ. Conservative therapy of interstitial cystitis. *Semin Urol* 1991;9:143–147.
23. Kirkemo AK, Miles BJ, Peters JM. Use of amitriptyline in the treatment of interstitial cystitis. *J Urol* 1989;141:846–848.
24. Gillespie L. Destruction of the vesicoureteric plexus for the treatment of hypersensitive bladder disorders. *Br J Urol* 1994;74:40–43.
25. Jacobson CE, Braash WF, Love JG. Presacral neurectomy for vesical pain. *Surg Gynecol Obstet* 1944;79:21–26.
26. Shanberg AM, Malloy T. Treatment of interstitial cystitis with neodymium:YAG laser. *Urology (Suppl)* 1987;29:31–33.

33

RADIATION CYSTITIS

CHARLES W. BUTRICK

KEY TERMS AND DEFINITIONS

Formalin therapy: Commonly used intravesical therapy for hemorrhagic cystitis. The formalin acts as a chemical cautery to the diffuse sources of bleeding that accompany hemorrhagic cystitis.

Glycosaminoglycan layer (GAG): Protective layer of the bladder made up of proteinaceous material produced by the uroepithelium. This protective coat plays an important role in antibacterial defenses and bladder impermeability. Radiation damages this coat in the majority of patients with radiation cystitis.

Hemorrhagic cystitis: A complication of radiation therapy that leads to fragile, abnormal vascularity of the mucosa such that when these vessels are damaged (often due to the insult of an episode of bacterial cystitis) significant hematuria can result, at times requiring hospitalization, surgery, and blood transfusions.

Hyperbaric oxygen therapy: Patients are placed in a hyperbaric oxygen environment for 90 to 120 minutes over several treatment sessions to induce a permanent improvement in oxygen tension within tissues that have been damaged by radiation. Typically used for patients with significant hemorrhagic cystitis.

Radiation cystitis: Radiation-induced damage to the bladder uroepithelium, blood vessels, and nerve supply that result in symptoms such as urgency, frequency, hematuria, and irritative voiding symptoms. This damage may be acute and resolve spontaneously or chronic with persistent symptomatology.

Sodium pentosanpolysulfate: Oral agent used to help correct the defective GAG layer seen in patients with radiation cystitis and hemorrhagic cystitis.

INTRODUCTION

In recent years there have been considerable advancements in the management of malignant disease utilizing sophisticated radiotherapeutic techniques. While these modern approaches have resulted in increased survival rates, their success must always be balanced against the potential of damage to the surrounding tissues. When treating pelvic malignancies the surrounding tissues that can suffer include the urologic tract, gastrointestinal tract, and the nerves that so richly innervate the pelvis. Ideally, cure of the malignant disease should be achieved with minimal functional or structural disruption to the normal tissues. Unfortunately, this ideal is rarely achieved and the resultant tissue damage to surrounding organs can at times result in radiation cystitis. The doses necessary for tumor control and that which will produce complications are very similar. Although patients with radiation cystitis generally present with predominantly urologic symptoms of dysuria, frequency, urgency, and hematuria, chronic pelvic pain (CPP) can be a significant problem. In patients with CPP and a history of radiation treatment for pelvic malignancy, obviously it is important to evaluation for radiation cystitis.

ETIOLOGY

Radiation produces the most destruction during the mitotic phase of the cell cycle, and therefore it affects rapidly dividing cells to a greater extent than more slowly regenerating cells. Cells lining the epithelium of the bowel and urogenital systems are mitotically very active and therefore at risk for the damaging effects of radiation. Early radiation reactions include depletion and denudation of the uroepithelial cells of the bladder and its thick layer of proteoglycan and glycoprotein (GAG layer). This protective coat plays an important role in antibacterial defenses and bladder impermeability (1). Bladder injury following radiation therapy can be mild and transitory, moderate or severe. Important factors that alter the susceptibility of the bladder to radiation injury include dose of radiation and duration of therapy. Additional factors that also are important include level of tissue oxygenation, invasion of tumor, infection, systemic disease, and concomitant cytotoxic drugs. It is rare to find significant changes in the bladder with less than 5,000 rads delivered over the routine 5-week time frame. As radiation dosage increases, so does the rate of urologic complications (Table 33.1) (2–4).

TABLE 33.1. UROLOGIC COMPLICATIONS WITH INCREASING DOSES OF RADIATION THERAPY

Authors of Articles	Comb Dose	Number of Patients	Percent with Urologic Complications
Kottmeier and Gray (2)	<8,000	329	5.5
	8,000–9,000	21	10
	>9,000	17	29
Perez et al. (3)	<8,000	648	4
	>8,000	162	11
Pourquier et al. (4)	<7,000	370	7.5
	>7,000	254	20

In 1983, the Radiation Therapy Oncology Group published a grading system that provides a meaningful rating system for radiation complications (Table 33.2) (5). Grades 1 and 2 should be classified as anticipated treatment-related reactions, not complications of therapy. If these mild symptoms persist for more than 1 month after the completion of therapy, then they also are considered complications of therapy.

Hemorrhagic cystitis is a serious complication of high-dose radiation therapy and can be a life-threatening complication. Hemorrhagic cystitis can present as acute or insidious vesical bleeding, sometimes requiring blood transfusions, hospitalization, and surgical intervention. A reliable estimate of the incidence of hemorrhagic cystitis following pelvic radiation therapy is difficult to determine. Various authors have reported incidences of 2% to 9%. Villasanta (6) reported a 7.8% incidence of hemorrhagic cystitis after radiation therapy with a mean interval of 23 months from the beginning of therapy to the onset of hemorrhagic cystitis. Levenback et al. (7) demonstrated a 6.5% incidence of hemorrhagic cystitis with a 58-month mean interval time to onset; they also demonstrated a 2.3% risk of hemorrhagic cystitis so severe that death occurred or surgical intervention was needed. Important clinical characteristics include the frequent occurrence of urinary tract infections as a cofactor in the initiation of the hematuria and that cystoscopy rarely demonstrates recurrent or metastatic disease to be an etiologic factor in a patient's hematuria.

PATHOLOGY

In 1933 Dean (8) described three types of bladder reaction to radiation: acute, subacute, and chronic. The early changes represent those changes associated with direct cellular damage, whereas the later changes are the result of the repair process involving particularly the connective tissue and blood vessels of the submucosal layers of the bladder.

Early Histopathology. The first tissue response is congestion of the submucosal capillaries with edema of the submucosa as described by Hueper et al. (9) This is followed by the development of degenerative changes in the epithelium. As these epithelial changes progress, desquamation of the epithelium can occur, resulting in superficial ulceration with a covering of fibrin and leukocytes. Perivascular lymphocytic infiltration surrounds dilated capillaries, and submucosal hemorrhages are frequently seen.

Late Histopathology. After cessation of radiation therapy, many of these early changes regress, but the persistence of vascular changes is noted in the majority of patients. Capillary proliferation and formation of ectatic vessels is seen, yet other capillaries show narrowing of their lumens due to subendothelial fibrosis. The epithelium may return to normal, or it may exhibit varying degrees of atrophy or ulceration depending largely on the response of the fine vasculature and connective tissue underlying the epithelium. The extent and rapidity of healing are also dependent upon the presence or absence of associated infection, the bladder being much more prone to infection under the circumstances of a disrupted epithelial lining.

There is a slow progressive obliterative arteritis that interferes with blood supply to the uroepithelium and the adjacent tissues. These vascular changes are responsible for the atrophy and even necrosis of the epithelium with ulcer-

TABLE 33.2. GRADING OF COMPLICATIONS OF PELVIC RADIATION THERAPY

Grade 1	Minor symptoms requiring no treatment
Grade 2	Symptoms respond to simple outpatient management, lifestyle not affected
Grade 3	Distressing symptoms altering patient's lifestyle. Hospitalization required for diagnosis or minimal surgical treatment (e.g., urethral dilation)
Grade 4	Major surgical intervention required (e.g., cystectomy, colostomy, etc.) or prolonged hospitalization required
Grade 5	Fatal complications

ation and formation of fissures and/or fistulas. These radiation-induced fistulas typically occur within the first 2 years after therapy. It is the slow progression of these vascular changes that results in many of these late sequelae of radiation therapy. Additionally, the autonomic nerve supply involving the sensory and motor function of the lower urinary tract and the distal ureter is frequently involved in the radiation induced damage. This may involve direct damage to the nerve and can also be the result of the vascular changes seen in the viscera.

Approximately 50% of patients with postradiation bladder complications will suffer from hemorrhagic cystitis. Radiation injury results in the development of obliterated endarteritis with resultant telangiectasia, submucosal hemorrhage, and fibrosis of smooth muscle and the interstitium of the bladder wall. Ischemic changes result in hypoxic tissue breakdown at the mucosal level, thus resulting in ulceration and bleeding.

SYMPTOMS OR HISTORY

The acute phase of radiation cystitis can begin 3 to 6 weeks after the initiation of radiation therapy and is often indistinguishable from the more common acute hemorrhagic cystitis of bacterial origin. The subacute symptoms start 6 months to 2 years after therapy and often result in more significant symptoms and complications. Chronic changes are typically the result of a very low capacity, fibrotic bladder with mucosal ulcerations, and at times fistula formation. Radiation-induced fistulas typically occur within the first 2 years after the initiation of therapy. It is always important to distinguish this from the recurrence of a tumor at the site of the fistula in the evaluation of any patient who presents with a postradiation therapy fistula.

Acute Radiation Cystitis. The symptoms of acute radiation cystitis are those of bacterial irritation, including frequency, urgency, suprapubic pain, dysuria, and urge incontinence. Hematuria with or without pain is often seen and is typically self-limiting, which is not always the case in the patients with hemorrhagic cystitis during the chronic or late stages of radiation cystitis. In Kottmeier's series, minimal symptoms were present in 8% of patients undergoing radiation therapy for cervical cancer (2). In this group of patients with symptoms, the symptoms resolved in 83%. Bourne et al. (10) have shown that the incidence of chronic complications was 8% in patients who were symptomatic in the acute phase of therapy as compared to only 3% in patients who were initially asymptomatic.

Chronic Radiation Cystitis. Typical symptoms of chronic radiation cystitis include urgency, frequency, nocturia, suprapubic pain, and pressure. Late complications of radiation therapy generally occur 6 to 24 months after the completion of therapy. These complications include (a) a contracted fibrotic bladder with resultant urgency, frequency, and irritative voiding symptoms and (b) hemorrhagic cystitis. The onset of clinically significant hematuria typically parallels the onset of nonhemorrhagic radiation cystitis symptoms, occurring approximately 39 months after completion of radiation therapy (11). DeVries and Freiha (12) have categorized the degree of hematuria into three groups: *mild hematuria*, not requiring transfusion or surgical intervention; *moderate hematuria*, requiring less than six transfusions and bladder irrigations for clot retention and bleeding; *severe hematuria*, requiring multiple transfusions and significant intravesical and surgical intervention. Cheng and Foo (13) demonstrated that 21% of patients with hemorrhagic cystitis will have severe hemorrhagic cystitis with a prolonged course of therapy that will result in death in 44% of these cases. Frustrating was the fact that 78% of those deaths occurred in patients with no evidence of recurrent cancer. Thus, they died from the therapy that cured them of their cancer.

Additional complications include ureteral stenosis and vesicovaginal fistula.

SIGNS OR EXAMINATION

Patients with CPP and radiation cystitis usually show tenderness suprapubically unless other serious complications such as fistula formation have occurred. Similarly, pelvic examination shows atrophic, thinned, and stenotic changes of the upper vagina unless other more serious complications are present. The anterior vagina under the bladder may be particularly tender. It is important to exclude any evidence of recurrence of cancer in patients with pain and suspected radiation cystitis.

DIAGNOSTIC STUDIES

The irritative bladder symptoms suggest bacterial cystitis so a urine culture must be obtained so that any infection present can be identified. Urine cytology and urinalysis are also indicated. Radiographic studies are generally not necessary unless there is a suspicion of recurrent cancer or of fistula formation.

Cystoscopy is essential to confirming the diagnosis. During the acute stage, cystoscopic findings include marked mucosal edema and diffuse erythema with prominent submucosal vascularity. Cystoscopic appearance of the chronic phase of radiation cystitis differs in that the bladder mucosa has patches of extreme pallor separating areas of intense erythema with petechia. Occasionally, uroepithelial ulceration is present. Bladder capacity and compliance are frequently reduced.

In patients with hemorrhagic cystitis, cystoscopically the mucosa demonstrates multiple hyperemic telangiectatic areas with significant edema and multiple bleeding points. The mucosa is extremely friable, and touching the hyperemic areas with the tip of the cystoscope results in immediate bleeding.

During cystoscopy, a careful evaluation for malignancy is required. Bladder washings are ideal during the cystoscopic evaluation, but we must remember that postradiation uroepithelium can be difficult to interpret at the time of cytopathologic analysis. Bladder biopsies should be avoided unless absolutely required because of an inordinately high incidence of postbiopsy fistulas at the biopsy site.

DIAGNOSIS

The diagnoses that may be differentiated from radiation cystitis are interstitial cystitis, irritable bladder syndrome, and bacterial cystitis. The clinical history of radiation treatment, cystoscopic findings, and results of urinalysis and urine culture usually are sufficient to eliminate the presence of these other diseases in women with CPP and irritative bladder symptoms.

TREATMENT

Medical Treatment

The majority of bladder symptoms can be treated medically. Concurrent infections markedly worsen bladder symptomatology and may induce an episode of serious hemorrhagic cystitis. Appropriate antimicrobials are given to treat acute infection. Additionally, chronic low-dose antibiotics may be necessary to prevent rapid reinfection of the damaged tissue.

The urgency, frequency, and irritative voiding symptoms are some of the most frustrating complaints that patients with radiation cystitis must face. Anticholinergics such as Ditropan, Detrol, or Imipramine help to relieve these symptoms with varying degrees of success. Pyridium is sometimes useful for relieving dysuria. General measures that are of benefit include a low acid diet, alkalinization of the urine, and decreased consumption of caffeine.

Correction of hypoestrogen-induced atrophy with vaginal estrogen cream is beneficial if estrogen vaginal cream is not contraindicated. In fact, Liu et al. (14) found that high-dose intravenous therapy with conjugated estrogen followed by 5 mg per day of oral conjugated estrogen had a profoundly positive effect on five patients with severe hemorrhagic cystitis with a total resolution of hematuria. The use of estrogen has been considered to be relatively contraindicated in patients with a history of endometrial cancer, but now even this is controversial.

Parsons et al. (15) have demonstrated that all patients with symptoms of radiation cystitis have a positive response to a potassium sensitivity test. Radiation-induced damage to the uroepithelium results in a defective glycosaminoglycan (GAG) layer of the bladder. This disruption in the protective GAG layer results in an increase in mucosal permeability which results in potassium ions and other irritative substances actually passing through the mucosa into the mucosal layers. Urine is actually found to be toxic to cultured uroepithelial cells that lack the protection that is offered by the GAG layer. Sodium pentosanpolysulfate (Elmiron) supplements the deficient GAG layer and has been found to benefit patients with radiation cystitis (16) and hemorrhagic cystitis (17).

Additional approaches to the irritative symptoms of chronic radiation cystitis involve many of the same intravesical therapies that have been used in the treatment of interstitial cystitis. These include intravesical dimethyl sulfoxide (DMSO) and intravesical saline with 100 mg of hydrocortisone. Cocktails using various combinations of drugs can also be used. My preference is a combination of 10,000 units of heparin, 40 mg triamcinolone acetate, 20 mL of 1% lidocaine. These intravesical therapies provide varying degrees of success in reduction of the patient's urgency, frequency, and nocturia, but none of them with a success of greater than 50%. This is particularly true in those patients who are found to have a significantly contracted bladder volume, which of course is due to fibrosis and the resultant decreased bladder compliance that occurs after high-dose radiation therapy.

The first step in management of patients with hemorrhagic cystitis must be to rule out a bacterial cystitis, because this is so often a contributing insult to the onset of hematuria. Mild hematuria can also be managed by adequate hydration, empiric antibiotics, and close observation for symptoms of clot retention. If clot retention occurs or blood transfusions are required, then hospitalization for cold saline bladder irrigation with a three-way Foley catheter and transfusions are all that is needed. If hematuria does not resolve, cystoscopy is indicated to rule out the slight possibility of recurrence of malignant disease as the source of the hematuria. As previously noted, biopsies should only be done when absolutely indicated because of the high incidence of fistula formation. Gentle fulguration of bleeding points can at times be helpful. But due to the frequent findings of diffuse friable hyperemic mucosa, fulguration attempts are often futile. Levenback et al. (7) showed that 70% of patients who respond to these simple measures will not require readmission for recurrent episodes of hemorrhagic cystitis but that 30% will have recurrent episodes of hematuria and it often results in a life-threatening condition that requires more aggressive intravesical and surgical intervention.

Formalin instillation is a commonly used technique requires that a cystogram be done prior to instillation of the toxic substance to rule out ureteral reflux. Formalin is so toxic that if ureteral reflux occurs, papillary necrosis can result as well as ureteral stenosis. Approximately 100 to 150 mL of a 1% solution of formalin is placed in the bladder and retained for 15 to 30 minutes. The details of the technique of formalin instillation are nicely described by Fair (18). General or regional anesthesia is required due to the pain induced by the chemical cauterization within the bladder that the formalin induces. Bleeding usually stops within 1 to 3 days; but if it persists, a second application can be administered. While some authors have recommended a higher concentration of formalin, Dewan et al. (19) demonstrated a higher complication rate with no improvement in therapeutic response. This study showed an overall success rate of 89% in patients with significant hemorrhagic cystitis. While the response rate was quite good, the cost for this was a major complication rate of 31% overall (only 13% of patients suffered a major complication when the formalin concentration did not exceed 1%). These complications included ureteral stenosis (secondary to ureteral reflux), decreased bladder capacity requiring diversion, and the development of vesicovaginal fistulas approximately 6 weeks after therapy. At a concentration of 4% using the Fair technique of instillation, the major complication rate was 100%. If ureteral reflux is identified, then ureteral catheterization with balloon occlusion of the distal ureter can be undertaken if formalin is to be used.

Because the main pathophysiology of radiation-induced hemorrhagic cystitis is the vascular insufficiency and resultant tissue hypoxia that causes necrosis, the use of hyperbaric oxygen—at least theoretically—is very appealing. Hyperbaric oxygen is thought to increase tissue oxygenation and neovascularization of the bladder wall. This neovascularization of the bladder has been shown to increase tissue healing, and this angiogenesis is essentially permanent with long-term follow-up (4 years after hyperbaric oxygen therapy) still demonstrating a persistence of improved tissue oxygen levels to near-normal levels (20). Twenty to sixty sessions of hyperbaric oxygen are required, each lasting 90 to 120 minutes. While complications are possible, they are very rare. Success rates vary between 60% and 88%, and recurrence of hemorrhagic cystitis is only 4% (21,22). The cost of therapy is $10,000 to $15,000; and because of the length of therapy required to resolve the hematuria, it is not ideal in patients with active bleeding. If bleeding should become excessive during the initial phases of therapy, cystoscopy with fulguration is often successful in providing enough time to complete the course of hyperbaric oxygen therapy.

In a preliminary report, Liu et al. (14) stated that they used high-dose intravenous conjugated estrogens (1 mg/kg) for two doses within a 24-hour time frame. This resulted in a marked decrease in hematuria, typically seen within 8 hours of initiation. After the initial doses, high-dose oral estrogen (5 mg/day) was used and recurrence of relatively mild hematuria was seen in only one of the five patients so treated. It is thought that conjugated estrogens correct the hematuria by decreasing the fragility of the mucosal microvasculature of the bladder.

Surgical Treatment

In more severe cases of life-threatening hemorrhagic cystitis that have not responded to the approaches outline above, more aggressive therapy will be required. The best "salvage" therapy is yet to be determined. Interruption of the internal iliac or superior vesical arteries by radiologic embolization have produced inconsistent results. Emergency urinary diversion with cystectomy is theoretically appealing, but the morbidity and mortality is so great that it is generally not acceptable. Urinary diversion alone is inadequate because there is no guarantee of resolution of hematuria. Cheng and Foo (13), however, advocate bilateral percutaneous nephrostomy as an adjunct in life-threatening hematuria because it breaks the vicious cycle of bleeding with resultant clot retention and bladder distention. If those patients respond well with resolution of bleeding yet persist to have the symptoms of a small contracted bladder or vesicovaginal fistula (whether or not these problems are due to complications of radiation therapy or from the treatment with formalin), then performing an ileal diversion in a nonemergent situation is much more acceptable although morbidity is still quite high.

While unusual, vesicovaginal fistulas represent a catastrophic complication of radiation therapy. Fistulas occur in 0.5% to 7% of patients and are most common in those patients treated for gynecologic malignancies such as cervical cancer (23). They occur within the first 2 years after therapy and are more common in patients who have undergone radiation as salvage therapy after recurrence is seen following the patient's initial therapy. A careful evaluation to rule out a tumor recurrence (both local and metastatic) is therefore important in patients who present with a postradiation fistula. This is particularly true if the fistula developed after a history of nonexcessive radiation doses or if it occurs later than the initial 2 years post therapy. An important point concerning the management of these fistulas is that surgical repair should be delayed approximately 12 months after their development. This is not only so that one can verify that there is no evidence of local or distant recurrent cancer, but it also gives time for the fistula to stabilize and mature; i.e., for all devitalized tissue to slough. One must also remember that if this high degree of destruction is seen at the anterior vaginal wall, then a similar degree of destruction has potentially occurred at the posterior vaginal wall. Therefore, the possibility of simultaneously occurring vesicovaginal and rectovaginal fistulas should be considered.

KEY POINTS

Differential Diagnoses

- Interstitial cystitis
- Bacterial cystitis
- Irritable bladder
- Bladder cancer or carcinoma *in situ*
- Recurrent pelvic cancer

Most Important Questions to Ask

- Is there a history of radiation therapy for a pelvic cancer?
- Did the symptoms start after the radiation treatment?
- Is there significant blood in the urine?

Most Important Physical Examination Findings

- Atrophic and stenotic changes in the vagina
- Tenderness of the anterior vaginal under the bladder
- Suprapubic tenderness

Most Important Diagnostic Studies

- Cystoscopy
- Urinalysis
- Urine culture

Treatments

- Antimicrobials
- Anticholinergics such as Ditropan, Detrol, or Imipramine
- Pyridium
- Low-acid diet
- Alkalinization of the urine
- Decreased consumption of caffeine
- Vaginal estrogen cream
- Sodium pentosanpolysulfate (Elmiron)
- Intravesical dimethyl sulfoxide
- Conjugated estrogens

REFERENCES

1. Hurst RE, Roy JB, Parsons CL. The role of glycofaminoglycans in the normal bladder physiology and the pathophysiology of interstitial cystitis. In: Sant GR, ed. *Interstitial cystitis.* Lippincott-Raven, Philadelphia: 1997, 93–100.
2. Kottmeier HL, Gray MJ. Rectal and bladder injuries in relation to radiation doses in carcinoma of the cervix. *Am J Obstet Gynecol* 1981;74(6):1294–1303.
3. Perez CA, Breaux S, Bedwineck JM, et al. Radiation therapy alone in the treatment of carcinoma of the uterine cervix II. Analysis of complications. *Cancer* 1984;54:235–246.
4. Pourquier H, Delard R, Achille E, et al. A quantified approach in the analysis and prevention of urinary complications in radiotherapeutic treatment of cancer of the cervix. *Int J Radiat Oncol Biol Phys* 1987;13:1025.
5. Pilepich MV, Pajak T, George SW, et al. Preliminary report on phase three PTOG studies of extended field irradiation in carcinoma of the prostate. *Am J Clin Oncol (CCT)* 1983;6:485–491.
6. Villasanta U. Complications of radiotherapy for cancer of the uterine cervix. *Am J Obstet Gynecol* 1973;114:717–726.
7. Levenback C, Eifel PJ, Burke et al. Hemorrhagic cystitis following radiotherapy for stage IB cancer of the cervix. *Gynecol Oncol* 1994;55:206.
8. Dean AL. Injury of the urinary bladder following irradiation of the uterus. *Am J Obstet Gynecol* 1933;25:667–676.
9. Hueper WC, Fisher CV, deCarvagjal-Forero J, et al. The pathology of the experimental roentgen in dogs. *J Urol* 1942;47:156.
10. Bourne RG, Kearsley JH, Grove WD, et al. The relationship between early and late gastrointestinal complications of radiation therapy for carcinoma of the cervix. *Int J Radiat Oncol Biol Phys* 1983;9:1445–1450.
11. Lanciano RM, Martz K, Montana GS, et al. Influence of age, prior abdominal surgery, fraction size and dose on complications and radiation therapy for squamous cell cancer of the uterine cervix: a pattern of care study. *Cancer* 1992;69:21–24.
12. DeVries CR, Freiha FS. Hemorrhagic cystitis: A review. *J Urol* 1990;143:1–9.
13. Cheng C, Foo KT. Management of severe chronic radiation cystitis. *Ann Acad Med* 1992;21:369.
14. Liu YK, Harty JI, Steinbock GS, et al. Treatment of radiation or cyclophosphamide induced hemorrhagic cystitis using conjugated estrogens. *J Urol* 1990;144:41–43.
15. Parsons CL, Stein PC, Dibair M, et al. Abnormal sensitivity to intravesical potassium in interstitial cystitis and radiation cystitis. *Neurourol Urodyn* 1994;13:515.
16. Parsons CL. Successful management of radiation cystitis with sodium pentosantolsulfate. *J Urol* 1989;136:813–814.
17. Hampson SJ, Woodhouse RJ. Sodium pentosanpolysulfate in the management of hemorrhagic cystitis: experience with fourteen patients. *Eur Urol* 1994;25:40–42.
18. Fair WR. Formalin in the treatment of masses hemorrhage: techniques, results and complications. *Urol J* 1974;3:573–576.
19. Dewan AK, Mohan MG, Ravi R. Intravesical formalin for hemorrhagic cystitis following irradiation of cancer of the cervix. *Int J Gynecol Obstet* 1993;42:131–135.
20. Marx RE, Johnson RP. Problem wounds in oral and maxillofacial surgery: the role of hyperbaric oxygen. In: Davis JC, Hunt TK, eds. *Problem wounds: the role of oxygen.* New York: Elsevier, 1988:70–75.
21. Norkool DM, Hampson NB, Gibbons RP, et al. Hyperbaric oxygen therapy for radiation induced hemorrhagic cystitis. *J Urol* 1993;150:332.
22. Bevers RF, Bakker DJ, Kurth KH. Hyperbaric oxygen treatment of hemorrhagic radiation cystitis. *Lancet* 1995;346:803–805.
23. Green TH, Jr. Urologic complications of radical pelvic surgery in radiation therapy. In Coppleson M, ed. *Gynecologic oncology: fundamental principles and clinical practice,* vol 2. Edinburgh: Churchill-Livingstone, 1981:979.

34

UROLITHIASIS

C. PAUL PERRY

KEY TERMS AND DEFINITIONS

Colic: Acute, intermittent, visceral pain that fluctuates with smooth muscle peristalsis.

INTRODUCTION

The smooth muscle of the renal pelvis and the ureter are a functional syncytium. A primary pacemaker in the renal pelvis coordinates the ureteral peristalsis. Ureteric activity is modulated primarily by sympathetic efferent stimulation and secondarily by diuresis (Fig. 34.1). The motor innervation is supplied by the renal, aortic, superior hypogastric, and inferior hypogastric plexus. The parasympathetic input is limited to indirect stimulation by detrusor activity, which spreads from the bladder into the lower ureter. Sympathomimetics stimulate and sympathetic blocking agents inhibit ureteric peristalsis (1). Afferent C fibers are present along with these autonomic motor nerves and refer pain to the corresponding T_{12}–L_{1-2} dermatomes. Chronic urolithiasis may result in chronic pelvic pain by prolonged visceral nociceptive signals producing central sensitization.

ETIOLOGY

The idea that acute pain is the result of uncoordinated spasms from the obstructed ureteral segment is no longer thought to be true. Complete obstruction of the ureter is followed by increase in the intraluminal pressure and a reduction in urine flow. Frequent waves of low amplitude and ineffective peristalsis result. The colic is from local distention, irritation, and ischemia. These acute episodes, if recurrent or prolonged, may produce chronic pelvic pain that can be mistaken as genital in origin.

The sharing of segmental innervation by the ureter, the duodenum, and the jejunum produces disordered bowel motility during renal colic. In addition to this viscerovisceral reflex, viscerocutaneous and visceromotor reflexes occur at the spinal cord level. These reflexes are responsible for the referred chronic pelvic pain syndromes produced by chronic urolithiasis (Chapter 55). The dermatome referral patterns usually involve the iliohypogastric, the ilioinguinal, and the genitofemoral nerves (1).

PATHOLOGY

Cutaneous and muscle hyperalgesia can be produced experimentally by artificial ureterolithiasis in rats (2). The degree of sensitization appears to be a function of the duration and intensity of the visceral afferent barrage. This sensitization occurs in dorsal column neurons of the spinal cord. Electrophysiologic measurements indicate that the recurrent visceral pain triggers central neuronal changes, which in

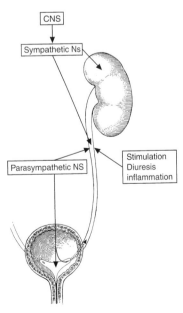

FIGURE 34.1. The innervation of the kidney, ureter, and bladder. A primary pacemaker in the renal pelvis coordinates the ureteral peristalsis. Ureteric activity is modulated primarily by sympathetic efferent stimulation and secondarily by diuresis.

turn are largely responsible for the occurrence and maintenance of referred hyperalgesia (3).

HISTORY

Patients presenting with chief complaints of chronic pelvic pain should be screened for history of recurrent urolithiasis. The ureteral obstruction would be ipsilateral to the corresponding pelvic pain. Multiple episodes of colic or prolonged visceral pain that was poorly relieved would be expected. The distribution would be in the dermatome segments previously discussed.

EXAMINATION

Cutaneous hyperalgesia can be elicited by gently brushing the skin over the affected area. Abdominal wall trigger points will often be present.

DIAGNOSTIC STUDIES

Imaging studies will be negative. An intravenous pyelogram should be done to rule out persistent urolithiasis. The most common areas of identification of calculi associated with pelvic pain are illustrated in Fig. 34.2. Differential nerve blocks of the iliohypogastric, ilioinguinal, and gen-

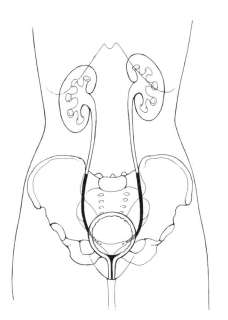

FIGURE 34.2. The areas where calculi associated with pelvic pain are generally located are shown by the shaded areas of the ureters and urethrovesical area.

itofemoral nerves may confirm the viscerosomatic referral by alleviating the pain.

TREATMENT

Neuropathic pain is often benefited by tricyclics and antiepileptic drugs. Repetitive nerve blocks can desensitize the spinal receptor neurons and break the pain cycle (Chapter 55). Muscle spasm may respond to physical therapy or specific anti-spasmodic medications. As in all neuropathic pain, the success of treatment depends on accurate diagnosis and aggressive pain relief. The greater the duration of symptoms, the less likely complete relief.

KEY POINTS
Differential Diagnoses

- Persistent urolithiasis
- Unilateral adnexal pathology
- Uncomplicated muscle spasms
- Uncomplicated abdominal wall trigger points

Most Important Questions to Ask

- Any history of urolithiasis?
- How many episodes on the affected side?
- How long before pain relief was obtained with each episode?

Most Important Diagnostic Studies

- Intravenous pyelogram for persistent urolithiasis
- Check for abdominal wall trigger points
- Check for cutaneous hyperalgesia
- Differential nerve blocks

Treatments

- Tricyclics and antiepileptic medications
- Repetitive nerve blocks

REFERENCES

1. Bach D. The treatment of ureteric colic and promotion of spontaneous passage. In: Schneider H-J, ed. *Urolithiasis: therapy, prevention.* New York: Springer-Verlag, 1986:75–83.
2. Giamberardino MA, Valente R, de Bigontina P, et al. Artificial ureteral calculosis in rats: behavioural characterization of visceral pain episodes and their relationship with referred lumbar muscle hyperalgesia. *Pain* 1995;61:459–469.
3. Giamberardino MA, Vecchiet L. Central neuronal changes in recurrent visceral pain. *Int J Clin Pharm Res* 1997;17:63–66.

35

DISCORDANT URINATION AND DEFECATION AS SYMPTOMS OF PELVIC FLOOR DYSFUNCTION

CHARLES W. BUTRICK

KEY TERMS AND DEFINITIONS

Anismus: Obstructive defecatory symptoms due to poor relaxation of the puborectalis muscle and in some patients paradoxical contractions of the puborectalis muscle during attempts to evacuate the rectum.

Biofeedback: Tool to measure physiologic processes (typically EMG activity for muscle biofeedback) so that the patient can develop better control and/or function; a type of neuromuscular reeducation.

Botulinum-A toxin: Toxin that inhibits the release of acetylcholine at the neuromuscular junction. It has been used in patients with detrusor–sphincter dyssynergia and occasionally in patients with localized myofascial pain.

Centralization of pain: Metabolic and neuropathic changes in the spinal cord, resulting from prolonged noxious stimuli to the spinal cord, that can result in persistent pain that is neurologically maintained even when the original insult has been eradicated.

Detrusor–sphincter dyssynergia: Lack of normal coordination between the urethral sphincteric mechanism and the bladder due to a known neurologic lesion (e.g., multiple sclerosis or spinal cord injury).

Discordant voiding: Voiding mechanism that demonstrates a lack of the normal coordination between the bladder and urethral sphincteric mechanism. Discordant voiding can be due to a known neurologic lesion or can be functional in nature (i.e., nonneurogenic).

Myofascial pain syndrome: Pain disorders associated with a localized group of muscles that, due to dysbehaviors or injury, characteristically demonstrate excessive muscle tension, pain, and trigger points.

Neuromodulation: Any modality of therapy that attempts to directly improve central processing of afferent stimuli and improve the regulatory reflexes within the spinal cord.

Pelvic floor tension myalgia: One of the terms used for myofascial pain syndromes involving the pelvic floor musculature; includes levator syndrome, pelvic floor spasticity syndrome, coccygodynia, or piriformis muscle syndrome.

Pelvic neuropathic hypersensitivity syndrome: Centralization of pain at the sacral spinal cord, with spinal cord windup and neurogenically mediated and maintained pain, and end-organ dysfunction of the pelvic tissues/organs innervated by the sacral nerves.

Spinal windup: Central nervous system-mediated enhanced response to afferent stimuli; a process of flawed gating of the noxious stimuli that occurs as a result of up-regulation of the spinal cord. Spinal windup is due to metabolic changes (especially within the dorsal horn) that occur as a result of prolonged noxious stimuli.

Trigger point: Seen in patients with myofascial pain syndrome. Identified as an exquisitely tender 3- to 6-mm nodule within a taut band. With palpation the trigger point will reproduce not only the patient's pain, but also the referral pattern of that pain.

INTRODUCTION

Clinicians who care for patients with chronic pelvic pain syndromes such as interstitial cystitis, vulvar vestibulitis, and dyspareunia notice a tendency for these problems to coexist in the same patient. Overlapping symptoms often lead to overwhelming patient complaints that the physician is frequently unable to explain. Because the symptoms are seemingly out of proportion to the physical findings, the patients are often thought to be somatizing. Why else would a patient with interstitial cystitis also develop problems of vestibulitis and dyspareunia and only a few weeks later start developing symptoms associated with functional bowel disease? And how else would one explain pain associated with intercourse that lasts for several hours after the completion of sexual relations and sometimes even worsens for 12 to 48 hours after attempted or completed intercourse? This chapter reviews some of the theories concerning such pain syndromes and also illustrates that, through an understanding of the neuropathology involved, the cause of chronic pelvic pain and successful therapies can be determined for many of these patients. In addition, it emphasizes that one of the largest structures in the pelvis, the pelvic floor musculature, is often not considered in the differential diagnosis of pelvic pain and is even less frequently treated.

The myofascial component of the pelvic floor is called upon in all aspects of life. When we stand we require that the muscles fight gravity. When we sit, we sit on them. And when we hold in urine, flatus, or feces we ask for continuous control for hours, yet they must relax to allow normal voiding and defecation at a moment's notice. They are traumatized with childbirth and pelvic surgery and, to a lesser degree, every time a woman has intercourse. Additionally, the complex functions of these muscles are not inherent processes that we are born with; instead they are learned during the early years of childhood. The pelvic floor musculature is a somatically innervated structure that has both autonomy and volitional control. We are born without this volitional control, and it must be learned independently because we are neither taught how to use our pelvic floor nor that pelvic floor muscle function should be maintained through regular exercise. All skeletal muscles have Golgi apparatus that provide proprioception so that one can be aware of the state of muscular tone at any time and at any location in the body. Yet one-third of women have no awareness whatsoever of their pelvic floor muscles. It should come as no surprise that when an insult occurs to the muscles or to the nerves involved in pelvic floor muscle control, or when any inflammatory process occurs within the pelvis, these events can result in pelvic floor myofascial pain and dysfunction. Reiter and Gambone (1) studied 183 women with chronic pelvic pain after nondiagnostic laparoscopy and found myofascial pain to be the most common somatic cause of their pain. Similar observations are reported for patients with vulvodynia or vestibulitis (2–4), or chronic urgency/frequency syndrome or interstitial cystitis (5–8). The key to successful therapy for many of these patients is the diagnosis and treatment of the pelvic floor muscle dysfunction and the myofascial component of their chronic pain.

ETIOLOGY

For the bladder to function properly there must be a normally functioning nervous system that interprets sensory input concerning volume of urine, assesses social acceptability to void, and orchestrates a series of complex events that must be coordinated and amplified. The pelvic floor muscles are intimately involved in this voiding mechanism. If they do not relax, voiding can be inadequate, obstructive,

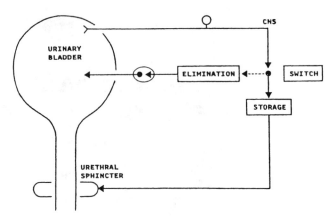

FIGURE 35.1. Micturition Reflex. Diagram illustrating the anatomy of the lower urinary tract and the switchlike function of the micturition reflex pathway. During urine storage a low level of afferent activity activates efferent input to the urethral sphincter. A high level of afferent activity induced by bladder distention activates the switching circuit in the central nervous system (CNS), producing firing in the efferent pathways to the bladder, inhibition of the efferent outflow to the sphincter, and urine elimination. (From Raz S. *Female urology,* 2nd ed. Pennsylvania: W.B. Saunders Co., 1996, with permission.)

intermittent, or even not possible. These neurologic functions are occurring on an ongoing basis throughout the day and night, so abnormalities in these nerve pathways frequently result in clinical and subclinical changes in bladder function. Because of this the bladder is often a very sensitive messenger of abnormalities in the sacral reflexes.

The function of the lower urinary tract during storage and voiding is governed by a complex set of both central and peripheral neuronal reflex mechanisms. These reflexes require the constant input from afferents arising from the bladder and the urethra and are modulated by higher centers including the frontal lobes of the cerebral cortex, the hypothalamus, and the pontine micturition center (9). The control center for these reflex pathways resides in the sacral cord. It is here that an "on/off switch" allows for the reciprocal relationship between the bladder and the urethral outlet, thus allowing their primary functions of storage and voiding to occur smoothly (Fig. 35.1)

Afferent Pathways

Bladder afferent nerves send information concerning fullness and discomfort to the portion of the central nervous system involved in initiating the micturition reflex. These afferents are of two types: small myelinated A-delta fibers and unmyelinated C-fibers. A-delta fibers transmit signals from mechanoreceptors that detect bladder fullness and wall tension. At the initiation of micturition this afferent signal becomes strong enough to activate the brainstem micturition center, which also inhibits the spinal guarding reflexes (see below). The C-fibers are primarily involved in transmitting signals that arise from noxious stimuli and painful sensations (e.g., urinary tract infections or chemical irritative conditions). C-fiber bladder afferents also have reflex functions to facilitate or trigger the voiding mechanism (10). C-fiber bladder afferents have been implicated in the triggering of certain types of bladder hyperactivity, including uninhibited contractions associated with multiple sclerosis or spinal cord injuries. They also are implicated in patients with bladder neck obstructions who have symptoms of urgency/frequency and/or urge incontinence (e.g., postretropubic urethropexy obstruction) (11). This is an important finding because it explains the development of the *de novo* detrusor instability of postretropubic urethropexy patients and explains why even with correction of the obstruction by urethrolysis many patients continue to have urgency/frequency and urge incontinence. Despite correction of the anatomic obstruction, the neuropathology can persist. This is an example of neural plasticity. Additionally, patients with urgency/frequency syndrome (interstitial cystitis) frequently complain of obstructed voiding with the clinical findings of tense pelvic floor muscles that do not relax completely. A cascade of events starts with an insult induced activation of the C-fibers which in turn induces constant urgency. The patient responds by initiating the dysbehavior of chronic pelvic floor muscle tightening as she vigorously works to "hold in" her urine. This dysbehavior is at times hard to overcome and thus functional obstruction occurs. Intravesical capsaicin, a C-fiber neurotoxin, has been shown to block detrusor hyperreflexia (12) and to reverse the irritative symptoms in patients with urgency/frequency syndrome (interstitial cystitis) (13,14). Thus an imbalance in the bladder afferents can be the cause of urologic symptoms and treatment of these neurologic imbalances often results in resolution of the symptoms.

Guarding Reflexes

The bladder is a unique viscera because it is governed by both voluntary control mechanisms, via the pudendal nerve action on urethral sphincter function (70% of which is derived from the action of the levator muscles), and involuntary or autonomic mechanisms. A number of important reflexes contribute to the storage and elimination of urine and modulate the voluntary control of micturition (15). These reflexes or pathways provide many functions, but one of the most important is the coordination between the bladder and the urethra. Coordination is important to allow the sphincter to open just prior to the onset of volitional voiding, yet to be closed at all other times. These are referred to as guarding reflexes.

There are two guarding reflexes that protect patients from stress urinary incontinence. A sympathetic efferent pathway that leads to the proximal urethra mediates the first. This is an excitatory reflex that contracts the urethral smooth muscle with cough or exercise, yet is suppressed during normal voiding. Any process that increases the sympathetic tone to the bladder neck can result in difficulty in initiating bladder neck opening. There is a significant amount of histochemical data demonstrating that most patients with the diagnosis of interstitial cystitis can be shown to have sympathetic nerve proliferation (16) and an increase in those neuropeptides that are believed to be mediators of a sympathetic response. It is this finding that has led many authors to describe interstitial cystitis as a syndrome similar to reflex sympathetic dystrophy (17). Additionally, lumbar sympathetic blocks result in a 90% likelihood of total and prolonged pain-free intervals in patients with interstitial cystitis (18).

A second guarding reflex is triggered by bladder afferents that synapse with sacral interneurons that in turn activate urethral external sphincter efferent neurons that then travel down the pudendal nerve. Central modulating pathways originating from the cerebral cortex and pontine micturition center inhibit both of these guarding reflexes during normal voiding.

Micturition Reflexes

Normal micturition requires two additional reflexes that result in a sustained contraction (allowing adequate bladder emptying) and coordination between the bladder and the urethral sphincteric mechanism. Bladder afferents (both A-delta and C-fibers) synapse with interneurons in the sacral spinal cord that then synapse with bladder preganglionic (efferent) parasympathetic neurons and also with urethral parasympathetic efferent neurons. This establishes two important reflexes for micturition. The first is a positive reflex (bladder reflex) that results in sustained contraction, and the second is an inhibitory reflex that results in relaxation of the smooth muscle of the proximal bladder neck. Many factors can modify these micturition reflexes. Both sets of reflexes can be modulated by a number of centers in the cerebral cortex and brainstem to either inhibit or stimulate voiding mechanisms.

In young kittens, perineal stimulation results in voiding; removal of this stimuli (separation of the mother cat from the kitten) can result in total urinary retention (19). Yet in adult cats this reflex is lost. In fact, in adult animals and humans, perineal stimulation results in inhibition of the micturition reflex (20). This reflex is used clinically in women who are treated with functional electrical stimulation for detrusor instability (21). Reactivation of these primitive reflexes often results in clinical symptoms of urgency and frequency that can further result in C-fiber-induced uninhibited detrusor contractions. This same C-fiber activation can result in the initiation and maintenance of vulvitis–vestibulitis and/or urgency–frequency symptoms. The control center for these reflexes resides in the sacral cord and involves the dorsal horn and the interneuron pool of spinal cord neurons. The sphincter motor nucleus (Ornuf's nucleus) is also within the same area of the sacral cord and is responsible for urethral sphincteric activity.

Voiding Dysfunction

Normal micturition requires a coordination of the parasympathetic, sympathetic, and somatic nervous systems to process information and initiate a series of events in a carefully orchestrated process that is constantly being modulated by the multiple areas within the central nervous system responsible for bladder function. Much of this regulation of the voiding function takes place within the sacral cord. When this complex process is disrupted, abnormal voiding symptoms quickly develop. In fact, interrupted micturition is a very sensitive measure of the neurologic integrity of the sacral cord.

Normal voiding requires the relaxation of the urethral sphincteric mechanism that includes the levator muscles, the external urethral sphincter, and the smooth muscle component of the bladder neck. The bladder neck component is not as significant in women as it is in men. This relaxation is quickly followed by a detrusor contraction that must be of significant strength and duration to effectively empty the bladder. The initial step in initiating normal voiding is frequently found to be abnormal in patients with urologic, gynecologic, gastrointestinal, or neurologic disorders (Table 35.1). While history can often identify these patients, the objective evidence of an instrumented pressure flow study with electromyographic (EMG) evaluation of the levator muscle function can more accurately delineate and verify the clinical diagnosis of discordant voiding.

The term detrusor–urethral dyssynergia is commonly misused. The International Continence Society has attempted to provide a standard terminology for use in describing and studying bladder function (22). Detrusor–urethral dyssynergia should be used to describe the simultaneous contraction of both the detrusor and the urethra. In adults, it generally should be reserved for patients with known neurologic disease such as multiple sclerosis or suprasacral cord injury. Patients with true neurogenic

detrusor–urethral dyssynergia demonstrate no electrical silencing (no decrease in EMG activity) with the onset of voiding. Instead, EMG activity increases before and during the up slope of the detrusor contractions, and generally EMG activity decreases during the down slope. Another pattern that is sometimes referred to as pseudodyssynergia is seen in patients without *obvious* neurologic lesions. This pattern demonstrates electrical silencing at the onset of voiding, yet there is an increase in EMG activity at the peak or slightly after the onset of the down slope of the detrusor contractions. This increase in EMG activity can be either continuous or intermittent. Many authors have described this latter pattern and have demonstrated subtle neurologic abnormalities such as sympathetic hypersensitivity (23). Because of the confusion in terminology and difficulty in interpreting the multichannel pressure flow studies (which are not available to all clinicians), it is best to use the term *discordant voiding* to describe the various symptoms and urodynamic observations. Additionally, as our understanding of the subtle neurologic changes (theoretically the cause of the majority of functional voiding abnormalities) increases, the distinctions between patients who have "neurogenic abnormalities" and those who do not are not as clear. Therefore, discordant voiding is a term that encompasses both neurogenic and nonneurogenic voiding dysfunctions.

Two additional groups of micturition disorders should also be discussed. The first is nonneurogenic neurogenic bladder, which is a term coined by Hinman in 1971 (24,25). This syndrome involves childhood urinary incontinence, recurrent urinary tract infections and bowel disorders of constipation, and fecal incontinence similar to functional bowel disease. The pathophysiology of this syndrome is now understood to involve significant discordant voiding and frequently uninhibited bladder contraction. It has been observed repeatedly by clinicians that many adult patients with urgency–frequency syndrome, chronic pelvic pain, and/or vulvodynia have a history of discordant voiding, and therefore dysfunctional pelvic floor muscles, that dates back to childhood. While this may represent a reactivation of abnormal micturition reflexes

TABLE 35.1. CLINICAL DIAGNOSES ASSOCIATED WITH DISCORDANT VOIDING

Gynecologic Disorders	Urologic Disorders	Gastrointestinal Disorders	Neurologic Disorders
Chronic pelvic pain	Urethral syndrome	Functional bowel disease	Multiple sclerosis
Endometriosis	Urgency/frequency syndrome	Anismus	Spinal cord injuries
Vestibulitis	Insterstitial cystitis	Anal fissures	(typically suprasacral)
Vulvodynia	Recurrent urinary tract infections	Proctalgia fugax	Neurosyphilis
Dyspareunia	Nonneurogenic neurogenic bladder		Central nervous system HIV
Vaginismus	Idiopathic urinary retention		Spondylotic myelopathy
Posthysterectomy syndrome	Prostatodynia		Spinal tumors
	Childhood incontinence		Cerebrovascular accident
	(fecal and urinary)		(especially frontal lobe
			and basal ganglia)

and pelvic floor dysbehaviors, it is more likely that these patients had subclinical dysfunction that was well compensated for but that became less well compensated for due to a variety of reasons. The second group to be discussed here includes those neurologically intact patients who void by Valsalva alone—that is, without any evidence of detrusor contraction. These patients are thought to have an intact micturition reflex, but they have not learned how to "turn it on." It is generally accepted that there can be an overinhibition of the micturition reflex by an overactive guarding reflex. This is best demonstrated in patients with idiopathic urinary retention who also lack pelvic floor control. Understanding the neuropathology of the last two groups of patients has made it clear that pelvic muscle dysbehavior can induce central (both upper modulating centers and at the sacral cord level) abnormalities in the neurologic balance of lower urinary tract function and control. Thus, pelvic floor dysbehavior induces dysregulation of the sacral cord reflexes that in turn affects bladder function—that is, storage and elimination.

Pelvic Floor Muscle Dysfunction

The evolution of bladder control is a gradual process that occurs during the early years of childhood and is typically completed by the age of three. During these formative years of developing conscious control, the brain and the sacral reflexes are very plastic or moldable and are therefore very susceptible to being disrupted by "abnormal" behavior. There are many reasons for the development of abnormal behavior during this time. Inappropriate postponing of voiding with prolonged pelvic floor muscle tightening and overbearing parents who induce stress and anxiety surrounding the toileting process are two of the most common avoidable circumstances. Particularly stressful events, whether emotional or physical (e.g., childhood sexual abuse, emotional or physical trauma), also lead to pelvic floor muscle dysfunction. In these situations the dysfunction arises due to abnormalities in the modulating pathways originating from the suprapontine areas. This in turn affects the function of the sacral cord center.

It is debatable whether these modulating pathways can induce negative effects on a normally balanced sacral cord or if the sacral cord reflexes must first be marginally dysfunctional or primarily unbalanced. If the former situation were true, then one would expect a much higher incidence of pelvic floor dysfunction and pelvic pain syndrome in patients who have been victimized by sexual abuse or emotional trauma during their formative years. However, an alternative explanation would be that some patients who experience this type of emotional trauma have an exaggerated response with heightened modulation.

While neural plasticity slows after age 10, this same process of abnormal pelvic floor muscle behavior resulting in abnormal neural reflexes certainly can also occur in adults. There exists a significant body of literature demonstrating in laboratory animals and humans that events and/or certain behaviors can result in changes in the processing and modulation of afferent input to the central nervous system, and that changes in the central nervous system result in both sensory and motor dysfunctions that are responsible for many of the pain syndromes seen in patients (26–29). Examples of these will be discussed later in the chapter.

Neuroplasticity and Pelvic Floor Muscle Dysfunction

It is well known that a large nociceptive barrage of afferent activity delivered anywhere within the spinal cord can have a destabilizing effect on neuronal circuits. These spinal cord changes can result in permanent dysregulation of central processing of sensory information. This principle is well established and is referred to as spinal cord *windup* (27). Metabolic changes within the spinal cord (particularly the dorsal horn) occur as a result of this increased nociceptive activity. There is a cascade of neural events that culminates in neurogenically mediated and maintained inflammation (30–33) so that even if the initial insult is abolished, the metabolic changes can persist. When the changes persist, it is known as centralization of pain. Phantom limb pain is a classic example. These changes within the spinal cord ultimately contribute to dysfunction, hyperalgesia, and pain involving tissues at that spinal cord level (34). This destabilizing effect frequently expands into levels both above and below the initially affected level. This is referred to as expansion of receptive fields (Fig. 35.2).

Pelvic neuropathic hypersensitivity syndrome is a concept proposed by R. Schmidt (35). It represents the same concepts of centralization of pain, spinal cord windup, and neurogenically mediated and maintained pain as was described above except for that it applies specifically to the sacral cord and those tissues innervated by the sacral nerves. Clinical manifestations of the end-organ dysfunction and sensory abnormalities include urgency/frequency syndrome, vulvodynia, pelvic floor muscle dysfunction, and pelvic floor myofascial pain. This neuropathic response results in neurogenically induced inflammation, hypersensitivity, and dysfunction involving the urethra, the bladder, the vestibule, and the pelvic floor musculature. As this neuropathic process expands up and down the cord and centralization and spinal windup progress, pelvic floor spasticity worsens, as does the pain. Thus, pelvic floor muscle dysfunction and myofascial pain syndrome can be caused by, and maintained by, this process of pelvic neuropathic hypersensitivity. Clinical manifestations of pelvic floor muscle dysfunction and myofascial pain are discussed in detail later in this chapter, but key

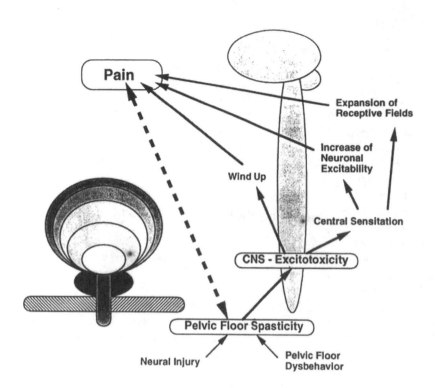

FIGURE 35.2. Cycle generating and supporting pelvic pain. *CNS*, central nervous system. (From Zermann DH, Ishigooka M, Doggweiler R, et al. Neurologic insights into the etiology of genital urinary pain in men. *J Urol* 1999;161:903–908, with permission.)

findings include lack of pelvic muscle awareness, poor relaxation, tender pelvic floor muscles, and discordant voiding. In those patients with subclinical preexisting pelvic floor muscle dysfunction, this process of sacral cord up-regulation can often turn the subclinical condition into a significant clinical one.

The three basic origins for pelvic noxious afferent stimuli that can result in sacral cord windup (up-regulation of the sacral cord reflexes) are pelvic floor dysbehaviors, direct pelvic floor muscle trauma, and other painful and/or inflammatory pelvic visceral disorders (Fig. 35.3).

Dysbehaviors include prolonged pelvic floor muscle tension such as inappropriately avoiding bladder emptying, postural stresses such as short leg syndrome, or occupational problems such as standing with most of the weight on one leg for many hours at a time. The chronic misuse of the levators results in myofascial pain syndrome with the development of trigger points, muscle shortening, and decreased range of motion with resultant muscle dysfunction and pain. This pain syndrome is often misdiagnosed for years and results in a prolonged bombardment of the sacral nerve's dorsal horn with noxious afferent stimuli (36). Stress

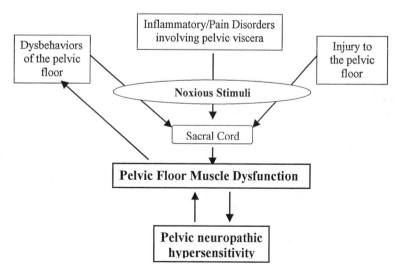

FIGURE 35.3. Origins of pelvic neuropathic hypersensitivity.

also results in the dysbehavior of increased muscle tension throughout the body as well as within the pelvic floor muscles. Frequently, a patient's history will correlate with the fact that an increase in stress results in increasing symptoms of voiding dysfunction as well as an increase in the perception of pain.

Injury to the pelvic floor is commonly seen in women as a result of a traumatic delivery. These patients often give a history of urinary retention after delivery. This is frequently due to traumatically induced pelvic floor spasticity. Additional examples of direct muscle trauma include straddle injuries, direct coccygeal trauma such as falling "on the tailbone," and pelvic surgery. Urinary retention postoperatively is often secondary to poor pelvic floor muscle relaxation due either to direct muscle trauma or to the problems of postoperative pain related to surgical wounding. This in turn results in overstimulation of the sacral nerve reflexes (e.g., guarding reflexes) and thus the secondary problem of inability to relax the pelvic floor muscles (see below). The problem of postoperative urinary retention is often blamed on "swelling," yet there is no evidence to support this contention.

The third cause of pelvic floor muscle dysfunction is a reflexive increase in the guarding reflex that is induced by any pain process. Chronic inflammatory or pain syndromes can be a major source of noxious afferent input to the spinal cord. Examples include endometriosis, primary vulvodynia, ulcerative colitis, and recurrent urinary tract infections. The noxious stimuli slowly induce an up-regulation in the delicate balance of regulatory sacral reflexes (e.g., guarding reflexes), and therefore pelvic floor muscle dysfunction can develop. This of course can result in voiding dysfunction, urgency/frequency syndrome, functional bowel disease, and other end-organ abnormalities. Many authors (2,37–40) have demonstrated evidence suggesting a neuropathic process in each of these pain syndromes. It is important to realize that many patients with these inflammatory and painful conditions experience the slow development of multiorgan pain and dysfunction. Multiorgan involvement suggests the expansion of receptive fields that occurs in patients with a spinal windup process. Multiorgan involvement is a criterion that many physicians use to define chronic pain syndrome, but it might better be used to help identify patients with sacral cord up-regulation (Fig. 35.4).

It is extremely important to identify and treat pelvic floor muscle dysfunction for several reasons. It can often be one of the primary sources of symptoms and, as noted previously, may be the primary insult to the delicate balance of the sacral regulatory circuits, or it can be seen as a result of sacral cord dysregulation. Failure to treat will typically end in the failure of "traditional therapies." If an up-regulated sacral cord is suspected, therapy must include a neurophysiologic approach that is likely to rely on neurolytic drugs such as amitriptyline, neuromuscular reeducation such as biofeedback, and neuromodulation via sacral nerve stimulation. Additionally, further insult to the pelvis in a patient with already up-regulated sacral cord reflexes can result in worsening of the spinal windup phenomena due to an increase in noxious stimuli. A large nociceptive barrage of afferent activity delivered to the central nervous system as a by-product of surgical wounding can be destabilizing to neuronal circuits and can thus be a cause of further spinal windup (Fig. 35.5). The risk of spinal windup increases if the neural regulatory pathways are already abnormal (i.e., clinical or subclinical symptoms of pelvic floor dysfunction and/or chronic pelvic pain syndromes). If surgical intervention is required in these patients who already suffer from compromised sacral reflexes, then all efforts must be taken to prevent a further barrage of noxious stimuli to the sacral nervous system. This is an ideal situation for the use of preemptive anesthesia to prevent a worsening of the neuropathic process that is already established in these patients.

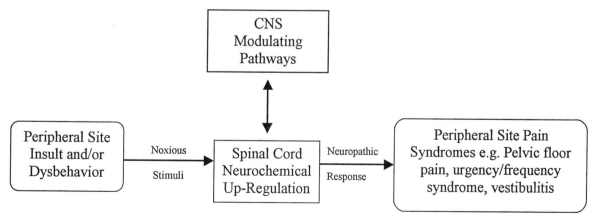

FIGURE 35.4. A possible mechanism for the development of multiorgan pain involvement with sacral cord up-regulation.

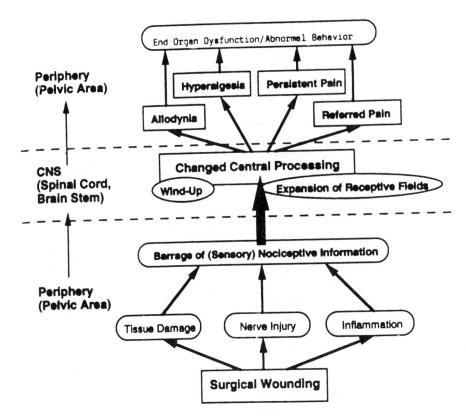

FIGURE 35.5. Chain of neurophysiological events following surgical wounding. (From Zermann DH, Ishigooka M, Doggweiler R, et al. Postoperative chronic pain and bladder dysfunction: windup and neural plasticity—do we need a more neurourological approach to pelvic surgery? *J Urol* 1998;160:102–105, with permission.)

HISTORY AND SYMPTOMS

Identification of pelvic floor muscle dysfunction can often be aided by taking a careful history. Key questions should be asked that address the voiding mechanism. The symptoms of pelvic floor muscle dysfunction include hesitancy to void ("shy bladder") and a slow intermittent urinary flow. In patients with mild dysfunction these symptoms are intermittent in nature and are typically seen during flares of their urologic and gynecologic symptoms such as urgency/frequency syndrome and/or vestibulitis. If one asks the patient about episodes where she might be required to "hold her urine" for a long time (such as at work or on a trip where bathroom access is limited) she might report that under those circumstances hesitancy becomes particularly pronounced. This history is frequently seen in women with preexisting or subclinical pelvic floor muscle dysfunction. It is the intermittent nature of this symptom that demonstrates to both the patient and the clinician that the symptom of abnormal voiding is truly functional in nature rather than being an anatomic obstruction. Pelvic floor muscle dysfunction should be suspected in all patients with dyspareunia, but especially in those who report a persistence of pelvic pain that lasts for many hours after intercourse or who report that sexual relations result in a prolonged flare of their baseline symptoms.

Frequently the prolonged muscle tension and dysfunctional activity within the pelvic muscles results in the development of a myofascial pain syndrome. Here the pelvic floor muscles become tender with trigger points (these are points of maximal tenderness that are easily identified on pelvic examination). Myofascial pain is seen in 56% of patients referred to my office for evaluation of urgency/frequency syndrome (interstitial cystitis). The constant urge to void induces a "hold" mechanism that results in prolonged pelvic floor muscle tension. This dysbehavior frequently leads to the development of a true myofascial pain syndrome. The etiology of myofascial pain syndrome is summarized in Fig. 35.6 (41). Gentle pressure on tender pelvic floor muscles often induces the urge to void, which should signal to the clinician that abnormal interpretation of afferent stimuli is taking place. This again represents a disruption of the sacral nerve function related to the process of expansion of the receptive fields as mentioned earlier. The development of pelvic floor myofascial pain in patients with pelvic floor muscle dysfunction is called pelvic floor tension myalgia (42). Additional terms used for pelvic floor tension myalgia (or its subgroups) include levator syndrome, coccydynia, piriformis syndrome, and spastic pelvic floor syndrome. This myofascial pain syndrome is commonly seen as a component of pain in many patients with chronic pelvic pain, urgency/frequency syndrome, and vestibulitis.

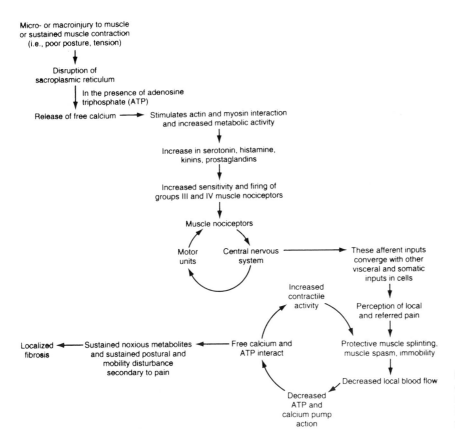

FIGURE 35.6. Pathophysiology of myofascial pain syndromes. (From *Chronic Pelvic Pain.* Steege JF, Metzger DA, Levy BS, eds. Pennsylvania: W.B. Saunders Co., 1999, 252, with permission.)

Patients with pelvic floor myofascial pain report symptoms of pelvic pain that are typically described as pressure, heaviness, or an achy feeling in the suprapubic, vaginal, or rectal area. This symptom in patients often results in a referral for "prolapse" symptoms, yet there is no evidence of support defects. Pain often is reported as bilateral or unilateral (with right being more commonly reported than left) in the lower quadrant. While both pelvic floor myofascial pain and prolapse are worse while standing, only prolapse symptoms resolve in less than 10 minutes of lying down. Sitting makes pelvic floor tension myalgia worse because the pelvic muscles are tender and only padded seating is tolerated. Because of this, patients often report that prolonged car rides result in flares of their symptoms. Pain during and for many hours after intercourse is another classic example of pelvic floor myofascial pain. Depending on which pelvic floor muscles are primarily involved, the pain can radiate into the groin, the buttocks, or the upper thigh.

PHYSICAL EXAMINATION

Clinical evaluation of the pelvic floor begins with simple observation of pelvic floor muscle activity during the process of squeezing and relaxation. This is a very important step in evaluation and is often quiet revealing. It can be compared to watching a patient walk to determine if there are any disturbances of gait. A brief lesson to help the patient understand the desired muscle action is often beneficial. The patient is asked to lift and squeeze as if to hold in flatus or urine. Patients with pelvic floor muscle dysfunction often have so much muscle tension at "rest" that they are unable to produce more contractile strength and certainly cannot relax completely. This is identified by failure to show closure of the genital hiatus, failure to lift the perineum, or failure to demonstrate the normal puckering of the anal verge at time of pelvic floor contractions. If relaxation is seen, it is often partial and sometimes can be seen as a discordant behavior that occurs in "steps." Because the baseline state of the pelvic floor is often tense, these patients typically do not demonstrate an anal wink despite having an intact sacral nerve reflex. Thus the absence of anal wink reflex is not related to a neurologic injury, but instead it is due to the abolishment of this reflex due to their tense pelvic floor muscles not being able to contract further upon stimulation. In patients with significant pelvic floor tension, instability can be seen with close observation. Fasciculations in the pelvic floor muscles can have the appearance of subtle twitches, and the clinician can see the intermittent closure of the genital hiatus or a puckering of the anal verge with these twitches. A lubricated cotton-tip applicator placed into the vaginal vault can aid in visual demonstration of pelvic floor function and instability. These fasciculations cannot be perceived by the patient, but often can easily be felt by the examiner with palpations of the pelvic floor muscles or visually as noted above. These fasciculations are easily demonstrated with EMG studies of the pelvic floor.

At this time a single finger is placed gently in the vagina and again the patient is instructed to squeeze and relax the pelvic floor (Fig. 35.7). The ability to rapidly squeeze the pubococcygeus muscle in a coordinated manner is assessed. Poor recruitment (i.e., slow lifting of the levator) is often appreciated in patients with pelvic floor muscle dysfunction. The ability to relax the levator plate is then assessed, and again speed of descent and completeness of relaxation is evaluated. The duration of maximal squeeze and the amount of lift produced are also evaluated. I typically grade these findings on a scale of 0 to 4, but other scales have been described (43,44). All these scales are subjective and have not yet been validated.

There are two common patterns of presentation. The first is usually seen in patients with the most severe and longest duration of symptoms. It includes a relatively thick, immobile, pelvic floor with a significant increase in baseline tone, little lift of the pelvic floor muscles during an attempted squeeze, and incomplete or very little pelvic floor relaxation on command to relax these same muscles. These patients generally have nearly total lack of pelvic floor muscle awareness and often will attempt to hold their breath or push when asked to squeeze their pelvic floor. The second common pattern seen in patients is a somewhat blunted pelvic floor muscle awareness and a slightly increased base-

line tone. While these patients can produce a good lift on attempting to squeeze these muscles, the relaxation phase is significantly dysfunctional. Relaxation is either (a) incomplete in its degree (decreased range of motion), (b) perceived to occur in "steps," or (c) discordant. At times while relaxation is nearly complete it is quickly followed by an immediate increase back to the original elevated baseline tone. These changes can be subtle, but careful evaluation of both normal and abnormal tone will prove that a careful dynamic pelvic floor evaluation is enlightening in nearly all patients with chronic pain.

Normally, the vaginal vault and its underlying levator muscles should form a smooth cylindrical configuration with complete relaxation. Those patients with incomplete relaxation have an obvious V configuration, and typically the examining finger can be advanced and dropped over a ridge that represents the inferior border of the levator plate. The finger drops over this border and onto the coccygeus muscle. If relaxation is complete, this V configuration is not seen and the inferior "shelf" is not felt.

The examination thus far should have been pain-free and should have been performed with very light touch. At this point in the exam determining the degree of pelvic floor muscle tenderness becomes important so that the examiner can ascertain if a myofascial component to the pain exists. This is done by applying gentle pressure to the levator muscles and assessing whether or not the patient's reported pain is reproduced. Also an evaluation for trigger points must be undertaken. Because most patients with myofascial pain involving the pelvic floor are tender along the lateral border of the levator ani (this is where the levator muscles insert onto the arcus tendineus levator ani), pressure is first applied medially and slowly swept laterally. Active trigger points are identified by finding an exquisitely tender area that is often palpable as a small 3- to 6-mm nodule within a taut band that will reproduce the patient's referral pattern reported in her description of pain. Nodules that do not reproduce the patients reported referral pattern and are minimally tender are referred to as inactive or latent trigger points. Latent trigger points can become active by increased neural stimulation such as would occur with centrally mediated efferent activity. Additional stressors that increase the likelihood of latent trigger points becoming active include physical trauma, pelvic muscle tension with muscle fatigue and overuse, emotional stress, and cold temperature, to name a few.

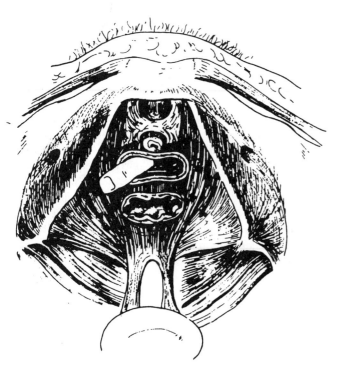

FIGURE 35.7. Transvaginal palpation of the perivaginal muscles from above. (From Laycock J. Clinical evaluation of the pelvic floor. Schüssler B, Laylock J, Norton P, Stanton S. *Pelvic floor re-education: principles and practice.* New York: Springer-Verlag, 1994, 43, with permission.)

DIAGNOSTIC STUDIES

Objective identification of pelvic floor muscle dysfunction is obtained by various techniques (Table 35.2). White et al. (45) described the EMG characteristics in patients with the clinical diagnosis of vulvar vestibulitis (Fig. 35.8). They found that 88% had at least three of five EMG characteristics that are compatible with pelvic floor muscle dysfunction. These five characteristics (listed in order of prevalence)

TABLE 35.2. TECHNIQUES TO IDENTIFY PELVIC FLOOR MUSCLE DYSFUNCTION

EMG evaluation (needle or surface electrodes)
   Resting tone
   Dynamic functional assessment
Urethral pressure profilometry
   Static maximal urethral closing pressure
   Urethral instability
Uroflowmetry
Defecography

included: (a) elevated and unstable resting baseline activity, (b) poor recovery, (c) poor post contraction relaxation with elevated and unstable baseline, (d) spasms on sustained contractions and evidence of muscle fatigue, and (e) poor contractile strength (i.e., poor recruitment). Glazer used a vaginal surface EMG to record pelvic floor activity. Others have used rectal surface EMGs, vaginal or rectal EMG probes, patch electrodes on the skin, and fine-needle electrodes. The vaginal sensor used by Glazer is easily obtained (P6050, Thought Technology Ltd. Montreal, Quebec, Canada or 211.202, Dantech Medical, Santa Clara, CA). Signals have a 99% correlation with data produced by invasive fine-needle electrodes.

Fowler described a unique finding using concentric needles in the urethral sphincter muscles in women with "idiopathic" urinary retention (46). This finding can easily be heard during EMG studies as a complex repetitive discharge with decelerating bursts. In patients with idiopathic severe voiding dysfunction and this unique EMG finding, two characteristics are seen: (a) nonrelaxing pelvic floor muscles and (b) excellent response to sacral nerve neuromodulation

(75% of patients have nearly total resolution according to Dirk et al. (47)).

Urodynamic evaluation offers two methods of evaluating pelvic floor muscle function. Urethral pressure profilometry is commonly abnormal in patients with the clinical diagnosis of interstitial cystitis, urethral syndrome, and voiding dysfunction. Gajewski and Awad (48) found that the mean maximal urethral closing pressure in female patients with interstitial cystitis was 116 cm of water versus 70 cm of water in a same age control group. These same authors also found that female patients with interstitial cystitis had a mean maximal flow rate of 16 mL/sec, and this was at the 12th percentile when compared to controls and corrected for voided volume.

While multiple authors (49,50) have described the high urethral pressures in patients with urethral syndrome, another abnormality that is commonly seen is urethral instability. This urodynamic abnormality is manifested by wide fluctuations of urethral pressure during two-channel urethral cystometric evaluation. This definition has not been standardized by the International Continence Society, but it is loosely defined as fluctuations in the urethral pressure between 15 and 20 cm of water from the mean. It is typically associated with the syndrome of urgency/frequency, but has also been seen in patients with vestibulitis and voiding dysfunction. Because the majority of urethral closing pressure is abolished by pudendal block, these findings are thought to represent abnormalities in levator tone and/or levator function (51). Normal patients can demonstrate similar fluctuations in urethral pressure, and the actual parameters to determine what is normal versus abnormal have yet to be determined. I feel we can safely say that urethral instability is likely a manifestation of pelvic floor instability. In symptomatic patients, this represents a component of the patient's

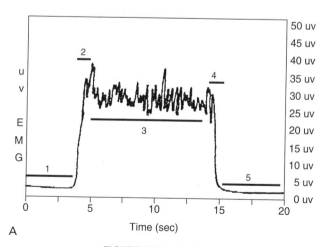

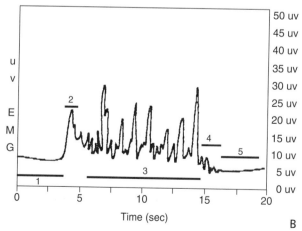

FIGURE 35.8. A: Typical nonmorbid EMG pelvic floor responses. Characteristics: (1) low resting baseline with good muscle stability, (2) good recruitment with clear demarcation between rest and contraction, (3) strong contraction with no fatigue (sustained contraction), (4) abrupt fall from contraction to resting baseline (relaxation), and (5) low resting baseline with good muscle stability after contraction. **B:** Pelvic EMG activity for typical vulvar vestibulitis. Characteristics: (1) elevated and unstable resting baseline, (2) poor recruitment, (3) spasm on sustained contraction and fatigue, (4) poor recovery, and (5) postcontraction baseline remains elevated, with high amplitude and instability.

pathology; that is, it demonstrates pelvic floor muscle dysfunction. In patients who are asymptomatic, this may represent a warning sign of subclinical pelvic floor muscle dysfunction and thus may have prognostic significance.

Evaluation of pelvic floor muscle dysfunction by uroflowmetry was discussed earlier in this chapter, but will be reviewed briefly here. For a uroflow to actually represent the patient's normal voiding mechanism it should be done at a volume at which the patient would normally void (this is referred to as functional volume). Ideally, this should be greater than 200 mL to accurately evaluate maximal flow rates. It should be done in a private setting to reduce problems of "performance anxiety." Even if an instrumented pressure flow study is done, the private setting is still quite important. After the patient has voided, she should be asked if she felt that that episode of voiding was representative of her normal voiding pattern.

As described earlier, an instrumented pressure flow study with recording of pelvic floor EMG activity is the most accurate in determining the etiology and severity of a patient's voiding dysfunction, but a simple uroflow is an important screening tool to evaluate pelvic floor muscle function during voiding. A screening uroflow will be abnormal in approximately one-third of patients who report no abnormalities in voiding. For some patients their abnormal voiding pattern has been in essence their "normal voiding pattern" for most of their life. A normal flow curve at time of uroflow imagery is a bell-shaped curve that is slightly shifted to the left. Peak

flow rate should be greater than 20 mL/sec, and any patient with a peak flow rate of less than 15 mL/sec should be considered as having an abnormal maximal flow rate assuming that the volume was greater than 200 mL. An intermittent, multipeak pattern is classic for patients with incomplete and inconsistent pelvic floor muscle relaxation. This pattern and others are demonstrated in Fig. 35.9 (52).

When a patient's symptoms primarily affect her posterior compartment, then one would expect symptoms of obstructed defecation, painful bowel movements, and perirectal pain. Clinically, these patients often have a history of anal fissures and hemorrhoids and state that their stools are elongated with a very small caliber, that is, "pencil-like." This compilation of symptoms mandates evaluation of the defecatory mechanisms via defecography. Using a barium paste the patient is asked to evacuate her rectum during a fluoroscopic evaluation while sitting on a radiolucent commode. The normal process of defecation requires relaxation of the puborectalis (the portion of the levator muscle that forms a sling under the distal rectum). With relaxation, the anal rectal angle should become more obtuse, allowing the bolus of fecal material to easily pass. In patients with obstructed defecatory symptoms due to poor relaxation of the puborectalis muscle, the angle remains acute and the puborectalis muscle can be seen indenting the posterior rectum during attempts to evacuate. This is called anismus, and failure to relax the puborectalis muscle causes the symptom of obstructed defecation (53).

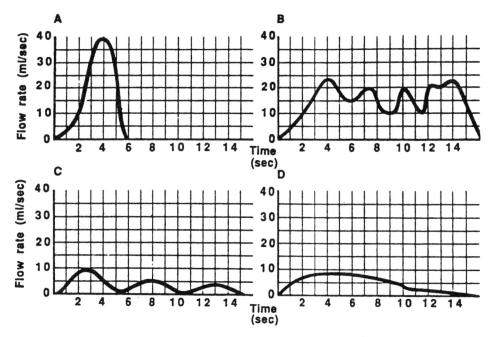

FIGURE 35.9. Graphic representation of various uroflow patterns. **A:** Superflow commonly seen with poor urethral resistance. **B:** Interrupted pattern due to intermittent sphincter activity. **C:** Interrupted stream during straining to void. **D:** Abnormal flow rate characteristic of detrusor outlet obstruction. (From Karram MM. Manometric investigation: urodynmics: In Benson JP, ed. *Urodynamics in female pelvic floor disorders: investigation and management.* New York: W.W. Norton and Co., 1992, p. 107, with permission.)

Patients with this type of pelvic floor muscle dysfunction can also have problems with urologic or gynecologic symptoms as previously discussed, but certainly the defect can occur as an isolated dysfunction involving only the puborectalis. This type of isolated dysfunction is believed to be primarily due to a dysfunction at the level of S4 versus the other problems that represent dysregulation at the level of S3. This information represents observational data from patients undergoing neuromodulation for these types of disorders.

DIFFERENTIAL DIAGNOSIS

Urinary retention with associated symptoms compatible with voiding dysfunction can be caused by many mechanisms. Clinicians must always consider a transient cause if the retentive history is acute. Causes of transient acute urinary retention include fecal impaction, medications, urinary tract infections, acute delirium, and psychogenic problems. Medications that can cause urinary retention include those that decrease bladder contractility (anticholinergics, antispasmodics, calcium channel antagonists, phenothiazine, and tricyclic antidepressants). Additionally, medications that increase resistance at the level of the bladder outlet can cause acute urinary retention. These include alpha-adrenergic agonists, L-dopa, and amphetamines.

When a patient reports a lengthy history of urinary retention, the differential diagnosis can best be conceptualized by considering two basic types: obstructive and decreased bladder contractility. Common causes of obstruction include severe prolapse with kinking of the urethra, iatrogenic obstruction such as after a retropubic urethropexy, or obstruction from intrinsic compression of the urethra secondary to a gynecologic mass such as cervical cancer, an incarcerated retroverted uterus, or a vaginal or urethral neoplastic process. An important point to consider is that patients often present with complaints compatible with prolapse (i.e., pressure, heaviness) when they actually have pelvic floor tension myalgia and have no evidence of significant support defect. Therefore, when patients complain of symptoms of prolapse and obstructive voiding, it is important to examine them while they stand up so that the true extent of their "prolapse" can be seen. Additionally, in patients with significant prolapse that results in kinking of the urethra, the obstructive voiding can be alleviated simply by reducing the prolapse. By having patients perform a uroflow with a pessary in place or at times even simply reducing the prolapse with 4 × 4s rolled and placed into the vault, the voiding parameters seen on uroflow should markedly improve. If they do not, then pelvic floor dysfunction and not prolapse may be the cause of the patient's voiding problems (assuming that adequate detrusor contractility is demonstrated). It is important to point out that women rarely have urethral stenosis as a cause of voiding dysfunction. While urethral dilations have been a traditional therapy for this problem, any obstruction

is functional in nature and not truly anatomic in the majority of women. The actual prevalence of urethral stenosis that is clinically significant is thought to be 1 per 1,000 women who are symptomatic.

If no obvious lesion is found that could be the cause of obstruction, then dysfunctional voiding should be considered. Within this group, a significant neurologic lesion must always be considered in the differential diagnosis. When a patient demonstrates classic detrusor–sphincter dyssynergia without a history of spinal cord injury or myelitis, multiple sclerosis or Parkinson's disease must always be considered. One must remember that the initial symptoms of multiple sclerosis often present in women in their twenties though forties and that 5% of them will see their primary care physician with urologic complaints as the first sign of this devastating disease. Referral for appropriate neurologic evaluation is required. If the initial evaluation is negative, but the neurologic symptoms continue to progress, then reevaluation is sometimes required in order to demonstrate the classic radiologic findings.

Decreased bladder contractility is most often neuropathic in origin and is frequently associated with decreased bladder sensation and the subsequent chronic overdistention. Common neuropathies associated with impaired contractility include cauda equina lesions, pelvic plexus injury, and peripheral neuropathies such as diabetic cystopathy and Shy–Drager syndrome. Hypotonic or atonic bladders are typically associated with chronic obstruction (anatomic or functional), radiation cystitis, or a significant lower motor neuron lesion such as cauda equina injury. Impaired contractility is also seen in elderly patients with urge incontinence who are found to have detrusor hyperactivity with impaired contractility.

TREATMENT AND MANAGEMENT

Because minor voiding dysfunctions can be intermittent and generally asymptomatic, the discussion that follows centers around symptomatic patients. A very basic concept of pain management involves the identification and treatment of all sites of ongoing pain. This means that true infectious pathogens should be treated (e.g., bacterial cystitis or vaginal candidiasis should be identified and treated if they exist). Factors that exacerbate inflammatory components should likewise be treated. This includes the use of estrogen vaginal cream for patients who are hypoestrogenic (postmenopausal women or women on birth control pills), topical steroids for patients with inflammatory vestibulitis (who have not already demonstrated failure to this therapy), and therapy for patients with urgency/frequency syndrome (e.g., DMSO, heparin, Elmiron).

As previously discussed, a common component of pelvic pain syndrome is pelvic floor dysfunction and pelvic floor tension myalgia. It is so common that failure to treat this component results in significant rate of failure of therapy.

Basic goals for therapy are to decrease baseline muscle tension, decrease myofascial pain, and improve pelvic floor muscle function. Clinically, this should result in improved urinary flow, less hesitancy, and a decrease in the manifestation of their pain syndrome.

Neuromuscular Reeducation

Improvement in pelvic floor function can be achieved using various approaches to pelvic floor reeducation. In patients with minor dysfunction, simple patient education concerning the normal function of the pelvic floor and normal pelvic floor muscle awareness is vital. It is important to emphasize that the pelvic floor muscle should normally be at rest and not actually "held tight." Teaching the patient pelvic floor relaxation techniques is the key to this neuromuscular reeducation. I refer to this as "reverse Kegel" because the key is teaching the patient to relax the pelvic floor musculature and not squeeze as is taught in standard Kegel exercises.

An important part of the management of patients with chronic pelvic pain syndrome is to give them tools that can be incorporated into their daily routine to prevent flares and therefore decrease their overall pain. This empowerment gives patients a sense of control over their pain. These tools include soaking in a hot bath two or three times per day for at least 15 minutes and using a soft pillow when sitting on a firm, hard surface. Patients should attempt to avoid sitting for longer than 15 minutes at a time (especially on a hard chair without getting up to walk and stretch their pelvic muscles and lower extremities). They are taught to wear loose-fitting clothing and avoid using tampons.

With a little education, patients can quickly develop an "awareness" of their pelvic muscles. Therefore, they must not limit their reeducation to a session of reverse Kegel, but instead they must also "check" their muscle status several times throughout the day. This is most easily done by relaxing the pelvic muscles "as if to pass flatus." If the perineum is perceived to drop significantly, then the patient's pelvic floor muscles were tense. The reader is encouraged to review the tools and exercise techniques discussed in further detail in the patient handout provided in Appendix A.

Biofeedback

Biofeedback involves tools of various types that measure and demonstrate physiologic processes such as heart rate, blood pressure, or muscle contraction. The gold standard for pelvic floor biofeedback involves the use of EMG-guided biofeedback. Its use by Glazer in the management of vestibulitis demonstrates the success that is available with this technique. In the early 1990s, it was generally thought the pelvic floor muscle dysfunction seen in

patients with vestibulitis was secondary to the pain of the vestibulitis. Therefore, treatment and correction of the pelvic floor instability would not be helpful for the primary complaint of pain associated with vestibulitis. However, Glazer's initial results demonstrated that biofeedback alone was very beneficial in the treatment of vestibulitis and the associated symptoms of urgency/frequency syndrome, functional bowel disease, and chronic pelvic pain. Glazer et al. (2) have characterized the pelvic floor EMG findings in patients with vestibulitis. There is an ongoing study by Rounazi et al. (53) to evaluate the best method to identify patients with pelvic floor muscle tension abnormalities. Preliminary results from this study show that digital examination is not as accurate as EMG assessment of tone, function, and instability.

The protocol for biofeedback in patients with pelvic floor muscle dysfunction and chronic pelvic pain syndromes generally involves at least a 20-minute session once or twice per day. Each session requires the use of an EMG biofeedback unit. The EMG sensor is typically in the form of a vaginal probe, yet intrarectal probes or surface electrode patches in the vulvar area can be used instead (Fig. 35.10). Formal biofeedback should continue for at least 3 months with follow-up throughout to assess the progress and assist the patient with any technical problems or concerns during the therapy session. Success rates vary depending upon which symptom is looked at as the end point, and most studies to date are uncontrolled. For vestibulitis, pain was reduced an average of 86% in women who completed an average of 16 weeks of biofeedback (2). Pelvic floor relaxation therapy has been shown to be beneficial for adolescents with recurrent urinary tract infections (UTIs) and ureteral reflux, with an impressive 83% demonstrating a resolution of UTIs and seven out of eight demonstrating resolution of ureteral reflux (54). Anismus (sometimes call nonrelaxing puborectalis syndrome) is best treated with EMG-guided biofeedback due to a success rate that sur-

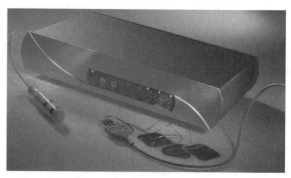

FIGURE 35.10. Biofeedback unit for treatment of pelvic flow muscle tension abnormalities. (Photo, courtesy of Laborie Medical, 1999.)

passes 80%. One of the real advantages of biofeedback is its low cost, minimal morbidity, and high success rate. But for most patients with chronic pelvic pain syndrome, it represents just one of the tools to be used. Multicomponent therapy is almost always required.

Physical Therapy

While the goal of biofeedback is to reestablish the proper dynamic behavior of the pelvic floor musculature, frequently the pathology involves more than just dysbehavior. When patients have manifestations of a true myofascial pain syndrome involving the pelvic musculature, direct physical therapy to these muscles is required. It is only with treatment of the myofascial pain syndrome that normal coordinated dynamic and resting behavior can be reestablished.

Physical therapists trained in the care of patients with chronic pelvic pain syndrome and pelvic floor tension myalgia have several unique tools to offer. The first and most important is direct soft tissue work. This approach was first eluded to by Theile in his use of internal massage therapy, which is referred to as Theile massage (55). His technique involved the performance of transrectal levator massage. Theile reported a 60% cure rate with an additional 35% improvement in patients with coccygodynia treated with 11 sessions of weekly levator massage. Physical therapists typically use a transvaginal, slowly progressive massage technique called myofascial manipulation or myofascial release. A muscle that has been in a high-tension state has shortened myofibrils that must physically be lengthened and/or stretched. That lengthening and/or stretching is the goal of myofascial manipulation. Improving the range of motion of these pelvic muscles is another goal that is addressed not only with internal soft tissue work, but also with passive stretching exercises. This is particularly beneficial for patients with piriformis muscle pain.

Most reports of therapy for pelvic floor tension myalgia-type syndromes involve a combination of modalities used by the physical therapist. An additional therapy includes ultrasound and/or heat therapy. Ultrasound has been shown to increase muscle temperature to a depth of 5 cm from the surface. The physiologic effect of this includes an increase in collagen tissue extensibility, improved blood flow, improved nerve conduction velocity, increased pain threshold, increased enzymatic activity, and improved contractile activity of skeletal muscles. Myofascial manipulation is usually augmented by being administered after ultrasound therapy. Sinaki et al. (42) described a 31% rate of complete resolution of symptoms of pelvic floor tension myalgia and another 38% with moderate or marked improvement when treatment consisted of a combination of myofascial manipulation, diathermy, and relaxation exercises.

If a trigger point persists in being painful and therefore has not responded to the interventions mentioned above,

then trigger point injection therapy is indicated. An active trigger that does not resolve with heat and soft tissue work will often limit the benefit of physical therapy because the pain will limit the amount of stretching and work that the muscle will tolerate. A trigger point injection will therefore allow a patient to continue to progress with therapy and thus avoid a plateau at only a partial response. Trigger point injections and/or pudendal blocks also provide quick relief of an episode of flare without resorting to narcotic therapy.

The technique of pelvic floor trigger point injection is similar to any trigger point injection. After the vagina is minimally prepped with an antiseptic, the trigger point is carefully identified and the transvaginal placement of a spinal needle is positioned at the trigger point with the help of the patient's response to identify when the needle is within the trigger point. The injection I most commonly use is 3 mL of 0.5% of lidocaine or ropivacaine with epinephrine. After the trigger point is injected, the clinician should provide massage to the area. If the trigger point injection is successful, massage should now be painless. If multiple trigger points are found, a pudendal block with 10 mL of 0.5% bupivacaine with epinephrine can be very beneficial rather than the injection of multiple trigger points. A series of trigger point injections 2 to 3 days apart is often beneficial with demonstration of lengthening pain-free periods far beyond the pharmacologic benefits of drug use. Rarely will I do more than three to five trigger point injections because if resolution is not obtained at that point, then it is rarely obtained with further injections.

Establishing a good relationship with a physical therapist that specializes in pelvic floor syndromes and knows how to work with pelvic floor tension myalgia and pelvic floor dysfunction is one of the most important steps in developing a practice that can manage chronic pelvic pain patients. That physical therapist should not only provide the modalities mentioned above, but should also be able to provide EMG-guided biofeedback as was mentioned previously. Once the pain has resolved and normal pelvic floor function has been reestablished, strengthening exercises can be initiated for patients with complaints of urinary incontinence. It is very important that strengthening exercises are not used until the pain and dysfunction have been alleviated.

Electrogalvanic Stimulation

This is a modality of therapy used in physical therapy for many types of myofascial pain syndromes. It can be applied across the sacrum or across the vulvar area with surface electrodes. It is now more commonly applied with a hand-held or self-retained vaginal or rectal probe and is frequently referred to as functional electrical stimulation. While the exact protocol for stimulation is yet to be determined, the majority of studies with positive results use a frequency of 80 to 100 Hz for 15- to 20-minute sessions at least once per week. Stimulation of spastic muscles results in muscle fasciculation and subsequent muscle fatigue. Suppression of the motor neuron and modulation of the sacral cord reflexes are also thought to be involved (56,57). Several uncontrolled studies show excellent to good results in 43% to 91%, with fair to poor results in 9% to 52%. Recurrence of pelvic floor myofascial pain syndrome was seen in as many as 33%, yet resolution of symptoms could be reestablished with reinstitution of therapy (58). For patients who fail to respond or for whom a significant recurrence occurred that did not respond to follow-up therapy, significant associated pathology could at times be found. This must always be considered in the management of any patient with chronic pelvic pain that appears not to respond to appropriate therapy.

Successful therapy requires that you do not overstimulate an already dysfunctional or spastic muscle. Initial sessions should be at a low amplitude that is slowly increased in intensity and duration. Additionally, this type of intervention lends itself to be combined with EMG-guided biofeedback that is extremely important. My preference is 10 minutes of biofeedback followed by 10 to 15 minutes of electrical stimulation at 100 Hz for patients with pelvic floor tension myalgia and pelvic muscle dysfunction.

Neuromodulation

The central nervous system is composed of a delicately balanced set of neural reflexes that have a built-in predisposition for instability. When these reflexes become disrupted within the sacral cord, then instability and imbalances develop. Instability can involve the bladder (urge incontinence), urethra (urethral syndrome), pelvic floor (pelvic floor dysfunction and pain with elimination abnormalities), and the vestibule (vestibulitis). Sacral nerve stimulation, frequently referred to as neuromodulation, provides an alternative mode of therapy that attempts to reestablish the balance of sacral cord reflexes in sensory pathways, thus eliminating symptoms of urge incontinence, urgency/frequency syndrome, voiding dysfunction, and pelvic pain.

Neurostimulation techniques were first applied in the 1960s and were later (since the mid-1980s) applied to the management of patient's refractory to traditional therapies for bladder dysfunction. Since then, over 1,000 patients have had their symptoms treated with sacral nerve stimulation. Their outcomes have resulted in FDA approval for the marketing of the Medtronic Interstim system of urinary control for the treatment of urge incontinence, urgency/frequency syndrome, and nonobstructive urinary retention. One of the real advantages to this intervention is that it involves a two-step procedure in which the first step is a *trial stimulation* (a simple office procedure) done to verify the efficacy and optimize the parameters of stimulation. Once efficacy has been demonstrated, then and only then will a surgically implanted electrode and pulse generator be placed. Thus, the patient and the physician are able to experience the degree of improvement in symptoms prior to a surgical procedure. If improvement in symptoms of at least 50% is not obtained, then a surgical implant is not done. During the performance of the percutaneous stimulation procedure (test stimulation) an insulated spinal needle is placed in the S3 foramen and the response to this stimulation is evaluated (Fig. 35.11). The ideal response involves the contraction of the levator muscle, with the patient reporting a gentle pulling sensation in the area of the perineum. Minor adjustments in the position of the insulated spinal needle can result in significant changes in the clinical response. This stimulation is typically most beneficial if done in the ipsilateral position if the patient has any lateralizing symptoms or findings. A trial stimula-

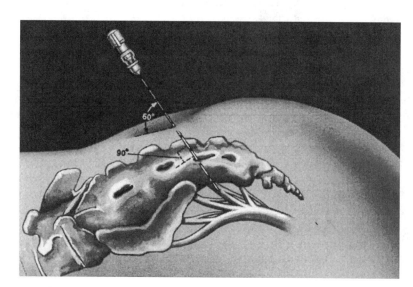

FIGURE 35.11. Percutaneous test stimulation needle placement for sacral neuromodulation. (From Medtronic Neurological. *Interstim continence control therapy.* Minneapolis, MN, p. 31, with permission.)

tion can also be done at the S4 foramen, but 75% of the time the best response is seen at the S3 level. Once the best site is determined (based upon the patient's response during the first step of trial stimulation), a wire electrode is placed and the spinal needle is removed. An external pulse generator is then connected to the wire electrode, and a three- to seven-day trial of stimulation is started. Voiding or bladder diaries are kept to compare preprocedure and postprocedure (during the trial stimulation) values of voided volumes, frequency, and postvoid residuals (when intermittent catheterization is required). When pain (originating from the pelvis, bladder, urethra, levator muscles) is a significant component of the patient's symptoms, then visual analog scales (0 to 10 scales) should be used to assess the patient's degree of pain resolution during the period of trial stimulation.

If improvement of at least 50% in the patient's symptoms is seen, then an electrode is surgically implanted in the same foramen as where the successful temporary wire electrode was located (Fig. 35.12). The implantable pulse generator is then placed in a subcutaneous pouch positioned just below the belt line in the upper gluteal area. This surgical procedure typically requires a 1- to 2-day hospitalization, and in approximately 75% of patients the results of surgical implantation matches or surpasses the clinical result seen during the period of trial stimulation.

The Medtronic Interstim system for urinary control was evaluated in a multicenter prospective randomized trial at study centers in the United States, Canada, and Europe. Specifically, 171 patients with severe nonobstructive urinary retention and 220 patients with severe urgency/frequency

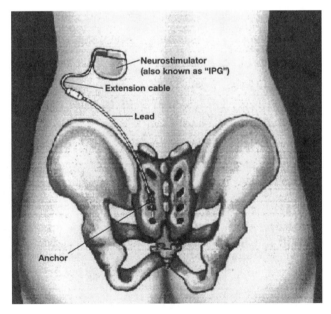

FIGURE 35.12. Posterior view of a typicallly implanted system (abdominal neurostimulator placement). (From Medtronic Neurological. *Interstim continence control therapy.* Minneapolis, MN, p. 38, with permission.)

syndrome (interstitial cystitis) unresponsive to conventional therapy were enrolled (59). In those patients with nonobstructive urinary retention who had a positive response to test stimulation, there was a total elimination for the need of clean intermittent self-catheterization in 61% and at least a 50% reduction in volume at time of catheterization for an additional 16% at 1-year follow-up. In those patients with urgency/frequency syndrome that had a positive test stimulation and went on to be implanted, there was a significant reduction in the number of voids, increased volume voided per void, and a decrease in the degree of urgency as compared to the control group. Sixty-four percent of implanted patients at 1 year were felt to have a clinical success as defined by a 50% reduction in the number of voids per day, or a reduction to less than eight voids per day. Eighty-two percent felt that there was an improvement in urgency with a documented increase in voided volumes. Quality of life scores (FF-36) were markedly improved in seven of eight conceptual areas (not in the area "role emotional"). Other authors have reported similar results with smaller numbers of patients (60–63). Part of this multicenter study was to evaluate the response to turning off the neural stimulation after 6 months of therapy. Discontinuation of stimulation resulted in a return to baseline urologic symptoms within 2 weeks for the majority of patients. This was done to demonstrate that the therapeutic benefits were truly in the administration of the neuromodulating current and not due to any other consequences of this intervention.

Adverse events involving the test stimulation most commonly revolved around migration of the wire electrode (11%). Because of this, Medtronic has redesigned the wire electrode, and migration is extremely rare. Approximately 2% of patients complained of pain at the site of the wire electrode, but all symptoms resolved at the removal of the wire. Only 0.1% (one patient) required surgical intervention to remove a sheared-off tip of the wire electrode.

The implantation procedure resulted in problems requiring surgical revision in 33% of patients. These included pain (29.7%), lead migration (8.4%), wound infection (6.1%), adverse changes in bowel function (3%), and technical problems (3.3%). Ninety-one percent of these adverse events were resolved with surgical revision. Since the submission of these data, Medtronics has redesigned the electrode, and lead migration has been significantly reduced. Additionally, the pulse generator had previously been implanted in the abdominal wall. Now that it is being placed in the gluteal area, pain and technical problems are being seen less frequently.

With prolonged nerve stimulation, the fear of nerve damage has not been realized. Chronic stimulation of a peripheral nerve can result in damage, but this adverse effect is seen at a high frequency of stimulation and is not seen on the basis of amplitude of stimulus. Typical initial programming parameters involved in Interstim therapy would be 10 to 20 Hz with a pulse width of 210 μsec and an amplitude of 2 to 4 mA. Battery life varies based upon amplitude of current applied and other programming parameters but ranges between 7 and 10 years.

Neuromodulation of the sacral cord via S3 or S4 nerve stimulation represents a significant advancement in the management of patients with urge incontinence, urgency/frequency syndrome, and nonobstructive voiding dysfunction. The demonstration of efficacy in this difficult group of patients should reemphasize to clinicians that dysregulation of the sacral cord reflexes is at the root of many of our patients' complaints. Neuromodulation represents a new tool that will markedly improve the quality of life for many of our patients when more traditional therapies have failed. Additionally, it offers the distinct advantage of a simple office procedure done to test the efficacy of neuromodulation before deciding to commit to a more significant surgical intervention.

Botulinum-A Toxin

Botulinum-A toxin is an inhibitor of acetylcholine release at the neuromuscular junction and is principally used in the management of focal dystonia, spasms, and spasticity (e.g., strabismus). Botulinum-A toxin has been endoscopically injected into the urethral striated sphincter for the treatment of detrusor–sphincter dyssynergia due to suprasacral cord disease—that is, an upper motor neuron lesion. Patients with this type of neurologic defect often have chronic urinary retention, chronic UTIs, and high intravesical pressure with the potential for vesicoureteral reflux and renal damage. Success, as measured by a decrease in residual urine and decreased frequency of intermittent catheterization and/or need for indwelling catheter, is seen in greater than 80% of patients (64,65). Clinical response was temporary due to the pharmacologic effect on the neuromuscular junction and the duration of response varied between 2 and 9 months, dependent on the dose used and protocol followed.

Botulinum-A toxin has been used in a 7-year-old girl with discordant voiding (66). Although this child did not have a upper motor neuron lesion, she was reported to have fetal alcohol syndrome. Marked improvement in her problems of recurrent UTIs and bed wetting were seen, but no duration or long-term data were available in this case report.

Botulinum-A toxin has also been used for isolated levator muscle pain with good results. The injection site was chosen based upon needle EMG identification of the most active site within the muscle (67).

These preliminary reports are very interesting, but at this time Botulinum-A toxin should be considered only for patients with upper motor neuron lesions or who have failed sacral nerve stimulation therapy (sacral nerve stimulation therapy is typically not beneficial in the majority of patients with an upper motor neuron lesion).

Patient Education

A critical step in management is patient education. Once patients understand the neuropathic cascade of events that have resulted in their chronic pain and dysfunction, they can better grasp the importance of a multicomponent treatment plan and will be more compliant with the demands of therapy. This plan will frequently involve neuromuscular reeducation (biofeedback), physical therapy, neurolytic drugs, and at times direct neuromodulation of the disrupted neural function. When treated appropriately with the correct mix of therapies, most of these patients will experience a significant decrease in their symptomatology and a significant increase in their quality of life.

KEY POINTS

Most Important Questions to Ask

- Is there urinary hesitancy ("shy bladder") and a slow intermittent urinary flow?
- Is urinary hesitancy a particularly prominent problem if you are required to "hold your urine" for a long time (such as at work or on a trip where bathroom access is limited)?
- Is there pain with intercourse or persistence of pelvic pain for many hours after intercourse?
- Is there pressure, heaviness, or an achy feeling in the suprapubic, vaginal, or rectal area?
- Is pain worse while standing, or resolved within 10 minutes of lying down?
- Does sitting make the pelvic pain worse?
- Doe the pain radiate into the groin, the buttocks, or the upper thigh?

Most Important Physical Examination Findings

- Observation of pelvic floor muscle activity during the process of squeezing and relaxation, showing inability to produce more contractile strength and relax completely
- Failure to show closure of the genital hiatus; failure to lift the perineum or to demonstrate the normal puckering of the anal verge at time of pelvic floor contractions
- Fasciculations in the pelvic floor muscles
- Inability to rapidly squeeze the pubococcygeus muscle in a coordinated manner
- Relatively thick, immobile, pelvic floor with a significant increase in baseline tone
- Trigger points of the levator muscles

Most Important Diagnostic Studies

- EMG testing of resting tone and dynamic functional assessment (needle or surface)
- Utethral pressure profilometry

- Uroflowmetry
- Defecography

Treatments

- Neuromuscular reeducation
- Biofeedback
- Physical therapy
- Pelvic floor trigger point or pudendal block
- Electrogalvanic stimulation
- Neuromodulation
- Botulinum-A toxin
- Patient education

APPENDIX A: PATIENT INFORMATION: THERAPY FOR RELIEF OF PELVIC FLOOR PAIN (PELVIC FLOOR TENSION MYALGIA)

Your pelvic floor muscles are a group of muscles at the base of the pelvis. In addition to supporting the bladder, they close the urethra, rectum, and vagina. These muscles lie just inside the pelvis. We typically learn to control muscles during the first few years of life when we become toilet-trained. Unlike the abdominal muscles, they are not easy to feel and it is important for patients to try to develop a mental awareness of their pelvic muscles. The pelvic floor muscles attach to the tailbone, wrap along the side toward the hips, and extend to the front of the pelvis near the pubic bone.

The pelvic floor muscles can become very painful if they are tightened for a long period of time. People often tighten these muscles as a result of injury to the pelvis such as a straddle injury, a difficult vaginal delivery, hemorrhoid surgery, or extensive pelvic reconstructive surgery. Additionally, some people never learn to relax their muscles totally, and often they give a history of a lifelong problem of frequency, urgency, and recurrent UTIs and/or chronic constipation. Another common symptom associated with this diagnosis is the problem of burning discomfort at the entrance to the vagina, often misdiagnosed as a chronic yeast infection. This muscle tightness may become a subconscious habit causing the symptoms on a continuous basis that I have outlined above. These instructions will help you learn how to keep the pelvic muscles relaxed.

During the period of treatment:
- Try to keep your surroundings quiet so that you can concentrate on relaxation therapy.
- Enjoy quiet, relaxed reading instead of watching television.
- Try to get 8–9 hours of good sleep each night and take naps if possible during the day (your physician might give you medication if necessary to help induce a good relaxed sleep if your body needs medication).
- Take warm tub baths to help your relaxation efforts, lying in the bath tub with knees up.
- Avoid wearing tight clothing, avoid using tampons, and avoid sitting longer than 15 minutes at a time (particularly sitting in a hard seat or riding in the car for a long distance).

A technique to relax pelvic muscles:
- The purpose of these exercises is to help you feel and become aware of your pelvic muscles so that you can develop the "awareness" of muscle tension and muscle relaxation and most importantly, to develop the control so that you can reestablish normal pelvic muscle function.
- Placing your hand in the vaginal area with the middle finger resting on the surface of the skin between the vagina and the rectum is the easiest place to feel these muscles in action. Developing a mental awareness of the degree of muscle tension and the ability to relax these muscles is the key to your successfully eradicating this problem.
- In order to feel your pelvic muscles relax, pretend you are relaxing your muscles to allow the passage of rectal gas. There should be an obvious descent or relaxation that your finger will feel and that your mind will become aware of.
- It is important that you do not bear down or strain to make your pelvic muscles descend, but instead allow them to relax on their own.
- Squeezing your muscles (i.e., Kegel squeeze) should demonstrate this same area of tissue between the vagina and rectum elevating or pulling up inside you. Because our emphasis is not on improving the ability to squeeze, but instead on the ability to relax these muscles, the squeeze should only be long enough so that we can induce the awareness of muscle tension and then quickly and completely relax these muscles.
- Relaxation should progress in a three-step fashion, imagining yourself walking down three steps one at a time on a flight of stairs. Thus: squeeze once, relax three times, then squeeze again, and relax three more times.
- Your goal is to keep your muscles relaxed at all times while you are involved in your everyday activities. Therefore, frequently be aware of your rectal and vaginal muscles and attempt to relax them (as if to pass gas) and you will often find that you were tense and did not realize it. Your goal, of course, is to "check" your pelvic floor muscles and find them already relaxed.
- During the first few days at home you may be able to keep your muscles relaxed only while lying down. Later on, you will be able to stay relaxed while standing and/or sitting.
- At first, you might want to sit with layers of towels or a cushion under your side or buttocks to keep pressure off of your buttocks if you have a job that requires that you sit for quite some time. Never use a rubber ring.
- Practicing muscle relaxation may not bring immediate relief, but over time it may help to reduce your pelvic floor pain.

Additional therapies include the following:

- Certain muscle relaxant medications.
- Physical therapist often will use biofeedback, electrical stimulation, ultrasound heat treatment, and internal muscle massage.
- Trigger point injection (where specific extremely tender spots within the pelvic muscles are injected with Novocaine).
- Nerve blocks to actually block the nerves responsible for muscle tension.
- An office procedure where a wire is placed along the nerves going to the pelvic muscles. After placement of this wire, a very mild electrical current is used to stimulate the nerve that will make these muscles relax for you. This type of therapy is called Interstim therapy, and a 50% success rate is seen in patients who have failed all other therapies.

REFERENCES

1. Reiter R, Gambone J. Non-gynecologic somatic pathology in women with chronic pelvic pain and negative laparoscopy. *J Reprod Med* 1991;36:253–259.
2. Glazer H, Rodke G, Swencionis P, et al. Treatment of vulvar vestibulitis syndrome with electromyographic biofeedback of pelvic floor musculature. *J Reprod Med* 1995;40:283–290.
3. Jones K, Lehr S. Vulvodynia: diagnostic techniques and treatment modalities. *Nurse Pract* 1994;19:34–46.
4. Pomerantz E. Vulvodynia: etiology and treatment strategies. *J Obstet Gynecol Phys Ther* 1994;18:10.
5. Chaiken D, Blaivas J, Blaivas S. Behavioral therapy for the treatment of refractory interstitial cystitis. *J Urol* 1993;149:1445–1448.
6. Whitmore KE. Self care regimes for patients with interstitial cystitis. *Urol Clin North Am* 1994;21:121–130.
7. Summitt RL. Urogynecologic causes of chronic pelvic pain. *Obstet Gynecol Clin North Am* 1993;30:685–698.
8. Webster DC. Sex and interstitial cystitis: explaining the pain and self care. *Urol Nurs* 1993;13:4–11.
9. deGroat WC. Neuroanatomy and neurophysiology: innervation of the lower urinary tract. In: Raz S, ed. *Female urology,* 2nd ed. Philadelphia: WB Saunders, 1996:28–42.
10. Kruse MN, deGroat WC. Spinal pathways mediate coordinated bladder/urethral sphincter activity during reflex micturition in normal and spinal cord injured neonatal rats. *Neurosci Lett* 1993;152:141.
11. Chai TC, Gray ML, Sterrs WD. The incidence of a positive ice water test in bladder outlet obstructed patients: evidence for bladder neural pasticity. *J Urol* 1998;160:34–38.
12. Das A, Chancellor MB, Watanabe T, et al. Intravesical capsaicin in neurologic impaired patients with detrusor hyperreflexia. *J Spinal Cord Med* 1996;19:190–193.
13. Lazzeri M, Beneforti P, Benaim G, et al. Intravesical capsaicin for treatment of severe bladder pain: a randomized placebo controlled study. *J Urol* 1996;156:947–952.
14. Cruz F, Guimaras M, Silva C, et al. Desensitization of bladder sensory fibers by intravesical capsaicin has long lasting clinical and urodynamic effects in patients with hyperactive or hypersensitive bladder dysfunction. *J Urol* 1997;157:585–589.
15. deGroat WC, Araki I, Vizzard MA, et al. Developmental and injury induced plasticity to the micturition reflex pathways. *Behav Brain Res* 1997;92:127.
16. Hohenfellner M, Nunes L, Schmidt RA, et al. Interstitial cystitis:

17. Irwin PP, Galloway N. Interstitial cystitis: the neurovascular perspective. In: Sant GR, ed. *Interstitial cystitis.* Philadelphia: Lippincott-Raven, 1997:129–135.
18. Irwin PP, Hammonds W, Galloway N. Lumbar epidural blockade in the management of pain in interstitial cystitis. *Br J Urol* 1993;71:413–416.
19. deGroat WC. Changes in the organization of the micturition reflex pathways of the cat after transsection of the spinal cord. In: Zeraa RP, Grafstein B, eds. *Cellular mechanisms for recovery from nervous system injury: a conference report. Exp Neurol* 1981;71:22.
20. deGroat WC, Vizzard MA, Araki I, et al. Spinal interneurons and preganglionic neurons in sacral autonomic reflex pathways. In: Holstege G, Bandler R, Saper C, eds. *Emotional motor systems. Progress in brain research,* New York: vol. 107. Elsevier, 1996:97–111.
21. Ohlsson BL, Fall M, Frankenbers S. Effects of external and direct pudendal nerve maximal electrical stimulation in the treatment of the uninhibited overactive bladder. *Br J Urol* 1989;64:374–380.
22. Walters MD, Karram MM. The standardization of terminology of lower urinary tract function recommended by the International Continence Society. In: Walters MD, Karram MM, eds. *Clinical urogynecology.* St Louis: Mosby, 1993:430–446.
23. Parsons KF, Turton MB. Urethral supersensitivity and occult urethral neuropathy. *Br J Urol* 1980;52:131–137.
24. Hinman F Jr. Non-neurogenic neurogenic bladder, read at annual meeting of American Urologic Association, Chicago, Illinois, May 1971.
25. Hinman F Jr. Non-neurogenic neurogenic bladder (the Hinman syndrome)—15 years later. *J Urol* 1986;136:769–777.
26. Elabbady A, Hassouna MM, Elhilali MM. Neural stimulation for chronic voiding dysfunction. *J Urol* 1994;152:2076–2080.
27. Chai TC, Gray ML, Steers WD. The incidence of a positive ice water test in bladder outlet obstructed patients: evidence for bladder neural plasticity. *J Urol* 1998;160:34–38.
28. Zermann DH, Ishigooka M, Doggweiler R, et al. Postoperative chronic pain and bladder dysfunction: windup and neural plasticity—do we need a more neurourological approach to pelvic surgery? *J Urol* 1998;160:102–105.
29. Zermann DH, Ishigooka M, Doggweiler R, et al. Neurologic insights into the etiology of genital urinary pain in men. *J Urol* 1999;161:903–908.
30. Kobierski LA. Cytokines and inflammation in the central nervous system. In: Borsook D, ed. *Molecular neurobiology of pain: progress in pain research and management,* vol 9. Seattle: IASP Press, 1997:45.
31. McMahon SB, Bennett DC, Koltzenburg M. The biologic effects of nerve growth factor on primary sensory neurons. In: Borsook D, ed. *Molecular neurobiology of pain: progress in pain research and management,* vol. 9. Seattle: IASP Press, 1997:59.
32. Doyle CA, Palmer JA, Munglani R, et al. Molecular neurobiology of pain: progress in pain research and management, vol 9. Borsook D, ed. *Molecular neurobiology of pain: progress in pain research and management,* vol. 9. Seattle: IASP Press, 1997:145.
33. Cerbero F. Mechanisms of visceral pain: past and present in visceral pain. In: Gebhart GF, ed. *Progress in pain research and management,* vol 5. Seattle: IASP Press, 1995:25.
34. Codderre TJ, Katz J, Vaccarino AL, et al. Contributions of central neuroplasticity to pathologic pain: review of clinical and experimental evidence. *Pain* 1993;52:259–285.
35. Schmidt Richard. Personal communication, 1999.
36. Travell JG, Simons DG. *Myofascial pain and dysfunction. The trigger point manual.* Baltimore: Williams and Wilkins, 1983.
37. Turner MLC, Marinoff SC. Pudendal neuralgia. *Am J Obstet Gynecol* 1991;165:1233–1236.
38. Mayer EA, Gebhart GF. Functional bowel disorders and the vis-

ceral hyperalgesia hypothesis. In: Mayer X, Raybould Y, eds. *Basic and clinical aspects of chronic abdominal pain.* New York: Elsevier, 1993:3.

39. Steers WD, Tuttle JB. Neurogenic inflammation and nerve growth factor: possible roles in interstitial cystitis. In: Sant GR, ed. *Interstitial cystitis.* Philadelphia: Lippincott-Raven, 1997:67.
40. Brookoff D. The causes and treatment of pain. In: Sant GR, ed. *Interstitial cystitis in interstitial cystitis.* Philadelphia: Lippincott-Raven, 1997:177–192.
41. Costello K. Myofascial syndrome. In: Steege JF, Metzger DA, Levy BS, eds. *Chronic pelvic pain: an integrated approach.* Philadelphia: WB Saunders, 1998:251.
42. Sinaki M, Merritt JL, Stillwell GK. Tension myalgia of the pelvic floor. *Mayo Clin Proc* 1977;52:717–722.
43. Laycock J. Clinical evaluations of the pelvic floor. In: Schussler B, Laycock J, Norton P, et al, eds. *Pelvic floor reeducation: principles and practice.* New York: Springer-Verlag, 1994:42–48.
44. DeRidder D, Vermeulen C, DeSmet E, et al. Clinical assessment of pelvic floor dysfunction in multiple sclerosis: urodynamic and neurologic correlates. *Neurourol Urodyn* 1998;17:532–542.
45. White G, Ven M, Jantos M, et al. Establishing the diagnosis of vulvar vestibulitis. *J Reprod Med* 1997;42:157–160.
46. Fowler CJ, Kirby RS. Electromyography of urethral sphincter in women with urinary retention. *Lancet* 1986;1(8496):1455–1457.
47. Dirk DR, Ben VC, Luc B. Sacral nerve stimulation for female urinary retention: two year follow-up. Abstract, submitted to the FDA by Medtronics, Inc., 1998.
48. Gajewski JB, Awad SA. Urodynamic evaluation. In: Sant J, ed. *Interstitial cystitis.* Philadelphia: Lippincott-Raven, 1997:169–172.
49. Brubaker LT, Sand PK. Urinary frequency and urgency. *Obstet Gynecol Clin North Am* 1989;16:883–896.
50. Weil A, Miege B, Rattenberg R, et al. Clinical significance of urethral instability. *Obstet Gynecol* 1986;68:106–110.
51. Raz S, Smith R. External sphincter spasticity syndrome in female patients. *J Urol* 1976;151:433–446.
52. Karram MM. Manometric investigation: urodynamics. In: Benson JP, ed. *Female pelvic floor disorders: investigation and management:* New York: WW Norton, 1992,100.
53. Rounazi L, Poloueczky M, Glazer HI. Submitted for publication.
54. DePaepe H, Hoebeke P, Renson C, et al. Pelvic floor therapy in girls with recurrent urinary tract infections and dysfunctional voiding. *Br J Urol* 1998;81(Suppl 3):109–113.
55. Theile GH. Coccygodynia and pain in the superior gluteal region: down the back of the thigh; causation by tonic spasm of the levator ani, coccygeus, and piriformis muscles and relief by massage of these muscles. *JAMA* 1937;109:1271–1275.
56. Nicosia JF, Abcarian H. Levator syndrome: a treatment that works. *Dis Colon Rectum* 1985;28:406–408.
57. Chancellor MR, deGroate WC. Hypotheses on how sacral nerve stimulation works for the treatment of detrusor overactivity and urinary retention. Submitted for publication.
58. Altringer W, Deziel BJ. Levator ani syndrome. In: Brubaker LT, Saclarides TJ. *The female pelvic floor: disorders of function and support.* Philadelphia: FA Davis, 1996:146–150.
59. Medtronic Neurological, Minneapolis, MN. Data submitted to FDA, 1998.
60. Thon WF, Baskin LS, Jonas U, eds. Neuromodulation of voiding dysfunction and pelvic pain. *World J Urol* 1991;9:138.
61. Elabbady AA, Hassouna MM, Elhilali MM. Neural stimulation for chronic voiding dysfunction. *J Urol* 1994;52:2076.
62. Shaker HS, Hassouna M. Sacral root neuromodulation in idiopathic non-obstructive chronic urinary retention. *J Urol* 1998;159:1476–1478.
63. Dijkema HE, Weil EHJ, Mijs PT, et al. Neuromodulation of sacral nerves for incontinence and voiding dysfunction. *Eur Urol* 1993;24:72.
64. Schurch B, Hauri D, Rodic B, et al. Botulinum-A toxin as a treatment of detrusor–sphincter dyssynergia: a prospective study of 24 spinal cord injury patients. *J Urol* 1996;155:1023–1029.
65. Petit H, Wiart L, Gaujard E, et al. Botulinum-A toxin: treatment for detrusor–sphincter dyssynergia in spinal cord disease. *Spinal Cord* 1998;36:91–94.
66. Steinhardt GF, Naseer S, Cruz OA. Botulinum toxin: novel treatment for dramatic urethral dilation associated with dysfunctional voiding. *J Urol* 1997;58:190–191.
67. Benson Tomas. Personal communication, 1999.

36

URETHRAL DIVERTICULUM

CHARLES W. BUTRICK

KEY TERMS AND DEFINITIONS

Diverticulectomy: Classic surgical procedure to excise a urethral diverticulum and close the resultant defect.

Pseudodiverticulum: A suburethral extension of the urethral mucosa through a suburethral fascial defect. While clinically there appears to be a typical urethral diverticulum, this is in fact a new class of diverticuli that requires a different approach to their successful repair.

Skenes gland cyst: The most commonly misdiagnosed suburethral mass.

Spence procedure: Simple outpatient surgical procedure to eradicate a distal urethral diverticulum. Major advantages of technical ease, high success rate, and rare complications.

Urethral diverticulum: Typically symptomatic, but at times asymptomatic, suburethral mass that requires careful evaluation prior to surgical intervention. They can be congenital, infectious, or iatrogenic in their origins.

Voiding cystourethrogram: Radiologic evaluation that depends on the filling of the diverticulum during the voiding phase of the study.

INTRODUCTION

Since the first female urethral diverticulum was described by Hey in 1805 (1), the frequency of diagnosis has been steadily increasing. Increased physician awareness of this problem and improved diagnostic techniques are two primary factors that have contributed to the increasing incidence of diagnosis. As recently as 1953, Novack reported that "this (urethral diverticula) is a relatively rare condition and no gynecologist will see more than a few in a lifetime" (2). It took the development of positive pressure urethrography by Davis and Scian (3) in 1956 to demonstrate that urethral diverticuli are relatively common (up to 3% of asymptomatic women) and can often be seen in patients with persistent lower urinary tract symptoms (up to 40% of patients with chronic urgency/frequency syndrome will have a urethral diverticulum). They are not commonly a cause of chronic pelvic pain (CPP), but occasionally a

woman with a diverticulum will have CPP as a component of her symptomatology or the diverticulum will be a contributor to or component of the woman's pain milieu.

ETIOLOGY

Multiple theories exist concerning the etiology of urethral diverticuli. They can be divided into three categories: congenital, infectious, and traumatic (Table 36.1). To date, only a small number of congenital lesions have been seen, and these typically present as a cystic lesion in the periurethral area of a newborn. The etiology of these lesions includes remnants of Gartners duct (4), faulty union of primal folds (5), and vaginal wall cysts of müllerian origins (6). The most common congenital diverticulum seen in a child under 4 years of age is an ectopic ureter that implants in the urethra or the periurethral tissue (7).

Most patients with urethral diverticuli acquire them and present between the ages of 30 and 50. These acquired urethral diverticuli are a result of an infectious process that was first described by Routh in 1890 (8) and further described by MacKinnon et al. in 1959 (9). The pathophysiology of

TABLE 36.1. ETIOLOGIES OF URETHRAL DIVERTICULI

Congenital Urethral Diverticuli
Gartners duct remnants
Faulty union of primordial folds
Cell nests
Congenital dilation of periurethral cysts
Urethral insertion of ectopic ureter
Infectious Urethral Diverticuli
Infection of periurethral glands with rupture into urethral lumen
Traumatic Urethral Diverticulum
Prior diverticulectomy
Anterior colporrhaphy
Needle bladder neck suspension
Repeated catheterization

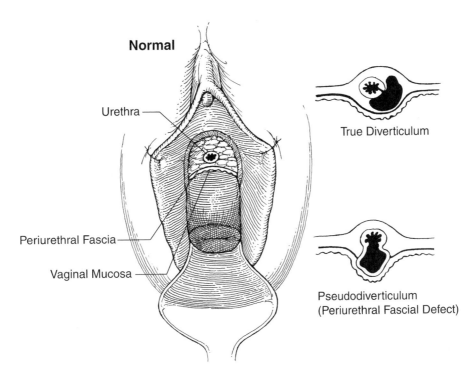

FIGURE 36.1. Urethral diverticulum. Upper figure illustrates normal urethral anatomy; lower two figures illustrate true urethral diverticulum and pseudodiverticulum. Note that a true diverticulum has intact periurethral fascia, whereas pseudodiverticulum has a periurethral fascial defect.

these acquired lesions begins with an infection of the periurethral glands with inflammation and subsequent obstruction. This obstruction leads to abscess formation that subsequently ruptures into the urethral lumen. Common offending organisms include gonococci, *Escherichia coli*, *Chlamydia*, and *Trachomatis*.

Leng and McGuire (10) have proposed an additional category which is traumatic in origin. They described this diverticulum to be a pseudodiverticulum. Although this is less frequent than the typical diverticulum, it represents an iatrogenic defect in the suburethral fascia and its management requires repairing this defect; therefore, preoperative identification is imperative. This can occur as a result of either a prior bladder neck suspension (retropubic or transvaginal needle suspension) or a prior urethral diverticulectomy. In both these circumstances there has been a potential disruption of the suburethral fascia with a herniation of the urethral mucosa through this fascial defect, the result being a pseudodiverticulum (Fig. 36.1). The importance of this new category of urethral diverticuli is in its preoperative identification so that appropriate surgical therapy can be undertaken (see Table 36.2). During the surgical repair of a pseudodiverticulum, meticulous correction of the fascial defect is the desired surgical goal. Leng and McGuire (10) have suggested that in those patients with concomitant stress incontinence or where the defect is particularly large, a suburethral sling is ideally suited to help support the surgical repair of this fascial defect and correct the concomitant stress urinary incontinence.

TABLE 36.2. DISTINGUISHING CHARACTERISTICS OF TRUE URETHRAL DIVERTICULUM VERSUS PSEUDODIVERTICULUM (10)

True Diverticulum	Pseudodiverticulum
No prior urethral surgery	History of urethral surgery
Chronic recurrent symptoms of urgency, dysuria, dyspareunia,and dribbling	Relatively few voiding symptoms
Chronic lower urinary tract infections	More likely to have concomitant stress incontinence
Narrow-neck ostium at times not readily apparent on radiography or cystoscopy	Cystoscopy demonstrates a broad-mouth ostium with apparent distention of the urethral lumen

From Leng WW, McGuire EJ. Management of female urethral diverticulum: a new classification. *J Urol* 1998;160:1297–1300, with permission.

SYMPTOMS OR HISTORY

The most common symptoms seen in patients with urethral diverticula are those of recurrent urinary tract infections. These symptoms include urgency, frequency, and dysuria. Additionally, pelvic pain and dyspareunia are not uncommonly seen (Table 36.3) (11). Urinary incontinence and postvoid dribbling occur in 30% to 70% of patients with urethral diverticuli (12,13).

SIGNS OR EXAMINATION

The majority of urethral diverticuli are located in the middle or distal third of the urethra (this distribution correlates with the location and distribution of the periurethral glands) (14). Physical findings are a tender suburethral mass in 10% to 12% of patients and suppurative material that can be expressed from the urethra in approximately 7% of cases (15,16). As noted earlier, it is not uncommon to find a diverticulum that originates posteriorly and extends anteriorly to almost encircle the entire urethra. Davis and Telinde (17) found that 63% of their cases of diverticuli were suspected due to physical findings. Up to 10% of patients have calculi within the diverticuli; and when calculi are present, they are often associated with significant tenderness and chronic infections. One should always consider the diagnosis of urethral diverticuli in a patient with persistent urinary tract symptoms with or without the findings of a suburethral mass. However, a high index of suspicion is the key to diagnosis in symptomatic patients due to the relatively high incidence of negative physical findings in patients who are found to have radiologic evidence of diverticuli.

TABLE 36.3. PRESENTING SYMPTOMS IN PTS* WITH URETHRAL DIVERTICULA (11)

Symptom	Number of Patients[a]	Percentage
Vaginal dryness	68	10
Dysuria	381	56
Frequency/urgency	387	57
Recurrent infections	190	28
Dyspareunia	136	20
Urethral pain	127	19
Hypogastric pain	46	7
Postvoid pain or dribbling	127	19
Hematuria	119	18
Stress incontinence	187	28
Urge incontinence	15	2
Urethral discharge	18	3
No symptoms	14	2

*PTS, pelvic floor trauma symptoms.
[a]In the nine series a total number of 676 patients were studied, many of whom presented with more than one symptom. From Leach GE, Bavendam TG. Female urethral diverticulum. *Urology* 1987;30:407, with permission.

DIAGNOSTIC STUDIES

Positive-pressure urethography using a Davis or Tratner catheter is the gold standard in radiologic evaluation for urethral diverticuli (Fig. 36.2). The double-balloon catheter occludes the urethra at the bladder neck and the external urethral meatus so contrast instilled through a lumen located between the two occluding balloons fills the urethra and any urethral diverticulum that has an ostium in communication with the urethral lumen. Voiding cystourethrography is another commonly used radiographic test; but because it depends on the chance filling of the diverticulum during voiding, it is less reliable and demonstrates only 65% of urethral diverticuli that can be seen by positive-pressure urethography. Noncommunicating suburethral masses such as Skenes glands cysts or retention cysts cannot be imaged with either technique. Up to 10% of diverticuli also contain calculi; and when these are present, they improve the diagnostic accuracy of x-ray diagnostic studies.

High-resolution magnetic resonance imaging (MRI), especially using intravaginal coils, appears to be one of the best minimally invasive techniques to evaluate the extent and location of urethral diverticula, because retropubic anatomy can be accurately delineated. It does not have the potential artifact or discomfort that is frequently associated with positive-pressure urethography. This is important also because not all periurethral masses are diverticuli that can be filled with contrast media using double-balloon radiologic techniques.

With the development of high-resolution sonographic transducers, transvaginal sonography has become a valuable technique for the evaluation of any suburethral mass (18,19). A combination of transvaginal, transperitoneal, and transurethral sonography is as effective as voiding cystourethrography in identifying urethral diverticula (20). Additionally, sonography more completely delineates the morphology of the diverticula, including the location of the ostium, the number of diverticula, the presence of any loculations, and whether the diverticulum is filled with debris. One study of sonography showed that 60% of the urethral diverticuli wrapped around at least half of the urethral circumference (18). The sensitivity of sonography may be improved by having the patient void just prior to the study so that the diverticulum will fill with urine and be more easily seen. Sonography is also able to image structures that do not communicate with the urethral lumen, such as periurethral or Skenes gland cysts or solid masses such as a periurethral leiomyomas. Sonography may also be useful during the surgical repair of urethral diverticula to verify complete resection. At the present time, transurethral sonography is a research tool and is too costly to be used on a regular basis.

Urodynamic testing is indicated in patients with stress urinary incontinence, especially prior to any surgical treatment. Although the urethral pressure profile may show a

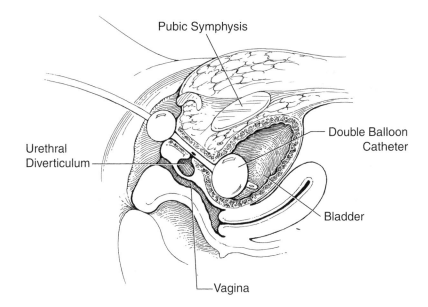

Pubic Symphysis

Double Balloon
Catheter

Urethral
Diverticulum

Bladder

Vagina

FIGURE 36.2. Illustration of catheter placement for positive-pressure urethography in the radiologic evaluation for urethral diverticuli. The double-balloon catheter occludes the urethra at the bladder neck and the external urethral meatus, so contrast instilled through a lumen located between the two occluding balloons fills the urethra and the urethral diverticulum via the ostium that is in communication with the urethral lumen.

dip in urethral pressure when the transurethral catheter is brought across the ostium of the diverticulum (21,22), urodynamic evaluation is not a reliable diagnostic approach. The major benefits of urodynamic testing in a woman with a urethral diverticulum are to show if there is concomitant genuine stress urinary incontinence and assist in determining the exact location of the diverticulum. If a complex dissection around the sphincteric mechanism is required, concomitant stress incontinence may be alleviated at the time of the surgical treatment of the urethral diverticulum.

The best test for diagnosing urethral diverticula is unclear. Voiding cystourethrography is a simple radiologic test, but it has a false-negative rate of approximately 35% (23). With double-balloon retrograde studies the false-negative rates are thought to be approximately 10%, and these studies only delineate diverticuli and are not be helpful in the evaluation of a suburethral mass that does not communicate with the urethra. Additionally, positive-pressure urethography is technically challenging and is often uncomfortable for patients who have significant urethral tenderness. Urethroscopy is sometimes useful; Robertson reports that multiple ostia can be found in up to 50% of patients evaluated by urethroscopy. However, this is an invasive approach, and it is easy to fail to visualize the ostium and miss the diagnosis. Transvaginal sonography is a simple, minimally invasive technique that adds significantly to the evaluation of patients with suspected urethral diverticuli and in the evaluation of any patient with a suburethral mass. In more complex cases—for example, when there is evidence of diverticuli located within the proximal urethra—a high-resolution MRI is often helpful. When vaginal coils can be used, MRI has superb resolution in the periurethral area and may represent the best approach to

delineate the full extent and the number of diverticuli. If MRI using intravaginal coils is not available, transvaginal sonography in the hands of an experienced radiologist may be the best approach to the evaluation of urethral diverticuli and suburethral masses.

To summarize, in a patient whose clinical presentation by history and/or physical examination is suggestive of a urethral diverticulum, a simple screening study such as a transvaginal sonogram of the urethra is very helpful. Further information can be gained by performance of a double-balloon positive pressure urethrogram or by transurethral sonography if it is available. High-resolution MRI is ideally suited for the more complex case or proximal urethral diverticulum that can be more difficult to delineate on routine evaluation. Urethroscopy is best reserved for use at the time of surgical intervention to further delineate the morphology of the diverticulum and the location of its ostium in reference to the urethra and the bladder neck. In addition, this intraoperative evaluation verifies that you are not dealing with a pseudodiverticulum. Any patient with complaints of incontinence should be evaluated preoperatively by urodynamic testing so that appropriate surgical interventions can be planned.

DIAGNOSIS

There are a number of periurethral lesions that can present in a manner similar to that of a urethral diverticulum. Most present as periurethral masses and may be mistaken as a urethral diverticulum if there is a lack of familiarity with the differential diagnosis of periurethral masses.

A *urethral caruncle* is a common lesion in postmenopausal, hypoestrogenic women. The exact incidence is not known, but in postmenopausal women it is the most common lesion located at the urethral meatus. Urethral caruncles present as a soft exophytic lesion, typically arising from the inferior margin of the meatus. At times it will be erythematous, hemorrhagic, and pedunculated. If symptomatic, it presents with dysuria, hematuria, and dyspareunia. When treated conservatively with Sitz baths and topical estrogen vaginal cream, resolution is typically seen within 4 to 6 weeks. However, when this does not occur all tissue should be excised and examined histologically to rule out dysplasia or an occult carcinoma (24).

Mucosal prolapse represents a circumferential eversion of the distal urethral epithelium and occurs in two distinct populations: prepubertal black girls and postmenopausal white women. Chronic Valsalva maneuvers, as with chronic voiding dysfunction or chronic constipation, and the changes associated with hypoestrogenic atrophic vaginitis result in a separation of the muscular lamina of the urethral wall and the urethral mucosa. Presenting symptoms include hematuria, urethral bleeding, irritative voiding symptoms, and at times a painless urethral mass. Demonstration of complete circumferential eversion of the urethral mucosa is the key finding on physical examination. This mucosa is often edematous, friable, and occasionally ischemic. Management with Sitz baths and topical estrogen usually results in resolution within 4 to 6 weeks.

A *Skenes gland abscess* presents as a painful mass eccentric and lateral to the urethral meatus. Additional symptoms include dysuria, dyspareunia, and obstructive voiding. Pressure on the tender, erythematous, fluctuate mass will at times express fluid and suppurative material from the ductal opening just inside the urethral meatus. Because of this eccentric position, consideration of the lesion actually being a prolapsed ureterocele (typically seen in young, prepubescent women) mandates an intravenous pyelogram (IVP) prior to surgical excision.

Prolapse of a ureterocele should be considered primarily in the differential diagnosis of periurethral masses in prepubescent girls, but it has been reported in four adults (25). A ureterocele may prolapse through the meatus, or it may arise at a location external to the meatus. The prolapse may also be intermittent in nature. Symptoms include hematuria, interrupted urinary stream, urinary retention, and pain. The definitive test in delineating this unusual congenital abnormality is an IVP. In addition to the ectopic ureter, 90% of patients will also show an ipsilateral duplication.

Paraurethral inclusion cysts arise from either urethral or vaginal wall cysts. They also may represent remnants of the mesonephric system and are typically asymptomatic lesions that do not require intervention. Solid periurethral lesions have been described and include *fibromas, leiomyomas,* and various *malignant lesions* including *squamous cell carcinoma, adenocarcinoma,* and *transitional cell carcinoma.* Leiomyomas can occur anywhere within the submucosa of the vagina because this is a layer made up of fibromuscular tissue and leiomyomas are benign smooth muscle tumors. While often asymptomatic, these lesions can produce dyspareunia and obstruction of the genital or urinary tracts. These lesions are usually solitary in nature. Solid vaginal and periurethral lesions can be identified by transvaginal ultrasound and because of the potential for malignancy in a solid lesion, excision is always required.

Lesions in anterior vaginal wall can arise from either the vaginal or the urethral tissues. Cysts arising within the vaginal wall are classified according to their histologic appearance: mesonephric origins (i.e., Gartners duct remnants), endometriotic origins (often with pronounced hemorrhagic changes), and epidermoid origins (i.e., stratified squamous lining which is usually from areas of prior trauma). These cysts are typically asymptomatic but can cause obstructive and irritative urinary symptoms. It is essential that these lesions be evaluated to rule out urethral diverticuli. Gartners duct cysts occur in 1% of all women and are diagnosed by their typical location on the anterolateral aspect of the anterior vaginal wall. There is a tendency for Gartners duct cysts to be on the left side. While it is rare, occasionally ureteral ectopia into the cyst can be seen thus requiring upper tract assessment to verify normal ureteral position and renal function.

MANAGEMENT OR TREATMENT

Medical Treatment

The mainstay of therapy for urethral diverticuli is surgical. However, asymptomatic urethral diverticuli without evidence of stones or tumors do not require surgical intervention. Occasionally, small symptomatic diverticuli will respond to minimal intervention, thus avoiding the trauma and potential complications of surgery. These therapies include antibiotics for 10 to 14 days, gentle urethral dilation, and vaginal estrogen cream in patients who demonstrate atrophy of the lower urogenital tract.

Surgical Treatment

There are several surgical procedures that have been described for the treatment of symptomatic urethral diverticuli. Most symptomatic diverticuli are treated with either the Spence procedure or a classic diverticulectomy. Tancer et al. (26) have advocated a partial ablation procedure with excellent results. Spencer and Streem (27) have recommended an endoscopic technique with a pediatric resectoscope in cases of diverticuli of the roof of the urethra, which is a very unusual location for a urethral diverticulum. Lapides has described a technique of transurethral sauceration in patients who have had multiple recurrent diverticuli that have failed previous surgical intervention (28).

Spence Procedure

This is the procedure of choice when the diverticulum is located in the distal third of the urethra (29). The more distal, the easier this technique is to accomplish. The Spence procedure is simply a marsupialization of the diverticulum into the meatus. It can be performed as an outpatient procedure under local anesthesia, and postoperative catheterization is not required. To perform the procedure, one blade of a pair of a Metzenbaum scissors is placed into the urethra with the tip at the ostium of the diverticulum while the other blade of the scissors is placed along the anterior wall of the vagina under the urethra and diverticulum. The tissue between the blades thus includes the floor of the urethra, the diverticular wall, and the vaginal mucosa overlying the diverticulum (Fig. 36.3). Cutting this tissue opens the diverticulum. Then its edges are approximated to the vaginal mucosa; so that it is marsupialized in such a way that the urethral meatus and the diverticulum become one structure. The end result is a large meatoplasty. Within 2 months this usually retracts, giving the appearance of a relatively normal urethral meatus. There are no significant complications with this procedure other than mild stress incontinence, which occurs in less than 2% of cases. This readily responds to simple nonsurgical therapy. Because of its ease, its 100% success rate, and its very low complication rate, the Spence procedure is the procedure of choice for distal urethral diverticuli.

Diverticulectomy

Classic surgical resection of a diverticulum is the procedure of choice for those lesions in the mid or proximal one-third of the urethra. Because of the proximity of the muscular and neurologic components of urinary continence, a careful historical and urodynamic evaluation is mandatory in order to develop a surgical management plan that will not result in postoperative incontinence. The procedure begins with a submucosal injection of 0.5% bupivicaine with epinephrine to aid in the dissection. Dissection is often difficult due to the normal fusion of the suburethral tissues to the vaginal mucosa, the associated inflammation and infection, and the tendency of the diverticulum to partially surround the urethra or extend up toward the bladder base. Basic principles of fistula surgery prevail—that is, adequate dissection and closure in a layered technique with minimal tissue tension. With these principles in mind, the ideal dissection attempts to locate the diverticular sac and proceeds between the sac and the periurethral fascia. Preservation of this fascia allows its use in a layered, tension-free closure. To facilitate this dissection, many authors advocate a small incision in the diverticular sac. Then a small pediatric or Fogarty catheter can be inflated within the diverticulum. This allows gentle traction and facilitates the dissection of the diverticular sac from the periurethral fascia. Once good exposure of the diverticulum is obtained, the sac can be opened further to delineate the ostium. At this point the sac is resected and closure is begun. First the urethral defect is closed with a fine absorbable suture followed by reapproximation of the periurethral fascia that was recovered from the dissection of the diverticular sac. If available, normal periurethral fascia on each side of the urethra can often be added to this closure. A fine, delayed-absorbable suture is used for this closure. Finally, the vagi-

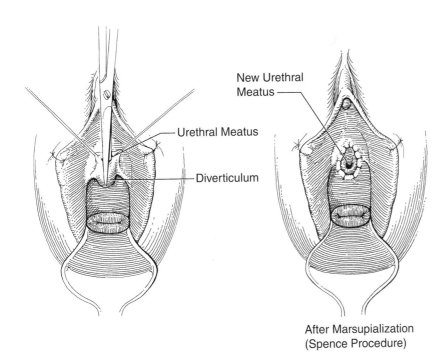

New Urethral Meatus

Urethral Meatus

Diverticulum

After Marsupialization (Spence Procedure)

FIGURE 36.3. The Spence procedure. This is a marsupialization of the diverticulum into the meatus. It can be performed when the diverticulum is in the distal third of the urethra. One blade of a pair of a Metzenbaum scissors is placed into the urethra with the tip at the ostium of the diverticulum, and the other blade of the scissors is placed along the anterior wall of the vagina under the urethra and diverticulum. Cutting this tissue opens the diverticulum. Then its edges are approximated to the vaginal mucosa; so that the urethral meatus and the diverticulum become one structure. The end result is a large meatoplasty. Within 2 months this usually retracts, giving the appearance of a relatively normal urethral meatus.

nal mucosa is closed with interrupted sutures verifying that the defect is hemostatic before the final closure. With complex repairs, closing the vaginal tissue using a "double-breasted" flap technique has the theoretical advantage of avoiding overlying suture lines (Fig. 36.4). Postoperatively, a transurethral catheter is left in place for 7 to 14 days, with the duration of bladder drainage based on the complexity of the case and the "tissue quality." In complicated cases a postoperative voiding cystourethrogram can be used to verify no extravasation of contrast material at the site of reconstruction.

Adjuncts to diverticulectomy include perioperative antibiotics, good lighting, irrigation (especially in cases where the diverticulum is filled with purulent material), and iris scissors or other small delicate scissors for dissection. Siegel (18) has suggested the intraoperative use of transurethral sonography so that complex, loculated or encircling diverticuli can be carefully evaluated prior to and at the end of the clinical resection of diverticuli. With intraoperative transurethral sonography it may be possible to verify total resection of the diverticulum. This is particularly important in patients who have had a recurrent diverticulum or are presenting with a particularly complex diverticulum.

Diverticulectomy can have a complication rate as high as 17%. The most common complication is recurrent urinary tract infections, which is reported in 5% of patients. Urethrovaginal fistulas occur in 4% of cases. Persistent or recurrent diverticuli complicate 4% of cases. Postoperative stress incontinence is seen in at least 2% of patients, with those having diverticuli involving the area of the proximal urethra being at greatest risk for postoperative stress incontinence (30). If surgical treatment is done without a thorough preoperative evaluation of symptoms of incontinence, then postoperative stress incontinence may be as high as 12% to 15% (31,32).

To avoid this complication, it is important to thoroughly evaluate the type and degree of any incontinence preoperatively. Recent studies report incontinence rates in patients with urethral diverticuli to be as high as 32% to 71%. The evaluation of stress urinary incontinence preoperatively allows a surgical approach that will eliminate the stress incontinence and the diverticulum. This evaluation will occasionally demonstrate urge incontinence or detru-

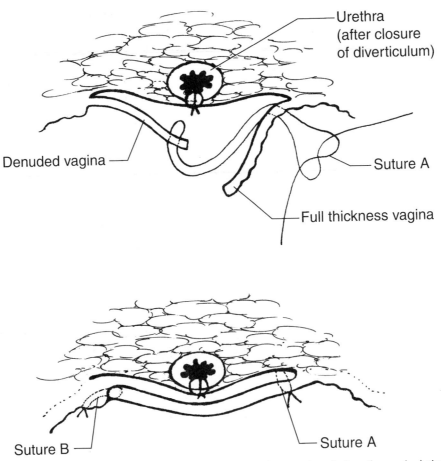

FIGURE 36.4. Double-breasted flap closure. With complex repairs, closing the vaginal tissue using a double-breasted flap technique has the theoretical advantage of avoiding overlying suture lines.

TABLE 36.4. DIFFERENTIAL DIAGNOSIS OF PERIURETHRAL MASSES (33)

Differential Diagnosis of Meatal/Perimeatal Lesions

Lesion	Location	Presentation	Comments
Caruncle	Inferior to meatus	Asymptomatic or dysuria/pain with ischemic mucosal changes	Postmenopausal age group
Skenes gland abscess	Inferior and lateral to meatus	Painful; orifice of duct visible at urethral meatus	—
Mucosal prolapse	Circumferential mucosal prolapse	Pain and dysuria; ischemic mucosal changes	Young girls or postmenopausal women
Prolapsed ureterocele	Submeatal or prolapsed through meatus	Glistening mucosa; may be ischemic; may be asymptomatic	IVP[a] to evaluate upper tract status

Differential Diagnostic Considerations for Urethral and Anterior Vaginal Wall Lesions

Lesion	Location	Symptoms or Physical Findings	Cystoscopic and Radiographic Findings	Comments
Urethral diverticulum	Anterior vaginal wall, midline	Urinary tract infection, dysuria, dyspareunia, postvoid dribbling, cystic mass	Orifice of diverticulum visible on urethral floor, voiding cystourethrography opacifies lesion	May be multilocular
Vaginal wall cyst	Anterior vaginal wall, midline or eccentric	Cystic mass may be multiloculated	Absence of or extrinsic compression	—
Gartners duct cyst	Anterolateral vaginal wall	Cystic mass	Absence of or extrinsic compression, IVP may indicate ectopic ureteral drainage	Rule out ureteral ectopia before excision
Leiomyoma; hamartoma	Vaginal wall	Solid mass	None or extrinsic compression	Rule out malignancy

[a]IVP, intravenous pyelogram.
From Dmochowski RR, Ganabathi K, Zimmern PE, et al. Benign female periurethral lesions. *J Urol* 1994;152:1943, with permission.

sor instability. This knowledge allows aggressive postoperative treatment of uninhibited detrusor contractions so they do not disrupt the surgical repair. Patients with mild genuine stress incontinence who have a large diverticulum in the proximal half of the urethra are at great risk for developing a worsening of their stress incontinence after the urethral diverticulectomy. Because of this, many authors advocate surgical treatment specifically for genuine stress incontinence at the time of removal of the diverticulum. This is especially important in patients who manifest significant urethral hypermobility preoperatively. By performing a simultaneous bladder neck suspension and classic diverticulectomy in patients who had both genuine stress incontinence and a diverticulum, Dmochowski et al. (33) showed a postoperative stress incontinence in only 1 out of 22 patients. Leng and McGuire (10) recommend placement of a fascial sling due to its higher long-term success rate for the treatment of stress incontinence and its benefit in treating the fascial defect described in patients with large pseudodiverticuli.

KEY POINTS

Differential Diagnoses

- Urethral caruncle
- Urethral mucosal prolapse
- Skenes gland abscess
- Prolapse of a ureterocele
- Paraurethral inclusion cysts
- Fibroma
- Leiomyoma

- Squamous cell carcinoma
- Adenocarcinoma
- Transitional cell carcinoma
- Gartners duct cyst
- Endometriotic cyst
- Epidermoid cyst

Most Important Questions to Ask

- Do you have urgency or frequency of urination?
- Do you have pain with urination?
- Do you have pain with intercourse? If so, when does this happen?
- Do you have dribbling of urine after voiding?

Most Important Physical Examination Findings

- Tender suburethral mass
- Suppurative material expressed from the urethra

Most Important Diagnostic Studies

- Positive-pressure urethography using a double-balloon catheter
- Voiding cystourethrography
- High-resolution magnetic resonance imaging
- Transvaginal sonography
- Urodynamic testing (with stress urinary incontinence)

Treatments

- Antibiotics for 10 to 14 days
- Gentle urethral dilation
- Vaginal estrogen cream
- Spence procedure
- Diverticulectomy
- Partial ablation procedure

REFERENCES

1. Hey W. *Practical observations in surgery.* Philadelphia: Jay Humphries, 1805.
2. Novack R. Editorial comments. *Obstet Gynecol Surv* 1953; 8:423.
3. Davis HJ, Cian LG. Positive pressure urethrography: a new diagnostic test for urethral diverticuli. *J Urol* 1956;75:753–757.
4. Johnson CM. Diverticula and cysts and of the female urethra. *J Urol* 1938;39:506–516.
5. Vanhoutte JJ. Ureteral ectopia into a Wolffian duct remnant presenting as a urethral diverticulum in two girls. *Am J Roentgenol Radium Ther Nucl Med* 1970;110:540–545.
6. McMahon SJ. Congenital diverticulum of the female urethral. *J Urol* 1946;55:69–72.
7. Ward JN, Patel NP, Levengood RW. Ectopic urethral ureter in the adult female. *Surg Gynecol Obstet* 1976;143:770–774.
8. Routh A. Urethral diverticula. *Br Med J* 1890;1:361.
9. MacKinnon M, Pratt JA, Pool TL. Diverticulum of the female urethra. *Surg Clin North Am* 1959;39:953–962.
10. Leng WW, McGuire EJ. Management of female urethral diverticulum: a new classification. *J Urol* 1998;160:1297–1300.
11. Leach GE, Bavendam TG. Female urethral diverticulum. *Urology* 1987;30:407–415.
12. Bass JF, Leach GE. Surgical treatment of concomitant urethral diverticula and stress incontinence. *Urol Clin North Am* 1991; 18:365–375.
13. Swierzewski SJ III, McGuire EJ. Pubovaginal sling for treatment of female stress urinary incontinence complicated by urethral diverticulum. *J Urol* 1993;149:1012–1014.
14. Leach GE, Bavendam TG. Female urethral diverticula. *Urol* 1987;30:407–415.
15. Davis BL, Robinson DG. Diverticula of the female urethra: assay of 120 cases. *J Urol* 1970;104:850–853.
16. Hajj SN, Evans MI. Diverticula of the female urethra. *Am J Obstet Gynecol* 1980;136:335–338.
17. Davis HJ, Telinde RW. Urethral diverticula: assay of 121 cases. *J Urol* 1958;80:34–39.
18. Siegel CL, Mittleton WD, Teesey SA, et al. Sonography of the female urethra. *Am J Roentgenol* 1998;170:1269–1274.
19. Lee TG, Keller FS. Urethral diverticulum: diagnosis by ultrasound. *Am J Roentgenol* 1977;128:690–691.
20. Baert L, Willemen P, Oyen R. Endovaginal sonography: new diagnostic approach for urethral diverticula. *J Urol* 1992;157: 464–466.
21. Bhatia NN, McCarthy TA, Ostergard DR. Urethral pressure profiles of women with urethral diverticuli. *Ob/Gyn* 1981;58: 375–378.
22. Bright TC. Urethral pressure profile: current concepts. *J Urol* 1977;118:418–422.
23. Drutz HP. Urethral diverticula. *Obstet Gynecol Clin North Am* 1989;16:923–929.
24. Marshall PC, Uson AC, Melicow MM. Neoplasms and caruncles of the female urethra. *Surg Gynecol Obstet* 1960;110:723–733.
25. Miller MAW, Cornaby AJ, Nathan MS, et al. Prolapsed ureterocele: a rare vulvar mass. *Br J Urol* 1994;73:109–110.
26. Tancer NL, Nooppan MM, Pierre-Louis C, et al. Suburethral diverticulum treated by partial ablation. *Obstet Gynecol* 1983;62: 511–513.
27. Spencer WF, Streem SB. Diverticulum of the female urethral root managed endoscopically. *J Urol* 1987;138:147–148.
28. Lapides J. Transurethral treatment of urethral diverticula in women. *Trans-American Association GU Surg* 1979;70:135–137.
29. Spence HM, Duckett JW. Diverticulum of the female urethra: clinical aspects and presentation of a single operative technique for care. *J Urol* 1970;104:432–437.
30. Ginsburg DF, Genadry R. Suburethral diverticulum in the female. *Obstet Gynecol Surv* 1984;39:1–7.
31. Ward JN, Draper JW, Tovell HM. Diagnosis and treatment of urethral diverticula in the female. *Surg Gynecol Obstet* 1967;127: 1293–1300.
32. Lee RA. Diverticulum of the urethra: clinical presentation, diagnosis and management. *Clin Obstet Gynecol* 1984;127:490–498.
33. Dmochowski RR, Ganabathi K, Zimmern PE, et al. Benign female periurethral lesions. *J Urol* 1994;152:1943–1951.

37

CHRONIC URETHRAL SYNDROME

FRED M. HOWARD

KEY TERMS AND DEFINITIONS

Acute urethral syndrome: Painful and frequent urination of less than 3 weeks' duration. It is distinguished from acute cystitis in that a voided urine is sterile or has less than 100,000 microorganisms per milliliter.

Chronic urethral syndrome: Persistent or recurrent dysuria and frequency, with associated pelvic pain, suprapubic pain, dyspareunia, or urinary urgency and negative cultures of urine and urethra.

INTRODUCTION

Chronic urethral syndrome is characterized by persistent or recurrent dysuria and frequency, with associated pelvic pain, suprapubic pain, dyspareunia, or urinary urgency. Acute urethral syndrome is similarly characterized by painful and frequent urination, but the duration is less than 3 weeks. Both acute and chronic urethral syndromes are distinguished from acute cystitis in that a voided urine is sterile or has less than 100,000 microorganisms per milliliter with either urethral syndrome. Acute and chronic urethral syndromes appear to be quite different diseases, without any specific relationship to one another. Acute urethral syndrome does not precede, precipitate, or predispose to chronic urethral syndrome. With antibiotic therapy a specific infectious etiology for acute urethral syndrome can generally be determined and a cure can be effected. Urine cultures are sterile with chronic urethral syndrome, and usually no specific etiology is found. In spite of many recommended therapies, cure is often difficult to obtain.

Dysuria and frequency account for more than 5,000,000 office visits per year in the United States. Most of these patients have acute cystitis or acute urethral syndrome. What percentage have chronic urethral syndrome is not known.

ETIOLOGY

An etiology for chronic urethral syndrome is usually not found. Cultures are uniformly negative, but there is evidence that at least in some cases infection may have an underlying role. This is not particularly surprising because the urethra has an important role in prevention of ascending bacterial infection (1). Normally, in the distal urethra there are an average of six to eight species of bacteria, but in the proximal urethra there are none. The mid-urethra has a high-pressure zone that functions as a mechanical barrier to bacterial ascent. Additionally, the posterior urethral glands produce mucus that serves as a barrier by trapping bacteria and by activity of immunoglobulin A. Evidence of chronic inflammation or infection in chronic urethral syndrome is suggested by the progressive structural and inflammatory changes that are sometimes found histologically in the periurethral glands. However, these structural and inflammatory changes are not always present, suggesting that even if chronic infection has a role, it is not the only etiology.

In many cases of chronic urethral syndrome, urethral spasm and irritability of the external urethral sphincter can be urodynamically demonstrated (2). Both the smooth and skeletal muscles of the urethra are involved in this spasticity. Concomitant pelvic floor spasm or tension may also occur. Several voiding abnormalities may result: (a) high resting urethral tone, (b) increased mean and maximal urethral closure pressures, (c) inability to voluntary relax the urethra, (d) incomplete funneling of the bladder neck, (e) distal urethral narrowing, and (f) intermittent urinary flow patterns. These changes account for many of the symptoms of chronic urethral syndrome, particularly dysuria, frequency, and postcoital voiding dysfunction. Pain may occur due to urethral spasticity and coincident stimulation of the pelvic muscle spindles with increased pelvic floor tension. Increased pelvic floor tension may result in pelvic muscular dysfunction and dyspareunia. Prolonged spasticity and increased tone may produce periurethral, urethral, or levator ani muscle fatigue with resultant chronic pelvic pain. However, none of this addresses the underlying cause of the urethral spasticity and irritability. It has been suggested that high tone of the pelvic floor musculature and external urethral sphincter can be due to introital infections, urethral infection, urethral diverticulae, hemorrhoids, anal fissure, vaginitis, pelvic inflammatory disease, or traumatic intercourse (3). How much these etiologies contribute to pain with chronic urethral syndrome is not clear.

Biopsychosocial factors influence the course of the disease and potentially could have an etiologic role. Another hypothesis is that due to anatomic, physiologic, or psychologic factors, some women are susceptible to repetitive urethral trauma with intercourse, and this plays the causative role in establishing urethral syndrome and producing its symptoms (4).

SYMPTOMS OR HISTORY

The classic symptoms of chronic urethral syndrome are urinary urgency, frequency, sensation of incomplete emptying, suprapubic pain, and dysuria (4). Other symptoms of chronic urethral syndrome include postvoiding fullness and incomplete voiding, urge or stress incontinence, voiding difficulties (especially postcoitally), suprapubic pain, low back pain, pelvic pain, or vaginal pain (Table 37.1). Dysmenorrhea is not present with chronic urethral syndrome. Dyspareunia is common with chronic urethral syndrome and generally localizes to the anterior vagina. Coitus also often causes voiding dysfunction, burning dysuria, or urgency (4). A history of treatment of recurrent urinary tract infections without documentation of positive cultures is typical with chronic urethral syndrome. Nocturia may be present, but is usually limited to the early nighttime.

SIGNS OR PHYSICAL EXAMINATION

A pelvic examination is essential in the evaluation of chronic urethral syndrome. Palpation should start with a gentle single finger evaluation of the vulva and vagina, including palpation of the urethra, trigone, and bladder base. Tenderness of the anterior vagina at the urethra and bladder base is almost always present with chronic urethral syndrome (4). The tenderness elicited classically mimics the

TABLE 37.1. SYMPTOMS OF PATIENTS WITH CHRONIC URETHRAL SYNDROME

Dominant Symptoms	Percentage
Frequency	65
Dysuria	60
Urgency	60
Dyspareunia	45
Postcoital voiding dysfunction	45
Postvoiding fullness	40
Nocturia	40
Abdominal pain	35
Suprapubic pain	25
Incontinence	25
Vulvodynia	25

patient's pain with coitus. Gentle massage of the urethra should be done. With chronic urethral syndrome, this usually only causes the pain already described. However, it also may yield a discharge, suggesting gonococcal or chlamydial infection. Inspection of the cervix for mucopurulent cervicitis may also suggest a chlamydial infection. These infections are not a component of chronic urethral syndrome, but it is important that they be adequately treated prior to further evaluation or treatment of the woman with chronic pelvic pain (CPP) and suspected chronic urethral syndrome.

Pubococcygeal muscle tenderness is often present. Suprapubic tenderness is occasionally found, but is not a consistent finding. The remainder of the pelvic examination is usually normal, with absence of uterine or adnexal tenderness.

DIAGNOSTIC STUDIES

A microscopic examination of a midstream urine for leukocytes and bacteria is basic. Urine cultures, as well as cultures or antigen tests of the urethra and cervix for gonorrhea and chlamydia, are also indicated. Recent studies suggest that polymerase chain replication (PCR) testing of urine for chlamydia is also worthwhile. Biochemical urine tests are useful for diagnosing cystitis. A positive nitrite test correlates with bacteriuria of 100,000 or more per milliliter. A positive leukocyte esterase test implies pyuria of eight or more leukocytes per cubic millimeter.

Because women with chlamydial or gonococcal urethral infections tend to have pyuria, it is particularly important that evaluations for chlamydia and gonorrhea be done in patients with sterile pyuria. More than two-thirds of women with pyuria and sterile urine have chlamydia (1). Conversely, it is quite uncommon for women with chlamydial urethritis not to have pyuria and a negative urine culture. Only 5% of women with symptoms of acute urethral syndrome without pyuria have chlamydia. These evaluations are necessary to rule out sexually transmitted diseases, cystitis, and acute urethritis in the woman thought to have chronic urethral syndrome.

Passage of a urethral catheter is characteristically painful in women with chronic urethral syndrome. This may suggest urethral syndrome or a pelvic floor muscle etiology. Muscle spasm of either urethral or pelvic floor muscles may make passage of a catheter difficult and painful (5).

Urodynamic studies may be useful in patients with chronic urethral syndrome. (Table 37.2) These studies can identify patients with abnormal voiding patterns due to dyssynergic voiding. Voiding and electromyographic studies reveal prolonged or intermittent voiding patterns and hyperactivity of the pelvic floor and/or external urethral sphincter. Mean urinary flow rates are notably decreased (less than 15 mL/sec; normal is greater than 15 mL/sec) and

TABLE 37.2. THE MOST FREQUENTLY OBSERVED URODYNAMIC FINDINGS WITH CHRONIC URETHRAL SYNDROME

Test	Chronic Urethral Syndrome	Normal
Mean urinary flow rate	<15 mL/sec	>15 mL/sec
Mean flow time	35–80 sec	<30 sec
Maximum urethral closure pressure	105 cm water	50 cm water
Residual volume	<50 mL	<50 mL

mean flow times are increased (35 to 80 sec; normal is less than 30 sec) with intermittent and prolonged flow rate patterns (Figure 37.1) (4,6). Maximal urethral closure pressure is increased by twofold over normal in women with chronic urethral syndrome (105 cm water compared to controls of 50 cm water) (2). In some cases these high urethral pressures may be decreased by pudendal anesthetic blocks (3). In spite of the common symptom of incomplete emptying, women with chronic urethral syndrome do not have an increase in residual volume. Maximal intravesical pressure is normal (12 to 60 cm water), as is functional bladder capacity (350 to 800 mL) (2). Detrusor instability is usually not found by regular or provocative cystometry (2,4). Not all patients with clinical evidence of chronic urethral syndrome have urodynamic abnormalities.

Radiographic studies are not generally indicated in the evaluation of chronic urethral syndrome. However, to rule out urethral diverticula in the differential diagnosis of chronic urethral syndrome, radiographic urethrography is sometimes useful (6).

Endoscopic evaluation is useful in women with suspected chronic urethral syndrome. In many of these patients, urethroscopy shows erythema, exudate, cystic dilation of periurethral glands, and inflammatory fronds throughout the urethra. Exudate is often demonstrable (4). It may also demonstrate incomplete funneling of the bladder neck and distal urethral narrowing. In CPP patients with chronic urethral syndrome, urethroscopy invariably reproduces their pain symptoms. Passing a urethral catheter may often produce similar excessive pain. Cystoscopy is normal, with no increase of bladder trabeculations (2).

DIAGNOSIS

Chronic urethral syndrome is generally a diagnosis of exclusion, necessitating a high index of suspicion in women with suggestive symptoms (Table 37.3) (6). It is often misdiagnosed as chronic or recurrent urinary tract infection. For this reason it is important that urine cultures be obtained prior to repeated antibiotic therapy. Such cultures will show at least 100 colonies per milliliter of a uropathogen in cystitis or acute urethral syndrome, but will be negative in chronic urethral syndrome. Repeated empiric antibiotic treatment of women with chronic urethral syndrome may delay accurate diagnosis and make subsequent therapy difficult.

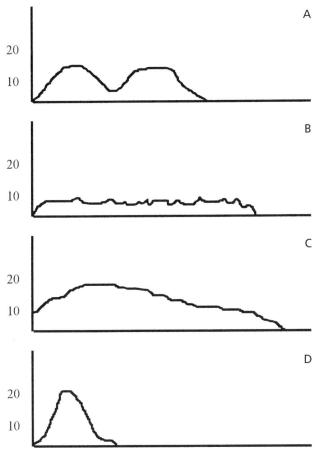

FIGURE 37.1. Urinary flow rate patterns in women with chronic urethral syndrome; **(A)** Interrupted; **(B)** Wavy; **(C)** Prolonged; and **(D)** Normal.

TABLE 37.3. BASIC CRITERIA FOR THE DIAGNOSIS OF CHRONIC URETHRAL SYNDROME

1. Symptoms of urgency, frequency, dysuria, and suprapubic pain.
2. Absence of urinary tract infection.
3. Absence of pyuria (≤5 white blood cells per high-power field)
4. Normal cystourethroscopy except for urethral pain with catheterization.
5. Absence of bladder instability.

Irritable bladder syndrome (Chapter 31) and interstitial cystitis (Chapter 32) present with similar chronic irritative urinary tract symptoms to those of chronic urethral syndrome. Dysuria is rarely present with either of these two syndromes, but is common with chronic urethral syndrome. Both irritable bladder syndrome and interstitial cystitis usually present with nocturia and pain on bladder filling, symptoms not common with urethral syndrome. Nocturia, when present with urethral syndrome, is usually early nighttime frequency related to sensory dysfunction of the urethra or bladder. In contrast, the nocturia of interstitial cystitis is due to a limited bladder capacity that causes consistent voiding throughout the night (6). Pain with interstitial cystitis is usually suprapubic, may radiate to the low back or groin, and is often relieved by voiding. Dyspareunia is common with interstitial cystitis, irritable bladder syndrome, and chronic urethral syndrome. Tenderness of the urethra and bladder base is usually found with urethral syndrome, but is infrequent with irritable bladder or interstitial cystitis. Cystoscopic findings are normal with irritable bladder syndrome and urethral syndrome, whereas glomerulations or Hunners ulcer are found with interstitial cystitis.

Urethral diverticulum may sometimes present with similar symptoms to urethral syndrome, including dyspareunia, pelvic pain, urgency, and frequency. Usually, urethral diverticula can be diagnosed by the presence of a suburethral tender mass or by visualization with cystourethroscopy or cystourethrography.

Pelvic floor pain syndrome (Chapter 45) may present with similar dysuria, dyspareunia, and voiding dysfunction, but urgency and frequency are not characteristic of pelvic floor pain. Physical examination usually distinguishes it from chronic urethral syndrome.

MANAGEMENT OR TREATMENT

Numerous treatments are used for chronic urethral syndrome, including antibiotics, bladder neck opening, internal urethrotomy, urethral dilation, local steroid injections, estrogens, tranquilizers (muscle relaxants), and psychiatric therapy. Frequently, the choice of treatment is based on tra-

dition or empiric trial and error. Specific treatment based on a defined potential etiology seems most appropriate, but often no such etiology can be found.

A common and reasonable initial treatment for women with chronic urethral syndrome is suppression with antibiotics, such as nitrofurantoin, timethoprim-sulfamethoxazole, or doxycycline, and/or urethral dilation. Dilations usually are to 36 to 38 French, done three times at biweekly intervals (1). Antibiotic suppression is usually done for 3 to 6 months (6). There is some evidence that these treatments are effective, both individually and combined. However, they probably work best in cases that show urethroscopic evidence of urethral inflammation. Antibiotics probably work via eradication of chronic, occult bacterial infection. Urethral dilations may open obstructed and inflamed periurethral glands, allowing drainage of inflammatory exudate and bacteria. Urethral dilation also has been shown in one study to increase peak and mean urine flow rates, but these changes were not seen with antibiotic treatment or with placebo (Table 37.4) (7). In this comparative study of urethral dilation (to 36 to 38 French with bladder pillar local anesthetic block every 2 to 3 weeks for three treatments) versus tetracycline (500 mg q.i.d. for 10 days) versus placebo (q.i.d. for 10 days), urethral dilation gave the best results. Twenty patients were assigned to each group and after completion of treatment, 4 (20%) were asymptomatic in the placebo group, 10 (50%) were asymptomatic in the tetracycline group, and 15 (75%) were asymptomatic in the dilation group. The study was not blinded or randomized. However, it suggests that the number-needed-to-treat (NNT) for dilation is two and the NNT for tetracycline is three. Subsequently, six of the ten patients unresponsive to tetracycline responded to urethral dilations, while one of the five patients unresponsive to dilations responded to tetracycline treatment.

In cases of chronic urethral syndrome with urodynamic studies showing evidence of external urethral sphincter spasm, diazepam at 2 to 6 mg per day for 2 to 5 months has been effective (8). Phenoxybenzamine hydrochloride, 10 to 40 mg per day, is an alternative effective treatment for this group of patients. Smooth muscle relaxants such as prazosin or dibenzyline used alone or combined with a skeletal muscle relaxant like valium can also be used in patients with

TABLE 37.4. RESULTS OF A TRIAL OF URETHRAL DILATION VERSUS TETRACYCLINE VERSUS PLACEBO IN THE TREATMENT OF CHRONIC URETHRAL SYNDROME IN 60 PATIENTS, COMPARING PEAK FLOW RATES (PFR), MEAN FLOW RATES (MFR), AND RESIDUAL VOLUMES (RV) BEFORE AND EIGHT WEEKS AFTER TREATMENT, AND RELIEF OF SYMPTOMS AFTER TREATMENT

Treatment	PFR Before	PFR After	MFR Before	MFR After	RV Before	RV After	Symptom Relief
Placebo	15 ± 6	16 ± 2	6 ± 3	7 ± 3	25 ± 17	28 ± 16	4 (20%)
Tetracycline	16 ± 4	19 ± 4	6 ± 2	7 ± 3	29 ± 14	25 ± 11	10 (50%)
Dilation	14 ± 5	19 ± 4	5 ± 3	9 ± 3	48 ± 31	20 ± 12	15 (75%)

urethral muscle spasm. As the external urethral sphincter is innervated by the pudendal nerve, pudendal nerve block has also been used with some success (3).

Behavioral modification may also be helpful in patients with urethral sphincter spasm. Monitored relaxation and contraction of the pelvic floor (levator muscles) may lead to reestablishment of voluntary control of the urethral sphincter and cessation of involuntary spasm. Establishing a regular voiding schedule is also helpful. Physical therapy, including pelvic floor biofeedback and electical stimulation treatments, may be a worthwhile component of this approach.

Surgical treatments for chronic urethral syndrome have not been adequately evaluated. Currently, surgical therapies are best done in research protocols and not advised for widespread use.

Unfortunately, many women with chronic urethral syndrome are misdiagnosed and undergo unneeded surgical evaluation or treatment. For example, in one case series one-fourth of patients had undergone total abdominal hysterectomy and bilateral salpingo-oophorectomy, one-fourth diagnostic laparoscopy, and one-eighth ovarian cystectomy before the diagnosis of chronic urethral syndrome was established (4).

KEY POINTS

Differential Diagnoses

- Chronic or recurrent urinary tract infection
- Irritable bladder syndrome
- Interstitial cystitis
- Urethral diverticulum
- Pelvic floor pain syndrome

Most Import Questions to Ask

- Do you have frequency or urgency of urination?
- How often do you urinate during the day?
- Do you feel you must hurry to get to the toilet to void?
- How often do you awake at night to void and at what times?
- Does it seem like your bladder empties completely when you void?
- Do you have pain when you urinate?
- Do you have pain with intercourse?
- It is difficult for you to void after intercourse?
- How often have you been treated for bladder infections in the past 1 to 2 years?

Most Important Physical Examination Findings

- Tenderness of the anterior vagina at the urethra and bladder base
- Pubococcygeal muscle and suprapubic tenderness
- Absence of uterine or adnexal tenderness

Most Important Diagnostic Studies

- Urinalysis and urine culture
- Cultures, PCR, or antigen tests of the urethra and cervix for gonorrhea and chlamydia
- Cystourethroscopy
- Urodynamic testing

Treatments

- Antibiotic treatment or suppression with nitrofurantoin, timethoprim-sulfamethoxazole, or doxycycline for 3 to 6 months
- Urethral dilation to 36 to 38 French, done three times at biweekly intervals
- Diazepam, prazosin, dibenzyline, or phenoxybenzamine hydrochloride for two to five months
- Pudendal nerve block
- Behavioral modification with biofeedback and/or pelvic floor stimulation, with monitored relaxation and contraction of the pelvic floor and an established regular voiding schedule

REFERENCES

1. Gravett MG. Acute urethral syndrome. *Contemp Obstet Gynecol* 1991;April:25–29.
2. Barbalias GA, Meares EM Jr. Female urethral syndrome: clinical and urodynamic perspectives. *Urology* 1984;23:208–212.
3. Raz S, Smith RB. External sphincter spasticity syndrome in female patients. *J Urol* 1976;115:443–446.
4. Summitt RL, Ling FW. Urethral syndrome presenting as chronic pelvic pain. *J Psychom Obstet Gynaecol* 1991;12(Suppl):77–86.
5. Bavendam TG. Irritable bladder—a commonsense approach. *Contemp Obstet Gynecol* 1993;April:70–7.
6. Summit RL Jr. Urogynecologic causes of chronic pelvic pain. *Obstet Gynecol Clin North Am* 1993;20:685–698.
7. Bergman A, Karram M, Bhatia NN. Urethral syndrome: a comparison of treatment modalities. *J Reprod Med* 1989;34:157–160.
8. Kaplan WE, Firlit CF, Schoenberg HW. The female urethral syndrome: external sphincter spasm as etiology. *J Urol* 1980;124:48–49.

38

ABDOMINAL WALL AND PELVIC MYOFASCIAL TRIGGER POINTS

JAMES E. CARTER

KEY TERMS AND DEFINITIONS

Active myofascial trigger point: A myofascial trigger point that causes a clinical pain complaint; to be distinguished from a latent myofascial trigger point.

Attachment trigger point: A trigger point at the musculotendinous junction and/or at the osseous attachment of the muscle; identifies the enthesopathy caused by unrelieved tension characteristic of the taut band that is produced by central trigger point.

Central myofascial trigger point: A myofascial trigger point that is closely associated with dysfunctional endplates and is located near the center of muscle fibers.

Enthesitis: Traumatic disease occurring at the insertion of muscle where recurring concentration of muscle stress provokes inflammation with a strong tendency toward fibrosis and calcification.

Enthesopathy: Disease process at musculotendinous junction and/or where tendons and ligaments attach into bones or joint capsules; characterized by local tenderness and may, in time, develop into enthesitis.

Flat palpation: Examination by finger pressure that proceeds along the muscle fibers at a right angle to their length, while compressing them against a firm underlying structure, such as bone. It is used to detect taut bands and trigger points.

Jump sign: A general pain response of the patient, who winces, may cry out, and may withdraw in response to pressure applied on a trigger point. This term has been used erroneously to describe the local twitch response of muscle fibers to trigger point stimulation.

Key myofascial trigger point: A trigger point responsible for activating one or more satellite trigger points. Clinically, a key trigger point is identified when inactivation of that trigger point also inactivates the satellite trigger points.

Latent myofascial trigger point: A myofascial trigger point that is clinically quiescent with respect to spontaneous pain and is painful only when palpated. It may have all of the other clinical characteristics of an active trigger point and always has a taut band that increases muscle tension and restricts range of motion.

Local twitch response: A transient contraction of a group of muscle fibers (taut band) that traverse a trigger point. It occurs in response to stimulation (usually by snapping, palpation, or needling) of the trigger point, or sometimes of a nearby trigger point.

Myofascial pain syndrome (myofascial syndrome): The sensory, motor, and autonomic symptoms caused by myofascial trigger points. This term is sometimes confusingly used to mean a regional pain syndrome of any soft tissue origin.

Myofascial trigger point (clinical definition): A hyperirritable spot in skeletal muscle that is associated with a hypersensitive palpable nodule in a taut band. This spot is painful on compression and can give rise to characteristic referred pain, referred tenderness, motor dysfunction, and autonomic phenomena. Types of myofascial trigger points include active, associated, attachment, central, key, latent, primary, and satellite. Any myofascial trigger point is to be distinguished from a cutaneous, ligamentous, periosteal, or any other nonmuscular trigger point. It is always tender, prevents full lengthening of the muscle, weakens the muscle, refers a patient-recognized pain on direct compression, mediates a local twitch response of muscle fibers when adequately stimulated, and, when compressed within the patient's pain tolerance, produces referred motor phenomena and often autonomic phenomena, generally in its pain reference zone, and causes tenderness in the pain reference zone.

Myofascial trigger point (etiological definition): A cluster of electrically active loci, each of which is associated with a contraction knot and a dysfunctional motor endplate in skeletal muscle.

Pincer palpation: Examination of groups of muscle fibers with a pincer grasp between the thumb and fingers. The fibers are rolled between the tips of the digits to detect taut bands, to identify trigger point nodules and tender points, and to elicit a local twitch responses.

Primary myofascial trigger point: A central myofascial trigger point apparently activated directly by acute and chronic overload or repetitive overuse of the muscle in which it occurs, not as a result of trigger-point activity in another muscle.

Referred (trigger point) pain: Pain that arises in a trigger point, but is felt at a distance, often remote from its source. The pattern of referred pain is reproducibly related to its site of origin. The distribution of referred trigger point pain rarely coincides entirely with the distribution of a peripheral nerve or dermatomal segment.

Satellite myofascial trigger point: A central myofascial trigger point that was induced neurogenically or mechanically by the activity of a key trigger point. Identification as a satellite trigger point usually is confirmed by simultaneous inactivation of the satellite when the key trigger point is inactivated. A satellite trigger point may develop in the zone of reference of the key trigger point, in an overloaded synergist that is substituting for the muscle harboring the trigger point (key muscle), in an antagonist countering the increased tension of the key muscle, or in a muscle linked apparently only neurogenically to the key trigger point.

Screening palpation: Digital examination of a muscle to determine the absence or presence of palpable bands and tender trigger points using flat and/or pincer palpation.

Snapping palpation: A fingertip is placed against the tense band of muscle at right angles to the direction of the band and then suddenly pressed down while it is drawn back, so as to roll the underlying fibers under the finger. The motion is similar to that used to pluck a guitar string, except that the finger does not slide over the skin but moves the skin with it. To most effectively elicit a local twitch response, the band is palpated and snapped at the trigger point, with the muscle positioned to eliminate slack.

Spasm: Increased tension of a muscle, with or without shortening, due to nonvoluntary motor nerve activity. Spasm is identified by motor unit potentials that cannot be terminated by voluntary relaxation.

Strain: Tissue and physiologic reaction to prolonged stress.

Stretch: Any procedure that elongates the muscle fibers. With trigger points, the goal of the procedure is to release the increased muscle tension by elongating the shortened sarcomeres of contraction knots.

Stress: (a) A physical or psychologic overload that produces a tissue or psychologic reaction. (b) The resisting force set up in a body as a result of an externally applied force. (c) A force that tends to produce distortion.

Taut band: The group of tense muscle fibers extending from a trigger point to the muscle attachments. The tension of the fibers is caused by contraction knots that are located in the region of the trigger point. Reflex contraction of the fibers in this band produce the local twitch response.

Trigger-point pressure release: Application of slowly increasing, nonpainful pressure over a trigger point until a barrier of tissue resistance is encountered. Contact is maintained until the tissue barrier releases, then pressure is increased to reach a new barrier to eliminate the trigger-point tension and tenderness. Trigger-point pressure release replaces the term ischemic compression.

Trigger-point release: Release of muscle tension by inactivating the trigger points that are causing the taut bands.

INTRODUCTION

The abdominal wall was recognized in 1926 as a primary source of abdominal pain (1). Chronic myofascial pain syndromes were first organized in a clinically useful way in 1952 (2). Although the incidence of myofascial trigger points (MTrPs) among patients with chronic pelvic pain is not known, the prevalence of myofascial trigger points among patients complaining of pain anywhere in the body ranges from 30% to 93%; for example, among patients with chronic craniofacial pain it is 55%, and for those with lumbar–gluteal pain it is 21% (3). In one study of 177 chronic pelvic pain patients, trigger points (TrPs) generated the majority of the pain experienced in 90% of the patients. In 131 (74%) patients, abdominal wall trigger points were found, with needle localization uniformly identifying the source as fat and fascial planes above the aponeurosis (4). In 71%, focal pain areas were found in the vaginal wall, particularly in the paracervical area, consistent with Frankenheuser's plexus. In 500 patients I have treated for chronic pelvic pain, 15% were found to have primarily myofascial TrPs (attachment, latent, or active) at sites including the abdominal rectus, obliques, levator ani, obturator internus, piriformis, iliopsoas, and adductors muscles as well as their musculoskeletal attachments (5).

Myofascial trigger points also occur in individuals without pain complaints. Among 200 asymptomatic young adults, focal tenderness representing latent trigger points were found in the shoulder girdle muscles of 54% of the females and 45% of the male subjects (6). In another study, 100 asymptomatic control subjects were examined for latent trigger points in the lumbogluteal muscles. Latent trigger points were found in the following muscles: quadratus lumbarum (45% of patients), gluteus medius (41%), iliopsoas (24%), gluteus minimus (11%), and piriformis (5%) (7).

The incidence of trigger points appears to be slightly higher in women, although they are clearly found in both sexes. In one report, myofascial pain syndrome occurred in 30% of women aged 20 to 40, 6% of whom presented with symptoms severe enough to require treatment (8). Pain has been shown to increase during the second week of the menstrual cycle, which suggests a hormonal influence. Patients 30 to 49 years old appear to have the highest prevalence of trigger points that subsequently decrease with age, as does activity and muscle stress (8). In a general sense, myofascial pain syndrome appears less common in laborers than in sedentary workers, which may imply a protective effect of daily vigorous activity, although a study of this using consistent trigger point definitions has not yet been performed.

PHYSIOLOGY AND PATHOLOGY

It appears that the critical abnormality in a trigger point is a neuromuscular dysfunction at the motor end point of an extrafusal skeletal muscle fiber, implying that myofascial pain caused by TrPs is a neuromuscular disease (Fig. 38.1) (3). The core features of myofascial TrPs are identified electrophysiologically by characteristic spontaneous electrical activity and histologically by contraction knots. Both phenomena apparently result from the excessive release of the neurotransmitter acetylcholine from the nerve terminal of the motor endplate (9). The characteristic referred pain and local twitch response of myofascial TrPs are dependent on spinal cord mechanisms. The taut band of skeletal muscle fibers is caused by many microscopic contraction knots in the endplate zone and relates to excessive release of acetylcholine in abnormal end-

plates (3,10). Spontaneous electromyographic (EMG) activity occurs at minute sites in a myofascial TrP region, but no such activity occurs at adjacent nontender sites. Both spikes and continuous low-amplitude action potentials can be recorded from an active myofascial TrP, and mostly only low-amplitude noise-like potentials can be found in latent myofascial TrPs. The etiological definition of a central myofascial TrP is a cluster of electrically active loci, each of which is associated with a contraction knot and a dysfunctional motor endplate in skeletal muscle.

A two-channel needle EMG method was developed that demonstrated that the 1- to 2-mm nidus of TrPs contains electrically active muscle fibers, while adjacent muscle fibers remain electrically silent. The active TrPs of patients with myofascial pain syndrome show significantly greater needle EMG activity than latent TrPs of normal controls (11,12). A sensitive locus is a minute site, which initiates a local twitch response when the stimulating needle penetrates it rapidly (10). An active locus is a minute site from which spontaneous electrical activity can be recorded if the recording needle approaches the site slowly and gently. It is demonstrated by physiology research to be an abnormal endplate. Histologic studies on the rabbit show a nerve fiber

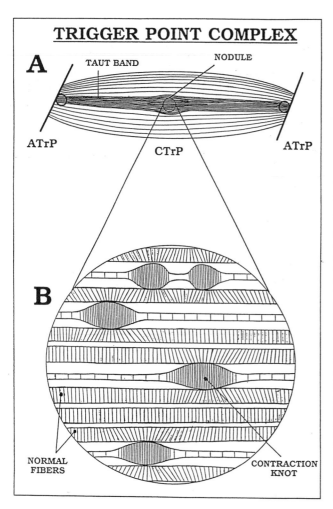

FIGURE 38.1. A credible pathogenesis of myofascial trigger points and its clinical consequences. Schematic of a trigger point complex of a muscle in longitudinal section. The schematic identifies three regions that can exhibit abnormal tenderness. It also illustrates contraction knots that most likely make a trigger point feel nodular, cause the taut band, and mark the site of an active loci. **A:** The central trigger point (CTrP), which is found in the endplate zone, contains numerous electrically active loci and contains numerous contraction knots. The local tenderness of the CTrP is centered in the nodule. A taut band of muscle fibers extends from TrP to the attachment at each end of the involved fibers. The sustained tension that the taut band exerts on the attachment tissues can induce a localized enthesopathy that is identified as an attachment TrP (ATrP). The local tenderness of the enthesopathy at the ATrP is identified by a circle. **B:** This enlarged view of part of the central TrP shows the distribution of five contraction knots. The vertical lines in each muscle fiber identify the relative spacing of its striations. The space between two striations corresponds to the length of one sarcomere. Each contraction knot identifies a segment of muscle fiber experiencing maximal contracture of its sarcomeres. The sarcomeres within one of these enlarged segments (contraction knot) of a muscle fiber are markedly shorter and wider than the sarcomeres of the neighboring normal muscle fibers, which are free of contraction knots. In fibers with these contraction knots (the lower three individual knots), the sarcomeres in the part of the muscle fiber that extends beyond both ends of the contraction knot are elongated and thin compared to normal sarcomeres. At the top of this enlarged view is a pair of contraction knots separated by an interval of empty sarcolemma between them that is devoid of contractile elements. This configuration suggests that the sustained maximal tension of the contractile elements in an individual contraction knot could have caused mechanical failure of the contractile elements in the middle of the knot. If that happened, the two halves would retract, leaving an interval of empty sarcolemma between them. In patients, the CTrP would feel nodular as compared to the adjacent muscle tissue, because it contains numerous "swollen" contraction knots that take up additional space and are much more firm and tense than uninvolved muscle tissues. (From Simons DG, Travell JG, Simons LS. *Travell and Simons, Myofascial pain and dysfunction: the trigger point manual*, vol 1, 2nd ed. Baltimore: Williams and Wilkins, 1999:70, with permission.)

in the immediate vicinity of a spontaneous electrical activity locus. Active loci are mostly distributed in the myofascial TrP region, always in the endplate zone. Needle contact is commonly associated with local and referred pain (10).

The myofascial TrP mechanism is closely related to spinal cord integration. When the input from nociceptors in a TrP receptive field persists (pain from an active myofascial TrP), central sensitization in the spinal cord may develop and the receptive field corresponding to the original dorsal horn neuron may be expanded to other neurons (referred pain). Through a central mechanism, new myofascial TrPs or satellite myofascial TrPs may develop in the referred zone of the original myofascial TrP. The key myofascial TrP is the initial myofascial TrP produced shortly after injury (or overloading). If the original condition is not appropriately managed, myofascial TrPs may propagate to other sites of the body (usually the referred zone). Inactivation of a key myofascial TrP may suppress satellite myofascial TrPs. A local twitch response or referred pain is mediated by the spinal cord in response to stimulation of a nociceptive sensitive locus that may be in the immediate vicinity of an active locus at a dysfunctional endplate.

A proposed pathogenesis (Fig. 38.2) of myofascial TrPs is that intracellular calcium in the involved muscle fibers may be excessively released in response to excessive acetylcholine release by a dysfunctional motor endplate. This dysfunction can be caused by trauma or abnormal stress. The abnormally increased calcium causes uncontrolled shortening activity and increased metabolism. The muscle fiber shortening produces a histologically demonstrable contraction and impairs local circulation, which causes a loss of oxygen

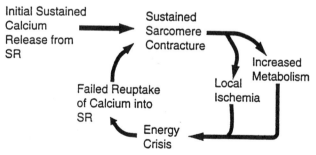

FIGURE 38.2. Schematic of the energy crisis hypothesis, which postulates a vicious cycle of events that appears to contribute significantly to myofascial TrPs. The function of the sarcoplasmic reticulum (SR) is to store and release ionized calcium that induces activity of the contractile elements, which cause sarcomere shortening. With initiating events such as trauma, a marked increase in the release of acetylcholine can result in excessive release of calcium from the sarcoplasmic reticulum. This calcium produces maximal contracture of a segment of muscle, which creates a maximal energy demand and chokes off local circulation. The ischemia interrupts energy supply, which causes failure of the calcium pump of the sarcoplasmic reticulum completing the cycle. (From Simons DG, Travell JG, Simons LS. *Myofacial pain and dysfunction: the trigger point manual,* vol 1, 2nd ed. Baltimore: Williams and Wilkins, 1999:71, with permission.)

and nutrients applied to the region. The resultant energy crisis completes a vicious cycle.

The taut band is the direct result of multiple contraction knots (Fig. 38.1). Taut bands commonly exist in pain-free individuals associated with latent TrPs. Those who are more prone to develop taut bands are also more likely to develop active myofascial TrPs. A latent myofascial TrP may develop in a taut band in response to acute or chronic muscle stress and to stressful life events combined with genetic predisposition. Further mechanical stress and other aggravating factors may cause a latent myofascial TrP to become active. The active myofascial TrP may recover spontaneously (if further overload is avoided), may persist without progression, or may be aggravated with increased pain intensity and spread to other sites, if perpetuating factors are present and are allowed to persist.

To summarize, the primary central TrP abnormalities are associated with individual dysfunctional endplates in the endplate zone (or motor point). This dysfunction produces a local energy crisis that results in sensitization of local nociceptors. This dysfunction can produce contraction knots that ultimately then produce a nodule and a taut band of tense muscle fibers. The attachment TrPs result from the sustained increased tension of these muscle fibers at the attachment point. This sustained tension can produce enthesopathy with swelling and tenderness where the muscle fibers attach to an aponeurosis, tendon, or bone. Some muscles have sufficient separation between the muscle fiber-to-tendon attachment and tendon-to-bone attachment that one end of the muscle may have two distinctly different attachment TrPs.

Perpetuating Factors

Perpetuating factors act clinically like a missing link that converts acute muscle syndrome into a chronic pain syndrome (8). These factors may be systemic or mechanical. Systemic factors increase irritability of the skeletal muscles throughout the body. Mechanical factors overload and aggravate TrPs in specific muscles. A patient with chronic pain due to myofascial TrPs usually has one or more perpetuating factors. Prior to activation of a TrP, existing perpetuating factors often cause negligible symptoms.

The presence of significant perpetuating factors is confirmed by a poor response to a trial of specific myofascial therapy applied to the muscle or muscles causing the myofascial pain. Although the initial response may be good, the symptoms return in hours or, more often, in days. Lack of any response to a therapeutic trial also may mean that treatment was applied to a latent TrP and not to the active TrP that was responsible for the pain (8).

Systemic Perpetuating Factors

Major systemic factors include enzyme dysfunctions because of nutritional inadequacy, metabolic and endocrine dysfunction, chronic infection, and psychologic stress. Anything that interferes with energy metabolism of the muscle tends to increase muscle irritability. The vitamin inadequacies that most commonly perpetuate myofascial TrPs are insufficient B complex vitamins, particularly B_1, B_6, B_{12}, and folic acid. Other nutritional inadequacies that perpetuate TrPs are low levels of potassium and calcium, as well as insufficiencies of major minerals such as zinc, copper, iron, and other essential trace minerals (8).

A vitamin serves as a coenzyme, and in its absence a metabolic step performed by an apoenzyme is blocked. For relevant vitamins, serum levels within or below the lower quartile of the normal range are more likely to perpetuate TrPs (3). The prevalence of unrecognized hypovitaminosis is distressingly high. In a randomly selected municipal hospital population, 105 of 120 patients (88%) had abnormally low levels of one or more of 11 vitamins, and over one-half were low in two or more vitamins. Serum folate was the most common vitamin deficiency and was low in 45% of the patients. There was a history of inadequate dietary intake in only 39% of the patients with hypovitaminosis. Moreover, hypovitaminosis was clinically apparent in only 38% of the entire group (13).

The B-complex vitamins and vitamin C are water-soluble. Thiamine (B_1) insufficiency causes loss of vibration sense at progressively more distal sites on the lower and upper extremities. The need for thiamine depends on the rate of energy expenditure, and muscles are energy engines. B_1 is leached out of food during washing and is destroyed in boiling. Pyridoxine (B_6) is an essential coenzyme for more than 60 apoenzymes in human metabolism. It activates phosphorylase, which releases glucose from glycogen, an essential part of muscle metabolism. B_6 suffers substantial losses during cooking and is quickly destroyed by ultraviolet light (sunlight) and oxidation. Cobalamin (B_{12}) and folate are interdependent and play an essential role in the synthesis of deoxyribonucleic acid (DNA), which is required for the maturation of erythrocytes and for oxygen transport. Vitamin C (ascorbic acid) prevents ecchymosis in those patients receiving injection therapy. It is essential to normal muscle function. Adequacy helps to reduce postexercise soreness and stiffness.

The fat-soluble vitamins A, D, and E are stored in fat and can reach toxic levels. Above-normal serum vitamin A levels are a source of increased muscle irritability.

Gout, anemia, low electrolyte levels, and hypoglycemia increase muscle irritability and aggravate symptoms caused by trigger points. So do the endocrine disorders of hypometabolism and estrogen deficiency. Monosodium urate crystals of gout tend to deposit in areas of local injury or of metabolic distress such as trigger points. Patients with gouty diathesis respond to treatment only when their hyperuricemia is under control. Vitamin C in relatively large amounts (1 to 4 g per day) is an effective uricosuric agent. The hyperirritability of myofascial TrPs subsides remarkably with uricosuric therapy in most patients with serum uric acid levels that are in the excessive or even in the high normal range. The presence of low electrolyte levels of ionized calcium and potassium can disturb muscle function by increasing muscle irritability. Serum ionized calcium is the essential measure. Total calcium correlates poorly with the level of serum ionized calcium. The presence of hypoglycemia intensifies metabolic distress in muscles and clearly aggravates myofascial trigger points. Therapy by stretch or injection is best deferred when patients are hypoglycemic. Patients with hyperinsulinemia, insulin resistance, and polycystic ovary syndrome are prone to hypoglycemic episodes. The underlying medical condition of the hyperinsulin state must be addressed to remove the perpetuating factor of hypoglycemia.

Hypometabolism, or thyroid inadequacy, describes a condition of someone whose serum levels of thyroid hormones are in the low euthyroid range, or just below the "normal" two standard deviation limit. The level of thyroid-stimulating hormone (TSH) may or may not be increased. Patients who are clearly hypothyroid have thyroid hormone levels below normal and an elevated TSH. Patients with myofascial pain syndrome often arrive untreated for their slightly low thyroid function because they have only mild symptoms of hypothyroidism and borderline low, or low normal, thyroid hormone levels. These patients are more susceptible to myofascial TrPs and obtain only temporary pain relief with specific myofascial therapy. The increased irritability of their muscles and poor response to therapy are greatly improved by supplemental thyroid if they have no other major perpetuating factor (14). Muscle pain, stiffness, weakness, muscle cramps, and pain on exertion are commonly cited manifestations of hypothyroidism. Hypothyroidism, detected with T3, T4, free T4, TSH, and/or TRH stimulation tests, was identified in 10% of 96 patients with chronic myofascial pain. Chronic autoimmune thyroiditis is a common disorder causing the majority of cases of hypothyroidism. At autopsy, prevalence rates of thyroiditis are as high as 15% in women and 5% in men. One-half of individuals with serum TSH levels greater than 5 mIv/L and 80% of those with TSH levels of greater than 10 mIv/L had thyroid antibodies characteristic of thyroiditis (15). I have found positive circulating thyroid antibodies (antimicrosomal and thyroid peroxidase) in patients with normal levels of TSH and free T4 with symptoms of hypothyroidism and TrPs which did not respond until thyroid treatment was provided. Measurement of circulating thyroid antibodies is recommended for patients with muscle pain, stiffness, weakness, or muscle cramps even with normal TSH and free T4.

Chronic viral disease, bacterial infection, and parasitic infections can also perpetuate TrPs. During any systemic viral illness including colds and the flu, the irritability of myofascial TrPs is likely to increase markedly. Chronic bacterial infection tends to exacerbate muscle irritability.

Mechanical Activating and Perpetuating Factors

One-time traumatic occurrences can activate TrPs but are not responsible for perpetuating them. Situations that cause repeated or chronic muscular overload can activate TrPs and then perpetuate them. The mechanical stresses that tend to activate myofascial TrPs acutely include wrenching movement, automobile accidents, falls, fractures (including chip fractures), joint sprains, dislocations, or a direct blow to the muscle (3). Active TrPs may also develop gradually due to chronic overload and strain. Synergistic muscles overloaded by substituting for an involved muscle or in sustained contraction to protectively splint an involved muscle are likely to develop secondary TrPs. A muscle immobilized in the shortened position for prolonged periods tends to develop active TrPs. Nerve compression favors the development of TrPs in the muscles supplied by the compressed nerve root.

Structural inadequacies, postural stresses, constriction of muscle and vocational stress due to poor ergonomics and repetitive movements are all mechanical perpetuating factors for TrPs. Two common and closely related structural inadequacies are a short leg and a small hemipelvis (Figs. 38.3 and 38.4). Short leg syndrome can cause a tilted pelvis when standing and can result in a compensatory scoliosis that is maintained by sustained muscular effort and is a potent perpetuating factor for TrPs in those muscles. A small hemipelvis can tilt the sacral base when the subject is standing or seated, similarly producing a compensatory scoliosis.

Short upper arms (in relation to torso height) leave the shoulders without adequate support in most seated positions. This leads to overloaded shoulder elevator muscles. It also produces compensatory distorted postures that can overload torso muscles and perpetuate their TrPs. The short first, long second metatarsal variation causes muscle imbalance that can extend from the leg to the head and perpetuate TrPs in those muscles. The long second metatarsal throws the foot off balance as a result of a knife-edge support during toeoff. This instability disturbs the gait and overloads lower extremity muscles. This can result in pain in the gluteus medius muscle and therefore low back and pelvic pain (3).

Myofascial TrPs are perpetuated by prolonged constricting pressure on a muscle such as a tight belt around the waist compressing the paraspinal, abdominal obliques, transversus abdominis, pyramidalis and rectus abdominis muscles. Lack of movement, especially when a muscle is in the shortened position, tends to aggravate and perpetuate myofascial TrPs. This commonly occurs when people sleep in a position that places the muscle in its shortest length, when the muscle cannot be moved through its full range of motion due to a fracture or articular disease, in individuals who do not change position regularly when seated (such as on long flights, auto trips, or bus trips), when patients have acquired habits of guarding against movements due to pain, or because they have been advised to restrict movement.

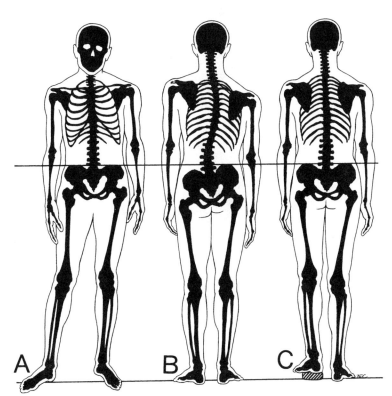

FIGURE 38.3. Skeletal asymmetry due to a shorter left leg. **A:** To compensate, the patient stands on the shorter leg, placing the longer leg forward and slightly to the side. This levels the pelvis. **B:** Tilted pelvis, functional scoliosis, and titled shoulder girdle access when the patient stands with the feet nearly together. **C:** The discrepancy in length is corrected by adding the precise full-correction heel lift under the shorter left leg. This levels the pelvis with the feet nearly together. (From Simons DG, Travell JG, Simons LS. *Myofacial pain and dysfunction: the trigger point manual*, vol 1, 2nd ed. Baltimore: Williams and Wilkins, 1999:931, with permission.)

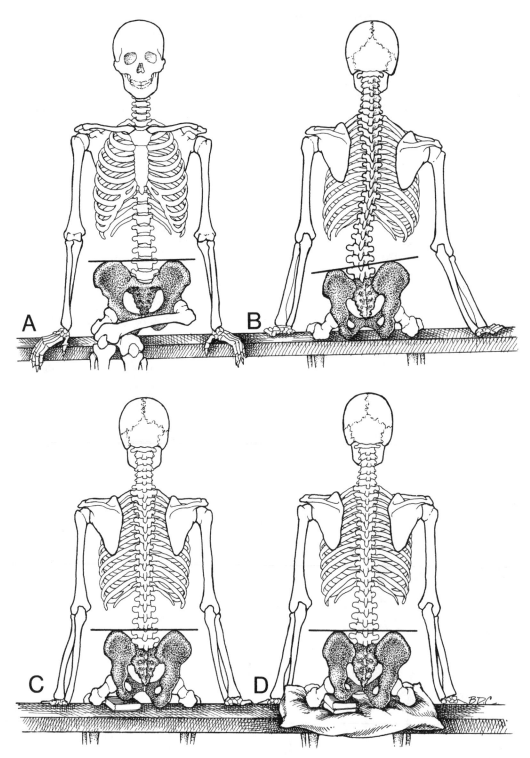

FIGURE 38.4. Effects of skeletal asymmetry due to a smaller hemipelvis on the left side are demonstrated by sitting on a flat level wooden bench. **A:** Crossing the leg on the short side over the opposite knee helps to level the pelvis. **B:** The tilted pelvis causes compensatory scoliosis, which tilts the shoulder girdle axis. **C:** A butt-lift levels the pelvis on a hard surface. **D:** On a soft cushion, a thicker butt-lift is required to provide the same correction as that obtained on a hard surface. (From Simons DG, Travell JG, Simons LS. *Myofacial pain and dysfunction: the trigger point manual*, vol 1, 2nd ed. Baltimore: Williams and Wilkins, 1999:932, with permission.)

Frequent repetitive movement can overload muscles and can initiate and perpetuate TrPs. TrPs are frequently activated by tasks that require repetitive use of the same muscles in the same way for long periods of time, such as the repetitive movements required in competitive swimming (breast stroke with frog leg kick), soccer, gymnastics, ballet, cheerleading, and horseback riding.

Much difference of opinion is generated by the question, "Is the chronic pain an expression of the patient's psychological dysfunction or is the pain driving the patient crazy?" If an organic cause of the pain is not obvious, it is tempting to conclude that the symptoms are psychogenic or behavioral in origin. This may relieve the health care professional but not the patient. Patients who suffer a serious chronic myofascial pain syndrome that is undiagnosed and ineffectively treated are strongly impacted psychologically. The ensuing depression aggravates the pain and reinforces uncertainty and a sense of hopelessness. The most important service one can render these patients is to recognize their treatable myofascial pain and make an unambiguous diagnosis with a convincing demonstration and explanation of active TrPs. As patients learn self-treatment and self-management techniques, they gain control of the pain; the pain no longer controls them and victimizes their lives. I have found that patients who receive TrP injections in pelvic floor muscles affected by TrPs respond with near amazement and profound gratitude with expression such as "You have found my pain" when the TrP is palpated, followed by "I no longer feel the pain" after the TrP is injected. Patients with chronic untreated myofascial pain syndrome usually require psychologic assistance and medication to help them with the depression and anxiety that frequently accompany any chronic pain syndrome.

SYMPTOMS OR HISTORY

To properly evaluate a patient with chronic musculoskeletal pain requires a review of medical records, a chronology of life and medical events, and a review of all medications taken and their effects. The exact distribution of the pain should be obtained on a body form on which the examiner and patient maps the specific pain patterns. A review of body systems should ensure that a significant medical problem is not overlooked. A sleep history is obtained, especially what disturbs sleep and sleep position. A dietary history should be obtained to ensure that there are no dietary deficiencies. A careful work, recreation, and sports history is fundamentally important. It is helpful for the patient to keep a written record of any onset of pain throughout the day and to relate it to activities at the time. Myofascial TrPs may cause constant pain, intermittent pain, or no pain. Patients in constant pain caused by TrPs are usually unaware of activities that aggravate the pain. They already have such

intense pain that they do not perceive an increase and thus cannot distinguish what makes it worse. They may be aware of tenderness at the TrP, but may not distinguish a change in their referred pain when pressure is applied to the TrP, partly because the TrP is so hypersensitive that minimal pressure reaches local pain tolerance. Most patients with active TrPs experience intermittent pain that is characteristically aggravated by specific movements and may be alleviated at least temporarily by a certain position. These patients may have some relatively pain-free days. They can usually identify what activities make them worse and what position or situation provides relief. Latent TrPs give no primary pain clues and must be identified by postural changes, muscle dysfunction, and physical examination.

The onset of pain following activation of the TrP due to muscle overload can be delayed as long as 12 to 20 hours. If the patient is subject to recurrence of severe episodic pain every few days, one should consider the possibility of episodic hypoglycemia. In this case, onset of pain should relate to eating and/or exercise and the patient can be tested for overreaction to a glucose tolerance test. Many patients with insulin resistance and resulting episodic hypoglycemia have concurrent polycystic ovary disease.

When asked "Do you remember the day your pain started?," most patients with TrPs respond with a clear affirmative or a fuzzy negative. Myofascial pain may start abruptly or gradually. Sometimes, the pain was felt at the moment of stress. Other patients remember feeling "something happened" or hearing "a snap" at the moment of stress, but the pain developed gradually several hours later. I have found acute-onset events associated with pelvic TrPs in women to include: adductor attachment TrPs resulting from forced positioning in ballet (splits); adductor attachment TrPs resulting from strenuous soccer movements; abdominal rectus, abdominal obliques, transversus abdominus, and pyramidalis attachment TrPs resulting from intensive abdominal contraction exercise; levator ani TrPs resulting from split-level falls (such as would occur stepping into an elevator which was positioned some inches below the floor level); obturator internus and adductor TrPs sustained after vigorous "frog leg" kicks in swimming competition; multiple pelvic muscle TrPs sustained from "picket fence" type injuries (missed frog leg style jump over fire hydrant at age 6 resulting in sustained TrPs treated at age 23; fall onto top-edge of open cabinet door at age 8 treated at age 21); and multiple TrPs sustained from falls and repetitive activities involved in horseback riding and cheerleading activities. If the source of strain is not obvious, the patient must help to identify it.

An essential part of the history is to determine in detail which activities and postures aggravate the pain and which ones relieve. Characteristically, pain symptoms are closely related to the activity of, or the demands on, the involved muscle (3,16).

MONTHLY PAIN CALENDAR

Day of cycle	1	2	3	4	5	6	7	8	9	10	11	12	13	14	15	16	17	18	19	20	21	22	23	24	25	26	27	28	29	30	31
Date																															
Gynecological																															
Menses																															
Medications																															
Cramps–pelvic																															
Cramps–other																															
Pelvic pain–left																															
Pelvic pain–right																															
Pelvic pain–low middle																															
Pelvic pain–other																															
Painful sexual intercourse																															
a. during																															
b. after																															
Gastrointestinal																															
Painful bowel movement																															
a. before																															
b. during																															
c. after																															
Genitourinary																															
Urinary problems																															
a. pain																															
b. urgency																															
c. frequency																															
Psychological Assessment																															
Depression																															
Anger																															
Anxiety																															
Musculoskeletal																															
Backache																															
General aches/pains																															
Myofascial																															
Abdominal wall pain																															

Menses:
0 - None
10 - Extremely heavy

Grading of symptoms and/or complaints:
0 - No symptoms
10 - Symptoms as severe as the worst I have experienced

For medications, list the initials and medication used.

By completing these forms, permission is given for use of this data in an anonymous manner for evaluation, research and publication.

FIGURE 38.5. Monthly pain calendar. (From Carter JE. *Chronic pelvic pain: diagnosis and treatment.* Golden, CO: Medical Education Collaborative, 1996:28, with permission.)

Myofascial TrP pain is characteristically aggravated by:

1. Strenuous use of the muscles, especially in the shortened position.
2. Passively fully stretching the muscle.
3. Pressure on the TrP.
4. Placing the involved muscle in a shortened position for a prolonged period.
5. Sustained or repeated contraction of the involved muscle.
6. Cold, damp weather, viral infections, and periods of marked nervous tension.
7. Exposure to a cold draft, especially when the muscle is fatigued.

Myofascial TrP pain is decreased by:

1. A short period of rest.
2. Slow, steady passive stretching of the involved muscles.
3. Moist heat applied over the TrP.
4. Short periods of light activity with movement.
5. Specific myofascial therapy.

The patient may report limitation of motion and increased stiffness that is worse in the morning and recurs after periods of overactivity or immobility in the day. This stiffness is apparently due to the abnormal tension of the palpable bands and to tension-induced sensitivity of the taut-band muscle fibers. The patient may complain of weakness with certain movements. The muscle learns to limit the force of the its contraction below its pain threshold of the central and attachment TrPs.

A history of immobilization in a shortened position for prolonged periods or of nerve or nerve root compression is consistent with a diagnosis of TrPs.

I have found the use of a series of five forms for acquisition of information to be very useful in the evaluation of patients with chronic musculoskeletal pain pretreatment and posttreatment (17,18). The five forms are (a) monthly pain calendar (Fig. 38.5), (b) symptoms check list (Fig. 38.6), (c) pain questionnaire (Fig. 38.7), (d) pain mapping (Fig. 38.8), and (e) psychologic assessment (Fig. 38.9). The addition of the Beck depression inventory to these forms is a useful adjunct to identify patients for whom psychologic treatment should be provided (19).

A pain map can be helpful in identifying areas of referred pain. Referred pain patterns are the key to identifying which muscle or muscles are most likely to be causing the myofascial pain. *Accurately* drawn referred pain patterns are the initial key to locating the trigger points. When pain involves several parts of the body, it is important to number the pain areas in the sequence of their appearance, to distinguish between pains that occur at different times, and to group together those that are experienced together in association with an activity or position. A pain distribution that is completed on a body form shows the referred pain patterns of that individual's TrPs. A knowledge of the pattern of pain referral from myofascial TrPs is essential.

Abdominal Oblique Muscles

These TrPs are capable of initiating somatovisceral responses, including projectile vomiting, anorexia and nausea, intestinal colic, diarrhea, urinary bladder and sphincter spasm, and dysmenorrhea (Fig. 38.10). When such visceral symptoms occur with abdominal pain and tenderness, the combination can closely mimic acute visceral disease, especially appendicitis, cholelithiasis, endometriosis, and endometritis.

Abdominal TrPs on one side frequently cause bilateral pain. Active TrPs located in the musculature of the lower lateral abdominal wall may refer pain into the groin. Active TrPs along the upper rim of the pubis and the lateral half of the inguinal ligament may lie in the lower internal oblique muscle and possibly in the lower rectus abdominus. These TrPs can cause increased irritability and spasm of the detrusor and urinary sphincter muscles, producing urinary frequency, retention of urine, and groin pain. When needled, such TrPs often refer pain to the region of the urinary bladder. TrPs in the superficial layer of the lateral abdominal wall musculature also may be a source of chronic diarrhea.

Rectus Abdominus and Pyramidalis Muscles

TrPs in the lower rectus abdominus about halfway between the umbilicus and the symphysis pubis may be a source of dysmenorrhea (Fig. 38.11). A TrP in the lateral border of the right rectus abdominus in the regions of McBurney's point half way between the anterior superior iliac spine and the umbilicus is likely to produce symptoms closely simulating those of acute appendicitis. A TrP just above the pubis may cause spasm of the detrusor and urinary sphincter muscles.

Quadratus Lumborum Muscle

Referred pain from TrPs in the quadratus lumborum muscle is projected posteriorly to the region of the sacral iliac joint and the lower buttock, sometimes anteriorly along the crest of the ileum to the adjacent lower quadrant of the abdomen and the groin, and to the greater trochanter (Fig. 38.12). Satellite TrPs that develop in paraspinal muscles or in the posterior section of the gluteus minimus may cause pain that extends to the groin, vulva, or in a sciatic distribution (20).

Iliopsoas

Referred pain from myofascial TrPs in the psoas major muscle extends along the spine ipsilaterally from the thoracic region to the sacroiliac area and sometimes to the upper

SYMPTOMS CHECKLIST

Symptoms Checklist	**Grade**	**Comments**

GYNECOLOGICAL
1. Painful periods
2. Painful ovulation
3. Painful intercourse
4. Other abdominal pain
5. Heavy bleeding with period
6. Irregular periods
7. Chronic yeast

GASTROINTESTINAL
1. Painful bowel movement - with menses
2. Painful bowel movement - anytime
3. Urgency with bowel movement
4. Blood in stool
5. Bloating
6. Constipation/diarrhea
7. Nausea/vomiting

MYOFASCIAL/MUSCULOSKELETAL
1. Lower back pain
2. Pain with certain movements/activities

URINARY TRACT
1. Pain with urination
2. Frequency of urination

PSYCHOLOGICAL
1. Stress
2. Depression
3. Anxiety
4. Anger
5. PMS - three worst symptoms
    A. _____
    B. _____
    C. _____

For symptoms: Grade 0 - No Symptoms
                  Grade 10 - Symptoms (pain, etc.) as severe as the worst I have experienced

FIGURE 38.6. Symptoms check list. (From Carter JE. *Chronic pelvic pain: diagnosis and treatment.* Golden, CO: Medical Education Collaborative, 1996:29, with permission.)

PAIN QUESTIONNAIRE

Date: _____   Name: _____

Age: _____   G: _____   P: _____   LMP: _____   Cycle day: _____

1. Pain Location
   (List each different
   location and number it)

2. Date First Noticed

3. Events Preceding Pain

4. Pain Description
   (Adjectives that patients
   use to describe typical
   pain and list cycle days)

5. Pain Intensity
   (Rate each pain

PAIN LOCATION	ONSET	EVENTS PRECEDING	DESCRIPTION	RATE PAIN FROM 0-10

6. Overall interference of pain with life (zero to 10)

   Work   School   Social   Childcare   Sports and   Relationships   Other:
                         Activities   Exercise

   _____   _____   _____   _____   _____   _____   _____

7. Description of things that:

   INCREASE PAIN   **DECREASE PAIN**
   Intercourse   Yes   No   Lying down   Yes   No
   Bowel movement   Yes   No   Heating pad   Yes   No
   Urination   Yes   No   Hot bath   Yes   No
   Physical activities Yes   No   Medication   Yes   No
   Other: Yes   No   Other: Yes   No

8. Prior treatment or medical workup:

   Surgeries: _____   Date: _____   Diagnosis: _____

   GI Studies: _____   Date: _____   Diagnosis: _____

   Other: _____

9. Use of medication:

   DATES: **EFFECTIVENESS:**
   A.
   B.
   C.
   D.

10. Current symptoms other than pain:

    A. Bleeding
    B. Bowel problems/nausea
    C. Headache
    D. Fatigue
    E. Other

FIGURE 38.7. Pain questionnaire. (From Carter JE. *Chronic pelvic pain: diagnosis and treatment.* Golden, CO: Medical Education Collaborative, 1996:30, with permission.)

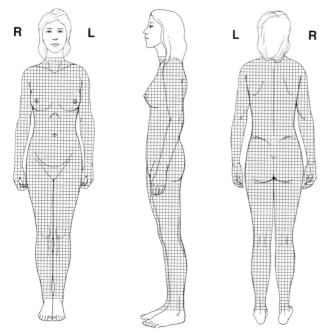

FIGURE 38.8. Pain mapping. (From Carter JE. *Chronic pelvic pain: diagnosis and treatment.* Golden, CO: Medical Education Collaborative, 1996:31, with permission.)

buttock (Fig. 38.13). Pain is referred similarly from the iliacus, and often also to the anterior thigh and groin. Pain referred from TrPs in the iliopsoas muscle form a distinctive vertical pattern ipsilaterally along the lumbar spine. It usually also includes the groin and upper anteromedial aspect of the thigh on the same side. Unilateral iliopsoas TrPs cause primarily low back pain.

Pelvic Floor Muscles

TrPs in muscles of the posterior half of the pelvic floor, including the sphincter ani, superficial transverse perinei, levator ani, and coccygeous muscles, refer poorly localized pain (Fig. 38.14). Patients are often uncertain whether to call it tailbone, hip, or back pain. They frequently complain of pain with intercourse, sometimes so severe that intercourse is intolerable. The pain is centered in the region of the coccyx, but often includes the anal area and the lower part of the sacrum. Both the levator ani and the coccygeous muscles typically refer pain to the region of the coccyx. This referred pain is often referred to as coccygodynia, although the coccyx itself is usually normal and not tender. Because the levator ani is the muscle commonly involved, pain in the region of the coccyx is also called the levator ani syndrome. The TrPs in the anterior half of the pelvic floor muscles, the ischiocavernosus, and the bulbospongiosus are likely to refer pain to the vagina. Vaginal pain can also arise from TrPs in the levator ani and has been reproduced by pressure on the tender sites in that muscle.

Obturator Internus Muscles

These TrPs can also result in pain in the vagina as well as pain in the anal and coccygeal region, and they may have a spillover pattern to the upper portion of the posterior thigh (Fig. 38.14). The obturator internus can cause pain and a feeling of fullness in the rectum and some pain referred down the back of the ipsilateral thigh, a condition also found with piriformis muscle involvement.

Anal and Vaginal Sphincter Muscles

Patients with TrPs in the sphincter ani muscle complain primarily of poorly localized aching pain in the anal region and may experience painful bowel movements. TrPs in the ischiocavernosus, bulbospongiosus, and transverse perinei muscles can cause dyspareunia, particularly during entry, and aching pain in the perineal region. Isolated entry dyspareunia has been found in women who give a history of "picket fence" type injuries experienced as children and are found to have TrPs in the bulbospongiosus, superficial transverse perinei, and ischiocavernosus muscles.

Myofascial TrPs in the coccygeous muscle cause pain referred to the coccyx, hip, or back. This pain limits sitting. TrPs in this muscle are likely to cause myofascial back ache late in pregnancy and early in labor (20).

TrPs in the scar tissue occurring in the vaginal cuff following hysterectomy have been described (4). These TrPs are usually associated with additional TrPs in the vaginal wall. The pain is usually described by the patient in terms of a familiar condition such as "ovarian pain," "menstrual cramps," or "bladder spasms." Nonmyofascial TrPs have reported in the tissues over the sacrum (4). These TrPs reproduced the pain the patient was reporting and responded to injection therapy.

Gluteus Maximus Muscle

Referred pain patterns of TrPs in the gluteus maximus muscle are located in the superior medial portion of the muscle, the lower midportion overlying the posterior surface of the ischial tuberosity, and the most medial inferior portion (Fig. 38.15). Referred pain from the TrPs in this muscle rarely projects to any distance from the buttock region. The symptoms from TrPs in this muscle commonly include restlessness and pain on prolonged sitting, increased pain when walking uphill in a bent-forward posture, and pain induced by swimming the crawl stroke (20).

Gluteus Medius Muscle

Referred pain from the gluteus medius muscle is commonly identified as low back pain. Its three TrP regions together refer pain and tenderness primarily along the posterior crest of the ileum, to the sacrum, and to the posterior and lateral

RELATED HISTORY FORM

A. Experience with other medical people or family/friends?
   (Ex: Have you seen other doctors? What did they tell you?)

B. How are you coping with pain currently?

C. Do you have any history of a major episode of depression?

D. Current symptoms of depression?   Yes   No

   (Underline appropriate words and explain below)

   Mood disturbances   Loss of pleasure in activities
   Feelings of hopelessness   Feelings of worthlessness
   Low energy   Loss of appetite
   Sleep disturbance   Thoughts/plans of suicide

E. Any history of sexual abuse? _____ What ages? _____
   By whom? _____

   Has anyone ever touched you in any way that made you feel uncomfortable? _____
   What ages? _____ By whom? _____

   Has anyone ever asked you to touch them when you did not want to? _____
   What ages? _____ By whom? _____

FIGURE 38.9. Related history form. (From Carter JE. *Chronic pelvic pain: diagnosis and treatment*. Golden, CO: Medical Education Collaborative, 1996:32, with permission.)

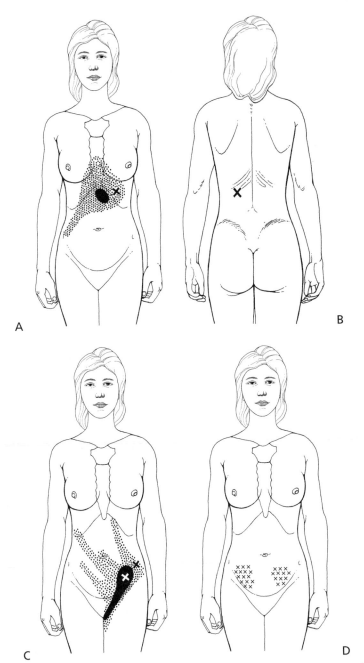

FIGURE 38.10. Referred pain patterns and visceral symptoms of trigger points (XX) in the oblique abdominal muscles. **A:** "Heartburn" from an attachment trigger point in the external oblique muscle overlying the anterior chest wall. **B:** Projectile vomiting and belching from the "belch button," which is usually located in the posterior abdominal wall musculature and may be on either side. **C:** Groin as well as chiefly lower-quadrant abdominal pain, referred from trigger points in the lower lateral abdominal wall musculature on either side. **D:** Diarrhea from trigger points in the lower abdominal quadrant. (Simons DG, Travell JG, Simons LS. *Myofacial pain and dysfunction: the trigger point manual*, vol 1, 2nd ed. Baltimore: Williams and Wilkins, 1999:942, with permission.)

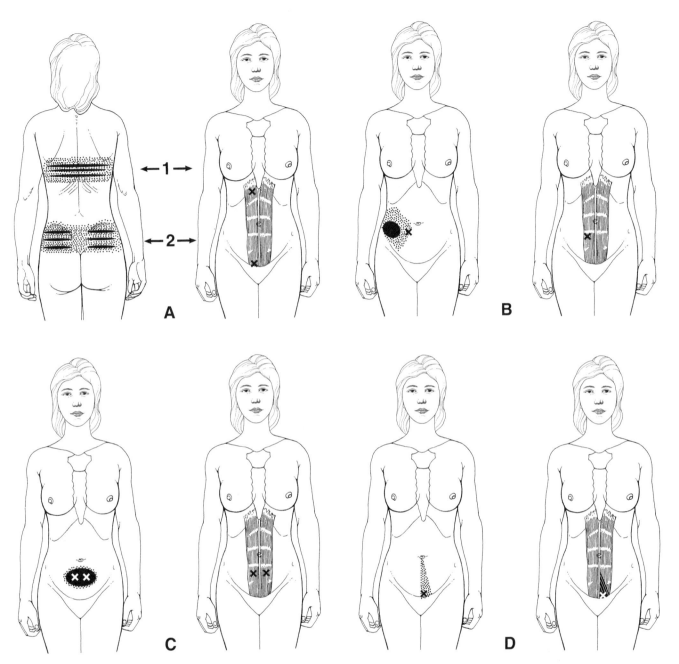

FIGURE 38.11. Referred pain patterns and visceral symptoms of trigger points (XX) in the rectus abdominus and pyramidalis muscles. **A:** Bilateral pain across the midback, precordial pain and/or feeling of abdominal fullness, nausea and vomiting can be caused by trigger point (1) in the left or right upper rectus abdominus. A similar pattern of bilateral low back pain is referred from an attachment trigger point (2) in the caudal end of the rectus muscle on either side. **B:** Lower right quadrant pain and tenderness simulating appendicitis may occur in the region of McBurney's point due to a nearby trigger point in the lateral border of the rectus abdominus. **C:** Dysmenorrhea may be greatly intensified by trigger points in the lower rectus abdominus muscle. **D:** Referred pain pattern of the pyramidalis muscle. (From Simons DG, Travell JG, Simons LS. *Myofacial pain and dysfunction: the trigger point manual,* vol 1, 2nd ed. Baltimore: Williams and Wilkins, 1999:944–945, with permission.)

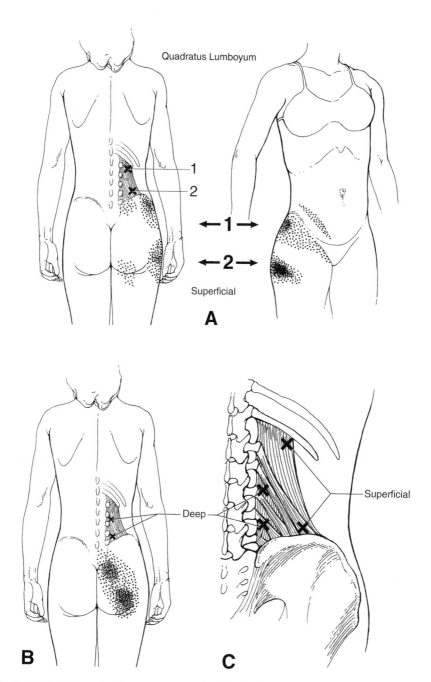

FIGURE 38.12. Referred pain patterns of TrPs (Xs) in the quadratus lumborum muscle. Solid black denotes an essential pain pattern and stippling represents a spillover pattern. **A:** Pain patterns of superficial (lateral) TrPs that are palpable (1) below and close to the 12th rib, and (2) just above the iliac crest. **B:** Pain patterns of deep (more medial) TrPs close to the transverse processes of the lumbar vertebrae. The more cephalad deep TrPs refer pain to the sacroiliac joint; more caudal TrPs refer pain low in the buttock. **C:** Examples of locations of TrPs in the quadratus lumborum muscle. (From Travell JG, Simons DG. *Myofacial pain and dysfunction: the trigger point manual*, vol 2, 1st ed. Baltimore: Williams and Wilkins, 1992:30, with permission.)

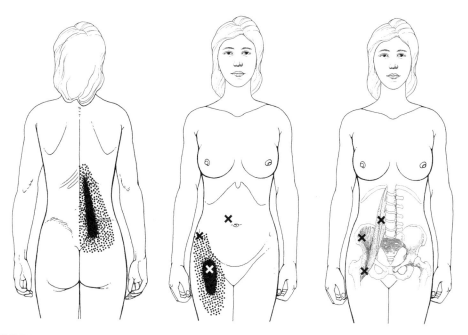

FIGURE 38.13. Pattern of pain referred from palpable myofascial trigger points (XX) in the right iliopsoas muscle. The essential pain reference zone and the spillover pattern are shown in solid black surrounded by stippling. (From Travell JG, Simons DG. *Myofacial pain and dysfunction: the trigger point manual*, vol 1, 1st ed. Baltimore: Williams and Wilkins, 1992:90, with permission.)

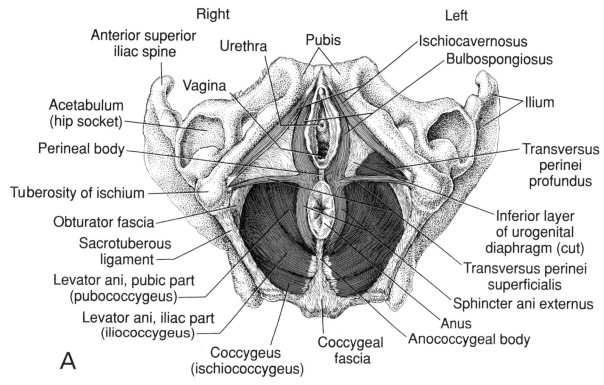

FIGURE 38.14. A: Pelvic floor muscles as seen from below in the supine female subject. The muscles of the pelvic diaphragm and the associated pelvic muscles are visualized. On the subjects left side, part of the deep fascia of the urogenital diaphragm has been cut and removed to reveal the transversus perinei profundus muscle. (From Travell JG, Simons DG. *Myofacial pain and dysfunction: the trigger manual*, vol 2, 1st ed. Baltimore: Williams and Wilkins, 1992:13, with permission.)

(continued on next page)

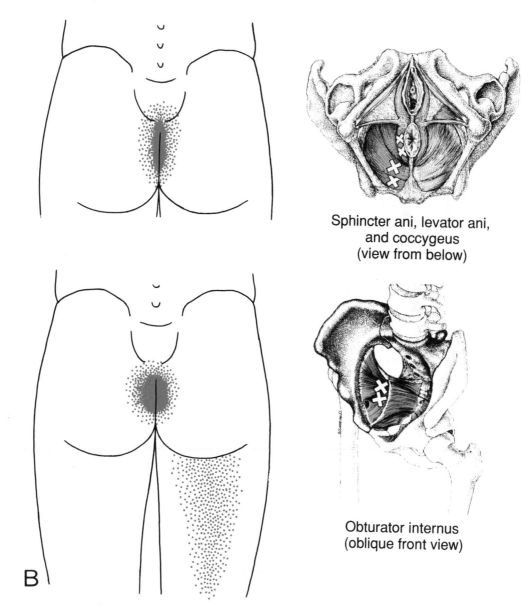

Sphincter ani, levator ani,
and coccygeus
(view from below)

Obturator internus
(oblique front view)

FIGURE 38.14. *(Continued)* **B:** Patterns of referred pain generated by trigger points (XX) (A) in the right sphincter ani, levator ani, and coccygeous muscles and (B) in the right obturator internus muscle. Pain referred from the muscle sometimes spills over to include the posterior proximal region of the thigh. (From Travell JG, Simons DG. *Myofacial pain and dysfunction: the trigger point manual*, vol 2, 1st ed. Baltimore: Williams and Wilkins, 1992:112, with permission.)

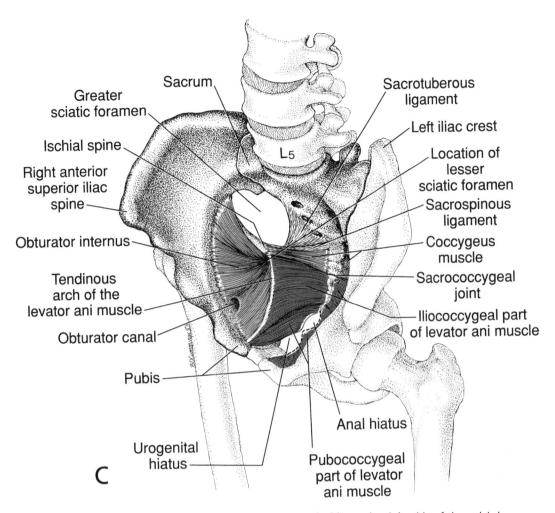

FIGURE 38.14. *(Continued)* **C:** Pelvic floor muscles palpable on the right side of the pelvis by intrapelvic examination with the patient lying on the right side. The muscles are seen obliquely from above and diagonally from the left side looking down inside the pelvis. (From Travell JG, Simons DG. *Myofacial pain and dysfunction: the trigger point manual*, vol 2, 1st ed. Baltimore: Williams and Wilkins, 1992:114, with permission.)

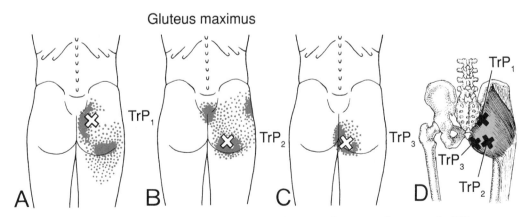

FIGURE 38.15. Referred pain patterns of TrPs (Xs) in the gluteus maximus muscle. TrPs are located in **(A)** the superior medial portion of the muscle (TrP 1), **(B)** lower midportion overlying the posterior surface of the ischial tuberosity (TrP 2), **(C)** the most medial inferior portion (TrP 3), and **(D)** location of TrP 1, TrP 2, and TrP 3 in the gluteus maximus muscle. (From Travell JG, Simons DG. *Myofacial pain and dysfunction: the trigger point manual*, vol 2, 1st ed. Baltimore: Williams and Wilkins, 1992:133, with permission.)

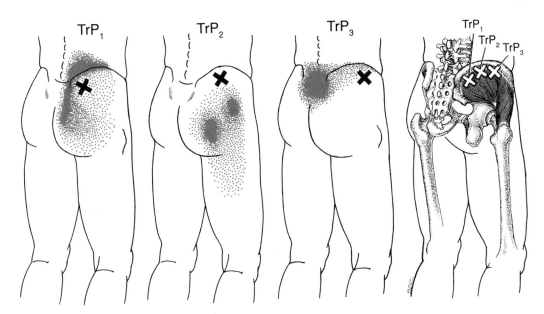

FIGURE 38.16. Pain patterns referred from TrPs (Xs) in the right gluteus medius muscle. The essential pain pattern is solid and the spillover pattern is stippled. The most medial TrP 1 refers pain primarily to the crest of the ilium, to the region of the sacral iliac joint, and to the sacrum. The TrP 2 area is located more cephalad and laterally, and it refers pain caudally to the buttock and to the upper thigh posteriorly and laterally. The most anterior TrP 3 occurs less often and refers pain bilaterally over the sacrum and into the lowest lumbar region. (From Travell JG, Simons DG. *Myofacial pain and dysfunction: the trigger point manual*, vol 1, 1st ed. Baltimore: Williams and Wilkins, 1992:151, with permission.)

aspect of the buttock (Fig. 38.16). Pain and tenderness may extend to the upper thigh. Myofascial TrPs in this muscle cause symptoms of pain when walking, when lying on the back or on the affected side, and when sitting slouched down in a chair (20). When the posterior fibers of the gluteus medius harbor TrPs, secondary TrPs are likely to develop in the piriformis and the posterior part of the gluteus minimus.

Gluteus Minimus Muscle

The referred pain from TrPs in the anterior part of the gluteus minimus extend over the lower lateral buttocks, down the lateral aspect of the thigh, knee, and leg to the ankle (Fig. 38.17). The TrPs from the posterior fibers in this muscle have a similar but more posterior pattern that projects pain over the lower medial aspect of the buttocks and down the back of the thigh and calf. The TrPs in this muscle cause symptoms of pain in a characteristic pattern, especially when arising from a chair or when walking.

Piriformis, Obturator Internus, and Other Short Lateral Rotators

The piriformis muscle causes as much distress by nerve entrapment as it does by projecting pain from TrPs. Referred pain from a TrP in the piriformis muscle may radiate to the sacroiliac region, laterally across the but-

tock, and over the hip region posteriorly and to the proximal two-thirds of the posterior thigh (Fig. 38.18). Symptoms may be caused by referral of pain from the TrPs in the muscle, by nerve entrapment, and/or by vascular compromise when neurovascular structures are compressed by the muscle against the rim of the greater sciatic foramen and by sacroiliac joint dysfunction. The myofascial pain component of this syndrome includes pain in the low back, buttock, and posterior thigh. It usually is increased by sitting, standing, and walking. Patients may report pain (and paresthesias) in the lower back, groin, perineum, buttock, hip, posterior thigh and leg, foot, and during defecation in the rectum. Symptoms are aggravated by sitting, by a prolonged combination of hip flexion, adduction, and medial rotation, or by activity. The patient may complain of dyspareunia (16,20).

TrPs in the piriformis and obturator can be activated by any unaccustomed overload. Catching oneself in a fall, twisting sideways while bending and lifting a heavy weight, forceful rotation with the body weight on one leg, and repetitive strains such as occurs in weight-bearing abduction exercises can activate and perpetuate TrPs in the piriformis and obturator internus. The muscle strain of overcorrection of a lower-limb length inequality can activate latent piriformis TrPs (20). Driving a car with a foot in place on the accelerator for long periods or sitting on one foot are activities that can activate piriformis TrPs.

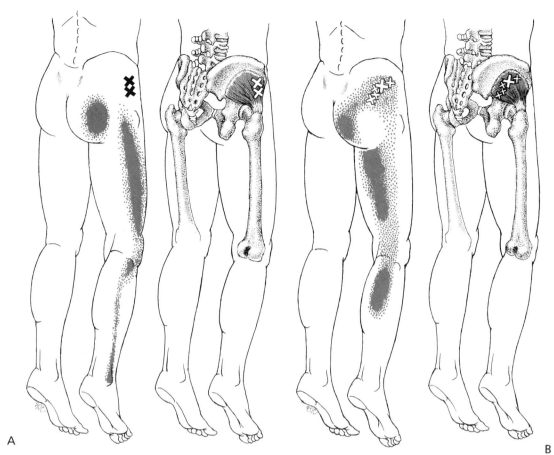

FIGURE 38.17. **A:** Pattern of referred pain from TrPs (Xs) in the anterior portion of the right gluteus minimus muscle. The essential pain pattern is solid and the spillover extension found when the muscle is more severely involved is stippled. **B:** Composite pain pattern referred from TrPs in the posterior part of the right gluteus minimus muscle. The essential pain pattern is solid and the spillover pattern is stippled. The large X marks the most common location of TrPs in the posterior part of this muscle. The most anterior small x lies at the junction of the anterior and posterior portions of this muscle. (From Travell JG, Simons DG. *Myofacial pain and dysfunction: the trigger point manual*, vol 2, 1st ed. Baltimore: Williams and Wilkins, 1992:169, with permission.)

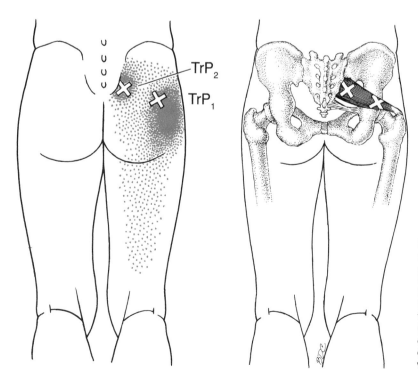

FIGURE 38.18. Composite pattern of pain referred from trigger points (TrPs) (Xs) in the right piriformis muscle. The lateral X (TrP 1) indicates a lateral attachment TrP location. The stippling locates the spillover part of the pattern that may be felt as less intense pain than that of the essential pattern (solid). Spillover pain may be absent. (From Travell JG, Simons DG. *Myofacial pain and dysfunction: the trigger point manual*, vol 2, 1st ed. Baltimore: Williams and Wilkins, 1992:188, with permission.)

335

Tensorfasciaelatae Muscle

Referred pain and tenderness in the tensorfasciaelatae muscle concentrate in the anterior lateral thigh over the greater trochanter and extend down the thigh toward the knee. Symptoms include pain deep in the hip and down the thigh as far as the knee. The pain prevents walking rapidly or lying comfortably on the side of the TrPs.

Sartorius Muscle

The specific TrPs of the sartorius produces surprising bursts of superficial sharp or tingling pain. Patients with upper sartorius TrPs may have symptoms of entrapment of the lateral femoral cutaneous nerve.

Pectineus Muscle

Myofascial TrPs in the pectineus muscle produce a deep seated aching pain in the groin immediately distal to the inguinal ligament (Fig. 38.19). The pain may also cover the upper part of the anteriomedial aspect of the thigh. The deep groin pain may also extend medially to the region where the adductor magnus attaches to the pelvis. After TrPs in the three other adductors or the iliopsoas have been inactivated, the pectineus is uncovered as the cause of persistent deep seated groin pain especially during weight bearing activities that cause abduction of the thigh. Pectineus muscle TrPs are likely to result from tripping or falling. Unaccustomed sexual activity that involves vigorous adductor activity can be responsible for activating pectineus TrPs. A sudden, vigorous,

adduction-flexion while performing gymnastic exercises may overload the muscle, especially when it is already fatigued. Another activity that can stress the muscle is horseback riding, when the rider uses the thighs, rather than the legs and feet, to grasp the horse. I have evaluated patients with persistent deep-seated groin pain who gave histories of the above activities (including ballet) and whose complaints were resolved only after inactivation of pectineus TrPs.

Rectus Femoris Muscle

The usual location of TrP in the rectus femoris is at the hip level, high on the thigh just below the anterior inferior iliac spines. However, the pain is felt at the knee in and around the patella.

Adductor Longus and Adductor Brevis Muscles

TrPs from these two muscles project pain both proximally and distally. Pain is experienced deep in, and proximal to, the groin and in the anteriomedial portion of the upper thigh (Fig. 38.20).

Adductor Magnus Muscle

The relatively common myofascial TrP location in the mid portion of adductor magnus muscle refers pain upward into the groin below the inguinal ligament and also downward over the anteriomedial aspect of the thigh nearly to the knee (Fig. 38.21). This groin pain is described as deep, almost as if

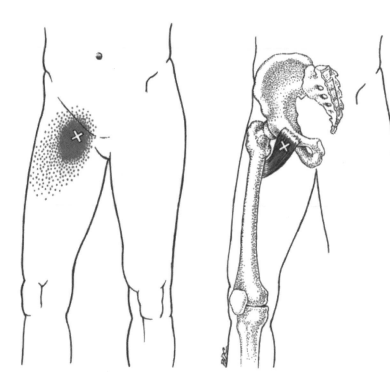

FIGURE 38.19. A pattern of pain referred from a TrP (X) in the right pectineus muscle, seen from in front and slightly from the medial side. The essential referred pain is solid and the occasional spillover pain is stippled. (From Travell JG, Simons DG. *Myofacial pain and dysfunction: the trigger point manual*, vol 2, 1st ed. Baltimore: Williams and Wilkins, 1992:237, with permission.)

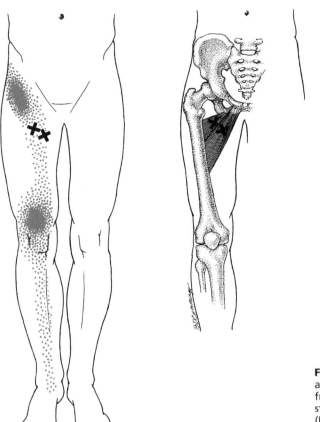

FIGURE 38.20. Anterior view of the right adductor longus and adductor brevis muscles and the composite pain pattern, referred from TrPs (Xs) in these two muscles. The essential pain pattern is solid; stippling indicates occasional extension to a spillover pain pattern. (From Travell JG, Simons DG. *Myofacial pain and dysfunction: the trigger point manual*, vol 2, 1st ed. Baltimore: Williams and Wilkins, 1992:291, with permission.)

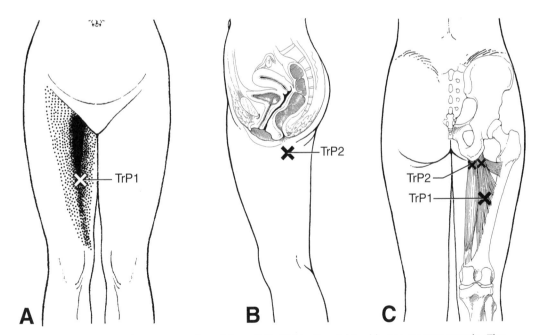

FIGURE 38.21. Pain pattern referred from TrPs (Xs) in the right adductor magnus muscle. The essential pattern is solid; stippling locates occasional extension of the referred pain in a spillover pattern. **A:** Anterior view of the referred pain pattern from the mid-thigh TrP region. **B:** Mid-sagittal view showing the intrapelvic pain pattern referred from the TrP region. These TrPs are found in the most proximal portion of the ischiocondylar part of the adductor magnus medial to or deep to the gluteus magnus muscle. **C:** Posterior view, anatomy of the muscle and location of common attachment TrPs and a central TrP. (From Travell JG, Simons DG. *Myofacial pain and dysfunction: the trigger point manual*, vol 2, 1st ed. Baltimore: Williams and Wilkins, 1992:292, with permission.)

it might be in the pelvis, but the patient is unable to identify pain in any specific pelvic structure. Pain referred from TrPs in the more proximal region of the adductor magnus is usually described as a generalized internal pelvic pain, but may be identified as including the pubic bone, vagina, rectum, or bladder. The pain may be described as shooting up inside the pelvis and exploding like a firecracker (20). Patients frequently have difficulty positioning the lower limb comfortably at night. They usually prefer to lie on the opposite side with the thigh horizontal and slightly flexed at the hip, as when a pillow is placed between the knees and the legs.

In some patients with TrPs in adductor magnus, symptoms occur only during sexual intercourse. I have found patients whose primary complaint has been pain with intercourse who had adductor magnus TrPs originating from stressors including ballet, gymnastics, horseback riding, skiing, and snow boarding. The pain with intercourse resolved after treatment of the adductor magnus TrPs.

TrPs in the adductor muscles can also be activated by sudden overload such as when someone slips on ice and resists spreading the legs apart when trying to recover balance. Adductor magnus TrPs can be activated by long bicycle trips, and a latent TrP can be reactivated by simple missteps such as off of a curb. Adductor TrPs can be perpetuated by sitting in a fixed position while driving on a long auto trip or while sitting for long periods in a chair with the hips acutely flexed and one thigh or leg crossed over the other knee.

Gracilis Muscle

The gracilis attaches to the lower rim of the outside of the pelvis at the junction of the body of the pubis and the inferior pubic ramus (Fig. 38.22). Attachment TrPs from

the gracilis occur in patients active in gymnastics and ballet.

SIGNS OR PHYSICAL EXAMINATION

The common clinical characteristics of an active myofascial TrP include the following:

- Compression of the myofascial TrP elicits local and referred pain that is similar to the patient's usual clinical complaint (pain recognition) or it may aggravate the existing pain.
- Snapping palpation compression across the muscle fibers at the TrP may elicit a local twitch response (LTR) (a brisk contraction of the muscle fibers in the vicinity of the taut band).
- Rapid repeated insertion of a needle into a myofascial TrP consistently elicits a LTR.
- Painfully restricted stretch range of motion of the involved muscle is present.
- The muscle with a myofascial TrP may be weak due to inhibition caused by pain or caused reflexly from a TrP in another muscle.
- Patients may have associated localized autonomic reflex phenomena including vasoconstriction, pilomotor response, ptosis, and hypersecretion (3).

An active TrP is one that produces a pain complaint such as spontaneous pain or pain in response to movement, whereas a latent myofascial TrP is a localized spot that produces discomfort only in response to compression. Spot tenderness, pain recognition, and taut bands are the most reliable signs and the minimal criteria needed to identify a

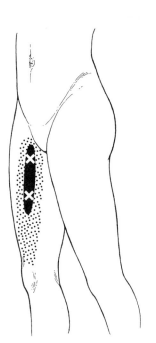
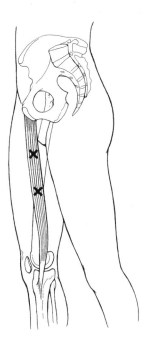

FIGURE 38.22. Medial view of the composite pain pattern referred from TrPs in the right gracilis muscle. Solid denotes the essential pain pattern, and stippling indicates the occasional spillover pattern. (From Travell JG, Simons DG. *Myofacial pain and dysfunction: the trigger point manual*, vol 2, 1st ed. Baltimore: Williams and Wilkins, 1992:293, with permission.)

myofascial TrP, while referred pain and local twitch response are most useful as confirmatory signs of myofascial TrPs.

Clinically, the TrP is identified as a localized spot of tenderness in a nodule in a palpable taut band of muscle fibers. When TrPs are palpated, the pain is felt locally in the TrP area and is usually referred to other, more distant areas known as zones of reference (3,22). Its location is usually constant and reproducible, and it does not follow a dermatomal or nerve root distribution. Palpation of the affected muscle by applying sustained deep pressure is the method used most frequently in the diagnosis of TrPs. Exquisite focal tenderness of the TrP is identified by the jump sign—a vocalization by and withdrawal of the patient. This localized spot tenderness is an essential feature of a TrP. Active TrPs are identified when patients recognize the pain that is induced by applying pressure to a TrP as "their" pain. The taut band fibers usually respond with an LTR when the taut band is accessible and when the TrP is stimulated by properly applied snapping palpation. The taut fibers respond consistently with the LTR when the TrP is penetrated by a needle.

Restricted stretch range of motion and palpable increase in muscle tenseness (decreased compliance) are more severe in more active TrPs. Muscles with active myofascial TrPs have a restricted passive (stretch) range of motion because of pain. An attempt to passively stretch the muscle beyond its limit produces increasingly severe pain because the involved muscle fibers are already under substantially increased tension at rest length. When the TrP is inactivated and the taut band is released and enthesopathy subsides, range of motion returns to normal. When a muscle with an active TrP is strongly contracted against fixed resistance, the patient feels pain. Weakness is generally a characteristic of a muscle with active myofascial TrPs, but the magnitude is variable from muscle to muscle and from subject to subject.

The presence of a taut band containing hypersensitive muscle fibers of harder-than-normal consistency is a typical finding. The stringlike or ropelike taut band can be palpated if the muscle is sufficiently superficial. The tense fibers that comprise the palpable band are most easily distinguished from the normally pliable fibers surrounding them by extending the muscle gently just short of, or to the onset of, resistance. I have found this to be especially true of the levator ani muscles. Criteria for a clinical diagnosis of TrPs as the source of myofascial pain are summarized in Table 38.1.

Three kinds of palpation are used: flat palpation, pincer palpation, and deep (probing) palpation. Flat palpation is used for relatively superficial muscles that have only one surface accessible for palpation. Pincer palpation is used when both sides of the muscle are accessible and the belly of the muscle can be grasped between the digits. Deep palpation must be used for deep muscles with considerable tissue between them and the skin. Flat palpation is performed with the use of the fingertip and employs the mobility of the overlying tissue to slide the patient's skin across the muscle fiber.

TABLE 38.1. CRITERIA FOR A CLINICAL DIAGNOSIS OF TRPS AS THE SOURCE OF MYOFASCIAL PAIN

1. Taut band palpable (if muscle accessible).
2. Exquisite spot tenderness of a nodule in a taut band.
3. Patient's recognition of current pain complaint by pressure on the tender nodule (identifies an active TrP).
4. Painful limit to full stretch range of motion.

Confirmatory Observations:
1. Visual or tactile identification of local twitch response.
2. Imaging of a local twitch response induced by needle penetration of a tender nodule.
3. Pain or altered sensation (in the distribution expected from a TrP in that muscle) on compression of the tender nodule.
4. Electromyographic demonstration of spontaneous electrical activity characteristic of active loci in the tender nodule of a taut band.

I find that for palpation in the vaginal area, the flat palpation technique is most appropriate. The levator ani muscles demonstrate ropy structures (taut bands) that are easily felt as they roll into the finger. The sensation of applying snapping palpation across the taut band can be compared to what plucking a violin or guitar string embedded in the muscle might feel like. In a muscle that has many central TrPs, five or six such bands or cords may lie in such close proximity to one another that they seem to merge. Using snapping palpation, multiple cords in the very broad levator ani muscles are frequently found. In addition, attachment TrPs are also a frequent occurrence in the levator ani muscles.

Localized tenderness that is elicited only when the finger pressure is directed in one specific direction is compatible with the diagnosis of either a central or an attachment TrP if pressure elicits pain recognized by the patient as her pain complaint. Additional evidence, such as restricted stretch range of motion and characteristic referred pattern, is helpful in making the diagnosis. Sufficient pressure on an active TrP will almost always elicit withdrawal, wincing, or vocalization by the patient when the levator ani muscles are palpated.

When the abdomen is examined for myofascial TrPs, the supine patient should take a deep breath using diaphragmatic (abdominal) breathing and hold the breath to passively stretch these muscles and to increase their sensitivity to palpation (3). To evaluate for lateral abdominal TrPs, the patient lies on the contralateral side and holds a similar deep breath.

External Oblique

Attachment TrPs to the external oblique muscle are found along the lower border of the rib cage and along the line where this muscle attaches to the iliac crest. I have found attachment points associated with the external oblique at its attachment to the iliac crest, particularly in patients who have been very active in such sports as soccer and gymnastics. In addition to examining the abdomen of the supine patient by flat palpation, the patient's hips may be flexed to slacken the abdominal muscles so that the abdominal wall in the flank area (external, internal obliques, and transversus muscles) can be grasped between the fingers and thumb.

Internal Oblique

To find attachment TrPs in the internal oblique the examiner presses down against the upper edge of the pubic arch, not on the flat anterior surface of the pubis. These TrPs feel like small buttons, or short bands at the region of attachments of the internal oblique fibers. I have found TrPs in this area in patients who have been active, especially in ballet and gymnastics. These patients have frequently undergone laparoscopies for evaluation and treatment of this pain without success.

Rectus Abdominus

TrPs are frequently found in the middle or lower portions of the rectus abdominus, especially along its lateral border and at its attachment to the pubic bone. I have found TrPs in this region in patients who have performed repetitive abdominal muscle training exercises.

Quadratus Lumborum

Active TrPs shorten the muscle and can thus distort pelvic alignment, elevating the pelvis on the side of the tense muscles. When the patient with active quadratus lumborum TrPs is standing, the pelvis is likely to tilt downward on the side opposite to the affected muscle. The lumbar spine usually exhibits a functional lumbar scoliosis that is convex away from the side of the involved quadratus lumborum Side bending is restricted toward the pain-free side.

Two common and closely related structural inadequacies are a short leg and a small hemipelvis (Figs. 38.3 and 38.4). Short leg syndrome can cause a tilted pelvis when standing and can result in a compensatory scoliosis that is maintained by sustained muscular effort and is a potent perpetuating factor for TrPs in those muscles. I have found compensatory scoliosis with associated short leg syndrome occurring in patients with underlying TrPs in the paraspinal, quadratus lumborum, iliopsoas, levator ani, and obturator internus muscles. Resolution of the TrPs in these associated muscles together with a lift for the short leg has resulted in correction of the functional scoliosis. The primary complaint of these patients is frequently dyspareunia.

A small hemipelvis can tilt the sacral base when the subject is standing or seated, similarly producing a compensatory scoliosis. The small hemipelvis can be corrected with a butt lift frequently for lasting relief of low back and pelvic

pain and sometimes head, neck, and shoulder pain due to myofascial TrPs. Short upper arms (in relation to torso height) leave the shoulders without adequate support in most seated positions. This leads to overloaded shoulder elevator muscles. It also produces compensatory distorted postures that can overload torso muscles and perpetuate their TrPs. The short first, long second metatarsal variation causes muscle imbalance that can extend from the leg to the head and perpetuate TrPs in those muscles. The long second metatarsal throws the foot off balance as a result of a knife-edge support during toeoff. This instability disturbs the gait and overloads lower-extremity muscles. This can result in pain in the gluteus medius muscle and therefore low back and pelvic pain.

To identify lower-limb length inequality, note that frequently one side of the patient is slightly smaller than the other. One lower limb is shorter than the other, the same side of the pelvis is smaller, and that side of the face is smaller. When asked, many patients remember having been told that one leg was shorter than the other at a previous exam. On observing these patients, they may walk with a tilt or lurch to one side; when standing they are likely to assume a short leg stance. That is, they stand with body weight on the shorter limb and the foot of the longer limb forward with the knee slightly flexed or with the longer limb placed diagonally to the side. The spine then curves to orient the head upright and level the eyes. If the inequality is slight, less than $1/2$ inch, a C-shaped scoliosis is likely to develop, causing the shoulder to rise on the side of the short leg. With a greater inequality, the scoliosis is often S-shaped, and the low shoulder may be on the side of the short leg. First, examine the patient for quadratus lumborum TrPs and, if present, inactivate them. Any TrP shortening of the quadratus lumborum is likely to produce a misleading result. For examination, the undressed patient should stand with the back to the examiner and with both knees straight, preferably facing a full length mirror. The feet are brought together and an estimate of length difference is made quickly by palpating the iliac crest and the posterior superior iliac spines. An approximate correction is placed promptly beneath the shorter limb, making sure that the patient finds that it comfortable. Add correction until the pelvis and shoulders are level and the spine is straight. Correction of as little as 3 mm (1/8 inch) can make an impressive difference in TrP irritability. I have found that TrPs in the levator ani and transverse perinei and in the attachments for the adductor muscles will resolve with injection therapy but recur if leg length correction is not made and if a functional scoliosis is not resolved by inactivation of quadratus lumborum and iliopsoas TrPs. Frequently, these patients will complain of severe pain with intercourse and vaginal and vulvar burning. The lower-limb inequality is one of the more frequent perpetuating factors for levator ani TrPs resulting in severe dyspareunia and even dysmenorrhea.

Examination for lower-limb length inequality with the patient supine can give the impression of a shorter limb on the side of an involved quadratus lumborum muscle. TrPs in the quadratus lumborum muscle are easily overlooked because almost all of this muscle lies anterior to the paraspinal muscle mass and is inaccessible from the posterior approach of a routine back examination. Examination for quadratus lumborum TrPs begins by palpating for the lateral edge of the paraspinal mass, the 12th rib, and the crest of the ilium. This is best performed with the patient positioned on her side. The muscle is examined for tenderness by applying deep pressure superior to the crest of the ilium and anterior to the paraspinal muscles. A second region is examined along the inner crest of the ilium where many of the iliocostal fibers attach. This flat palpation locates taut bands with tender spots in those fibers. Patients with quadratus lumborum TrPs and functional scoliosis also will have levator ani TrPs that are only responsive to treatment after the quadratus lumborum TrPs have been inactivated.

Iliopsoas Muscle

Patients with active TrPs that shorten the iliopsoas muscle significantly are likely to stand with the weight on the uninvolved limb and the foot of the involved limb forward with the knee bent slightly to lessen iliopsoas tension. When asked to bend forward while standing, they lean farther to the involved side through approximately the first 20 degrees of trunk flexion. Patients with active or latent iliopsoas TrPs tend to walk with a stooped posture, have a forward tilt to the pelvis, and exhibit hyperlordosis of the lumbar spine. The supine patient can be checked for shortening of the iliopsoas by testing the hip for extension range of motion with the thigh positioned over the end of the examining table.

In the supine patient, pressure can be exerted on the psoas musculotendinus junction and on iliacus muscle fibers by pressing against the lateral wall of the femoral triangle. Pain from TrPs in this part of the muscle is referred to the low back and usually to the anterior medial aspect of the thigh and to the groin. A second TrP can be identified if one palpates the proximal fibers of the iliacus muscle inside the iliac crest of the pelvis to the aponeurosis of the external abdominal oblique muscles. The patient must relax the abdominal muscles and must be positioned so that the skin of the abdominal wall becomes slackened. Fingers reach inside the crest of the ilium starting in the region behind the anterior superior iliac spine and slide back and forth parallel to the iliac crest while pressing against the bone, palpating across the fibers of the iliacus muscle. Palpation reveals taut bands and their associated spot tenderness. Pain evoked from these TrPs is likely to refer to the low back and the sacral iliac region. Many patients with TrPs in the iliopsoas and also in the abdominal muscles have been subjected to laparoscopies (which were negative) in a search for endometriosis or adhesions by physicians who are not familiar with the condition of myofascial TrPs.

The psoas muscle can be palpated indirectly through the abdominal wall. The patient must be comfortable, and the abdominal wall must be relaxed. The psoas major is palpated for tenderness along the entire length of the lumbar spine. Tenderness can usually be elicited at approximately the level of the umbilicus or slightly lower.

Endometriotic implants in the peritoneum overlying the iliopsoas muscle have been identified by this author as a perpetuating cause of iliopsoas TrPs. Only by treatment of the endometriosis has it been possible to then effect complete resolution of the identified iliopsoas TrP pain. It is frequently necessary to provide treatment for iliopsoas TrPs after complete excision of endometriotic lesions in order to achieve a complete relief of the pain experienced by these patients.

Pelvic Floor Muscles (Bulbospongiosus, Ischiocavernosus, Transversus Perinei, Sphincter Ani, Levator Ani, Coccygeous, and Obturator Internus)

Patients with TrPs in the pelvic floor musculature are likely to walk somewhat stiffly and sit down cautiously, often on one buttock close to the edge of the chair seat. The patient shifts sitting position frequently; and, after prolonged sitting, the act of rising from the chair often causes obvious pain and requires increased effort. If the obturator internus harbors active TrPs, the stretch range of motion will show some restriction. The clinician tests this in the supine position by looking for restricted medial rotation of the thigh with the hip straight. It is also helpful to screen for a tilted pelvis and for pelvic asymmetries in patients with pelvic floor muscle TrPs.

For the purpose of locating myofascial TrPs within the pelvis, the pelvic muscles can be considered in three categories: perineal muscles, pelvic floor muscles, and pelvic wall muscles.

The perineal muscles—the transverse perinei, bulbospongiosus, and ischiocavernosus—are the most superficial and contribute some support to the pelvic floor. Usually only the ischiocavernosus and transversus perinei superficialis muscles are identifiable by external palpation if they have taut bands and tender TrPs. This exam is best performed with the patient in lithotomy position with the feet in stirrups. The ischiocavernosus lies close to and along most of the length of the perineal margin of the pubic bone below the pubic symphysis. On vaginal examination, taut bands become evident when compressed by flat palpation against the margin of the pubic bone at the distal vaginal level and at right angles to the direction of the muscle fibers.

The pelvic floor muscles commonly affected with TrPs are the sphincter ani, levator ani, and coccygeous muscles.

If the patient has TrPs in the anal sphincter, insertion of the finger can be distressing. Internal hemorrhoids can perpetuate TrPs of the anal sphincter. In the presence of excessive sphincter contraction or tenderness the patient may bear down on the rectum to enhance relaxation of the sphincter ani as the clinician slowly inserts the examining finger directly into the anal orifice. The finger first encounters the external and then the internal sphincter ani. The finger should be withdrawn to halfway along the sphincters, and pressure should be gently applied to the muscle at every 1/8 of the circle. When the finger locates tenderness in one direction, the muscle is explored to determine where the spot of maximum tenderness occurs. An associated taut band may be identified.

To examine the levator ani, recall that the most medial and anterior portion of the pubococcygeous muscle loops around the urogenital tract and serves to constrict the vagina in women. The most posterior portion of pubococcygeous (the puborectalis) loops around the rectum at the level of the external ani sphincter. The iliococcygeous part of the levator ani forms a sling between the ilium and coccyx that supports the pelvic floor and pulls the coccyx inward. Palpation of the levator ani starts by feeling the ends of the muscle fibers for tenderness. The examiner moves the finger across the midbelly of the muscle from the region of the perineal body to the middle of the sacrospinous ligament, feeling for local tenderness and taut bands indicative of TrPs. By sweeping the finger from side to side through an arc of 180 degrees at successfully higher levels, the examiner can palpate all of the fibers of the levator ani and of the coccygeous muscle. It is necessary to inactivate TrPs in the ischiocavernosus, bulbospongiosus, and transverse perinei muscles prior to attempting the examination of the levator ani. In addition, patients with significant TrPs in the levator ani frequently require inactivation of those identified in the superficial one-third of the vaginal musculature, prior to continuing with examination of the middle one-third and deep one-third.

Tender spots in the lateral portion of the levator ani below this muscle's tendinous arch may be due to TrPs in the underlying obturator internus. Lateral rotation of the extended thigh against resistance activates the obturator internus. If the TrP is in the obturator internus, the increase in muscle tension will identify the contracting muscle. The obturator internus can also be identified by having the patient abduct the flexed thigh against resistance, a maneuver easily performed while the patient is in stirrups with the examiner providing the resistance with one hand while pressing against the TrP through the vagina with the other. I have found this maneuver to be indispensable in distinguishing levator ani from obturator internus TrPs.

The coccygeous muscle is palpable mainly at the level of the sacrococcygeal joint. Much of the muscle lies between the examining finger and the underlying sacrospinous ligament. Against this firm ligament, taut bands and their TrPs are usually readily identified by palpation across the muscle fibers. The gluteus maximus attachments to the outer margins of the sacrum and coccyx correspond closely to the coccygeous muscle's attachments on the inner margins of these bones. Tenderness along the margin of the coccyx suggests tenderness of either (a) levator ani musculotendinous junctions, (b) coccygeous musculotendinous junctions, or (c) a sacrococcygeous ventralis muscle.

The pelvic wall muscles include the obturator internus and piriformis as well as the sacrococcygeous ventralis (if present). When running the finger around the lateral wall of the pelvis above the tendinous arch of the levator ani from the ischial spine to the pubis, any observed tender spots or taut bands are in the obturator internus. Examination of the exit point of the obturator internus from the pelvis through the lesser sciatic foramen (below the tip of the ischial spine beneath the tendinous arch) is a critical point to determine if TrPs are present in the obturator internus muscle.

Patients with piriformis TrPs, when seated, tend to squirm and frequently shift position. They are likely to have difficulty crossing the involved thigh with the other knee when asked to do so. Tenderness of the piriformis muscle can be detected through the gluteus maximus for most of its length. Its medial end is accessible to nearly direct palpation by rectal or vaginal examination (Fig. 38.23). Its location is determined by drawing a line from the uppermost border of the greater trochanter through the sacroiliac end of the greater sciatic foramen. The medial end of the piriformis can be palpated within the pelvis by the vaginal route if the examiner has a long finger. The piriformis muscle lies just cephalad to the transversely oriented sacrospinous ligament, which can be felt as a firm band stretching between the sacrum and the ischial spine. A bimanual examination with one hand pressing externally on the buttock while the other hand palpates internally can also be performed. The greater sciatic foramen presents an unmistakable soft spot to which palpation pressure from one finger outside the pelvis can be transmitted to another finger inside the pelvis. To confirm identification of the piriformis muscle, the examiner palpates for contractile tension in the muscle while having the patient attempt to abduct the thigh by lifting the uppermost knee.

The bulbospongiosus and levator vaginae portions of the levator ani muscles also are examined for TrPs by gentle pincer palpation at about the middle of each lateral wall of the introitus. When present, taut bands are clearly delineated, are tender, and can contain TrPs that usually reproduce the patient's pain complaint. In addition, these myofascial TrPs weaken the muscles. Their strength can be assessed by having the patient squeeze the examining finger. TrPs can also be assessed by gentle palpation with a Q-tip against the perineal and vaginal tissues.

The coccygeal region and coccygeous muscle are more difficult to palpate from the vagina than from the rectum because one must palpate through two layers of rectal mucosa and one of vaginal mucosa. An optimum localiza-

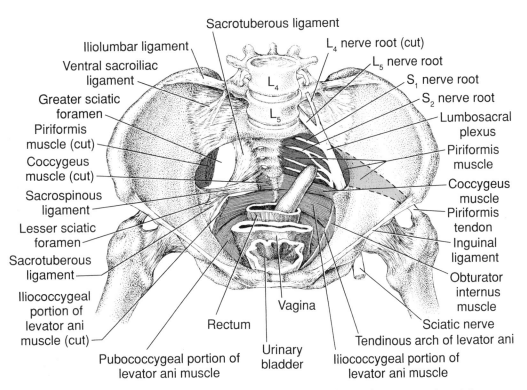

FIGURE 38.23. Internal palpation of the left piriformis muscle via the rectum, viewed from inside and above. The sacrospinous ligament (covered by the coccygeous muscle) is the last major transverse landmark identified by the palpating finger before it reaches the piriformis muscle. The sacrospinous ligament attaches cephalad mainly to the coccyx, which is usually easily palpated and mobile. The posterior wall of the rectum and the S2 and S3 nerve roots lie between the palpating finger and the piriformis muscle. (From Travell JG, Simons DG. *Myofacial pain and dysfunction: the trigger point manual*, vol 2, 1st ed. Baltimore: Williams and Wilkins, 1992:200, with permission.)

tion of all of the intrapelvic musculoskeletal structures requires both rectal and vaginal examinations.

Gluteus Maximus

Patients with active TrPs in the gluteus maximus muscle when seated shift position frequently to relieve pressure on their TrPs. Tightness of the muscle is tested in the supine patient by bringing the knee toward the opposite axilla and medially rotating the thigh at the hip. Normally the thigh should rest firmly against the chest at full range of motion. Gluteus maximus TrPs can reduce this range by as much as 35 degrees. Taut bands in this superficial gluteal muscle are relatively easy to palpate, and local twitch responses are vigorous and often visible. TrPs can also occur in the gluteus medius and gluteus minimus muscles.

Pectineus Muscle

The pectineus muscle can be located by first palpating the upper border of the symphysis pubis. Two or three centimeters lateral to the symphysis is the pubic tubercle, to which the medial end of the inguinal ligament attaches. When the thigh is placed in moderate abduction without flexion, the adductor longus muscle should be palpable if not visible. The adductor longus and brevis muscles lie parallel to, and are immediately medial and deeper than, the pectineus. The pectineus muscle attaches to the crest of the superior ramus of the pubic bone just inferior to the medial portion of the inguinal ligament. By palpating lateral to the pubic tubercle, the anterior edge of the superior ramus of the pubic bone is readily felt. The lateral distal part of the pectineus muscle lies deep to the femoral neurovascular bundle. The artery courses down the middle of the femoral triangle. Its pulsation is readily palpable in most patients. The TrPs in the pectineus muscle are located just distal to the superior ramus of the pubis. After TrPs in the three other adductors or in the iliopsoas have been inactivated, the pectineus may be uncovered as the cause of persistent deep-seated groin pain.

Adductor Longus, Adductor Brevis, Adductor Magnus

Active TrPs in the adductor longus and adductor brevis restrict abduction of the thigh. The one-third of the adductor longus that is closest to the pelvis is best examined by pincer palpation. Because the adductor brevis underlies the longus, it is reached only by deep flat palpation. The adductor magnus is accessible to subcutaneous palpation only in the proximal portion of the posterior medial aspect of the thigh. This narrow triangle is bordered by the ischial tuberosity and pubis proximally, the semimembranous and

semi-tendinous muscles behind and the gracilis anteriorly (Fig. 38.24) TrPs in the pectineus and adductor muscles frequently occur in patients with a history of vigorous physical activity such as soccer and ballet.

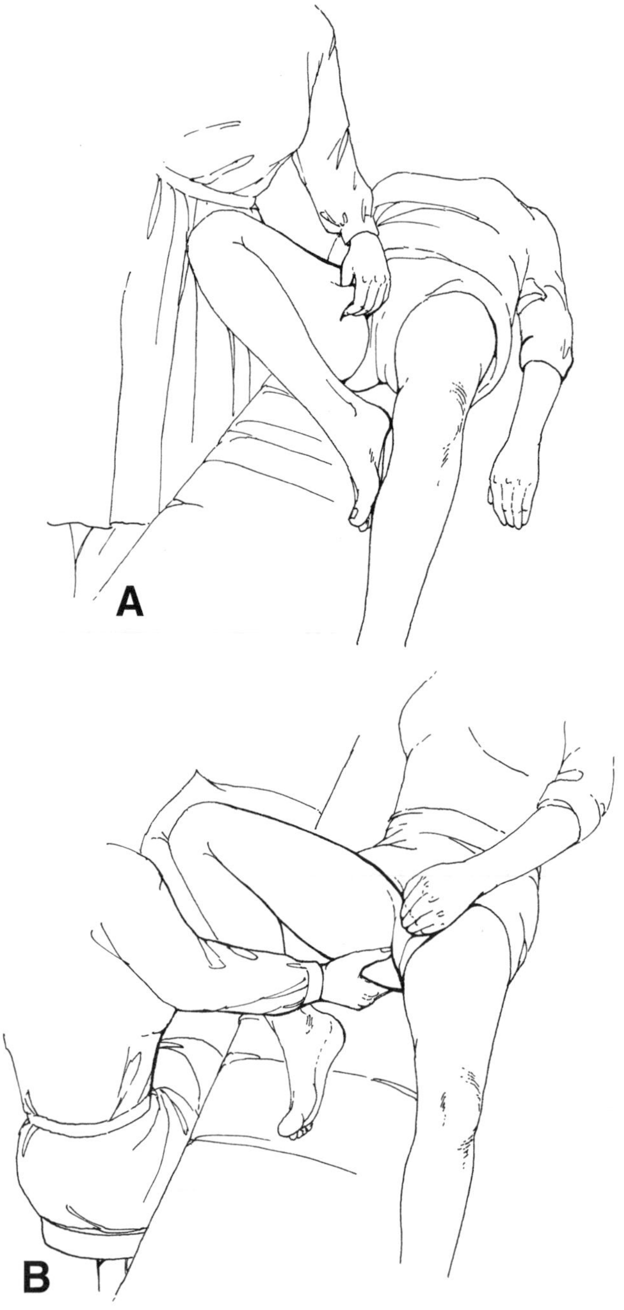

DIAGNOSTIC STUDIES

One reason for the neglect of myofascial TrPs, misdiagnosis, and often ineffective treatment has been the absence of an objective method of diagnosis. For TrPs alone, laboratory studies such as x-ray, computerized tomography, magnetic resonance imaging, and blood tests are normal. Nerve conduction and routine electromyographic studies are also frequently normal.

Surface Electromyography

TrPs are known to cause distortion or disruption of normal muscle function. Functionally the muscle with the TrP evidences a threefold problem: It exhibits increased responsiveness, delayed relaxation, and increased fatigability, which, together, increase overload and reduce work tolerance. In addition, the TrP can produce referred spasm and referred inhibition in other muscles.

I have found that intravaginal electromyographic (EMG) recordings of patients with levator ani TrPs consistently shows hypertonus in the resting state and decreased excursion compared to normal with attempted maximal contraction. In addition, the fast twitch fibers activate more slowly and the slow twitch fibers show rapid degradation of activity. These EMG readings are obtained with internal surface sensors. Needle EMG studies of patients with TrPs employing a special technique have shown characteristic electrical activity and active loci of the TrPs. Histologic examination of TrPs in canine muscles has shown contraction knots.

Pressure Algometry

Pressure algometry is a diagnostic tool used to quantify the sensitivity of myofascial trigger points and identify abnormal tenderness. It provides a useful method to assess the outcomes of different treatments. Localized tenderness can be quantified by measurement of pressure threshold, which is defined as the minimum pressure that elicits pain.

Needle Electromyography

Spontaneous low-voltage motor endplate "noise" activity as well as high-voltage spike activity is present when myofascial TrPs are present. The source of high-voltage spikes alone can be ambiguous. When the endplate noise activity is observed, it a strongly confirmatory finding and is an invaluable research tool.

FIGURE 38.24. Examination for proximal TrPs in the right adductor muscles. **A:** Adductor longus and adductor brevis by examined pincer palpation. The knee is supported against the operator to ensure voluntary relaxation while these muscles are placed on moderate stretch for examination. **B:** Proximal end of the adductor magnus, examined by flat palpation against the underlying ischium posterior to the adductor longus, adductor brevis, and gracilis muscles. (From Travell JG, Simons DG. *Myofacial pain and dysfunction: the trigger point manual,* vol 2, 1st ed. Baltimore: Williams and Wilkins, 1992:306, with permission.)

Blood Testing

Vitamin B$_{12}$ is essential for normal fat and carbohydrate metabolism (including muscles). Folates are also critical for normal muscle function. Chronic myofascial pain patients should be tested routinely for both of these vitamins. B$_{12}$ is commonly deficient, especially in strict vegetarians. Folic acid is found in small amounts in many foods, particularly leafy green vegetables, and is largely destroyed by processing and cooking. Patients taking a daily total of more than 10,000 international units of vitamin A should have their serum levels tested.

Normal erythrocyte sedimentation rate and C reactive protein tests help to eliminate the possibility of chronic infection.

Diffuse muscle tenderness may be the major physical finding in mild hypothyroidism. Measurement of serum creatine kinase (CK) and cholesterol, both of which become elevated in hypothyroidism, may be useful. The TRH stimulation test produces an abnormal elevation of TSH in hypothyroidism and may be useful in the diagnosis of mild hypothyroidism. Measurement of TSH, free T4, thyroid peroxidase antibodies, and thyroglobin antibodies (from Hashimoto's thyroditis) are used to evaluate these patterns. Mild hypothyroidism can also be the result of impaired peripheral utilization despite adequate circulating thyroid hormone.

Utrasound Imaging

High-resolution ultrasound has been used to visualize a local twitch response. This test, however, requires the examiner to insert a needle into the TrP in order to elicit the twitch response.

DIFFERENTIAL DIAGNOSIS

The differential diagnosis of diseases that produce symptoms that are commonly caused by or may mimic the pain caused by abdominal muscle TrPs includes articular dysfunctions, fibromyalgia, appendicitis, peptic ulcer, gallstone colic, colitis, painful rib syndrome, intractable dysmenorrhea, enigmatic pelvic pain syndrome caused by abdominal wall TrPs, and urinary tract disease (1). This author has found that the differential diagnosis also includes chronic endometritis and endometriosis. Additional differential diagnostic considerations include hiatal hernia, gastric carcinoma, chronic cholecystitis or ureteral colic, inguinal hernia, hepatitis, pancreatitis, gynecologic pathology, diverticulosis, umbilical hernia, thoracic ridiculopathy, upper lumbar ridiculopathy, costal chondritis, epilepsy and rectus abdominus hematoma. Articular dysfunctions associated with abdominal TrPs include pubic and innominate dysfunctions and depressed lesions of the lower half of the rib cage on the side of involvement.

Sacroiliac joint displacement, malignant neoplasm, neurogenic tumors, and local infection can mimic the piriformis syndrome. A herniated intervertebral disc will generally result in absence or marked weakness of the Achilles tendon reflex and motor denervation shown by electromyography. Slowing of conduction velocity in the sciatic nerve to the pelvis suggests piriformis entrapment. Inactivation of the piriformis muscle TrPs relieves the limp and the buttock and posterior thigh pain of myofascial entrapment origin. Spinal stenosis should be considered when the pain and pelvic wall tenderness are bilateral. Piriformis syndrome may develop secondary to sacral iliac arthritis (20).

Patients with obturator nerve entrapment may present with pain similar to pectineus TrPs. The obturator and genitofemoral nerves may cause pain or tingling in the groin or in the medial thigh when they become entrapped. About half of the patients who have an obturator hernia develop symptoms of entrapment of the obturator nerve: pain and/or tingling and paresthesias down the medial surface of the thigh to the knee. Entrapment of the genitofemoral nerve can be caused by excessively tight clothing over the inguinal ligament.

Pubic stress symphysitis seen in distance runners and persons who compete in contact sports causes pain in the region of the symphysis pubis.

Three conditions associated with chronic overload of the adductor muscles must be considered: pubic stress symphyisitis (osteitis pubis), pubic stress fracture (avulsion stress fracture of the pubic bone), and adductor insertion avulsion syndrome.

Examination of patients with pubic stress symphysitis reveals focal tenderness of the pubic symphysis bilaterally and pain on abduction and extension of the thighs. This may be accompanied by adductor TrPs. Confirmatory findings include radiographic evidence of sclerosis and irregularity of the pubic bone at the symphysis and scintigraphic evidence of increased radionuclide uptake at the symphysis. Shearing action on the symphysis is the cause of symphysitis. Stress fractures of the inferior pubic ramus usually at the junction with the ischial ramus occur in 1% to 2% of runners. Adductor insertion avulsion occurs at the insertion of the adductor muscles due to stress. The referred pain from adductor longus TrPs may be mistaken for the pain of osteoarthritis of the hip (20).

Fibromyalgia

Subjects identified as having fibromyalgia must satisfy the criteria of the American College of Rheumatology, specifically giving a history of widespread pain and tenderness at 11 of 18 tender points on digital palpation. Widespread pain must have been present for at least 3 months. A considerable number of fibromyalgia patients also have myofascial TrPs. Distinguishing myofascial TrPs and fibromyalgia is relatively simple when the myofascial TrPs are acute, but can be much more difficult when the myofascial TrPs have evolved into a chronic pain syndrome through neglect or inappropriate treatment. Clinical features distinguishing myofascial pain due to TrPs from fibromyalgia include the following: TrPs are local or regional, whereas pain from fibromyalgia is widespread and general; TrPs show focal tenderness, whereas fibromyalgia shows widespread tenderness; the muscle with TrPs feels tense (taut bands), whereas the muscle of fibromyalgia feels soft and doughy; the muscles with TrPs have restricted range of motion, whereas muscles involved in fibromyalgia are hypermobile; and with TrPs there is an immediate response to injection, whereas fibromyalgia shows a delayed or poor response to injection. Twenty percent of patient with TrPs also have fibromyalgia, whereas 72% of patient with fibromyalgia have active TrPs (3). In fibromyalgia patients, locations other than tender point sites are as tender at all three depths of tissue (cutaneous, subcutaneous, and intramuscular) as are their tender point sites. Non-TrP sites in myofascial patients measure the same high pain thresholds as corresponding sites in normal subjects. Fibromyalgia patients are abnormally tender almost everywhere. Myofascial pain patients are abnormally tender only at sharply circumscribed TrP sites and specific sites of referred tenderness.

Articular Dysfunction

Pain in articular dysfunctions that require manual mobilization is commonly caused by TrPs. In the segmental vicinity of an osteopathic lesion (vertebrae with evidence of articular dysfunction) there is decreased pain thresholds, increased sympathetic activity, and facilitation of motor pathways. The muscle dysfunction component and the articular dysfunction component of musculoskeletal pain syndrome should be addressed when both are present. The increased tension of TrP taut bands in their facilitation of motor activity can maintain displacement stress on a joint while abnormal sensory input from the dysfunctional joint can reflexly activate the TrP dysfunction. The two conditions can aggravate each other.

Abdominal Pathology

Myofascial pain syndromes must be distinguished from peripheral nerve injuries, hernias, abdominal pain of spinal origin, spontaneous rectus sheath hematoma, and visceral pain that can result in abdominal wall pain (24).

TREATMENT AND MANAGEMENT

Acute myofascial pain due to TrPs caused by a clearly identifiable strain of one muscle can usually be fully relieved and normal function restored. Usually, the longer the period between the acute onset of pain and the beginning of TrP treatment, the greater the number of treatments that will be required over a longer period of time (3). Patients who have had a stable pattern of referred TrP pain for months or longer, without extension to other muscles, are likely to respond better to treatment than patients with progressively more severe symptoms. When the pain has spread with successively more muscles involved, multiple perpetuating factors must be eliminated before specific myofascial therapy can provide sustained relief.

It is important to consider whether the TrPs being treated are central TrPs in the endplate zone of the muscle or are attachment TrPs located where the muscle attaches to its aponeurosis (tendon) or bone. Stretching (lengthening) inactivates central TrPs, but may tend to aggravate the overloaded muscle attachments. The attachment TrPs are more likely to respond to manual therapy that is directed to the regions where central TrPs are located and therapy that concentrates on relieving the strain of the attachments caused by the TrP-induced shortening of the taut fibers. Because the attachment TrPs are the result of tension from the taut bands of the central TrPs, inactivation of the central TrP is essential. On the other hand, reducing the sensitivity of the attachment TrPs may greatly facilitate inactivation of the central TrPs. Recovery of full function may involve more than just TrP inactivation and relief of pain. If the muscle has learned dysfunction that restricts both its length and coordination during functional activities, it must be retrained to normal function.

If after treatment the patients returns pain-free with complete restoration of full range of motion and the prior TrP sites are no longer abnormally tender, the treatment was successful. If the pain relief was complete for some hours or days, one can assure the patient that a muscular cause of the pain is present and that it can be relieved, at least temporarily. However, repeated treatment without first resolving the perpetuating factors that make the TrPs so hyperirritable is likely to be fruitless. A major effort should then focus on identifying and eliminating the perpetuating factors. If careful comparison of a current pain pattern with the patterns of the patient's previous visits shows a distinct improvement and if some of the muscles previously treated no longer contain tender TrPs, this represents satisfactory progress. In this case one set of TrPs has been inactivated, but the absence of that pain has unmasked the referred pain pattern of the next most active TrP. Without the accurately recorded pain patterns for comparison, the clinician and the patient might overlook the progress being made.

Trigger Point Release

Techniques of TrP release include spray and stretch, voluntary contraction and release methods, TrP pressure release, deep stroking massage, and TrP injections (3,9,20,23,25,26).

Spray and Stretch

Spray and stretch is the single most effective noninvasive method to inactivate acute TrPs. A single muscle syndrome of recent onset frequently responds with full return of pain-free function when two or three sweeps of spray are applied while the muscle is being extended gently to its full stretch length. This spray and stretch technique does not require the precise localization of the TrP that is needed for injection; it requires only identification of where the taut bands are located in the muscle to ensure that those fibers are released. The essential therapeutic component is the stretch, but the spray reduces tension-sensitive tenderness of the enthesopathy to facilitate stretch release of the muscle tension. Spray and stretch is especially useful immediately after TrP injection during the period that the local anesthesia remains. This combination procedure helps to inactivate any residual TrP activity and to attain full stretch range of motion.

To be effective for releasing TrP tension and recovering full-strength range of motion, the vapocoolant must be released as a fine stream and not as a disbursed spray. Either Fluori-Methane (Gebauer) or ethyl chloride may be used. Ethyl chloride is excessively cold, flammable, and a lethal anesthetic. If it is used, it must be handled with care. Because it is a fluorocarbon mixture, a suitable substitute for Fluori-Methane is being developed.

By reproducing the referred pain with digital pressure on the TrP, the clinician assists the patient to more fully understand why treatment is directed primarily to the tender region in the muscle and not primarily to the region of the pain complaint. I have found this technique very helpful in treating the pain described by patients as severe pain on one side of the vulva, which is in fact arising from attachments of the adductor muscles and which responds to spray and stretch techniques for the adductor muscles in the regions of their central TrPs.

Spray and Stretch Techniques

The patient should be comfortable, warm, and well-supported so that the involved muscle is fully relaxed. To effectively stretch a muscle, one end of it must be anchored so that the operator can help move the other end to take up any slack in the muscles. Figures 38.25, 38.26, and 38.27 summarize the steps in the technique for the abdominal and adductor muscles. Sweeps of spray are continued over the complete pain pattern to begin releasing muscle tension before taking up the slack to lengthen the muscle toward its stretch position. The spray procedure can be repeated until full normal muscle length is achieved. Any given area of skin should be covered only two or three times before rewarming. After the skin is rewarmed, several cycles of full active range of motion complete one spray and stretch treatment of that muscle.

Frosting of the skin can occur when one spot is sprayed too long (about 6 secs), and this should be avoided. However, the closer the bottle is held to the skin, the warmer is the stream of vapocoolant on impact. If the skin is hyper-sensitive to cold, hold the bottle close to the skin and move the jet stream across the skin rapidly. Usually the bottle can be held about 12 in. from the skin and slow, even sweeps at about 4 in./sec are spaced to provide a slight overlap of the tracks of wet spray. Two or three superimposed sweeps are usually the maximum before the skin must be rewarmed. Spray may be especially effective in quieting attachment TrPs, and the stretch may be specific for the release of central TrPs. The value of spray and stretch may lie in the fact that both kinds of TrPs need to be relieved and that this technique addresses both. The vapocoolant spray is remarkably effective for chilling the skin to numb it for painless TrP injections.

Lengthening the contracted sarcomeres of the contraction knots by gentle sustained stretch with augmentation techniques apparently induces gradual reduction in the overlap between actin and myosin molecules and reduces the energy being consumed. When the sarcomeres reach full stretch length, there is minimal overlap and greatly reduced energy consumption. This breaks an essential link in the energy crisis vicious cycle. The key to treating TrPs is to lengthen the muscle fibers that are shortened by the TrP mechanism. Initially the operator should gently lengthen the muscle until there is a rapidly increasing resistance to further movement (the barrier) and then hold that degree of tension. As unhurried, rhythmic intermittent sweeps of vapocoolant are applied, the gentle pressure is maintained to keep the muscle stretched to the barrier. As the muscle "gives up" and releases its tension, the operator smoothly takes up the slack to reestablish a new stretch position that again engages the barrier. After completing full stretch, the return to resting length must be smooth and gradual.

The stretch technique can be performed by any method that gently stretches (lengthens) a muscle with TrPs and increases its pain-free range of motion. It is often possible with a newly activated TrP to inactivate it immediately by simply passively, slowly stretching the muscle without spray. The release can be expedited when stretch is combined with augmentation maneuvers such as coordinated exhalation, postisometric relaxation, contract–relax, and reciprocal inhibition (actively assisting passive stretch). The muscle may be elongated by moving the joints it crosses or by direct manual traction applied to the muscle itself.

Direct stretch release is performed by placing two hands near the attachments of the muscles and gently separating them until a tissue barrier is encountered. This tension elongates the muscle and the associated connective tissues. This stretch release is preceded by prespraying with vapocoolant.

The most important poststretch (or postinjection) procedure is to have the patient actively perform three full cycles of the range of motion that fully lengthens and fully shortens each muscle that was treated. A program of home stretch exercises is important. Posttreatment muscle sore-

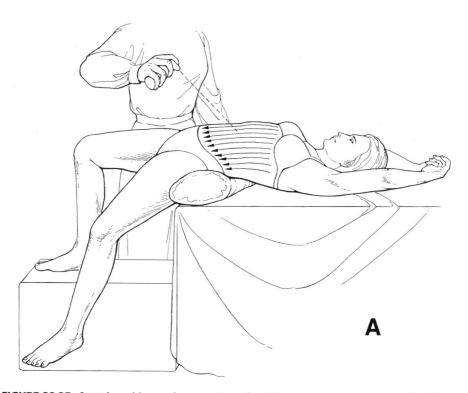

FIGURE 38.25. Stretch position and spray pattern for TrPs in abdominal muscles on the left side of the body with follow-up range of motion. **A:** The patient lies supine with the hip joint at the edge of the treatment table and with the lower limb extending over the end of the table. The hips are padded with a pillow. The arms are raised and one lower limb is supported on a stool or a chair seat. The lower limb on the treatment side at first is supported by the stool or by the therapist in order to allow gradual stretch. After the operator initially applies vapocoolant with sweeps in the caudal direction, the patient allows the lower limb on the treatment side (left) to hang free and takes a very deep, slow breath, allowing the downward moving diaphragm to strongly protrude the relaxed abdominal musculature. This is a critical step to stretch the abdominal muscles effectively. As the patient completes the inhalation and begins to slowly exhale, sweeps of spray are applied in a caudal direction and extend to the attachment of the iliopsoas (because that muscle often also has TrPs and is stretched by this procedure.) The procedure should be repeated for the contralateral abdominal muscles. **B:** Bilateral knee-to-chest position that unloads stress that might have been placed on the lumbosacral spine. The patient assumes this position after release of the muscles on both sides of the abdomen. In this position, the abdominal muscles are fully shortened when the patient gently and fully exhales. To restore full functional range of motion, the patient should gently alternate between the fully stretched and fully shortened position three times, one leg at a time. Return from the fully stretched position may require assistance to avoid muscle overload at first. (From Travell JG, Simons DG. *Myofacial pain and dysfunction: the trigger point manual*, vol 2, 2nd ed. Baltimore: Williams and Wilkins, 1992:960, with permission.)

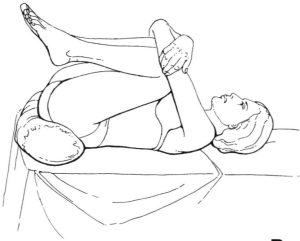

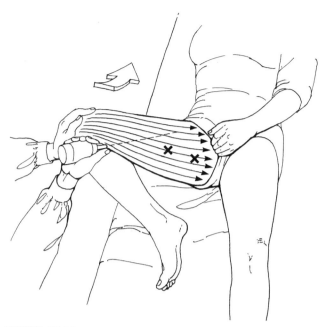

FIGURE 38.26. Stretch position and intermittent cold pattern for TrPs in the right adductor magnus muscle with the patient lying supine. The X's mark frequent, central, and attachment location of these TrPs. The intermittent cold pattern extends upward from the patella covering the entire muscle in parallel sweeps. The thick arrow shows the direction of pressure downward toward the floor and cephalad to increase the abduction–flexion passive stretch on this muscle. (From Travell JG, Simons DG. *Myofacial pain and dysfunction: the trigger point manual*, vol 2, 1st ed. Baltimore: Williams and Wilkins, 1992:308, with permission.)

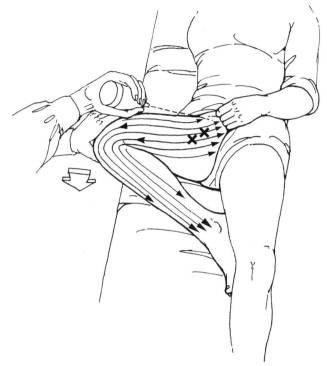

FIGURE 38.27. Stretch position and intermittent cold pattern for TrPs in the right adductor longus and adductor brevis muscles. A vapocoolant spray or an application using ice first covers the muscle and its proximal referred pain pattern with upward parallel sweeps, and then it is applied downward over the distal pain reference zone, including the knee, shin, and ankle. As the adductor muscle tension release, the thigh and knee drop down towards the table (thick arrow). Sweeps of intermittent cold also cover the thigh anteriorly and laterally to release any tension of the vasti of the quadriceps femoris. The right foot is successively moved up the thigh for additional stretch. (From Travell JG, Simons DG. *Myofacial pain and dysfunction: the trigger point manual*, vol 2, 1st ed. Baltimore: Williams and Wilkins, 1992:309, with permission.)

ness is reduced by applying moist heat (a hot pack) for a few minutes immediately after spray and stretch (or injection).

Voluntary Contraction and Release Methods

These methods basically employ voluntary (active) contraction followed by relaxation. The reduction in muscle stiffness (tension) following a contraction provides an increase in range of motion during the period of relaxation. Included among these techniques are contract–relax, postisometric relaxation, a combination of postisometric relaxation and reciprocal inhibition, hold–relax, and many muscle energy techniques.

Postisometric Relaxation

The basic concept of postisometric relaxation (PIR) is to contract the tense muscle isometrically against resistance and then encourage it to lengthen during a period of complete voluntary relaxation. PIR begins by having the patient perform a gentle isometric contraction of the tense muscle at its maximum pain-free length while the clinician stabilizes that part of

the body to prevent muscle shortening. After holding this contraction for 3 to 10 sec, the patient is instructed to "let go" and to relax the body completely. Reciprocal inhibition can also be incorporated to enhance the release of tight muscles.

Reciprocal Inhibition

To invoke reciprocal inhibition, the muscles that oppose the muscle that is being stretched are voluntarily contracted to actively assist the stretching movement. Thus, the muscle to be stretched is reciprocally inhibited.

Contract–Relax

Contract–relax is a gentle, voluntary, minimally resisted contraction of the tight muscle. The contraction is followed by relaxation to permit passive elongation of the muscle to a new stretch length.

Hold–Relax

Hold–relax consists of isometric contraction of the tight muscle followed by relaxation, but not by elongation of the tight muscle. Hold–relax is commonly combined with manual techniques applied directly to the muscle, such as deep-stroking massage and TrP pressure release. I have found that hold–relax and contract–relax techniques combined with biofeedback using a computerized EMG system with an intravaginal probe has been helpful in the release of TrPs in the pelvic floor muscles.

Trigger Point Pressure Release

Trigger point pressure release employs the barrier release concept. The patient learns what optimal pressure feels like for subsequent self-treatment. To apply TrP pressure release, the clinician lengthens the muscle to the point of increasing resistance within the comfort zone and then applies gentle, gradually increasing pressure on the TrP until the finger encounters a definite increase in tissue resistance (engages the barrier). At that point, the patient may feel a degree of discomfort but should not experience pain. This pressure is maintained but not increased until the clinician senses relief of tension under the palpating finger. The palpating finger increases pressure enough to take up the tissue slack and to encounter (engage) a new barrier (the finger "follows" the releasing tissue). The clinician again maintains only light pressure until more of the muscle tension releases ("lets go") under the finger. TrP pressure release is particularly well suited to muscles like the levator ani and obturator internus when applied by a clinician with a high manual skill. Patients frequently complain of discomfort during initial treatment using this technique, and skillful vocal reassurance is helpful in assisting the patient to cope with this discomfort.

This barrier release approach may fail to afford relief because (a) the TrP is too irritable to tolerate any additional mechanical stimulation, (b) the operator misjudged the pressure required to reach the barrier, (c) the operator pressed too hard, causing pain and autonomic responses with involuntary tensing by the patient, and (d) the patient has perpetuating factors that make the TrPs hyperirritable and resistant to treatment. In some cases, I have found it necessary to provide TrP injections with local anesthetic into the pelvic floor muscles to enhance the effectiveness of TrP pressure release.

Deep-Stroking Massage and Other Massage

Deep-stroking massage (stripping massage) is an effective way to inactivate central TrPs when using a direct manual approach. The muscle to be treated is completely relaxed and lengthened to the barrier (without pain). The skin is lubricated. The thumbs of both hands are placed so that they trap a taut band between them at the band's TrP. As the digits encounter the nodularity of the TrP that is caused by its contraction knots, pressure is exerted to engage the restrictive barrier. Tissue release occurs as the nodularity "gives" to some extent. The stroking massage is continued along the length of the remaining taut band to the attachment of that band. The next massage stroke proceeds in the reverse direction starting on the nodule to further release the contractured sarcomeres. Another technique is to apply pressure on the TrP with paired digits and slowly separate them away from the TrP. The taut band is then trapped between each pair of digits (one pair on each hand).

Strumming Massage

The strumming finger runs across the taut bands at the level of the TrPs over the nodules from one side of the muscle to the other. The operator's finger pulls perpendicularly across the muscle fibers rather than along the length of the fibers. This method applies specifically to central TrPs. When the nodule of the TrP is encountered, light contact is maintained at that point until the operator senses tissue release under the finger. Relaxed deep coordinated abdominal breathing by the patient facilitates general relaxation during the exhalation phase. This technique is particularly applicable to the pelvic floor muscles, which permit direct palpation of the muscle through only a thin layer of mucosa.

Biofeedback

Glazer et al. (27) reported this approach in patients with longer-term moderate to severe chronic introital dyspareunia and tenderness of the vulvar vestibule. Patients underwent EMG evaluation of the pelvic floor muscles. They were then provided with portable EMG biofeedback instrumentation and instructions on the conduct of daily at-home biofeedback-assisted, pelvic-floor muscle rehabilitation exercises. Patients were instructed to perform a contract–relax exercise program at home. After an average of 16 weeks of practice, the electrical activity during maximum-effort contractions of pelvic floor muscles increased 95% and resting electrical activity levels (spasm) decreased 68%. Muscles at rest were more stable, with EMG reading changing from a highly fluctuating to a nearly flat-line level. Subjective reports of pain decreased an average of 83% using visual analog scales. Twenty-two of 28 patients who had abstained from intercourse resumed intercourse by the end of the treatment. Six-month follow-up indicated maintenance of therapeutic benefits.

I have found that the addition of EMG-controlled biofeedback in the office at 1-week intervals, with the patient performing the exercises for 15 min on a computerized EMG-controlled system, followed by 15 min of neuromuscular stimulation and a second 15 min biofeedback session, supplemented by a pelvic floor trainer used at home, to be a helpful adjunct to treatment of patients with levator ani TrPs and associated pain with intercourse.

Heat and Cold

It appears that central TrPs are more responsive to warmth and that attachment TrPs are more responsive to cold. However, no controlled study is known that has explored the effectiveness of heat versus cold when applied to TrPs as therapy.

Microamperage

The whole field of cutaneous stimulation procedures to treat underlying TrPs needs critical investigation to resolve whether there is effectiveness in these techniques and, if so, why are they effective.

Therapeutic Ultrasound

Clinically, many therapists find the application of ultrasound an effective means of inactivating TrPs. One technique starts with 0.5 W/cm^2 and uses a slow dwell technique with a circular motion that completes one circle in 1 or 2 sec. The circle is small enough to provide a small overlap over the TrP in the center of the circle.

High-Voltage Galvanic Stimulation

The use of high-voltage galvanic stimulation is common practice among some therapists as a primary modality for treatment of TrPs. Clinical experience suggests that one effective technique is to increase the intensity of cyclic electrical stimulation to the point of gentle muscular contraction. The wave-form characteristic of this kind of electrical stimulation is relatively high frequency brief spikes of at least 150 V with very rapid rise times and no duration of peak voltage.

Transcutaneous Electrical Nerve Stimulation

Transcutaneous electrical nerve stimulation (TENS) is well established as one means of obtaining temporary, sometimes prolonged, pain relief. It is not a treatment modality for myofascial TrPs. I have had success using interferential stimulation at a low frequency (0 to 100 Hz) for control of pain from TrPs. The interferential unit uses a carrier current frequency of 4,000 Hz that is delivered to the electrodes and penetrates comfortably through the different tissue layers with the treatment frequency incorporated. The system modulates at different frequencies allowing different tissue layers to be treated. The modulated frequencies for pain control are between 0 and 100 Hz and are controlled by the patient. This allows the patient to target a specific area of pain at deeper levels than allowed by a TENS unit.

Neuromuscular Stimulation

This author has found the use of neuromuscular stimulation with an intravaginal probe at settings; frequency of 125 Hz, pulse width of 200 microsec, and amplitude to tolerance (15–40 milliamperes) very effective in treating pelvic floor muscle trigger points—especially when preceded and followed by biofeedback under EMG control. A frequency of 50 Hz with pulse width of 250 millisec is also effective.

Trigger Point Injection

I have found TrP injection of the pelvic floor muscles to be a reliable, safe, and effective technique for the treatment of pelvic floor TrPs. It is especially effective in demonstrating to the patient that there is a technique that provides them the hope for successful therapy.

Generally, the injection of a local anesthetic without corticosteroid or adrenaline is recommended. Dry needling also can be effective but results in more postprocedure soreness. Under special circumstances only, one can inject botulinum toxin A. Treatment using injection of a local anesthetic or dry needling depends on mechanical disruption and inactivation of the active loci in that TrP. One Trp site has a highly variable number of active loci that must be inactivated, and all of the loci in one TrP can be needled or injected with one skin penetration. When a local anesthetic is used, one should inject only a small amount (less 3 mL) at any one location within the TrP. When reporting TrP injections, for each injection the clinician should specify the muscle injected, whether it was a central TrP or an attachment TrP, and the type and amount of solution.

Identification and injection of key TrPs can produce impressive results. I have found that injection of one or two abdominal TrPs and/or one or two pelvic floor TrPs is frequently sufficient to demonstrate to the patient the effectiveness of the treatment program, which is then undertaken with a combination of TrP injection, manual techniques, biofeedback, interferential and microcurrent techniques. I prefer a mixture of lidocaine HCl 1% mixed with sodium bicarbonate 8.4% (50 mEq/50 mL). This combination is mixed 9 mL of 1% lidocaine to 1 mL of sodium bicarbonate just prior to injection for maximum effectiveness. This combination decreases the discomfort of the first sensation that the patient sometimes experiences with a lidocaine injection and also increases the effectiveness of the anesthetic medication. At any one session, no more than 20 mL equivalent of a 1% lidocaine solution is given. This provides a reasonable safety margin to avoid complications that can occur if too much local anesthetic solution is given. Solutions of stronger than 1% become increasingly and significantly myotoxic. Longer-acting anesthetic tend to be more myotoxic than shorter-acting ones. Epinephrine severely increases myotoxity without conferring any appreciable clinical advantage when injecting TrPs.

With 0.5% procaine, accidental injection of 2 mL into an artery or vein creates no problem if adequate hemostatis is applied to the vessel. Injection with the same strength solution near a nerve causes only mild sensory loss for a maximum of about 20 mins, which is well-tolerated if the patient is previously warned that this might happen. Procaine is the least myotoxic among the local anesthetic that are commonly injected. Pain sensation following nerve block reappears in 19 min after 1% procaine and in 40 min after 1% lidocaine. Procaine is not rapidly absorbed from mucus membranes. Procaine selectively affects small, usually unmyelinated, fibers as compared to large myelinated nerve fibers and thus blocks pain perception more than voluntary motor control. Procaine 0.5% is not commercially available, and therefore it is produced by diluting one part of 2% procaine solution with three parts of an isotonic saline solution.

Isotonic saline injection also has been used with good therapeutic results. Corticosteroids offer no advantage in the treatment of central TrPs. On the other hand, the nerve sensitization of attachment TrPs is the result of chronic mechanical stress, which may produce aspects of an inflammatory reaction that would be responsive to corticosteroids. The common practice of relieving the pain of enthesopathy with injection of corticosteroids supports this as a possibility. The definitive treatment for attachment TrPs is inactivation of the central TrPs responsible for them. However, prompt reduction in the tenderness and irritability of the region of enthesopathy at the attachment TrP is therapeutically beneficial to the patient's comfort, facilitates stretch release of related central TrPs, and most likely helps to reduce the irritability of corresponding central TrPs.

The patient should be recumbent for the TrP injection. It is then easier to adjust muscle tension so that the bands containing TrPs stand out in a background of relaxed muscle fibers. For internal pelvic TrPs, standard stirrups with the patient in dorsolithotomy position are adequate, but at times a frog-leg position is more comfortable for the patient.

The increased capillary fragility characteristic of a low serum vitamin C level can cause excessive bleeding. At least 500 mg of timed-released vitamin C three times daily is recommended for a minimum of 3 days prior to injection of TrPs. The patient should take no aspirin for 3 days before TrP injection.

The needling must be sufficient to reach the contraction knots in the TrP to disrupt them. For all TrPs up to the midpoint in the vagina, this author has found a 30-gauge, 1-in. needle to be sufficient to reach the TrPs of the levator ani. For deeper TrPs, a standard trumpet guide with an appropriate small-bore pudendal or spinal needle can be used. For difficult-to-reach TrPs deep in the vagina or TrPs in which an angle is required, the trumpet guide from a standard pudendal set may be curved at an appropriate angle with the use of a standard pipe-bending tool (28). This author has found this technique an ingenious and simple method for reaching TrPs in all muscle and fascial attachments surrounding the vaginal tube. A 30-gauge needle is 0.30 mm, and a 25-gauge needle is 0.50 mm in size. I try to avoid the use of any needle larger than 25 gauge for injection through the vaginal mucosa because of tissue bleeding that may ensue. If bleeding occurs, the placement of a lubricated tampon into the vagina for a period of several minutes has always been sufficient to tamponade the bleeding. For abdominal wall TrPs, a 22-gauge

needle (0.70-mm diameter) provides an accurate feel for the texture of the tissue being penetrated by the needle tip. However, the thinner 27-gauge (0.40-mm) needles cause less tissue damage with each penetration and are well-suited to a fast-in, fast-out technique. For thick subcutaneous muscles, such as the gluteus maximus or deep paraspinal muscles, in nonobese persons a 21-gauge 2-in. needle is usually necessary. The needle should be long enough to reach the TrP without inserting the needle to its hub.

The patient should be warned that successful needle contact with a TrP may produce a flash of distant pain and will likely cause the muscle to twitch. The referred pain pattern of the TrP reassures the clinician and the patient as to the importance of inactivating that TrP.

Localization of a TrP is done mainly by the clinician's sense of feel, assisted by patient expressions of pain and by visual observation of local twitch response. The TrP is identified by gentle palpation for a taut band in the muscle, next for a firmer nodule in the taut band, and then for exquisite taut spot tenderness of the nodule. The tender spot in the nodule is also the most responsive spot for eliciting of local twitch response by snapping palpation or by needle insertion.

For abdominal wall TrPs, the TrP can be fixed for injection by pinning it down midway between two fingertips in either side of the TrP. The needle can then be aimed halfway between the fingers. For pelvic floor muscle TrPs, this author has found it more effective to palpate the TrP with one finger and then to position the finger so that the center of the fingernail is pointing at the TrP, with the TrP at the same level as the fingernail and the finger pressing against the soft muscle tissue next to the TrP. The needle is then advanced along the nail so that it is not possible to accidentally penetrate the clinician's glove and skin. For deeper TrPs the use of the trumpet guide is essential.

Attachment TrPs are identified as spots of marked tenderness and usually some palpable induration in the region of the muscle attachment. Attachment TrPs may be found along the pelvic bones associated with both (a) pelvic floor muscles internally and (b) adductor and other leg and abdominal muscles external to the pelvis. The region of tenderness is injected with anesthetic to provide relief. It is essential to minimize bleeding from the tissues involved and in order to do so continuous pressure should be applied with the examining fingers. Recently activated (acute) myofascial TrPs that have no perpetuating factors or additional tissue damage because mechanical injury to other tissues should resolve with one or two injections. This is especially true if, after injection, the patient is trained and then performs exercises to maintain full range of motion of the involved muscles. When both central TrPs and attachment TrPs are present, both sites must be injected (Fig. 38.28). When there are multiple active TrPs in functionally related muscles, there is a distinct advantage to inactivating them as a group. I have found that 5 and even 10 injections at one visit for both central TrPs and attachment TrPs of the pelvic floor muscles are sometimes

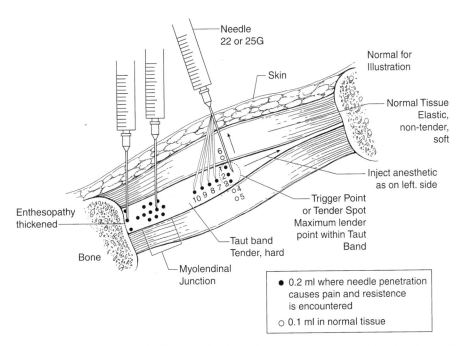

FIGURE 38.28. Needling and infiltration that, in addition to the trigger point, extends over the myotendinal junction and enthesopathy at attachment to the bone. (From Fischer AA. New approaches in treatment of myofascial pain. *Phys Med Rehabil Clin North Am* 1997;8:153–160, with permission.)

required for effective therapeutic response. Each injection requires no more than 2 mL of anesthetic solution.

Stretch following TrP injection is an integral part of that treatment. Immediately following injection (before the effect of injected anesthetic has worn off) the patient should *actively and slowly* move each muscle injected through its *full* range of motion three times, reaching its fully shortened and its fully lengthened position during each cycle. I have found it helpful to have patients perform EMG-controlled biofeedback (Kegel) exercises immediately following injection therapy of the pelvic floor or to have the patient's physical therapist perform stretch treatments for the affected muscles immediately following injection therapy. If two or three treatments by injection fail to produce lasting improvement of the TrPs in a muscle, repeated injections are rarely the answer. The perpetuating factors that are making the TrPs so irritable must be identified and managed.

Exercise to lengthen the involved muscles is the key to sustained relief of myofascial pain. Improving conditioning (exercise tolerance or stamina) and increasing strength of a group of muscles reduces the likelihood of their developing TrPs. However, in patients with remaining active TrPs, conditioning and strengthening can further activate the TrPs, encourage substitution by other muscles, and aggravate symptoms. These exercises, however, render latent TrPs less prone to reactivation if properly based at a gradual rate of progression. When the patient is experiencing rest pain for a considerable part of the time, the TrPs are very active and rarely respond favorably to any-

thing more than gentle release and moist heat. As the TrPs are inactivated, and rest pain fades, a carefully selected, gradual exercise program is needed to improve conditioning and endurance. The program should start with lengthening exercises, not shortening ones. Isotonic exercises in which the muscle moves against a uniform force is preferred to isometric exercises.

Injection of TrPs in the right rectus abdominus muscle is demonstrated in Fig. 38.29, injection in the external abdominal oblique muscles is shown in Figure 38.30, and that in piriformis is shown in Fig. 38.31.

Multiple sessions of TrP injections may be required for chronic pelvic floor myofascial pain. It has been this author's experience that these injections are best given on a daily or every other day schedule followed or preceded by physical therapy of the same TrPs. Physical therapy appears to be most effective if attachment TrPs have been treated prior to the manual treatment of central TrPs. The use of corticosteroid injections has been of some value for attachment TrPs. The duration of relief following injection of TrPs gradually increases with successive injections (29).

The treatment of myofascial pain syndrome by TrP injections is a most satisfying part of a clinician's armamentarium for the treatment of chronic pelvic pain. This author's practice is replete with the almost immediate feedback of satisfied patients whose comments are as follows: "I have been bedridden for 1 year with severe pain, have undergone two surgeries without success and in 3 weeks I am walking, my horrible pelvic pain is gone, and I can look

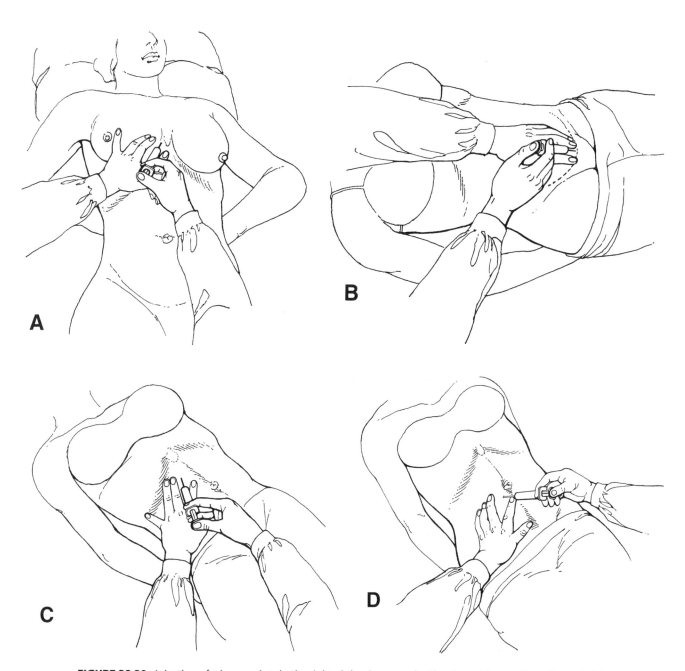

FIGURE 38.29. Injection of trigger points in the right abdominus muscle. The dotted line outlines the xyphoid process in parts (**A, C,** and **D**). In (**B**), the dotted line outlines the upper border of the inguinal ligament and pubis. **A:** In the paraxyphoid space, with close attention to the depth of needle penetration. **B:** In the suprapubic region. The pyramidalis muscle also lies in this region, but the needle is directed cephalad to inject it. **C:** Along the lateral border of the muscle, just above the umbilicus. **D:** In the lower rectus abdominous adjacent to McBurney's point. (From Travell JG, Simons DG. *Myofacial pain and dysfunction: the trigger point manual*, vol 1, 2nd ed. Baltimore: Williams and Wilkins, 1992:964, with permission.)

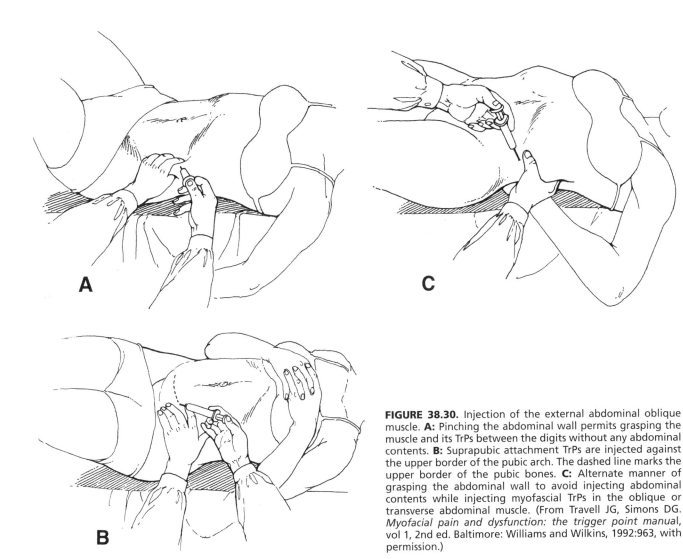

FIGURE 38.30. Injection of the external abdominal oblique muscle. **A:** Pinching the abdominal wall permits grasping the muscle and its TrPs between the digits without any abdominal contents. **B:** Suprapubic attachment TrPs are injected against the upper border of the pubic arch. The dashed line marks the upper border of the pubic bones. **C:** Alternate manner of grasping the abdominal wall to avoid injecting abdominal contents while injecting myofascial TrPs in the oblique or transverse abdominal muscle. (From Travell JG, Simons DG. *Myofacial pain and dysfunction: the trigger point manual*, vol 1, 2nd ed. Baltimore: Williams and Wilkins, 1992:963, with permission.)

forward to a future" (23-year-old ballet student with severe attachment TrP pain from the adductor muscles centered in the left side of her groin and central TrPs in the adductor muscles as well as attachment TrPs of the abdominal rectus and obliques and central TrPs in each of those; treatment protocol for 3 weeks with almost daily visits to physical therapy and the clinician for TrP treatments).

"My husband and I had intercourse for the first time in 1 year, and it was pain-free. Prior to this treatment, when we attempted intercourse it felt like he was hitting a wall and we could not accomplish this and it was extremely painful" (34-year-old patient with severe levator ani and obturator internus central TrPs resulting from 6 months of recumbency due to a prolonged illness). Three sessions of injections into TrP in the levator ani muscles were required for sustained and complete relief of pain with intercourse. The patient also had paraspinal TrPs creating constant and severe back pain that resolved with spray and stretch and interferential therapy and manual techniques.

"My last period was pain-free and I did not notice that the flow was going to start, compared to the disabling pain I used to experience which had me bedridden and using two codeine every 4 hours" (23-year-old competitive swimmer with obturator internus TrPs as well as levator ani central TrPs and attachment TrPs of the adductors who had also experienced a "picket fence" fall onto the edge of a kitchen cabinet door at age 6; successful treatment required 4 TrP injection sessions and 15 manual physical therapy sessions for treatment of both central and attachment TrPs throughout the pelvic floor muscles and associated adductor muscles as well as treatment of a functional scoliosis and short leg syndrome).

With pelvic floor muscle TrPs, one of the most common perpetuating physical factors is the short leg syndrome, which, if not treated, results in continued reactivation of the TrPs. Another common perpetuating metabolic factor is thyroid dysfunction, including the presence of antithyroid antibodies in patients who by lab studies are euthyroid.

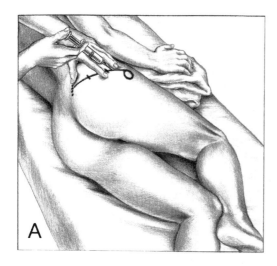

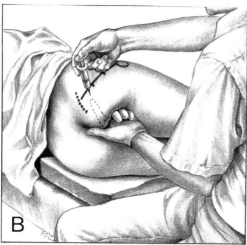

FIGURE 38.31. Injection of the TrPs in the right piriformis muscle. The open circle locates the greater trochanter; the dotted line indicates the palpable margin along the edge of the sacrum; and the solid line, marked in thirds, overlies the upper (cephalad) margin of the piriformis muscle. **A:** Injection of TrP1 using the usual completely external approach. **B:** Injection of TrP 2 using bimanual technique. The left hand locates the TrP tenderness via intrapelvic palpation and the right hand directs the needle toward the fingertip. (From Travell JG, Simons DG. *Myofascial pain and dysfunction: trigger point manual*, vol 2, 1st ed. Baltimore: Williams and Wilkins, 1992:207, with permission.)

Treatment of underlying thyroid disorder has been critical to the success of the treatment program for the myofascial TrPs. To treat hypothyroidism, levothyroxine (T4) is given at 1.7 µg per kilogram of body weight. In persons over the age of 50, the replacement dose needed may be less and the starting dose should be 0.025 to 0.05 mg of levothyroxine daily. In patients with peripheral resistance to thyroid hormone, the eventual dose of T4 needed to normalize function can be quite high. The maintenance dose is monitored by measuring serum TSH with the target range of 0.5 to 2.5 mIU/L. A steady state of serum T4 is not reached for about 4 weeks after initiation of therapy. T4 is physiologically converted to T3 at rates that are determined by the state of the individual, primarily by a process of deiodination of extrathyroidal T4. The most physiologic means of providing T3, therefore, is to give thyroxin and to the let the bodily needs regulate the rate of conversion of T4 to T3. In some individuals, however, peripheral conversion of T4 to T3 may be impeded and provision of T3 in addition to T4 may result in an improved sense of well-being.

When thyroid insufficiency is present, thyroid supplementation results in serum cholesterol decrease, basal metabolism or basal temperature normalization, decrease in irritability of the muscles, and return of normal energy and stamina. Before starting treatment with thyroid hormone, it is important that the patient have an adequate vitamin B_1 level. Because thyroid hormone increases metabolism, and thiamine requirements are metabolism-dependent, thyroid therapy can convert an undesirable vitamin B_1 inadequacy to a serious vitamin B_1 deficiency. The patient can first be given a sufficient supplement of vitamin B_1 to establish a safe level (25 to 100 mg three times daily, for at least 2 weeks before starting thyroid medication). Thiamine in a reduced dosage should be continued during thyroid therapy.

Another common perpetuating metabolic factor is insulin resistance (hyperinsulinemia) diagnosed by an increased fasting C peptide or by an abnormal 3-hr glucose tolerance test after a 75-g glucose challenge (a flat glucose response, a hypoglycemic glucose response, or a hyperglycemic glucose response). Treatment of the underlying hyperinsulinemia with dietary instructions and in some cases, metformin, has been critical to the success of the treatment program for the myofascial TrPs in these patients.

Folate and vitamin B_{12} insufficiency can also be a perpetuating factor. An initial oral supplement of 2 mg of folic acid three times daily should elevate the folate level to mid-normal range within 2 to 3 weeks. A 0.5-mg daily dosage should maintain this blood level. Supplementation should include both of these vitamins, not only one of them. Daily 1-mg oral supplemental vitamin B_{12} usually restores the serum level to midlevel within 4 to 6 weeks.

Nonmyofascial TrPs also can exist in apparently normal skin, scar tissue, fascia, ligaments, and periosteum. Cutaneous TrPs generally result in sharp, stinging, moderately severe pain referred either locally or remotely to the skin. Skin TrPs are found by pricking the skin with a needle, exploring for a sensitive spot that reproduces the patient's symptoms. The symptoms are relieved by repeated intercutaneous injections, but only if they are made precisely at the skin TrP. Scar TrPs refer burning, prickling, or lightning-like jabs of pain. Scar TrPs can often be inactivated by intracutaneous injection with local anesthetic solution. In refractory cases, the addition of a soluble steroid to the local anesthetic solution used for injection of the scar TrP can be effective. Nonmyofascial TrPs are also found in fascia, ligaments, and joint capsules. Periosteal TrPs can refer pain just as muscles do. Clinically, the periosteum can be a potent source of referred pain. Relief of this referred pain may be obtained by injecting the periosteal TrPs analogous to the relief obtained by injecting myofascial or cutaneous TrPs.

TrPs and Acupuncture

The distinction between TrPs and acupuncture points for the relief of pain is blurred. There is a high degree of correspondence (71%) between published locations of TrPs and classic acupuncture points for the relief of pain. Frequently the acupuncture points selected for the treatment of pain is actually a TrP.

KEY POINTS

Most Important Questions to Ask

- Was there any traumatic event associated with the onset of the pain?
- Have you participated in any activities that would acutely or repetitively overload the pelvic and/or abdominal muscles such as gymnastics, soccer, ballet, competitive swimming, aerobics, or cheerleading?

Most Important Physical Examination Findings

- TrPs in a taut band that, when compressed, reproduces the patient's pain complaint.
- Mechanical perpetuating factors such as poor posture, a leg length inequality, a small hemipelvis, or pelvic articular dysfunction.

Most Important Diagnostic Studies

- Evaluation for systemic perpetuating factors, especially metabolic conditions such as thyroid abnormalities, insulin resistance, and vitamin inadequacy.

Differential Diagnosis

- Fibromyalgia
- Hernias
- Visceral pain
- Spontaneous rectus sheath hematoma
- Endometriosis
- Pelvic infections

Treatments

- Postisometric relaxation
- Release by activation of antagonists
- TrP release/massage
- Spray and stretch techniques
- Electrical stimulation (interferential, microcurrent)
- TrP injection therapy
- Follow-up physical therapy
- Active limbering exercises
- Regular lengthening and strengthening home exercises.

ACKNOWLEDGMENT

The author deeply appreciates the assistance of Dr. David G. Simons, who reviewed this chapter. I am grateful and forever indebted for his teaching and selfless sharing of knowledge.

REFERENCES

1. Carnett JB. Intercostal neuralgia as a cause of abdominal pain and tenderness. *Surg Gynecol Obstet* 1926;42:625–632.
2. Travell J, Rinzler SH. The myofascial genesis of pain. *Postgrad Med* 1953;11:425–434.
3. Simons DG, Travell JG, Simons LS. *Travell and Simons, Myofascial pain and dysfunction: the trigger point manual,* vol I, 2nd ed. Baltimore: Williams and Wilkins, 1999:1,038 pp.
4. Slocumb JC. Neurological factors in chronic pelvic pain: trigger points and the abdominal pelvic pain syndrome. *Am J Obstet Gynecol* 1984;149:536–543.
5. Carter JE. Surgical treatment for chronic pelvic pain. *J Soc Laparoendosc Surg* 1998;2:129–139.
6. Sola AE, Rodenberger ML, Gettys BB. Incidence of hypersensitive areas in posterior shoulder muscles. *Am J Phys Med* 1955;34:585–590.
7. Fröhlich D, Fröhlich R. Das piriformissyndrom: eine häufige differentialdiagnose des lumboglutäalen schmerzes (Piriformis syndrome: a frequent item in the differential diagnosis of lumbogluteal pain). *Manuelle Med* 1995;33:7–10.
8. Simons DG, Simons LS. Chronic myofascial pain syndrome. In: Tollison CD, ed. *Handbook of pain management,* 2nd ed. Baltimore. Williams and Wilkins, 1994:556–577.
9. Simons DG. Diagnostic criteria of myofascial pain caused by trigger points. *J Musculoskel Pain* 1999;7:111–120.
10. Hong C-Z, Simons DG. Pathophysiologic and electrophysiologic mechanisms of myofascial trigger points. *Arch Phys Med Rehabil* 1998;79:863–872.
11. Simons DG. Clinical and etiological update of myofascial pain from trigger points. *J Musculoskel Pain* 1996;4:93–121.
12. Hubbard DR. Chronic and recurrent muscle pain: pathophysiology and treatment, and review of pharmacologic studies. *J Musculoskel Pain* 1996;4:123–142.
13. Baker H, Frank O. Vitamin status in metabolic upsets. *World Rev Nurtr Diet* 1968;9:124–160.
14. Gerwin R. A study of 96 subjects examined both for fibromyalgia and myofascial pain. *J Musculoskel Pain* 1995;3:121.
15. Dayan CM, Daniels GH. Chronic auto-immune thyroiditis. *N Engl J Med* 1996;335:99–107.
16. Pace JB, Nagle D. Pyriform syndrome. *West J Med* 1976;124:435–439.
17. Carter JE. *Chronic pelvic pain: diagnosis and management.* Golden, CO: Medical Education Collaborative. 1996:27 pp.
18. Carter JE. Laparoscopic treatment of chronic pelvic pain in 100 adult women. *J Am Assoc Gynecol Laparosc* 1995;2:255–262.
19. Beck AT, Speer RA. *Beck depression inventory,* New York: Harcourt Brace and Javanovich, 1987.

20. Travell JG, Simons DG. Myofascial pain and dysfunction. *The trigger point manual,* vol 2. Baltimore: Williams and Wilkins, 1992:607.
21. Travell J. Identification of myofascial trigger point syndromes: a case of atypical facial neuralgia. *Arch Phys Med Rehabil* 1981; 62:100–106.
22. Hong C-Z, Chen YN, Twehous D, et al. Pressure threshold for referred pain by compression on the trigger point and adjacent areas. *J Musculoskel Pain* 1996;4(3):61–79.
23. Fine PG, Milano R, Hare BD. The effects of myofascial trigger point injections are naloxone reversible. *Pain* 1988; 32:15–20.
24. Gallegos NC, Hobsley M. Abdominal wall pain: an alternative diagnosis. *Br J Surg* 1990;77:1167–1170.
25. Feinberg BI, Feinberg RA. Persistent pain after total knee arthroplasty: treatment with manual therapy and trigger point injections. *J Musculoskel Pain* 1998;6(4):85–95.
26. Hong C-Z. Lidocaine injection versus dry needling to myofascial trigger point: the importance of the local twitch response. *Am J Med Rehabil* 1994;73:256–263.
27. Glazer HI, Rodke G, Swencionis C, et al. Treatment of vulvar vestibulitis syndrome with electromyographic biofeedback of pelvic floor musculature. *J Reprod Med* 1995;40:283–290.
28. Kotarinous R. *Clinical Management of myofascial trigger points associated with pelvic pain: a tool for precise internal injections.* The American Uro-Gynecologic Society, Annual Meeting, New Orleans, 1996.
29. Hong C-Z, Simons DG. Response to treatment for pectoralis minor myofascial pain syndrome after whiplash. *J Musculoskel Pain* 1993;1:89–131.

39

LUMBAR VERTEBRAL DISEASE

C. PAUL PERRY

KEY TERMS AND DEFINITIONS

Ankylotic: A joint rendered immobile by degenerative changes.

Cauda equina: The collection of spinal nerves that descend from the lower part of the spinal cord and occupy the vertebral canal below the cord.

Discogenic: Pain arising from pathology of the intervertebral disc.

Lumbar spondylosis: Degenerative joint disease affecting the lumbar vertebrae and intervertebral discs, causing pain and stiffness.

Osteoarthritis: A noninflammatory joint disease characterized by hypertrophy of bone at the margins with degeneration of the articular processes, pain and immobility.

Osteoporosis: Reduction in the trabecular bone mass with resultant painful vertebral fractures of the crush type.

Radicular pain: Pain produced by inflammation or compression of a spinal nerve root at that portion of the root which lies between the spinal cord and the intervertebral canal.

Spondylolisthesis: Forward displacement of one vertebra over another, usually the fifth lumbar over the body of the sacrum or the fourth lumbar over the fifth.

Spondylosis: Degenerative changes due to osteoarthritis.

INTRODUCTION

Low back pain and pelvic girdle dysfunction are well-described phenomena in pregnancy (1). Chronic pelvic pain is rarely seen from lumbar vertebral pathology in the nonpregnant patient. However, radicular pain from lumbar nerve root irritation or compression may present in the L_{1-2} distribution (Chapter 55). Discogenic low back pain may originate in the L_{1-5} intervertebral spaces and may be mistakenly attributed to pelvic visceral pathology. This pain is usually constant, unilateral, and aggravated by movement. It will often be lancinating, burning, or constantly aching.

It may be located in the iliohypogastric, ilioinguinal, genitofemoral, or lateral femoral cutaneous distribution.

ETIOLOGY

The lumbar vertebral bodies serve as conduits for the spinal cord, cauda equina, and lumbar sensory and motor nerves. The spinal cord usually ends at the level of L_1. The central vertebral canal and the lateral vertebral foramen are sites of most nerve compressions due to their bony encasements (Fig. 39.1). Mechanical root lesions may be caused from disc protrusion, osteophytes, facet joint degeneration, fracture of inferior articular processes, or spondyloysis with spondylolisthesis (2). Lumbar nerve root compression may also occur in the central vertebral canal with chronic adhesive arachnoiditis, entrapment of a root descending in the narrow lateral recess (superior facet syndrome), lumbar spinal stenosis, or intradural tumor compressing the cauda equina (Fig. 39.2) (2).

The anterior (sensory) and posterior (motor) divisions unite within the intervertebral portion to the nerve root canal and exit the foramen as a single motor–sensory spinal nerve. The sensory division goes to a dorsal root ganglion, and a peripheral extension of this then goes to join the motor root to form the spinal nerve. These lumbar spinal nerves are located in the body of the psoas muscle forming the lumbar pelvic plexus. The L_1 root of the lumbar plexus gives rise to the iliohypogastric, ilioinguinal, and genitofemoral nerves. The genitofemoral nerve also receives input from L_2. L_2 also contributes to the obturator nerve, as do L_3 and sometimes L_4. The femoral nerve is formed by contributions from L_{2-4}. The lateral femoral cutaneous nerve is formed by L_{2-3}. Thus, lumbar pelvic plexus injuries may result in a mixed motor–sensory deficit, pure sensory deficit, or pure motor deficit depending on the location of the lesion (3).

Discogenic pain may originate from herniation of the nucleus pulposus with nerve root compression or with degeneration of the disc. Degeneration of a disc leads to centripetal growth of nerve fibers into the disc. Higher lev-

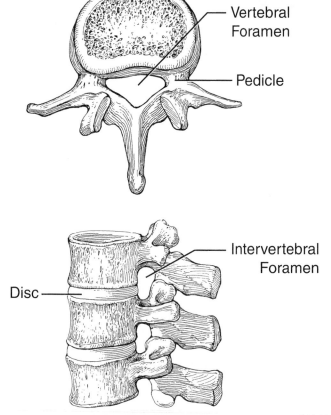

FIGURE 39.1. Illustration of lumbar vertebra, pointing out vertebral canal, intervertebral foramen, and disc.

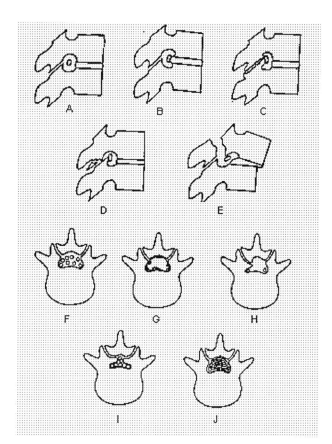

FIGURE 39.2. Nerve root lesions. **A:** Normal nerve root, disc, and vertebrae. **B:** Disc protrusion and osteophytes. **C:** Facet joint degeneration. **D:** Fracture of inferior articular process. **E:** Spondylolysis with spondylolisthesis. **F:** Normal configuration of the spinal canal and cauda equina. **G:** Chronic adhesive arachnoiditis and atrophic roots. **H:** Entrapment of a root descending in narrow lateral recess. **I:** Lumbar spinal stenosis due to spondylosis. **J:** Intadural tumor compressing the cauda equina.

els of substance P have been demonstrated in the painful discs (4). Disc degeneration may be considered a part of the normal aging process, but makes the vertebral canal more vulnerable to stenosis. The onset of stenosis is slow with symptoms described as heaviness, soreness, or weakness in the legs. Trauma to the intervertebral joints and ligaments often causes acute pain localized to the back or referred pain to the buttocks, groin, or legs. This pain may occur without nerve root compression. Nerve root compression may be present if associated with disc rupture, bony or ligamentous root entrapment, or adhesive radiculitis. Root entrapment by bone is more common over age 50, whereas disc rupture is more common under 50. A disc rupture also usually occurs only at one segmental level (5).

Osteitis deformans (Paget's disease) is a metabolic bone breakdown with remodeling by weaker bone. It is more common in women over 40 years of age. The resulting bone may be thickened, weaker, and misshapen. Paget's disease of the spine may result in stenosis of the neural canal with claudication from neural compression. Osteogenic sarcoma is 30 times more common in women with Paget's (5).

Multiple sclerosis may rarely present as abdominal or pelvic pain. Even more unusual is unilateral pain associated with multiple sclerosis. This disease is of neuroinflammatory nature and produces a broad range of symptoms including ataxia, choreoathetosis, hemianopia, and bladder dysfunction (6).

HISTORY

Patients with lumbar vertebral pathology presenting as chronic pelvic pain will have some component of back pain. The pain may be accompanied by motor deficit. The somatic pelvic nerve distribution may be interpreted as originating from the pelvic viscera (Chapter 55). A history of traumatic back injury may be present. Older women with osteoarthritis or osteoporosis should be suspect.

The pain can be severe or moderate in intensity. It may be described as sharp, lancinating, and associated with movement of the lower extremities or trunk. The longer the pain persists, the more diffuse, constant, and burning it will become. Muscle weakness from guarding or motor deficit may be seen.

EXAMINATION

Palpation of the lumbar spine in search of tenderness is helpful to localize potential sites of nerve compression from lumbar vertebral disease. Several physical medicine signs have been developed to confirm lumbar pathology (7).

Schober Test to Estimate Lumbar Function. With the patient standing, a mark is made on the middle of the back at the level of the posterior iliac spine (L_5) and a point 10 cm above. The increase in distance between these two points is measured on maximum anterior flexion of the lumbosacral spine. The normal flexion is more than 3 cm. In conditions such as ankylosing spondylitis, the flexion will be reduced to less than 3 cm.

Straight Leg Raising to Test for Spinal Nerve Root Disorders. The examiner grasps the ankle while the knee is held in extension. The lower limb is lifted until pain is elicited. If this is painful, one must differentiate between hamstring pain and sciatic nerve pain. Hamstring pain involves only the posterior thigh, whereas sciatic pain extends all the way down the leg.

Lasegue Test. The leg is lowered slightly from the painful position on straight leg raising. The foot is dorsiflexed to stretch the sciatic nerve to reproduce pain. If the patient does not experience pain when the foot is dorsiflexed but there is pain during the straight leg maneuver, this may indicate tight hamstrings rather than nerve root pathology.

Reverse Straight Leg Raising/Femoral Nerve Stretch Maneuver. With the patient lying prone, the knee is flexed 90 degrees. The hip is extended with the pelvis fixed to the table. Anterior thigh radicular pain is considered a positive test.

Crossed Straight Leg Raising. With the patient lying supine, the unaffected limb is lifted with the knee held straight. In the presence of a herniated disc, this maneuver will exacerbate the pain in the affected limb and also cause sciatic pain in the unaffected limb, the spinal cord, and the meninges.

DIAGNOSTIC STUDIES

Plain radiographs will adequately illustrate gross bony abnormalities such as vertebral fractures, osteophytes or severe osteoporosis. Computerized tomographic (CT) scans and magnetic resonance imaging (MRI) studies along with myelogram or discography may be needed to diagnose more subtle areas of nerve root compression or tumors. Bone densities are helpful in preventive care of osteoporosis and to follow the progress of its therapy.

Nerve conduction studies are useful to delineate mixed motor–sensory deficits when weakness or loss of deep tendon reflexes is noted. Peripheral nerve blocks may be done to diagnose iliohypogastric, ilioinguinal, and genitofemoral involvement of L_{1-2} (Chapter 55).

TREATMENT

Initial treatment of nerve compression is rest, analgesia, and avoidance of physical activities that aggravate the pain. A lumbar brace may be beneficial. Muscle relaxants may be required to treat the spasms if present. Heat usually will help in the treatment of these spasms; but in severe cases, baclofen may be necessary. Bedrest should be tried in an attempt at spontaneous resolution as swelling and compression subsides. If pain does not resolve, MRI or CT scan should help delineate the nerve root involved. Epidural steroid injection may treat the pain successfully and allow time for further spontaneous resolution.

Surgical decompression of a compromised nerve root is warranted by progression of the neurologic deficit or by intractable pain. Lumbar root compression is usually treated by a posterior surgical approach. Removal of any disc, bone, or thickened ligament distorting the involved root is the goal. Postoperative epidural scar encasement of the root may be a cause for failure of disc surgery. Pain of chronically damaged roots does not respond to these basic measures. Repeated exploration and decompression of traumatized roots is usually futile. Symptomatic lumbar spinal stenosis is an indication for surgical decompression of the involved levels. Rarely, a single level of stenosis can be relieved by limited surgery; but far more often, laminectomies and foramenotomies are required at multiple levels between L_2 and the sacrum. Chemonucleolysis has not been as successful to relieve the signs of nerve root compression and has fallen into disuse. The complications from this type decompression can be formidable including anaphylaxis to the chymopapain, discitis, and neural toxicity.

Chronic radicular pain that persists after surgery may respond to transcutaneous electrical nerve stimulation (TENS) or percutaneous electrical nerve stimulation (PENS). Lysis of epidural adhesions under the operating microscope may yield about 50% long-term success. Intrathecal use of hyaluronidase has not received widespread attention, but it may offer some relief to patients with persistent postoperative radicular pain.

KEY POINTS

Differential Diagnosis

- Peripheral neuropathies from distal nerve entrapment
- Visceral pathology

- Multiple sclerosis
- Paget's disease
- Compression in the central vertebral canal
- Compression in the intervertebral canal

Most Important Questions to Ask

- Any history of trauma?
- Any predisposing factors for osteoporosis (endocrine, genetic, or metabolic)?
- Any muscle spasms or weakness?
- Did back pain precede the pelvic pain?

Most Important Physical Examination Findings

- Point tenderness over lumbar vertebrae
- Pain intensification on straight leg raising
- Schober test
- Lasegue test
- Reverse straight leg raising test
- Crossed straight leg raising test
- Absence of pelvic visceral tenderness
- Decreased deep tendon reflexes
- Cutaneous paresthesia

Most Important Diagnostic Studies

- Lumbosacral radiograph
- CT or MRI imaging
- Discography

- Myelography
- Nerve conduction studies
- Bone densitometry

Treatments

- Bedrest
- Back brace
- Baclofen for muscle spasms
- Epidural steroid injection
- Surgical decompression
- Surgical or chemical lysis of adhesions

REFERENCES

1. Ostergard HC, Zetherstrom G, Ross-Hansson E. Back pain in relation to pregnancy. *Spine* 1997;24:2945–2950.
2. Dubuisson D. Nerve root damage and arachnoiditis. In: Wall PD, Melzak R, eds. *Textbook of pain,* 3rd ed. New York: Churchill Livingstone, 1994:711–735.
3. Kline DG, Hudson A. *Nerve injuries: operative results for major nerve injuries, entrapments, and tumors,* Philadelphia: WB Saunders, 1995:324–327.
4. Coppes MH, Marani E, Thomeer RT, et al. Innervation of "painful" lumbar discs. *Spine* 1997;2:2342–2350.
5. Riczo DB. Spinal dysfunction in the female. *Orthop Phys Ther Clin North Am* 1996;1:47–69.
6. Boivie J. Central pain. In: Wall PD, Melzak R, eds. *Textbook of pain,* 3rd ed: New York: Churchill Livingstone, 1994:893–895.
7. Shankar K. *State of the art reviews: physical medicine and rehabilitation: physiatric anatomic principles.* Philadelphia: Hanley and Belfus, 1996:641–642.

40

FAULTY POSTURE
AND CHRONIC PELVIC PAIN

JOAN S. BROWN

KEY TERMS AND DEFINITIONS

Active myofascial trigger point: A myofascial trigger point that causes a clinical pain complaint; it is always tender, prevents full lengthening of the muscle and weakens it, refers a patient-recognized pain on direct compression, mediates a local twitch response of muscle fibers when adequately stimulated, and, when compressed within the patient's pain tolerance, produces referred motor phenomena and often autonomic phenomena and causes tenderness in the pain reference zone (16).

Anterior tilt (of the pelvis): Anterior tilt rocks the cephalad portion of the pelvis (crest of the ilium) anteriorly, tending to increase lumbar lordosis (6).

Biofeedback: The technique of using feedback of a normally automatic bodily response to a stimulus in order to acquire voluntary control of the response (2).

Contranutation: Anterior torsion of the sacroiliac joint or posterior rotation of the sacrum on the ilium on one side; occurs when the anterior superior iliac spine (ASIS) is lower and the posterior superior iliac spine (PSIS) is higher on the one side; iliac bones move apart and the ischial tuberosities approximate; limited by tension of the anterior and posterior sacroiliac ligaments (1,3).

Fascia: Fascia may be described as consisting of three layers:

- *Superficial:* Attached to the undersurface of the skin; is loosely knit, fibroelastic, areolar tissue.
- *Deep:* Tougher, tighter, more compact; can be described as compartmentalizing the body; envelopes and separates muscle; surrounds and separates internal visceral organs; contributes greatly to the contour and form of the body.
- *Subserous:* Loose, areolar tissue that covers all the internal visceral organs (2).

Flatback: Decreased pelvic inclination to 20 degrees and a mobile lumbar spine (1).

Inflare: Anteriorly rotated ilium (1).

Instability: Usually present with guarding (hypertonicity) and trigger points in the muscles that support the hypermobile articulations, as well as in the muscle groups that share peripheral and nerve root innervation with the pathologic structures (4).

Latent myofascial trigger point: A myofascial trigger point that is clinically quiescent with respect to spontaneous pain; painful only when palpated (16).

Lordosis: An anteroposterior curvature of the spine that places the lumbar spine in extension, with the convexity of the curve anterior (6).

Massage: Movement of soft tissues, usually manually but sometimes mechanically (2).

Mobilization: The attempted restoration of full painless joint function by passive movements to the patient's tolerance, in voluntary or accessory range; patient is at all times able to stop the movement if so desired (2).

Muscle energy technique: Involves the voluntary contraction of the patient's muscle in a precisely controlled direction, at varying levels of intensity, against a distinctly executed counterforce applied by the therapist or operator; used to correct biomechanical malalignments (2).

Muscle tone: A continuous state of mild contraction of muscles, dependent on the integrity of nerves and their central connections, and the muscle's properties of contractility, elasticity, ductility, and extensibility (4).

Myofascial release: A combined technique of treatment using soft tissue technique, muscle energy, and craniosacral technique; combines soft tissue changes, faulty body mechanics, and altered reflex mechanisms in both diagnosis and treatment; also described as the three-dimensional application of sustained pressure and movement into the fascial system in order to eliminate fascial restrictions; used to reduce pain and increase tissue mobility and flexibility (2,6,10).

Myofascial trigger point: A hyperirritable spot in skeletal muscle that is associated with a hypersensitive palpable nodule in a taut band; spot is painful on compression and can give rise to characteristic referred pain, referred tenderness, motor dysfunction, and autonomic phenomena; underlying muscle pathology such as abnormal posture and stiffened joints that prevent normal muscle resting length may cause trigger points (4,16).

Nutation: The backward rotation of the ilium on the sacrum; if this occurs only on one side, the anterior superior iliac spine (ASIS) is higher and the posterior superior iliac spine (PSIS) is lower on that side; the iliac innominate bones move together and the ischial tuberosities move apart; the result is an apparent or functional short leg on the ipsilateral side; nutation is limited by the anterior sacral ligaments, the sacrospinous ligament, and the sacrotuberous ligament (1,3,10).

Outflare: A posteriorly rotated ilium (1).

Posterior tilt: Cephalad portion of the pelvis (crest of the ilium) is rocked posteriorly, tending to flatten the lumbar spine or decrease the lumbar lordosis (6).

Posture: The relative disposition of the body at any one moment; the body readying for the next movement; a composite of the positions of the different parts of the body at the same time (1,2).

- Correct: The position in which minimum stress is applied to each joint (1).
- Faulty: Any position that increases the stress to the joints (1).

Range of motion: The extent of movement (usually in degrees) of an anatomical part at a joint (16).

Scoliosis: A deformity in which there is one or more lateral curvatures of the lumbar or thoracic spine; a scoliosis may be nonstructural (functional) or structural (1,6).

Spasm: Increased tension with or without shortening of a muscle owing to nonvoluntary motor nerve activity; it is identified by motor unit potentials that cannot be terminated by voluntary relaxation (16).

Strain and counterstrain: The technique of spontaneous release by positioning; used to increase joint mobility and decrease muscle spasm (2,17,37).

Stretching: The application of a sustained force to one part of the body; done to distract or lengthen the soft tissue and its attachments (2).

Swayback: Increased pelvic inclination to approximately 40 degrees and increased thoracolumbar curvature (kyphosis) (1).

Traction: A sustained or rhythmically intermittent force, manual or mechanical, to the longitudinal axis of the body part (2).

Trigger point pressure release: Application of slowly increasing, nonpainful pressure over a trigger point until a barrier of tissue resistance is encountered; contact is maintained until the tissue barrier releases, and pressure is increased to reach a new barrier to eliminate the trigger point tension and tenderness (formerly called ischemic compression).

Upslip: A dysfunction characterized by the upward displacement of an innominate bone in relation to the sacrum (also called shear) (6).

INTRODUCTION

Posture is a reflection of the positions that one takes through a lifetime. It is the way we stand, sit, rest, work, and sleep. It is how we present ourselves to the world and the results of how we have handled life, or accepted its abuses. Posture is rather like history, because it tells a story and is not static. How the practitioner uses this information may determine the direction of treatment and the results of care of the chronic pelvic pain (CPP) patient.

Posture is defined as, "the relative disposition of the body at any one moment. It is a composite of the positions of the different joints of the body at that time" (1). It encompasses the position that the body assumes in preparation for the next movement (2). Correct posture is the body position in which minimum stress is applied to each joint with the successful use of the least muscle activity to maintain this position (1). Faulty postures are those positions that increase the stress to the joints and use excessive muscle activity (1). Viewed this way, posture is a mechanical state and when body mechanics are altered in a way that is less functional, the end result is dysfunction and pain (3). As a guideline, the accepted "ideal postural alignment" is the standing posture that allows a straight line beginning at the ear to pass through the ear lobe, the cervical bodies, the superior aspect of the shoulder, the mid-thoracic region, the lumbar bodies, just posterior to the hip joint and finally just anterior to the lateral malleolus (1).

A "typical pelvic pain posture" with exaggerated lumbar lordosis and thoracic kyphosis may be found in 75% of the women with CPP (4). This faulty posture is a contributing cause of weak, deconditioned muscles allowing for imbalances in the pelvis with formation of trigger points and hypertonicity, and, as a result, pelvic pain (4,5). A physical therapist can contribute to the care of many patients with CPP through a complete postural evaluation and examination, and comprehensive treatment of musculoskeletal dysfunction.

ETIOLOGY AND PATHOLOGY OF POSTURAL DYSFUNCTION

Postural dysfunctions may be genetic or structural, and arise from accidents or injuries, self-esteem problems, obesity, work positions, pregnancy and childbirth, disorders related to aging, and other medical disorders and illnesses. The typical spinal dysfunctions are *lordosis, swayback, flatback, roundback,* and *scoliosis* (1,6). For this discussion we will add *short leg syndrome.*

The *typical pelvic pain posture (TPPP)* mentioned earlier presents with: (a) anterior pelvic tilt of the pelvis, (b) increased lumbar lordosis, (c) increased thoracic kyphosis, and (d) anterior line of gravity to the pelvis and knees (3,7). Poor posture places strains on all elements of the body—the joints, muscles, and ligaments (4). For example, lordosis, a major component of TPPP, increases the pelvic angle from an average of 30 to 40 degrees inclination. To accommodate to these changes, the hip flexors, iliopsoas, and tensor fascia latae shorten and the abdominal muscles weaken because their angle of pull has been disturbed (1,4,8). The piriformis muscles shorten and the coccygeus muscles stretch (9). Posteriorly, the thoracolumbar fascia shortens, decreasing the ability of the lumbar spine to flex and allowing shortening of the spinal extensors (4,7). Hip range of motion is also affected.

Pregnancy and some seated breast feeding positions may disturb posture (10). Multiple pregnancies within short periods of time increase the risk of postural dysfunction. With pregnancy and menstruation there is a release of relaxin. This may increase the discomfort of conditions that have been dormant or increase the discomfort from a disorder that caused only slight or infrequent discomfort (4,5). Relaxin relaxes and softens tissue in the pelvic girdle and lumbar region, causing laxity in the capsuloligamentous structures that support the articulations of the lumbar spine, pelvis, and hips (4). For example, the normal 4 mm width at the symphysis pubis increases to 9 mm by parturition and becomes a less stable joint (11). These changes increase the ease of injury. The ligamentous laxity lasts for 6 to 12 weeks or more after delivery. Soft tissue changes also occur during pregnancy, with shortening of the iliopsoas, piriformis, hamstrings, and other hip musculature. Weakness develops because of stretch in the scapular adductors, the abdominals, and the gluteals along with the levator ani group and other pelvic floor muscles (12). The anterior tilt of the pelvis increases as does the lumbar lordosis. Pregnancy may be a possible cause of TPPP. As pregnancy advances, the center of gravity moves anteriorly over the hip or acetabulum. This increases lumbar lordosis and causes some of the changes that are typically seen with TPPP (12). There may be a tendency for tissue to remain in the new shortened or stretched state after childbirth, leading to the characteristic problems with TPPP (7,10). All of these pregnancy effects, although temporary, may cause permanent pelvic asymmetries and pubic, sacral, lumbar, or thoracic problems if attention is not paid to strengthening the weakened structures (11–13). Pubic separation may occur during childbirth and when untended may cause loss of motion in the hip, ilium position changes, muscle length and tone alterations, and gait disturbance. Pain and postural dysfunction may result from such changes (7,10,14).

The sitting position during breast feeding continues the postural tensions in the spine because of a position of flexion with some rotation. A nursing pillow helps but is often not used. Tissue at this time is still lax and increased thoracic kyphosis may be a result. This position is assumed not only in nursing but as the new mother cares for the baby (11).

The postural dysfunction associated with increased thoracic kyphosis and lumbar lordosis is generally known as *swayback*. The angle of pelvic inclination is 40 degrees in the lordotic posture, an anterior tilt position. The addition in this case is the increased thoracic kyphosis. Here the spine shows an increased angularity at the lumbosacral angle. In order to maintain balance or center of gravity, the thoracic spine then flexes on the lumbar spine, resulting in an increase in both curves. This results in hypertonicity or shortening in the upper abdominals, iliopsoas, rectus femoris, and lower lumbar extensors, and weakness in the lower abdominals, hip, and lower thoracic extensors (1). There is a loss of hip extension, as well.

In the *flatback* condition, the angulation of the pelvis is reduced to 20 degrees, a posterior tilt position (1). This is accompanied by shortened lower abdominals. Weakness in the gluteals and lumbar erector spinae muscles is found. The sacrum is often held in extension with decreased mobility. This condition best relates to a "slumped" sitting posture that causes strain to the ligaments and muscles attaching to the ischial spine such as the iliococcygeus, coccygeus, and the sacrospinous ligament (15).

Scoliosis occurs when there are one or more lateral curvatures in the lumbar or thoracic spine. It may be structural or functional (1,6). Structural scoliosis may be caused by a short leg, a wedging of vertebrae, or other such anomalies. Functional scoliosis may be the result of macrotrauma (such as a fall on one side of the back or hip, or a severe whiplash to the entire spine) or repetitive microtrauma (such as may occur from working with the body rotating unilaterally for hours). With scoliosis there is ipsilateral tightness and shortening of the quadratus lumborum muscles, abdominal obliques, erector spinae, and iliopsoas, with the contralateral muscles frequently on stretch. Scoliosis varies markedly in degrees of severity and in the regions of curvature and rotation involved. The curvature may be noted to be a compensated S curve or a noncompensated C-shaped curve. The patient may have any one of the preceding dysfunctions, as well.

The *short leg syndrome* refers to the discomfort and symptoms caused by an inequality in leg lengths. The inequality usually must be over half an inch. It causes a pelvis that is lower on the short leg side, which the patient attempts to correct by altering the position of either leg. The end result may be fatigued and painful muscles, sacral and pelvic tilt with muscles that are stretched and shortened, and possibly a change in the angulation of the lumbar spine (16–18). The pain accompanying this disorder occurs generally in the back, SI joint, hip, lower extremity, and groin (7,18). The pain is usually incurred by irritation to the quadratus lumborum muscle from repetitive injury or trauma and from imbalance (17,19). This short leg can cause lumbar spine angulation, increased pelvic tilt and increased sacral tilt (16). Scoliosis is usually present with a substantial leg length discrepancy (7). The false impression of a short leg is noted when there is significant lateral lumbar muscle hypertonicity, thus hiking the ilium and giving the appearance of decreased leg length. This is not handled in the same manner as true short leg syndrome, as it is a spine disorder. When the muscles are relaxed, the legs appear of equal length. The small hemipelvis also has findings that may be confused with short leg syndrome, but is actually an asymmetry caused by differences in the size of each side of the pelvis (17). The leg lengths are actually equal and the imbalances are generally a lateral distortion noted on sitting and standing, usually toward the smaller side.

Issues of growth and development during childhood can also have an etiologic role. Children who are growing faster than their peers may change their posture to appear shorter (1). Many young women develop breasts early or are much larger than the average girl and thus round their shoulders and hunch forward to appear smaller breasted. This can cause irritation at the thoracolumbar junction with resultant nerve irritation to the subcostal nerve, or increased lordosis, either of which can lead to pelvic pain in the future. Self-esteem problems in youth also set a pattern and design for the adult posture.

The Pelvic Connection

Pelvic pain may be a result of musculoskeletal dysfunction more frequently then generally believed (4,7,12,20,21). To understand this better it is worthwhile to go over the muscoskeletal and neurological components of the pelvis.

Through evolution, we have altered the mechanics of our world and our posture. This has not necessarily been all that positive for women. We birth babies with very large craniums. We stand erect, which increases the intraabdominal pressure and causes the muscles that were intended to support the pelvic viscera to rotate anteriorly, along with the pubic symphysis (22). It is no surprise that our pelvic floor musculature becomes so abused.

The support mechanisms of our pelvic viscera include the axis of the bony pelvis, the pubocervical fascia and ligament, and the pelvic floor musculature (22). When one aspect of this support system is disturbed, the function of the others is compromised.

The Bony Pelvis

The major job of the bony pelvis, aside from being a supportive structure for viscera, is to allow us to move. The pelvis transfers the weight bearing forces from the spine to the sacroiliac articulations and symphysis pubis and through the hips to the lower extremities. The forces from the lower extremities then reverse this process as the ground is struck. This is the body's shock absorbing system. This

function of the sacroiliac (SI) joint and the symphysis pubis sets it apart from other joints (1,7).

Mobility in the SI joint is greater in the female than in the male. This mobility decreases with advancing age (6,7). The symphysis pubis is a mobile, cartilaginous joint. Although the motion in this joint is small, it does have superior and inferior motions during gait and one leg standing. It is an important part of gait and with each step, strong shearing forces are imparted onto the pubic symphysis. During pregnancy, this normally well-supported joint becomes lax because of hormonal changes (2,7). A change in width of over two times the normal 3 to 4 mm may occur during pregnancy (11,23). At the time of menstruation and even menopause, there also may be a relaxation in the pelvic ligaments (4,5,11).

Injury or dysfunction of these bony joints changes the mechanics of standing, sitting, and walking. The body's response to this alteration eventually may be pain. These changes generally appear in the way that the individual moves and carries her body. Weakness in the attached muscles may allow disorder or dysfunction to occur and alter motion. Postural accommodations then occur.

The Muscles Relative to the Spine and Pelvis

The relationship between the spine and the bony pelvis is directly affected by its physical attachments to muscle, fascia, and nerves. This includes the abdominal muscles; the extensors and rotators of the thoracic and lumbar spine; the flexors, extensors, and rotators of the hips; the muscles of the pelvic floor; and, less directly, the muscles of the external genitalia and the urogenital diaphragm (7). By understanding the position, function, and innervation of these muscles, we can understand how they influence postural dysfunction, and their complicity in producing pelvic pain.

Multifidus

Originates from the post aspect of the sacrum, the PSIS, mamallary processes of all lumbar vertebra, and the articular process of the last cervical vertebrae. Inserts into the spinous processes of the vertebra from L5 to the axis (24).

- Action: Extension and rotation of the vertebral column (16,24).
- Innervation: Adjacent spinal nerves (16).
- Painful regions: Thoracolumbar; abdomen, medial to the ASIS and distal to the costal border; SI joint, buttock, and coccyx.

Piriformis

Originates from the inner or anterior surface of the sacrum with some fibers attaching to the margin of the sciatic foramen at the capsule of the SI joint and some fibers to the sacrotuberous or sacrospinous ligament. It attaches laterally by inserting into the greater trochanter medially at its superior border. Its tendon is accompanied by the obturator internus and the gemelli (2,6,24). The piriformis muscle passes from the inner surface of the pelvis through the greater sciatic foramen with nerves and blood vessels, and if it is swollen, hypertonic, or just very large, compression of these nerves and vessels may occur (6).

- Action: Primarily external rotation of the hip; may abduct the hip when the hip is in 90 degrees of flexion; stabilizes the hip and may place a strong oblique force on the sacrum (2,6,14,25). When the femur is fixed, it exerts an anterior force on the sacral base (7).
- Innervation: S1 or S2 (2,6).
- Painful regions: Low back; lateral to the sacrum; posterolateral aspect of the hip; pain in the buttock, coccyx, posterior thigh, leg and foot; inguinal region; dyspareunia; pain on defecation and any symptoms caused by pressure on those nerves exiting through the greater sciatic foramen along with this muscle (6,25–27).

Quadratus Lumborum

The iliocostal fibers attach to the crest of the ilium and iliolumbar ligament and insert into the lower border of the twelfth rib for about one half its length. The iliolumbar fibers travel between the iliac crest and the transverse processes of the upper four lumbar vertebra and extend medially to the intercostal fibers.

- Action: It is a stabilizer of the lumbar spine; in the upright position, it controls side bend to opposite side; lateral flexor of thoracolumbar spine; bilaterally extends lumbar spine and assists forced exhalation when coughing.
- Innervation: Adjacent thoracolumbar spinal nerves, from T12 to L4 (6,24).
- Painful regions: May be deep, aching, or sharp; occurs in the crest of the ilium, side of lower abdomen, outer aspect of groin, greater trochanter (hip pain), outer aspect thigh, SI joint, upper sacral region, lower buttocks, low back, anterior thigh. Tension in this muscle can hold the SI joint in a dysfunctional position. The "missed" quadratus lumborum disorder has been labeled as "failed surgical back syndrome" (6).

Iliopsoas

The psoas muscle arises from the anterior bases and inferior borders of the transverse processes of the lumbar vertebra by five slips and also from the sides of the bodies and intervertebral discs of the last dorsal and all lumbar vertebrae. It then passes down across the brim of the pelvis where it eventually attaches to the lesser trochanter of the femur. It receives with it all the fibers of the iliacus muscle to form the iliopsoas muscle. The iliacus attaches to the upper two-thirds of the inner surface of the iliac fossa, completely lining its wall. It then joins the fibers of the psoas to attach to the lesser trochanter and has some fibers that attach independently to the adjacent femur (11,24).

- Action: Hip flexion; probable extension of the lumbar spine (increased lordosis) when standing; assists with flexion when bending forward and during straight legged

"sit-up" exercise; may assist in abduction of the thigh; this muscle is significant in maintaining upright posture; the iliacus may stabilize hip extension (6,11).
- Innervation: Branches of the lumbar plexus; spinal nerves of L2-L4 (6,24).
- Painful regions: Low back, anterior thigh, lower quadrant abdomen lateral to the rectus abdominis, sacrum, proximal medial buttock, groin and difficulty getting up from a deep chair (6,7).

Rectus Abdominis

Originates from the crest of the pubis and attaches to the cartilage of the fifth, sixth, and seventh ribs (6,24).

- Action: Support of the abdominal viscera; forward flexion of the spine; very effective in gait, especially uphill; assists in maintenance of normal lordotic curve (6).
- Innervation: Seventh to the twelfth Intercostal nerves (6,24).
- Painful regions: Thoracolumbar region (T7-T12), the sides or middle abdomen, low back and SI joint, throughout the abdomen or in one quadrant and may be noted from the iliac fossa to genitalia; there may be diarrhea, spasms in the urinary sphincter, indigestion or nausea, dysmennorhea, or discomfort mimicking peptic ulcers (6,7,28).

External Obliques

Originates from the anterior inferior aspect of the lower eight ribs and travels diagonally downward to attach into the abdominal aponeurosis and then into the linea alba, the crest of the ilium and the pubis (6,24).

- Action: Flexion of the vertebral column; increase of intraabdominal pressure; spinal rotation and lateral flexion. These muscles along with the other abdominal wall muscles assist to pump venous blood from the abdominal region; assists in maintenance of normal lordotic curve (6).
- Innervation: T8-T12; eighth–twelfth intercostal nerves, branches of the iliohypogastric and ilioinguinal nerves (24).
- Painful regions: Heartburn; along the inguinal ligament, throughout the abdomen from the inferior border of the pubis to the groin and genitalia and proximal hip adductors; pain may be very deep and simulate pain from the pelvic organs (6,29).

The muscles of the hip—the flexors, extensors, adductors, abductors and rotators—also exert forces on the pelvis and through the pelvis to the spine. Hip adductors create a downward force on the pelvis. Therefore, with the femur fixed, they allow for increased anterior rotation to the innominates (7). The gluteals (hip extensors) work with the abdominals to maintain appropriate tilt of the pelvis and hip flexors create anterior torsion on the ilium (7).

Obturator Internus

This muscle originates from the inner surface of the obturator membrane where it surrounds and covers the greater part of the obturator foramen as it attaches to the rim. As it exits from the pelvis through the lesser sciatic foramen, it makes a right angle bend around the grooved surface between the spine and the tuberosity of the ischium. Finally, it inserts onto the greater trochanter, near but below the piriformis muscle. This exit area leaves very little room for increased size of this muscle and the obturator, like the piriformis, shares its pathway with other vessels (6,24).

- Action: External rotation when the hip is in extension and assists in abduction when the hip is flexed. This is not a muscle that functions as a pelvic floor muscle but just happens to live there (6).
- Innervation: One nerve, with fibers from L5-S2 or S2-S3 (6,24).
- Painful regions: Posterior to the greater trochanter (hip pain), upper portion of the posterior thigh, anococcygeal region, genitalia; pain and fullness in the rectum (6).

Levator Ani Complex

The pelvic floor is composed of muscles whose functions are supportive and protective. These muscles are called the *levator ani complex* or the pelvic diaphragm. This group of muscle forms a broad, thin body that arises anteriorly from the inner surface of the pubic bone, posteriorly from the base of the ischial spine, covers one-half to two-thirds of the obturator internus muscle and almost all the obturator foramen and then attaches to the last two segments of the coccyx. Individually, these are the *pubococcygeus, iliococcygeus,* and *coccygeus* muscles (6,24). Dysfunction of these muscles may be incurred by prolonged sitting, birthing without the assistance of gravity (supine), pelvic or sacral torsion, and from injury, which alters the muscle attachments and decreases the ability to function optimally. This can occur with falls, landing on the sacrum or coccyx, or with a pelvic shear force, such as an uncontrolled "split" or stepping off a ledge unexpectedly.

Pubococcygeus

Originates from the superior ramus of the pubis to the last two segments of the coccyx; the anterior fibers serve as a sphincter for the vagina and the more posterior form a sling around the rectum.

Iliococcygeus

Originates from the inner surface of the spine of the ischium to the opposite side of the muscle in a median fibrous raphe; attaches to the anterior margin of the obturator membrane or to the pubic bone just medial to the margin of the membrane; attaches then to the last two segments of the coccyx (6,24)

- Action: Pubococcygeus and iliococcygeus—form the pelvic diaphragm to support the viscera; oppose sudden increases in intraabdominal pressure; support and elevate the pelvic floor; constrict the vagina and rectum (6).
- Innervation: S4 spinal nerve (6,24).

- Painful regions: Low back, posterior thigh, hip, sacrum, coccyx, rectum, pelvic floor, vagina, buttock, suprapubic, lower abdominal quadrants; dyspareunia; sitting and laying down may be uncomfortable (6,22,26,30).

Coccygeus

This pelvic floor muscle originates at the ischial spine and fibers of the sacrospinous ligament and attaches to the last segment of the sacrum and the lateral margins of the coccyx (6,24).

- Action: Pulls the coccyx forward and supports it after it has been pushed back for defecation or childbirth; may stabilize the SI joint. Some believe that the coccygeus muscle can exert much force in sacral rotation. Thereby, when in spasm, it would promote sacral torsion (6,31). This is disputed by anatomists who claim that the muscle is not strong enough to exert that kind of force. That "pelvic muscles of the living bear little resemblance to those of the dead" further enhances the argument for the actions of the coccygeus in sacral dysfunction (22).
- Innervation: S4-5 spinal nerves (6,24).
- Painful regions: Hip, low back, sacrum, coccyx, pelvic floor, vagina, posterior thigh (6,26,30,31).

Bulbospongiosis

This muscle is sometimes called the bulbocavernosis or the sphincter vaginae. It attaches anteriorly to the corpora cavernosa clitoris, crossing over the body of the clitoris and compressing the deep dorsal vein. Posteriorly it attaches to the perineal body. It then meets with the external anal sphincter and transversus perinei superficialis.

- Action: In the woman constricts the opening of the vagina and contributes to erection of the clitoris by compressing the deep dorsal vein
- Innervation: Second, third, and fourth sacral nerve via the perineal branch of the pudendal nerve
- Painful regions: Painful intercourse, vagina, perineum, and adjacent urogenital structures, in the female (6)

Ischiocavernosis

This is the lateral border of perineum next to the bony ridge of the anterior pubic ramus. It extends from the symphysis pubis to the ischial tuberosity. It ends in an aponeurosis that blends with the crus clitoris, above and anteriorly and below and posteriorly it anchors to the crus clitoris and the ischial tuberosity.

- Action: To maintain erection of the clitoris
- Innervation: Second, third, and fourth sacral nerve via the perineal branch of the pudendal nerve
- Painful regions: Perineum and adjacent urogenital structures (6)

Mild or moderate strength changes in the pelvic floor may lead to imbalances within the pelvis or abdominal wall

(29). Weakness or asymmetries in the pelvis or abdominal wall may then lead to alterations in the mechanics of an individual's posture. Just as weakness or hypertonicity in the lumbar spine can undermine the ability of the levator ani to function optimally, so can a disorder of the levator ani place more stress on the lumbar spine. Without symmetry and mobility, we are prime for dysfunction.

THE ASSOCIATED NERVE

Subcostal Nerve

The subcostal nerve from T12 descends inferiorly and medially and innervates the cutaneous area of the mons pubis (32). Thus, alteration at the thoracolumbar junction may affect sensation and comfort in the pubic region.

Lumbar Plexus

Nerves also become contributory or causative agents when disturbed in function or position. Arising from the lumbar plexus, L1-L4, are the iliohypogastric, ilioinguinal, lateral femoral cutaneous, femoral, genitofemoral, and obturator nerves. From the point of exit at the spine to the terminal point in the muscle or tissue, any alterations, injury, or compressive force encountered by the nerve may cause a disorder in the region supplied by that nerve.

The nerves of the lumbar plexus exit the spine just anterior to the quadratus lumborum muscle and travel without and within the psoas muscle. The *iliohypogastric nerve* actually pierces the internal oblique muscle and runs between both the internal oblique and external oblique before it innervates the skin above the pubic bone at the mons pubis. This nerve innervates surrounding muscle, as well. It has a lateral cutaneous branch that innervates the posterolateral gluteals (24,32,33).

The *ilioinguinal nerve* runs just inferior to the iliohypogastric. It is positioned between the transversus abdominis muscle and the internal obliques. Then it moves through the external obliques and inguinal canal and ends 2 cm lateral to the pubic tubercle (24,32,33). This nerve runs along the psoas muscle and may actually pass through its belly (6,33). The ilioinguinal nerve innervates the mons pubis and the anterior aspect of the labia majora, and it also innervates the cutaneous aspect of the anteromedial thigh and surrounding musculature (32). Entrapment of this nerve at the ASIS has resulted from loss of motion at the hip or exaggeration of the anterior pelvic tilt (34).

From L2-3 comes the *lateral femoral cutaneous nerve*. It runs behind the psoas, anterior to the quadratus lumborum over the iliacus, and under the inguinal ligament (24,32). It exits through the lacuna musculorum with the iliopsoas and the femoral nerve. There is little room through this passage for accommodation of inflamed, irritated, hypertrophied, or hypertonic tissue (6). The entrapment area of this nerve is

thought to be the point where the nerve pierces the inguinal ligament in the fascia lata (35). Entrapment is unique to pregnancy with the nerve becoming entrapped as it passes over the inguinal ligament. This is usually owing to a leg length discrepancy (12). The *lateral cutaneous nerve* innervates the cutaneous region of the anterior and lateral thigh as well as the lateral buttocks (32). With the lordotic posture, the lateral femoral cutaneous nerve may be stretched and thus be further compromised at the ASIS (36).

The *femoral nerve* is one of the largest nerves in the body and arises from the lumbar plexus. This nerve is also associated with the psoas muscle and courses through the muscle itself. It leaves the psoas and travels through the iliopsoas groove and underneath the inguinal ligament, then goes through the same restricted foraminal region as the psoas and the *lateral femoral cutaneous nerve* as it separates into more branches (6). This innervates the anteromedial thigh and associated muscles (psoas, iliacus, sartorius, pectineus quadriceps femoris) (32).

The *genitofemoral nerve,* from L1-2 follows the psoas on its anterior surface and continues anteriorly as it reaches the iliac crest. It becomes two branches, the femoral and the genital. The femoral branch innervates the cutaneous region of the upper anterior thigh and the genital branch refers to the mons pubis (6,24,32,33).

The *obturator nerve* arises from L2, 3, and 4. It emerges from the medial border of the psoas muscle, entering the pelvis just under the iliac vessels and superficial to the SI joint. It travels through the obturator notch into the obturator canal along with the obturator vein and artery. It innervates the cutaneous area on the medial thigh and the adductor muscles (6,24,32).

The psoas muscle is a connection between the spine and the pelvis and the support structure for the nerves of the anterior trunk, pelvis, and thighs. A dysfunction or injury to this muscle can affect the functions of the nerves that course along and move through the psoas muscle. Ilioinguinal and obturator nerve damage is frequently noted postsurgery and can cause irritation and inflammation to the psoas muscle (35). Muscle or nerve may be cause or effect.

Sacral Plexus

The sacral plexus arises from L4-5 and S1 through S5 (6,32). It is the nerve source for the levator ani, the piriformis, obturator internus, coccygeus, the ischiocavernosis, bulbospongiosis, the gemelli, and the quadratus femoris (6,24,32,33). This area has been labeled a "pain in the rear" (6). The nerve that frequently lives up to that title is the largest nerve in the body, the *sciatic nerve*. The sciatic nerve originates from L4, 5, S1, 2, and 3 and is a combination of the tibial nerve and the common peroneal nerve. As it leaves the spine, it moves through the gluteal region and generally appears at the inferior border of the piriformis, just posterior to the obturator internus muscle tendon (32). In a small percentage of individuals, the sciatic nerve may actually run through the belly of the piriformis muscle in whole or in part (6). This can be a potential problem. The nerve exits to the lower extremities through the greater sciatic foramen, a very uncompromising area that accommodates several vessels (6,24,32). The sciatic nerve innervates the muscles of the posterior thigh and most of the muscles of the leg and foot (6).

The *pudendal nerve* also exits through the greater sciatic foramen. It emerges from the sacral plexus and after moving through the greater sciatic foramen it immediately turns and goes around the spine of the ischium, thus moving into the perineal area through the lesser sciatic foramen. After it has entered the pudendal canal, it gives of one or more rectal nerves. It also gives a branch to the underside of the levator ani (6,24,32). The pudendal nerve innervates the bulbocavernosis, ischiocavernosis, the sphincter urethrae membranacea muscles, the external ani sphincter muscles, the skin of the posterior thigh, the labia majora, and the clitoris. Innervation of these structures is essential to sexual functioning (6).

The *superior* and *inferior gluteal nerves* innervate the gluteal muscles. The inferior gluteal nerve specifically innervates the gluteus maximus muscle. These nerves also go through the greater sciatic foramen. Chronic compression of these nerves is a major problem and results in buttock, groin, and posterior thigh pain (6,32).

Faulty posture standing, sitting, and in motion, repetitive emotional and physical stresses, poor work positions, and injuries such as falls, auto accidents, surgery, and childbirth can all influence the length, position, and condition of surrounding tissue and vascularization of the nerve. Entrapment neuropathy may result.

SYMPTOMS AND HISTORY

The location, timing, onset, and character of pain are important. It is necessary to be thorough in this part of the history because patients often will tell only of pain that they believe is relevant to the clinician's specialty. For example, they often will not tell their gynecologist about pain that they believe to be unrelated to "female troubles" (2).

It is important to ask about injuries, including childhood injuries, even mild ones (Table 40.1).Injuries during childhood may leave a lasting impression on the body. Injury to the psoas muscle with resultant spasm has been noted to alter the pelvic joint orientation in children and cause an increase in the lumbar lordosis (1,11). Falls off horses, swings, fences, gymnastics, dance and other activities affect the pelvic structures, lumbar spine, SI joint, hips, discs, and joint capsules (26).

Injuries as an adult are important also. Trauma from falls, auto accidents, sports, or exercise are most commonly encountered. Following microtrauma or macrotrauma, the connective tissue of the body tightens and balance is disturbed (7). Muscle length changes begin, fascial restrictions

TABLE 40.1. POSSIBLE CAUSES OF POSTURAL DYSFUNCTION (1,4,7,10,15,16,26,35,46)*

Childhood injuries
Structural malormation (e.g., scoliosis, short leg syndrome, small hemipelvis)
Ergonometrically undesirable work station positions
Recreational attitudes and form
Frequent wearing of high heels
Sedentary lifestyle
Constant sitting, especially with poorly designed chairs and sofas
Constant driving with poor support for back
Pregnancy
Breast feeding positions
Trauma (i.e., falls, auto accidents, sports- or exercise-related)
Poor breathing patterns utilizing upper chest and not diaphragm
Illness or disorders (e.g., emphysema, asthma, chronic fatigue syndrome, and fibromyalgia)
Surgical adhesions
Pelvic laxity

*For all references, please refer to end of chapter.

occur, and normally relaxed structures become tense as body mechanics continue to alter. An unexpected step down, or even the frequent "splits" performed by dancers, gymnasts, and cheerleaders may initiate imbalances in the pubic symphysis, with pubic shearing or pubic symphysis subluxation. This joint is poorly protected. It depends on the balance between the abdominal and the thigh muscles (14). Falls and direct trauma to the coccyx or SI region may produce the symptoms of coccydynia, including pain symptoms of the entire pelvic floor (7,26,37). Labor and delivery may also be a cause of coccygeal trauma (7–9,11,26). Hypertonicity of the pelvic floor muscles from any trauma may be a reason for or a cause of dyspareunia as well as painful elimination (7,11,29). There may be inability to sit comfortably. Surgery may similarly be considered a trauma, and a possible cause of postural dysfunction, so a thorough history of surgical procedures and any complications is important. Autopsies revealed pelvic adhesive disease in 50% to 80% of women who have had pelvic surgery (38). Resultant muscle weakness, postsurgery, also should be a red flag as causative of postural dysfunction and resultant pelvic pain.

History of pregnancy and breastfeeding may be significant. As previously discussed, the hormonal, weight, and postural changes of pregnancy may be a cause of permanent postural dysfunction and pelvic pain.

History about the woman's work and lifestyle is important. Working in ergonomically undesirable positions may contribute to pain, as may sedentary lifestyle, frequent wearing of high heels, and constant driving with poor back support. Poor sleeping positions, with no pillow, too firm a pillow, a poor mattress, flat on the abdomen, or sitting up while reading or watching television, may be contributory. A history of poor sleep or inadequate sleep may also be important because sleep is the time that the body uses for most healing. When people do not sleep well minor discomforts seem to intensify and fatigue decreases the ability of the muscles to support properly.

Medical illness such as emphysema, asthma, chronic fatigue syndrome, or fibromyalgia can affect posture.

A history or worsening of pain premenstrually and menstrually may suggest postural musculoskeletal dysfunction rather than reproductive tract disorders. The hormonal changes during the luteal and menstrual phases of the menstrual cycle are similar to those of pregnancy, although to a lesser degree. The production of relaxin causes ligamentous laxity, allowing for increased mobility in supporting structures and increased stress on joints, with resultant inflammation and pain (4,5,11). Severe premenstrual or menstrual pain may have an underlying musculoskeletal or postural cause that will respond to correction and strengthening.

Pain caused by pubic dysfunction may be felt in the SI joint, pubis, lumbar region, lower abdomen, or pelvic floor. It may increase with menses, defecation, and activities such as stair climbing (7,10,11). Iliosacral motion, hip external rotation, and gait are affected (7,8,14). It is the motion that occurs at the transverse axis of the symphysis pubis that allows for the normal forward and backward iliac motion during ambulation (14).

It may be useful to ask about activities that may lead to unilateral standing, such as holding a child on one hip frequently, lifting objects on one side all the time, limping, or increased weight bearing on one leg.

SIGNS AND PHYSICAL EXAMINATION

The examination starts while the history is being taken (Table 40.2). The examiner should notice if the patient is shifting in her seat, putting weight on her hands to decrease the pressure on her buttocks, sitting in a slumped position with her body weight behind rather than on her ischial tuberosities, very tense, maintaining crossed legs, leaning to one side as she sits or seeming to favor one side, or standing so as to avoid sitting.

During the physical assessment it is necessary that the patient is disrobed or wearing minimal cover-up items (11,39). In each position of the examination—standing, sitting, supine, prone, and lithotomy—assessment includes observation, evaluation of range of motion (ROM), and palpation. Initially it is not necessary to measure ROM exactly, but rather to determine if ROM has been lost and if ROM is equal on both sides. Palpation is done in all positions during the examination, but this is usually done most comfortably and findings are generally reproducible and most likely in the supine, prone, and lithotomy positions.

Normal muscles are not tender and do not refer pain to firm palpation. Thus, with the use of firm pressure one can determine areas of distress that otherwise may not be described. When you palpate a point of intense discomfort you may be identifying a "myofascial trigger point" or a "hyperirritable spot in skeletal muscle" (16). An active myofascial trigger point "is always tender, prevents the full lengthening of the muscle, weakens the muscle, refers a patient-recognized pain on direct compression, mediates a local twitch response of muscle fibers when adequately stimulated, and, when compressed within the patient's pain tolerance, produces referred motor phenomena and often autonomic phenomena, generally in its pain reference zone, and causes tenderness in its pain reference zone" (16). The results of these trigger points in themselves may be weakness, generalized pain, localized pain, referred pain, poor patterns of movement, poor posture, or lessening of postural control (16,26). When a muscle is healthy and has sufficient blood flow, normal flexibility, and normal strength, it does not develop trigger points. Microtrauma and macrotrauma, whether repetitively or acutely induced or because of sustained muscle activation, cause trigger points that are painful and may refer pain (16,26,40). Postural dysfunction as an end result of microtrauma or macrotrauma causes and perpetuates trigger points (17,26). Trigger points are numerous in many CPP patients. When several are present, a comprehensive musculoskeletal physical therapy evaluation is warranted.

Palpation may also reveal the nerve irritability and entrapment syndromes discussed earlier, that may also be the results of dysfunctional posture (3,4,7,26).

Standing

Gait is evaluated by having the patient walk briskly back and forth in the room. Particular note is taken of the following:

1. Are their steps of equal distance?
2. Is there a limp or constant protective motion present?
3. Is body weight shifted more to one side?
4. Is one leg externally or internally rotated?

Gait with unequal length of steps or limp may indicate sacral nutation, a short leg, a pubic shear, a torsioned ilium, a lumbar spine dysfunction, significant hypertonicity in trunk or hip muscles, or hip dysfunction (i.e., bursitis) (1,7,10). Unequal weight bearing between extremities while standing or during gait should also be looked for and may suggest short leg, sacral torsion, a small hemipelvis, a pubic shear, scoliosis, or lumbar problem (e.g., disc disease or neuropathy) (1,10).

Standing posture is evaluated with the patient in a relaxed position with the feet shoulder width apart. The examiner should first stand back in order to get full perspective. A closer, detailed evaluation is then performed with the examiner seated. Anteriorly, the examiner should determine if the shoulders are level, if the patient can stand on one leg, if the

TABLE 40.2. SUMMARY FORM FOR THE PHYSICAL ASSESSMENT OF POSTURE

Gait
1. Are steps of equal distance?   Yes___ No___
2. Is there a limp or constant protective motion present?   Yes___ No___
3. Is body weight shifted more to one side?   Yes___ No___ Right___ Left___
4. Is one leg externally rotated?   Yes___ No___ Right___ Left___
5. Is one leg internally rotated?   Yes___ No___ Right___ Left___

Standing Examination
Anterior
1. Are the shoulders level?   Yes___ No___
                                                                     Right___ Left___: High___ Low___
2. Can the patient stand on one leg?   Yes___ No___ Right___ Left___
3. Are the arms hanging equidistant from the body?   Yes___ No___
                                                                     Right: In___ Away___
                                                                     Left: In___ Away___
4. Are the anterior superior iliac spine's (ASIS) level?   Yes___ No___
                                                                     Right___ Left___: High___ Low___
5. Is the umbilicus centered?   Yes___ No___ Right___ Left___
6. Is there equal weight on both legs?   Yes___ No___
                                                                     Increased weight: Right___ Left___
7. Is one knee consistently bent or rotated?   Yes___ No___ Right___ Left___

Posterior
1. Are the sacral sulci level?   Yes___ No___
                                                                     Right___ Left___: High___ Low___
2. Is there a difference in their depth on palpation?   Yes___ No___
                                                                     Right: Ant.___ Post.___
                                                                     Left: Ant.___ Post.___
3. Are iliac crests level?   Yes___ No___
                                                                     Right___ Left___: High___ Low___
4. Are the greater trochanters level?   Yes___ No___
                                                                     Right___ Left___: High___ Low___
5. Are gluteal folds equal?   Yes___ No___
                                                                     Right___ Left___: High___ Low___
6. Are the knee creases level?   Yes___ No___
                                                                     Right___ Left___: High___ Low___
7. Is there hypertonicity noted in the lumbar extensors?   Yes___ No___ Right___ Left___
8. Is a scoliosis present?   Yes___ No___
9. Is decreased muscle mass in one LE or buttock present?   Yes___ No___ Right___ Left

Lateral
1. Is there a forward head?   Yes___ No___
2. Is the thoracic kyphosis increased or flattened?   Normal___ Increased___ Flat___
3. Is the lumbar lordosis increased or flattened?   Normal___ Increased___ Flat___
4. PSIS and ASIS angle—anterior or posterior pelvic tilt.   Normal___
                                                                     Right ASIS: Ant.___ Post.___
                                                                     Left ASIS: Ant.___ Post.___

Sitting Examination
1. Are iliac crests level?   Yes___ No___
                                                                     Right___ Left___: High___ Low___

Supine Examination
1. Are both pubic bones level at the symphysis pubis?   Yes___ No___
                                                                     Right___ Left___: High___ Low___
2. Are the ASIS equidistant from the center line of the body?   Yes___ No___
                                                                     Right___ Left___:
                                                                     Smaller distance
3. Are the ischial tuberosities equal?   Yes___ No___
                                                                     Right___ Left___: Closer to coccyx
                                                                     Right___ Left___: More posterior

arms are hanging equidistant from the body, if there appears to be equal weight on both legs, if one knee is consistently bent or rotated, if the umbilicus is centered, and if the anterior superior iliac spines (ASIS) are level. The assessment of the ASIS is performed by placing the examiner's thumbs, pointing at each other, on the tip of each ASIS. Posteriorly, the examiner should initially determine if the sacral sulci are level and if there is a difference in their depth on palpation. The sacral sulci are examined by sitting and using the thumbs to define the landmarks and to check for symmetry. Next the iliac crests are examined with the palmar surfaces of the index and middle fingers of each hand on the highest points of the iliac crests, using medial and inferior pressure to secure good accurate localization. If the iliac crests are not level, a simple assessment to determine if the patient has the "short leg syndrome" and may benefit from a shoe or heel lift can be done by placing one or more magazines under the leg that appears to be shorter to see if this makes the patient more comfortable. Assessment is then repeated without the magazines. Using the lift the examiner can see if there is any decrease in the scoliosis associated with the leg length discrepancy. If the lift increases the lateral curvature of the spine, it is not advisable. If lifts are to be prescribed, lifts up to 1/2 in. are usually sufficient initially. They should not be of magnitude to cause a sudden radical change in body position. The next part of the posterior evaluation is to see if the greater trochanters are level, which is done by using the thumb tips or index fingertips to press into the hip joints perpendicular to the limbs. Then the examiner determines if the gluteal folds are equal, if the knee creases are level, if a scoliosis is present, if there is asymmetry of muscle mass present, particularly the buttocks, or if there is unilateral or bilateral hypertonicity noted in the lumbar extensors. Hypertonicity in the lumbar extensors is apparent when there is more bulk of muscle noted along the lumbar spine or appearance of increased muscle tension on one side.

The lateral evaluation of standing posture consists of seeing if there is a forward head, if the thoracic kyphosis or lumbar lordosis is increased or flattened, and checking the angle of the PSIS and ASIS to determine whether there is anterior or posterior pelvic tilt. For the evaluation of pelvic tilt the seated examiner places a thumb tip on the most superior aspect of the ASIS and, while maintaining that position, places the other thumb tip on the PSIS. There should be a slight anterior tilt of the pelvis with the ASIS being about 1/4 in. lower then the PSIS. If the difference appears to be over 1/4 in. it suggests there is abnormal pelvic tilt.

A stance with one leg externally rotated may result from a shorter leg, a hip rotator muscle dysfunction, or pubic separation or strain (1,6,7,18). If one leg is held internally rotated it may indicate a contranutation at the SI joint or pubic obliquity (1,3). Shoulders held unevenly can be owing to a cervical or thoracic spine disorder, shoulder dysfunction, scoliosis, short leg, or unilateral shortening or

hypertonicity of trunk musculature such as quadratus lumborum and iliopsoas.

ROM evaluation starts by having the patient slowly march in place. Pain on either side may indicate symphysis pubis or sacral involvement with instability or torsion (1,11). Then with the knees straight the patient is asked to slowly bend forward, attempting to reach her toes. Reversal of lordosis should occur (4,7). If not, this may indicate hypertonus or shortening of the erector spinae and iliopsoas muscles, shortening of spinal fascia, sacral dysfunction, a disc problem, and so on. The patient need not touch her toes, but should have comfortable, free motion as she bends forward. At reaching her maximum bend, she should not have pain. Then you should place your thumbs at the PSIS and have the patient lean slowly forward as in the previous step. Note the position of your thumbs; if one thumb moves upward during this motion then it indicates a SI joint restriction (10). Next have the patient lean to one side slowly and then the other. Note where her fingertips reach along the side of her leg so you can determine symmetry of motion. If one side is markedly limited, there is probably quadratus lumborum muscle spasm on the opposite side and a scoliosis, a small hemipelvis, or a short leg may be present. Then have the patient lean back, avoiding motion at the knees. Difficulty with extension may be caused by stenosis, shortening or hypertonicity of the rectus abdominis, or even sacral torsion or hypomobility.

Sitting

Next sitting posture is evaluated. If the iliac crests were asymmetrical standing, they should be reevaluated. This may determine if the problem is a short leg or a small hemipelvis. Seated behind the patient with palmar surfaces of index and middle fingers of each hand on the highest point of the iliac crests, use medial and inferior pressure to move inward and to secure good contact and determine if the height of ilia bilaterally are level. Also the spine is reexamined. If scoliosis was present standing and remains when sitting, we have excluded the lower extremity as the cause. If there is still a lateral curvature present and a lower ilium, then attempt to place a cushion or some magazines under the buttock on the lower ilium side. See if that reduces the scoliosis or generally feels better. That will help determine if the patient has a small hemipelvis. Sitting may then be more comfortable for this patient with the addition of a small pad under one buttock.

ROM in hip rotation is evaluated in the sitting position with the knees bent to 90 degrees and no hip hike during testing. To check external rotation bring the heel of the foot toward the opposite knee. Of course, this is done bilaterally. Internal rotation is evaluated by bringing the ankle away from the body laterally, without straightening the knee or changing the position of the trunk. ROM should be 35 to 45 degrees and equal on both sides. Hip rotation is affected by a shortening of the external rotators, sacroiliac dysfunction, and hip disease. Loss of hip motion is common in women with pelvic pain when a musculoskeletal factor is involved (1,7,20).

Supine

Examination of supine posture starts by determining if both pubic bones are level at the symphysis pubis. With the tips of the index and middle fingers of both hands find the pubic bones at the symphysis, then move superiorly until your fingertips drop off the pubis. Move laterally until securely against the pubic bones. Each hand should be a similar distance from the symphysis. Next in the examination is to visually check whether the ASIS are equidistant from the center line of the body. Then the patient is asked to bend her knees while still supine to see if the ischial tuberosities are equal. To do this, the examiner stands at the edge of the table at the patient's feet and reaches forward to place thumbs on the base of both ischial tuberosities, and uses the position of the thumbs to determine if the tuberosities are equally separated from the coccyx in the vertical plane and level off the table in the horizontal plane (1,2,4,5,7,10,11,14,18,20).

Palpation is performed with the patient lying on a treatment table comfortably, using moderate and sustained pressure to identify trigger points in the following areas:

1. Along the rectus abdominis muscles from the lower rib cage to the pubic bone
2. Suprapubically (abdominals)
3. Lateral from the umbilicus and diagonally inward (psoas)
4. Just distal to the ASIS and under the ilium (iliacus)
5. At the lateral pubis (adductors)
6. At the posterolateral distal ribs (quadratus lumborum)
7. At the lateral crest of the ilium (quadratus lumborum)

Diastasis recti may be easily observed by having the patient tense her rectus abdominis muscles (head or leg raises help), but sometimes palpation is necessary to make the diagnosis. Diastasis recti is a separation of the rectus abdominis at the linea alba. If significant it decreases the ability of the abdominal muscles to support the viscera and decreases the synergistic effect that the abdominals have with the pelvic floor muscles (7). This may allow increased anterior pelvic tilt of the ilium, because the now stronger erector spinae are shortened. There is a diminished ability of the abdominal muscles to maintain posture and to protect the pelvis from increased intraabdominal pressure (26). If this separation is greater than two finger widths it is considered significant (7). Pain may be noted in the low back or pubis (26). Diastasis rectii is a common occurrence during the second and third trimester of pregnancy.

Prone

Palpation for trigger points is also done in the prone position. You should palpate at the following sites:

1. Tip of the coccyx
2. At the ischial tuberosities, move the thumbs medially and superiorly on a diagonal to reach the levator ani
3. At the mid-lateral edge of the sacrum (piriformis)
4. At the sacroiliac joints
5. At the lumbosacral joint
6. At the lumbar and thoracolumbar paraspinals

Lithotomy

Observation may reveal evidence of pelvic floor relaxation with genital prolapse, a possible result of the strain on the pelvic floor ligaments and fascia as a result of childbirth. If this tissue does not return to normal, genital prolapse may occur with muscle splinting and hypertonicity occurring as protection and support for this widened levator hiatus (22,26).

The musculoskeletal assessment in the lithotomy position consists mostly of palpation. As with other positions, careful evaluation for possible trigger points should be performed. The following areas must be evaluated:

1. Pubic arch (these points may be exquisitely tender and should be pressed gently)
2. Levator ani, including the pubococcygeus and the iliococcygeus
3. Coccygeus
4. Obturator Internus
5. Sacrotuberous ligament
6. Coccyx

Assessment of muscular function is also performed. While your finger is inserted in the vagina ask the patient to attempt to pull your finger inward toward her chest. If she is unable to even get started, you may put some pressure or a quick stretch on each of the four quadrants, while asking for the same motion. After all four quadrants have been checked, then ask again for a full pull inward. She should have better proprioception by this time. In some patients, it is beneficial to use two digits and do a gentle stretch to facilitate muscle contraction. During this evaluation check for symmetry of motion, general strength, endurance, and ability to relax. Frequently patients can produce an excellent contraction, but are unable to release and the levator ani remain in a perpetual state of contraction. Be sure that there is not substitution with gluteal and abdominal muscles. Some lower abdominal muscle contraction may occur because these muscles of the pelvis will work in synergy.

Malfunction of the pubococcygeus muscle or the entire levator ani complex alters the position and support of the pelvic floor. This directly affects the position of the sacrum on the ilium and at the L5-S1 region of the spine. Hypertonicity of the levator ani may be experienced therefore as back pain, or back pain may the result of the altered pull of these pelvic floor muscles on surrounding tissue and joints.

It is also important to assess the tone of the external vaginal muscles. The inability of the muscles surrounding the vagina to either contract or relax after a contraction presents a musculoskeletal dysfunction that may cause many problems in sexuality and in activities of daily living. Chronic hypertonus of the bulbospongiosis may be seen in patients complaining of painful intercourse.

Weakness or hypertonicity of the obturator internus directly relates to the functioning of the piriformis muscle. The symbiotic relationship between the two is apparent with the type of pain and limitation of motion that this patient describes.

The position of the coccyx should be palpated. After injury the coccyx may deviate to one side, or may be held in a position of extreme flexion or extension (11). Depending on the position that the coccyx and sacrum have assumed, there may be distinct alterations in the lordotic curve of the lumbar spine and the tilt of the pelvis.

With this initial assessment of posture, there are a number of findings that serve as "red flags" suggesting postural dysfunctions (Table 40.3). Such dysfunctions may directly or indirectly produce pelvic pain via alterations of the mechanics of functional posture. A full physical therapy evaluation should be performed before making final diagnoses (41). A physical therapy evaluation by a therapist who specializes in gynecologic physical therapy may assist in determining any mechanical problems, the causative lesions associated with them, and may recom-

mend appropriate treatment cases of nongynecologic pelvic pain (42).

DIAGNOSTIC STUDIES

Plain film radiographs are sometimes useful to rule out fractures, infections, ankylosing spondylitis, tumors, and so on. Occasionally they may identify other structural abnormalities, as well as bony changes in density or texture. Computerized tomography (CT) gives higher resolution and may often be more appropriate than plain x-rays to evaluate for structural abnormalities. Bone scans with radioactive tracers are sometimes useful in cases of suspected infection, fractures (especially stress fractures), and tumors. Magnetic resonance imaging (MRI) is better at visualizing soft tissue and may soon supplant other imaging modalities for diagnostic evaluation. It is now commonly used to evaluate possible spinal disc pathology, ligamentous tears, spinal cord tumors, osteochondritis, and many central nervous system (CNS) disorders. It remains expensive.

Ultrasound, which is commonly used in other areas of evaluation of CPP, is not especially useful in musculoskeletal evaluation (1). Needle electromyography may be indicated when weakness in a limb is noted and positive results can determine the presence of nerve entrapment.

DIFFERENTIAL DIAGNOSIS

Although a woman with CPP certainly may have visceral, systemic, and musculoskeletal disorders all as contributors to her pain, it is often difficult to tease out these disorders from one another and determine their importance, or lack of importance, in a given patient (Tables 40.3 and 40.4). The following are some of the characteristics from the history and physical examination that may help in this differential (8,11,38).

1. No related history of injury
2. Can not be altered with change in position
3. May have insidious or gradual onset
4. Rest does not alter the pain.
5. Migrating pain rather than localized in one area of the body
6. Symptoms that cannot be reproduced or increased by positions or movement
7. Nonspecific pain
8. Fever
9. Recent weight gain or loss
10. No loss of motion
11. No noticeable postural anomalies
12. No response to physical therapy

TABLE 40.3. THE MOST COMMON MUSCULOSKELETAL SYMPTOMS AND DIAGNOSES IN WOMEN WITH CHRONIC PELVIC PAIN

Scoliosis with pelvic myalgia
Sacral dysfunction
Short leg syndrome
Iliopsoas and quadratus lumborum irritability
Levator ani and obturator internus hypertonicity (pelvic floor muscle spasm)
Pelvic floor weakness
Groin pain as initial complaint
Pain with intercourse (dyspareunia with pelvic floor muscle spasms)
Low back pain
Postural hypotonia with pelvic floor laxity
Long-term pain that has not responded to surgery, medications, or psychological care
Depression from the unresolved pain and lack of control of the situation

TABLE 40.4. DIFFERENTIAL DIAGNOSES RELATIVE TO MUSCULOSKELAL SYSTEM AND POSTURE

Disorder	Musculoskeletal Symptoms	Possible Postural Dysfunction (Refs)
Cystitis and urethritis	Low back pain, pelvic pain, lower abdominal pain, dyspareunia, urinary, frequency or urgency	None from short-term disorder (38)
Hypothyroidism	Back pain, myalgias, stiffness, headache, fatigue, muscular/joint edema, poor peripheral circulation, slowed reactions, proximal muscle weakness, constipation	"Dowager's hump" (fatty deposit over C7), altered thoracic kyphosis, altered lumbar lordosis (38)
Spinal cord tumors	Muscle weakness/atrophy, back pain groin or leg pain	Alterations to spinal curves as disease progresses (38)
Systemic lupus erythematosis	Myalgias, arthritis, headaches, peripheral neuritis, spinal pain	Postural alterations caused by joint and muscle pain, weakness, or deconditioning (8,38)
Fibromyalgia	Widespread myalgias, tendinitis, headache, trigger points, stiffness, paresthesia, swelling, urinary urgency, fatigue, widespread pain, pelvic pain, specific tender points	Alteration in thoracic and lumbar curves from change in activities, fatigue, and weakness. Poor posture may be contributing factor (10, 26, 38)
Pregnancy	Low back/sacral pain, groin and lower extremity pain, sacroiliac joint pain	Increased lumbar lordosis, anterior tilt pelvis, ligamentous laxity (12, 38)
Uterovaginal prolapse	Low-grade back pain, suprapubic/groin pain, dyspareunia	Not causative of postural changes (2, 38)
Dysmenorrhea	Severe cramping pain	Not causative of postural changes (38)
Endometriosis	Rectal pain, sacral/coccygeal pain, nonspecific pelvic/abdominal pain	Postural changes from tissue sensitivity and adhesions. Muscle hypertonicity incurred because of pain and position changes (38)
Gynecologic surgery	Sacroiliac pain, abdominal pain, low back pain	Postural changes from tissue alteration (scar), irritation of SI joint from lithotomy position (5, 38, 46)
Diverticulitis	Pain left lower abdomen	Not causative of postural anomalies (38)
Childbirth	Low back/sacral/pubic pain, pain in coccyx, pelvic floor distress, urinary incontinence	Increased lumbar lordosis, sacral malposition, anterior tilt pelvis, pubic subluxation (8, 10, 11, 38)
Musculoskeletal sprain/strain of Thoracic Lumbar Sacral Sacroiliac Coccygeal Pubic	Buttock/side pain, posterior thigh/calf pain, abdominal pain, buttock/hip pain, pain over sacrum/rectum, dyspareunia, rectal pain, pain on elimination, urinary incontinence, dysmennorhea, pelvic floor/ genital pain, visceral pain (ovaries, uterus, etc.)	Altered anterior/posterior curves, altered lateral curves, uneven hip position, altered trunk muscle balance, (4,8,38,49)
Disc disorder of Thoracic Lumbar Lumbosacral	Pain with movement, stiffness, back pain with/without leg pain, pain posterior buttock, unilateral discomfort (generally), difficulty sitting, paresthesia, lower extremity weakness, tingling in feet or legs, lateral trunk pain, discomfort in lower abdomen, pain in coccyx, trigger points present, achy, cramping pain, may be autonomic nervous system involvement	Protective scoliosis, reduced/increased lumbar lordosis (As time passes other spinal compensations will occur) (4, 8, 11, 38)
Sacral or pubic disorder	Pain posterior sacroiliac joint, medial buttock pain, pelvic pain, visceral pain, sacroiliac joint pain, dysmennorhea, pain with intercourse, painful sitting, pubic pain, low back pain, headaches, pain with walking/stair climbing, trigger points present	Increased or flattened thoracic kyphosis, increased or decreased lumbar lordosis, iliac crest height inequality, appearance of short leg, protruding abdomen, hyperextension of one or both knees, umbilicus off center (8, 38)

TABLE 40.4. *(Continued)*

Disorder	Musculoskeletal Symptoms	Possible Postural Dysfunction (Refs)
Hip pathology	Hip/groin/pubic pain, low back/sacroiliac pain, lower extremity pain, anterior thigh pain	Effect on the iliopsoas muscle can effect thoracic and lumbar positions, protective mechanisms causing pelvic obliquity and sacral torsion (7, 38)
Trunk and pelvic floor muscle hypotonicity or hypertonicity	Side and abdominal pain, rib pain, shoulder/scapular pain, visceral pain, constipation, low back/thoracic pain, pubic trigger points, abdominal wall trigger points, tender muscles on pressure, urinary disturbance, painful intercourse, dysmenorrhea, pain anterior/lateral thighs, genital sensitivity, autonomic nervous system irritation	Increased or flattened thoracic kyphosis, increased lumbar lordosis, forward head, rounded shoulders, unequal iliac crest height, protruding abdomen, weakened gluteal muscle, hyperextended knees or knee, typically, anterior pelvis
Sprain/dislocation/fracture of coccyx	Inability to sit on both buttocks at the same time, tenderness at coccyx, low back pain, pain on defecation, painful menstruation, stepping up may be painful	May not demonstrate posture change or anomaly (8, 11)

TREATMENT AND MANAGEMENT

Physical therapy may be indicated in many patients suffering from pelvic pain, either as sole treatment or as combined treatment with more invasive, potentially complicated surgical or medical treatments. One study of patients with CPP noted that 94% reported backache, 71% dyspareunia, 74% had left inguinal pain, 52% malaise, 70% headaches, and 56% insomnia. Almost all of the patients had undergone surgery for their pain. It was found that with a team approach and addition of physical therapy, their treatments were highly successful (43). The therapist's role and goals are to restore functional, painless range of motion. Restoration of full or functional motion may be a crucial factor in reversing the downward-spiraling cycle in which the patient is caught.

Documentation of a full postural analysis at initial evaluation allows for objective monitoring of changes with treatment. The gynecologic physical therapist documents both internal and external tissue responses. A plan for treatment is created from the information gathered (4,7,17,44). Initial treatment attempts to decrease the pain. The therapist may choose to use modalities such as microcurrent electrical stimulation, ultrasound, or heat to initiate treatment and prepare tissue to allow the use of manual techniques to continue either mobilizing or stretching the body more efficiently and comfortably, and thus return motion to a hypomobile region. Mobilization techniques encompass broad varieties and patterns of motion to free a joint or to relax soft tissue. The patient is instructed in stretching and pain-relieving exercises and positions to continue at home. Strength and endurance exercises accompany the treatment when the pain is tolerable. These are increased as appropriate. Strength and endurance are essential factors in stabilizing any area of hypermobility and altering poor postural habits. Time must be allowed to discuss work and home, and to assist the patient in altering positions and activities that may be causing irritation.

Treatment is most beneficial when the external work on the body is performed first, because in many cases the external muscles or torsions initiated the problem. Then the internal structures are addressed. The therapist enters vaginally and accesses trigger points and fascial restrictions. Exercises may be performed internally with the therapist feeling the strength of contraction and using her finger as a stimulus for increased kinesthetic awareness. Internal myofascial release, ischemic compression, or massage are all done to increase the tissue vascularity and decrease restrictions. Mobilization is initiated as the tissue relaxes. Joint positioning may be attempted using various techniques to alter pubic symphysis subluxations or shears, coccyx and sacral dysfunctions, and even to reduce pressure at the lumbosacral junction. Therapeutic exercise, electrotherapy, and the various manual techniques all can be done internally, thus allowing direct access to those tissues that are the weakest, most inflamed, or most hypertonic.

Table 40.5 summarizes some of the treatment modalities that can be used in the treatment of postural and musculoskeletal pain.

These women have heard the worst: "It's all in your head." "You will have to live with it." "You may have to have more surgery (10)." They have had changes that have altered their everyday lives. Even their relationships have suffered. This type of pain and frustration may very well lead to depression. The confusion, invalidations, and evaluations by others, as well as the difficulty in doing everyday tasks leads the patient to feel tired, frustrated, and introverted (11,40,45). As the patient begins to first feel positive changes occurring, she will begin to take more and more responsibility for her own heal-

TABLE 40.5. SUMMARY OF SOME OF THE PHYSICAL THERAPY MODALITIES (2,4,6,7,10,16,17,19,21,26,37,39,47,48)*

Manual techniques: to increase joint motion, relax tissue, increase vascularization, and stretch shortened muscle, fascia, and scar tissue
    Ischemic compression or now revised as "trigger point pressure release"
    Mobilization
    Myofascial release
    Manipulation
    Stretching
    Massage
    Muscle energy
    Strain and counterstrain
    Spray and stretch
Electrical stimulation
    Microcurrent (Electro-Acuscope System): Microamperage: subthreshold—no muscle contraction but will work at the cellular level for healing and decrease in inflammation
    Interferential current: Milliamperage: no muscle contraction used to decrease inflammation and pain
    TENS: Milliamperage: mild sensation with no muscle contraction used for pain decrease
    High-voltage pulsed galvanic: high amperage to allow for muscle contraction, used frequently to exhaust the muscle and allow for relaxation
Therapeutic exercise
    Strengthening (correction of imbalances)
    Stretching
    ROM
    Fitness (aerobics)
    Postural
    Frequently to assist in exercising, tools may be used:
    Foam roll: This as it sounds—a long styrofoam log. The patient relaxes on this log and performs a series of exercises that the therapist has chosen. The exercises may be used to stretch or strengthen or usually both. The patient utilizes this roll as a part of their home exercise program and is advised to continue this regimen for life.
    Swiss ball: These large balls come in many sizes to allow for the individual to sit or lie over the ball, prone or supine. Again the therapist designs a program of exercises to be used while in various positions on the ball. This also is done as a home program.
    Theraband: This is a wide rubber or plastic, stretchable band. It has varying degrees of elasticity to allow for differing resistance. It is also used to assist with resistive exercises for strengthening with a home program.
Heat and cold
    Heat is used to relax tissue, increase the circulation and reduce pain.
    Cold is used for desensitization, numbing, and reduction of inflammation.
Ultrasound
    Allows use of high frequency sound waves (vibrational energy) to penetrate tissue with heat and massage and probable molecular chemical changes, relaxing the activity level of skeletal muscle
Postural and body mechanics education
    Correction with lift for short leg syndrome when beneficial
    Ergonometric assists for home and work
    Instruction in body mechanics
    Postural direction pertaining to ADLs
Biofeedback
    The use of relaxation techniques, muscle reeducation and EMG to allow the patient to feel or hear his or her body as it relaxes or stresses. Patients learn what is needed to control or improve body reactions. In a patient with poor coping skills, education will be stressed.

*For all references, please refer to end of chapter.

ing; as she learns self-management she will become more responsible for herself (19). In many cases, when the pain is treated and no longer present, the depression vanishes (26). She will once more extrovert and join her family and society. To see this happen is also a wonderful experience. We as healthcare providers can be a part of this cycle.

KEY POINTS

Most Important Questions to Ask

- Where is your pain? Is that all of it?
- Are there other areas that create discomfort at times?
- When was the first time that you noticed the pain?

- Have you had pain similar to that in the past?
- Have you had injuries in your lifetime (e.g., falls, auto accidents), perhaps many years ago?
- Have you been involved in activities where you may have fallen or hurt yourself without giving it much thought (e.g., roller blading, gymnastics, dance, etc.)? People forget injuries frequently or may place less importance on them.
- What type of work do you do?
- What positions do you work in most of the time?
- What stresses, physical and emotional, are present on the job or related to it?
- When do you get discomfort (i.e., time of day; during an activity)?
- Has your pain increased in the last few days, weeks, months?
- What makes it worse and what eases the pain?
- What activities have you stopped or changed because of this discomfort?
- Have your sleep patterns changed?
- What do you do for recreation?
- When did you have your last baby? How was the delivery?
- What surgical procedures have you had?

Most Important Physical Examination Findings

- Unequal length of steps or limp
- Unequal weight bearing between extremities while standing or during gait
- A stance with one leg externally rotated
- One leg held internally rotated
- Shoulders held unevenly
- Inability to stand on one leg
- Arms not equidistant from the torso
- Umbilicus off center
- Standing with a knee bent to shorten or equalize
- Asymmetrical deepness of the sacral sulci
- Uneven sacral sulci
- Iliac crests that are not level
- Greater trochanters that are not level
- Unequal gluteal folds
- Knee creases that are not level
- Hypertonicity in lumbar extensors
- Scoliosis
- Decreased muscle mass in buttocks or lower extremity
- Changes in the normal spinal curves—forward head, increased or decreased thoracic kyphosis, or lumbar lordosis
- ASIS higher on one side and lower on the other
- Bilateral anterior pelvic tilt
- Diastasis rectii
- Uneven pubis
- ASIS distance from the center line of the body not equal
- Ischial tuberosities uneven
- Sitting very uncomfortable as shown by constant shifting in the seat, leaning to one side as sitting or seeming to favor one side, or standing so as to avoid sitting

- Putting weight on the hands to decrease the pressure on the buttocks
- Sitting in a slumped position with the body weight behind rather than on the ischial tuberosities
- Palpation of trigger points
- Abnormal coccygeal position
- Genital prolapse

Most Important Diagnostic Studies

- X-rays
- Ultrasound
- Computerized tomography
- Bone scan
- Magnetic resonance imaging
- Needle electromyography

Treatments

- Manual techniques
  Ischemic compression or "trigger point pressure release"
  Mobilization
  Myofascial release
  Manipulation
  Stretching
  Massage
  Muscle energy
  Strain and counterstrain
  Spray and stretch
- Electrical stimulation
  Microcurrent
  Interferential current
  TENS
  High-voltage pulsed galvanic
- Therapeutic exercise
  Strengthening (correction of imbalances)
  Stretching
  ROM
  Fitness (aerobics)
  Postural
- Heat, cold
- Ultrasound
- Postural and body mechanics education
  Correction with lift for short leg syndrome when beneficial
  Ergonometric assists for home and work
  Instruction in body mechanics
  Postural direction pertaining to ADLs
- Biofeedback

REFERENCES

1. Magee DJ. *Orthopedic physical assessment*, 3rd ed. Philadelphia: Saunders, 1997.
2. Greenman P. *Principles of manual medicine*. Baltimore: Williams & Wilkins, 1989.

3. MacConkey-Sandalcidi D. *Sacroiliac dysfunction and pelvic floor involvement.* Presentation American Physical Therapy Assoc., Combined Sections Meeting, 1998.

4. Baker PK. Musculoskeletal origins of chronic pelvic pain: diagnosis and treatment. *Obstet Gynecol Clin NA* 1993;20:4.

5. Ryder RM. Chronic pelvic pain. *Am Fam Phys* 1996;54:7.

6. Travell JG, Simons DG. *Myofascial pain and dysfunction: the trigger point manual, the lower extremities.* vol. 2. Baltimore: Williams & Wilkins, 1992.

7. Baker PK. Musculoskeletal problems. In: Steege JF, Metzger DB, Levy BS. *Chronic pelvic pain: an integrated approach.* Philadelphia: Saunders, 1998:215–240.

8. Saunders HD. *Evaluation, treatment and prevention of musculoskeletal disorders.* Minneapolis: Viking Press, 1985.

9. Hunter W, Zehlman AL. Abdominal [pain from strain of intrapelvic muscles] (Letter). *Clin Orthop* 1970;71:279–280.

10. Barnes JF. *Myofascial release, the search for excellence.* P.T. and Rehabilitation Services, Inc., 1990.

11. Grieve GP. *Common vertebral joint problems.* London: Churchill Livingstone, 1985.

12. George S. Preparing the nest. *Adv Dir Rehab* 1998;7:8.

13. Paris SV. Physical signs of instability. *Spine* 1985;10:3.

14. Mitchell F, Moran P, Prizzo N. *An evaluation and treatment manual of osteopathic muscle energy procedures.* Valley Park: Mitchell, Moran & Prezzo Assoc., 1979,27–225.

15. Paradis H, Morganoff H. Rectal pain of extrarectal origin. *Dis Colon Rectum* 1969;12:306–312.

16. Simons DG, Travell JG, Simons LS. *Myofascial pain and dysfunction: the trigger point manual,* vol. 1. *Upper half of body,* 2nd ed. Baltimore: Williams & Wilkins, 1999.

17. Gerwin RD. The management of myofascial pain syndromes. *J Musculoskel Pain* 1993;1(3/4):83–94.

18. Sicuranza BJ, Richards J, Tisdall LH. The short leg syndrome in obstetrics and gynecology. *Am J Obstet Gynecol* 1970;107:2.

19. Simons DG, Simons LS. Chronic myofascial pain syndrome. In: Tollison CD, Satterthwaite JR, Tollison JW, et al. *Handbook of pain management.* Baltimore: Williams & Wilkins 1994:556–571.

20. Sanfillippo JS, Smith RP. *Primary care in obstetrics and gynecology: a handbook for clinicians.* New York: Springer-Verlag, 1998.

21. Vulvar Pain Newsletter. *Demystifying physical therapy.* Vulvar Pain Foundation, 1996;(10).

22. Agosta A. The Etiology of Pelvic Relaxation Disorders. *Am Uro-Gynecol Soc Quart Rep* 1992;10:1.

23. Abramson D, Roberts SM, Wilson PD. Relaxation of pelvic joints in pregnancy. *Surg Gynecol Obstet* 1934;58:595–613.

24. Gray H. *Gray's anatomy.* Philadelphia: Running Press, 1974.

25. Retzlaff EW, Berry AH, Haight AS, et al. The piriformis muscle syndrome. *J Am Osteopath Assoc* 1974;73:799–807.

26. Costello K. Myofascial Syndromes. In: Steege JF, Metzger DB, Levy BS. *Chronic pelvic pain: an integrated approach.* Philadelphia: Saunders, 1998:251–266.

27. Pace JB et al. Piriform syndrome. *West J Med* 1976;124:435–439.

28. Mehta M, Ranger I. Persistent abdominal pain: treatment by nerve block. *Anaesthesia* 1971;26:330–333.

29. Bachman GA, Phillips NA. Sexual dysfunction. In: Steege JF, Metzger DB, Levy BS. *Chronic pelvic pain: an integrated approach.* Philadelphia: Saunders, 1998:77–90.

30. Lilius HG, Valtonen EJ. The levator ani spasm syndrome: a clinical analysis of 31 cases. *Ann Chir Gynaecol Fenn* 1973;62:93–97.

31. Malbohan IM et al. The role of coccygeal spasm in low back pain. *J Manual Med* 1989;4:140–141.

32. Rogers RM. Basic pelvic neuroanatomy. In: Steege JF, Metzger DB, Levy BS, et al. *Chronic pelvic pain: an integrated approach.* Philadelphia: Saunders, 1998:31–58.

33. Anderson J. *Grant's atlas of anatomy,* 8th ed. Baltimore: Williams & Wilkins, 1983.

34. Kopell HP, Thompson AL. *Peripheral entrapment neuropathies,* 2nd ed. Huntington, NY: Kreigha, 1976.

35. Benson JT. Neuropathic pain. In: Steege JF, Metzger DB, Levy BS, et al. *Chronic pelvic pain: an integrated approach.* Philadelphia: Saunders, 1998:241–250.

36. Paris SV. *Foundations of Clinical Orthpedics.* St. Augustine, FL: Institute Press, 1990.

37. Jones L. Strain and counterstrain. *Am Acad Osteop* 1991,11–39.

38. Goodman CC, Snyder TEK. *Differential diagnosis in physical therapy,* 2nd ed. Philadelphia: Saunders, 1995.

39. Steege JF. Pain after hysterectomy. In: Steege JF, Metzger DB, Levy BS. *Chronic pelvic pain: an integrated approach.* Philadelphia: Saunders, 1998:135–144.

40. Slocumb JC. Neurologic factors in chronic pelvic pain: trigger points and the abdominal pelvic pain syndrome. *Am J Obstet Gynecol* 1984;149:5.

41. Levy BS. Diagnostic studies. In: Steege JF, Metzger DB, Levy BS. *Chronic pelvic pain: an integrated approach.* Philadelphia: Saunders, 1998:101–105.

42. Levy BS. History. In: Steege JF, Metzger DB, Levy BS. *Chronic pelvic pain: an integrated approach.* Philadelphia: Saunders, 1998:59–66.

43. Peters AA, van Dorst E, et al. A randomized clinical trial to compare two different approaches in women with chronic pelvic pain. *Obstet Gynecol* 1991;77:740.

44. Moyer P. Physical therapy may relieve chronic pelvic pain. *Obstet Gynecol News* 1998.

45. Renaer M, Vertommen H, Nijs P, et al. Psychological aspects of chronic pelvic pain in women. *Am J Obst Gynecol* 1979;134:75.

46. Steege JF. Adhesions and pelvic pain. In: Steege JF, Metzger DB, Levy BS. *Chronic pelvic pain: an integrated approach.* Philadelphia: Saunders, 1998:115–125.

47. Metzger DA. Laparoscopy in Diagnosis. In: Steege JF, Metzger DB, Levy BS. *Chronic pelvic pain: an integrated approach.* Philadelphia: Saunders, 1998:107–114.

48. Slover R. *Chronic pelvic pain management: an anesthesiologist's approach.* The International Pelvic Pain Society, 1998,1–2.

49. Guerriero WF, Guerrierro CP, Eward D, et al. Pelvic pain, gynecic and nongynecic: interpretation and management. *So Med J* 1971;64:9.

41

FIBROMYALGIA

C. PAUL PERRY

KEY TERMS AND DEFINITIONS

Fibromyalgia syndrome: Chronic, diffuse painful muscles with chronic fatigue and dysautonomia.

Myofascial pain syndrome: The chronic pain produced by multiple trigger points without chronic fatigue or dysautonomia.

Tender points: Specific anatomical sites of muscle tenderness, the manifestations of which are pathognomic for fibromyalgia.

Trigger points: A painful focus of hyperirritable muscle or fascia, palpation of which produces a characteristic muscle twitch with a specific pattern of referred pain.

INTRODUCTION

Fibromyalgia syndrome (FMS) is a common, often misdiagnosed condition affecting millions of women. It is estimated that 2% to 6% of the population worldwide (including men and children) suffers from FMS (1). Because many women with FMS may present with chronic pelvic pain (CPP) with dysmenorrhea or dyspareunia, fibromyalgia should be considered in all patients with these complaints. Unlike other rheumatic diseases, which produce painful swollen joints, this syndrome is characterized by pain in the ligaments, tendons, and muscles. A spectrum of symptoms may be present along with the gynecologic complaints.

The American College of Rheumatology published its criteria for the diagnosis of fibromyalgia in 1990 (2). Their criteria include a history of widespread pain along with the finding of at least 11 out of a possible 18 specific tender points on physical exam (Fig. 41.1). The cutoff criterion of 11 or more tender points has a sensitivity of 88% and a specificity of 81%. FMS is a progressive disease; therefore, patients with early fibromyalgia may not initially meet these criteria. Other nonrheumatic symptoms encompass multiple organ systems (Table 41.1). These symptoms and syndromes may all share genetic predisposition and common etiologies.

ETIOLOGY

Disease expression may be influenced by genetic, inciting, and modulating factors. Several studies suggest that family members of fibromyalgia patients have a higher-than-expected rate of this condition. Although some studies suggest an autosomal dominant pattern, a polygenic pattern is most consistent with the clinical heterogeneity. Trauma (physical or psychological), stress, and infection have been suggested as possible factors that may initially incite the symptoms of FMS. Higher levels of physical fitness are credited with downmodulating the symptoms.

A solitary cause for fibromyalgia has thus far eluded investigators. The current theories may be divided into "peripheral" and "central" hypotheses (1).

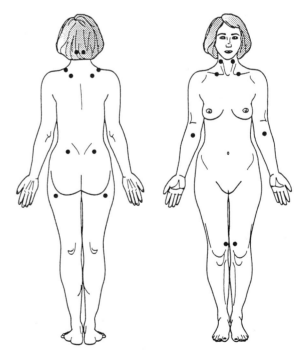

FIGURE 41.1. Figure showing eighteen of the specific tender points characteristic of fibromyalgia.

TABLE 41.1. MULTIPLE ORGAN SYSTEM MANIFESTATIONS OF FIBROMYALGIA

Chronic fatigue syndrome
Dysmenorrhea
Irritable bowel syndrome
Migraine headaches
Pelvic floor myalgia
Temporomandibular joint syndrome
Tension headaches
Vulvar vestibulitis

Peripheral Hypothesis

The presence of "ragged muscle fibers" in the tender points of patients with FMS has been proposed as a histological marker. More recent studies have failed to confirm these findings.

Muscle biopsies may show a significant difference biochemically. A decrease in muscle high-energy phosphates and tissue oxygenation is documented in these muscular tender points. Magnetic resonance spectroscopy demonstrates low intramuscular ATP levels at exhaustion after exercise. However, the preponderance of evidence suggests that this biochemical marker represents an effect rather than the cause. It may simply be evidence of muscle disuse (1).

Central Hypothesis

Most recent data suggest that it is unlikely that FMS is a pathological process localized in tender points. It is now known that pain in FMS is not isolated to the documented tender sites; diffuse peripheral nociception can be documented. FMS patients are differentiated from controls by testing their pain threshold or tolerance anywhere on the body. Visceral nociception is also increased, which may be responsible for the clinical observations of increased dysmenorrhea, irritable bowel, noncardiac chest pain, and so on. A central nervous system (CNS) mechanism not only explains the high incidence of nonmusculoskeletal symptoms in a variety of organs and tissues, but also the affective disorders and neurological features of FMS.

Neurotransmitter abnormalities have been implicated. A deficiency of inhibitory neurotransmitters such as serotonin, norepinephrine, and endogenous opioids could explain the increased peripheral nociception. These substances are responsible for the descending inhibitory pathways, which inhibit pain.

Substances that have a pronociceptive effect are called excitatory neurotransmitters. These compounds play a leading role in "pain sensitization" in animals that is very reminiscent of FMS. These include the excitatory amino acids (acting at the *N*-methyl-D-aspartate receptor) and tachykinins (substance P). Patients with FMS are known to have a higher level of substance P in their cerebrospinal

fluid (CSF) than normal controls. Other neurotransmitters, such as nerve growth factor and dynorphin A, have also been implicated (3).

Other factors that may be responsible for the CNS abnormalities seen in FMS include neuroendocrine abnormalities, autonomic nervous system dysregulation, hypothalamic-pituitary-adrenal dysregulation, and immune system dysfunction. There is evidence that each, or all, of these systems are involved.

Clauw in 1995 proposed an integrated hypothesis in an attempt to explain these various clinical, neurophysical, and psychological observations (1). Further research is necessary to prove this unifying theory of etiology. Ultimately, the effect on the female reproductive tract will be explained by whatever mechanisms are involved in the production of FMS.

SYMPTOMS

Chronic pelvic pain is very common in women affected with FMS. Frequently, their symptoms of dysmenorrhea or dyspareunia may overshadow all other complaints. The patients may even attribute all of their other complaints as originating from their reproductive tracts. Therefore, a thorough review of systems during the history is necessary to raise the suspicion of FMS.

Pain is the hallmark of FMS. It is common for one specific area to dominate (hips, legs, coccyx, etc.). Most patients describe it as an "aching" or "sore" pain. Some may relate that they feel as if they have the flu perpetually. The painful areas always involve the muscles, but may localize to sites of tendinous attachment to the bone and be mistaken for arthritis; however, arthritis is not present in patients with FMS. The discomfort is usually worse as the day progresses, but can be worse when first arising in the morning. There may be occasional chest, jaw, or leg pain. Earaches (temporomandibular joint pain) and headaches at the base of the skull are common.

Pelvic pressure, aching after intercourse, and dyspareunia may be manifestations of muscle tenderness and spasm. Patients may describe it as a sensation of fullness or "something filling the vagina." Penetration dyspareunia will be present if vestibulitis is associated with the FMS (Chapters 12,21). Urinary frequency, nocturia, and pain with a full bladder may be present because of interstitial cystitis, which is more common in patients with FMS (4).

Fatigue is often the most debilitating symptom of FMS. Some patients perceive it as a lack of muscle endurance. Most will describe it as a lack of physical energy. Chronic fatigue syndrome (CFS) is usually associated with FMS. Recent studies show that chronic fatigue syndrome may be present without FMS (5).

Sleep disturbance is common with FMS and may be partly responsible for the chronic fatigue. Stage IV is the

TABLE 41.2. LOCATION OF TENDER POINT AREAS USED IN THE DIAGNOSIS OF FIBROMYALGIA

Name	Location
Occiput	Insertion of occipital muscles into base of the skull
Low cervical	Cleidomastoid over anterior part C5–7 intertransverse process
Trapezius	Midpoint of upper border of muscle belly
Supraspinatus	Above scapular spine at medial border
Second rib	Pectoralis major just lateral to the second costochondral junction
Lateral epicondyle	Extensor origin about 2 cm distal to the lateral epicondyle
Gluteal	Gluteal muscles origin over upper outer quadrant of buttocks
Greater trochanter	Gluteal muscles insertion posterior to the trochanteric prominence
Knee	Vastus medialis just above the joint

Each of the tender points is bilateral and at least 11 of 18 must be present to support the diagnosis.

TABLE 41.3. MEDICATIONS THAT ARE HELPFUL IN THE MANAGEMENT OF FIBROMYALGIA

Analgesics and antiinflammatories
  Ibuprofen
  Tizanidine hydrochloride
  Celecoxib
  Tramadol hydrochloride
  Propoxyphene hydrochloride
Antidepressants
  Fluoxetine hydrochloride
  Paroxetine hydrochloride
  Sertraline hydrochloride
  Bupropion hydrochloride
  Citalopram hydrobromide
  Fluvoxamine maleate
  Nefazodone hydrochloride
  Mirtazapine
Hypnotics
  Trazodone hydrochloride
  Nortriptyline hydrochloride
  Amitriptyline hydrochloride
  Clonazepam

most restful stage of sleep and, as with many other pain syndromes, has been found to be disordered in most patients with FMS. Persistent sleep disturbance also is known to produce increased muscle pain.

Other symptoms may be reported, such as poor circulation to the hands or toes, tingling in the legs or hands, leg cramps, abdominal bloating with diarrhea or constipation, muscle tremors, bladder spasms, or blurred vision.

EXAMINATION

The elicitation of pain with slight pressure (4 kg) over at least 11 of the 18 designated sites (Fig. 41.1) confirms the diagnosis of FMS (Table 41.2) (2). These *tender points* differ from *trigger points* in etiology and degree. Trigger points are always painful, plus they manifest palpable bands, twitch responses, referred pain, and restricted range of motion unique to this type of myofascial pain syndrome (Chapter 38) (6). However, it is possible to find trigger points in the same muscle groups that are examined for the classic tender points of fibromyalgia.

There are no laboratory or imaging studies diagnostic for FMS.

TREATMENT

The treatment of FMS requires a multidisciplinary approach. Physical, psychological, and medical treatments are required. The patient and her family must be educated about this disease. Reassurance is necessary because many patients feel that the progressive nature of this syndrome will cause them to become invalids.

The avoidance of aggravating factors must be taught. Cold, fatigue, sedentary state, overactivity, anxiety, and poor sleep can exacerbate the symptoms of FMS. Exposure to inhalants, as found in new fabrics or paints, may worsen symptoms.

Helpful modulating factors include a warm and dry climate, hot showers and local heat, modest physical activity, general relaxation, naps, and restful sleep.

Physical therapy techniques are an integral part of relief for FMS patients. General physical conditioning programs are helpful to prevent exacerbations by exertion. Pool therapy with water aerobics in a heated pool is ideal. Deep tissue massage and heat therapy may be helpful. For localized pain, TENS units may be beneficial. Injections, as are done for trigger points, will often alleviate the more painful areas.

Medical therapy consists of pain control, reduction of inflammation, hypnotics to improve sleep, and antidepressive therapy (Table 41.3). Tricyclic antidepressants and nonsteroidal antiinflammatory drugs (NSAIDs) are often helpful. Patients with FMS may be exquisitely sensitive to medications. The lowest possible dose should be initiated with titration to therapeutic levels and tolerance. Dependence-producing medications should be avoided if possible.

KEY POINTS

Differential Diagnosis (7)

■ Rheumatic
  Early rheumatoid arthritis
  Polymyalgia rheumatica
  Systemic lupus erythematosis
  Sjögren's syndrome
  Polymyositis/dermatomyositis
  Scleroderma

- Endocrine/metabolic
    - Hypothyroidism
    - Hyperparathyroidism
    - Hypoparathyroidism
    - Hypercalcemia
    - Alcoholic or metabolic myopathy
    - Hypokalemia
    - Osteomalacia
    - Paget's disease
- Neoplastic
    - Carcinomatosis
    - Multiple myeloma
    - Lymphoma
- Infectious
    - Human immunodeficiency virus infection
    - Viral hepatitis
    - Parasitic infections
    - Subacute endocarditis

Most Important Questions to Ask

- Are you often tired?
- Do you have any trouble sleeping?
- Do you have any cold intolerance?
- Is there a history of fibromyalgia in the family?
- Has there been any recent physical or emotional traumatic event?
- Do you exercise regularly?
- Is there sensitivity to multiple medication?
- Has any depression been noted?

Most Important Physical Examination Finding

- Tenderness in at least 11 of the 18 designated sites with 4 kg of pressure applied

Most Important Diagnostic Studies

- Sedimentation rate to rule out polymyalgia rheumatica (8)
- Rheumatoid factor to rule out early rheumatoid arthritis

Treatments

- Avoid aggravating factors
    - Cold
    - Physical or psychological stress
    - Fatigue
    - Poor sleep
    - Sedentary state
    - Seek modulating factors
    - Warm dry weather
    - Hot showers
    - Local heat
    - Massage
    - Relaxation therapy
    - Naps and restful sleep
- Analgesics
- Antiinflammatories
- Antidepressants
- Hypnotics

REFERENCES

1. Clauw DJ. The pathogenesis of chronic pain and fatigue syndromes, with special reference to fibromyalgia. *Med Hypotheses* 1995;44:369–378.
2. Wolfe F, Smythe HA, Yunus MB, et al. The American College of Rheumatology 1990 criteria for the classification of fibromyalgia. *Arthritis Rheum* 1990;33:160–172.
3. Russell IJ. Advances in fibromyalgia: possible role for central neurochemicals. *Am J Med Sci* 1998;315:377–384.
4. Clauw DJ, Schmidt M, Radulovic D, et al. The relationship between fibromyalgia and interstitial cyctitis. *J Psychiat Res* 1997;31:125–131.
5. Evengard B, Nilsson CG, Lindh G, et al. Chronic fatigue syndrome differs from fibromyalgia. No evidence for elevated substance P in cerebrospinal fluid of patients with chronic fatigue syndrome. *Pain* 1998;78:153–155.
6. Simmons D. Clinical and etiological update of myofascial pain from trigger points. *J Musculoskeletal Pain* 1996;4:93–121.
7. Clauw DJ. Fibromyalgia: more than a musculoskeletal disease. *Am Fam Phys* 1995;52:843–851.
8. Feinberg HL, Schrepferman CG, Sherman JD, et al. Steroid treatment of polymyalgia rheumatica. *Am J Pain Manage* 1995;5:52–54.

42

HERNIAS

JAMES E. CARTER

KEY TERMS AND DEFINITIONS

Broad ligament hernia: A rare internal hernia passing through a defect in the broad ligament of the uterus.

Direct inguinal hernia: A hernia that passes through the floor of the inguinal canal in Hesselbach's triangle. The hernia path does not enter the internal ring but may exit through the external ring.

Femoral hernia: A protrusion of preperitoneal fat or intraperitoneal viscus through a weak transversalis fascia into the femoral ring and the femoral canal.

Hernia: A protrusion of organs or parts thereof from their natural place in a cavity through an abnormal opening

Hernia of the linea alba (Epigastric Hernia): A protrusion of preperitoneal fat or a peritoneal sac with or without an incarcerated viscus through the linea alba. It usually occurs in the midline between the xiphoid process and the umbilicus.

Hernial defect: The abnormal opening or defect through which an organ or part could potentially protrude.

Hesselbach's triangle: As described in 1814 it is the area formed by the following boundaries: superolateral—the inferior (deep) epigastric vessels; medial—the rectus sheath (lateral border); inferior (or, the base)—the inguinal ligament. Most direct inguinal hernias occur in this area.

Incisional hernia: The abnormal protrusion of peritoneum through a separation of the edges of a musculoaponeurotic wound that may be fresh, recent, or old.

Indirect inguinal hernia: A hernia that leaves the abdomen through the internal inguinal ring and passes down the inguinal canal a variable distance with the round ligament. Occasionally, the sac may not reach the labia majora but may enter the abdominal wall through any cleavage plane between muscles; this is an interparietal hernia.

Internal supravesical hernia: A hernia that passes through the supravesical fossa of the anterior abdominal wall and remains within the abdomen, passing into spaces around the urinary bladder. It may instead protrude through the abdominal wall as a direct inguinal hernia, in which case it is called an external supravesical hernia.

Obturator hernia: An abnormal protrusion of preperitoneal fat or an intestinal loop through the obturator foramen alongside the obturator vessels and nerve.

Perineal hernia: The protrusion of a viscus through the floor of the pelvis (pelvic diaphragm) into the perineum. A hernial sac is present.

Sciatic hernia: A protrusion of a peritoneal sac and its contents through the greater or lesser sciatic foramen. It has also been called a "sacral sciatic," "gluteal," or "ischiatic" hernia.

Sliding indirect inguinal hernia: An indirect inguinal hernia that contains a herniated viscus that makes up all or some of the posterior wall of the sac. Most typically, sliding hernias involve the colon, but they can involve the bladder or the ovary and fallopian tube.

Spigelian hernia: A spontaneous protrusion of preperitoneal fat, a peritoneal sac, or a sac containing a viscus through the Spigelian zone (fascia) at any point along its length.

Spigelian zone or Spigelian fascia: The zone bounded medially by the lateral margin of the anterior lamina of the rectus sheath and laterally by the muscular fibers of the internal oblique muscle.

Sports hernia: A syndrome of weakness of the posterior inguinal wall that occurs in athletic women, causing chronic groin pain without a clinically recognizable hernia.

Umbilical hernia: When the umbilical scar in infants does not close completely or if it fails and stretches in later years, the abdominal contents protrude through the opening and constitute an umbilical hernia. Midline hernias abutting on the umbilicus superiorly and inferiorly are called paraumbilical hernias and are usually included in this group.

INTRODUCTION

Hernia (a word derived from the Greek, meaning "sprouting forth") has been defined, from the time of A. Cornelius Celsus (second century AD) to modern time as a protrusion of organs or parts thereof from their natural place in a cavity through an abnormal opening. Such a definition is unsatisfactory in that it does not cover those situations in which protruded parts have returned or have been returned, are held back by mechanical means, or have not yet protruded and only the potentiality of a protrusion may be recognized. Thus, it is the hernial defect, the opening through which a protrusion may occur, that characterizes hernias, not the protrusion of a viscus. Consistent with this, the designation of various hernias, in contrast to the commonly accepted definition of hernia, uses not the protruded viscus but the location or region in which a hernia can take place (1).

This chapter discusses the role in chronic pelvic pain (CPP) of the following hernias:

1. Hernias of the pelvic wall, perineum and pelvic floor that include sciatic hernia, obturator hernia, and perineal hernia
2. Groin hernias including direct inguinal hernia, indirect inguinal hernia, and femoral hernia
3. Hernias of the abdominal wall including epigastric hernia, umbilical hernia, spigelian hernia, and incisional hernia
4. Internal abdominal hernias including internal supravesical hernias and hernias through the broad ligament
5. Sports hernia
6. Pelvic floor support defects

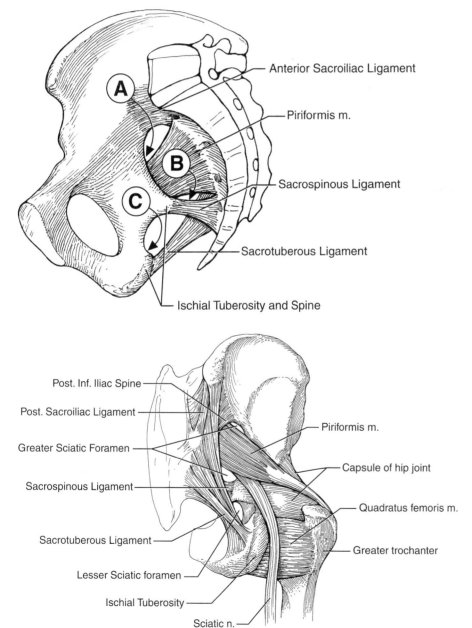

FIGURE 42.1. Sites of potential hernias through the sciatic foramina: **A:** supra piriformis sciatic hernia; **B:** infrapiriformis sciatic hernia; **C:** subspinous sciatic hernia through the lesser sciatic foramen.

SCIATIC HERNIAS

A sciatic hernia is a protrusion of a peritoneal sac and its contents through the greater or lesser sciatic foramen. It has also been called a "sacral sciatic," "gluteal," or "ischiatic" hernia (1). Sciatic hernias have been described as the rarest of all hernias (2). A search of the literature for the period 1966 to 1996 generated a total of 57 cases of sciatic hernia (3). Cases have been reported in children younger than 1 year of age, but most are found in adults between the ages of 20 and 60 years (4). In a recent series the mean age at diagnosis was 34 years (range 23 to 58).

In one study of women with chronic pelvic pain diagnosed and treated using laparoscopy, sciatic hernia was diagnosed in 20 of 1,100 (3). This gives an incidence of 1.8% in women with CPP requiring laparoscopic intervention. In 14 of the cases the hernia was right-sided, in five left-sided, and in one bilateral. This study suggests that sciatic hernia as a source of CPP has been underdiagnosed.

Etiology

Sciatic hernias are either congenital or acquired. Approximately 20% of sciatic hernias are present in infancy and are secondary to maldevelopment of the piriformis muscle or pelvic bones (5). More commonly adults present with an acquired weakness of the piriformis muscle. This can result from chronic increase in intraabdominal pressure owing to pregnancy, severe constipation, surgery, and trauma with weakness of the pelvic muscles and tissues. Atrophy of the piriformis muscle may be a predisposing factor for the sciatic notch hernias and may occur in women who have neuromuscular or hip disease (2). Tumors causing erosion or atrophy of the piriformis are also causative (2). These hernias are slightly more common in females, owing to their wider pelves and sciatic notches.

Pathology and Anatomy

Sciatic hernia is a protrusion from the pelvis of a peritoneal sac through the greater sciatic notch, above or below the piriformis muscle, or through the lesser sciatic notch (Fig. 42.1) (6). The piriformis muscle divides the greater sciatic notch into a supra and infrapiriformis area normally represented as slits between the pelvic muscle groups. The lesser sciatic foramen is bounded superiorly by the sacrospinous and inferiorly by the sacrotuberous ligaments.

The suprapiriformis hernia is by far the most common type. The hernia sac exits the pelvis above the piriformis along the course of the superior gluteal artery and nerve. The infrapiriformis hernia sac tracks a course with the inferior gluteal vessels, internal pudendal vessels, and sciatic nerve. It exits caudal to the piriformis but cephalad to the sacrospinous ligament. The subspinous hernia sac leaves the pelvis through the lesser sciatic foramen medial to the inter-

nal pudendal vessels and nerve and the sciatic nerve. It is bounded superiorly by the sacrospinous and posteriorly by the sacrotuberous ligaments. Any hernia that exits below the sacrotuberous ligaments is considered a perineal hernia (2).

Symptoms or History

Clinically, sciatic hernias present with pain originating in the pelvis. Patients may report ipsilateral posterior thigh or buttocks pain or both (3). Compression of the sciatic nerve may occur, causing pain to radiate down the posterior thigh that is aggravated by dorsiflexion. The pain may be confused with intermittent claudication (4). Intestinal or ureteral obstruction with or without strangulation is sometimes responsible for the first symptoms, as the small openings predispose the hernia to incarceration and strangulation. Symptoms of intestinal obstruction plus pain in the gluteal region point to a sciatic hernia. In addition to pain, the patient may complain of a mass. As the hernial defect enlarges, it may present as a mass just below the inferior border of the gluteus maximus muscle (Fig. 42.2) (2).

Physical Examination

As noted, sciatic hernias pass downward and may present under the lower border of the gluteus maximus muscle in the posteromedial aspect of the thigh (1). If such a palpa-

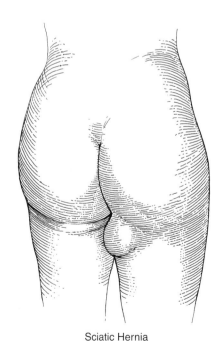

Sciatic Hernia

FIGURE 42.2. Possible clinical appearance of sciatic hernia. A sciatic hernia passes backward and downward to the buttock where it lies deep to the gluteus maximus muscle. The hernia usually contains small bowel, but colon, omentum, bladder, fallopian tube, ovary, Meckel's diverticulum, and even ureter have been reported.

ble, reducible mass is present and symptoms are aggravated by coughing and straining, a sciatic hernia should be suspected (2). However, because of the large gluteal muscle overlying the sciatic foramen and the piriformis muscle, sciatic hernias only are rarely evident on physical examination (3).

Diagnostic Studies

If the ureter herniates into the sciatic foramen it may give rise to a pathognomonic urographic appearance of a redundant, horizontally oriented ureter within a hernia sac that has been called a "curlicue ureter" (7). In frontal projection on excretory urography, the knuckle of herniated ureter passes lateral to the medial wall of the bony pelvis (Fig. 42.3) (8).

Computed tomography shows the contrast-filled ureter posterior, lateral, and craniad to the ischial spine, allowing the confident diagnosis of a ureteral hernia. In adults ureteral sciatic hernias tend to occur in women (8). It is important to differentiate the sciatic type of ureteral hernia from the inguinal herniation where the ureter has a vertical curlicue (7).

Although oblique x-ray studies, computed tomography, herniography, enterography, intravenous pyelography, and cystography may be helpful in the diagnosis of sciatic hernias, they are most often not diagnostic. Sciatic hernias are usually diagnosed during surgery. Laparoscopy aids in the diagnosis of hernias by providing excellent visualization of the pelvis. Intraabdominal pressure, created by insufflation, may be helpful in the detection of sciatic hernia through stretching the peritoneum to its limit of support (e.g., bone

or muscle). However, the sciatic hernia may be filled with the ipsilateral ovary or fallopian tube, leaving little room for distention of the peritoneum by intraabdominal carbon dioxide (3). In one laparoscopic series, all sciatic hernias contained the ipsilateral ovary alone or with its fallopian tube. For this reason and because of lack of general knowledge of sciatic hernias, a prior history of laparoscopic evaluation may not preclude the need for reevaluation. In a series of 20 patients with CPP and sciatic hernias, 14 had undergone 17 prior diagnostic laparoscopies by other surgeons without the diagnosis being made. Clearly, laparoscopy will assist in the definitive diagnosis and treatment of sciatic hernias only if the surgeon has a thorough knowledge of pelvic anatomy and its potential defects (3).

Differential Diagnosis

Lipoma, gluteal aneurysm, or abscess must enter into the differential diagnosis when a mass is present (1). In one series, 6 (30%) of 20 patients with sciatic hernia also had associated findings of endometriosis (1), adhesions (2), endometriosis and adhesions (1), indirect inguinal hernia (1), and indirect inguinal and umbilical hernia (1) (3).

Surgical Therapy

When there is evidence of bowel obstruction the hernia usually is approached through a lower midline abdominal incision. In the woman the bowel is seen entering the hernia behind the broad ligament. Even when an intestinal obstruction is present, the bowel usually can be reduced with light traction. When needed, the opening can be

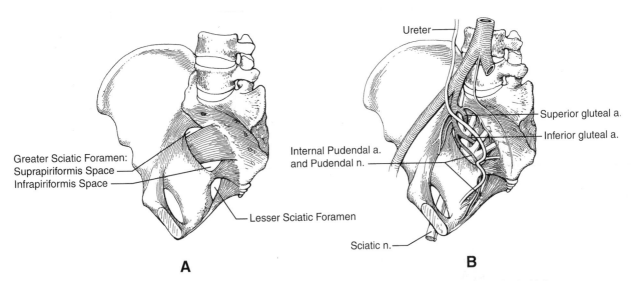

FIGURE 42.3. A: Oblique view of the pelvis from anteromedial shows relation to the ischial, sacrospinous ligaments. Piriformis muscle normally fills much of the greater sciatic notch. **B:** Same view with major arteries and nerves shows course of the herniated right ureter into infrapiriformis space of the greater sciatic notch.

dilated with a finger or else the piriformis muscle may be partially incised, taking great care to avoid the many nerves and vessels in the region. The sac then is everted and excised and the opening repaired by suturing the edges with monofilament polyamide or polypropylene suture. When this repair is not possible, the opening can be plugged with a rolled up strip of polypropylene mesh held in place with a few stitches. Larger defects should be covered with a sheet of polypropylene mesh (4).

A posterior or transgluteal method may be used for uncomplicated and reducible sciatic hernias diagnosed preoperatively. The gluteus maximus muscle is approached through a gluteal incision and is detached at its origin to expose the hernia. The sac is dissected free and opened. The contents are reduced and the sac is dealt with. The defect is closed using local tissues or polypropylene mesh (4).

When a sciatic hernia is approached laparoscopically, its contents are reduced and the peritoneum overlaying the sciatic hernia is elevated and transected transversely with endoscopic scissors. Using blunt dissection the obturator internus and coccygeus muscles are identified. A 6.0 × 12.5 cm piece of mesh material is folded and placed into the space created by the atrophic piriformis muscle. A second piece of mesh is trimmed to the size of the peritoneal defect and placed over the folded mesh. This overlying mesh is secured to the obturator internus fascia laterally and the coccygeus medially with a hernia stapler. The peritoneum overlying the mesh is closed using a hernia stapler (3). Using this technique 14 of 20 patients reported complete pain relief and six noted improvement over preoperative

symptoms with the median length of follow-up of 13 months (range 3 to 36) (3).

OBTURATOR HERNIAS

An obturator hernia is an abnormal protrusion of preperitoneal fat or an intestinal loop through the obturator foramen alongside the obturator vessels and nerve (9). Its relation to groin hernias is seen in Figure 42.4. Obturator hernias are the most common of the three types of pelvic hernias (sciatic, obturator, and perineal) and account for 0.07% of all hernias (10). Obturator hernia was first described in 1724 by Arnaud De Ronsil of France. Over 600 cases have been reported.

Obturator hernias have been reported in patients from 12 to 93 years of age, but greater than 80% of obturator hernias are found in thin, elderly women in the seventh or eighth decade of life. They are more common on the right (60%) and more common in women (6:1). They are bilateral in about 6% of cases. Associated other groin hernias are not uncommon (4). It is difficult to estimate the incidence of obturator hernias in women with chronic pelvic pain. However, because it has now been demonstrated that almost 2% of women with chronic pelvic pain in one series had sciatic hernias, and because obturator hernias are more common than sciatic hernias, it is reasonable to assume that obturator hernias may be significantly underdiagnosed in women with CPP and may occur in more than 2% of patients who require surgery for CPP (3,4).

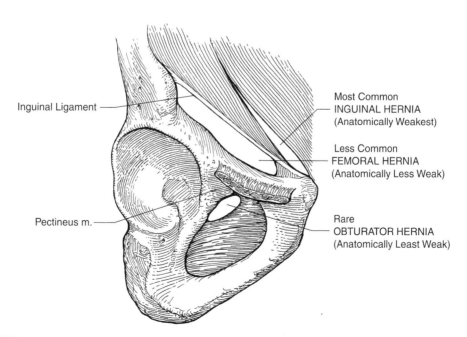

FIGURE 42.4. Surgical anatomy of the obturator region. Lateral view of the right side of the pelvis showing the sites of inguinal, femoral, and obturator hernias.

Etiology/Anatomy

The obturator canal is a tunnel 2 to 3 cm long, beginning in the pelvis at the defect in the obturator membrane. It passes obliquely downward to end outside the pelvis in the obturator region of the thigh. The canal is bounded above and laterally by the obturator groove of the pubis and inferiorly by the free edge of the obturator membrane and the internal and external obturator muscles. Through this canal pass the obturator artery, vein, and nerve. The opening of the obturator canal, located at the anterosuperior border of the foramen, is approximately 1 cm in diameter. Other than the obturator vessels and nerve, it is filled primarily with preperitoneal fat. In emaciated elderly people, loss of the fatty tissues leads to a larger space around the vessels and nerve, facilitating the formation of a hernia (11).

The obturator nerve is usually superior to the artery and vein. The nerve separates into anterior and posterior divisions as it leaves the canal. The hernial sac may follow either division of the nerve. The obturator artery divides to form an arterial ring around the foramen (9).

An obturator hernia consists of a peritoneal sac and may contain small or large intestine, appendix, omentum, bladder, ovary, fallopian tube, or uterus. The sac may pass completely through the foramen and come to rest on the obturator externus, covered by the pectineus muscle. In some instances it may pass between the fasciculi of the obturator externus muscle or may insinuate itself between the layers of the obturator membrane (Fig. 42.5) (1).

The formation of an obturator hernia begins with a "pilot tag" of retroperitoneal fat in the first stage, followed by the appearance of a peritoneal dimple in the second stage, into which a knuckle of viscus may be partially incarcerated (Richter's hernia) in the third stage. Pilot tags of preperitoneal fat have been found in the obturator foramen in up to 64% of female cadaver dissections (12). It is not known how many of these women suffered from CPP. The frequency of pilot tags in cadavers and the rarity of actual obturator hernias in patients suggests that most obturator hernias do not progress beyond the first and second stages of development (4).

Parity of greater than two births is implicated as causative secondary to relaxation of pelvic tissues. The female preponderance is also attributed to the wider pelvis and more oblique obturator canals. Chronic constipation is a risk factor in the elderly. Aging, loss of body weight, and chronic lung disease also are associated with obturator hernia.

Symptoms or History

Pain distributed along the obturator nerve and known as the Howship-Romberg sign is pathognomonic of an obturator hernia, but is by no means invariably present (1). Fifty percent of patients complain of this characteristic pain down the inner surface of the thigh, in the knee joint, and often in the hip joint as well. This represents pain from the cutaneous branch of the anterior division of the obturator nerve and is caused by compression of the nerve in the narrow and unyielding canal. In the elderly patient, this pain is often misinterpreted as arthritic in origin. The nerve also contains motor fibers, and compression may lead to weakness and wasting of the adductors and to loss of the adductor reflex in the thigh (9).

Symptoms of intestinal obstruction are the most common symptoms and occur in 88% of patients, usually in the form of acute obstruction with strangulation (9). In one reported series obturator hernias represented 1% (16 of 1,554) of all hernia repairs performed and 1.6% (16 of 1,000) of cases of mechanical and intestinal obstruction encountered during the same period, suggesting the diagnosis is most often made only after incarceration occurs (13).

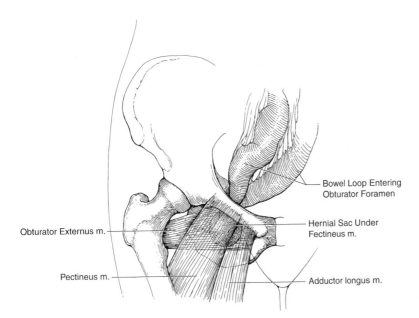

Obturator Externus m.

Pectineus m.

Bowel Loop Entering Obturator Foramen

Hernial Sac Under Fectineus m.

Adductor longus m.

FIGURE 42.5. Anatomic relations of obturator hernia.

In about 30% of patients there is a history of repeated attacks of intestinal obstruction that passed spontaneously. These are probably the result of intermittent compression of the small bowel in the hernia, followed by remissions (9).

Physical Examination

There is a palpable mass high in the medial aspect of the thigh at the origins of the adductor muscles in 20% of cases. The mass is best felt with the thigh flexed, adducted, and rotated outward. Patients rarely complain of a lump in the groin, because large obturator hernias are unusual and many of the patients are too elderly to notice it. Also, because obturator hernia is not always thought of in cases of intestinal obstruction, examination for this palpable lump frequently does not occur. Ecchymosis in the medial part of the groin below the inguinal ligament may occur because of seeping of blood-stained effusions from an infarcted hernia and bowel.

A tender mass may be palpable in the obturator area felt laterally on vaginal examination (Fig. 42.6) (4,9). In the dorsal position with the thigh flexed, adducted, and rotated outward so as to relax the pectineus, adductor longus, and obturator internus muscles a slight bulge may or may not be noticeable as a tender, tense mass in the

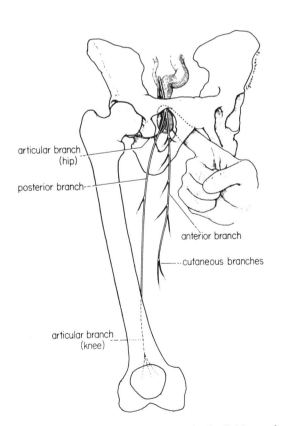

articular branch
(hip)

posterior branch

anterior branch

cutaneous branches

articular branch
(knee)

FIGURE 42.6. Compression of either or both divisions of the obturator nerve by the hernia may produce pain (Howship-Romberg sign). Palpation by vagina or rectum may confirm the presence of a hernia.

upper obturator region, the upper, inner part of the femoral (Scarpa's) triangle.

Diagnostic Studies

With incarceration, computerized tomography (CT) of the pelvis shows a low density mass between the obturator and pectineus muscles—containing air density in some cases and apparently different from the opposite (nonincarcerated) side—and dilated bowel (11). In one series CT led to a correct diagnosis in eight of nine cases of surgically confirmed obturator hernias in patients with symptoms of small bowel obstruction (11). In the one case where CT did not correctly diagnose obturator hernia, the scan focused on the upper abdomen and did not evaluate the pelvic area. Prior to signs and symptoms of obstruction, however, both clinical and imaging diagnoses are difficult.

Ultrasonography has been successful in the diagnosis of some cases but has resulted in questionable diagnosis in others (11). A small bowel series may occasionally demonstrate a knuckle of intestine in the obturator canal. Herniography has been shown to identify obturator hernias that may or may not be symptomatic (2).

Differential Diagnosis

The diagnosis is most likely if the four cardinal features of obturator hernias are present: the Howship-Romberg sign, intestinal obstruction, a history of prior attacks of obstruction, and a mass in the medial thigh. However, delay in diagnosis and treatment is still a common feature of obturator hernia and preoperative diagnosis is uncommon, occurring in as few as 10% of cases (14). The usual absence of external signs, such as inguinal mass, or characteristic signs that may help in early detection of obturator hernia contribute to this delay (11). The common symptoms of intestinal obstruction varies in severity. In many cases the initial symptoms are mild nausea, vomiting, and anorexia. Only one-third of the reported patients gave a history previous attacks of obstructive symptoms.

The differential diagnosis must take into consideration inguinal adenitis, psoas abscess, obturator neuritis, diseases of the hip joint, internal, perineal, and femoral hernias, and other causes of intestinal obstruction. Obturator hernias also may exist in association with a femoral hernia and contralateral obturator hernia. The general absence of preperitoneal fat and the weak supporting structures render such association not surprising (4).

Surgical Treatments

Surgical treatments via the abdominal, femoral, and inguinal routes have been described. The abdominal route is preferred because of the frequent necessity for an intestinal resection by the time the hernia has been diagnosed (1).

The midline extraperitoneal approach is the best method for dealing with an obturator hernia when the diagnosis has been made preoperatively. It allows good exposure of the internal opening of the obturator canal without interfering with the abdominal contents and risking intraabdominal adhesions. An incision is made from the umbilicus to the pubis in the midline, without breaching the peritoneum, which is peeled off the bladder in the midline, and also laterally to expose the superior pubic ramus and the obturator internus muscle. The sac is seen as a projection of peritoneum passing into the obturator canal. It is incised at its base. The contents are reduced into the peritoneal cavity, the sac is transected at the neck, and the peritoneal defect is closed. The sac is extracted from the canal by traction or by an artery forceps, which is passed down into the sac to grasp the distal end and to extract the sac by inversion. The internal opening of the obturator canal is closed with a continuous monofilament nylon suture, taking bites of the tissues around it, such as the periosteum of the superior pubic ramus and the fascia of the internal obturator muscle. Care must be exercised not to injure the obturator nerve and vessels. Alternatively, a sheet of prosthetic mesh may be laid down to cover the area and tack down around its edges. The peritoneum is allowed to return to the pelvic wall, and the abdominal incision is closed (4).

The midline transperitoneal approach is the most common method for repair of obturator hernia, because most cases are unexpectedly encountered during laparotomy for intestinal obstruction of unknown cause. Reduction by gentle traction on the loops of bowel is often successful. This attempt may be augmented by pressure on the hernial sac over the medial aspect of the thigh. Extraction of the bowel can be made easier by carefully incising the sharp edge of the obturator membrane. Care must be taken to identify and avoid injury to the obturator nerve (4).

A laparoscopic approach to the preperitoneal prosthetic herniorrhaphy is possible (15). Seven obturator hernias were repaired laparoscopically in a series of 290 laparoscopic preperitoneal hernia repairs. However, "technical complications" affected 5% of the patients. Continued scrutiny and critical review is suggested before widespread acceptance of the laparoscopic procedure (15).

The high incidence of recurrence bilaterally and difficulty with clinical diagnosis may warrant bilateral repair, even when only a unilateral hernia is evident (14).

PERINEAL HERNIAS

A perineal hernia is the protrusion of a viscus through the floor of the pelvis (pelvic diaphragm) into the perineum. A hernial sac is present (Fig. 42.7) (1,16). Perineal hernias are also called pelvic hernias, ischiorectal hernias, pudendal hernias, posterior labial hernias, subpubic hernias, hernias of the Pouch of Douglas, and vaginal hernias. Scarpa, in

1821, first reported a case, but de Garengeot is supposed to have seen one in 1731 (4). The condition is considered extremely rare, and fewer than 100 cases have been reported (2). Primary perineal hernias are spontaneously occurring hernias. They occur most commonly between the ages of 40 and 60 years and are five times more common in women than in men. Secondary or postoperative hernias may occur following abdominoperineal resection of the rectum and related procedures (4).

Etiology

Primary perineal hernias occur more frequently in women because of the broader female pelvis and attenuation of the pelvic floor during pregnancy. Other factors are obesity, ascites, and recurrent pelvic floor infection. Secondary perineal hernias are incisional ones through the reconstructed pelvic floor in patients who have had extensive pelvic surgery. They are seen in approximately 1% of abdominoperineal resections and 3% to 10% of pelvic exenterations, usually occurring within 1 year of the surgery (2).

Anatomy

Anatomically, two types of perineal hernia are described, anterior and posterior, depending on their relationship to the transversus perinei muscles (Figs. 42.7 and 42.8) (4). A primary perineal hernia may be an anterior or posterior hernia. An anterior hernia protrudes through the urogenital diaphragm into the triangle formed by the bulbocavernosus muscle medially, the ischial cavernosus muscle laterally, and the superficial transverse perineal muscle inferiorly. Anterior hernias occur only in women (16). They have been variously called pudendal, labial, lateral, or vaginal-labial.

Posterior perineal hernias occur in both women and men, but are more frequent in women. The hernia enters between the rectum and the uterus and passes posterior to the broad ligament and lateral to the uterosacral ligament. It may pass through the levator ani muscle or between it and the iliococcygeus muscle, or even directly through the iliococcygeus muscle. It may remain in the midline and pass forward to press into the vaginal wall or backward into the rectum. It may also lie in the ischiorectal fossa below the lower margin of the gluteus maximus muscle and may be confused with a sciatic hernia.

Anterior perineal hernias contain intestine or bladder. Posterior perineal hernias may contain omentum, small bowel, or rectum. The hernias have a wide neck and usually soft borders with no rigid fibrous ring, so that incarceration or strangulation are rare (4).

A lateral pelvic hernia has also been described. In this case the peritoneal sac passes through a gap in the line of origin of the levator ani muscle from the fascia of the internal obturator muscle. It passes anteriorly into the labia majus or posteriorly into the ischiorectal fossa (4).

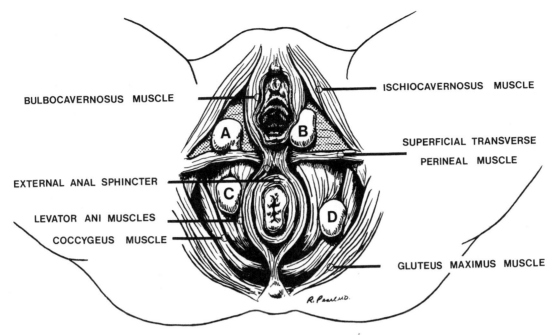

FIGURE 42.7. The female perineum seen from above showing possible sites of perineal hernias. A primary perineal hernia may occur anterior or posterior to the superficial transversus perineal muscle. An anterior hernia protrudes through the urogenital diaphragm into the triangle formed by the bulbocavernosus muscle medially, the ischial cavernosus muscle laterally, and the superficial transverse perineus muscle inferiorly. Anterior hernias occur only in woman. A posterior perineal hernia may merge between component muscle, bundles of levator ani muscle, or between that muscle and the coccygeus muscle, midway between the rectum and the ischial tuberosity.

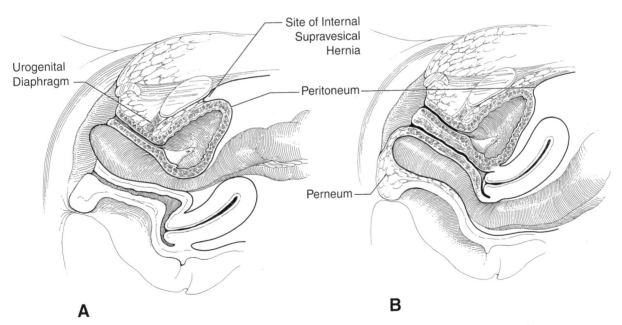

A   **B**

FIGURE 42.8. The course of anterior and posterior perineal hernias in the woman—sagittal section of the female pelvis. **A:** Course of the anterior perineal hernia. The sac passes between the urinary bladder and the vagina to reach the surface of the perineum. **B:** Course of a posterior perineal hernia. The sac passes between the vagina and rectum to reach the surface of the perineum.

Symptoms or History

The patient may complain of a soft protuberance that is easily reduced when the recumbant position is assumed. Symptoms are usually mild. In cases of anterior hernia, minor urinary discomfort may have been noted. In cases of posterior hernias in which the mass may assume a large size or even protrude below the lower edge of the gluteus maximus muscle, sitting may be difficult or impossible. A dragging sensation may be felt on standing or straining. Rarely, constipation may be attributed to the hernia. A posterior hernia protruding into the posterior wall of the vagina may interfere with labor (4).

Physical Examination

Physical examination may reveal a soft and easily reducible mass with a cough impulse. The direction in which it reduces indicates the anatomic nature of the hernia. Strangulation is rare because the hernial defect is usually large and bounded by soft and often atrophied muscle. If strangulation occurs, local pain, swelling, and signs of inflammation develop, together with the signs and symptoms of intestinal obstruction. The hernia then becomes tender and irreducible (4).

Diagnostic Studies

Bimanual, rectal, and vaginal examinations help to differentiate perineal hernia from rectocele or cystocele. Plain abdominal films or a barium enema with postevacuation views may confirm the presence of the hernia. Computed tomography or herniography can be used to diagnose difficult cases (2). Although not well-studied, defecography should be helpful in differential diagnosis.

Differential Diagnosis

The differential diagnosis for perineal hernia includes cystocele, rectocele, perineal abscess, lipoma, fibroma, and polyps. Rectal prolapse must sometimes be differentiated from a perineal hernia. The two may coexist, with the perineal hernia appearing anterior to the prolapsed rectum. Surgical exploration is usually the only definitive way to make the diagnosis.

Surgical Treatment

Three options are available for surgical repair: abdominal, perineal, or combined abdominal-perineal approach. The abdominal approach is preferable because it allows better exposure of the anatomy of the defect and a more secure repair. The abdomen is opened through a midline subumbilical incision. The bowel disappears through a defect in the pelvic floor and usually can be reduced easily. Occasionally, mild traction or even outside pressure on the hernia may be needed. The empty sac is everted and excised. Small defects can be closed by interrupted sutures of monofilament polyamide or polypropylene. If the atrophied muscle tissue is used for the repair, the recurrence rate is high. Recurrence can be avoided by using a sheet of prosthetic nonabsorbable mesh to reinforce the repair. It is laid on the pelvic floor of the region to cover the repair and is tacked down by nonabsorbable monofilament sutures. When the defect is large and the edges are thinned and friable, they cannot be approximated. In these cases, a synthetic nonabsorbable mesh prosthesis is sutured to cover the defect. The rectovesicle pouch then can be eliminated by a series of sutures (4).

With secondary or postoperative hernias, reinforcement of the pelvic floor is often required with free fascial grafts, synthetic mesh, or tissue grafts consisting of muscle, omentum, or mesenteric leaf. Prosthetic mesh may be sutured to the sacroperiosteum posteriorly below the level of S3. Anteriorly, it can be sutured to the vaginal apex. If the uterus is still present, the defect can be obliterated by suturing the retroflexed uterus to the sacrum. Muscle flaps from the rectus abdominis, gluteus, gracilis, and bulbocavernosus muscles have also been described in the repairs of the pelvic floor (2).

GROIN HERNIAS

The groin has been defined as that portion of the anterior abdominal wall below the level of the anterior superior iliac spines. In this area a hernia may protrude forming a visible and usually palpable swelling (Fig. 42.9). Three types of hernia—direct inguinal, indirect inguinal, and external supravesical—may emerge through the abdominal wall by way of the external inguinal ring above the inguinal ligament. A fourth type, femoral hernia, emerges beneath the inguinal ligament by way of the femoral canal. These four hernias make up 90% of all hernias.

An indirect inguinal hernia leaves the abdomen through the internal inguinal ring and passes down the inguinal canal a variable distance with the round ligament. Occasionally, the sac may not reach the labia majora but may enter the abdominal wall through any cleavage plane between muscles. This is an interparietal hernia (17).

A sliding indirect inguinal hernia contains a herniated viscus that makes up all or some of the posterior wall of the sac. Typically, sliding hernias involve the colon, but they can involve the bladder, and, in the woman, the ovaries and uterine tube (17).

A direct inguinal hernia passes through the floor of the inguinal canal in Hesselbach's triangle, which is covered by the transversalis fascia and aponeurosis of the transversus abdominis muscle. The hernia path does not enter the internal ring but may exit through the external ring (19). Hesselbach's triangle as described in 1814 is formed by the following boundaries: superolateral—the inferior (deep) epigastric vessels; medial—the rectus sheath (lateral border); inferior (or, the base)—the inguinal ligament (Fig. 42.10). Most direct inguinal hernias occur in this area (17).

trude through the abdominal wall as a direct inguinal hernia.

INGUINAL HERNIAS

The incidence of inguinal hernias in adults in the Western hemisphere is 10% to 15%. The male to female ratio is 12:1. The incidence is 5% to 8% in patients 25 to 40 years of age. Hernias are present in greater than 45% of men at 75 years of age and older. Over 700,000 groin hernia operations are performed annually in the United States (4).

The incidence of inguinal hernias in women with CPP is not known. The most common hernias in women are inguinal (indirect or direct) and femoral, just as in men. However, femoral hernias are relatively more common in women than men, accounting for 20% of all groin hernias found in women. Indirect inguinal hernias are congenital, and direct inguinal and femoral hernias are considered acquired (4). External and internal views of the locations of these hernias are shown in Figure 42.11.

Etiology

During embryologic development, the round and ovarian ligaments in the woman are distinguishable by the eleventh week, once Mullerian duct fusion has occurred. The processus vaginalis, a diverticulum of the peritoneal cavity, also appears at this period of gestational development. The processus vaginalis is patent in 80% to 94% of newborns studied at autopsy. This rate steadily decreases with age as closure continues until adulthood, when 15% to 30% of autopsies show a patent processus vaginalis. Most closures of the processus appear to occur before the age of 2 years. Why many women with patent processus vaginalis remain asymptomatic can only be speculated. Although a patent processus vaginalis is held to be the prime cause of indirect

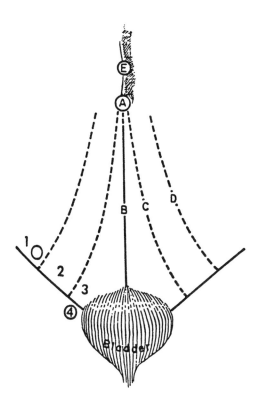

FIGURE 42.9. Diagram of the fossa of the anterior abdominal wall and their relation to the sites of groin hernias: **A:** Umbilicus. **B:** Median umbilical ligament (obliterated urachus). **C:** Medial umbilical ligament (obliterated umbilical arteries). **D:** Lateral umbilical ligament containing inferior (D) epigastric artery. **E:** Falciform ligament. Sites of possible hernias: (1) lateral fossa (indirect inguinal hernia); (2) medial fossa (direct inguinal hernia); (3) supravesical fossa (supravesical hernia); and (4) femoral ring (femoral hernia).

A femoral hernia is a protrusion of preperitoneal fat or intraperitoneal viscus through a weak transversalis fascia into the femoral ring and the femoral canal (18). An external supravesical hernia and its contents pass through the supravesical fossa of the anterior abdominal wall and pro-

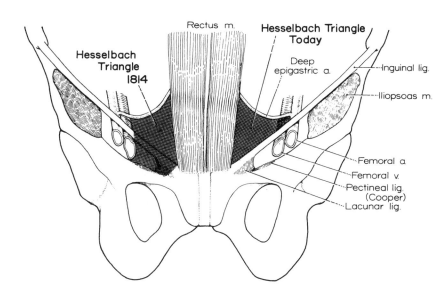

FIGURE 42.10. The triangle described by Hesselbach in 1814 is slightly larger than the triangle accepted today as defining the area where the direct inguinal hernia is most likely to occur.

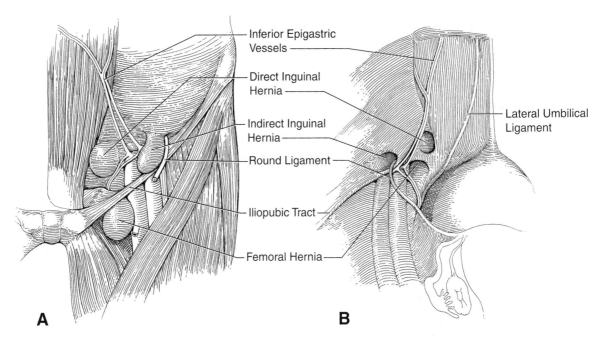

A   **B**

FIGURE 42.11. A: Three types of groin hernia and some important landmarks: 1, inguinal ligament; 2, femoral artery; 3, indirect hernial sac; 4, direct hernial sac; 5, femoral sac; 6, inferior epigastric vessels; 7, lateral umbilical ligament. (From Rowe JS Jr, Skandalakis JE, Gray SW. Multiple bilateral inguinal hernias. *AM Surg* 193;39:269, with permission.) **B:** Internal view of the groin demonstrating anatomic landmarks for the identification of direct and indirect inguinal hernia and femoral hernia.

inguinal hernia, almost all other mammals have a permanently patent processus vaginalis and only rarely suffer from inguinal hernia. It is assumed that three factors are involved in generating inguinal hernias: the presence of a preformed sac, repeated elevations in the intraabdominal pressure, and weakening of the body muscles and tissues with time. Raised intraabdominal pressure such as that which occurs during pregnancy can make a hernia appear for the first time. Other conditions that predispose to hernia development include prematurity, low birth weight, family history, peritonitis, liver disease with ascites, abdominal wall defects, connective tissue disease, ventriculoperitoneal shunts, and continuous ambulatory peritoneal dialysis.

Enormously high intraabdominal pressures are generated when an individual coughs or strains, but the abdominal wall usually maintains its integrity in spite of preformed weak areas, notably the transversalis fascia and the internal inguinal ring. This is generally explained on the basis of a "shutter mechanism." The muscles of the abdominal wall must contract to raise the intraabdominal pressure. As the external oblique muscle contracts, it becomes tense and presses on the weak posterior wall of the inguinal canal and so reinforces it and also tends to pull the inguinal ligament upward (i.e., convex cranially). At the same time the muscular arch passing over the round ligament also sharply contracts, and as its fibers shorten, the arch is straightened out and comes to lie on or close to the raised inguinal ligament, and so protects the weak posterior wall of the canal. As this "shutter" comes down, it passes in front of the internal ring and so counteracts the pressure on the ring from inside the

abdomen. The very act of contraction of the abdominal muscles in coughing or straining, which tends to blow out the internal ring and the transversalis fascia, automatically, and at the same time, brings into play mechanisms that prevent the occurrence of this damage. Animals that walk on all four limbs rarely suffer from inguinal hernia. The change to the upright posture may have reduced the mechanical efficiency of the shutter mechanism that leads to a greater propensity to develop inguinal hernias in humans (4). The assumption of an upright posture in humans has resulted in the development of a true anterior abdominal wall rather than two anterolateral walls, as are found in quadrupeds. The result of these changes is to increase the distance between the inguinal ligament and the arch of the transversus abdominis and internal oblique muscles. The iliofemoral vessels are displaced laterally. The inguinal shutter mechanism has thus become less efficient than in quadrupeds. Evolution for bipeds has created a region of weakness in the groin at risk for hernia (4).

Another major factor involved in the etiology of inguinal hernia, weakening of the muscles and fascias of the abdominal wall, occurs with advancing age, lack of physical exercise, adiposity, multiple pregnancies, and loss of weight and body fitness, as may occur after illness or operation. It has been suggested that abnormalities in the structure of collagen, such as a reduction in polymerized collagen and a decrease concentration of hydroxyproline, leads to a loss of lining between the collagen fibers. This mechanism is important in some cases, especially in cases of repeated recurrent hernia and perhaps in cases of familial tendency to hernia (4).

Clearly, the cause of hernia is multifactorial. In the case of indirect hernia, a preformed sac (patent processus vaginalis) is present, but bowel is prevented from entering by efficient muscular action. A sudden and unusually high increase in intraabdominal pressure may be sufficient to overcome this protective mechanism, and a hernia may quite suddenly appear. This may be seen in the case of fit young individuals who perform a strenuous physical act that they are not accustomed to doing. In persons weakened by age, adiposity, illness, chronic cough, constipation, and urinary obstruction, the protecting mechanisms deteriorate until they are no longer able to prevent the bowel from entering the preformed sac (4).

In direct hernia, there is no preformed sac; in fact there is no real peritoneal sac at all. Because of the factors mentioned previously, the protective mechanisms fail. The weakened transversalis fascia, on its own, cannot withstand the repeatedly raised intraabdominal pressure and stretches, ballooning out in front of the advancing bowel, or simply tears and allows the peritoneum-covered bowel to pass through it.

Anatomy

Contraction of the transversus abdominis muscle causes a shutter-like approximation of the muscle and its tendon to the inguinal ligament (see previous discussion). The interposition of a strong musculotendinous wall reinforces thin transversalis fascia covering the indirect and direct inguinal rings. A descending barrier of transversus abdominis muscle and tendon during exercise bolsters transversalis fascia in the groin and helps prevent herniation through the inguinal rings (Figs. 42.12 and 42.13) (17,18,19).

There exists in the groin a myopectineal opening between the abdomen and the thigh (Fig. 42.14) (19). The myopectineal orifice is bounded by the rectus sheath medially, internal oblique and transversus abdominis muscle superiorly, the iliopsoas muscle laterally, and pubis inferiorly. The orifice is spanned by the inguinal ligament, traversed by the round ligament and iliofemoral vessels, and covered on its inner surface by transversalis fascia. The myopectineal orifice is the site through which all inguinal and femoral hernias must pass to present on the anterior surface. All hernias result from a defect in this orifice. For this reason the entire myopectineal orifice must be addressed for any comprehensive repair of a groin hernia (19).

That part of the transversalis fascia medial to the inferior epigastric vessels is known as Hesselbach's triangle, which is bounded by the vessels laterally, the conjoined tendon and rectus sheath superiorly, and the inguinal ligament inferiorly. Indirect inguinal hernias pass through the internal ring lateral to the inferior epigastric vessels, and direct hernias bulge forward medial to the vessels, through Hesselbach's triangle, pushing the attenuated transversalis fascia ahead of them while emerging through a tear in the fascia (4).

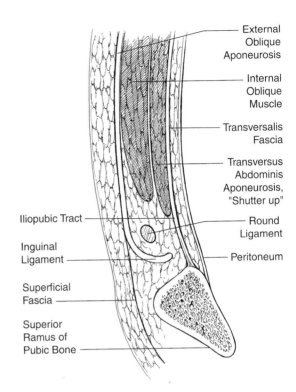

FIGURE 42.12. Transversus abdominis, internal oblique muscles—"shutter up."

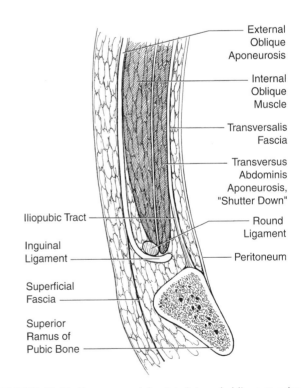

FIGURE 42.13. Transversus abdominis, internal oblique muscles—"shutter down."

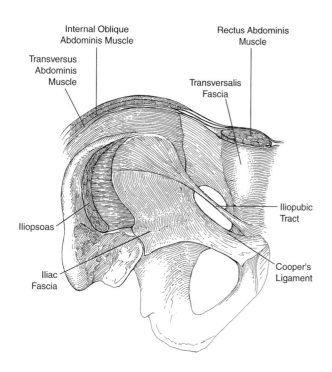

FIGURE 42.14. Myopectineal orifice.

Symptoms or History

In exceptional cases there can be a rapid onset, even within hours or 1 or 2 days, of an "acute" inguinal hernia (usually indirect) following sudden, unexpected, unusual exertion and accompanied by pain and possibly by ecchymosis in the inguinal region. In the usual case, the patient may feel some discomfort in the groin and notice a small bulge above the inguinal crease when coughing or straining that immediately subsides. As the hernia develops, it appears when the patient stands and reduces when she lies down. As it grows larger, it may not reduce spontaneously when she is lying down, and the patient learns to reduce it manually. In the early stages when the hernia is stretching and tearing the tissues of the abdominal wall, the patient may complain of much discomfort and pain in the region, especially when walking or straining. Later, when the hernia is established, the complaints usually are concerned with the presence of an unaesthetic bulge in the groin area that interferes with walking and other activities and causes a heavy dragging sensation. Patients often complain of an unpleasant sickening feeling in the pit of their stomachs when they are straining. This may be a result of tension on the mesentery as the bowel is forced down into the hernia. Also, traction on nerves in the region of the hernia detected may cause symptoms in the distribution of that nerve.

The hernia may be incarcerated or irreducible because of adhesions between the sac and the contents or because of adhesions between the loops of bowel and omentum, especially in longstanding hernias in which the matted mass of contents cannot pass through the relatively narrow hernial orifice. Bowel and omentum may be caught by pressure on the edge of the hernial orifice, leading to interference with its blood supply and to strangulation of the hernial contents. In such cases an obvious emergency manifests itself with extreme pain and signs of intestinal obstruction and later signs of gangrenous bowel (4).

Physical Examination

Clinical examination reveals a bulge that increases in size and turgor with coughing and that usually can be reduced (a gurgling sound is produced) when the patient is supine. Smaller hernias only may be visible as a bulge when the patient coughs. When the patient stands, a cough impulse can be felt at the tip of the finger after introducing it into the inguinal canal through the external ring by invagination (4).

An indirect hernia is sausage- or pear-shaped and lies parallel to the inguinal ligament. After reduction it reappears more laterally and runs down above the inguinal ligament. A direct hernia is more rounded, more medial, bulges forward, and tends not to go down into the labial area. After reduction it reappears in a forward direction. When an indirect hernia is present, a finger inserted through the external ring into the inguinal canal will pass laterally and upward of the internal ring. In the case of the direct hernia, the finger will pass directly backward into the abdomen through the opening in the transversalis fascia. When the hernia is reduced and the examiner applies manual pressure over the internal ring and requests the patient to stand and cough, an indirect hernia will not reappear, whereas a direct hernia will immediately bulge forth. These signs are not always clear-cut. A longstanding, large indirect hernia stretches the internal ring until it occupies most of the transversalis fascia; its appearance is no different from that of a direct hernia. A small direct hernia protruding through a narrow tear of the transversalis fascia appears clinically like an indirect hernia. The differentiation is of academic interest only. The true nature of the hernia is revealed at operation and is handled accordingly (4).

An incarcerated hernia is soft and nontender, but irreducible. A strangulated hernia is tense, swollen, tender, and irreducible and becomes red, edematous, and inflamed (4).

Diagnostic Studies

Herniography can be performed for the diagnosis of inguinal hernia. Radiopaque contrast material is injected intraperitoneally and the patient is maneuvered through various positions in an attempt to introduce the material into an actual or potential hernial sac that can be demonstrated radiographically. This technique reveals true or potential hernial sacs, but it has failed to gain popularity because of the ease with which most hernias can be diagnosed by simple clinical means. It may be of some use in specially selected cases, for instance, to confirm or exclude the presence of an inguinal hernia in a patient complaining of unexplained groin pain (4).

Laparoscopically, an indirect inguinal hernia is evident as an opening adjacent to the round ligament (Fig. 42.15).

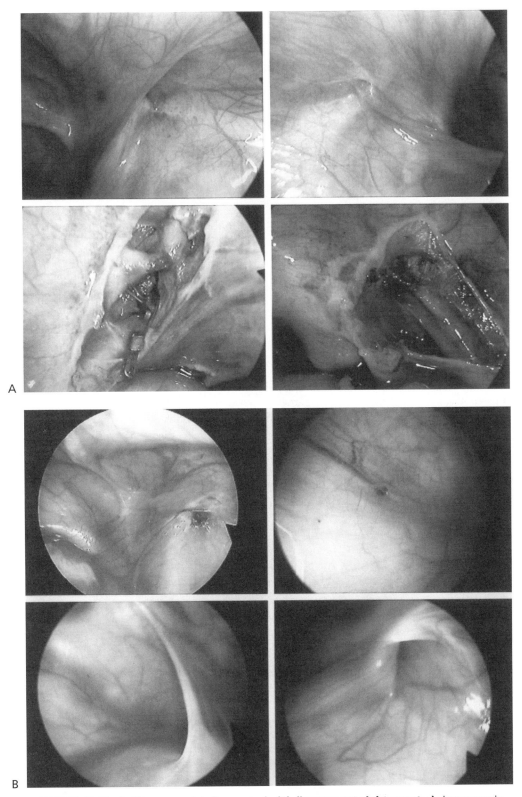

FIGURE 42.15. A: (Uppermost left quarter); (B) (lowermost right quarter): laparoscopic views of right indirect inguinal hernias

However, a direct or femoral hernia may not be clearly seen until the peritoneum is opened. These hernias are usually found after dissecting the preperitoneal fat. A direct inguinal hernia can sometimes be clearly seen as a defect or indentation in the peritoneum in the area of Hesselbach's triangle (19). If it is not clear, the peritoneum in Hesselbach's triangle can be grasped and pulled cephalad, and a redundant peritoneum or sac identified (20).

Differential Diagnosis

The diagnosis of inguinal hernia in the adult is usually not difficult, but occasionally it may have to be differentiated from femoral hernia or from enlarged inguinal lymph nodes owing to lymphogranuloma venereum, cat scratch fever, or involvement with primary malignant disease, such as lymphoma, or with secondary carcinomatous deposits. If the patient's complaint is localized pain, this may indicate an area of separation of fascial layers through which an actual herniated viscus has not yet protruded. This pain could be from separation of the fascial fibers, trapping of preperitoneal fat in the fascial separation, from tearing of the muscle fibers, or from traction on nerves in the vicinity of the hernial defect. The diagnosis of a fascial defect may be difficult if the viscus has not yet passed through. Even laparoscopic examination may be unrevealing unless the peritoneal layer is opened and the defect searched for. Thus the differential diagnosis of occult hernias in the inguinal area includes all conditions of inflammation, torsion, and peritoneal, fascial, or muscular irritation that can exist in the same region.

Surgical Treatment

The surgical repair of the inguinal hernia in modern times has its foundations in the work of the Italian surgeon, Eduardo Bassini (1844–1924), who devised a method of hernia repair that utilized a three-layer reconstruction of the inguinal floor. Bassini recommended a "triple layer" approximation of the internal oblique muscle, transversus abdominis muscle, and transversalis fascia to the inguinal ligament. However, the recurrence rate for a "Bassini" operation in most hands was about 5% to 10%. Irving Lichtenstein described a "tension-free" repair for the inguinal hernia in the early 1970s. Lichtenstein maintained that the hernia recurrence rate could not be improved until the tension inherent in approximating tissues for inguinal floor reconstruction was eliminated. To perform a "tension-free repair" Lichtenstein utilized a sheet of prosthetic mesh to reconstruct the inguinal floor. A bridge of synthetic material was used to cover the direct and indirect inguinal ring rather than forcibly approximate muscle and fascia to the inguinal ligament, as in Bassini's repair. In 1986 Lichtenstein reported a recurrence rate of just 0.7% in a series of 6,321 consecutive herniorrhaphies (17,19).

Although these procedures are readily performed through open techniques, the laparoscopic approach to the

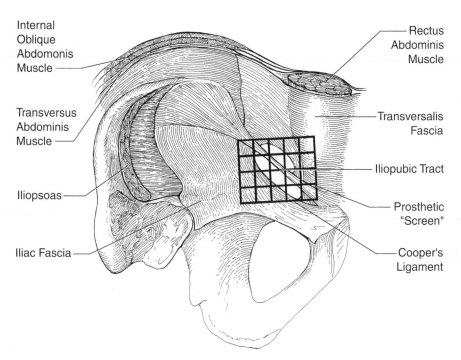

FIGURE 42.16. The goal of laparoscopic hernioplasty is to cover all potential defects of the myopectineal orifice with a prosthetic screen.

groin hernia repair offers the ability to (a) expose fully and reconstitute the entire myopectineal orifice, (b) examine easily and repair bilateral groin hernias, and (c) perform a thorough intraabdominal examination at the time of hernioplasty. All groin hernias, regardless of presentation, must pass through the myopectineal orifice. The goal of laparoscopic groin hernia repair is to place a large prosthetic screen permanently over the myopectineal window of the groin. The prosthesis is sized to cover and overlap all potential defects in the myopectineal orifice (Fig. 42.16) (19). A preperitoneal placement of graft is preferred to lessen the possibility of reaction with intraabdominal content. Placing a large graft over the myopectineal orifice allows groin hernias to be treated relative to their site of origin, a "deep" inguinal repair, rather than their site of presentation. The myopectineal orifice is completely covered and the effect of the shutter mechanism reconstituted (19).

FEMORAL HERNIAS

A femoral hernia is a protrusion of preperitoneal fat or intraperitoneal viscus through a weak transversalis fascia into the femoral ring and the femoral canal (Fig. 42.17) (18). In clinical practice, one encounters about one femoral hernia for every 10 inguinal hernias. They are four times more common in women than men and account for one-third of abdominal wall hernias in women. They are almost as frequent as inguinal hernias. Femoral hernias are twice as common on the right and are bilateral in about one out of 15 cases. It is not unusual for individuals to develop a femoral hernia who have had a previous repair of an inguinal hernia. The femoral hernia may have been present but missed at the time of the first operation or may have developed later on the basis of the same etiology. About one-third of femoral hernias strangulate (4).

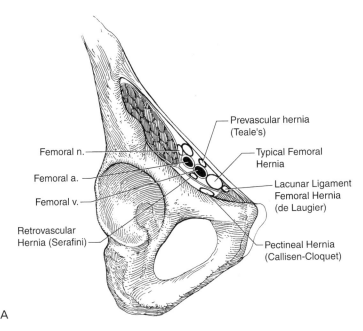

Prevascular hernia (Teale's)

Femoral n.

Femoral a.

Femoral v.

Retrovascular Hernia (Serafini)

Typical Femoral Hernia

Lacunar Ligament Femoral Hernia (de Laugier)

Pectineal Hernia (Callisen-Cloquet)

A

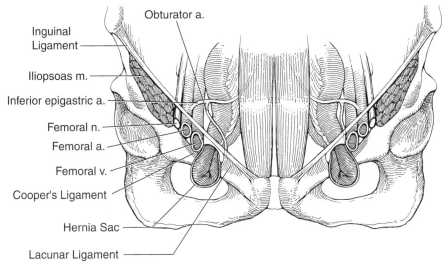

Obturator a.

Inguinal Ligament

Iliopsoas m.

Inferior epigastric a.

Femoral n.

Femoral a.

Femoral v.

Cooper's Ligament

Hernia Sac

Lacunar Ligament

B

FIGURE 42.17. A: Femoral hernia. Typical and atypical pathways taken by the femoral hernia sac. Note the possible relations to the femoral artery (A) and femoral vein (V). **B:** Femoral hernia. The left half of the drawing shows an aberrant obturator artery passing medial to the hernia sac, making it dangerous to incise the lacunar ligament. The right half of the drawing shows an aberrant obturator artery passing lateral to the hernial sac, making it safe to incise the lacunar ligament.

Etiology

The etiology of femoral hernias is probably not congenital. There is no evidence of a preformed sac. These hernias usually appear after middle age, suggesting that natural weakening of the tissues and loss of elasticity is the basic cause. They are more common in multiparous women (4).

Anatomy

The transversalis fascia emerges above from behind the musculoaponeurotic arch of the internal oblique and the transversus abdominis muscles and passes down to attach to the pectineal ridge. In this way it closes off the area between the inguinal ligament and the superior pubic ramus and separates the abdomen from the thigh. This area is mainly filled by the iliopsoas and pectineus muscles and the femoral artery, vein, and nerve passing from the abdomen to the thigh. At its most medial end, there exists a potential canal, the femoral canal, through which the common type of femoral hernia emerges. It is bounded anteriorly by the inguinal ligament, medially by the lacunar part of the inguinal ligament, posteriorly by the pubic ramus and the pectineal ligament, and laterally by the femoral vein and sheath. The canal is filled by loose areolar tissue and femoral lymph nodes. With weakening of the transversalis fascia closing the canal, the peritoneal sac of the femoral hernia transverses the narrow confines of the rigid canal and passes into the loose subcutaneous area of the thigh. Here it is able to expand and pass forward to bulge below the inguinal ligament. It may even pass upward to cross the inguinal ligament. The sac is covered with extraperitoneal fat and con-

tains either small bowel, omentum, or both. The sac is relatively large compared to the narrow neck, which has no room to expand, so that striangulation is common (4).

Symptoms or History: Femoral Hernia

The patient may notice a small reducible lump in the medial aspect of the groin. Symptoms of intestinal obstruction may be the first presentation. Femoral hernias do not appear to otherwise be a frequent cause of pelvic pain.

Physical Examination

Femoral hernias can be easily overlooked if small. The diagnosis can usually be made on finding a soft tumor at the femoral fossa and by ascertaining the location of the tumor below the inguinal ligament and lateral to the pubic tubercle.

Diagnostic Studies

If a femoral hernia is not evident by physical examination but is suspected by symptoms, a laparoscopy can be performed. A femoral hernia is usually seen below the iliopubic track and above Coopers ligament just medial to the iliac vein (Fig. 42.18) (20). If a femoral hernia is not readily visible, a gentle push with a blunt instrument reveals weakness in the peritoneum (19,20).

Differential Diagnosis

In diagnosing a femoral hernia, reducible or not, one must exclude also inguinal adenitis, lipoma, varicosities of the

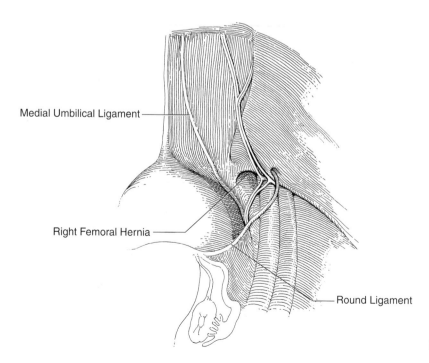

Medial Umbilical Ligament

Right Femoral Hernia

Round Ligament

FIGURE 42.18. Right femoral hernia.

saphenous vein, psoas abscess, obturator hernia, hydrocele of the femoral sac, hydatid cyst, dermoid cysts, and myofascial conditions such as trigger points (1,4).

Surgical Treatment

Repair of the femoral hernia through the open approach requires a skin incision, division of the external oblique aponeurosis, elevation of the round ligament, and separation of it from the posterior wall. This is followed by incision of the internal oblique and transversus abdominis muscles. The transversalis fascia is then incised and the preperitoneal space is identified. Blunt dissection of the preperitoneal space directs the surgeon to the neck of the hernia sac. The unopened sac is gently pushed upward through the femoral canal into the inguinal canal. The femoral hernia has now become a direct hernia and is repaired in the standard fashion for direct inguinal hernias (8).

A laparoscopic approach to the femoral hernia is also possible. The femoral hernia is treated in the same manner by placement of a nonabsorbable mesh to occlude the myopectineal orifice as previously described on the section on inguinal hernias (9).

HERNIAS OF THE LINEA ALBA (EPIGASTRIC HERNIAS)

Hernias of the linea alba are protrusions of preperitoneal fat or a peritoneal sac with or without an incarcerated viscus that occur in the midline between the xiphoid process and the umbilicus (Fig. 42.19). The linea alba is wider above the umbilicus and more prone to penetration. In the usual hernia of the linea alba, preperitoneal fat bulges through a small defect in the linea alba. Less commonly, the defect enlarges and a peritoneal sac is present. The sac may be empty or contain omentum or small or large intestine. Such a hernia is covered by skin, subcutaneous fat, and peritoneum (21).

Hernias of the linea alba are uncommon, with an incidence estimated at 0.4% to 1% of all hernias. They are three times more common in men than women, and most common between the ages of 20 and 50 years. Although they are usually located above the umbilicus, hernias of the linea alba can also occur below the umbilicus. They occur just to the right or left of the midline (4).

Etiology

Hernias of the linea alba occur because of a congenital defect, a rise of intraabdominal pressure, adiposity, or weakening of the muscles in adults. They are more frequent in people with a wide linea alba (diastasis of the recti muscles). They possibly occur because of a lack of fibers at the midline decussation, which allows preperitoneal fat to herniate between the gaps.

As a result of a weakness of the fascial wall, hernias of the linea alba protrude where ventral cutaneous blood vessels emerge. At the right of the midline they usually contain fat of the falciform ligament and at the left preperitoneal fat or a preperitoneal lipoma.

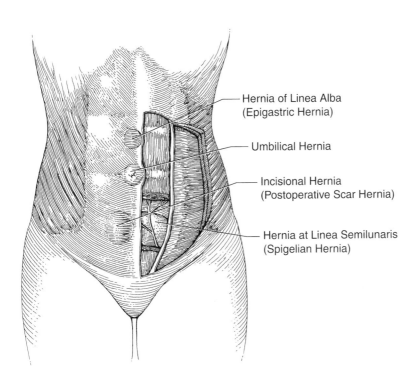

Hernia of Linea Alba
(Epigastric Hernia)

Umbilical Hernia

Incisional Hernia
(Postoperative Scar Hernia)

Hernia at Linea Semilunaris
(Spigelian Hernia)

FIGURE 42.19. Ventral hernia showing hernias of the linea alba, umbilical hernia, incisional hernia, and Spigelian hernia.

Symptoms or History

Most hernias of the linea alba are symptom-free and are discovered only on routine physical examination. Occasionally they may cause colicky pain, a "dragging" sensation in the epigastrium, nausea, dyspepsia, and even vomiting (1). The pain of epigastric hernia is exacerbated by exertion and relieved by rest in the supine position. The smaller hernias may become painful because of strangulation of the preperitoneal fat nipped by the sharp fascial edges of the opening. Omentum in the sac may strangulate, in which case the hernia may become swollen, painful, and tender, and the overlying skin may redden (4).

Physical Examination

The typical examination reveals a smooth, rounded, slightly tender lump usually above, but sometimes below, the umbilicus to the right or the left of the linea alba. In obese people this finding may be lost in the depths of subcutaneous fat.

Diagnostic Studies

History and physical examination should be sufficient to provide the diagnosis of hernias of the linea alba. Abdominal wall ultrasound or CT scan may assist if the diagnosis is in doubt.

Differential Diagnosis

History and physical findings are generally sufficient to make the diagnosis, but surgical findings definitively confirm a hernia of the linea alba. A differential diagnosis based on symptoms may include peptic ulcer, cholelithiasis, and hiatus hernia.

Surgical Treatment

Operative repair is effected by removal of fat, ligation of the neighboring vessels, and suture or imbrication of the fascial layers (1,21).

UMBILICAL HERNIAS

When the umbilical scar in infants does not close completely or if it fails and stretches in later years, the abdominal contents protrude through the opening and constitute an umbilical hernia (Fig. 42.19). Midline hernias abutting on the umbilicus superiorly and inferiorly are called paraumbilical hernias and are usually included in this group. The incidence of umbilical hernia at birth ranges from 10% to 30%. Premature infants have a 70% incidence of umbilical hernias. The majority of congenital umbilical hernias close spontaneously during the first few years of life. Some may continue to constrict and close through 10 years of age. The incidence of umbilical hernia in the adult is unknown. It is three times more common in women (4).

Etiology

When the cord is ligated at birth, the arteries and vein thrombose and the umbilical ring contracts and closes by scar tissue. If this process is halted before complete closure of the umbilical ring a congenital umbilical hernia results. The cause of umbilical hernia in adults is unknown, as is its possible relationship to the presence of an umbilical hernia in childhood. It occurs more frequently in middle-aged women and is often associated with fair to gross adiposity and with multiple pregnancies. Raised intraabdominal pressure acting on the weakened and stretched scar tissue of the umbilicus are probably important factors in causation (4).

Pathology

The defect in the abdominal wall is usually 2 to 5 cm in diameter but large openings are also common. The opening is often relatively narrow compared to the size of the sac, which may be large, long, and multi-loculated, protruding forward and downward even to overhang the pubis. The hernia also may spread in all directions, burrowing into the subcutaneous fat. These hernias usually contain only omentum, but transverse colon, loops of small bowel, and even stomach may enter as the hernia grows (4).

Symptoms and History

Most umbilical hernias are symptomatic. Patients with small umbilical hernias often complain of quite severe pain in the region, especially when coughing or straining. Larger hernias are uncomfortable because of their weight dragging on the abdomen. Skin over the hernia is stretched and becomes very thin and may be ulcerated by pressure necrosis. In obese women, the combination of sweaty moisture, warmth, and friction causes large areas of ulceration and weeping dermatitis.

Physical Examination

A protrusion in the umbilicus is usually easily recognized. The protrusion increases when the patient coughs or strains.

Diagnostic Studies

Although physical examination is sufficient for the diagnosis of umbilical hernia, ultrasound or CT scan can be utilized to further visualize the defect.

Differential Diagnosis

Patients with small umbilical hernias complain of quite severe pain in the region, especially when coughing or straining. Other sources of pain in this region can include paraumbilical hernias, hernias of the linea alba, esophagitis, gastroenteritis, gastritis, peptic ulcer disease, and cholelithiasis.

Surgical Treatment

For small umbilical hernias, the umbilical cicatrix need not be excised. A curved incision, concave cranially, is made around the inferior aspect of the hernia and the skin crease between the hernia and the abdominal wall. The end-flap with umbilical cicatrix is raised by incising the subcutaneous fat. After exposure, the neck of the sac is circumscribed along the edge of the hernial opening so that it may be lifted away from the abdominal wall. The bowel is returned to the peritoneal cavity and the omentum and the sac are excised. The opening is closed transversely with monofilament polypropylene sutures.

SPIGELIAN HERNIAS (HERNIAS AT THE SEMILUNAR LINE)

A Spigelian hernia is a spontaneous protrusion of preperitoneal fat, a peritoneal sac, or a sac containing a viscus through the Spigelian zone or fascia at any point along its length (Fig. 42.20). The zone is bounded medially by the

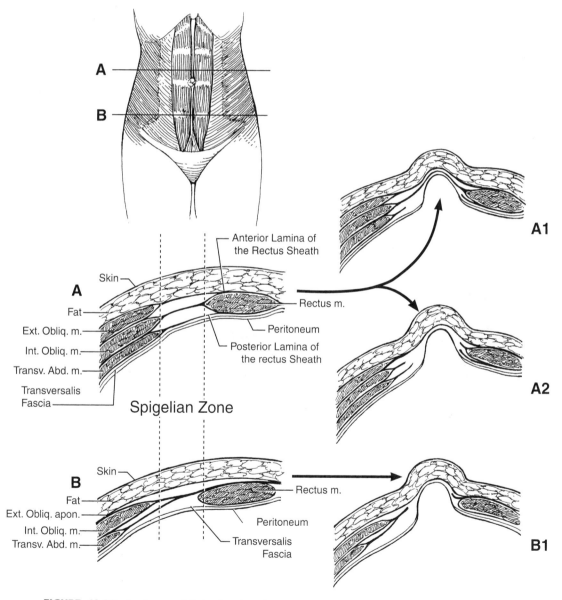

FIGURE 42.20. Anatomy of Spigelian hernia. **A:** Diagram of cross-sections of the anterior abdominal wall, above and below the semicircular line. The extent of the Spigelian fascia or zone is indicated. **B:** Herniation usually begins with preperitoneal fat passing through defects in the transversus abdominis (A1) and internal oblique (A2) aponeuroses. Notice that the aponeuroses of the external oblique muscle remains intact and with the skin forms the covering of the hernia. A1. Tranversus abdominis broken. A2. Transversus abdominis and internal oblique broken. B1. Transversus abdominis and internal oblique broken.

lateral margin of the anterior lamina of the rectus sheath and laterally by the muscular fibers of the internal oblique muscle.

The incidence of Spigelian hernia is not known, although almost 1,000 cases have been described in the literature. Mean age is 50 years and the ratio of women to men is 1.4:1. The hernia occurs on the right side more than the left at a ratio of 1.6:1. Most of the hernias are located below the level of the umbilicus. Patients have ranged in age from 6 days old to 94 years of age. Incarceration has occurred in 21% of reported cases. In most cases the hernia was located between the musculoaponeurotic layers of the anterior abdominal wall (4).

Etiology

The insertions of the transversus abdominis and internal oblique muscles into the rectus sheath are a series of microbundles of muscle and microtendons in a parallel arrangement, with gaps between them that are filled by fibrofatty septae. The usual protective gridiron arrangement of the abdominal wall musculature does not exist here; therefore, factors such as aging of the tissues, obesity, increased abdominal pressure owing to coughing, constipation, sudden lifting of a heavy weight and pregnancies may force the preperitoneal fat through the fibrofatty septae and thus cause a Spigelian hernia. Hernias occur particularly at the point where the semilunar and arcuate lines meet, between it is at this point that all the fibers of the transversus abdominis muscle pass in front of the rectus muscle. There is no posterior rectus sheath below this point. The rearrangement of the fibers at this point is believed to cause an area of functional weakness where the hernias can more easily occur. Almost all Spigelian hernias are interstitial (interparietal). As the hernia develops, preperitoneal fat pushes its way through the slit-like defects of the Spigelian fascia and the aponeuroses of the internal oblique muscle, dragging a protrusion of peritoneum with it (4).

Anatomy

The semilunar line of Spigel marks the lateral border of the rectus sheath and extends from the pubic tubercle to the tip of the costal cartilage of the ninth rib. The semicircular line (arcuate line, fold or line of Douglas) marks the caudal end of the posterior lamina of the aponeurotic rectus sheath, below the umbilicus and above the pubis. This Spigelian zone is composed of the aponeuroses of the external oblique, internal oblique, and transversus abdominis muscles between these muscles and the lateral border of the rectus muscle. The Spigelian fascia is formed by the approximation and fusion of the internal oblique and transversus abdominis aponeuroses. If the fusion of these aponeuroses is loose, a "zone" rather than a fascia is formed. The external oblique aponeurosis remains intact over a Spigelian hernia. The Spigelian fascia is widest between the umbilical plane above and the interspinous (ilium) plane below. The majority of Spigelian hernias occur here (Fig. 42.20). A fully developed Spigelian hernia is covered by peritoneum, transversalis fascia, aponeurosis of the external oblique muscle, and skin. In some cases, the hernia passes through the transversus abdominis aponeuroses only (22).

Spigelian hernias are usually less than 2 cm in diameter but occasionally larger hernias are seen. The small peritoneal sacs are usually empty, but the larger ones may contain omentum, small or large bowel, or even part of the stomach wall (4).

Symptoms and History

Patients complain of pain, a lump, or both at the site of herniation. The pain is sharp and constant or intermittent, or there is a dragging, uncomfortable feeling. With strangulation of any hernial contents, the pain is severe and constant and associated with symptoms and signs of complete or partial intestinal obstruction (4).

Physical Examination

When a mass is present along the semilunar line, especially in the region below the umbilicus, the diagnosis is easier. The mass may be reducible, after which the hernial defect in the fascia may be felt. There is usually tenderness present in the region of the defect. The palpable mass of the Spigelian hernia, whether it is subcutaneous or interstitial, usually persists during abdominal contraction (4).

Diagnostic Studies

Ultrasound diagnosis is accurate in 86% of cases of Spigelian hernia. A combination of ultrasound and tangential radiographs can improve the diagnosis. If the hernia is reduced and no mass is palpable, ultrasound scanning will show a break in the echogenic shadow of the semilunar line corresponding to the fascial defect. Whether or not the hernia is palpable, if it is not reduced, the hernial sac and contents will be demonstrated passing through the defect in the Spigelian fascia and lying in an interstitial or subcutaneous plane. Scanning by thin section CT can also confirm the presence of a Spigelian hernia (4).

Differential Diagnosis

When the hernia is incarcerated and irreducible it may be confused with lipoma, desmoid tumor, hematoma of the rectus sheath, or even an appendiceal abscess. When there is no incarceration it may be confused with a myofascial trigger point. Spigelian hernia may be an elusive diagnosis and may mimic other intraabdominal conditions.

Surgical Treatment

If the hernia is approached by laparotomy, a transverse or oblique skin incision is made over the lump or over the fascial defect. A subcutaneous hernia immediately reveals itself, but more commonly the hernia is interstitial and the external oblique muscles must be split in the line of its fibers to demonstrate the sac. The sac is freed from the surrounding tissues down to the neck, opened, and the contents reduced back into the peritoneal cavity. Some adhesions between the contents and the sac wall may have to be freed and after that the sac may be excised or inverted. The defect in the fascia of the transversus abdominis and the internal oblique muscle is closed with a continuous suture of monofilament polyamide or polypropylene. The defect in the external oblique muscle is similarly repaired (4).

Laparoscopic repair of Spigelian hernia was reported in 1992 and is similar to repair of an inguinal hernia (23). The peritoneum and transversalis fascia are incised, preperitoneal dissection is performed, and the hernia content reduced. Sufficient circumferential dissection of the hernia is performed to allow placement of a prosthetic mesh with adequate overlap of the hernia defect. The graft is secured with staples or tacks and the peritoneum closed with absorbable running suture (22,23).

INCISIONAL HERNIAS

An incisional hernia is the abnormal protrusion of peritoneum through a separation of the edges of a musculoaponeurotic wound. The wound may be fresh, recent, or even old. The peritoneal sac may or may not contain a viscus.

Incisional hernias are common after open surgical procedures and occur in 0.5% to 14% of abdominal operative procedures. Incarceration is present in about one-third of those cases that present for repair (19). Five percent of incisional hernias occur within 2 weeks, nearly 70% within the first year, and 97% within 5 years of surgery (4).

Incisional hernias also occur after laparoscopy with the risk of herniation through a 12-mm trochar site (3.1%) approximately 13-fold greater than that for a 10-mm trochar site (0.23%) (24). Laparoscopic incisional hernias can be prevented best by mass closure of the fascia and peritoneal layers under direct laparoscopic vision. With one reported technique, a conical needle guide is used to direct the needle and suture and maintain a pneumoperitoneum. A needle point suture passer introduces the suture through the muscle, fascial, and peritoneal layers and then retrieves it through the opposite side. The suture is then tied over the muscle layer but under the skin and subcutaneous fat. In this manner laparoscopic port sites from 5 to 20 mm can be completely closed and secured so that neither bowel nor omentum can enter the wound site (25).

Etiology

Infection, obesity, postoperative strain, inadequate suture material, and nerve injury are some of the etiologic factors of incisional hernias. Hernias after laparoscopy may occur because of the difficulty in closing fascia at the port sites, especially in obese patients (26).

Wound herniation is more common in elderly patients, in men, in the obese, in patients undergoing bowel surgery, and in patients with incisions greater than 18 cm. Postoperative complications, particularly chest infection, abdominal distention, and wound infection are significant factors associated with herniation. A higher proportion of patients whose wounds were closed with absorbable polyglycolic acid had incisional hernias compared to those whose closure technique was with nylon in a mass closure method. Forty-eight percent of patients with wound sepsis went on to develop an incisional hernia (4).

Although transverse incisions take more time and cause more bleeding than do vertical incisions, they result in slightly fewer incisional hernias. Postoperative herniation occurs more often in vertical incisions because of contractions of muscles pulling on the edges of the wound. Healing without incisional hernia or a disfiguring scar results with the absence of tension on sutures, with little or no pressure or dead space, and with good debridement, hemostasis, irrigation, and skin approximation (27).

Symptoms and History

Incisional hernias with a narrow neck and large sac are at risk of strangulation; those with a wide neck are a nuisance but not usually a danger. Patients may have no complaints or may complain of nausea, vomiting, or protrusion at an incision site. They may complain of intermittent pain or a dragging sensation. If they have herniated small bowel they may complain of distention and severe abdominal pain.

Physical Examination

When the patient is asked to lift the legs off the examination couch, to sit up, or to cough, a small bulge may be seen through the wound. A hernia may present with an apparent large unsightly bulge through the wound site without pain. Palpation of the wound site may allow reduction of the hernia and the fascial defect may become apparent.

Diagnostic Studies

The diagnosis of herniation into an incision site can be made by CT scan or ultrasonography. In patients with intermittent symptoms in whom a Richter's hernia is suspected, CT scan will very accurately demonstrate the loop of small bowel above the fascia. Omental herniations have also occurred, especially in laparoscopic procedures with their smaller incision sites. These can also be detected by CT scan (26).

Differential Diagnosis

The differential diagnosis of incisional hernia includes myofascial pain, adhesions causing intermittent small bowel obstruction, and bowel or pelvic conditions in the underlying region of the previous incision.

Surgical Treatment

It is not possible to describe the technique for every incisional hernia approached in an open technique. A good knowledge of the anatomy of the anterior and lateral abdominal wall is a must for a good repair (27).

Incisional hernias can be approached in a laparoscopic manner. Hernia reduction is accomplished and the abdominal wall defect is measured by palpating its external boundaries and viewing these maneuvers laparoscopically. The boundaries are marked with skin pencil on the anterior abdominal wall. These marks are used as a template to determine the dimensions and size of a prosthetic graft that will be used to cover and overlap the defect. If the hernia screen is not to be positioned in a preperitoneal position, it is advisable to employ materials with the least propensity for adhesion formation. Expanded polytetrafluoroethylene (ePTFE) creates a minimal amount of adhesion when placed as an onlay graft in the abdomen. Staples or tacks may be used to secure the graft in position. To anchor a large ePTFE graft it is recommended that fascial sutures be used to fix the graft permanently at four cardinal points (19).

INTERNAL SUPRAVESICAL HERNIAS

A supravesical hernia sac and its contents pass through the supravesical fossa of the anterior abdominal wall (Fig. 42.21). It may then protrude through the abdominal wall as a direct inguinal hernia (external supravesical hernia), or may remain within the abdomen, passing into spaces around the urinary bladder (internal supravesical hernia). Internal supravesical hernias are rare (28).

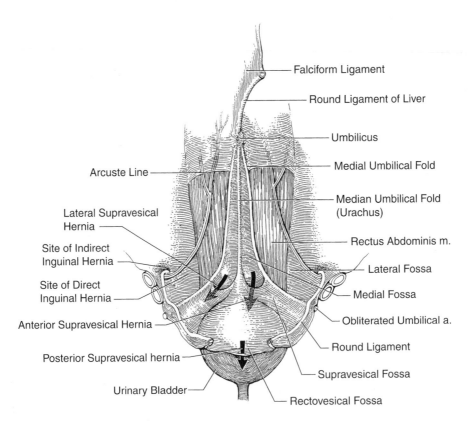

FIGURE 42.21. Surgical anatomy of internal supravesical hernia. The anterior portion of the abdominal wall viewed from the posterior surface. Internal supravesical hernias result from the loss of integrity of the transversus abdominis muscle and the transversalis fascia. Also, these hernias pass downward as direct inguinal or femoral hernias. About half of direct inguinal hernias originate in the supravesical fossa between the middle umbilical ligament and the medial umbilical fold.

Etiology

A supravesical hernia anterior to the bladder forms as a result of failure of the integrity of the transversus abdominis aponeurosis and the transversalis fascia, both of which insert on the pectineal ligament of Cooper.

Anatomy

The posterior surface of the anterior abdominal wall contains three shallow fossae on either side of the midline. The midline is marked by the median umbilical ligament, the adult remnant of the urachus of the fetus. The lateral fossa is bounded medially by the inferior epigastric artery and is the site of the internal inguinal ring through which may pass indirect inguinal hernias. The medial fossa lies between the inferior epigastric artery and the medial umbilical ligament (obliterated umbilical artery). It is the site of direct inguinal hernias. The supravesical fossa lies between the median umbilical ligament and the medial umbilical ligaments. It partially overlies Hesselbach's triangle. Although all internal supravesical hernias by definition start in the supravesical fossa, their subsequent course is variable. The anterior retropubic and lateral hernias pass into the retropubic space of Retzius between the pubis and the bladder. The invaginating type pushes in the anterior bladder wall and is very rare. The posterior hernias enter the space between the bladder and the uterus and are also rare (Fig. 42.22) (28).

Symptoms and History

Patients with supravesical hernias have complaints similar to those with direct and indirect inguinal hernias. In addition, those with anterior supravesical hernias may have complaints of urgency, decreased bladder capacity, and pain in the suprapubic area. Symptoms of urgency and pressure may occur in cases of posterior supravesical hernias.

Physical Examination

In 50% of internal supravesical hernias, the findings are consistent with direct inguinal hernias. Anterior supravesical hernias present with tenderness over the bladder and posterior supravesical hernias present as tenderness on vaginal examination between the uterus and the bladder.

Diagnostic Studies

Ultrasound and CT scan may confirm the existence of an internal supravesical hernia.

Differential Diagnosis

Direct inguinal hernias and conditions that create bladder discomfort and irritability must be distinguished from this hernia.

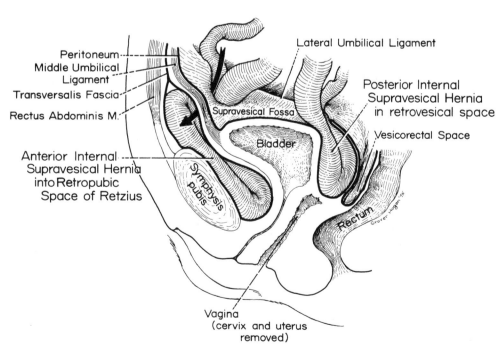

FIGURE 42.22. Surgical anatomy of internal vesical hernias.

Surgical Treatment

Surgical repair of the internal supravesical hernia requires reduction of the hernia and inversion of the hernia sac, followed by ligation and excision of the sac and closure of the peritoneal defect with prolene mesh (28).

BROAD LIGAMENT AND INTERNAL HERNIAS

Herniations through a defect in the broad ligament of the uterus are rare. The incidence of such internal hernias through the broad ligament is not known. A hernia through the broad ligament may occur as a result of tearing of the broad ligament at the time of a tubal ligation or other surgical procedure performed in the vicinity of the broad ligament.

Other internal hernias may be congenital or may develop as a result of adhesion formation or surgical intervention. Adhesions may create bands of tissue through which bowel or omentum can pass and then be trapped.

Anatomy

The broad ligament is a triangular mesentery of the uterus, tubes, and ovaries that extends from each lateral uterine side to the lateral pelvic wall. Medially, the broad ligament envelops the uterus. The upper free part is related to the tubes (mesosalpinx) and ovaries (mesovarium), and the lower fixed part is attached to the levator ani muscles through a special formation, the cardinal ligament. The broad ligament has thin vascular areas through which a viscus may pass (1,29).

Symptoms and History

Patients with internal hernias complain of symptoms of intermittent bowel obstruction with bloating, generalized abdominal pain, and discomfort. There may be a past history of a surgical procedure performed in the vicinity of the broad ligament.

Physical Examination

During times of partial obstruction patients will have signs similar to a Richter's hernia with abdominal tenderness and guarding, abdominal distention, decreased bowel sounds, and decreased evidence of peristalsis.

Diagnostic Studies

CT scan and upper gastrointestinal with small bowel follow-through studies are helpful. Definitive diagnosis can be made only at laparoscopy or laparotomy.

Differential Diagnosis

All causes of intermittent small bowel obstruction symptoms must be considered in the diagnosis.

Surgical Treatment

Surgical intervention can be by laparoscopy or laparotomy. At surgery the hernia is reduced carefully and the defect is closed with absorbable, nonreactive suture.

SPORTS HERNIAS

Sports hernia is a cause of chronic groin pain in athletic women. A sports hernia can be considered a syndrome of weakness of the posterior inguinal wall that causes chronic groin pain without a clinically recognizable hernia.

Chronic groin pain in sports women is a complex diagnostic and therapeutic problem. Groin injuries account for 5% of those attending a sports injury clinic but are responsible for much longer proportion of time lost from competition and work (30).

Etiology

Theories of etiology of the condition of chronic groin pain caused by stretching and tearing of the transversalis and conjoint tendon have been described. The first implicates a reduction in internal rotation of the hip joint. An inward twisting then produces a shearing force across the pubic symphysis from adductor pull. This leads to stress on the inguinal wall musculature perpendicular to the lie of the fascia and muscle fibers. The stretching of the transversalis and the tearing from the inguinal ligament account for the pain. The anatomical defects in the wall compound the problem. This theory accounts for both the common finding of the adductor muscle pain and the presence of osteitis pubis. The injury is most likely to be an overuse syndrome. An alternative theory is that it is simply a chronic stretching of the posterior inguinal wall owing to excess demands and aggravated by the anatomy of the region.

Pathology

There is a weakening of the transversalis fascia with separation from the conjoint tendon. The internal ring is dilated, often with the inferior epigastric vessels clearly visible. There may be a small knuckle of peritoneum seen at the internal ring (30).

Symptoms and History

The groin pain may be of insidious onset or a sudden tearing sensation. In the early stages of a sports hernia the pain gives rise to aching during the evening following competition or training. As the sports hernia progresses the discomfort begins to appear toward the end of training. As the problem progresses the pain comes on earlier and is more severe such that it is impossible to stride or turn quickly without a stab of pain. The pain typically is worse on one side but radiates laterally and across the midline, down the inside of the thigh into the adductor area, and can cause pain on sexual intercourse. Some patients complain of pain in the perineum and up into the abdomen (30). The pain disappears on prolonged rest, only to recur with the same intensity on resumed training.

Signs or Examination

The best time to perform the examination is after a return to exercise and a return of the pain. Adductor stretch is usually painful with tenderness around the belly and origin of the group. The patient will recognize that the tendon as palpated is not the source of the pain. The symphysis pubis is tender. The pain is worse over the pubic tubercle of the affected side. The area around the external inguinal ring is tender. When the mid-inguinal canal is palpated, the patient usually confirms that the pain is both worst there and is aggravated by coughing. A slight cough impulse can be felt in some cases (30).

Diagnostic Studies

Herniography and computed tomographic herniography can be performed. The objective is to provide an accurate diagnostic test, but also by injecting local anesthetic with the contrast to attempt to discover the source of pain. A positive study is the appearance of a distention of the peritoneal folds, indicating a general stretching out of normal fascial layers (30).

Differential Diagnosis

The differential diagnoses of groin pain include nerve entrapment, snapping hip syndrome with psoas bursitis, psoas tendon stretch, spondylolisthesis of the fifth lumbar vertebra (L5), early osteoarthritis, simple adductor strain or tendinitis, and osteitis pubis.

Surgical Treatment

Using a standard parainguinal approach the transversalis fascia and conjoint tendon are carefully assessed. The repair reconstitutes the internal ring and is performed with plication of transversalis fascia. The plication is then covered with nonabsorbable suture apposing the conjoint tendon to the inguinal ligament using a darn technique (30). Using this technique 80% of patients with sports hernia return to full activity. A distention of the posterior inguinal canal wall musculature, an early type of direct hernia, is a source of chronic groin pain and can be surgically corrected by the technique described. Other techniques of standard hernia repair can also achieve success in the treatment of sports hernia.

PELVIC FLOOR SUPPORT DEFECTS

Pelvic support defects (urethrocele, cystocele, uterine prolapse, enterocele, and rectocele) have been thoroughly discussed in Chapter 20. However, for purposes of completeness the basic concept of pelvic support defects will be summarized here.

All support defects involve some break in the continuity of support from one or more layers of the pelvic floor. In the uppermost layer (connective tissue), a break can contribute to the occurrence of a urethrocele, cystocele, uterine prolapse, or enterocele. These hernias can occur with intact levator ani muscles and a good urogenital diaphragm. In the bottom layer (urogenital diaphragm and perineum), an isolated break can result in a rectocele and a deformed perineum. Again, the other two layers may remain intact. In the middle layer (levator ani and coccygeus muscles) alone, a weakness or tear does not result in a specific hernia or prolapse. However, because these muscles support the layer above, any major weakness or tear predisposes to the development of a urethrocele, cystocele, uterine prolapse, or enterocele (29).

Urethrocele, cystocele, uterine prolapse, enterocele, and rectocele all occur as a result of some weakness of the tissue supporting the floor of the female pelvis. When a loss of the integrity of the supporting tissue occurs, one or more extraperitoneal viscera are pushed outward; the defect is then named according to the viscus so displaced (29). All of the visceral structures rest on or are contained within the floor of the abdominal pelvic cavity. They will not fall out; they are always pushed out by pressure from within.

KEY POINTS

Differential Diagnosis

- Hernias may be a more common cause of CPP than generally recognized and should generally considered in the differential diagnosis when pain is relatively localized and consistent in location.
- A history of intermittent bowel obstruction should suggest the possibility of a hernia as a cause of CPP.
- In patients with nausea and vomiting suggesting small bowel obstruction, other causes such as gastritis, hiatus hernia, esophagitis, gastroenteritis, peptic ulcer disease, and cholelithiasis must be ruled out.

- The diagnosis of the fascial defect may be difficult if the viscus has not yet passed through.
- When hernias present as a bulge or mass, depending on their locations, one must consider in the differential lipoma, gluteal aneurysm, abscess, adenopathy, psoas abscess, fibroma, varicosities of the saphenous vein, hydrocele of the femoral sac, hematoma of the rectus sheath, and polyps.
- Other neuromuscular conditions such as nerve entrapment, snapping hip syndrome with psoas bursitis, psoas tendon stretch, spondylolisthesis of the fifth lumbar vertebra (L5), early osteoarthritis, simple adductor strain or tendinitis, osteitis pubis, and myofascial trigger points can be difficult to differentiate from a hernia prior to a significant bulge or defect.

Most Important Questions to Ask

- Does your pain radiate to the buttocks or posterior thigh?
- Is your pain intermittent?
- Are you experiencing pain in the inner aspect of the thigh?
- Have you noticed a soft mass in the pelvic area that increases with cough but is easily reduced?
- Did the pain come on suddenly?
- Does the pain recur with exercise or lifting?
- Do you feel a small lump in the groin area that enlarges with stress, with straining?
- Is the pain made worse by exertion and relieved by rest in the supine position?
- Is the pain increased with coughing and straining?
- Do you experience bladder irritation and experience a protrusion over the bladder?
- Have you had previous surgery in the area of the tubes or uterus or ovary or any previous abdominal surgery?
- Did the pain begin after athletic training and has it now become so severe that striding or turning quickly is impossible without a stab of pain?

Most Important Physical Examination Findings

- A reducible mass is most consistent with a hernia.
- A hernia ring is often tender.
- A palpable defect identifiable with the patient in the standing position
- A protruding lump with cough

Most Important Diagnostic Studies

- Computerized tomography
- Herniogram
- Ultrasound
- Laparoscopy

- Upper gastrointestinal series with small bowel follow-through

Treatments

- Hernias are most definitively treated by surgical repair with permanent suture or mesh.
- Many hernias can be repaired either laparoscopically or by laparotomy.

REFERENCES

1. Netter FH, Iason AH, Pansky B. Hernias. In: Oppenheimer E, ed. *The Ciba collection of medical illustrations.* Summit, New Jersey CIBA: 1962:204–218.
2. Cali RL, Pitsch RM, Blatchford GJ, et al. Rare pelvic floor hernias: report of a case and review of the literature. *Dis Colon Rectum* 1991;25:604–612.
3. Miklos JR, O'Reilly MJ, Saye WB. Sciatic hernia as a cause of chronic pelvic pain in women. *Obstet Gynecol* 1998;91:998–1001.
4. Abrahamson J. Hernias. In: Zinner MJ, Schwartz SI, Ellis H, eds. *Maingot's abdominal operations.* Stanford, CT: Appleton & Lange, 1997:479–580.
5. Zimmerman LM, Anson DJ. *Anatomy and surgery of hernia.* Baltimore: Williams & Wilkins, 1953:352.
6. Skandalakis JE. Sciatic hernia. In: Skandalakis JE, Gray SW, Mansberger AR, et al, eds. *Hernia surgical anatomy and technique.* New York: McGraw-Hill, 1989:168–173.
7. Beck WC, Baurys W, Brochu J, et al. Herniation of the ureter into the sciatic foramen ("curlicue ureter"). *JAMA* 1952;149:441–442.
8. Spring DB, Vandeman F, Watson RA. Computed tomographic demonstration of ureterosciatic hernia. *AJR* 1983;141:579–580.
9. Skandalakis JE. Obturator hernia. In: Skandalakis JE, Gray SW, Mansberger AR, et al, eds. *Hernia surgical anatomy and technique.* New York: McGraw Hill, 1989:174–184.
10. Bjork KJ, Mucha P, Cahill DR. Obturator hernia. *Surg Gynecol Obstet* 1988;167:217–222.
11. Ijiri R, Kanamaru H, Yokoyama H, et al. Obturator hernia: the usefulness of computed tomography in diagnosis. *Surgery* 1996;119:137–140.
12. Singer R, Leary PM, Hofmuyr N. Obturator hernia. *So Afr Med J* 1955;29:73–75.
13. Lo CY, Lorentz TG, Lau PWK. Obturator hernia presenting as small bowel obstruction. *Am J Surg* 1994;167:396–398.
14. Bergstein JM, Condon RE. Obturator hernia: current diagnosis and treatment. *Surgery* 1996;119:133–136.
15. Tucker JG, Wilson RA, Ramshaw BJ, et al. Laparoscopic herniorrhaphy: technical concerns in prevention of complications and early recurrence. *Am Surg* 1995;61:36–39.
16. Skandalakis JE. Perineal hernia. In: Skandalakis JE, Gray SW, Mansberger AR, et al, eds. *Hernia surgical anatomy and technique.* New York: McGraw-Hill, 1989:185–206.
17. Skandalakis JE. Inguinal hernia. In: Skandalakis JE, Gray SW, Mansberger AR, et al, eds. *Hernia surgical anatomy and technique.* New York: McGraw-Hill, 1989:77–146.
18. Skandalakis JE. Femoral hernia. In: Skandalakis JE, Gray SW, Mansberger AR, et al, eds. *Hernia surgical anatomy and technique.* New York: McGraw-Hill, 1989:1–384.
19. Kavic MS. *Laparoscopic hernia repair.* The Netherlands: Harwood Academic Publishers, 1997, 117.
20. Daoud I. General surgical aspects. In: Steege JF, Metzger DA,

Levy BS, eds. *Chronic pelvic pain: an integrated approach.* Philadelphia: W.B. Saunders 1998, 364.

21. Skandalakis JE. Hernias of the anterior abdominal wall. In: Skandalakis JE, Gray SW, Mansberger AR, et al, eds. *Hernia surgical anatomy and technique.* New York: McGraw-Hill, 1989:1–384.

22. Skandalakis JE. Spigelian hernia. In: Skandalakis JE, Gray SW, Mansberger AR, et al, eds. *Hernia surgical anatomy and technique.* New York: McGraw-Hill, 1989:1–384.

23. Carter JE, Mizes C. Laparoscopic diagnosis and repair of Spigelian hernia: report of technique. *Am J Obstet Gynecol* 1992;166:77–78.

24. Kadar N, Reich H, Liu CY, et al. Incisional hernias after major laparoscopic gynecologic procedures. *Am J Obstet Gynecol* 1993; 168:1493–1495.

25. Carter JE. A new technique of fascial closure for laparoscopic incisions. *J Laparoscop Endoscop Surg* 1994;4:143–148.

26. Boike GM, Miller CE, Spirtos NM, et al. Incisional bowel herniations after operative laparoscopy: a series of 19 cases and review of the literature. *Am J Obstet Gynecol* 1995;172: 1726–1733.

27. Skandalakis JE. Internal supravesical hernias. In: Skandalakis JE, Gray SW, Mansberger AR, et al, eds. *Hernia surgical anatomy and technique.* New York: McGraw-Hill, 1989:1–384.

28. Skandalakis JE. Incisional hernia. In: Skandalakis JE, Gray SW, Mansberger AR, et al, eds. *Hernia surgical anatomy and technique.* New York: McGraw-Hill, 1989:1–384.

29. Richardson AC. Pelvic hernias. In: Skandalakis JE, Gray SW, Mansberger AR, et al, eds. *Hernia surgical anatomy and technique.* New York: McGraw-Hill, 1989:1–384.

30. Hackney RG. The sports hernia: a cause of chronic groin pain. *Vr J Sp Med* 1993;27:58–62.

43

NEOPLASIA OF THE SPINAL CORD OR SACRAL NERVES

C. PAUL PERRY

KEY TERMS AND DEFINITIONS

Cauda equina: The collection of spinal roots that descend from the end of the spinal cord and occupy the vertebral canal below the level of L5.

Conus medullaris: The cone-shaped end of the spinal cord located at the level of the upper lumbar vertebrae.

Intramedullary: Originating from within the spinal cord.

Leptomeningitis: Inflammation of the pia (innermost covering) and arachnoid (middle covering just under the dura) of the spinal cord.

Nervi vasorum: Sympathetic afferent innervation of the blood vessels responsible for some of the pain produced by spinal cord neoplasia.

Paresthesia: An abnormal sensory perception, such as burning or prickling.

Radicular pain: Pain produced by inflammation or compression of a spinal nerve root at that portion of the root that lies between the spinal cord and the intervertebral canal.

Syringomyelia: A progressive cavitation of the spinal cord, which sometimes follows traumatic injury.

INTRODUCTION

Tumors involving the spinal cord or cauda equina are a rare cause of chronic pelvic pain. However, if diagnosis is missed or delayed, the results may be permanent and devastating. Neoplasms may be divided into primary or metastatic. Compression, distortion, or invasion of the lumbosacral nerves may elicit symptoms mistakenly attributed to primary visceral pathology. Symptoms may initially be unusual and subtle. Dysfunction of pelvic visceral and somatic nerves could be expected with T2-L2 or S2-4 involvement.

PATHOLOGY

Reports of primary spinal cord tumors include neurocytomas, astrocytomas, oligodendrogliomas, ependymomas, Schwannomas, neurofibromas, and melanocytomas (1–4). Metastatic tumors to the spinal cord, producing symptoms of spinal nerve injury, commonly include pulmonary, breast, lymphoma, colorectal, melanoma, or renal cell (5). Osteosclerotic myeloma, sacrococcygeal germ cell tumors, and paragangliomas can produce less common metastatic lesions (6–8). Sacral lesions may also be produced by an upper central nervous system (CNS) lesion that gravitates down to the cord and cauda equina (9).

Spinal cord neoplasia can be extradural, intradural, or intramedullary. Symptoms of an extradural tumor evolve over days or weeks. Once these symptoms are well established, even laminectomy may fail to restore function. Lung and breast cancers are the most frequent causes of extradural tumors, followed by lymphomas.

Intradural (extramedullary) tumors develop more chronically over months to years. They often produce radicular pain.

Intramedullary tumors also evolve over months to years. Regional or radicular pain is usually absent. Because symptoms result from intrinsic compression, sensory or motor dysfunction may start far below the level of cord involvement. This is explained by the lamination of sensory and motor fibers in the tract itself, the largest and longest fibers being affected first (10).

SYMPTOMS

Symptoms of spinal cord neoplasia may be divided into five categories: (a) pain, (b) motor abnormalities, (c) sensory abnormalities, (d) reflex and muscle tone abnormalities, and (e) urinary bladder dysfunction (11).

Pain

Three types of pain are seen in patients with spinal cord disease: local, radicular, and diffuse. Local pain is the most common type of pain. A ring of bone and ligaments, all of which are pain sensitive (except the ligamentum flavum), surrounds the cord. Pain may be sensed in the back, hips, or lower extremities. Pain directly over the lesion may also be mediated by the nervi vasorum of the blood vessels or can arise from involvement of the intrinsic pain pathways of the spinal cord. Pain may evolve over days, months, and years.

Radicular pain is rarely seen without local pain. This pain usually will not extend into the toes like paresthesias commonly do.

Diffuse aching or burning pain is occasionally seen in patients with spinal cord disease. The pain may occur in the buttocks, feet, and legs. This type of pain is often associated with significant impairment of pain perception in the involved areas.

Motor Abnormalities

Some motor abnormality is present in practically all disorders of the spinal cord. Weakness reflects cessation of function of more than 50% of descending motor pathways or more than 50% of anterior horn cells. Progressive weakness evolving over hours or days is seen in extradural tumors. With lesions of the cauda equina, atrophy and fasciculations are sometimes not as evident as with cervical lesions. This is probably owing to concealment of muscle by subcutaneous fat in the legs. Also, intrinsic foot muscle weakness causes less functional impairment than intrinsic hand muscle weakness. Therefore, the patient may not notice this weakness until it is very advanced.

Sensory Abnormalities

Paresthesias are "positive" sensory manifestations produced by malfunctioning, but not destroyed nerves. The patient may describe tingling, buzzing, or a feeling of "pins and needles." Sensations of cold or warmth or itch are less common and may indicate involvement of the dorsal horn or spinothalamic tract axons that convey pain and temperature. Paresthesias produced by lesions of the cauda equina are perceived in the lower extremities and feet.

"Negative" symptomatology such as numbness indicates a conscious lack of sensation in some part of the body. The patient may describe this as a "deadness" sensation. These symptoms are probably indicative of a dorsal column lesion. Loss of vibratory and pinprick sensation may be noted.

Reflex and Muscle Tone Abnormalities

Tendon reflexes are depressed bilaterally in the lower extremities in patients with compressive lesions of the cauda equina. Unilateral loss of a single tendon jerk may be a sign of spinal root or cord disease. Reflex hyperactivity is eventually seen in almost all spinal cord diseases. Loss of the anal reflex (S2-4) is indicative of sacral root involvement.

Urinary Bladder Dysfunction

Bladder dysfunction is an early sign of involvement of the conus medullaris or the sacral roots of the cauda equina at the junction of the lumbar and sacral spine. The most reliable historical sign is urinary incontinence. Decreased compliance and hyperactive detrusor stretch reflexes cause symptoms of urgency, frequency, and incontinence. S3 is the predominant innervation of the pelvic floor and the main autonomic (parasympathetic) supply of the detrusor muscle. Only a cystometrogram or urodynamics test can diagnose early disturbances of micturition. Because this is an important clue of initial spinal cord injury by neoplastic lesions, it should be done at first suspicion (12).

PHYSICAL EXAMINATION

The dermatomal distribution of the patient's pain, tenderness, and paresthesias should be documented. Deep tendon reflexes of the lower extremities and their symmetry is noted. Anal and bulbocavernosus reflexes may be abnormal. Pinprick and vibratory sensation of the perineum and lower extremities should be tested.

DIAGNOSTIC STUDIES

Cystometrogram or urodynamics are used as a general screen. If there is normal bladder function and reflexes, sacral nerve compromise is unlikely. Magnetic resonance imaging (MRI) is the most sensitive diagnostic study available to diagnose spinal cord neoplasia. It may be augmented by CT scan, myelogram, or plain radiography.

DIAGNOSIS

After ruling out visceral etiologies for the chronic pelvic pain (CPP), other rare causes of pain such as spinal cord lesions may be considered. Pathology producing insults to the cord or cauda equina (excluding neoplasms) include: (a) inflammatory, (b) trauma, (c) bony abnormalities, and (d) nontraumatic myelopathies.

Inflammatory Diseases of the Spinal Cord

Viral diseases affecting the spinal cord are caused by infection with neurotropic viruses (e.g., rabies, acute anterior poliomyelitis, herpes zoster, and herpes B encephalomyelitis). The bacterial infections of the subarachnoid space around the brain and spinal cord are well known. Extradural abscess is seen from neighboring sources of infection, such as osteomyelitis of the spine, penetrating wounds, or metastatic spread from a distant infection. *Staphylococcus aureus*, *Diplococcus pneumoniae*, and *Pseudomonas pyocyanea* are the most common organisms cultured from extradural abscesses. Tuberculosis may produce ischemia of the cord by inflammatory arteritis or extrinsic pressure from osteitis. Fungal infections may produce leptomeningitis or compression by an inflammatory mass. The most common fungal infections include *Cryptococcus hominis, Histoplasma capsulatum, Coccidioides immitis,* and *Aspergillus fumigatus.* These infections are usually only seen in the immunocompromised patients. Parasitic infections by cysticercosis, hydatid disease, and schistosomiasis have been reported (13).

Trauma

Traumatic injury to the spinal cord may produce progressive cavitation and symptoms long after the acute changes have stabilized. This is called posttraumatic syringomyelia. The central part of the cord is the most affected and progressively higher levels of the cord may become involved (13).

Bony Abnormalities

Osteitis deformans (Paget's disease), osteoarthritis, intervertebral disc protrusion, and vertebral canal stenosis may cause lumbosacral nerve injury with chronic pain mistaken for visceral origin (Chapter 39).

Nontraumatic Myelopathies

Nontraumatic injuries of the spinal cord include autoimmune diseases such as multiple sclerosis and transverse myelitis. Arteriovenous malformations may compress the sacral nerves and produce pain in the back, lower abdomen, hips, and lower extremities. Vascular occlusion by atheromatous plaques or emboli may lead to spinal cord lesions difficult to differentiate clinically from neoplastic symptoms (13).

TREATMENT

Neoplasia of the spinal cord and sacral nerves is rare and difficult to diagnose. In one study of malignant spinal cord compression, delay in diagnosis was the most common reason for poor functional outcome (15). Decompression can best be accomplished by combining radiotherapy for shrinkage of the tumor with steroid therapy to reduce swelling and inflammation. Surgical resection is reserved for benign tumors or those malignant neoplasms that offer the best hope of cure with the least deficit after extirpation.

KEY POINTS

Differential Diagnosis

- Inflammatory lesions: viral, bacterial, fungal, and parasitic

- Posttraumatic syringomyelia
- Bony abnormalities: osteitis deformans, osteoarthritis, intervertebral disc protrusion, and vertebral canal stenosis
- Nontraumatic myelopathies: multiple sclerosis and transverse myelitis

Most Important Questions to Ask

- Is there a back pain component to the CPP?
- Is the pain radicular or diffuse?
- What quality is the pain: burning, prickling, and so on?
- Is there any history of a primary malignancy?
- Any immunosuppressive medications taken?
- Any muscle weakness?
- Any difficulty with walking?
- Any urinary incontinence?
- Any numbness?

Most Important Physical Examination Findings

- Presence, absence, or asymmetry of deep tendon reflexes of lower extremities
- Vibratory sensation deficits
- Pinprick sensation deficits
- Temperature sensation deficits
- Absent anal or bulbocavernosus reflex

Most Important Diagnostic Studies

- Cystometrogram or urodynamics
- Magnetic resonance imaging
- CT scan
- Plain radiograph of lumbosacral area

Treatments

- Radiotherapy
- Steroid administration
- Surgical extirpation

REFERENCES

1. Stapleton SR, David KM, Harkness WF, et al. Central neurocytoma of the cervical spinal cord (letter). *J Neurol Neurosurg Psychiatry* 1997;63:11.
2. Breningstall GN, Nagib MG. Chronic compulsive foot rubbing. *Clin Pediatr* 1996;35:411–413.
3. McLaughlin MP, Marcus RB, Buati JM, et al. Ependymoma: results, prognostic factors and treatment recommendations. *Int J Radiat Oncol Biol Phys* 1998;40:845–850.
4. Glick R, Baker C, Husain S, et al. Primary melanocytomas of the sinal cord: a report of seven cases. *Clin Neuropathol* 1997;16:127–132.
5. Schiff D, O'Neill BP. Intramedullary spinal cord metastases:

clinical features and treatment outcome. *Neurology* 1996;47:
906–912.

6. Benito-Leon J, Lopez-Rios F, Rodriguez-Martin FJ, et al. Rapidly
deteriorating polyneuropathy associated with osteosclerotic
myeloma responsive to intravenous immunoglobulin and radiotherapy. *J Neurol Sci* 1998;158:113–117.

7. Smithers BM, Theile DE, Dickinson IC, et al. Malignant sacrococcygeal germ cell tumour in an adult. *Aust NZ J Surg* 1996;66:
185–189.

8. Paleologos TS, Gouliamos AD, Kourousis DD, et al. Paragan-
glioma of the cauda equina: a case presenting features of increased
intracranial pressure. *J Spinal Disord* 1998;11:362–325.

9. Lee TT, Landy HJ. Spinal metastases of malignant intracranial
meningioma. *Surg Neurol* 1998;50:437–441.

10. Adams RD, Salam-Adams M. Chronic nontraumatic diseases of
the spinal cord. *Neurol Clin* 1991;9:605–623.

11. Woolsey RM, Young RR. The clinical diagnosis of disorders of
the spinal cord. *Neurol Clin* 1991;9:573–583.

12. Watanabe T, Vaccaro AR, Kumon H, et al. High incidence of
occult neurogenic bladder dysfunction in neurologically intact
patients with thoracolumbar spinal injuries. *J Urol* 1998;159:
965–968.

13. Hughes JT. Neuropathology of the spinal cord. *Neurol Clin*
1991;9:551–571.

14. Dawson DM, Potts F. Acute nontraumatic myelopathies. *Neurol
Clin* 1991;9:585–603.

15. Husband DJ. Malignant spinal cord compression: prospective
study of delays in referral and treatment. *BMJ* 1998;317:18–21.

44

MONONEUROPATHY AND NERVE ENTRAPMENT

AHMED M. EL-MINAWI
FRED M. HOWARD

KEY TERMS AND DEFINITIONS

Allodynia: Pain owing to a stimulus that does not normally provoke pain.

Dysesthesia: An unpleasant abnormal sensation, whether spontaneous or evoked.

Hyperalgesia: An increased response to a stimulus that is normally painful.

Hyperesthesia: Increased sensitivity to stimulation, excluding the special senses.

Hyperpathia: A painful syndrome characterized by an abnormally painful reaction to a stimulus, especially a repetitive stimulus, as well as an increased threshold.

Hypoalgesia: Diminished pain in response to a normally painful stimulus.

Hypoesthesia: Decreased sensitivity to stimulation, excluding the special senses.

Mononeuropathy: A peripheral neural disease that arises from focal involvement of a single nerve trunk.

Neuralgia: Pain in the distribution of a nerve or nerves.

Neuropathy: A disturbance of function or pathological change in a nerve.

Nerve entrapment: The most common variant of mononeuropathies seen in chronic abdominopelvic pain; specific form of pressure neuropathy caused by naturally occurring angulation or compression by adjacent tissues or iatrogenically secondary to surgical procedures.

Paresthesia: An abnormal sensation, whether spontaneous or evoked, that is not unpleasant.

INTRODUCTION

The causes of chronic abdominopelvic pain do not necessarily lie within the viscera but can also arise from the skin, subcutaneous tissues, muscles, bone, and nerves. Because of referred pain, such parietal pain may be misinterpreted by the patient and physician as having its origin in visceral disease (1). This occurs not uncommonly with neuropathies and nerve entrapment, both of which are problems that may contribute to chronic abdominopelvic pain in some women.

A mononeuropathy is a peripheral neural disease that arises from focal involvement of a single nerve trunk. Multiple factors may be important in its production, such as direct trauma, compression, or stretch and entrapment. Manifestations of mononeuropathies may (a) be pansensory, (b) reflect mainly large afferent fiber involvement with deficits of vibratory and proprioceptive sense, areflexia, and sensory ataxia with or without tingling dysesthesias, or (c) reflect mainly small afferent fiber involvement with numbness and cutaneous hypesthesia to pinprick and temperature stimuli, often with painful burning dysesthesias (2).

Nerve entrapment neuropathies are the most common variant of mononeuropathies seen in chronic abdominopelvic pain. Entrapment neuropathies are regarded as specific forms of pressure neuropathy. The peripheral nerves may be injured by mechanical pressure or ischemia at the points where they pass through anatomic canals or beneath tight ligamentous or fascial bands. These causes may either be naturally occurring, such as angulation or compression by adjacent tissues, or iatrogenic secondary to surgical procedures (3).

ANATOMY

To properly understand the etiology and pathophysiology of peripheral nerve mononeuropathies requires some knowledge of the anatomy of the nerves that are most commonly afflicted in women with chronic abdominopelvic pain. The lower abdomen and the pelvis are supplied by the lumbar plexus, the sacral plexus, and the pelvic autonomic plexus.

The Lumbar Plexus

The lumbar plexus is positioned to the side of the first four lumbar vertebrae. It is formed by the ventral rami of spinal nerves L1-L4 and some fibers from T12. The nerves that arise from the lumbar plexus innervate structures of the lower abdomen, pelvis, and medial portions of the lower extremity (Table 44.1) (4). Any of the branches of the plexus may be involved in entrapments, but the most common are the iliohypogastric and ilioinguinal (5).

The *iliohypogastric nerve* is the uppermost branch of the plexus and is larger than the ilioinguinal. The majority of its fibers are derived from L1 with the remainder from T12 and occasionally T11. It emerges from the upper lateral margin of the psoas major to run parallel to the twelfth thoracic nerve and anterior to the quadratus lumborum. At the crest of the ilium it pierces the transversalis muscle to run between it and the internal oblique muscle. It then divides into its two terminal branches, the iliac and the hypogastric nerves, which supply the hypogastric and suprapubic skin. It also gives off some muscular branches along its course, supplying the transversalis as well as the internal and external obliques (4,6).

The *ilioinguinal nerve* is the second branch of the lumbar plexus and is smaller than the iliohypogastric. Its fibers arise mainly from L1 but at times it receives some fibers from T12. It occasionally forms a common trunk of considerable length with the iliohypogastric. The nerve is parallel to the iliohypogastric at first and follows a similar course to reach the intermuscular cleft between the internal oblique and transversalis muscles. In its final course it enters the inguinal canal, from which it emerges either through the external abdominal ring or through the external pillar of the ring. It also gives off muscular branches along its course (4,6).

The *genitofemoral nerve* originates from two roots, the first of which arises from the loop between L1 and L2 and contains fibers from both, whereas the other arises directly from L2. It consists mainly of sensory fibers with a few muscular fibers. It runs within the fascial lining of the abdominal cavity by piercing the psoas muscle and fascia near their medial border opposite the third or fourth lumbar vertebra. It then descends under the peritoneum on the surface of the psoas major and crosses obliquely behind the ureter. At a variable distance from the inguinal ligament it divides into its terminal genital and femoral branches. The genital branch usually contains fibers from L1. It passes downward on the inner margin of the psoas major, crosses the external iliac artery and proceeds to the posterior wall of the inguinal canal, which it enters by piercing the transversalis fascia. It traverses the inguinal canal with the round ligament to reach the labia majora. The femoral branch is mostly composed of fibers from L2. It passes downward along the anterior surface of the psoas major, lateral to the genital branch and enters the thigh by passing beneath the inguinal ligament. This branch is the cutaneous nerve to the femoral triangle. The genitofemoral nerve can have considerable variation. For example, the two parts may arise as separate offshoots from the lumbar plexus or it can be partially absent, with the missing fibers integrated into the ilioinguinal nerve (4,6).

The *lateral femoral cutaneous nerve* arises from the posterior aspect of the lumbar plexus receiving fibers from L2 and, to a lesser extent, L3. It passes downward and outward beneath the lateral margin of the psoas major and over the iliacus muscle, through the iliac fossa, lying under the iliac fascia. It passes under the inguinal ligament in a fibrous tunnel after crossing the deep circumflex iliac artery 1 cm medial to the anterior superior iliac spine. It may course over or under the tendinous origin of the sartorius muscle. It descends into the thigh deep to the fascia lata and divides into anterior and posterior terminal branches. Anatomical variations can occur.

The *femoral nerve* is the largest branch of the lumbar plexus, arising from L1, L2, L3, and L4. After passing obliquely downward and outward it runs posterior to the psoas major and then emerges from the middle of the lateral margin of that muscle. It continues between the outer edge of the psoas and the medial edge of the iliacus, covered by the iliac fascia as far as the inguinal ligament. It passes underneath the inguinal ligament to enter the anterior portion of the thigh. During its course in the abdomen it is separated from the femoral vessels by the psoas major, but it gradually approaches them until it lies in apposition to the femoral sheath in the femoral triangle. Near the inguinal ligament the femoral nerve gives off several branches, including muscular branches and two main divisions. The anterior or superficial division is mainly cutaneous in distribution, whereas the deep division is mainly motor.

The *obturator nerve* arises in most instances from L2, L3, and L4, but occasionally L2 is missing entirely or it may receive contributions from L1 or L5. The roots unite to form the nerve within the psoas major, then it passes downward to emerge from the medial margin of the psoas opposite the

TABLE 44.1. THE NERVES OF THE LUMBAR PLEXUS AND THEIR AREAS OF INNERVATION

Nerve	Spinal Component	Sensory Innervation
Iliohypogastric	T12-L1	Lower abdomen, suprapubic area
Ilioinguinal	L1	Lower abdomen, pubic area, labium majus, upper median thigh
Genitofemoral	L1 and L2	Labium majus, inguinal area, upper median thigh
Lateral femoral cutaneous	L2 and L3	Anterolateral and posterior thigh
Femoral	L2–L4	Anterior thigh, medial aspect of leg
Obturator	L2–L4	Medial aspect of thigh
Saphenous	L3–L4	Medial aspect of leg

pelvic brim. It then passes along the anterolateral wall of the pelvis above the obturator vessels until it leaves the pelvis via the obturator canal. While still in the obturator foramen or shortly thereafter, it divides into its terminal anterior and posterior branches, and a branch to the obturator externus.

The Sacral Plexus

The sacral plexus is formed by a portion of L4, all of L5, and considerable portions of S1 through S4. The plexus lies largely on the pyriformis muscle and is covered by fascia of the pelvic wall. The lumbar contributions together form the lumbosacral cord, which emerges from the medial margin of the psoas major, passes downward over the brim of the pelvis, and joins the plexus. The first and second sacral nerves pass out of their foramina, laterally and anterior to the pyriformis, and divide into anterior and posterior branches. The third sacral nerve likewise divides but into upper and lower branches, with the former becoming part of the sacral plexus and the latter joining the pudendal plexus (Table 44.2).

The *pudendal nerve* arises from the second, third, and fourth sacral nerves. The main source is from S3 and there may also be contributions from S1. It passes between the pyriformis and cocygeus to leave the pelvis via the greater sciatic foramen, underneath the great sciatic nerve. It then passes forward accompanying the internal pudendal artery and the nerve to the obturator internus, crossing the base of the lesser sacrosciatic ligament till it reaches the spine of the ischium. It passes through lesser sacrosciatic foramen internal to the pudendal artery and enters the ischiorectal fossa, giving off the inferior hemorrhoidal nerve. The main nerve trunk then passes forward through a fascial tunnel (Alcock's canal) in the obturator fascia on the outer wall of the ischiorectal fossa. Within the canal it gives rise to one or more inferior rectal nerves. On reaching the anterior segment of the fossa, near the base of the triangular ligament, it divides into its terminal branches, the perineal nerve and the dorsal nerve of the clitoris (4,6). The former innervates the muscles of the superficial space of the urogenital triangle as well as the muscles of the deep perineal compartment.

The *sciatic nerve* is formed by fibers from the anterior rami of L4, L5, S1, S2, and S3. It is the largest nerve in the

TABLE 44.2. THE BRANCHES OF THE SACRAL PLEXUS

Collateral branches
Muscular
Superior gluteal
Inferior gluteal
Small sciatic nerve
Perforating cutaneous
Terminal branches
Pudendal nerve
Great sciatic nerve

human body and is comprised of the common peroneal and tibial nerves. It passes through the greater sciatic foramen below the piriformis muscle to enter the gluteal region. In this area it sends branches to the obturator internus, gemelli, and quadratus femoris muscles, the main external rotators of the thigh.

ETIOLOGY AND PATHOPHYSIOLOGY

Causes of compression neuropathies in the abdominopelvic area may be pressure, stretch, angulation, adaptive changes in tone and length of pelvic musculature, or iatrogenic. The incidence of compression neuropathies of individual peripheral nerves is increased if the patient suffers from generalized peripheral neuropathy, as occurs with renal failure, alcoholism, or diabetes (2).

The compression may be acute, continuous, or intermittent. *Acute nerve compression* that is insufficient to damage a nerve fiber but obliterates its vascular supply will lead to a reversible ischaemic conduction block. Generally speaking, the postischemic paresthesias are usually more pronounced than those occurring at the time of compression. On the other hand a more severe form of acute compression injury is a focal demyelination. The myelin is displaced outward from the site of compression, in a manner similar to intussusception, into the adjacent myelin segment.

In vivo inspection of the involved nerve at time of operation in humans has revealed narrowing at the site of *chronic nerve compression* with expansion on the proximal side mainly. Observational studies of the actual histopathology of chronic nerve compression and entrapment are lacking in humans but have been performed on animal models. These have suggested that in severely affected fibers paranodal demyelination and distal fiber degeneration occur with a progressive axonal atrophy (7).

Stretch injury is another mechanical cause of neuropathies. This most commonly occurs during labor and delivery, but may also occur inadvertently by retraction during abdominopelvic or perineal procedures. Although mild traction may only produce a transient reversible conduction block, excessive traction can cause damage to a considerable length of the nerve. The exact pathological picture is still disputed, but in general there is rupture of some fibers with or without accompanying rupture of the perineurium (8).

The pain in entrapment syndromes can be explained from an anatomical and neurophysiological viewpoint. Whenever a nerve is damaged, whether by entrapment or external trauma, regeneration of nerve endings may result. These regenerated endings, known as sprouts, are exquisitely sensitive to stimuli including mechanical, chemical, and thermal. They may become ectopic foci of nerve impulses that arise by mechanical or other stimulation. The nerve's function thus switches from a conductor to a generator of impulses (9,10).

As previously stated, a number of factors may be responsible for the various mononeuropathies encountered. *Trauma* to a nerve may be the cause of neuropathy. Trauma may result from occupational injury, surgery, childbirth, or skeletal fractures or dislocations. Occupational trauma may cause excessive pressure on a specific nerve during work that may lead to a neuropathy of that nerve. Examples include the development of sciatica in women with desk jobs, femoral nerve neuralgia in nuns who kneel during prayer, and peroneal nerve palsy in models (11,12). Surgical abdominopelvic procedures, such as appendectomies, hernia repairs, and others, may lead to injury of nerves in the vicinity of the wound or surgical field. Improper positioning of a patient's legs during delivery or difficult labor may result in trauma to the nerves of the lumbosacral plexus of nerves (12). Trauma to the lumbar spine, particularly the fourth or fifth segments, may lead to sciatica. Fractures of the pelvis or head of the femur may injure the sacroiliac plexus, the femoral nerve, or the sciatic nerve (12).

Toxins may occasionally have a role in the occurrence of a neuropathy affecting the abdominopelvic region. Rarely, following antirabies treatment, neuroparalytic accidents localized primarily in the spinal nerve roots may occur. A localized allergic neuropathy to an insect sting may also occur (12,13).

Neoplasms may also cause mononeuropathies. Neurofibromas and ganglioneuromas are examples of nerve tumors arising from the nerve sheath and nerve fiber, respectively, that may lead to a neuritis. Kaposi's sarcoma may also lead to multiple mononeuropathies. Lymphomas, including Hodgkin's disease, may directly infiltrate nerve roots and plexuses, with the lumbosacral plexus being particularly prone (12).

Compression or *entrapment* are common causes of neuropathies of the lumbosacral plexus. Each nerve has its own set specific of conditions under which compression may occur. The iliohypogastric, ilioinguinal, genitofemoral, and lateral femoral cutaneous nerves are the commonest branches of the lumbar plexus to be involved in nerve entrapment neuropathies. In most cases these are complications of a variety of abdominal surgical procedures, but they can also be associated with an inflammatory process. The most frequently cited surgical procedures associated with neuropathies are appendectomy, inguinal herniorraphy, laparoscopic hernia repairs, bladder needle suspension procedures, Pfannenstiel incisions, and, occasionally, midline infraumbilical incisions (5,14–17). Recently, nerve entrapment has been reported as a complication of gynecologic laparoscopic procedures also (18). The nerve may be injured by incision with subsequent neuroma formation, incorporation by suture in a closure, or tethering in the scar of healing (16).

The *iliohypogastric nerve* may become entrapped following low transverse muscle-splitting incisions such as done for appendectomy, Pfannenstiel incisions, use of self-retaining retractors, and hernia repairs. With Pfannenstiel incisions it most often occurs when the incision is extended laterally past the fascial aponeurosis to include the medial edge of the internal oblique muscle where the nerve runs (16). In a recently reported case following laparoscopic oophorectomy the entrapment was owing to too-wide a deployment of a fascial closure device to control bleeding from a 12-mm lateral suprapubic trocar site (10).

Ilioinguinal nerve entrapment is the most commonly seen and best described. It may rarely occur spontaneously as a result of entrapment between the transverse and the oblique internal muscle, but most often is a consequence of herniorraphies, appendectomies, Pfannenstiel incisions and needle suspension procedures for stress incontinence. This nerve is most vulnerable at its exit from the superficial inguinal ring (14,15,19).

Genitofemoral neuralgia was relatively unknown among surgeons until the past decade. Until 1987 only 28 cases had been reported in the world's literature, the first having been reported by Magee in 1942 (20). It is a documented complication following appendectomies, inguinal herniorraphy, lower quadrant blunt trauma and, in one instance, attributed to constricting blue jeans (21). Fibrous adhesions, resulting from previous surgery in the vicinity of the nerve or from blunt trauma, usually entrap small branches and twigs of this nerve (14).

Lateral femoral cutaneous neuropathies were first described in 1895 by Roth, who coined the term *meralgia paresthetica*, in addition to Bernhardt and Freud separately (22–24). The most common entrapment locations are at the site of penetration of the deep fascia to reach the skin and at the point of passage from the pelvis into the thigh. Additional aggravating factors include prolonged wearing of braces or tight corsets that cause continuous or intermittent pressure on the nerve. It is frequently seen in obese patients, presumably owing to greater stress on the structures around the inguinal ligament in addition to the possible nerve traction a large pannus may produce. Pregnancy, ascites and other causes of increased intraabdominal pressure may also be causes (12). After the widespread use of laparoscopic hernia repair the incidence of this complication has risen owing to entrapment of the nerve within the staples used to fix the polypropylene mesh to the abdominal wall peritoneum (25). Recent data show a 1 to 2 percent incidence of various entrapment neuralgias after open and laparoscopic herniorraphy (26).

Femoral neuropathies are usually the result of trauma. The commonest causes are compressing hematomas as a result of injury or bleeding disorders (12). It is uncommonly the complication of surgical procedures. In major pelvic surgery such as radical cystectomy or vaginal hysterectomy the compression may be direct or more frequently may be indirect from compression between the psoas muscle and lateral pelvic wall from retraction (27,28). Surgical retractors may also compromise the blood supply of the nerve and cause subsequent neuropathy. In addition to these causes, a syndrome of femoral nerve entrapment at the iliopectineal arch, analogous to carpal tunnel syndrome, was recently described in three cases (28).

Obturator nerve compression neuropathies are rarely seen. Compression by the fetal head during difficult deliveries or pressure from obturator hernias and intrapelvic tumors are the known causes.

Saphenous nerve compression, which can occur spontaneously at the fascia of the subsartorius or Hunter's canal, is also rarely associated with improper leg support during childbirth or perineal surgical procedures, both of which lead to compression against the medial femoral condyle.

Sciatic nerve compression or entrapment may sometimes be the cause of chronic pelvic pain in women. Pain from compression of the nerve at the sciatic notch has been described in women who horseback ride frequently (13). Pain may also occur with entrapment secondary to increased tone and shortening of the piriformis muscle (2). Less common causes are sacral fractures in older women with osteoporosis, intraoperative or postoperative complications of total hip arthroplasty and, in one case, a hematocolpos in a 15-year-old girl (29,30).

Pudendal neuralgia may occur anywhere along the course of the pudendal, but usually occurs within Alcock's canal where it is fixed in the obturator fascia. The relation of the nerve to the ischial spine also places it at risk of compression or stretching. Pressures generated during the second stage of labor may be sufficient to produce a permanent nerve injury if sustained for long enough. Pelvic floor descent of only 14 mm or more can cause stretch sufficient to produce neuropathy (10). Women who cycle or horseback ride for prolonged periods may be prone to pudendal neuralgia. It may be iatrogenic in nature also, for example, following vaginal sacrospinous colpopexy procedures (31).

SYMPTOMS AND SIGNS

As previously explained an injured or compressed nerve undergoes various changes leading to impairment of nerve conduction and neuropathologic signs and symptoms.

TABLE 44.3. GENERAL SYMPTOMS AND SIGNS THAT MAY OCCUR WITH NEURALGIAS

Sensory loss
Paresthesias
Dysesthesias
Hyperesthesia
Allodynia
Hyperpathia
Pain
Motor Loss
Autonomic disturbances

Patients with neuropathy may present with any combination of these symptoms and signs (Table 44.3).

Sensory Loss

In a peripheral neuropathy the loss of sensation may encompass all or only certain types of sensory modalities. Sensory loss usually is restricted to the area supplied distal to the injury, especially with nerve entrapment.

Paresthesias, Dysesthesias, Hyperesthesia, Allodynia, and Hyperpathia

Mononeuropathies, particularly of a mixed sensorimotor type, are frequently accompanied by tingling paresthesia or burning dysesthesia that are felt in the distribution area of the affected nerve as well as along its course. Ectopic impulses arising from the ischemic, or postischemic, nerve trunks cause these sensations and it is postulated that the ectopic impulses are of an *abnormal* spatiotemporal pattern, arising from a variety of different sensory units (32). Ectopic discharges may also arise in axonal sprouts in regenerating nerves. Hyperesthesia refers to an increased sensitivity to stimulation; a tactile or thermal stimulus that normally would not be uncomfortable may become painful or uncomfortable. Allodynia is the preferred term when describing pain owing to a normally nonnoxious stimulus; this is a common finding with neuropathy. Hyperpathia is an overreactive pain reaction in response to stimulus, especially a repetitive stimulus. This is usually seen following a nerve injury or during the recovery phase (33).

Pain

The onset and intensity of pain in a mononeuropathy is variable. It may occur immediately following the incident or anytime up to 2 weeks after the insult (5). Immediate, constant, burning pain is most often encountered with nerve entrapment in a tight suture or staple, swelling of a nerve within a restricted space, pressure from a rapidly growing hematoma, or direct external compression. A subacute onset is usually encountered with nerves involved in healing scars and in nerve injury arising from pressure of growing tumors or toxins. In some postoperative cases, after a period of time the suture cuts through the fascia and pulls on the entrapped nerve when the patient does certain movements.

The distribution of pain in a focal mononeuropathy is usually within the distribution area of the nerve, but may radiate widely in some cases. The type of pain sensation is also variable. Although intense burning pain is characteristic, in some cases pain may be dull, aching, and deep-seated or it may be superficial burning or stinging. The severity of pain can also be affected by movement in some types of nerve injuries (5).

Motor Loss

In addition to sensory loss, motor involvement may also occur because of injury or destruction of motor axons within the affected nerve. A conduction block may also occur. The pathology is usually myelinopathy at first and axonal injury in more severe cases (34). With myelinopathy no denervation atrophy occurs, whereas in axonal injury atrophy may be clinically evident within a few weeks.

Autonomic Disturbances

Although uncommon, autonomic disturbances may occur in some peripheral nerve disorders. An example is anhidrosis occurring in the cutaneous distribution of a peripheral nerve in mononeuropathy. This is caused by deficient sudomotor innervation and is more common in diabetic neuropathies (35). Another example may be the role of pudendal neuropathy in the etiology of fecal incontinence in rectal prolapse (36).

Evaluations of vasomotor and trophic changes, if present, are important components of the physical examination relative to these aspects of peripheral neuropathies. The relative warmth or coolness of the area, cyanosis or ruber, and changes in the skin are all telltale signs in the diagnosis of neuropathy of a specific nerve.

In cases of lower abdominal pain the examination should assess whether the pain is visceral or parietal by employing a test such as Carnett's (1).

Describing specific symptoms and signs of the neuropathies that are most often encountered in women with chronic abdominopelvic pain may allow a better understanding of the varied symptomatology. Neuropathies of the ilioinguinal, iliohypogastric, genitofemoral, lateral femoral cutaneous, and pudendal nerves are most relevant to a discussion of etiology in women with chronic abdominopelvic pain.

Iliohypogastric and Ilioinguinal Neuropathies

Neuropathy of the ilioinguinal nerve or iliohypogastric nerve is owing in almost all cases to nerve entrapment following abdominal wall surgery. As might be predicted from the neuroanatomy, there is significant overlap in the presentation of ilioinguinal and iliohypogastric neuropathies. The onset is often immediately postoperatively, but may also occur later. Pain, which is the main symptom, is invariably judged as coming from the abdomen and not from the skin. The patient may present with diffuse lower abdominal burning or lancinating pain in the area surrounding the surgical wound. In other cases pain may be localized or it may present along the course of the nerve and radiate to the labia or inner aspect of the thigh on the affected side (Fig. 44.1). Although pain is characteristically burning in quality, it also may be colicky, intermittently sharp and stabbing, continu-

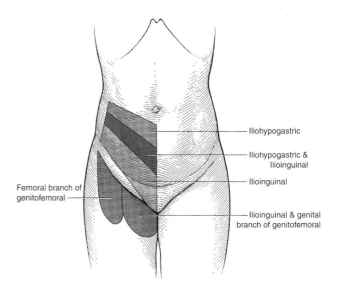

FIGURE 44.1. The distribution of pain with ilioinguinal, iliohypogastric, and genitofemoral nerve entrapments.

ously gnawing, or persistently dull and burning in quality. In addition the pain can be aggravated by movement, cough, or lifting movements of the ipsilateral leg. Hyperesthesia and hyperalgesia are usually present, whereas only a small number report hypoesthesia (13,15,17). Gait disturbances may occur because of pain and women usually cannot practice previous physical activities such as jogging. Tenderness may be present medial to the anterior superior iliac spine and over the point of entrapment (9,14,34). Tapping over the area of tenderness usually elicits pain (Tinel's sign). Communication between the iliohypogastric and ilioinguinal nerves and overlap in sensory distribution of both nerves may be present, so that entrapment of one nerve may result in a broader than expected set of signs and symptoms (14).

Genitofemoral Neuropathy

Neuropathy of the genitofemoral nerve usually produces constant or intermittent pain and paresthesias in the medial inguinal region. This is accompanied by pain radiating to the upper inner thigh and the labium majus. The pain is usually increased by standing, walking, stooping, and extension of the hip, and is relieved by recumbency. Hyperesthesia may be present in the distribution of the nerve and localized tenderness along the inguinal canal is usually present (14).

Lateral Femoral Cutaneous Neuropathy

Meralgia paresthetica is the name used for neuropathy of the lateral femoral cutaneous nerve. It often begins with pain in the flank or lower abdomen and the groin with radiating pain to the anterolateral thigh. Later this is accompanied by burning paresthesias and hyperpathia. Paresthesia or hypoesthesia may be present along the anteromedial aspect of the thigh. Symptoms are increased by prolonged standing or walking or sustained extension and adduction of the lower limb. Because of this the patient may hold the hip in flexion and external rotation. The onset of pain may be abrupt or over a period of time. As a postoperative complication, the pain usually appears immediately, whereas as a complication of pregnancy it usually appears in the latter half when the abdominal size increases greatly. The patient may have wasting of the quadriceps muscle if the nerve is severely affected, whereas diminution of the patellar reflex is present in mild cases (12,27).

Pudendal Neuralgia

Neuralgia of the pudendal nerve is classically described by Wilson and Kinnier as "mostly vague but sometimes well-defined pains, referred to the perineum ... perhaps with spread to groin, leg or abdomen.... Pain ... is often very severe and at times paroxysmal: the parts become extremely sensitive to touch, while light pressure may be frankly intolerable ..." (37). In addition, ipsilateral buttocks pain has been reported (30). Pudendal nerve injury may lead to motor dysfunction in the external anal sphincter causing fecal incontinence (10,36).

DIAGNOSTIC STUDIES

Electrophysiologic studies of nerve function may help in localization and assessment of severity of compression or entrapment neuropathies. Studies include determination of nerve conducting velocities of the sensory and motor fibers and needle electromyographic (EMG) studies. Conduction tests are more applicable in the study of motor neurons than sensory neurons. They are not very sensitive in detecting degeneration of small fibers or of a few large fibers in association with preservation of a great number of large fibers. They may be of value in documenting the existence of a generalized neuropathy that may predispose to compressive neuropathy (12). EMG studies may be helpful in determining whether muscular atrophy, if present, is owing to a neuropathic or myopathic disorder (10). Generally speaking they are of relatively low value in the neuropathies of the smaller branches of the lumbosacral plexus.

Quantitative evaluation tests of cutaneous sensation are sometimes useful because abnormalities of thermal discrimination and nociception may be present in difficult cases where no other motor or electrophysiologic changes are detected (10,12).

Nerve biopsies are generally reserved for diagnosis when peripheral neuropathy is suspected to be part of a more widespread disease process. When properly done, biopsies can be more sensitive than conventional electrophysiologic studies (12).

Radiographic techniques such as plain x-rays or computerized tomography (CT) may be helpful in revealing abnormalities in bones and joints or in visualizing retroperitoneal masses that may be compressing the affected nerve. Occasionally they may reveal a tumor of the affected nerve.

Local nerve block is a very useful technique in the diagnostic evaluation of nerve compression and entrapment (9,10,14–16,18,26). Injection of a local anesthetic at the point of maximal tenderness with subsequent improvement in pain or hyperalgesia is usually sufficient to implicate the nerve in pain causation. Failure of relief may point to a higher site of nerve irritation. Proper placebo control of the block should be implemented. The nerve block may be both diagnostic and therapeutic in many cases (14–16).

Ilioinguinal and Iliohypogastric Nerves

In nerve entrapment an electric shocklike sensation is elicited over the course of the nerve if the skin above the entrapment site is tapped (Tinel's sign). A local anesthetic nerve block is useful to diagnose entrapments of these nerves (Fig. 44.2). Sippo et al. describe their technique for local nerve block as follows:

> The patients were placed in a supine position, with the region from the umbilicus to the upper thigh exposed on the side involved. A 3-inch, 25-gauge spinal needle was guided with a gloved hand beneath the external oblique aponeurosis at a point 1-inch medial and 1-inch inferior to the anterior supe-

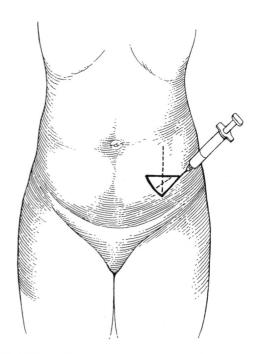

FIGURE 44.2. Local anesthetic nerve block of the ilioinguinal and iliohypogastric nerves.

rior iliac spine. With a 2:1 mixture of 0.5% bupivacaine and 1.0% lidocaine without epinephrine, 1 ml was deposited at this site. The needle was advanced toward the pubic tubercle, and on its withdrawal 3 ml of the mixture was injected with steady even pressure. Without removal of the needle, it was redirected such that, in three or more passes, a fan-shaped deposition of anesthetic was accomplished (16).

Of course, variations on this technique exist (14,15,18). Communicating fibers between the ilioinguinal and iliohypogastric nerves make a specific diagnosis difficult.

Genitofemoral Nerve

The genitofemoral nerve commonly has communicating fibers to the ilioinguinal nerve and differentiation can be done by doing separate nerve blocks. If a primary ilioinguinal nerve block fails to relieve the pain, then a paravertebral block of the L1 and L2 plexus should be done using 0.5% bupivacaine and 0.75% lidocaine with epinephrine 1:200,000.

Lateral Femoral Cutaneous Nerve

Lateral femoral cutaneous nerve entrapments are usually diagnosed by history, the sensory changes, and exclusion of other nerve entrapments. Nerve conduction studies cannot be conducted reliably (12). Differential blocks may be helpful, as the lateral femoral cutaneous nerve can be blocked via an inguinal ligament approach (Fig. 44.3).

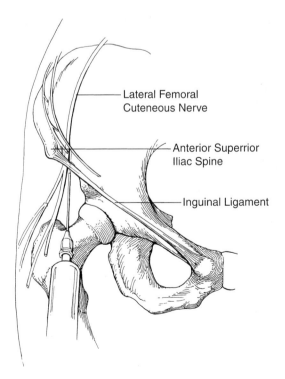

Lateral Femoral
Cuteneous Nerve

Anterior Superrior
Iliac Spine

Inguinal Ligament

FIGURE 44.3. Inguinal approach to local anesthetic nerve block of the lateral femoral cutaneous nerve.

Pudendal Nerve

Pudendal neuropathy presents with classic sensorimotor manifestations previously described. In patients with complete rectal prolapse and associated fecal incontinence, the condition should be suspected. EMG may reveal reduced activity in the external anal sphincter and the levator muscle. Pudendal nerve terminal motor latency (PNTML) assessment may also be done because it may be prolonged in patients with pudendal neuropathies owing to a stretch injury (38). One study of PNTML following normal vaginal deliveries showed that it is often pathologically high immediately following delivery but recovery occurs in most after a 3-month period (40).

DIAGNOSIS

A thorough evaluation of the patient with a neuropathy is needed to reach a proper diagnosis. In mononeuropathies of the lumbosacral plexus there is enough overlap in sensory distribution that symptoms alone may be misleading. A diagnostic triad for nerve entrapment neuropathies includes: (a) pain in the area supplied by the nerve, (b) sensory impairment in the distribution of the nerve, and (c) relief of pain by local anesthetic injection. These should be taken into account while doing the complete diagnostic work-up.

MANAGEMENT OR TREATMENT

Medical Treatment

The majority of nerve entrapments, especially those of the cutaneous nerves, resolve spontaneously over time. In cases where the pain is too severe or the condition persists, treatment is necessary and may be conservative or surgical.

Pharmacological drug therapy of neuropathy is indicated when entrapment or compression owing to surgical sutures or staples is not the cause. For example, in cases of work-related or obesity-related meralgia paresthetica, hydrocortisone injections medial to the anterior superior iliac spine may provide temporary relief. Medical therapy of pudendal neuralgia by CT-guided injection of antiinflammatory corticoid drugs is successful in abolishing pain in about one-third of cases. Unfortunately, the relief is not long-lasting and at 1-year the results are poorer (39).

Neuropathic pain is characteristically unresponsive to simple analgesics and often is refractory to opiate treatment. Tramadol, a synthetic centrally acting analgesic displaying both weak opioid and nonopioid properties, is a good initial approach to oral pharmacological treatment and has good efficacy, at least short-term (40). It is usually administered in doses of 50 to 100 mg every 4 to 6 hours. A typical daily dose for moderately severe pain is 200 mg.

The tricyclic antidepressants amitriptyline, imipramine, and desipramine are useful in the treatment of neuropathy in diabetic patients and in postherpetic neuralgia (Chapter 53) (41,42). However, side effects may limit effectiveness. For this reason, dosage is usually started at a low level, such as amitriptyline at 25 mg per day, and slowly increased to effective or intolerable doses (whichever comes first). Gabapentin, a structural analog of τ-aminobutyric acid, is also effective in the treatment of neuropathy in diabetic patients and in postherpetic neuralgia (43,45). Initial dosage is 300 mg times per day and it can be increased to 1,200 mg three times per day, based on intolerance and response. Other medications, especially phentoin, carbamazepine, mexiletine, and topical capsaicin, are also commonly used for the treatment of neuropathic pain, but there is less definitive evidence for their efficacy.

Nerve blocks using local anesthetics are both diagnostic and therapeutic in many instances. Patients sometimes have significant pain relief with multiple injections and require no further treatment. Often, however, pain relief is only temporary with nerve blocks and if surgical excision or decompression is a viable option then it is the preferred treatment. If surgery is not appropriate, then repeated blocks may be a reasonable option. For example, CT-guided pudendal nerve block has been used to treat patients with intractable pudendal neuralgia with some success (45,46).

Physiotherapeutic massage techniques and targeted muscle exercises may be of value in some cases of cutaneous nerve entrapments. These are most beneficial when the afflicted nerve is caught in the healing scar of an abdominal wound. Proper massage and myofascial manipulation techniques may increase the flexibility of the scar and prevent further pull on the entrapped nerve (47).

SURGICAL TREATMENT

Surgery is indicated when the pain does not respond to local anesthetic injection, is of intolerable severity, or is a cause significant morbidity. The actual procedure may be as simple as removal of a tight suture or a staple. In others it may involve neurectomy of a portion of the nerve that includes the entrapped segment (14). Surgery may not be effective in all cases, particularly when a central lesion exists.

Communicating fibers between the ilioinguinal and iliohypogastric nerves make a specific diagnosis and surgical treatment difficult. To differentiate them, separate local nerve blocks may be necessary. Once the proper nerve is identified surgical exploration can be done to confirm the diagnosis and treat the condition. Surgical exploration of the genitofemoral nerve, as classically described by Starling, is done via a transverse flank incision several centimeters above and lateral to the umbilicus and extending to the anterior axillary line. Muscles are divided if needed, the retroperitoneum identified and the psoas muscle and ureter identified. The nerve usually is seen along the medial edge of the psoas (14). More recently laparoscopic approaches have been described that can be used for surgical treatment of the condition (25,48).

KEY POINTS

Differential Diagnoses

- Direct nerve trauma
- Acute nerve compression
- Chronic nerve compression
- Stretch injury
- Nerve entrapment
- Nerve damage by toxins
- Neoplasms

Most Important Questions to Ask

- Was the onset of pain related to recent trauma or surgery in the region of the pain?
- Is there history of past trauma or surgery to this region?
- Is there any increase or decrease in sensitivity of the skin in the region of the pain?
- Is the pain affecting the patient's lifestyle or affecting her sleep pattern?
- Character of pain, duration, and any aggravating factors such as movement?

Most Important Physical Examination Findings

- Tinel's sign
- Sensory loss
- Hyperesthesia
- Allodynia
- Tenderness in the distribution of a specific nerve
- Motor loss
- Autonomic disturbances
- Carnett's test

Most Important Diagnostic Studies

- Nerve conduction velocities
- Needle electromyographic studies
- Quantitative evaluation tests of cutaneous sensation
- Nerve biopsies
- X-rays or computerized tomography
- Local anesthetic nerve blocks

Treatments

- Observation
- Analgesics
- Tramadol
- Tricyclic antidepressants
- Gabapentin
- Phenytoin, carbamazepine, mexiletine, and topical capsaicin
- Cryotherapy
- Nerve blocks using local anesthetics or corticosteroids or neurolytic agent
- Physiotherapeutic massage techniques and targeted muscle exercises
- Surgery removal of a tight suture or a staple
- Surgical neurectomy

REFERENCES

1. Gallegos NC, Hobsley M. Abdominal wall pain: an alternative diagnosis. *Br J Surg* 1990;77(10):1167–70.
2. Dawson DM, Hallett M, Millender LH. *Entrapment neuropathies,* 2nd ed. Boston: Little, Brown, 1991:196–197.
3. Melville K, Schultz EA, Dougherty JM. Ilioinguinal-iliohypogastric nerve entrapment. *Ann Em Med* 1990;19(8):925–929.
4. Warwick R, Williams PL. *Gray's anatomy.* Philadelphia: Saunders, 1973:1050–1053.
5. Seid AS, Amos E. Entrapment neuropathy in laparoscopic herniorraphy. *Surg Endoscop* 1994;8:1050–1053.
6. Dwight T, McMurrich JP, Hamann CA, et al., eds. *Human anatomy.* Philadelphia: Lippincott, 1923.
7. Baba M, Fowler CJ, Jacobs JM, et al. Changes in peripheral nerve fibers distal to a constriction. *J Neurol Sci* 1982;54:197.
8. Haftek J. Stretch injury of peripheral nerve. Acute effects of stretching on rabbit peripheral nerve. *J Bone Joint Surg* 1970;52B:354.
9. Hahn L. Clinical findings and results of operative treatment in ilioinguinal nerve entrapment syndrome. *Br J Obstet Gynecol* 1989;96(9):1080–1083.
10. Benson JT. Neuropathic pain. In: Steege JF, Metzger DA, Levy BS, eds. *Chronic pelvic pain. An integrated approach.* Philadelphia: Saunders, 1998, 241–250.
11. Guillain G, de Seze S, Bondin-Walter M. Etude clinique et pathogenizue de certaines paralies professionelles du nerf sciatique poplite externe. *Bull Acad Med Paris* 1934;111:633..
12. Dyck PJ, Low PA, Stevens JC. Diseases of peripheral nerves. In: Baker AB, Joynt RJ, eds. *Clinical neurology.* Philadelphia: Harper & Row, 1985:1–126.
13. Ross AT. Peripheral neuritis: allergy to honeybee stings. *J Allerg* 1930;10:382..
14. Starling JR, Harms BA, Schroeder ME, et al. Diagnosis and treatment of genitofemoral and ilioinguinal entrapment neuragia. *Surgery* 1987;102:581–586.
15. Miyazaki F, Shook G. Ilioinguinal nerve entrapment during needle suspension for stress incontinence. *Obstet Gynecol* 1992;80(2):246–248.
16. Sippo WC, Burghardt A, Gomez AC. Nerve entrapment after Pfannenstiel incision. *Am J Obstet Gynecol* 1987;157(2):420–421.
17. Hall PN, Lee AP. Rectus nerve entrapment causing abdominal pain. *Br J Surg* 1988;75(9):917–921.
18. El-Minawi AM, Howard FM. Iliohypogastric nerve entrapment following gynecologic operative laparoscopy. *Obstet Gynecol* 1998;91:871.
19. Kopell HP, Thompson WAL, Postel A. Entrapment neuropathy of the ilioinguinal nerve. *N Engl J Med* 1962;161:16–19.
20. Magee RK. Genitofemoral causalgia (a new syndrome). *Can Med Assoc J* 1942;46:326–329.
21. O'Brien MD. Genitofemoral neuropathy. *Br Med J* 1979;1:1052.
22. Roth VK. *Meralgia paresthetica.* Berlin: Karger, 1895.
23. Bernhardt M. Über isoliert im Gebeite des N. cutaneous femoris externus vorkommende parästhesien. *Neurol Cbl* 1895;14:242–248.
24. Freud S. Über die Bernhardt'sche Sensibiliätsstörung. *Neurol Cbl* 1895;14:491–492.
25. Eubanks S, Newman L 3rd, Goehring L, et al. Meralgia paresthetica: a complication of laparoscopic herniorrhaphy. *Surg Laparosc Endoscop* 1993;3(5):381–385.
26. Krahenbuhl L, Striffeler H, Baer HU, et al. Retroperitoneal endoscopic neurectomy for nerve entrapment after hernia repair. *Br J Surg* 1997;84(2):216–219.
27. Chen S-S, Lin ATL, Chen K-K, et al. Femoral neuropathy after pelvic surgery. *Urology* 1995;46(4):575–576.
28. Natelson SE. Surgical correction of proximal femoral nerve entrapment. *Surg Neurol* 1997;48(4):326–329.
29. Finiels H, Finiels PJ, Jacquot JM, et al. Fractures of the sacrum caused by bone insufficiency. Meta-analysis of 508 cases. *Presse Medicale* 1997;26(33):1568–1573.
30. London NJ, Sefton GK. Haematocolpos. An unusual cause of sciatica in an adolescent girl. *Spine* 1996;21:1381–1382.
31. Alevizon SJ, Finan MA. Sacrospinous colpopexy: management of postoperative pudendal nerve entrapment. *Obstet Gynecol* 1996;88(4) 2:713–715.
32. Ochoa JL, Torebjörk HE. Paraesthesiae from ectopic impulse generation in human sensory nerves. *Brain* 1980;103:835.
33. Merskey H, Albe-Fessard DG, Bonica JJ, et al. Pain terms: a list with definitions and notes on usage. *Pain* 1979;6:249.
34. Logigian EL. Neurologic disorders. In: Stein JH, ed. *Stein internal medicine,* 4th ed. St. Louis: Mosby, 1994.
35. Goodman JI. Diabetic anhidrosis. *Am J Med* 1966;41:831.
36. Shafik A. Role of pudendal canal syndrome in the etiology of fecal incontinence in rectal prolapse. *Digestion* 1997;58(5):489–493.
37. Wilson SA, Kinnier. In Bruce AN, ed. *Neurology,* 2nd ed. Baltimore: Williams & Wilkins, 1955:304.
38. Tetzschner T, Sorensen M, Lose G, et al. Pudendal nerve recovery after a non-instrumented vaginal delivery. *Int Urogynecol J Pelvic Floor Dys* 1996;7(2):102–104.
39. Amarenco G, Kerdraon J, Boujo P, et al. Treatments of perineal neuralgia caused by involvement of the pudendal nerve. *Revue Neurol* 1997;153(5):331–334.
40. Harati Y, Gooch C, Swenson M, et al. Double-blind randomized trial of tramadol for the treatment of the pain of diabetic neuropathy. *Neurology* 1998;50:1842–1846.
41. Kingery WS. A critical review of controlled clinical trials for peripheral neuropathic pain and complex regional pain syndromes. *Pain* 1997;73:123–139.
42. Max MB. Thirteen consecutive well-designed randomized trials show that antidepressants reduce pain in diabetic neuropathy and postherpetic neuralgia. *Pain Forum* 1995;4:248–253.
43. Backonja M, Beydoun A, Edwards KR, et al. Gabapentin for the symptomatic treatment of painful neuropathy in patients with diabetes mellitus: a randomized controlled trial. *JAMA* 1998;280:1831–1836.

44. Rowbotham M, Harden N, Stacey B, et al. Gabapentin for the treatment of postherpetic neuralgia: a randomized controlled trial. *JAMA* 1998;280:1837–1842.

45. Personal communication, John McDonald, MD, Columbus, OH, 1998.

46. El-Minawi AM, Howard FM. Computerized tomography-guided pudendal nerve block for chronic vulvar pain. Presented at the International Congress of Gynecologic Endoscopy. AAGL 27th annual meeting. Nov. 10–15, Atlanta, GA, 1998.

47. Kessler RM, Hertling D. *Management of common musculoskeletal disorder: physical therapy principles and methods,* 2nd ed. Philadelphia: Lippincott, 1990.

48. Perry CP. Laparoscopic treatment of genitofemoral neuralgia. *J Amer Assoc Gynecol Laparoscop* 1997;4:231–234.

45

PELVIC FLOOR PAIN SYNDROME

FRED M. HOWARD

KEY TERMS AND DEFINITIONS

Coccygeus: Pelvic floor muscle that originates at the ischial spine and fibers of the sacrospinous ligament and attaches to the last segment of the sacrum and the lateral margins of the coccyx; pulls the coccyx forward.

Coccygodynia: Term used by Thiele in his classic description of pain related to the coccyx and the muscles attached to the coccyx.

Levator ani: Complex of muscles that form the pelvic floor or pelvic diaphragm; composed of puborectalis, pubococcygeus, iliococcygeus.

Pelvic floor pain syndromes: Pelvic pain caused by or associated with pain and tenderness of one or more of the muscles of the "pelvic floor"—levator ani, coccygeus, or piriformis—or their associated fascia or insertions.

Piriformis: Muscle that is often considered part of the pelvic floor, although not technically so; originates from the inner or anterior surface of the sacrum and attaches laterally into the greater trochanter; externally rotates the hip.

INTRODUCTION

Most physicians, especially gynecologists, are accustomed to considerations of the pelvic floor related to relaxation defects. However, as a major component of the musculoskeletal system of the pelvis, the pelvic floor is not infrequently a contributor to chronic pelvic pain (CPP), and in some cases it may be the primary cause (1).

Pelvic visceral innervation and thereby pelvic pain generally arise from T10 to S4 spinal cord segments. Numerous musculoskeletal structures also have this innervation, and they may cause pelvic pain and low back pain (Table 45.1 and Chapter 40). There are a number of musculoskeletal dysfunctions that are reported to clinically correlate with CPP (Table 45.2). For this discussion, those specifically related to the pelvic floor are pertinent—for example, myalgia or spasm of the levator ani, coccygeus, or piriformis, and levator ani trigger points. However, it must be noted that considering these dysfunctions as iso-

TABLE 45.1. MUSCULOSKELETAL STRUCTURES INNERVATED BY T10 TO S4 THAT MAY CONTRIBUTE TO PELVIC PAIN (1)

Lumbar vertebrae
  Joint capsules
  Ligaments
  Discs
Hips
  Joints
  Ligaments
Muscle groups
  Abdominals
  Iliiopsoas
  Quadratus lumborum
  Piriformis
  Obturator internus and externus
  Levator ani
  Coccygeus

From Baker PK. Musculoskeletal origins of chronic pelvic pain. *Obstet Gynecol Clin North Am* 1993;20:719–742, with permission.

lated occurrences is undoubtedly artifactual, because the musculoskeletal synergy needed to maintain bipedal posture means that many structural dysfunctions probably occur concurrently to cause CPP related to the pelvic floor.

TABLE 45.2. MUSCULOSKELETAL DYSFUNCTIONS THAT ARE REPORTED TO CLINICALLY CORRELATE WITH CHRONIC PELVIC PAIN

Abdominal trigger points
Levator ani trigger points
Intrapelvic muscle strain
  Obturator internus
  Coccygeus
  Piriformis
Pelvic floor myalgia/spasm
  Levator
  Coccygeus
  Piriformis
Abdominal weakness
Gluteus maximus weakness
Anterior pelvic tilt
Leg length/pelvic postural asymmetry
Loss of hip range of motion
Lumbar joint dysfunction
Iliopsoas adaptive shortening

TABLE 45.3. SOME OF THE NAMES USED FOR PELVIC PAIN DUE TO THE PELVIC FLOOR

Levator ani syndrome
Levator (ani) spasm syndrome
Coccydynia
Proctalgia fugax
Proctadynia
Proctalgia
Coccygodynia
Pelvic floor myalgia
Piriformis syndrome
Diaphragma pelvis spastica
Tension myalgia of the pelvic floor

TABLE 45.4. INDIRECT CAUSES OF MUSCULAR SPASM AND PELVIC FLOOR PAIN SYNDROME

Inflammation
Gastrointestinal tract
  Cryptitis
  Ulcer
  Hemorrhoids
  Proctitis
  Anorectal abscess
  Anal fistula
Urinary tract
  Cystitis
  Urethritis
Reproductive tract
  Cervicitis
  Vaginitis
  Salpingitis
Trauma
Direct fall or kick
Childbirth
Pelvic surgery
Irradiation treatment
Fracture of coccyx
Rectal surgical scar
Musculoskeletal
Prolonged sitting
Poor posture
Herniation of vertebral disc
Neoplasms
Spinal cord
Retroperitoneal
Presacral and postsacral
Psychosomatic
Anxiety state
Hysteria

CPP due to pelvic floor dysfunction was probably first brought to "modern" attention by Thiele in the 1930s (2). He termed the syndrome "coccygodynia," but numerous other names have been used for pain thought secondary to the levator ani, coccygeus, and piriformis muscles of the pelvic diaphragm (3,4) (Table 45.3). The choice of nomenclature is sometimes a function of the primary location of the pain (e.g., anal) and sometimes a function of the physician's or clinician's specialty. Possibly *pelvic floor pain syndrome* may be a better, all-inclusive name.

Most often the pain with these syndromes is attributed to spasm or tension in one or more of the muscles. This spasm is thought to directly cause pain in the muscle and/or referred pain in the attachment to the sacrum, coccyx, ischial tuberosity, or pubic rami (4,5).

Pelvic floor pain syndrome (PFPS) occurs predominantly in women in their forties and fifties. For example, in the Mayo Clinic series of 94 patients, 83% were women (4). In a series of 144 cases presented by Smith (5), 73% were 40 to 60 years of age. Most of the patients have been treated for numerous other problems prior to the diagnosis of PFPS—for example, endometriosis, pelvic inflammatory disease, low back pain, lumbar disc disease, or degenerative joint disease. Many patients with this problem have had two or more laparoscopies and have had hysterectomies. A quote from Sinaki et al. (4) from their 1977 paper is illustrative of the bias of many physicians and the difficulty of diagnosis of PFPS: "Although rather simple, [the diagnosis] is usually obscured by a plethora of multiple, vague, and chronic physical complaints in a patient who is often neurotic."

ETIOLOGY

The direct cause of pain in PFPS is most likely spasm of one or more of the muscles of the pelvic diaphragm. Prolonged and repeatedly sustained muscular contraction leads to lactic acid formation with muscle fatigue and persistent pain (3). However, numerous problems have been proposed as indirect causes of this habitual or chronic muscular spasm (Table 45.4). In the 94 cases from the Mayo Clinic, a history of the following possible etiologic factors were noted: lower back or pelvic trauma without fracture or x-ray changes, 24; lumbar laminectomy, 12; irritable bowel syndrome, 5; hysterectomy, 19; poor posture, 35; deconditioned abdominal muscles, 32; and general muscle tenderness, 20. Many of the pathologies that contribute to PFPS are themselves sources of pain. The normal response to such pain may result in muscular contraction and spasm of the pelvic floor. However, in some cases this spasm persists and becomes itself a primary problem (6).

Abnormalities of posture are probably more important than generally appreciated in the etiology of this syndrome (Chapter 40). Many of the women are "slumpers" or "slouchers" who sit with pressure on the upper buttocks, coccyx, and base of the spine rather than on the ischial tuberosities. Prolonged sitting in this posture may result in fatigue and spasm of the supporting pelvic muscles (6).

Three muscles are partially inserted into the lateral border of the coccyx, the levator ani, coccygeus, and bundles from the gluteus maximus. These muscles tend to pull the coccyx anteriorly to its normal 120-degree angle to the sacrum (3). Slumping when sitting tends to flex the sacro-coccygeal joint, decreasing the angle to less than 120 degrees and increasing the pain of the PFPS. X-ray studies demonstrate this decreased angle in many patients with PFPS. In addition to slouching when sitting, many women with PFPS have other physical habits that cause asymmetric and excessive strain on the lumbar spine, abdomen, pelvis, and hips that may result in CPP: frequent periods of daily, prolonged sitting; unilateral standing patterns; sedentary lifestyles with poor muscular conditioning; and side or stomach sleeping (1). These habits may cause true mechanical strain on the joint capsules, ligaments, and muscles of the pelvis with pain as the consequence.

CPP of PFPS due to musculoskeletal dysfunction tends to be a disease of high-tech societies, where the majority of daily activities occur while sitting, not walking or standing. Long intervals of sitting cause adaptive changes in muscle length, strength, and tone, changes that result in abnormal postures (7). Normal or optimal posture is the position in which minimal muscle activity is required to overcome gravitational force and maintain erect bipedal stance or sit. The abnormal posture noted by Baker (1) was termed "typical pelvic pain posture" (TPPP). This is a kyphosis–lordosis usually, but occasionally just a marked lordosis (Fig. 3.3). TPPP is associated with a number of musculoskeletal dysfunctions:

- Stretch of the abdominals with resultant weakness and loss of tone
- Shortening of the thoracolumbar fascia
- Shortening of the posterior muscles of the trunk
- Compression of the posterior articulations of the lumbar spine
- Shortening of the iliopsoas muscles
- Increase of pelvic floor muscle tone

Baker (1) found these changes in 99 of 132 CPP patients.

Trigger points are a problem often noted in PFPS. Although not extremely well understood, trigger points appear to be associated with long-term changes in muscle length, probably representing the clinical manifestation of metabolic and mechanical strain on the muscle tissue (Chapter 38). The release of noxious or algesic substances may trigger musculoskeletal nociceptors to secondarily increase muscle tone or myofascial tension, even before the threshold for cognition of pain is reached. This increased tone, if localized, is a trigger point, and it may continue to release algesic substances, becoming a self-generating source of pain even after the initial insult has resolved.

Normal muscle tone is a fine balance, representing a continuous state of mild contraction dependent on (a) the integrity of nerves and their central connections and (b) the muscle's properties of contractility, elasticity, ductility, and extensibility. An increase of muscle tone is a common characteristic of most muscular dysfunctions. It appears to be the most common dysfunction associated with CPP due to musculoskeletal disorders. Most patients with PFPS have not only dysfunctional pelvic floor muscles, but also abdominal, lumbar spine, hip, and iliopsoas muscle dysfunctions. Each of these structures is capable of referring pain to the lower abdomen and pelvis (7).

TABLE 45.5. FACTORS THOUGHT TO AGGRAVATE PAIN IN PATIENTS WITH PELVIC FLOOR PAIN SYNDROME

Factor	Number	Percentage
Sitting for >1/2 hour	83	88
Tension (anxiety)	46	49
Bowel movements	31	33
Physical activity	28	30
Standing for >1/2 hr	15	16
Sexual intercourse	14	15
Lying supine	2	2
Nighttime	2	2

SYMPTOMS AND HISTORY

Symptoms are usually vague and poorly localized. Pain may be diffuse within the pelvis or more localized about the rectum or the anterior pelvis. In a significant number of patients the pain is unilateral. The pain is most often described as aching, throbbing, or heaviness. Similarly to patients with pelvic relaxation disorders, patients may describe the sensation as one of "everything falling out or dropping." Occasionally, it is described as pelvic pressure, but this sensation is more characteristic of pelvic relaxation defects than of spasm or tension of PFPS. The pain may be quite severe, and in some patients it has a characteristic of acute attacks that awake the patient from sleep with rectal pain ("proctalgia fugax") or vaginal pain ("colpalgia fugax"). Low back pain and radiation of pain to the sacrum at the area of insertion of the levator ani is not uncommon (greater than 80% of patients). Radiation to the hip and down the back of the thigh, like sciatica, may also be noted and is particularly characteristic of piriformis spasm.

Characteristically, the pain is not worsened by bowel movements (less than 33%), and only in a minority it is worsened by coitus (less than 15%). However, dyspareunia is a common symptom. Pain is increased by long sitting or prolonged standing in one position. Table 45.5 summarizes the aggravating factors noted in one series (4).

Characteristically, pain from spasm of the levator ani starts in the afternoon and becomes progressively worse. When the pain flares, it may be constant for days at a time. As previously noted, it sometimes occurs suddenly with a short duration.

The pain may mimic that due to diseases of the reproductive organs, with alterations and cyclic variations due to hormonal influences on the muscles, ligaments, and joints of the pelvis.

SIGNS AND PHYSICAL EXAMINATION

If PFPS is suspected, and in fact in all women with CPP, the initial portion of the pelvic examination should include a gentle, single finger palpation of the pelvic floor musculature to assess tone, sensation, and tenderness. The most common finding with PFPS is tenderness and spasm of one or more of the muscles of the pelvic floor. Digital pressure on the involved muscle characteristically reproduces or intensifies the patient's pain symptoms. It is not unusual for the tenderness to be unilateral.

The levator ani muscles are easily palpated during vaginal or rectal examination. They lie adjacent to the lateral vaginal walls just above the hymeneal ring. The medial margins of the muscles are slightly thicker than a standard pencil, running in an anteroposterior direction. Identification may be confirmed by having the patient contract her pelvic muscles. The anus simultaneously elevates when the levators are contracted. The bulbocavernous muscles lie distal to the hymeneal ring, allowing them to be easily differentiated from the levators (8).

The piriformis muscles are somewhat more difficult to palpate. Rectal examination may allow an easier evaluation than vaginal examination. With rectal examination, as one starts in the posterior midline and sweeps laterally and anteriorly, the rectal finger first passes over the piriformis, then the coccygeus and the levator ani muscles. The piriformis originates from the anterior surface of the sacrum and passes from the pelvis via the greater sciatic notch, and it may be palpated along this portion of its course. In the lithotomy position, if the patient is asked to abduct the thigh against resistance as the piriformis is palpated, there is exquisite tenderness of the muscle in cases of spasm or tension myalgia involving the piriformis.

In some patients with PFPS, there will also be tenderness of the coccyx, lateral sacrum, or sacrococcygeal ligaments.

DIAGNOSIS

The diagnosis of PFPS is by clinical history and physical findings. No imaging or laboratory evaluations are useful in establishing the diagnosis. However, because PFPS may not infrequently occur secondary to other pelvic pathology and pain, other evaluations may be needed to rule out diagnoses such as endometriosis or adhesions. This is especially true if PFPS does not respond to appropriate physical therapy and medical treatment.

It is important to also remember that other significant musculoskeletal dysfunctions may be associated with PFPS. A thorough musculoskeletal evaluation by a physical therapist or physiatrist is useful in patients with PFPS.

TREATMENT OR MANAGEMENT

The classic treatment for PFPS is Thiele's massage. This is done with the rectal finger, massaging the involved, tender muscles with a firm sweeping motion. Fifteen to twenty strokes, taking about 5 minutes, are done at each treatment. Treatments are repeated daily for 4 to 5 days, then every other day until improvement. Most often about six sessions are needed. The initial sessions are usually quite uncomfortable, and most patients note an exacerbation of pain after the first one or two treatments. I have found it most helpful to teach a physical therapist this technique, so that she may perform it as part of her overall treatment of patients with PFPS, rather than doing it myself as a solitary approach to treatment. Also, many women find it less unpleasant if the technique is modified to transvaginal massage rather transrectal.

Hot sitz baths may also be helpful, either as an adjunct to Thiele's massage or as an initial therapy prior to starting massage. Vaginal and rectal diathermy, ultrasound, bedrest, relaxation exercises, biofeedback training, analgesics, Kegel exercises, TENS unit, acupuncture, vaginal electrical stimulation, and infiltration with steroid and/or local anesthetic (especially if trigger points are present) are all treatments that are suggested for PFPS. There are no well-performed studies that allow a recommendation of any specific treatment modality or combination at this time. Coccygectomy is sometimes done for this syndrome; but it probably has little, if any, role in the modern management of the problem.

If an underlying etiology is found, then clearing that problem with appropriate therapy is likely to improve both the initial response and the duration of response. However, my bias is that most often the underlying etiology is postural, and this is not easy to correct. Because of this, physical therapy evaluation and treatment should be given serious consideration in all women with PFPS.

Finally, treatment with muscle relaxants, particularly diazepam, may be helpful for acute control of spasm and pain. McGivney and Cleveland treated 64 patients and obtained "marked" symptom relief in 51 patients with 3 weeks to 6 months of treatment with 10 to 30 mg per day of diazepam (3). Physical therapy was concurrently used. In my practice most patients with PFPS have had other significant problems as well, and treatment with diazepam has been less successful than McGivney's and Cleveland's experience. Physical therapy and frequent office visits with "counseling" sessions have been the most effective modalities in my experience.

REFERENCES

1. Baker PK. Musculoskeletal origins of chronic pelvic pain. *Obstet Gynecol Clin North Am* 1993;20:719–742.
2. Thiele GH. Coccygodynia and pain in the superior gluteal region. *JAMA* 1937;109:1271–1275.
3. McGivney JQ, Cleveland BR. The levator syndrome and its treatment. *South Med J* 1965;58:505–510.
4. Sinaki M, Merritt JL, Stillwell GK. Tension myalgia of the pelvic floor. *Mayo Clin Proc* 1977;52:717–722.
5. Smith WT. Levator spasm syndrome. *Minnesota Med* 1959; August;1076–1079.
6. Steege JF. Assessment and treatment of chronic pelvic pain. *Telinde's Operative Gynecology Updates* 1992;1:1–10.
7. King PM, Myers CA, Ling FW, et al. Musculoskeletal factors in chronic pelvic pain. *J Psychosom Obstet Gynaecol* 1991;12:87–98.
8. DeLancey JO, Sampselle CM, Punch MR. Kegel dyspareunia: levator ani myalgia caused by overexertion. *Obstet Gynecol* 1993;82: 658–659.

46

RECTUS ABDOMINIS PAIN

JAMES E. CARTER

KEY TERMS AND DEFINITIONS

Rectus abdominis pain or rectus syndrome: Somatic pain originating from the rectus abdominis musculature of the abdomen.

INTRODUCTION

The first clear description of abdominal pain originating from structures other than the viscera was provided in 1919 by Cyriax (1). He was convinced that in a number of cases "the diagnosis of referred pain of visceral disease is erroneous." He thought that such pains could be mimicked by lesions that affected the vertebra, ribs, or their associated muscles, or that they were the result of direct irritation of nerves in the intercostal spaces. By identifying conditions such as alterations in the normal vertebral curves, minor subluxation of vertebral bodies, and pressure on the peripheral portions of intercostal nerves, he was able to employ various mechanical treatments to correct the abnormalities and relieve his patient's symptoms (2).

Despite Cyriax's work, little attention was paid to the identification of parietal lesions until the observations of Carnett in 1926 (3). Carnett recognized diagnostic problems posed by abdominal wall lesions and maintained that abdominal pain could be caused by neuralgia affecting one or more of the lower six intercostal nerves. To distinguish this condition from intraabdominal diseases, he developed a simple test that, when positive, localized the origin of symptoms to the parietes rather than the viscera (2).

The segmental pattern of referred pain and other manifestations associated with visceral disease were reproduced by the injection of hypertonic saline into the interspinous ligaments (4). By injecting the interspinous ligament at the level of the first lumbar vertebra, pain could be produced which was both similar to that of renal colic and associated with the same somatic reflexes, such as muscular rigidity and retraction of the testes. All the features that we normally attribute to painful visceral disease could be derived from somatic structures lying in the appropriate dermatome.

Among patients who present with abdominal pain, female patients predominate. Even excluding gynecologic conditions, such as pelvic inflammatory disease, women still outnumber men by approximately 2:1. The average age of the patients with abdominal pain is 34 years (5). A large percentage of patients who present with abdominal pain have no identifiable cause for their complaint.

ETIOLOGY AND PATHOLOGY

The ability to define the site of a noxious stimulus becomes increasingly difficult as one passes through the deep tissues to the viscera. In contrast to the epicritic pain of cutaneous tissues, visceral and muscular conditions produce a dull aching pain that is felt more diffusely. At these deeper levels the site of the pain no longer provides an accurate guide to its origin. Parietal and visceral pain are frequently confused because of the phenomenon of referred pain. Referred pain is the somatic localization of sensory experiences evoked from the viscera. Referred abdominal pain results from the integration of nervous impulses rising in the two main divisions of the nervous system. The autonomic system provides visceral pain afferents via sympathetic nerves, and the somatic nervous system supplies the anterior abdominal wall with sensation via the lower six intercostal nerves. When a stimulus is applied to the viscera that is sufficiently great, pain is felt. However, because the viscera are not represented at a conscious level, the pain is not localized to a particular organ and is instead referred to the surface of the abdomen. It is referred to an area innervated by the same spinal cord segments that serve the affected viscus. According to the projection–convergence theory, visceral pain afferents entering the spinal cord converge with cutaneous pain efferents to end on a common neuron. The brain then interprets impulses reaching the common pathway as having come from the skin. The spinothalamic tract appears to be the most likely site for visceral and cutaneous afferents to converge. In this way, pain from the viscera and pain from the abdominal wall can be confused in terms of their origin by the patient and the diagnostician (2).

SYMPTOMS AND HISTORY

Features in the history that are important in the diagnosis of abdominal wall syndrome include (a) a relationship to abdominal surgery, (b) damage to muscle fibers following physical exertion, and (c) a long and fruitless search for visceral disease. Activities such as coughing, turning over in bed, or the lifting of heavy weights may all increase tension in the affected muscle groups and hence the discomfort of the abdominal wall pain. Generally, there is an absence of associated visceral symptoms, such as nausea, vomiting, diarrhea, or constipation, and of systemic symptoms, such as fever or chills.

SIGNS AND PHYSICAL EXAMINATION

Carnett's test is used to differentiate symptoms originating from the parietes from those arising from the viscera. The abdomen of the supine patient is palpated to elicit the area of tenderness. Then, with the palpating finger still located over the tender spot, the patient is asked to contract the abdominal muscles by raising the head from the examining table. Once the muscles are tensed, pressure is reapplied and the patient is asked if the pain has altered. If the cause of symptoms is intraabdominal, the tense muscles now protect the viscera and the tenderness should diminish. On the other hand, if the source resides in the abdominal wall, the pain will be at least as severe and, perhaps, increased (6).

False-positive diagnoses may arise when examining patients with conditions that have produced inflammation in the adjacent parietal peritoneum. This structure forms part of the anterior abdominal wall and therefore has a somatic nerve supply; tenderness will still be elicited on palpation after muscle contraction. The abolition of symptoms with local anesthetic strongly suggests a diagnosis of an abdominal wall origin for pain in these subjects (7).

In one study of 158 patients, 33% had a final diagnosis of appendicitis. Other visceral diagnoses included diverticulitis, peptic ulcer, pancreatitis, renal colic, and cholecystitis. This study showed a less impressive prognostic accuracy for a positive abdominal wall test, but confirmed that the test is positive in significantly more patients with nonspecific abdominal pain than with intraabdominal disease. This study supported the hypothesis that in up to 28% of patients with nonspecific abdominal pain, the pain arises in the muscles of the abdominal wall (8).

DIAGNOSTIC STUDIES

Figure 46.1 sets out an algorithmic approach to the diagnosis of abdominal wall pain. Although Carnett's test provides objective evidence of the diagnosis, the condition can often be suspected from features in the history (9).

DIAGNOSIS

Other causes of abdominal wall pain include iatrogenic peripheral nerve injuries, abdominal cutaneous nerve entrapment, hernias, myofascial pain syndromes, the rib tip syndrome, abdominal pain of spinal origin, and spontaneous rectus sheath hematoma (2).

Iatrogenic Peripheral Nerve Injuries

A prior surgical procedure is one of the commonest causes of abdominal wall pain (10). Where the incision directly involves a cutaneous nerve, subsequent entrapment of that nerve may occur either in a suture or in later scar formation. The ilioinguinal and iliohypogastric nerves are particularly at risk in lower abdominal incisions. In addition to Carnett's test, the following triad is diagnostic: (a) burning or shooting pains in the area supplied by the nerve; (b) impaired sensory function in the distribution of the nerve; and (c) relief of pain by infiltration with local anesthetic. Once recognized, treatment may be by local injection of steroids, local anesthetic or 5% phenol. Accurate placement of the injection is of paramount importance and may be improved by the use of a nerve stimulator. Should these measures fail, then exploration of the scar should be considered. The involved nerve is traced laterally to where it leaves the retroperitoneum and is then sectioned. The subsequent neuroma that forms generally produces no pain at this point. Cryoablation has also been used as a technique to reduce the pain from iatrogenic peripheral nerve injuries.

Abdominal Cutaneous Nerve Entrapment

A nerve entrapment syndrome may occur without prior surgical damage. Well-localized areas of abdominal tenderness may occur lying along the lateral margin of the rectus muscle. Such areas are produced at sites where the anterior cutaneous branch of an intercostal nerve passes through the rectus muscle to pierce its anterior sheath; in this position it may become intermittently compressed, producing pain that may mimic the pain normally associated with conditions such as biliary or renal colic. Patients suffering from this syndrome will obtain relief from local anesthetic injection. A resection of the relevant nerve as it emerges from the rectus muscle may be necessary (2,11).

Hernias

The majority of abdominal wall hernias are apparent on clinical examination, with the presence of a lump with an

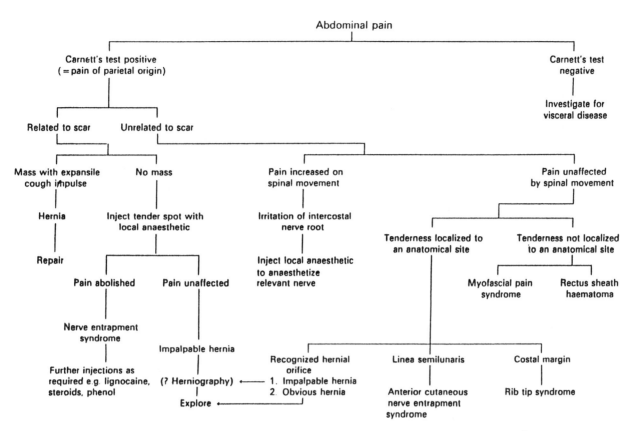

FIGURE 46.1. An approach to the diagnosis and management of abdominal wall pain. (From Gallegos NC, Hobsley M. The recognition and treatment of abdominal wall pain. *J R Soc Med* 1989;82:343–344, with permission.)

expansile cough impulse serving to make the diagnosis. However, some hernias elude detection, either because they are small or because the patient is obese. In cases where the diagnosis is suspected but clinically unconfirmed, additional investigation using radiography or ultrasonography may be helpful. Herniography, in which contrast medium is introduced into the peritoneal cavity, has been successfully used to reveal previously unsuspected inguinal hernias in patients with groin pain of uncertain origin and to detect impalpable interparietal lesions such as Spigelian hernias (3, 12,13). By traction of associated nerve, hernia may cause pain along a nerve distribution.

Myofascial Pain Syndromes

This group of syndromes is now well-described but continues to go unrecognized and remains poorly understood. The syndromes arise from the presence of trigger points in muscles or fascia. Such points are usually the result of antecedent trauma, and activity within them produces pain that may occur, for example, during muscle contraction. Diagnosis relies on finding the trigger spot, either by palpa-

tion or by eliciting certain physical signs such as a taut band of muscle fibers or localized twitch response when the involved part of the muscle is pinched. Treatment again rests on the acute injection of local anesthetic solution into the affected area. In some patients, several such areas may be present and require treatment (3,14,15) (Chapter 38).

The Rib Tip Syndrome

This syndrome, characterized by pain along the costal margin, is generated by the hypermobility of the eighth, ninth, and tenth ribs. These ribs do not articulate with the sternum but instead are bound to each other by a thin band of fibrous tissue. Should this fibrous attachment be divided, the rib may ride up and irritate the intercostal nerve to produce pain. The patient may be aware of a snapping or clicking sensation as the ribs move relative to one another, and the clinician can reproduce the symptoms by hooking his or her fingers under the costal margin and pulling upwards. Relief can be provided by anesthetizing the relevant intercostal nerve with local anesthetic; but if symptoms persist, rib tip resection may be necessary (16).

Abdominal Pain of Spinal Origin

The complex arrangement of musculoskeletal structures that make up the vertebral column, along with the close relationship that these bear to the nerve roots, can produce a variety of neurologic symptoms. When the normal anatomy is disturbed in such a way that the roots of the intercostal nerves are irritated, abdominal pain may result. In some cases the spinal origin of the pain will be made obvious by additional symptoms and signs, but in many patients with only minor degenerative disease the true etiology may escape identification. The diagnosis may be suspected by finding that the pain is aggravated by certain postures, by eliciting tenderness at the site of the pain which is increased by muscle contraction, and by observing posterior intercostal tenderness in the regions of the vertebral transverse processes. Intercostal nerve blocks have rendered pain-free 67% of those patients who had confirmed diagnosis of pain of spinal origin (2,17).

Spontaneous Rectus Sheath Hematoma

Spontaneous rectus sheath hematoma is a condition resulting from rupture of the epigastric vessels. The patient usually presents suddenly with well-localized abdominal pain associated with a tender nonpulsatile abdominal mass, usually in the lower abdomen. There is frequently a plausible precipitating factor such as local trauma, a bout of coughing, or anticoagulant therapy. The diagnosis can be confirmed on ultrasound examination, and a conservative approach to treatment can be adopted provided that the hematoma does not enlarge (18,19).

MANAGEMENT AND TREATMENT

Once an area of abdominal wall tenderness has been identified, its position is localized as accurately as possible with a single fingertip (20). Provided that the clinical picture suggests no other course of action, the tender spot is injected with a mixture of 1 mL 1% lignocaine and 25 mg hydrocortisone acetate using a 21-gauge needle. To start with, a small bleb is raised in the skin overlying the tender spot. The needle is then inserted, and its point is moved around in the tissues until the patient complains of pain that is similar to the original symptom. The injection is made into that point and into the immediately surrounding area. Eighty percent of correctly diagnosed patients are completely or partially relieved of their pain by this treatment. Prolonged relief of pain is provided for 67% of patients using an intercostal nerve block. Fifty-six percent of patients with parietal pain treated with local injections of 5% aqueous phenol are pain-free or improved at follow-up 3.5 years after treatment (21). In one study, treatment of abdominal wall trigger points was performed by placing a 22-gauge, 1.5-in. needle through the skin at the trigger point and slowly penetrating the fat pad until the needle tip reproduced the same sharp pain. The abdominal wall trigger points were found in fatty tissues above the fascia or along the margins of abdominal wall scar tissue. Injection of 3 to 5 mL of 0.25% bupivacaine stimulated sharp and at times severe pain followed by relief. All trigger points were blocked beginning with the most tender points up to a total dose of 50 mL. Additional trigger points of the vulva, vagina, cervix, and paracervical tissues were injected. Using these techniques a total of 89% of patients with abdominal pelvic pain syndrome reported relief or improvement in the pain such that no further therapy was required (22). The efficacy of injecting the parietes to relieve chronic abdominal symptoms has been well-demonstrated (23).

KEY POINTS

Differential Diagnoses

- Iatrogenic peripheral nerve injuries
- Abdominal cutaneous nerve entrapment
- Hernias
- Myofascial pain syndrome
- The rib tip syndrome
- Abdominal pain of spinal origin
- Spontaneous rectus sheath hematoma
- Appendicitis
- Other visceral diseases

Most Important Question to Ask

- Has the patient had a long and fruitless search for visceral disease?

Most Important Physical Examination Finding

- Persistence of the pain with pressure from the examining finger when the abdominal muscles are tensed (Carnett's sign)

Most Important Diagnostic Studies

- Abdominal wall ultrasonography
- Herniography
- Local anesthetic injections

Treatments

- Local anesthetic injections

REFERENCES

1. Cyriax EF. On various conditions that may simulate the referred

pains of visceral disease, and a consideration of these from the point of view of cause and effect. *Practitioner* 1919;102:314–322.

2. Gallegos NC, Hobsley M. Abdominal wall pain: an alternative diagnosis. *Br J Surg* 1990;77:1167–1170.

3. Carnett JB. Intercostal neuralgia as a cause of abdominal pain and tenderness. *Surg Gynecol Obstet* 1926;42:625–632.

4. Lewis T, Kellgren JH. Observations relating to referred pain, viscero-motor reflexes and other associated phenomena. *Clin Sci* 1939;4:47–71.

5. Adelman A. Abdominal pain in the primary care setting. *J Fam Pract* 1987;25:27–32.

6. Clearfield HR. Diagnosing parietal abdominal pain. *Hosp Pract* 1982;August:219–227.

7. Gallegos NC, Hobsley M. The recognition and treatment of abdominal wall pain. *J R Soc Med* 1989;82:343–344.

8. Gray WR, Dixon JM, Seabrook G, et al. Is abdominal wall tenderness a useful sign in the diagnosis of nonspecific abdominal pain? *Ann R Coll Surg Engl* 1988;70:233–234.

9. Gallegos NC, Hobsley M. Abdominal wall pain: an alternative diagnosis. *Br J Surg* 1990;77:1167–1170.

10. Stulz P. Peripheral nerve injuries resulting from common surgical procedures in the lower abdomen. *Arch Surg* 1982;117:324–327.

11. Applegate WV. Abdominal cutaneous nerve entrapment syndrome. *Surgery* 1972;71:118–124.

12. Ekberg O, Fork FT, Fritzdorf J. Herniography and atypical inguinal hernia. *Br J Radiol* 1984;57:1077–1082.

13. Holder LE, Schneider HJ. Spigelian hernias: anatomy and roentgenographic manifestations. *Radiology* 1974;112:309–313.

14. Simons DG, Travell JG. Myofascial pain syndrome. In: Wall PD, Melzack R, eds. *Textbook of pain.* Edinburgh: Churchill Livingstone, 1984:263–264.

15. Brown BR. Diagnosis and therapy of common myofascial syndromes. *JAMA* 1978;239:646–648.

16. McBeth AA, Keene JS. The rib-tip syndrome. *J Bone Joint Surg (Br)* 1975;57:795–797.

17. Ashby EC. Abdominal pain of spinal origin. *Ann R Coll Surg Engl* 1977;59:242–246.

18. Wyatt GM, Spitz HB. Ultrasound in the diagnosis of rectus sheath haematoma. *JAMA* 241:1499–1500.

19. Titone C, Lipsius M, Krakauer JS. Spontaneous hematoma of the rectus abdominis muscle: a critical review of 50 cases with emphasis on early diagnosis and treatment. *Surgery* 1972:568–572.

20. Choi YK, Chou S. Rectus syndrome: Another cause of upper abdominal pain. *Reg Anesth* 1995;20:347–351.

21. Mehta M, Ranger I. Persistent abdominal pain. *Anaesthesia* 1971;26:230–233.

22. Slocumb JC. Neurological factors in chronic pelvic pain: trigger points in the abdominal pelvic pain syndrome. *Am J Obstet Gynecol* 1984;149:536–543.

23. Melnick DG. Treatment of trigger mechanisms in gastrointestinal disease. *N Y State J Med* 1954;54:1324–1330.

47

ABDOMINAL EPILEPSY

AHMED M. EL-MINAWI

KEY TERMS AND DEFINITIONS

Abdominal epilepsy: Syndrome characterized by paroxysmal abdominopelvic pain often followed by tiredness, behavioral changes, and EEG abnormalities.

Polyserositis: A genetic disease affecting particular segments of the populace of the Mediterranean basin, including Arabs, Sephardic Jews, Turks, and Armenians. Typically, patients suffer bouts of fever accompanied by attacks of pain in one or more specific parts of the body or arthritic-like symptoms.

Porphyria: A group of inherited enzymatic disorders that affect the biosynthesis of heme and result in accumulation of porphyrins or their precursors.

INTRODUCTION

Abdominal epilepsy is a syndrome characterized by paroxysmal abdominopelvic pain often followed by tiredness, behavioral changes, and electroencephalographic (EEG) abnormalities. Most often the disorder occurs as short acute episodes, but it can be a chronic condition, particularly in the elderly (1). The dearth of information on the subject suggests that this a rare disorder, which, in fact, is not the case. Sporadic cases have been reported since the late nineteenth century, but it was not until the 1950s that it was fully described and named (2,3). The syndrome can afflict all age groups and does not occur "uniquely in children or young adolescents" as has been suggested (4).

ETIOLOGY AND PATHOPHYSIOLOGY

The pathophysiology of this disorder remains unclear. Stimulation of specific areas in the hypothalamus, brainstem, and cerebral cortex can result in a variety of visceral sensations. This is well-established in patients with temporal lobe seizures, in whom up to 20% experience a visceral aura preceding the motor seizure. These aural symptoms vary greatly, and they may be as simple as increased salivation or as serious as violent vomiting (4). The electrical discharges usually arise within the amygdala and are transmitted to the gastrointestinal tract via dense direct projections to the dorsal motor nucleus of the vagus. Sympathetic pathways from the amygdala to the gastrointestinal tract can also be activated via the hypothalamus (5).

Unlike temporal lobe seizures, abdominal epilepsy is an example of a convulsive equivalent state. Visceral symptoms may be the only sign of paroxysmal disturbance of cerebral electrical activity (4). However, it is not certain if the initial disturbance occurs in the brain. Several theories have been put forth to explain the relationship of the abdominal pain to brain electrical activity, based on the fact that the gastrointestinal tract is well represented in the epileptogenic regions of the limbic system (6):

1. Pain is central in origin and is referred to the abdomen.
2. Similarly to what occurs in temporal lobe seizures, bowel contraction occurs as a result of brain stimulation.
3. A primary gastrointestinal tract event, such as a bowel contraction, precipitates ictal discharges in the brain.

Based on the fact that all their patients were females, Peppercorn and Herzog (5) suggest a gender-based theory of neuroendocrine dysfunction as has been described in women with temporal lobe epilepsy. It is noteworthy that of 19 reported cases of abdominal epilepsy, 15 (79%) have been in females (1,2,5,7,8).

SYMPTOMS AND SIGNS

The syndrome of abdominal–visceral epilepsy is a recognized entity with a well-documented pattern of symptoms and signs that aid in diagnosis (Table 47.1). Nearly all patients with the syndrome complain of pain. The pain is usually paroxysmal, colicky, and nonradiating, and it is often in the periumbilical area, lower abdomen, or the right upper quadrant. In most cases, attacks last

TABLE 47.1. CRITERIA THAT AID IN DIAGNOSIS OF ABDOMINAL EPILEPSY

1. Paroxysmal abdominal pain
2. Exclusion of abdominal visceral pathology
3. Alterations of mental state during some of the attacks
4. Abnormal electroencephalographic tracing
5. Positive response to anticonvulsant therapy

only a few minutes, but multiple attacks may occur over the period of a day. Some patients complain of nausea during the episode. There may also be associated diarrhea, chronic constipation, or, particularly in children, cyclic vomiting (2,5,6,8).

A variety of behavioral and mental changes may occur during an attack, but it is rare for the patient to lose consciousness. States of confusion have been reported at the onset of an episode, whereas others have reported difficulty in remembering the event (4,5). Disorientation can occur, and patients have sensed complete disassociation from their surroundings during an attack. Lethargy and lassitude during the event are other complaints (2,5).

Headaches often occur, lasting the duration of the attack and for some time after. They have been described as pounding and usually unilateral. These are usually accompanied by dizziness, which is usually of short duration. Syncopal attacks have also been reported (1,2,4,5).

DIAGNOSIS

Criteria that aid in the diagnosis of this disorder are listed in Table 47.1. It is important to emphasize that the spectrum of gastrointestinal and central nervous system (CNS) manifestations need not all be present to make a diagnosis (2,5).

DIAGNOSTIC STUDIES

Most patients with this syndrome have an abnormal EEG (1). Although there is no stereotypical pattern of EEG abnormalities, the two most common patterns are:

- *Paroxysmal generalized dysrhythmia of slow activity*: This usually occurs episodically throughout the EEG record (1,2).
- *Paroxysmal spike-wave activity*: The spikes or sharp waves are most commonly localized over one or both temporal regions (1,2,4,5,7).

Sleep studies are of great importance and generally increase the incidence of case detection (5). At one time the presence of the so-called "14 and 6/sec positive spike pat-

tern" was considered to be diagnostic of abdominal epilepsy. This has been disputed because this was found in 50% of the normal young-adult and child population with EEG recordings showing light sleep drowsiness (1,4).

True abdominal epilepsy is relatively uncommon. Diagnosis must be made by exclusion of other causes and by adherence to rigid diagnostic criteria. After ruling out gastrointestinal disease, seizures, and other CNS disorders, the clinical should attempt to exclude other diseases that are commonly mistaken for abdominal epilepsy. Acute porphyrias and familial Mediterranean fever are two such entities.

Acute Porphyrias

The porphyrias are a group of inherited enzymatic disorders that affect the biosynthesis of heme and result in accumulation of porphyrins or their precursors. They most commonly manifest after puberty. The acute porphyrias, which include both neuroporphyrias and neurocutaneous porphyrias, are accompanied by acute and intermittent neurologic attacks whose manifestations mimic a variety of commonly occurring disorders and pose a diagnostic quagmire (9,10).

Autonomic dysfunctions manifest recurrently as abdominal pain, nausea or vomiting, tachycardia, and sweating (9). The abdominal pain is usually transient. Psychiatric manifestations include hysteria, anxiety, depression, phobias, and altered states of consciousness. Psychosis similar to schizophrenia may occur (10).

Diagnosis depends on the history, symptomatology, and measurement of porphyrins or precursors in urine or stool specimens. The Watson–Schwartz test is a qualitative screening test for porphobilinogen (PBG) in urine. Ideally, this should be done between attacks. With porphyria, PBG levels are twice normal. Quantitative tests such as ion-exchange chromatography give an accurate measurement of PBG levels (9).

Recurrent Polyserositis (Familial Mediterranean Fever)

This is a genetic disease affecting particular segments of the populace of the Mediterranean basin, including Arabs, Sephardic Jews, Turks, and Armenians. Due to immigration, it is now seen all over the world. Typically, the patients suffer bouts of fever accompanied by attacks of pain in one or more specific parts of the body and/or arthritic-like symptoms. There are no specific laboratory tests, and diagnosis is clinical. A variety of diagnostic criteria have been proposed over the years, but none are widely accepted. The most recent criteria proposed by Livneh et al. (11) have a sensitivity and specificity of 95% and 97%, respectively. This diagnostic approach depends on identification of a number of major and minor criteria (Table 47.2).

TABLE 47.2. SIMPLIFIED CRITERIA FOR THE DIAGNOSIS OF POLYSEROSITIS

Major Criteria (Typical Attacks)	Minor Criteria (Incomplete Attacks)
1. Peritonitis (generalized)	1. Chest pain
2. Unilateral pleuritis or pericarditis	2. Joint pain
3. Monoarthritis (hip, knee, ankle)	3. Exertional leg pain
4. Fever alone	4. Favorable response to colchicine

TREATMENT OF ABDOMINAL EPILEPSY

The prognosis for patients with this disease is good. As previously stated in the diagnostic criteria, there is almost always a positive response to anticonvulsant therapy. In fact, a therapeutic trial of anticonvulsants following an abnormal EEG leads to nearly complete abolition of both gastrointestinal and CNS manifestations. The most commonly employed drugs have been phenytoin and phenobarbital, but diazepam has also been used effectively. Zarling (1) reports complete resolution with a therapeutic serum level of phenytoin sodium of 14.4 μg/mL. Patients should be encouraged to continue maintenance anticonvulsant therapy, because recurrences have occurred after cessation of medication (1,5,8).

KEY POINTS

Differential Diagnosis

- Acute porphyria
- Polyserositis (familial Mediterranean fever)

Important Questions to Ask

- Was the attack associated with a feeling of disorientation or confusion?
- Did the patient feel fatigued or sleepy after the attack?
- Did the attacks end while on anticonvulsant therapy?

Important Physical Examination Findings

- Normal physical findings

Important Diagnostic Studies

- EEG tracing
- Sleep EEG tracing

Treatment

- Anticonvulsant drugs: phenytoin, phenobarbital, diazepam

REFERENCES

1. Zarling EJ. Abdominal epilepsy: an unusual cause of recurrent abdominal pain. *Am J Gastroenterol* 1984;79(9):687–688.
2. Douglas EF, White PT. Abdominal epilepsy: a reappraisal. *J Pediatr* 1971;78(1):59–67.
3. Moore MT. Abdominal epilepsy. *J Bras Psiqiat* 1952;1:5–32.
4. Babb RR, Eckman PB. Abdominal epilepsy. *JAMA* 1972;222(1):65–66.
5. Peppercorn MA, Herzog AG. The spectrum of abdominal epilepsy in adults. *Am J Gastroenterol* 1989;84(10):1294–1296.
6. Peppercorn MA, Herzog AG, Dichter MA, et al. Abdominal epilepsy: a cause of abdominal pain in adults. *JAMA* 1978;240(22):2450–2451.
7. Agrawal P, Dhar NK, Bhatia MS. Abdominal epilepsy. *Ind J Pediatr* 1989;56(4):539–541.
8. Mitchell WG, Greenwood RS, Messenheimer JA. Abdominal epilepsy. Cyclic vomiting as the major symptom of simple partial seizures. *Arch Neurol* 1983;40:251–252.
9. Tefferi A, Colga JP, Solberg LA, Jr. Acute porphyrias: diagnosis and management. *Mayo Clin Proc* 1994;69:991–995.
10. Burgovne K, Swarz R, Ananth J. Porphyria: reexamination of psychiatric implications. *Psychother Psychosom* 1995;64(3–4):121–130.
11. Livneh A, Langevitz P, Zemer D, et al. Criteria for the diagnosis of familial Mediterranean fever. *Arthritis Rheum* 1997;40(10):1879–1885.

48

ABDOMINAL MIGRAINES

JAMES E. CARTER

KEY TERMS AND DEFINITIONS

Abdominal migraine: A disorder that causes characteristic episodic abdominal pain that lasts for 1 hr or more, may or may not be associated with headache, almost always includes nausea, and characteristically ends when the individual falls asleep.

INTRODUCTION

Migraine is more than just a headache. Patients usually suffer from abdominal symptoms, such as vomiting, bloating, diarrhea, and abdominal pain. Though the symptomatology and pathophysiology of migraine headaches have been extensively studied, little attention has been paid to disturbances in the rest of the body during the migraine attack. In some patients, abdominal symptoms are more troublesome than the headache itself. The episodes of abdominal pain may be a cardinal symptom and may be a headache equivalent. Abdominal pain without headache may be common as a migraine equivalent in children, but the frequency of this phenomenon in adult migraineurs has not been ascertained (1).

The prevalence and clinical features of migraine headache and abdominal migraine were studied in a well-defined population of schoolchildren. Children with at least two episodes of severe headache or severe abdominal pain, attributed by the parents either to unknown causes or to migraine, were interviewed and examined. Ten percent of children fulfilled the International Headache Society's criteria for the diagnosis of migraine. Four percent of children had abdominal migraine. A population-based study of recurrent abdominal pain performed in 1993 showed that 2% of children 3 to 11 years of age satisfied the clinical features of abdominal migraine (2). Children with abdominal migraine have demographic and social characteristics similar to those of children with migraine headache. They also have similar patterns of associated recurrent painful conditions, trigger and relieving factors, and associated symptoms during attacks. Similarities between the two conditions are so close as to suggest they have a common pathogenesis (3). Abdominal migraine is associated with a mean of 3.7 days per year of school absence because of the recurrent abdominal pain. With a possible prevalence of 4% in children, it may represent a sizable clinical and social problem.

The concept of abdominal migraine as a disease entity has been debated since the start of the twentieth century. In 1922 three adult patients with abdominal migraine were described. Abdominal migraine was defined as a disorder comprising (a) personal or family history of typical migraine headache and (b) attacks of epigastralgia with nausea, vomiting, bile, and mucus, and occasionally with diarrhea in the absence of any definite abnormal signs on physical examination (4). The attacks lasted for a few days and began and ended rather abruptly with complete resolution between attacks.

In a study of 85 patients with nonorganic abdominal pain unresponsive to a high-fiber diet, a detailed analysis of the symptoms and family history suggested that in 19 the symptoms might have been caused by abdominal migraine. Six of the 19 had typical migraine-associated symptoms during the attack, characteristic abdominal pain in their family history, or a personal history of classic migraine headaches (5).

Childhood abdominal migraine is slightly more common in girls than in boys (1.2:1) and starts at a mean age of 7 years with two distinct peaks at ages 5 and 10 years. The prevalence rate of migraine headache in children with abdominal migraine is 24%, about twice the prevalence of migraine in the general childhood population (11%). Conversely, the prevalence rate of abdominal migraine in children with migraine is 9%, just more than twice the prevalence of 4% of abdominal migraine in the general childhood population (3).

Among adult migraineurs, 12 of 100 have recurrent attacks of abdominal pain (1). The mean age in this group is 30 years. All have a family history of migraine. Similar recurrent attacks of unexplained abdominal pain have not been observed in patients with tension headaches unless there is a family history of migraine (1).

ETIOLOGY

The observation that abdominal migraines are found in patients with migraine headaches and that headaches and abdominal pain occur together suggest that the attacks of abdominal pain are migraine equivalents. This is further supported by treatment responses abdominal migraine to migraine therapies. The observation that recurrent attacks of abdominal pain occur in migraineurs, but not in patients with tension headaches, also supports the suggestion that both migraine and abdominal pain may have a common etiology in these patients.

Further support of this concept comes from a study of 132 children with recurrent abdominal pain that led to the removal of a normal appendix. Follow-up was available on 90 of the patients, and 54 (60%) subsequently developed adult migraine headaches (6).

SYMPTOMS OR HISTORY

The history is of paramount importance in abdominal migraine, because the diagnosis depends on a history of typical symptoms and strong family history of typical migraine headache. There are no specific tests for the disorder.

Generally, pain with abdominal migraine is located in the upper half of the abdomen, but many patients have pain centered around the umbilicus, in the lower part of the abdomen, or poorly localized. It is dull or colicky in nature. An episode can last up to 72 hours, but characteristically it ends when the patient falls asleep. There is no impairment of consciousness during the attacks, but some patients fall asleep afterwards. Usually the patient awakens feeling much improved (7). A number of symptoms may occur in association with the abdominal pain, such as headache, pallor, anorexia, nausea, vomiting, dizziness, visual disturbances, focal paresthesias, and radiation into the limbs. Transient fever and diarrhea are uncommon but can occur with migraine. Patients characteristically have concurrent headaches or have alternating attacks of headaches and abdominal pain. Symptoms may occur up to several times per week, but do not usually occur on a daily basis. The pain resolves completely between attacks.

Attacks of pain with abdominal migraine are similar to attacks of migraine headache in that they commonly have triggering and relieving factors and have associated gastrointestinal, sensory, and vasomotor symptoms. It has been suggested that in almost all patients the attacks of abdominal pain appear first in childhood or early adult life and are self-limiting. In a large subgroup of children the abdominal pain is typically severe enough to disturb the child's normal daily activities. In children there can be episodic abdominal pain even in the absence of headache. Despite the recurrent nature of the condition, the children are healthy with normal growth and development. Because no obvious organic cause can be found, the condition has been termed *psychogenic* abdominal pain, although no psychologic differences have been found between these children and pain-free control children, or children with abdominal pain and known organic cause. Abdominal migraine or migraine equivalent should be considered in children with otherwise unexplained severe recurrent abdominal pain.

Also, abdominal migraine should be considered in adults with abdominal pain when symptoms are not typical of irritable bowel syndrome and organic disease has been excluded (8). There is significant controversy about the existence of abdominal migraine in adult populations. It has been stated that abdominal pain is not a feature of adult migraine unless provoked by vomiting, altered large bowel frequency, or rectal tenesmus (9).

PHYSICAL EXAMINATION AND DIAGNOSTIC STUDIES

There are no specific signs at physical examination or specific diagnostic studies for abdominal migraine. With a thorough evaluation, no cause for the abdominal pain can be readily identified.

DIAGNOSIS

Abdominal migraine as a clinical diagnosis continues to be a subject of controversy. The criteria for the diagnosis of abdominal migraine are that the pain is:

- Severe enough to interfere with normal daily activities
- Dull or colicky in nature
- Periumbilical or poorly localized
- Associated with any two of the following: anorexia, nausea, vomiting, pallor
- Of at least 1-hr duration with each attack
- Completely resolves between attacks (3)

Thus patients with mild symptoms that do not interfere with normal activities and with attacks of less than 1-hr duration are excluded from a diagnosis of abdominal migraine. Also patients who have burning abdominal pain and gastroesophageal reflux or peptic ulceration should be excluded. Those with pain associated with large bowel or renal disease or with a menstrual disorder are excluded. Patients who fulfill the above criteria for abdominal migraine, but also have problems with food intolerance, malabsorption, weight loss, or persistent symptoms between attacks of abdominal pain, should be excluded, too.

Some of the other potentially identifiable causes for recurrent abdominal pain include constipation, food or lactose intolerance, gastroesophageal reflux, peptic ulceration, duodenitis, Crohn's disease, urinary tract infections, and menstrual disorders (3). These diagnoses are discussed elsewhere in this text.

MANAGEMENT OR TREATMENT

Abdominal migraine may respond favorably to the use of antimigraine medical treatment. In one study in which 12% of migraineurs had recurrent attacks of abdominal pain (2), treatment was provided with ergotamine tartrate 0.25 to 0.5 mg subcutaneously or Cafergot orally for the pain. Some patients were treated prophylactically with Orgametil (lynestrenol), 5 mg daily, flumedroxone 10 mg daily, or cyproheptadine 4 mg daily for 2 to 18 months. With these treatments, 80% of the patient's were symptom-free during therapy (2). In children, pizotifen syrup has been utilized for the treatment of abdominal migraine with great success (10).

Abdominal migraine is well-recognized in children; but in spite of anecdotal reports, migraine is not well-established as a cause of abdominal pain in adults (11). Functional abdominal pain is usually classified as either irritable bowel syndrome or nonulcer dyspepsia. Some patients have intermittent abdominal pain associated with headache or other migraine symptoms, and in these patients a diagnosis of abdominal migraine should be considered. It is possible that some patients with functional abdominal pain have migraine presenting with few or even no associated migraine symptoms. There are only clinical criteria for diagnosing abdominal migraine, and research in this area is therefore very difficult. Nevertheless, some patients with functional abdominal pain may respond to antimigraine medication; and if their symptoms are suggestive, a trial of therapy may be desirable (11).

In an interesting study of 31 children with a median age of 12 years and suffering from migraine headaches, endoscopic evaluations showed 42% had esophagitis, 52% had gastritis of the corpus, 39% had antral gastritis, and 87% had duodenitis. Also, *Helicobacter pylori* colonization was found in 7 of the children. Overall, 29 of the 31 children had underlying inflammatory lesions that could explain their abdominal and gastrointestinal complaints (6). Ranitidine and tripotassium dicitratobismuthate, with or without antibiotics, were more effective than placebo in the management of this group of children with migraine. These data suggest that not all gastric symptoms such as nausea, vomiting, and recurrent abdominal pain associated with migraine are neurally mediated (6).

KEY POINTS

Differential Diagnoses

- Constipation
- Food or lactose intolerance
- Gastroesophageal reflux
- Peptic ulceration
- Duodenitis
- Crohn's disease
- Urinary tract infections
- Menstrual disorders, especially dysmenorrhea

Most Important Questions to Ask

- Is there a history of migraine headache as a child?
- Is there a history of recurrent abdominal pain as a child without a diagnosis?
- Is there occurrence of migraine headaches at the same or at other times than the recurrent abdominal pain?

Most Important Physical Examination Findings

- Abdominal migraine is a diagnosis of exclusion and can only be determined by the effectiveness of the therapy with migraine medications.

Most Important Diagnostic Studies

- Most important diagnostic studies are the gastrointestinal evaluation for other causes of abdominal pain such as positive findings of inflammation of the gastrointestinal tract, which, when treated, result in elimination of the migraine headache symptoms.

Treatments

- Treatments with antimigraine medications are therapeutic options.

REFERENCES

1. Lundberg PO. Abdominal migraine—diagnosis and therapy. *Headache* 1975;15:122–125.
2. Mortimer MK, Kay J, Jaron A. Clinical epidemiology of childhood abdominal migraine in an urban general practice. *Dev Med Child Neurol* 1993;35:243–248.
3. Abu-Arafeh I, Russell G. Prevalence and clinical features of abdominal migraine compared with those of migraine headache. *Arch Dis Child* 1995;72:413–417.
4. Brams WA. Abdominal migraine. *JAMA* 1922:78:26–27.
5. Long DE, Jones SC, Boyd N, et al. Abdominal migraine: A cause of abdominal pain in adults? *J Gastroenterol Hepatol* 1992;7:210–213.
6. Mavromichalis I, Zaramboukas T, Giala MM. Migraine of gastrointestinal origin. *Eur J Pediatr* 1995;154:406–410.
7. Sellman GL. *Pain management.* In: Nelson WE, Behrman RE, Kliegman RM, eds. *Nelson: Textbook of pediatrics,* 15th ed. Philadelphia: WB Saunders, 1996:287–298.
8. Long DE, Jones SC, Boyd N, et al. Abdominal migraine: a cause of abdominal pain in adults? *J Gastroenterol Hepatol* 1992;7:210–213.
9. Blau JN, MacGregor EA. Is abdominal pain a feature of adult migraine? *Headache* 1995;35:207–209.
10. Symon DNK, Russell G. Double blind placebo controlled trial of pizotifen syrup in the treatment of abdominal migraine. *Arch Dis Child* 1995;72:48–50.
11. Axon ATR. Abdominal migraine: does it exist? *J Clin Gastroenterol* 1991;13:615–616.

49

BIPOLAR DISORDERS

DANIEL M. DOLEYS
DANIEL C. LOWERY
FRED M. HOWARD

INTRODUCTION

Bipolar disorders are considered under the major heading of mood disorders in *Diagnostic and Statistics Manual-IV* (DSM-IV) (1). A patient is defined as having bipolar disorder if he or she has had a manic episode (Table 49.1) or a hypomanic (mild mania) episode, even if the patient has never had a depressive episode. This definition is supported by observational data on the course of the illness. Patients with bipolar disorders are differentiated into bipolar I disorder, bipolar II disorder, and bipolar disorder NOS (not otherwise specified). Bipolar I disorder is characterized by one or more manic or mixed episodes accompanied by a depressive episode. Bipolar II disorder is characterized by one or more major depressive episodes accompanied by at least one hypomanic episode. Bipolar disorder NOS includes disorders wherein information is inadequate or too contradictory to make a definitive diagnosis but suggests the presence of bipolarity. The lifetime prevalence of a bipolar I disorder has been estimated at 0.04% to 1.6%, and that of bipolar II has been estimated at 0.5%. Although no gender differences have been reported regarding bipolar I disorder, it appears as though bipolar II disorder is more common in women than in men.

The symbiotic relationship between depression and pain is categorically established. Whether this relationship is altered depending upon the type of depression (major depressive episode versus bipolar I versus bipolar II) or the severity of depression remains unclear. Furthermore, the relationship of these factors to patients suffering from chronic pelvic pain has received relatively little systematic investigation. In an effort to secure information for this chapter, two MedLine searches were conducted using key words "mental disorders and pelvic pain" and "bipolar disorder and pain." Twenty-nine articles from 1993 to 1998 were found under "mental disorders and pelvic pain" (these are listed in the appendix to this chapter). However, none of these articles specifically dealt with bipolar disorder and pelvic pain. Eighty-one articles were cited from

1966 to 1998 under "bipolar disorder and pain." None of the articles specifically discussed or utilized patients with bipolar disorder who have pain predominantly located in the pelvic region. The most common pain diagnosis or etiology was headache. Therefore, at this point in time, no statement can be made as to the specifics of a relationship between bipolar disorder and chronic pelvic pain in women. Whether there is a relationship similar to the one noted between unipolar depressive disorders and chronic pain (including chronic pelvic pain) has not been specifically evaluated. Systematic pain ratings and the administration of qualitative and quantitative testing such as the McGill Pain Questionnaire in women suffering from chronic pelvic pain during depressive and/or manic episodes is sorely needed.

ETIOLOGY

The relationship between pain and depression appears well established. Most studies have estimated that 30% to 60% of patients with mood disorder complain of pain (2). In addition, the most prevalent psychiatric diagnoses among patients with chronic pain are major depression and dysthymia. Some have indicated that the onset of depression predisposes a patient to the development of chronic pain. Others have noted depression to be a result. Independent of the order in which they appear, pain and depression seem to function in a synergistic fashion, each enhancing the magnitude of the other. Although the research literature clearly documents the relation between depression and pain, there appears to have been little work at specifically identifying those patients with a bipolar mood disorder in an effort to determine any differential response to experimental pain or treatment.

Several studies have been carried out in an attempt to evaluate the relationship between pain and depression. One might be tempted to hypothesize that depressed patients are more responsive to pain. This hypothesis has been tested in

TABLE 49.1. DSM-IV CRITERIA FOR A MANIC EPISODE

A. A distinct period of abnormally and persistently elevated, expansive, or irritable mood, lasting at least 1 week (or any duration if hospitalization is necessary).

B. During the period of mood disturbance, three (or more) of the following symptoms have persisted (four if the mood is only irritable) and have been present to a significant degree:
   1. Inflated self-esteem or grandiosity.
   2. Decreased need for sleep (e.g., feels rested after only 3 hr of sleep).
   3. More talkative than usual or pressure to keep talking.
   4. Flight of ideas or subjective experience that thoughts are racing.
   5. Distractibility (i.e., attention too easily drawn to unimportant or irrelevant external stimuli).
   6. Increase in goal-directed activity (either socially, at work or school, or sexually) or psychomotor agitation.
   7. Excessive involvement in pleasurable activities that have a high potential for painful consequences (e.g., engaging in unrestrained buying sprees, sexual indiscretions, or foolish business investments).

C. The symptoms do not meet criteria for a mixed episode (i.e., mixed manic and depressive symptoms are present, in which case a mixed episode is diagnosed).

D. The mood disturbance is sufficiently sever to cause marked impairment in occupational functioning or in usual social activities or relationships with others, or to necessitate hospitalization to prevent harm to self or others, or there are psychotic features.

E. The symptoms are not caused by the direct physiologic effects of a substance (e.g., a drug of abuse, a medication, or other treatment) or a general medical condition (e.g., hyperthyroidism).

Note: Manic-like episodes that are clearly caused by somatic antidepressant treatment (e.g., medication, electroconvulsive therapy, light therapy) should not count toward a diagnosis of bipolar I disorder.

the laboratory evaluating the response of depressed patients to various stimuli including electrical pain (3–9), thermal pain (10–12), pinprick and pressure pain (3,13), and cold pressor pain (13–15). Overall, the results of these studies show that patients with mood disorders tend to be less responsive to experimental pain than controlled subjects. Considering that the perception of pain involves both sensory and affective processes, it is unclear if the apparent analgesia seen in depressed patients is secondary to some sensory deficit or an affective impediment.

A study by Davis et al. (6) was one of the few to distinguish between the sensory and affective processes involved in pain perception utilizing patients divided into manic and depressed groups. An electrical stimulus, varying in intensity, was presented to the left forearm. Subjects rated the stimulus as noticeable, distinct, unpleasant, or very unpleasant. "Pain counts" were the total number of unpleasant or very unpleasant responses. The results showed that depressed patients as a group had fewer "pain counts" than control subjects. Furthermore, the level of stimulus that differentiated "distinct" from "unpleasant" was higher for depressed subjects than for controlled subjects. These findings were somewhat higher for depressed men than for depressed women. When considered separately, depressed women did not seem to differ significantly from nondepressed subjects. In the male population both "unipolar and bipolar" depressed patients demonstrated analgesia measured by pain counts, whereas only unipolar males showed a significant increase in the distinct/unpleasant response level and only bipolar males demonstrated significant analgesia to pain insensitivity measures.

Of the bipolar patients, 10 were actively manic. Women in the manic phase did not differ from controls in most cat-

egories, but they did appear to be more pain-responsive. Yet, there was some element of an analgesic pattern noted on measures of pain "insensitivity." On the other hand, men in the manic phase demonstrated an analgesic pattern in all four categories.

Fishbain (16) theorized that the manic state may be caused by an excess of endorphin activity, which may help explain the pain insensitivity observed in manic patients. If Fishbain's theory is correct, then displacing endorphins from their opiate receptor sites could ameliorate the manic symptoms. Researchers tested this hypothesis by administering to manic patients the drug naloxone hydrochloride, which displaces endorphins from their opiate receptor sites. After administering the drug, Janowsky et al. (17) reported acute, antimanic effects such as loss of hyperactivity, grandiosity, and pressure of thoughts and speech. Emrich et al. (18) and Davis et al. (6) were unable to reproduce these findings.

Overall the data show that depressed patients seem more analgesic than normal subjects to an experimental electrical stimulus. These findings are similar to those reported by others (3–5,10,11). Although the gender differences may be difficult to explain, studies have begun to delineate gender as a factor in pain sensitivity.

Regarding the sensory and affective processes of pain, Davis et al. (6) examined ratings for the barely noticeable electrical stimulus. No differences were found between depressed and control subjects except for those patients who appear to be in a manic phase. It was felt, therefore, that the results were more likely to be attributable to affective measures rather than a sensory impediment.

Clark and Mehl (12) evaluated the responsivity of psychiatric patients to a thermal stimulus. Some years later,

Dworkin et al. (2) reanalyzed the data, sorting the psychiatric patients into major depression or bipolar disorder. The experimental design involved the administration in a randomized sequence of stimuli 3 sec in duration at one of five intensities. Dworkin et al. found that patients with major depression and bipolar disorders were less responsive to the painful stimulus than were the controls. Patients with major depression did not differ from controlled subjects in sensory discrimination aspects of the task for lower intensity stimuli but had poor sensory discrimination for higher intensity stimuli. The bipolar disordered patients did not differ from controlled subjects in sensory discrimination at either high or low intensities but did show some element of analgesia to lower stimuli intensity levels.

Dworkin et al. (2) concluded that patients with major depression and controlled subjects differed significantly in sensory discrimination of painful stimuli but not in discrimination of nonpainful stimuli. The apparent insensitivity of depressed patients was not a result of some abnormal cognitive processing or poor attention. It was felt that both affective and sensory processes were involved. Gender analysis was precluded by the small sample size.

SYMPTOMS

Patients with bipolar disorder typically have histories of onset in young adulthood, most commonly in the second or third decade. Occasionally, there is a history of onset in childhood. Much less often the onset is later in life, even in the elderly years. Most often there is a history of recurrent episodes of illness, but there rarely is a history of only an isolated prior episode.

Symptoms develop over the course of days to weeks. With manic episodes there may be a history of precipitation by antidepressant therapy or sleep deprivation. During manic episodes, patients exhibit euphoria or irritability, increased energy, and decreased need for sleep. They are often intrusive, have increased sexual drive, and are impulsive. They often have inflated self-esteem, which may be delusional. Mood is usually elevated, and patients are infectiously cheerful and unselectively enthusiastic. However, the euphoria may easily reverse and the patient may suddenly become irritable, angry, or sad. This marked lability is a basic characteristic of mania. Patients may have brief periods of tearfulness, or even depression and suicidal ideation, even if the predominant mood is euphoric.

In some cases, patients may be predominantly irritable, paranoid, and dysphoric and may exhibit little or no euphoria or be euphoric only early in the manic episode. This dysphoric manic presentation sometimes leads to a misdiagnosis of depression or schizophrenia. The diagnosis of dysphoric mania in such cases is suggested by a past history of bipolar disorder, by the presence of other components of the manic syndrome such as increased energy and decreased need for sleep, and by the progression of the current episode.

Psychotic symptoms, such as delusions of special powers or hearing voices, are common during manic episodes. These symptoms are usually compatible with the elevated mood. However, some patients have florid psychotic symptoms, including bizarre delusions, that make it difficult to distinguish the illness for schizophrenia. Again, the correct diagnosis is based on the presence of typical manic symptoms, course of illness, and family history. Patients who have chronic psychotic symptoms superimposed on unipolar or bipolar disorder are often described as schizoaffective.

During depressive episodes, symptoms of patients with bipolar disorder are indistinguishable from those of patients with unipolar depression. The onset of either manic or depressive episodes tends to be acute. The rate of cycling between mania and depression varies widely among individuals, but often the episodes tend to become more frequent with age. Between episodes of depression and mania, the majority of patients are free of symptoms, but up to one-third may have some residual symptoms.

Corticosteroids, cocaine, amphetamines, phencyclidine, alcohol, and other drugs can cause disinhibition, expansive mood, irritability, emotional lability, and psychosis that can mimic acute mania. Therefore, a drug history and toxicology screen are important parts of the history and evaluation for mania.

SIGNS

Often speech is loud, rapid, pressured, and difficult to interrupt. On mental status examination, patients appear distractible, may not be able to stick to a topic, and may have flight of ideas. There may be evidence of marked mood lability.

DIAGNOSIS

There are no pathognomonic markers for bipolar disorder. Diagnosis is made on the basis of clinical presentation, the course of the illness, and a positive family history. Differentiation from other psychiatric disorders is not always easy, but is usually possible.

Schizophrenia may be confused with bipolar disorder, but even in the presence of florid psychotic symptoms or dysphoria, mania can generally be distinguished from schizophrenia. Whereas the onset of schizophrenia is usually insidious and the course chronic, mania is generally associated with an acute onset and episodic course. Acute exacerbations that may be superimposed on the chronic course of schizophrenia can cause some uncertainty. However, schizophrenic patients usually do not have prominent sleep disturbances or changes in appetite or energy. Delusions are more frequent and more bizarre with schizophrenia than with bipolar disorder. Schizophrenic patients typically have bland or flat affects. The family history is more likely to be significant for schizophrenia in schizophrenic patients and for mood disorder in bipolar disorder patients.

Personality disorders are not uncommon in women with chronic pelvic pain and are distinguished by unstable moods. Those with borderline or histrionic personality disorders may have symptoms similar to those of hypomania (mild mania) and depression. However, mood fluctuations are often extremely rapid and occur within hours, in contrast to bipolar disorder in which fluctuations are usually gradual and take days. Patients with personality disorders do not usually have vegetative symptoms of depression.

Bipolar disorder must also be differentiated from cyclothymic disorder, which has periods of depression but not of a degree that would qualify as major depressive episodes. Additionally, cyclothymic disorder differs from bipolar disorder in that it involves numerous periods of hypomanic symptoms of at least 2 years' duration which do not meet the criteria of a manic episode.

MANAGEMENT OR TREATMENT

Prompt treatment of bipolar disorder, especially with manic episodes, is crucial. Without prompt treatment, mania can cause poor judgment that endangers interpersonal relationships, jobs, possessions, and financial resources. Management of mania must include not only medication, but also protection from potentially harmful activities. Thus, initial management is usually best accomplished in a hospital. This may require the help of the patient's family because manic patients are often incapable of reasonable discussion and action.

Lithium is the drug of choice for the treatment of acute mania and for prophylaxis against both manic and depressive recurrences in patients with bipolar disorder. It is effective in 70% to 80% of cases of acute mania when therapeutic serum levels of approximately 1 mmol/L are achieved. Measurement of serum concentration is vital for effective management and treatment with lithium. Initial improvement may not occur until at least 14 days of treatment, and a full response may take 4 to 6 weeks. Because the response to lithium is slow, treatment with antipsychotic drugs (e.g., such as 10 mg/day of haloperidol) is necessary when mania is severe.

Before lithium is started, it is important to assess renal function with blood urea nitrogen (BUN) and creatinine levels. Thyroid function also needs to be evaluated, which can be done with measurement of thyroid-stimulating hormone level. If the woman is over 40 years of age or she has a history of cardiac disease, then an electrocardiogram should be performed. Clinically significant conduction disturbances due to lithium are rare, although sinus node dysfunction and sinoatrial block have been reported. Patients with preexisting sinoatrial node dysfunction should probably be treated with lithium only if they have a pacemaker.

Toxic lithium levels may occur with sodium depletion, so patients taking lithium should be instructed to maintain uniform salt intake. Diuretics and rapid weight-loss diets are best avoided, but if they are essential they require careful medical supervision. Also, care must be taken with over-the-counter medications such as nonsteroidal antiinflammatory drugs that may alter renal blood flow without careful monitoring of lithium levels. In adults with normal renal function, the initial dosage is 300 mg three times per day, but dosages as low as 150 mg/day should be used if the patient is elderly or has renal disease. Again it must be stated that safe and effective use of lithium can be monitored only by measuring serum levels. Levels are measured every 5 days and used to adjust the dosage to achieve a therapeutic level. For acute mania the therapeutic range is 1.0 to 1.2 mEq/L. For long-term prophylaxis, most physicians have recommended lithium levels in the range of 0.4 to 0.6 mEq/L to minimize side effects, but evidence suggests that in lithium-responsive patients, levels of 0.8 to 1.0 mEq/L are more effective. It is important to avoid lithium toxicity. Patients with serum levels of 2 mEq/L generally have serious toxic symptoms, and levels of 4 mEq/L or greater may produce permanent neurologic impairment or death. High serum levels should be treated aggressively, employing dialysis if necessary.

Poor therapeutic response to lithium treatment may occur in patients that are rapid cyclers, have dysphoric symptoms, have mixed symptoms of depression and mania, or have medical or psychiatric comorbidity. A history of prior mediocre response to lithium is also a predictor of poor response.

The majority of patients with bipolar disorder suffer recurrences. Lithium decreases the frequency and the severity of both manic and depressive recurrences in the majority of patients. It does not abolish all recurrences; and it particularly appears to be less effective for patients with a history of frequent recurrences, especially if they have more than three recurrences a year. In these rapidly cycling patients, it is important to rule out thyroid abnormalities. Trials of lithium should not be terminated too early, because some rapid cyclers will begin to show improvement only after a year of treatment. Rapid cycling occurs more commonly in women.

Approximately 30% of patients with bipolar disorder cannot tolerate or do not respond to lithium. The anticonvulsants valproate and carbamazepine appear to be effective alternatives to lithium for the treatment of acute mania and rapidly cycling patients, and they may act synergistically with lithium in some treatment-refractory cases. There is preliminary evidence that another anticonvulsant, valproic acid, may also be effective in the treatment of acute mania. Perhaps 5% of patients experience chronic unremitting symptoms despite treatment.

In treating rapid cyclers and patients with dysphoric mania, the use of antidepressants should be minimized if possible, because antidepressants can seriously worsen the clinical picture. A high percentage of patients have the onset of rapid cycling while being treated with antidepressants.

KEY POINTS

Differential Diagnoses

- Schizophrenia
- Thyroid disease
- Personality disorders
- Cyclothymic disorder
- Drugs or alcohol

Most Important Questions to Ask

- At what age did your symptoms first appear?
- Is there a family history of mood disorders or bipolar disorder?
- Have you been on antidepressant therapy or been sleep deprived?
- What is your mood like?
- Do you have special powers?
- Do you hear voices?
- Have you been taking any drugs or medications?
- How much alcohol do you drink?

Most Important Physical Examination Findings

- Flat or bland affect
- Flight of ideas
- Loud, rapid, pressured speech
- Distractibility
- Mood lability

Most Important Diagnostic Findings

- Toxicology screen
- Thyroid-stimulating hormone level

Treatments

- Lithium
- Haloperidol
- Valproate
- Carbamazepine
- Valproic acid

REFERENCES

1. American Psychiatric Association. *Diagnostic and statistical manual of mental disorders,* 4th ed. Washington, DC: *American Psychiatric Association,* 1994.
2. Dworkin RH, Clark CW, Lipsitz JD. Pain responsivity in major depression and bipolar disorder. *J Psychiatr Res* 1995;56:173–181.
3. Merskey H. The effect of chronic pain upon the response to noxious stimuli by psychiatric patients. *J Psychsom Res* 1965;8:405–419.
4. von Knorring L. An individual comparison of pain measures, averaged evoked responses and clinical ratings during depression and after recovery. *Acta Psychiatr Scand (Suppl)* 1974;255:109–120.
5. von Knorring L. An experimental study of visual averaged evoked responses (VAER) and pain measures (PM) in patients with depressive disorders. *Biol Psychol* 1978;6:27–38.
6. Davis GC, Buchsbaum MS, Bunney WE. Analgesia to painful stimuli in affective illness. *Am J Psychiatry* 1979;136(9):1148–1151.
7. Ben-Tovim DI, Schwartz MS. Hypoalgesia in depressive illness. *Br J Psychiatry* 1981;138:37–39.
8. Buchsbaum MS, Wu J, DeLisi LE, et al. Frontal cortex and basal anglia metabolic rates assessed by positron emission tomography with [^{18}F]2-dexocyglucose in affective illness. *J Affective Disord* 1986;10:137–152.
9. Adler G, Gattaz WF. Pain perception threshold in major depression. *Biol Psychiatry* 1993;34:687–689.
10. Hemphill RE, Hall KRL, Crookes TG. A preliminary report on fatigue and pain tolerance in depressive and psychoneurotic patients. *J Ment Sci* 1952;98:433–440.
11. Hall KRL, Stride E. The varying response to pain in psychiatric disorders: a study in abnormal psychology. *Br J Med Psychol* 1954;27:48–60.
12. Clark WC, Mehl L. Thermal pain: a sensory decision theory analysis of the effect of age and sex on d', various response criteria, and 50% pain threshold. *J Abnormal Psychol* 1971;78:202–212.
13. Stengel XY, Oldham AJ, Ehrenberg ASC. Reactions to pain in various abnormal mental states. *J Ment Sci* 1955;101:52–69.
14. Ward NG, Bloom VL, Dworkin S, et al. Psychobiological markers in coexisting pain and depression: toward a unified theory. *J Clin Psychiatry* 1982;43:32–41.
15. Otto MW, Doughter JJ, Yeo RA. Depression, pain and hemispheric activation. *J Nerv Ment Dis* 1989;177:210–218.
16. Fishbain DA. Pain insensitivity in psychosis. *Ann Emerg Med* 1982;11:11.
17. Janowsky D, Judd LL, Huey L, et al. Naloxone effects on manic symptoms and growth-hormone levels. *Lancet* 1978;II:320.
18. Emrich HM, Cording C, Piree S, et al. In: Usdin E, Bunney WE Jr, Kline NS. *Endorphins in mental health research.* New York: Macmillan, 1979:452–460.

DEPRESSION

JAMES E. CARTER
KEVIN M. KINBACK

KEY TERMS AND DEFINITIONS

Affective disorders: A spectrum of clinically significant mood disturbances ranging from depressive, or low states, to manic or high states.

Anhedonia: Loss of interest or pleasure in most activities for most days.

Biogenic amines: Neurotransmitters in the central nervous system, particularly the brain, which are responsible for normal cognitive and behavioral functioning.

Cognitive distortions: Automatic, defensive mechanisms that censor and prevent unconscious thoughts from reaching awareness. These can prolong or predispose to depression, and they are usually beyond voluntary control or even awareness.

Cytochrome P450: A system of many enzymes responsible for metabolism of drugs. Most notable among antidepressants are subtypes 2D6 and 3A4.

Depression: A state of significantly decreased emotional, psychologic, and social functioning, with neurovegetative symptoms, lasting at least 2 weeks. Anger, fear, and hopelessness become turned in upon the self, eventually producing or worsening biochemical changes.

Dysthymia: A form of mild but chronic depression, lasting at least 2 years.

Endogenous depression: Produced within a patient, arising *de novo* without apparent external stressors or triggers.

Exogenous depression: Originating outside an organ (brain) or patient, usually caused or triggered by stressful circumstances. These can be brief or chronic, severe or mild. Each patient has a particular threshold beyond which stressors will trigger depressive symptoms.

Hypomania: A state more activated and hyperactive than normal for a patient, but of insufficient severity to be considered mania.

Joint or conjoint therapy: Psychotherapy in which a therapist counsels two people together at the same time.

Mania: A state of abnormally elevated or expansive mood, lasting at least 1 week or requiring hospitalization. Often accompanied by overtalkativeness and increased goal-directed activity and is beyond the control of the patient.

Neurovegetative: The cluster of symptoms related to depressive changes in neurotransmitters, such as insomnia, hypersomnia, changes in appetite or weight, psychomotor retardation or excitation, and difficulties in memory or concentration.

INTRODUCTION

Medical illnesses have long been known to cause depressive episodes. This involves many complex factors, and such is also the case in the relationship between depression and chronic pelvic pain (CPP). Many questions persist as to whether and how depression and pain relate to each other. In CPP, as with any type of chronic pain, a certain state of depression may be expected, such as "burn-out" or moodiness. In more severe forms there is neurovegetative dysfunction, with cognitive distortions, which will in turn exacerbate physical symptoms or the perception of pain. This can create a "vicious cycle" that can amplify itself to devastating proportions if left untreated.

Depression comorbid in CPP can have a lifetime incidence as high as 65%, compared to only 25% overall in the general population of females (1,2). One study found a lifetime prevalence of depression in CPP patients of 65%, compared with only 17% in controls (1). Psychologic factors, such as learned coping skills, primary and secondary gain, and relational or family dynamics also play a key role in both the perception of pain and the course of the illness itself. Genetic and personality factors may also predispose toward or prolong an episode of depression. Other complications include dependence on and/or distrust of doctors, litigiousness, loss of occupational or social functioning, and substance abuse or dependence.

Depression is responsible for staggering morbidity in terms of lost occupational and other functioning and significant mortality. There are many forms of depression, ranging from a few symptoms of brief duration to many severe and incapacitating symptoms of full-blown major depression. Bipolar disorder is also a possibility, where patients have abnormally elevated moods, which can sometimes be associated with severe depressive episodes. Cyclothymia is a condition of exaggerated mood changes, which are more than normal but not as severe as bipolar disorder.

If untreated, some conditions may become chronic or may be highly resistant to future treatments. In general, however, depression is extremely responsive to treatment. We will highlight the various interwoven etiologic factors, diagnosis, and treatment options for various types of depression comorbid with pelvic pain.

ETIOLOGY

There are many theories as to the etiology of depression. It may be endogenous or exogenous in response to overwhelming or chronic stressors. There may be genetic mediation or predisposition to depression (3). These genetic links may lead to future correlation with treatment, because it is postulated that certain genetic and neurologic patterns may respond to particular treatments for depression and pain, whereas others may require significantly different treatments. Identifying these possible markers and subtyping them may lead to important prognostic and treatment considerations.

A prominent theory is the biogenic amine hypothesis, which theorizes abnormalities in neurotransmitter systems in the brain, including norephinephrine, serotonin, acetylcholine, dopamine, and gamma-aminobutyric acid (GABA). These same amines modulate neurovegetative symptoms of mood, as well as pain. For example, it has been shown that increasing serotonin reduces depression, as well as the perception of pain. In other studies, putting serotonin in cerebrospinal fluid (CSF) of animals helped reduce pain, whereas introducing norepinephrine increased pain perception (4). Such findings may explain some of the overlapping symptoms, as well as redundant pathologies. Newer research is being conducted regarding the role of other neurotransmitter systems in depression. These include other glutamates, *N*-methyl-D-aspartate, and substance P.

There are also many complex theories regarding depression and chronic pain. They postulate that either (a) the depression is primary to the pain, (b) the depression is secondary to pain, or (c) both occur concurrently. Primary depression has been noted to lead to increased reporting of pain, decreased pain threshold in the laboratory, and increased bodily preoccupation (5). Many experts believe that any type of chronic pain leads to a certain degree of depression, which may progress to clinical depression. In chronic pain, depression may develop as a "demoralization" due to the constant and relentless pain itself, as well as the stress on the brain's neurochemical homeostasis. One of the best ways to determine whether depression is primary or secondary is to investigate the time course. It would seem

that the onset of depression closely related in time to the onset of pain depression would more likely be secondary. A study of chronic back pain showed that 58% of depressive episodes began after the onset of pain, with 42% preceding the pain. Of course, temporality does not confirm causality, but most evidence suggests that chronic pain leads to chronic depression. Certain types of pain may be more predictive of depression than others: in one study, only neck–back and hip pain significantly predicted depression. Blumer and Heilbronn (6) proposed that chronic pain without an identified medical cause can actually be a variant of depression itself; they also proposed that pain is neither primary or secondary to depression, but a "synchronous expression of the disorder." Depression has also been found to be associated with sleep disorders, sexual victimization, endometriosis, physical abuse, hypochondriasis and somatization disorder, and substance abuse (1,7,8).

The "gate theory of pain" theorizes that many types of peripheral fibers transmit noxious nociceptive signals, which travel bidirectionally to and from the brain. Mediated mostly by serotonin and endorphins, motivational and affective states affect these signals (1). Thus, psychologic and emotional issues directly affect these neurotransmitter systems and nerve conduction, and they affect how the brain interprets and assigns meaning to these signals. This partially explains how pain control positively affects mood and how serotonergic antidepressants help mediate pain perception.

Nolan et al. (7) reported that of 72 patients with CPP, 51% had clinical depression, and 72% had sleep disorders. They also pointed out that subclinical depression is often overlooked and, when untreated, can worsen or prolong CPP. Emotional conflicts can become internalized and somatized, presenting as sleep disturbances, CPP, and depression. One definition of depression is "anger turned inward." Anger and frustration can increase the suffering of chronic pain (9). Women with this cluster of symptoms are frequently preoccupied and worried; they tend to keep their feelings and struggles to themselves, rather than acting out or becoming aggressive (7). It seems no coincidence that sleep, pain perception, and depression are all at least partially mediated by serotonergic neurons, which could be a unifying factor (4).

Cognitive distortions, including overgeneralizing, catastrophizing, selective abstraction, and personalization, increase the risk of CPP patients developing depression. Smith et al. (10) found that cognitive distortions were associated with increases in self-reported depression in patients with chronic pain.

In cases where no identifiable cause of CPP is found, patients often seek many opinions in an effort to prove that their pain is "real." These particular women are prone to substance abuse and can develop learned pain behavior as well as depression. Unless treated appropriately, this pattern can be inadvertently reinforced by well-meaning physicians

(4). Iatrogenic complications seem worse in patients whose CPP lacks adequate medical explanation, and these patients frequently seek increasingly more care, further propagating the cycle (11).

SYMPTOMS AND HISTORY

The symptoms of depression vary and occur as a spectrum that leads to a range of diagnostic categories (Fig. 50.1). Additionally, there is considerable overlap between depressive symptoms and pain symptoms, such as loss of pleasure or interest, sleep disturbances, altered self-image, change in appetite or weight, and excessive or inappropriate guilt. Virtually any form of depression can present concurrently with CPP.

There are three basis elements utilized in the diagnosis of all types of depression: (a) severity and number of symptoms; (b) duration and time course of symptoms; and (c) clinically significant distress or impairment of functioning. The "classic" form of depression is the major depressive episode. There are nine symptoms of a major depressive episode.

1. Sad or down mood, or tearfulness, most of every day.
2. Significant loss of interest or pleasure in nearly all activities (anhedonia).
3. Significant weight change of 5% in a month, either up or down.
4. Insomnia or hypersomnia daily.
5. Psychomotor agitation or retardation (which other people notice).
6. Lack of energy or daily fatigue.
7. Feeling worthless or experiencing inappropriate or excessive guilt.
8. Problems with decision making, thinking, or concentration.
9. Recurrent thoughts of death or suicide.

By definition, these symptoms must last at least 2 weeks and must include either (a) sad or blue mood or (b) the loss of interest or pleasure in nearly all activities. Another critical factor is that these symptoms must cause "clinically significant distress or impairment in social, occupational, or other important areas of functioning" (12). If someone complains of depressive symptoms yet denies any problems at work or in their marriage, family, and social life, the diagnosis is not likely to be major depression. The most severe

form of major depression presents with psychosis, which can be in the form of auditory, or less commonly visual, hallucinations or delusions. Depressive delusions are often about some aspect of self-condemnation and a need to be punished, or they have themes of hopelessness or nihilism. These indicate the need for immediate treatment and are risk factors for suicide. Fortunately, major depression with psychosis is rare in chronic pain patients (13).

The depressed patient seems to function in "low gear," meaning that positive or hopeful thoughts are ignored, and her focus turns exclusively to hopeless, negative, and pessimistic thinking. Attitudes toward pain, as well as actual perception and sensation of pain, change with the biochemical influence of depression. Although the threshold for pain tolerance varies widely among patients, the depressed woman complains of more frequent or more severe exacerbations of pain, or she presents with larger numbers of new findings. At times a clinician may embark on escalating pain control measures, with decreasing efficacy. This may be a clue to undiagnosed depression, and many times the patient's subjective complaints of pain can be greatly reduced with treatment of depression, even though the actual cause of the pain has remained unchanged. It is the perception and subjective experience of the patient that is the key to the level of pain control.

Bereavement or grief, including that caused by chronic pain and loss of functioning, must be distinguished from depression. Major depression is usually diagnosed if the symptoms are still active 2 months after the loss or the onset of pain. Other clues that point more to depression than to bereavement include thoughts of death, morbid preoccupation with worthlessness, severe psychomotor retardation, and ongoing and severe functional impairment (12). Often patients will just present with a severe, persistent "tiredness" or fatigue or will complain that they have "chronic fatigue syndrome." Further questioning often elicits symptoms that substantiate the diagnosis of depression.

Less severe than major depression, *adjustment disorder with depressed mood* has clinically significant impairment in social or occupational functioning that develops within 3 months after onset of a stressor and, with an acute episode, resolves within 6 months. Adjustment disorders can also present with anxiety or mixed anxiety and depression, as well as with disturbances of conduct. An adjustment disorder with depression in a patient with chronic pain is likely to become chronic, with symptoms persisting longer than 6 months. Thus while adjustment disorder is usually tran-

Depression	Adjustment	Major Depression	Dysthymia	Chronic	Recurrent	Bipolar
N.O.S. ———	Disorder with ———	Single episode ———	———	Major	——Major ———	Depression
(Atypical)	Depressed Mood			Depression	Depression	

FIGURE 50.1. Range of diagnostic categories of depression, arranged from mild to serious.

sient, in cases of chronic pelvic pain it is likely to progress to major depression, or at least chronic adjustment disorder with depression. These symptoms should be treated if they cause a noticeable impairment in functioning.

Depression not otherwise specified (depression NOS or atypical depression) is the least severe in the spectrum of depression and is very common. Depressive features are insufficient in number, severity, or duration to be considered a major depressive episode. This is often a prodrome of a future major depressive episode and is often a postpartum finding. At times it is difficult to distinguish depression NOS from adjustment disorder with depressed mood. Sometimes considered a "mild depression," it should be treated if it causes significant clinical impairments. Another form of depression NOS, called *premenstrual dysphoric disorder*, commonly varies with the menstrual cycle, with markedly depressed mood, marked anxiety, affective lability, and decreased interest in activities, which markedly interfere with functioning. This is also commonly called *premenstrual syndrome* (PMS).

Dysthymia or dysthymic disorder is depression that occurs on most days (more often than not) for at least 2 years. There also needs to be at least two of the following criteria: decreased or increased appetite; insomnia or hypersomnia; low energy or fatigue; low self-esteem; poor concentration or difficulty with decisions; or feelings of hopelessness. Because of the often insidious and chronic nature of these symptoms, they are easily overlooked, especially in the patient with CPP, so these patients should be routinely screened for dysthymia. Major depression can also be imposed on top of dysthymia, the so-called "double depression," but only if there has first been 2 years of dysthymia by itself (12).

Chronic major depression is major depression that does not spontaneously resolve in 12 to 24 months. These persistent symptoms are quite serious and lead to prolonged disability. This is commonly seen in patients with CPP. If treated, these patients may be refractory, or they may not have been able to complete an adequate trial of medication due to side effects.

Recurrent major depression is another depressive episode separated from the previous episode by at least 2 months without any significant symptoms. The risk of recurrent major depression is about 50% within the 5 years following the first episode of major depression. With each subsequent episode the risk increases further, with an incidence of over 80% for someone with three or more prior episodes. These episodes also increase in frequency, in a sort of "snowballing" effect. This risk also increases with age, because patients over 40 years of age are more prone to recurrent depression. Recurrent major depression should be treated with medication for at least 5 years, with serious consideration given to lifelong prophylaxis.

Bipolar depression is characterized by at least one episode of mania. This is also known as "manic depression" or the more recent term of "bipolar disorder." There are many varieties of bipolar disorder as well, and some patients are genetically predisposed to manic episodes. Mania is also a potential side effect of antidepressant treatment, especially in someone with prior manic or hypomanic episodes or who has a strong family history of mania. Manic episodes are basically the opposite of depression, and they are characterized by a distinct period or unusual and persistent elevation or expansion of mood (euphoria), or irritability, for at least 1 week. During this time, patients have at least three of the following: inflated self-esteem (grandiosity); less need for sleep; pressured or increased speech; flight of ideas or complaints of racing thought; increased goal-directed activity (sexual, social, occupational) or psychomotor agitation; or excessive involvement in pleasurable activities with potentially painful consequences (so-called "thrill-seeking," such as spending sprees, promiscuity, foolish investments, or other such schemes) (12). In rare cases, patients may present with a "mixed" presentation, with both depressive and manic symptoms at the same time.

With CPP and all forms of depression, collateral history is important, because patients may not be totally reliable in presenting either their pain symptoms or those of depression. They might tend to minimize symptoms for fear of stigmatization, or they may dread referral to a psychiatrist. Others might exaggerate their symptoms, either in fear they will not be taken seriously or for secondary gain, such as disability, extra attention, or sympathy. With the patient's permission, other "eyewitnesses" should be queried, and often they provide vital information regarding the patient's ability to actually function. These sources often include spouses, parents, children, fellow employees, or friends who may accompany patients to the office. It is extremely helpful when patients bring someone else along and they don't seem to mind when there are differences of opinion, although the physician may occasionally need to act as a referee. For example, someone might claim that they sleep little and have lost interest in eating and other activities. A spouse might observe that the patient actually sleeps most of the night and has only lost appetite or interest for certain things that are distasteful to the patient. Patients often misperceive the quality of their sleep and the extent of their disability due to pain, as well as depressive symptoms.

Prior treatment history and family history are also important in diagnosing depression in CPP. Because many neurotransmitter receptors are under genetic control, it has been noted that responses to specific agents follow specific patterns. For example, if a patient notes that a parent and two siblings have all suffered from depression and had a good response to nefazodone, then this agent is particularly likely to be effective in this patient. The patient should be asked to list previous attempts at treating depression, including specific medications, dosages, and duration. The clinician must know whether an adequate trial of each agent was given. The suggested clinical trial is 8 weeks at a medium to high dosage. Examples are 40 mg fluoxetine, 100 to 150 mg sertraline, 40 mg paroxetine, 300 to 400 mg buproprion, and 400 to 600 mg nefazodone.

Another useful tool is having the patient keep a journal or "mood diary." Patients should be asked to rate their depression on a scale of zero (nondepressed) to minus five (severely depressed) and record their daily overall moods on a calendar. They should also record their menses. Bipolar patients should also record their "up" phases on a scale of zero (nonmanic) to plus five (nearly out of control mania). If patients have "swinging moods," or those that vary greatly without known triggers within the course of a single day, they may want to record several numbers daily, along with the duration of each level of mood.

SIGNS AND PHYSICAL EXAMINATION

The diagnosis of depression in patients with CPP is mostly clinical and can be made based on the lists of symptoms presented above. Two of the most useful objective signs of depression available to the clinician are depressed affect and psychomotor retardation. From the diagnostic criteria noted above, it is vital to note that the depressed patient may be either noticeably slowed or agitated. Some depressed patients present with movements, thoughts, and speech in "slow motion." Others, less commonly, present as highly anxious and fidgety, and they may be unable to stop bouncing around in their chairs. You should note a patient's posture, gait, and speed of motion and speech. You may also query both the patient and any other source of information about motor changes.

Observation of affect is important. Depressed patients often appear haggard, sometimes with dark circles under the eyes, and appear ready to nap at any time. They rarely smile and don't respond to humor as expected. They take longer to answer questions and are less willing to elaborate on their answers. They might also appear highly worried or anxious and may be unable to stop talking about their symptoms. This can sometimes be confused with mania or hypomania.

DIAGNOSTIC STUDIES

Depression is a clinical diagnosis based on the criteria in the *Diagnostic and Statistical Manual of Mental Disorders*, 4th edition (DSM-IV), and there are no diagnostic laboratory findings. There are some associations, however, such as electroencephalographic abnormalities showing reduced non-rapid eye movement in stages 3 and 4 of slow-wave sleep, increased phasic rapid eye movement (REM) sleep, and total REM sleep. Functional and structural brain imaging, evoked potentials, neuroendocrine challenges, and the dexamethasone suppression test have also demonstrated some abnormalities, but not consistently enough to be clinically useful as widespread diagnostic tools (5).

Many patients falsely believe that there is a blood test that "proves a chemical imbalance in the brain," and they often ask for it. Although there have been many research correlations that support various biogenic amine hypotheses, there are currently no definitive tests for affective disorders in widespread clinical use. Some tests have shown depression in general to be directly correlated with biogenic amine deficiencies, as well as neuroendocrine dysregulation. Urinary and CSF levels of biogenic amines also vary with depression, but not consistently enough to be of clinical use (2). Some other studies used in research include positron emission topography (PET) scanning, single-photon emission computerized tomography (SPECT) scanning, and the dexamethasone suppression test (DST).

The hypothalamic–pituitary–adrenal axis is often disturbed in depression. The dexamethasone suppression test (DST), first used in 1960 to study Cushing's disease, is positive in some cases of depression. A dose of 1 mg of dexamethasone is given to a patient in the evening, and then several levels of cortisol are measured the next day. Depressed patients with positive DSTs show a failure to suppress cortisol release upon administration of dexamethasone. Some clinicians have attempted to show that normalization of this test is an indication to discontinue antidepressant treatment, but the results are inconclusive, because the test is false-positive in up to 10% of cases and can be confounded by a number of variables (2). Other tests including thyroid-releasing hormone (TRH), growth hormone, and somatostatin are also being investigated, with discordant data too inconsistent to be of clinical use.

Psychometric testing, using psychologic tests such as the Beck Depression Inventory (BDI), Hamilton Depression Test, and Minnesota Multiphasic Personality Inventory (MMPI), is useful to objectively pinpoint depressive symptoms. The Zung scale is a very rudimentary screening tool using the simple criteria for major depression and is easily given in the office within 5 minutes. Many clinicians use a simple checklist with symptoms of major depression which patients can complete in the waiting room. These tests are particularly useful when a patient is minimizing depressive symptoms or there is diagnostic uncertainty.

Standard tests to rule out other medical conditions are important, including thyroid-stimulating hormone, thyroxine, and triiodothyronine levels (TSH, T4, T3). If a patient remains refractory to several treatments, with normal or borderline thyroid tests, sometimes antithyroid antibody assays may be necessary to rule out subclinical hypothyroidism. Other tests include blood counts to rule out anemia and infection, renal and hepatic function tests, electrolytes, rapid plasma reagen (RPR) to rule out neurosyphilis, and human immunodeficiency virus (HIV) testing to rule out autoimmune deficiency syndrome (AIDS). A 12-lead electrocardiogram (ECG) is indicated in patients with known heart disease or in those over 40 years of age. Street drug as well as prescription drug abuse should be ruled out with a urine drug screen (UDS). In patients with any prior head trauma, interventricular shunting, any neurologic findings (including headaches), or persistent, unexplained symptoms of depression (especially with obsessions, compulsions, or psychosis), a brain imaging study such as computerized axial tomography (CAT) or magnetic resonance imaging (MRI) may be indicated. If occupational or other exposure dictates, testing for heavy metal exposure could be warranted. While these tests cannot "rule in" depression, they can rule out or reveal underlying medical conditions that may help alleviate depression when reversed.

DIFFERENTIAL DIAGNOSIS

Differential diagnosis of depression in patients with chronic pelvic pain includes the following:

- General medical conditions, such as thyroid dysregulation, poor pain control, infection, seizures, and so on
- Sleep disorders
- Substance abuse
- Coexisting personality disturbance
- Chronic psychotic disorders
- Malingering
- Posttraumatic stress disorder (PTSD)
- Bereavement
- Adjustment disorder

If there is a question whether pain or depression is primary, it may be helpful to initiate treatment with an antidepressant, as well as nonspecific therapies for the pain in the form of supportive encouragement. A dramatic response of both pain and depression to this therapy suggests that depression was primary. Psychometric testing can also help differentiate between primary and secondary depression, and it is especially useful for identifying underlying personality disturbances.

MANAGEMENT OR TREATMENT

Treatment of depression has become increasingly complex due to the explosion of research and the advent of dozens of medications for depression. Many of these agents have different modes of actions, yet all have roughly the same efficacy across large groups of people (2). The most effective treatment of depression and CPP is both multidisciplinary and multimodal. Rosenthal (1) points out four useful principles in addressing treatment in patients with CPP: (a) Take the patient seriously, (b) lay out expectations for treatment and enlist the patient's help, (c) reeducate the patient about her role and her illness as treatment progresses, and (d) assess the patient's psychosocial situation. Education in a supportive environment helps prepare patients to accept psychologic counseling, take antidepres-

sants, deal with prior abuse and underlying personality traits, and put their perceptions of pain into perspective (1). If the "usual" methods of pain control have failed, referral to a specialized pain clinic may be helpful, because they have access to treatments such as acupuncture, biofeedback, relaxation, trigger point injections, transcutaneous electrical nerve stimulation (TENS) units, nerve blocks, and implanted devices that either interferentially stimulate nerves or release pain medication.

Medical Treatment

The treatment of depression and CPP most familiar to physicians is pharmacologic (14). Antidepressant medications, particularly the tricyclics, have long been used for chronic headaches, arthritis, and other recurrent pain. There are discordant opinions about the usefulness of antidepressants for CPP alone (Chapter 56), but antidepressants are always indicated for clinically significant symptoms of depression regardless of cause, as long as the underlying cause is also treated. However, in many cases of secondary depression, the neurochemical imbalance seems to "take on a life of its own," and the vegetative symptoms persist for months after the underlying cause has been corrected.

Many antidepressants have complex effects on multiple neurotransmitter systems. For example, medications known to inhibit the uptake of norepinephrine or serotonin in the brain, such as imipramine or fluoxetine, reverse the symptoms of depression in most patients. In a given patient, it is impossible to predict whether the response to treatment will be greater with a serotonergic agent or an adrenergic agent. The overall efficacy of antidepressants is about 70% to 80%, with monoamine oxidase inhibitors being slightly higher. When one agent fails, however, many clinicians will switch to an agent of a different class, in hopes of inducing remission. Electroconvulsive therapy (ECT) has the highest therapeutic efficacy at approximately 90%. It is hoped that new and effective antidepressants, with unique actions and effects, will soon be available for clinical use.

The treatment for bipolar depression is quite different from major depression (sometimes called "unipolar" depression), and involves mood-stabilizing agents. Care must be taken to avoid precipitating a manic episode by using unopposed antidepressants in bipolar patients. In rare cases, patients may present with a "mixed" presentation, with both depressive and manic symptoms at the same time. This is very difficult to treat and is an indication for psychiatric referral.

Choosing an Antidepressant

Categories of antidepressants include tricyclics, selective serotonin reuptake inhibitors (SSRIs), monoamine oxidase inhibitors (MAOIs), and atypicals, such as desyrel, nefazodone, buproprion, venlafaxine, and mirtazepine. ECT is also of benefit, but is usually reserved for more severe or refractory cases.

Of the tricyclics, the tertiary amines, including doxepin, clomipramine, imipramine, amitriptyline, and nortriptyline, block serotonin reuptake more than they block norepinephrine. Doxepin and amitriptyline appear to be especially efficacious in mixed depression and pain (4). In general, lower doses of tricyclic antidepressants can be used for chronic pain, and pain relief occurs more quickly than the antidepressant response (15). For example, pain is usually improved with low doses of 10 to 25 mg of doxepin or amitriptyline given at bedtime. Other tricyclics in similar dosages may also be effective. If sedation is excessive, the next morning the dosage may be lowered or given slightly earlier than bedtime. These agents must be used cautiously in elderly women due to the risk of ileus, orthostatic hypotension and falls, and arrhythmias. It is prudent to check an ECG in patients who have preexisting arrhythmias or are over the age of 40 years.

SSRIs, which include fluoxetine, paroxetine, fluvoxamine, sertraline, and citalopram, have been used increasingly over the past 10 years. Tricyclics have fallen out of favor due to significant anticholinergic and antihistimine side effects. SSRIs also have side effects, mostly gastrointestinal, such as anorexia, nausea, weight loss or gain, and sexual—including decreased libido and anorgasmia. Headaches occasionally lead to discontinuation. A small percentage of patients become sedated or activated and have insomnia even with morning dosing. Fortunately, most of these side effects are transient and dose-related, and they can be avoided by using low starting doses and titrating up slowly as needed. Examples of starting dosages are 10 mg for fluoxetine and paroxetine, 12.5 or 25 mg for sertraline and fluvoxamine, and 5 to 10 mg of citalopram. If side effects occur, a reduction in dosage will usually help relieve them. If activation occurs, dosing should be in the mornings. If sedation occurs, bedtime dosing is best. Cytochrome P450 interactions should be kept in mind with the SSRIs, with sertraline having only a slight effect on the 2D6 system. Paroxetine and fluoxetine have the strongest inhibitory effect on the 2D6 system and increase serum levels of tricyclic antidepressants, some antiarrhythmia agents, and some antipsychotics, for example. Fluvoxamine strongly inhibits the 3A4 enzyme system and is contraindicated with astemazole, cisapride, and terfenadine. Antibiotics such as erythromycin and most antifungals also clear through this system, so dosages of SSRIs should be kept as low as possible to avoid drug interactions.

Of the atypical antidepressants, desyrel and mirtazepine are the most sedating, so bedtime dosing is indicated. Both agents can also cause weight gain. Desyrel does not typically have much efficacy as an antidepressant at dosages less then several hundred milligrams. Desyrel has been associated with ventricular ectopy and should be avoided in cases of known ventricular ectopic arrhythmias. Mirtazepine has

side effects that are *inversely* related to dosage. Many clinicians use a starting dose of 15 to 30 mg to avoid sedation that can occur at lower dosages. If insomnia is still a problem, or if weight gain is desired, the dosage should actually be reduced to obtain these side effects. The dose can be raised as high as 45 mg if needed. Nefazodone is an improvement of desyrel in that it does not have cardiac side effects, but it strongly inhibits the cytochrome P450 (CYP450) 3A4 isoenzyme and is contraindicated with astemazole, cisapride, and terfenadine. Also, doses of trazolobenzodiazepines such as triazolam and alprazolam should be lowered by one-half. Nefazodone is also associated with occasional dizziness, but is largely weight neutral—causing neither significant loss nor gain in most cases. Nefazodone comes in convenient starter sample packages containing 50-mg, 100-mg, and 150-mg tablets. The labeling indicates twice-daily dosing, but it can be given in one large bedtime dose if sedation is a problem. A good starting dose is 50 mg twice daily, increasing by 50 to 100 mg every 5 to 7 days. Unlike the tricyclics and SSRIs, nefazodone rarely causes sexual dysfunction. Buproprion also is not associated with sexual dysfunction, but has a slightly higher risk of seizures, about 4 per 1,000 at the top dose. Buproprion comes in two forms, immediate and sustained release. The sustained release form has fewer side effects, which can include headache, tremor, activation, anxiety, insomnia, and anorexia. Buproprion is more noradrenergic and has a slight effect on dopamine, and it may help improve low energy, memory, focus, and concentration. Buproprion has minimal CYP450 interactions. Venlafaxine has side effects and actions midway between the SSRIs and atypicals. It has only modest CYP450 interactions and side effects similar to SSRIs, but is usually well tolerated. It comes in both immediate and sustained release forms. The Achilles' heel of venlafaxine is hypertension, a dose-related complication that requires monitoring of blood pressure with each follow-up visit. A good starting dose is 37.5 to 75 mg daily, which may need to be raised by 37.5 or 75 mg every 5 to 7 days.

For buproprion and the tricyclics there is an upper limit of dosage. It is usually 250 to 300 mg for most of the tricyclics, 450 mg for immediate release buproprion, and 400 mg for sustained release buproprion, with doses always divided evenly twice or thrice daily to minimize seizure risk. For the SSRIs and atypicals, however, there is technically no upper limit. Some clinicians find supranormal doses of these agents to be helpful, but it is critical to watch for dose-related side effects and increased chances of drug interactions.

Monoamine oxidase inhibitors (MAOIs) are rarely prescribed due to severe dietary restrictions on tyramine, which can cause a severe hypertensive reaction. MAOIs can also cause the serotonin syndrome, a toxic surplus of serotonin in the CNS caused by overzealous administration of high doses or combinations of multiple serotonergic agents. This syndrome is characterized by weakness, confusion, and ataxia, and it can lead to serious consequences if not recognized and treated promptly. There are some MAOIs, such as meclobamide, that have reversible effects and do not require the dietary restrictions, but these are unfortunately not yet available in the United States.

ECT remains the single most effective treatment of depression overall and is also effective in depression comorbid with CPP. The only relative contraindication is increased intracranial pressure. There are no absolute contraindications. This is safely and effectively performed and is available in most major cities, but there is some stigma involved and insurance coverage can be tricky. A second opinion is always required, along with a medical evaluation and special informed consent. The main side effects are transient memory loss, headaches, and myalgia. Most patients do not experience significant or sustained memory impairment, except for the few hours after each treatment. The average course of ECT consists of 8 to 12 individual treatments, usually three times weekly. The response to ECT is more complete and comes faster than with most other agents.

Because there is equivalent efficacy among the newer antidepressants, the choice of agent may also be based on desirable side effects, such as sedation in the insomniac, weight gain in the anorexic, stimulation in the lethargic patient, or weight loss in the obese patient. Because side effects tend to wane with time, they may wear off when they are no longer indicated, which is an added bonus. If they persist and become countertherapeutic, the dosage can be adjusted or "antidotes" may be added later.

Time Course of Treatment

As noted above, there may be some amelioration in pain within a few days to a week, but the antidepressant response is often delayed by 2 to 4 weeks or longer. It does not make sense to raise the dosage by more than a small amount every 2 weeks or so, because it can take this amount of time for a response. Also because the pain is chronic and the depression is usually acute, there is a risk of alienating the patient with adverse effects that can lead to a refusal to try other agents. The first phase of treatment, called *initiation*, is getting the patient titrated on the medication, starting low and increasing slowly at first. This reduces the incidence of side effects and does not seem to delay the response significantly. It is best to prepare patients for a lengthy delay in response, to bolster compliance. If the response is more rapid, then the patient will be pleasantly surprised. Therapeutic dosages should be targeted for a minimum of 8 weeks on each agent before lowering the dose or switching, except in the case of significant side effects. If a patient can tolerate the lowest dosage of an agent without significant side effects, then the drug can be titrated upwards fairly rapidly for severe cases. Patients with severe depression, anorexia, and suicidal ideation should be treated more aggressively, titrating as rapidly as tolerated.

The next phase of treatment is called *continuation*. Once a satisfactory remission of symptoms is obtained, it is vital to continue the medications at the same dosage that brought about remission, without lowering for 8 to 12 months. Any interruption or reduction in dosage may result in exacerbation or recurrence of symptoms. Recent clinical experience and thinking suggest that refractoriness to a particular agent may result from interruption in treatment, particularly in patients over 40 years old. Given these factors, early treatment and compliance take on paramount importance.

The final phase of treatment is called *maintenance*. The risk of relapse within 5 years after a successfully treated episode of major depression is approximately 50%. The risk increases with each subsequent episode, and for up to two subsequent episodes the recommended length of treatment increases to 5 years. Further episodes, or three in women over 40, are in indication for lifelong antidepressant treatment.

Response to Treatment

Each antidepressant has a response rate of approximately 70%. A patient tolerating an adequate dose for 8 weeks without reduction of symptoms is a nonresponder. Some patients have partial response to the medication. The dosage can usually be increased to the upper limit of the usual dosage range in the hopes of bringing about a response with a single agent. For severely depressed and suicidal, agitated, pregnant, or psychotic patients, ECT may be a good early option.

Treating the Nonresponder

There are two ways to address the nonresponding patient. The first is to switch agents, either within a class or to another class of antidepressant. For patients with a good clinical response that loses its effect, or for side effects, such as gastrointestinal (GI) upset with an SSRI, another agent in the same class may be effective. If a patient has not responded to an adequate trial of one antidepressant, but tolerated it well, it may be prudent to switch to an agent in a different class. Some agents are more serotonergic, such as the SSRIs and venlafaxine, whereas others are more adrenergic, such as nortriptyline, buproprion, and other tricyclics. Some agents such as nefazodone, mirtazepine, and other tricyclics work on both systems. If a patient has not responded to a serotonergic agent, perhaps a more adrenergic agent would be more effective. When switching, the agents can be briefly overlapped in an exchange titration, or the first agent can simply be stopped before the second is starting. It is often helpful to reduce the dosage of the first agent while adding low dosages of the second agent in partial responders. This way, the partial response to the first agent is preserved, while awaiting a more effective response from the second agent. The physician should beware of drug interactions, particularly in the CYP450 system, when combining antidepressants of different classes.

The second way to treat the nonresponding patient is to augment the response by adding a second agent. This second agent may be another antidepressant in lower doses, usually from a different classification. Typical combinations are SSRIs and desyrel or low-dose tricyclics, or low-dose buproprion with SSRIs or tricyclics. The second agent may be another medication known to increase the effectiveness of antidepressants. These commonly include lithium, divalproex sodium, thyroxine, psychostimulants, buspirone, and occasionally antipsychotics. The newer atypical antipsychotics such as risperidone and olanzapine are preferred, due to their improved tolerability and lower tendency to cause tardive dyskinesia than the typical neuroleptics. A psychiatry consultation may be helpful in refractory cases, because augmentation in this fashion often requires additional monitoring with office visits, blood levels, and laboratory testing.

The ultimate tool for the nonresponder is ECT, which can be used for all types of depression. MAOIs are also a last resort, due to dietary restrictions, but are often effective when other agents have failed.

Cessation of Treatment

After a successful maintenance phase, medication should usually be tapered off gradually, over several months. The longer the maintenance, the longer the taper should last. Some antidepressants, including the tricyclics and SSRIs, have been associated with a discontinuation syndrome. This is more pronounced with agents having shorter half-lives, such as paroxetine and the tricyclics, intermediate with sertraline and fluvoxamine, and shortest with flouxetine. Discontinuation symptoms are usually either "flu-like," with myalgias, joint pain, nasal congestion, GI upset, and so on, or "pseudoneurologic," with shock-like sensations usually in the head, paresthesias, or strange visual phenomena. These should be explained to the patient ahead of time, and even as a precaution during maintenance, lest the patient inadvertently stop the medication abruptly. Discontinuation phenomena are usually self-limiting, lasting less than a week and rarely exceeding 3 weeks. They can be treated by restarting the antidepressant and tapering more slowly, or by brief doses of short-acting benzodiazepines, such as lorazepam. This syndrome usually resolves within 24 hours of treatment.

Another advantage a slow taper allows is time for both patient and physician to monitor for recurrence of symptoms. Theoretically, if there is still some antidepressant left in the system, then in the event of relapse a therapeutic level of antidepressant can be quickly reached, hopefully preventing the plunging levels that can lead to future refractoriness. The patient will also have a more rapid response to reinstitution of therapeutic dosages, rather than having to wait for onset of effect after a protracted period without medication.

If a patient relapses during a taper, she should return at once to the dosage that brought about remission and remain there for another full maintenance period. Taper can then again be attempted at the completion of maintenance, perhaps at a slower rate.

For patients who stop medication due to adverse effects or who are reticent to remain on maintenance, nonpharmacological treatments are recommended.

Nonpharmacological Treatments

Biofeedback and relaxation training therapy can be helpful, especially if a patient has an underpinning of high anxiety (1). Both group and individual psychotherapy with a broad-spectrum behavioral approach helps with stress management. Some patients may benefit from hypnosis, anxiety and anger management, cognitive therapy, activity management, and sex education. Early childhood issues and past abuses may need to be dealt with, along with any unresolved grief issues. Psychotherapy can help build coping skills, provide education about pain management, and identify stressors and triggers to pain. Therapy should involve concrete goal setting and behavioral modification techniques, with homework assigned to ensure productivity. Journaling of behaviors, feelings, external events, and their relation to pain symptoms can help identify triggers to pain. Occasionally, joint therapy or marital counseling is necessary as well (16).

Surgical Treatment

Psychosurgery is no longer indicated in depression, although it has been refined and is sometimes useful in obsessive–compulsive disorder and some movement disorders.

KEY POINTS

Differential Diagnoses

- General medical conditions, such as thyroid dysregulation, poor pain control, infection, seizures, and so on
- Sleep disorders
- Substance abuse
- Coexisting personality disturbance
- Chronic psychotic disorders
- Malingering
- Posttraumatic stress disorder (PTSD)
- Bereavement
- Adjustment disorder

Most Important Questions to Ask

- Screen for symptoms of depression, including
  Sad or down mood, or tearfulness, most of every day
  Significant loss of interest or pleasure in nearly all activities (anhedonia)

Significant weight change, either a 5% body weight gain or loss in a month

Insomnia or hypersomnia daily

Psychomotor agitation or retardation (which other people notice)

Lack of energy or daily fatigue

Feeling worthless or inappropriate or excessive guilt

Problems with decision making, thinking, or concentration

Recurrent thoughts of death or suicide

- Prior history of depression, suicide attempts, and response to prior treatment?
- Is medical workup complete to rule out medical causes of depression?
- Are there significant psychosocial stressors that could respond to psychotherapy?
- Is there a significant impairment in social, occupational, or personal functioning?
- Is chemical dependency a complicating factor?

Most Important Examination Findings

- Presence of suicidal ideation with intent, means, and plan
- Significant loss or gain in weight
- Significant problems in concentration, memory, or decision making
- Severe psychomotor retardation or agitation
- Severe disruption of sleep

Most Important Diagnostic Studies

- Basic laboratory studies to rule out:
- Anemia
- Endocrine abnormalities, especially thyroid; consider antithyroid antibodies
- Renal or hepatic compromise
- Vitamin B_{12} or folate deficiency
- Substance abuse
- Consider neuroimaging for refractory cases, or with neurologic signs.
- Some medications require ECG prior to use (tricyclics, lithium, desyrel in the elderly).
- Some medications require ongoing monitoring or hepatic function, CBC, thyroid (anticonvulsants, lithium).
- If comorbid dementia is present, or occupational exposure warrants, test for heavy metals.

Treatments

- Pain management clinics
- Biofeedback
- Relaxation training
- Individual and group therapy to deal with psychosocial stressors
- Grief or anger management
- Support groups for chronic pain

- Psychotropic medications, including:
- Tricyclics (amitriptyline, nortriptyline, desipramine, imipramine, doxepin)
- SSRIs (paroxetine, fluoxetine, fluvoxamine, citalopram, sertraline)
- Atypical antidepressants (venlafaxine, mirtazepine, nefazodone, desyrel, buproprion)
- Monoamine oxidase inhibitors (MAOIs) (isocarboxyzid, phenylzine)
- Electroconvulsive therapy (ECT)
- Combinations of medications, or augmentation for refractory patients
- Division of treatment into phases of initiation, continuation, and maintenance

REFERENCES

1. Rosenthal RH. Psychology of chronic pelvic pain. *Obstet Gynecol Clin North Am* 1993;20(4):726–742.
2. Kaplan HI, Sadok BJ, eds. *Comprehensive textbook of psychiatry/VI*, vols 1 and 2, Baltimore: Williams and Wilkins, 1995:2804 pages.
3. France RD, Houpt JL, Ellinwood EH. Therapeutic effects of antidepressants in chronic pain. *Gen Hosp Psychiatry* 1984;6:55–63.
4. Hendler N. Depression caused by chronic pain. *J Clin Psychiatry* 1984;45(3), Section 2:30–38.
5. Banks SM, Kerns RD. Explaining high rates of depression in chronic pain: a diathesis–stress framework. *Psychol Bull* 1996;119(1):98–110.
6. Blumer D, Helibronn M. Chronic pain as a variant of depressive disease: the pain-prone disorder. *J Nerv Ment Dis* 1982;170:381–406.
7. Nolan TE, Metheny WP, Smith RP. Unrecognized association of sleep disorders and depression with chronic pelvic pain. *South Med J* 1992;85(12):1181–1183.
8. Walker EA, Sullivan MD, Stenchever MA. Sexual victimization and chronic pelvic pain. *Obstet Gynecol Clin North Am* 1993;20(4):795–807.
9. Fernandez E, Turk DC. Clinical review, the scope and significance of anger in the experience of chronic pain. *Pain* 1995;61:165–175.
10. Smith TW, O'Keeffe JL, Christensen AJ. Cognitive distortion and depression in chronic pain: association with diagnosed disorders. *J Consult Clin Psychol* 1994;62(1):195–1989.
11. Kouyanou K, Pither CE, Rabe-Hesketh S, et al. A comparative study of iatrogenesis, medication abuse, and psychiatric morbidity in chronic pain patients with and without medically explained symptoms. *Pain* 1998;76:417–426.
12. Frances A, Pincus HA, First MB (Task force on DSM-IV). *Diagnostic and statistical manual of mental disorders*, 4th ed. (DSM-IV), Washington, DC: American Psychiatric Association, 1994:886 pages.
13. Robinson RG, Rabins PV, eds. Depression and chronic pain, Chapter 11 in *Depression and coexisting disease*, Medical Publishers, Inc., New York: Igaku-Shoin, 1989:242 pages.
14. Walker EA, Sullivan MD, Stenchever MA. Use of antidepressants in the management of women with chronic pelvic pain. *Obstet Gynecol Clin North Am* 1993;20(4):743–751.
15. Hahn MD, Jones MM, Carron H. Idiopathic pelvic pain, the relationship to depression. *Postgrad Med* 1989;85(4):263–270.
16. Kames LD, Rapkin AJ, Naliboff BD, et al. Effectiveness of an interdisciplinary pain management program for the treatment of chronic pelvic pain. *Pain* 1990;41:41–46.

51

FAMILIAL MEDITERRANEAN FEVER

JAMES E. CARTER

KEY TERMS AND DEFINITIONS

Familial Mediterranean fever: An inherited, recurrent, inflammatory disease of unknown cause, characterized by acute self-limited attacks of fever and peritonitis, and sometimes accompanied by pleuritis, arthritis, and erythematous skin lesions.

INTRODUCTION

Familial Mediterranean fever is largely restricted to ethnic groups originating in the Eastern Mediterranean area. Half of the reported cases are in patients of Sephardic Jewish ancestry, 20% are Armenian, and another 20% are of Turkish or Arabic descent. The remaining patients are of Italian, Greek, or Ashkenazi Jewish ancestry. The disease is familial and males predominate by a ratio of 3:1 (1).

ETIOLOGY

The etiology remains unknown. The recent identification of the chromosomal location of the gene associated with familial Mediterranean fever should assist in the eventual elucidation of the defect that underlies the disease (2).

PATHOLOGY

Pathologic findings in familial Mediterranean fever are those of nonspecific, acute inflammation. Neutrophil infiltration predominates in exudates recovered from the peritoneal, pleural, or joint spaces at the times of acute attacks. Serosal thickening and secondary adhesions may occur, which in the abdomen may lead to mechanical bowel obstruction (1).

CLINICAL PRESENTATION

More than 95% of patients experience abdominal pain and signs of peritonitis during acute attacks. Pain often begins in one quadrant and then becomes diffuse, sometimes with distention, rigidity, rebound tenderness, and ileus with nausea and vomiting. Pain may radiate to the back or to the shoulders. Pleuritic pain occurs during acute attacks in 75% of patients. Mild arthralgia is a common cause of febrile attacks. The duration and frequency of attacks vary considerably. Acute attacks typically last 24 to 48 hours and recur once or twice a month. Pregnancy is often associated with the remission of attacks, which resume postpartum. Familial Mediterranean fever is frequently complicated by amyloidosis and progressive renal failure (1).

As many as one-third of patients experience transient, well-circumscribed, painful erythematous areas of swelling on the lower leg, ankle, or the dorsum of the foot, which are 5 to 20 cm in diameter. Laboratory findings in familial Mediterranean fever are nonspecific. During acute attacks leukocytosis is present and the erythrocyte sedimentation rate is increased.

DIFFERENTIAL DIAGNOSIS

The diagnosis of familial Mediterranean fever is based primarily on clinical presentation and history. In individuals of appropriate ethnic background with typical recurrent, self-limited attacks, diagnosis is usually delayed because it is not considered. The major differential diagnoses includes appendicitis, pancreatitis, cholecystitis, and intestinal obstruction.

MANAGEMENT OR TREATMENT

Colchicine treatment is effective in familial Mediterranean fever. Prophylactic colchicine 0.6 mg orally two or three times a day prevents or substantially reduces the acute attacks of familial Mediterranean fever in 75% to 90% of patients. Some patients can abort attacks with intermittent courses of colchicine beginning at the onset of attacks (0.6 mg orally every hour for 4 hours and then every 2 hours for 4 hours and then every 12 hours for 2 days) (3).

KEY POINTS

Differential Diagnosis

- Appendicitis
- Pancreatitis
- Cholecystitis
- Intestinal obstruction

Most Important Questions to Ask

- What is your ethnic background?
- Are you experiencing recurrent self-limited attacks of pain?

Most Important Physical Examination Finding

- Signs of peritonitis during acute attacks beginning in one quadrant

Most Important Diagnostic Studies

- Leukocytosis and elevated erythrocyte sedimentation rate during attacks

Treatments

- Colchicine

REFERENCES

1. Wright DG. Familial Mediterranean fever. In: Bennett JC, Plum F, eds. *Cecil textbook of medicine.* Philadelphia: Saunders, 1996: 907–908.
2. Pras E, Aksentijevich I, Gruberg L. Mapping a gene causing Familial Mediterranean Fever to the short arm of chromosome 16. *NEJM* 1992;326:1509–1513.
3. Zemer D, Pras M, Sohar E. Colchicine in the prevention and treatment of amyloidosis of Familial Mediterranean Fever. *NEMJ* 1986;314:1001–1005.

52

PORPHYRIA

C. PAUL PERRY

KEY TERMS AND DEFINITIONS

Acute intermittent porphyria (AIP): An inherited deficiency of the hepatic enzyme porphobilinogen deaminase, which causes a build up of the heme precursors δ-aminolevulinic acid (ALA) and porphobilinogen (PBG). Abnormally high levels of these compounds are responsible for the pain and metabolic disturbances observed.

Heme: The porphyrin chelated with iron (Fe) that forms the basic building block for hemoglobin, cytochromes, catalase, and tryptophan pyrrolase. Disturbance of its biosynthesis is the metabolic error responsible for porphyria.

Porphyria: A group of diseases, consisting of inborn errors of metabolic production of porphyrins, that have neurological, cutaneous, or mixed neurocutaneous manifestations.

INTRODUCTION

Chronic pelvic pain (CPP), described as episodic, severely colicky with bloating, constipation, and nausea, may be caused by neurovisceral dysfunction produced by porphyria. Porphyria is derived from the Greek word "porphuros," which describes the purple-red crystalline porphyrins. In biological terms it applies to a group of compounds that are involved in energy capture and utilization. Chlorophyll in plants and heme in animals owe their green and red colors to this organic molecule. The metal binding capability (magnesium-chlorophyll, iron-heme) of porphyrins is central to most of its biological oxidation and oxygen transport functions (Figure 52.1).

   Heme biosynthesis is one of the essential pathways of life, and it occurs in all metabolically active animal cells. Hepatic tissue utilizes heme in the synthesis of hemoglobin, cytochrome P-450, catalase, cytochrome oxidase, and tryptophan pyrrolase. Each of the different types of porphyria diseases is linked to a deficiency in a specific enzyme in the heme biosynthetic pathway (Table 52.1). Consequently, there is an overproduction and increased

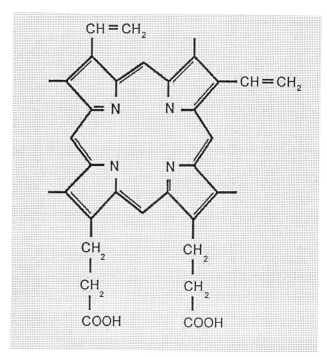

FIGURE 52.1. The structure of protoporphyrin IX, immediate precursor to heme, before iron (Fe) chelated.

excretion of the heme precursors formed prior to the enzyme defect (1).

ETIOLOGY

Stokvis reported the first case of acute intermittent porphyria (AIP) in 1889 (2). Since that time, eight more types of porphyria have been described and their specific enzymatic defect isolated (1). The various types are grouped by whether they involve the erythropoietic or hepatic cells. Another more clinically relevant classification is by their clinical manifestations, such as primarily neurologic, cutaneous, or both (Table 52.1). The majority of types of porphyria present as chronic dermatologic

TABLE 52.1. THE PORPHYRIAS

Type Porphyria	Inheritance	Organ	Enzyme Defect	Systemic Findings
Neuorporphyrias				
Acute intermittent porphyria	AD	Liver	Porphobilinogen deaminase	Abdominal pain and neurologic dysfunction; AA
Plumboporphyria or ALA	AD	Liver	ALA dehydratase	Very rare; neurologic complications; AA
Neurocutaneous Porphyrias				
Hereditary coproporphyria	AD	Liver	Coproporphyrinogen oxidase	Mild photosensitivity; AA
Variegate porphyria	AR	Liver	Protoporphrinogen oxidase	Visceral, cutaneous, and neurologic; AA
Cutaneous Porphyrias				
Congenital erythropoietic porphyria	—	Red cell	Uroprophyrinogen synthase bullae	Congenital light-induced
Porphyria cutanea tarda	AD	Liver	Uroporphyrinogen decarboxylase	Skin fragility; bullae
Erythropoietic protoporphyria	?	Red cell and liver	Heme Synthase	Light-induced erythema and purpura
Erythropoietic coproporphyria	?	Red cell	Very rare	Light-induced bullae
Hepatoerythropoietic	?	Red cell and liver	Very rare	Light-induced bullae

AA, acute attacks; AD, autosomal dominant; ALA, δ-aminolevulinic acid; AR, autosomal recessive.

problems and are not usually associated with undiagnosed CPP. The types of porphyria producing abdominopelvic pain without skin lesions include acute intermittent porphyria (AIP) and plumboporphyria. Only AIP occurs with sufficient frequency to be included in the differential diagnosis of CPP (3).

AIP is the most severe of the inherited porphyrias. The estimated prevalence of the disease is 1:1,000 to 1.5:100,000. It has a slight female preponderance. It is inherited as an autosomally dominant condition causing at least a 50% decrease in the activity of porphobilinogen deaminase. The genetic locus is on chromosome 11 and it shows great molecular heterogeneity. Although the penetrance is only 10% to 20%, acute attacks of AIP are disabling and can be life-threatening (4).

PATHOLOGY

Neuropathy involving both autonomic and somatic nerves accounts for the symptoms of porphyria. The pathogenetic mechanisms that lead to this neurological dysfunction have remained poorly understood. Current theories include: (a) δ-aminolevulinic acid acts as a neurotoxin, (b) neurotransmitters are disturbed secondary to hepatic heme deficiency, and (c) heme depletion in nerve cells affect function. There are numerous other proposed theories, as well (5). Axonal degeneration and central chromatolysis appear to be the most characteristic histopathologic lesions in porphyria. Muscle tissue shows neurogenic atrophy. Peripheral nerve shows segmental demyelination, axonal swelling, and fragmentation. The vagus nerve reveals demyelination and axonal loss. Sym-

pathetic ganglion cells exhibit chromatolysis. Degeneration of neurons in the spinal cord, cerebellum, brainstem, and hypothalamus has been described (6).

SYMPTOMS

AIP may remain dormant until the second or third decade of life. Drug ingestion, stress, concurrent illness, or change in hormonal milieu may precipitate a pain crisis. Drugs dependent on hepatic enzyme degradation are especially a threat, because this may overload a previously compensated system. This is such a common association that many consider AIP a "drug-induced" disorder. Among dangerous drugs, the worst offenders are barbiturates, hydantoins, and sulfonamides. Table 52.2 includes a partial listing of drugs and their relative risk (7).

The most compelling symptom for the patient is pain. Other visceral symptoms may include nausea, vomiting, bloating, bladder dysfunction, constipation, palpitations, diaphoresis, or anhydrosis. Confusion, psychiatric manifestations, and seizures can be present. Hyponatremia may result from inappropriate antidiuretic hormone syndrome. This results in coma and death if not recognized and treated. Muscle weakness, even to the point of compromised respiration, has been reported. Fever, tachycardia, orthostatic hypotension, and hypertension may be present as a result of autonomic dysregulation. Motor weakness, paresthesias, or dysesthesias are possible when sensory nerves are affected.

Some women manifest midcycle and premenstrual pain crises. This is often confused with the visceral pain produced by endometriosis (Chapter 14). They may be sub-

TABLE 52.2. DRUGS AND RELATIVE RISKS IN PORPHYRIAS

Known to Exacerbate Disease	Theoretically Risky	Believed to Be Safe
Aminoglutethimide	Alcuronium	Acetaminophen
Antipyrine	Allyl-containing compounds	Amitriptyline
Aminopurine	Amphetamines	Aspirin
Barbiturates	Bupivacaine	Atropine
Bemegride	Camphor	Bromides
N-butylscopolammonium bromide	Chloroform	Calcium salts
Barbamazepine	Clonazepam (large doses)	Chloral hydrate
Carbamazepine	Clonidine	Chlorpromazine
Carbromal	Colistin	Colchicine
Chloramphenicol	Dramamine	Corticosteroids
Chlordiazepoxide	Etidocaine	Dicumarol
Chloroquine	Etomidate	Digoxin
Chlorpropamide	Erythromycin	Diphenhydramine
Danazol	Felbamate	Droperidol
Dapsone	Furosemide	Fentanyl
Diazepam	Heavy metals	Gabapentin
Diclofenac	Hydralazine	Gallamine
Enflurane	Lamotrigine	Guanethidine
Ergot preparations	Lidocaine	Heparin
Estrogens	Mepivacaine	Hyoscine
Ethanol excess	Methychlothiazide	Ibuprofen
Ethchlorvynol	Metoclopramide	Insulin
Ethinamate	Metyrapone	Labetalol
Eucalyptol (in mouthwash)	Mitotane	Lithium
Glutethimide	Nalidixic acid	Mefenamic acid
Griseofulvin	Nortriptyline	Meperidine
Halothane	Pargyline	Methadone
Hydantoins	Pentylenetetrazole	Morphine
Imipramine	Phenoxybenzamine	Naproxen
Isopropylmeprobamate	Prilocaine	Neostigmine
Mephenytoin	Pyrrocaine	Nitrofurantoin
Meprobamate	Rifampicin	Nitrous oxide
Methyldopa	Sulfonylureas	Oxazepam
Methyprylon	Spironolactone	Pancuronium
Methsuximide	Terpenes	Paraldehyde
Nikethamide	Tiagabine	Penicillin
Novobiocin	Tranylcypromine	Phenothiazines
Oral contraceptives (high-dose)		Propoxyphene
Pentazocine		Propranolol
Phensuximide		Prostigmin
Phenylbutazone		Reserpine
Phenytoin		Streptomycin
Primidone		Succinylcholine
Progestogens		Tetracycline
Pyrazinamide		Thyroxine
Pyrazolone derivatives		
Succinimide		
Sulfonamides		
Theophylline		
Troxidone		
Valproate		

jected to multiple surgeries and hormonal manipulations without success. There is no evidence that low-dose contraceptives or pregnancy are a threat to these patients. Acute cystitis may be misdiagnosed because patients may notice discolored (red) urine with an acute attack. Bladder dysfunction and dysuria have been reported.

PHYSICAL EXAMINATION

Patients in pain crisis are in obvious distress. Dry mucous membranes, abdominal distension without rebound, and diffuse abdominal tenderness may be present. Bowel sounds are usually diminished. Low-grade fever is common. Neurological abnormalities may be present. Cranial or peripheral, sensory, and motor nerve deficits can be seen. Respiration may be compromised if the phrenic nerve is affected. Hand muscles may become atrophied with recurrent attacks (8).

Menstruation may be noted. Pelvic organs are diffusely tender, mimicking pelvic inflammatory disease and acute cystitis. A reddish tint to the urine may be mistaken for hematuria.

Mental confusion, somnolence, seizures, and obtundation also may be the presenting clinical manifestations. This could be the result of hyponatremia produced by inappropriate antidiuretic hormone syndrome, which is sometimes associated with AIP. Women are more vulnerable to this metabolic disturbance. The mortality rate is high if untreated (9).

DIAGNOSTIC STUDIES

Heme Biosynthesis and Laboratory Tests

The porphyrins are molecules produced along the heme biosynthetic pathway. Heme, which consists of protoporphyrin IX and iron (Fe), is most prevalent in erythrocytes and hepatic cells. Synthesis begins in the mitochondria where δ-aminolevulinic acid (ALA) is produced. This rate-limiting step is catalyzed by ALA synthase and is negatively regulated by the increased concentration of heme. Subsequent steps in heme biosynthesis occur in the cytoplasm where two ALA molecules condense to form porphobilinogen (PBG). This step is catalyzed by ALA dehydratase. Next, four molecules of PBG join to form hydroxymethylbilane. This step is catalyzed by PBG deaminase and is another rate-limiting step. Uroporphyrinogen is formed and then converted to coproporphyrinogen, which in turn is converted to protoporphyrinogen IX. The final step is the insertion of Fe into the protoporphyrinogen IX molecule to make heme (10).

In AIP, the inherited deficiency of *PBG deaminase* causes a decrease in heme production. Simultaneously, there is a buildup of the porphyrin precursors ALA and PBG. The diagnosis of AIP is dependent on the detection of increased levels of precursors ALA and PBG during acute attacks. If no elevations in these occur during an acute attack, AIP is not the etiology of the pain (10).

Rapid Bedside Screening Test

The two most commonly available tests to rapidly detect increased urinary heme precursors are the Hoesch test and the Watson-Schwartz test. The reagents used for these, when mixed with the urine from patients in pain crisis, produces a characteristic red pigment. These tests are not totally specific and depend on only elevated PBG. They are usually negative between attacks.

Confirmatory Tests

Quantitative tests for 24-hour excretion of ALA and PBG will confirm the diagnosis of AIP. Levels should be at least twice the normal ranges. The rate of return to normal of these metabolic products is variable and this quantitative test is invalid unless measured during an acute attack. Other more sophisticated tests are available, such as synthase enzyme levels, total plasma porphyrins, and genetic mapping. These are usually reserved to screen family members of those with clinical AIP to determine their heterozygous carrier state. This should be done for genetic counseling and to determine their risk for possible future attacks. Life-threatening illness may be avoided by limiting drug intake and maintaining a healthy diet (11).

Other diagnostic studies are not indicated. Pelvic ultrasound and flat and upright radiographs are likely to show dilated loops of bowel from the ileus. Serum sodium levels should be monitored to detect hyponatremia. Blood alcohol levels can be performed if there is a possibility of excess intake.

TREATMENT

Avoidance or withdrawal of any inducing drugs should be a priority. Adequate nutrition and hydration must be maintained. Good pain relief can usually be accomplished with meperidine or morphine with or without phenothiazines. Administration of carbohydrates represses the activity of hepatic ALA synthase, the so-called "glucose effect." At least 300 g of glucose is needed per day. Monitoring for hyponatremia or hypomagnesemia should be done and, if present, treated appropriately. If hypertension or tachycardia persists they are treated with propranolol. Neurologic evaluation should be done often and the clinician should be prepared to support respirations if paresis occurs. Gabapentin is probably the drug of choice for the treatment of seizures (7).

Hematin (Heme) Therapy for AIP

The presence of biologically available heme decreases the production of the precursor ALA by negative feedback. If unresponsive to general measures, the pain crisis of AIP may be ameliorated by the administration of commercially available heme (Panhematin; Abbott Laboratories, North Chicago, IL) in doses of 3 to 5 mg/kg of body weight every 12 to 24 hours (7).

Prevention of Attacks in Women

The best management of AIP is prevention. Patients with AIP should be advised to use as few drugs as possible. A moderate amount of carbohydrate should always be consumed, and starvation and fad diets should be avoided.

Infections, other stressors, and intercurrent illnesses should be aggressively sought and treated.

Some women with AIP suffer attacks almost every month during the luteal phase of their menstrual cycle. Low-dose oral contraceptives or parenteral gonadotropin releasing hormone agonists are now accepted as effective treatment for women with cyclical attacks. Progesterone administration may actually precipitate a pain crisis (7).

KEY POINTS

Differential Diagnosis

- Recurrent pelvic inflammatory disease
- Recurrent hemorrhagic cystitis
- Primary psychiatric disorders
- Recurrent intermittent bowel obstruction
- Diverticulitis
- Endometriosis
- Guillain-Barré syndrome

Most Important Questions to Ask

- Any family history of similar crises?
- Any recent drug or alcohol intake?
- Specifically, any exposure to barbiturates, hydantoins, or sulfonamides?
- Any progesterone therapy?
- What phase of the menstrual cycle does it usually occur?
- Age of first attack?
- Where is the pain located?
- Any numbness, tingling, or motor weakness?
- Any discoloration of urine?
- Any nausea, vomiting, constipation, or fever?
- Any change in perspiration or rapid heart rate?

Most Important Physical Examination Findings

- Hypertension, tachycardia, or diaphoresis
- Disorientation to person, place, and time
- Temperature elevation
- Abdominal or pelvic tenderness
- Abdominal distension
- Presence of menstruation
- Hypoactive bowel sounds
- Cranial nerves I to XII dysfunction
- Abnormal deep tendon reflexes

Most Important Diagnostic Studies

- Hoesch or Watson-Schwartz test
- Quantitative 24-hour urinary excretion of ALA and PBG

Treatments

- Withdrawal of any inducing drugs
- Good analgesia with meperidine or morphine
- At least 300 g of glucose per day
- Hydration
- Correction of hyponatremia or hypomagnesemia
- Gabapentin for seizures
- Respiratory support if necessary
- Phenothiazines for nausea or anxiety
- Hematin administration if unresponsive to general measures
- Prevention by eliminating drug exposure
- Prevention by eradicating luteal phase with oral contraceptives
- Prevention by abolishing luteal phase with parenteral gonadotropin releasing hormone agonist

REFERENCES

1. Moore MR. The biochemistry of the heme synthesis in porphyria and in the porphyrinurias. *Clin Dermatol* 1998;16:203–223.
2. Stokvis BJ. Over twee zeldzame kleurstoffen in urine van zieken. *Need Tijd Geneesk* 1889;13:409–417.
3. Steiner G, Arffa RC. Psoriasis, ichthyosis, and porphyria. *Int Ophthalmol Clin* 1997;37:41–61.
4. Petersen NE, Nissen H, Horder M, et al. Mutation screening by denaturing gel gradient electrophoresis in North American patients with acute intermittent porphyria. *Clin Chem* 1998;44:1766–1768.
5. Meyer UA, Schuurmans MM, Lindberg RLP. Acute porphyrias: pathogenesis of neurological manifestations. *Semin Liver Dis* 1998;18:43–52.
6. Suarez JI, Cohen ML, Larkin J, et al. Acute intermittent porphyria: clinicopathologic correlation: report of a case and review of the literature. *Neurology* 1997;48:1678–1683.
7. Kalman DR, Bonkovsky HL. Management of acute attacks in the porphyrias. *Clin Dermatol* 1998;16:299–306.
8. Gupta S, Dolwani S. Neurological complications of porphyria. *Postgrad Med J* 1995;72:8631–8632.
9. Perry CP. Syndrome of inappropriate antidiuretic hormone after laparoscopic-assisted vaginal hysterectomy. *J Amer Assoc Gynecol Laparoscop* 1994;1:273–275.
10. Tefferi A, Colgan JP, Solberg LA. Acute porphyrias: diagnosis and management. *Mayo Clin Proc* 1994;69:991–995.
11. Bonkovsky HL, Barnard GF. Diagnosis of porphyric syndromes: a practical approach in the era of molecular biology. *Semin Liver Dis* 1998;18:57–65.

53

HERPES ZOSTER NEURALGIAS

AHMED M. EL-MINAWI

KEY TERMS AND DEFINITIONS

Allodynia: Painful response to nonnoxious stimuli.

Hyperesthesia: Enhanced pain sensitivity or intensity to noxious stimuli.

Postherpetic neuralgia: Pain syndrome that may follow herpes zoster or shingles after the resolution of the cutaneous manifestations.

Varicella-zoster virus: Virus that causes chickenpox and shingles.

Zoster or shingles: A reactivation of the latent Varicella-zoster virus that results in a localized infection with skin lesions that follow the course of peripheral nerves.

Zoster-associated pain: Pain that is associated with herpes zoster either during acute infection or after resolution of skin lesions.

INTRODUCTION

Zoster, or shingles, is caused by the Varicella-zoster virus (VZV), which causes two clinically distinct diseases. The primary acute infection in a susceptible individual is varicella, or chickenpox. Reactivation of the latent virus within the same person, particularly when elderly, results in the more localized infection known as zoster, or shingles. The name shingles is derived from the Latin *cingulus*, meaning girdle, and refers to the peculiar nature of the skin lesions that follow the course of nerves and appear to encircle the body (1). A rarer type of reactivation can also occur, known as *zoster sine herpete*, characterized by pain without zosteriform rash (2).

The neuralgia accompanying herpes zoster (HZ) is either *acute-phase pain*, which is pain that occurs during the initial attack, or *postherpetic neuralgia* (PHN), pain that may follow the resolution of the cutaneous manifestations. PHN is usually a long-term chronic condition that may afflict the affected dermatome. Authors argue that patients with HZ feel pain as a continuum and that, despite the differing pathophysiologies of acute and postherpetic pain, the proper measurement of the pain should be in continuum (3,4). The recommended term, *zoster-associated pain* (ZAP), was coined by the International Herpes Management

Forum, but its drawback is that it does not properly indicate PHN, an indication that is important because the majority of patients who experience acute-phase pain do not develop chronic pain (5,6).

Because postherpetic neuralgia (PHN) is a separate disease, Johnson suggested that the best definition for PHN is, "... a continual or continuous severe pain, often with allodynia, persisting many months after shingles, and leading to a reduction in the quality of life" (7,8).

The annual incidence of HZ is estimated to be between 0.8 and 4.8 per 1,000 population (9,10). There is a direct relationship between the incidence of zoster and increasing age (11,12). The marked increase in the incidence of HZ with age supports the hypothesis that a strong cell-mediated immunity, which deteriorates with age, maintains the VZV in a latent state within the satellite cells of the posterior ganglion, and prevents its reactivation (9).

The incidence of PHN also increases with the age of the patient. The risk below age 50 is relatively negligible, but rises greatly after age 60. Individuals over 50 years of age have a 15- to 27-fold higher prevalence of PHN than those less than 50 (13). The risk of PHN lasting more than 1 month is 50% at age 60 (14).

There are also racial and gender differences in the occurrence of HZ. Blacks are one-fourth as likely as Whites to experience zoster (15). Although some authors report no gender-based influence in the occurrence of HZ, data from more recent reports challenge this and suggest a marked predominance of women (16). Recent data also suggest that PHN may occur somewhat more often in women (17).

If PHN develops after lumbosacral HZ, it can cause chronic pelvic pain (CPP). This appears, however, to be a rare cause of CPP in women in reported case series. At least a partial explanation for this is that published series of CPP patients deal primarily with women of reproductive age and the majority of patients affected with PHN are elderly (18).

ETIOLOGY AND PATHOPHYSIOLOGY

The VZV causes a primary varicella infection (chickenpox), usually in childhood, leaving the virus dormant in the dorsal root ganglion cells. For poorly understood reasons, the VZV can reactivate and move down the nerve toward the skin, producing the painful dermatologic condition of zoster or shingles. In around 20% of patients (reports range from 7% to almost 75%) after the initial zoster attack, PHN occurs (19,20). This is pain persisting beyond 4 weeks after the acute eruption of zoster. The etiology of this condition is perplexing. The risk of pain that lasts more than 12 months ranges from 2% to 20% (20,21).

Malignancy, HIV infection, radiation therapy and trauma have been suggested as risk factors, but there are little data on the effect on the incidence of PHN (8,12).

Various theories have been proposed for PHN. One of these suggests that ongoing inflammation causes the pain in PHN. Vafai et al. have detected proteins and DNA specific to VZV in mononuclear cell in patients with PHN months to years after the disappearance of the rash, as compared to 6 weeks in patients without PHN (22,23). They suggested that ongoing ganglial inflammation without rash was the basic cause of PHN pain. This theory is supported by histological studies of spinal nerve ganglia that reveal an inflammatory infiltrate of mononuclear cells around dying neurons in patients with PHN and intractable intercostal pain 1 year after an acute episode of zoster (24).

Others have attempted to link neurodegenerative changes in the afferent pathways to the pain of PHN by showing, for example, morphological changes, including atrophy in one case, in the dorsal horns of the spinal cord in subjects with PHN (25). It is suggested that such morphological central nervous system (CNS) changes caused by the VZV are reversible in HZ, but not in PHN (7). It has been suggested that multiple injuries at the peripheral and CNS levels are induced by an intense viral attack lead to PHN pain (20). In addition to damaged fibers discharging abnormally into the CNS and distorting naturally generated signals, afferent neurons may become abnormally sensitive to various stimuli. The abnormal barrage of impulses reaching the dorsal horn, in addition to the deafferentation, may lead to substantial changes in the excitability of the second-order neurons in the dorsal horn as well as possible inducement of new synaptic connections.

Positron emission tomography testing has shown a statistically significant decrease in thalamic activity contralateral to the symptomatic side in patients with chronic neuropathic pain, including postherpetic neuralgia, in comparison with normal subjects (26). This suggests that functional alterations in thalamic pain processing circuits may be an important component of chronic neuropathic pain.

SYMPTOMS AND SIGNS

Patients with HZ always have history of varicella except in the extremely rare cases of zoster following administration of varicella vaccine (27). The cutaneous eruption is usually preceded by pain in the affected dermatome up to 2 weeks prior, or by flulike symptoms and mild fever. Prodromal symptoms may include hyperesthesia, paresthesia, itching, or pain (1,19). The pain may be either burning, stabbing, or shooting, tends to be more severe in older patients, and does not correlate well with the extent of the eruption (28).

The occurrence of prodromal symptoms with HZ predicts PHN. Choo et al. reported that 46% of their patients with PHN lasting more than 30 days and 51% of those with PHN lasting more than 60 days had prodromal symptoms (13). Galil et al. reported that occurrence of opthalmic zoster increased the risk of a complication sevenfold (29).

The lesions are grouped vesicles on an erythematous base appearing in patches. The vesicles are clear first, becoming cloudy a few days later, then purulent, then drying and rupturing to form crusts. In immunocompromised individuals, bullous, chronic ecthymatous, and verruciform lesions are infrequently seen. The acute eruption, which is almost always unilateral and involves a single dermatome, lasts an average of 21 days.

The dermatomes most frequently affected in HZ are, in order of frequency, thoracic (55%), cranial (20%), lumbar (15%), and sacral (5%). Although lumbosacral involvement represents only 20% of the cases of HZ involvement, complications in this area, particularly PHN, may produce debilitating CPP in the affected patients. Although zoster and postherpetic neuralgia cause a relatively small number of the cases of CPP seen, the diagnosis can be challenging. Liesegang has reported that localization to the cervical and lumbosacral regions is characteristic of zoster in infants and children (30).

Complications, morbidity, and psychological problems can occur after an attack of HZ and specific syndromes may occur with different zoster-infected ganglia. *Herpes zoster opthalmicus* may lead to ulcerative zoster keratitis or a temporary or permanent Argyll-Robertson pupillary reaction. Involvement of the geniculate ganglion, and the facial and auditory nerves, may lead to the *Ramsay Hunt syndrome.* *Glossopharyngeal zoster* causes pharyngeal pain. *Vagal nerve* involvement can cause cardiac and gastrointestinal pain of sufficient intensity as to mimic myocardial infarction or acute abdomen. Involvement of the second to fourth *cervical nerves* may lead to ipsilateral paralysis of the hemidiaphragm (31).

Lumbosacral nerve involvement may lead to chronic pelvic conditions in the form of bladder and bowel dysfunction. Thiers and Sahn mention that symptoms similar to those associated with the passage of urinary stones may occur (1). Herpes zoster infection, particularly involving the distribution of the second and third sacral dermatomes, has been associated with bladder and bowel dysfunction, most commonly urinary retention. Tanikawa et al., in a case report of a 68-year-old woman with urinary retention and constipation secondary to sacral herpes zoster, stated that 47 cases had been reported in the Japanese literature prior to their case (32). Jensen and Walter report that the neurogenic bladder dysfunction in sacral herpes is reversible (33). They documented the gradual reversibility of motor paralysis of the detrusor muscle utilizing urodynamic studies. Persson and Melchior have also documented the transient quality of sacral herpes bladder dysfunction and note that symptoms and residual urine usually disappear within 2 to 3 weeks (34). In some cases anal sphincter tone may be impaired (35).

PHN is not a continuation of acute HZ, but a separate disease that is a complication of HZ (7). Although separate diseases, HZ usually gradually merges into PHN and presents the dilemma of determining the exact moment at which the term PHN can be applied, with most authors placing the onset at 1 to 3 months after disappearance of the rash (1,7,17,19,20,36). Despite this, some authors believe that a minimum of 6 months of pain duration is necessary, particularly if assessing the effect of a treatment (17). The clinical features seen in PHN patients appear to be very consistent, with some variation dependent on the site of previous zoster manifestation (Table 53.1).

Pain is the common denominator in all patients affected by PHN and is a prerequisite to the diagnosis. The chronic pain in the affected dermatome(s) is considered to be one of the severest types of pain, in addition to being one of the most difficult to treat (17). The character of PHN pain has been variously described as aching, burning, searing, scalding, stabbing, or lancinating. The pain is, in most cases, confined to the affected dermatome and is usually felt within the areas of lost or impaired sensation (20). The pain exhibits autonomic instability and its intensity is related to the emotional and physical state of the patient, with exacerbation occurring under stressful conditions and amelioration with relaxation (7,20,37). PHN affecting the lumbosacral area causes CPP, with lower back pain and suprapubic pain owing to bladder involvement. In some instances, the chronic pain may resemble that of ureteric spasms similar to that felt in case of urinary stones (1). Sciatic nerve involvement leads to chronic pain in the distribution of the nerve.

Recently, Chen and colleagues have suggested that a significant portion of the pain in PHN might be owing to myofascial trigger points arising as a result of zoster (36).

TABLE 53.1. THE CARDINAL FEATURES OF POSTHERPETIC NEURALGIA AND THEIR REPORTED INCIDENCE (7,17,19,20)

Feature	Incidence (%)
Pain	100
Allodynia	87–100
Sensory deficits	94–100

From Bowsher D. Pathophysiology of postherpetic neuralgia: towards a rational treatment. *Neurology* 1995;45(Suppl 8):S56–S57; Bowsher D. Postherpetic neuralgia and its treatment: a retrospective survey of 191 patients. *J Pain Symp Management* 1996;12(5):290–298; Goh CL, Khoo L. A retrospctive study of the clinical presentation and outcome of herpes zoster in a tertiary dermatology outpatient referral clinic. *Int J Dermatol* 1997;36(9):667–672; Nurmikko T. Clinical features and pathophysiologic mechanisms of postherpetic neuralgia. *Neurology* 1995;45(Suppl 8):S54–S53, with permission.

They reported two cases with clinical characteristics of PHN after HZ infection of the thoracic nerves. Both patients, in addition to having hyperesthesia, were found to have several tender myofascial trigger points of the intercostal muscles beneath the affected skin. Pressure on the myofascial trigger points caused referred pain in the intercostal space distal to the tender spot. Likewise, local twitch responses were elicited during injection of the spots. The 1% lidocaine injections caused an immediate decrease in hyperesthesia and pain intensity that lasted up to 2 weeks after the initial injection.

Allodynia, which is defined as pain produced by non-noxious stimuli, is present in greater than 90% of PHN patients (17). The most commonly seen type is mechanical or tactile allodynia. In most cases it is to moving rather than static stimuli (20,36,68). Low-intensity mechanical stimuli, such as the brushing of clothes against skin, stimulate rapidly adapting low-threshold $\alpha\beta$ mechanoreceptors and produce pain. An important sign is that the allodynia is suppressed by firm pressure, which stimulates slowly adapting low-threshold $\alpha\beta$ mechanoreceptors; as a result patients are often seen using bindings and pressure dressings over the affected areas (17). Thermal allodynia is sometimes present, usually to cold, which also exacerbates any indigenous pain in the affected dermatome (20).

Sensory deficits are also common in PHN patients. All modalities of sensation (warm, cold, touch, heat pain, pinprick, vibration, and two-point discrimination) are affected within the involved area (68). Up to 94% of patients may have sensory deficits (7). In addition to sensory manifestations, motor deficits are also reported (17).

Other signs or symptoms may be present. Changes in the emotional state of the patient often occur, with patients exhibiting higher state and trait anxiety and increased intolerance to pain (8). They also are more prone to depressive states and lower life satisfaction than patients who do not develop PHN, although one researcher believes that there may be psychosocial antecedents making these patients more prone to the development of chronic pain (38). Pigmentary changes and scarring of the skin may also occur in some patients (17).

DIAGNOSTIC STUDIES

Diagnoses of HZ and PHN rely mainly on clinical history and evaluation. Laboratory tests are rarely required but can be very helpful in differentiating the disease from herpes simplex, which may have a zosteriform distribution. However, herpes simplex affected patients often give a history of recurring attacks.

Viral culture from vesicular fluid is the most definitive method for diagnosis of HZ virus, but the drawback is the time needed, which may be up to 14 days (28). The Tzanck preparation or skin biopsy, which is positive in 50% to 80%

of cases, shows multinucleated giant cells, but cannot distinguish zoster from herpes simplex or varicella (1,27,28).

The modern rapid methods of diagnosis include immunoflourescence for detecting specific viral antibodies in serum in addition to direct immunofluorescence antibody staining of infected cells, which is a rapid and accurate method. Other, less commonly employed methods include gel diffusion and electron microscopical diagnosis, which is a rapid method (less than 30 min) when it is available (1,27,28).

TREATMENT

CPP as a result of HZ infection and subsequent PHN can not be totally prevented, but its incidence and severity can be decreased by early aggressive treatment of HZ. The treatment of HZ relies primarily on antiviral drugs and incidentally on immunomodulating agents, specific immunoglobulins, antiviral enzymes, and corticosteroids as well as analgesics.

Antiviral drugs have been in use for many years. Acyclovir (Zovirax) speeds rash healing, decreases viral shedding as well as causing earlier relief of pain (1,4,21,39,40). In addition it reduces the incidence of certain HZ opthalmicus-related intraocular complications (41). Dosage is 800 mg, five times daily, because lower doses of 400 to 600 mg, five times daily, have not been as effective, as only 20% of the dose absorbed orally (42). Adequate amounts of fluids must be taken by the patient. This is particularly important when the drug is used intravenously in immunocompromised patients, because it may lead to crystalluria and renal damage if not given slowly. The intravenous dose is usually 500 mg/m^2 every 8 hours for 7 to 10 days (21,27,43). A meta-analysis of randomized clinical trials of acyclovir to prevent postherpetic neuralgia showed an odds ratio 0.5 for the occurrence of "any pain" in the distribution of HZ rash at 6 months in adults treated with acyclovir. This suggests that treatment with 800 mg, five times daily, of oral acyclovir within 72 hours of onset of rash may reduce the chance of residual pain at 6 months by about 50% in immunocompetent adults (44).

Prednisone has been used with acyclovir based on data suggesting that prednisone has a significant antiinflammatory effect and reduces the risk of persistent pain (4,45,46). At least one randomized clinical trial in immunocompetent patients has shown accelerated crusting and healing, decreased time to cessation of acute neuritis, decreased time to return of uninterrupted sleep, and decreased time to cessation of analgesic therapy. There was no effect on the development of postherpetic neuralgia (47). The dosage of acyclovir was 800 mg, five times daily for 21 days, and the dose of prednisone was 60 mg per day for first 7 days, 30 mg per day for days 8 to 14, and 15 mg per day for days 15 to 21.

Because of the problems of bioavailability and dosage compliance, other antiviral drugs have been introduced. Valaciclovir (Valtrex), is the *l*-valyl ester of acyclovir, and is rapidly converted almost completely to acyclovir after oral administration of the drug, giving threefold to fivefold increases in acyclovir bioavailability. In at least one randomized clinical trial, valaciclovir significantly accelerated the resolution of herpes zoster associated pain at 7 and 14 days, as compared to acyclovir (42). Valaciclovir also resulted in a smaller proportion of patients having pain lasting for 6 months (19% versus 26%). It appears that valaciclovir is more effective in shortening the duration of PHN than acyclovir (43).

Netuvidine is a nucleoside analogue with the benefits of greater potency and better bioavailability. It is almost sevenfold more potent than acyclovir and has a significantly longer half-life of 14 to 20 hours (48,49). In a small clinical trial a dosage of 200 mg orally every 12 hours for 7 days caused rapid cessation of new lesion formation (48). The effect on long-term pain is unclear and one clinical trial reported it to be inferior to acyclovir in reducing pain duration (50).

Famciclovir is the oral form of the purine nucleoside analogue penciclovir. Famciclovir may reduce the severity of postherpetic neuralgia when compared with placebo (51). Sorivudine is an antiviral drug that inhibits replication of varicella zoster virus with enhanced oral bioavailability. The once-daily dose is one-hundredth that of acyclovir, and less than one-tenth of the doses of valaciclovir or famciclovir (52). A randomized clinical trial of sorivudine showed shortening of the mean time to full crusting and a reduction of the mean days that new lesions formed (53). Sorivudine therapy is superior to acyclovir, but undesirable fatal drug interactions have been reported. Sorivudine inhibits dihydropyrimidine dehydrogenase, which is required for the metabolism of 5-flouro-uracil (5-FU). As a consequence, toxic levels of 5-FU accumulate in the plasma and may lead to toxicity and mortality in patients using them together (54).

Additional treatments, which are usually reserved for immunocompromised and debilitated patients, are vidarabine and interferon. Vidarabine accelerates cutaneous healing and, if given within 72 hours of onset, prevents progression of lesion formation within the affected dermatome and causes slow regression of the disease in the area involved (21).

Tranquilizers and opioids are also helpful in the treatment of the acute pain of HZ and are of definite benefit in relieving the chronic pain of PHN. PHN has been treated traditionally using tricyclic antidepressants, especially amitriptylline (55–57). A recent randomized clinical trial by Bowsher involving patients 70 years of age or more with a diagnosis of HZ showed that 25 mg of amitriptyline daily for 90 days after diagnosis reduced pain prevalence by more than 50% (58). Based on this study there may be a benefit to the use of amitriptylline preemptively in combination with an antiviral drug in elderly patients diagnosed with HZ.

Tricyclic antidepressants, independent of their antidepressant action, are thought to actually produce an analgesic effect owing to potentiation of serotonin and nora-drenaline in the CNS (14). When antidepressant treatment is initiated, it should start with a low dose and be titrated upward. Elderly patients (over 65) should receive smaller starting doses than younger patients with incremental increase every 7 to 10 days, until either pain relief or intolerable side effects occur. The drugs are cumulative, and care should be taken to prevent overdosing (14). Some authors have recommended combinations of amitriptyline and perphenazine or chloroprothixene, because no single drug or combination of drugs is completely effective in eradicating the pain of PHN (1).

Although tricyclic antidepressants, sometimes combined with neuroleptics, are generally recommended for PHN treatment, opioids may be added if analgesia is inadequate. Their use, although controversial, has been of benefit in some types of chronic pain. Among the newer opioids being used is tramadol. This is a synthetic, centrally acting analgesic having both opioid and nonopioid analgesic activity. Its nonopioid component stimulates serotonin release at the spinal level in addition to inhibition of norepinephrine uptake. Tramadol may be particularly useful in cases where conventional antidepressants are contraindicated, as in obvious cardiovascular disease, and in patients where an antidepressant effect is not required (59).

Local methods of treatment are also available and encompass a variety of modalities. Local anesthetics have been used to relieve pain in PHN and acute HZ in a number of novel ways. These methods are of particular help in CPP owing to PHN. Manabe et al. have investigated the effects of a continuous epidural blockade on zoster associ-

ated pain as compared to intermittent epidural blocks (60). Patients received either intermittent epidural blocks (1% mepivicaine, 4 to 6 mL, three to six times per day) alone or in combination with acyclovir or vidarbine for 5 days. A third group was given continuous epidural 0.5% bupivicaine infusion (0.3 to 1.0 ml/hr) for 2 weeks. The continuous blockade patients had a significantly shorter duration of treatment than the other two groups because of greater relief of pain. Another study by Eide and colleagues studied the effect of continuous subcutaneous infusion of ketamine on nerve pain in PHN (61). Results showed that ketamine reduced allodynia 59% to 100% after 1 week, and wind-up pain was reduced by 60% to 100% after infusion of 0.05 mg/kg/h and 0.15 mg/kg/h, respectively, of the drug over a 1-week period. Itching and induration were the side effects, and were of sufficient magnitude to cease treatment of one patient. Topical local anesthetics such as lidocaine gel and EMLA cream (eutectic mixture of local anesthetics) have also been used, but appear to be of limited effect and should be considered as adjunctive measures (14). Other methods of local treatment include local nerve blocks and lumbar blockades. The latter is of great benefit in reducing the chronic pain associated with lumbosacral PHN (62).

Topical agents such as capsaicin, the active principle of hot chili pepper, are being used with increasing frequency. Capsaicin purportedly selectively stimulates unmyelinated C fiber afferent neurons, causing substance P release. Depletion of substance P in small primary afferents reduces, or abolishes, the transmission of painful stimuli to the higher centers (14). A review of the published clinical trials of capasaicin concluded that its potential benefits merited more research

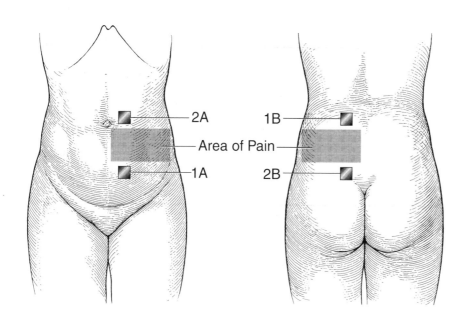

Electrodes 1A & 1B = Channel 1
Electrodes 2A & 2B = Channel 2

FIGURE 53.1. Placement of TENS electrodes for treatment of post-herpetic neuralgia abdominopelvic pain.

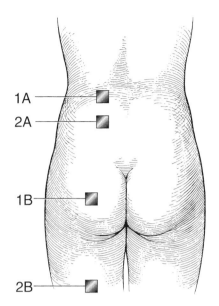 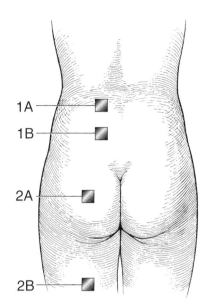

Electrodes 1A & 1B = Channel 1
Electrodes 2A & 2B = Channel 2

FIGURE 53.2. Placement of TENS electrodes for treatment of post-herpetic neuralgia sciatic pain.

and condoned its use as adjunctive therapy, because trials have shown that it is more efficacious than placebo (63).

Transcutaneous electrical nerve stimulation (TENS) has been used for chronic pain management for over two decades. From the theoretical point of view it seems an excellent solution to the chronic pain in lumbosacral involvement. Although anecdotal reports of its efficacy in postherpetic neuralgia have been published, very few studies have been conducted on its benefits in zoster or PHN (64). Wolf and colleagues published the results of TENS use in a group of 114 patients with chronic pain of various origins (65). The pulse width used was 100 μsec at a pulse rate of 50 to 100 pulses per second, applied at submotor threshold intensity during 30 to 45 minute sessions three to five times a week. Pain before and after was evaluated using the McGill Pain Questionnaire. Thirteen of 18 patients (72%) with peripheral neuropathy reported 60 percent relief of pain after therapy. Among this group, patients with postherpetic neuralgia responded most favorably to TENS. Figures 53.1 and 53.2 show electrode placements and treatment times for postherpetic neuralgia-induced chronic pain in the lower abdomen, pelvis, lower back, and thighs (66).

KEY POINTS

Differential Diagnoses

- Herpes simplex infection
- Other cause of neuropathy

Most Important Questions to Ask

- Is there a history of varicella and zoster?
- Is the pain burning, stabbing, or shooting?
- What is the distribution of the pain? (Is the pain in a dermatomal distribution?)
- Is there any problem with bladder and bowel dysfunction?

Most Important Physical Examination Findings

- Myofascial trigger points
- Allodynia, mechanical or tactile
- Sensory deficits to warm, cold, touch, heat pain, pinprick, vibration, and two-point discrimination
- Pigmentary changes and scarring of the skin

Most Important Diagnostic Studies

- Viral culture from vesicular fluid
- Tzanck preparation or skin biopsy
- Immunoflourescence testing for specific viral antibodies in serum or infected cells

Treatments

- Acyclovir (Zovirax)
- Prednisone plus acyclovir
- Valaciclovir (Valtrex)

- Netuvidine
- Famciclovir
- Sorivudine
- Tricyclic antidepressants, especially amitriptylline
- Opioids
- Epidural blockade
- Ketamine infusion
- Topical local anesthetics, such as lidocaine gel and EMLA cream
- Local nerve blocks
- Lumbar nerve blocks
- Capsaicin
- Transcutaneous electrical nerve stimulation

REFERENCES

1. Thiers BH and Eleanor ES. Varicella-zoster virus infections. In: Moschella SL, Hurley HJ, eds. *Dermatology,* 3rd ed. Philadelphia: Saunders, 3rd ed., 1992:797–805.
2. Gilden DH, Dueland AN, Devlin ME, et al. Varicella-zoster reactivation without rash. *J Infect Dis* 1992;166(Suppl 1): S30–34.
3. Wood MJ. How to measure and reduce the burden of zoster-associated pain. *Scand J Infect Dis* 1996;100(Suppl):55–58.
4. Wood MJ, Johnson RW, McKendrick MW. A randomized trial of acyclovir for 7 days or 21 days with and without prednisolone for treatment of acute herpes zoster. *N Engl J Med* 1994;330: 896–900.
5. International Herpes Management Forum. How can the burden of zoster-associated pain be reduced? Recommendations from the IHMF Management Strategies Workshop, Washington DC, 1995.
6. Boon RJ, Griffin DRJ. Efficacy of famciclovir in the treatment of herpes zoster. *Neurology* 1995;45(Suppl 8):S76–S77.
7. Bowsher D. Pathophysiology of postherpetic neuralgia: towards a rational treatment. *Neurology* 1995;45(Suppl 8):S56–S57.
8. Johnson RW. The future of predictors, prevention, and therapy in postherpetic neuralgia. *Neurology* 1995;45(Suppl 8):S70–S73.
9. Editorial. Herpes zoster. *Virus SA* 1996;5(3).
10. McGregor RM. Herpes zoster, chicken pox, and cancer in general practice. *Br Med J* 1957;1:84–87.
11. Hope-Simpson R. The nature of Herpes Zoster: a long term study and a new hypothesis. *Proc R Soc Med* 1965;58:9–20.
12. Donahue JG, Choo PW, Manson JE, et al. The incidence of Herpes Zoster. *Arch Int Med* 1995;155(15):1605–1609.
13. Choo PW, Galil K, Donahue JG, et al. Risk factors for postherpetic neuralgia. *Arch Intern Med* 1997;157(11):1217–1214.
14. Watson CP. The treatment of postherpetic neuralgia. *Neurology* 1995;45(Suppl 8):S58–S59.
15. Schmader K, George LK, Burchett BM, et al. Racial differences in the occurrence of herpes zoster. *J Infect Dis* 1995;171(3): 701–703.
16. Cerny Z. Changes in the incidence and clinical manifestations of herpes zoster. *Casopis Lekaru Ceskych* 1996;135(8):244–248.
17. Bowsher D. Postherpetic neuralgia and its treatment: a retrospective survey of 191 patients. *J Pain Symp Management* 1996; 12(5):290–298.
18. Bowsher D. Post-herpetic neuralgia in older patients. Incidence and optimal treatment. *Drugs Aging* 1994;5(6):411–418.
19. Goh CL, Khoo L. A retrospective study of the clinical presentation and outcome of herpes zoster in a tertiary dermatology outpatient referral clinic. *Int J Dermatol* 1997;36(9):667–672.
20. Nurmikko T. Clinical features and pathophysiologic mechanisms of postherpetic neuralgia. *Neurology* 1995;45(Suppl 8):S54–S55.
21. Whitley RJ. Therapeutic approaches to Varicella-zoster infections. *J Infect Dis* 1992;166(Suppl 1):S51–S57.
22. Vafai A, Wellish M, and Gilden DH. Expression of varicella zoster virus in blood mononuclear cells of patients with postherpetic neuralgia. *Proc Natl Acad Sci USA* 1988;85:2767–2770.
23. Gilden DH, Devlin M, Wellish M, et al. Persistence of varicella zoster virus DNA in blood mononuclear cells of patients with varicella or zoster. *Virus Genes* 1989;2(4):299–305.
24. Smith FP. Pathological studies of spinal nerve ganglia in relation to intractable intercostal pain. *Surg Neurol* 1978;10:50–53.
25. Watson CPN, Deck JH, Morshead C, et al. Post-herpetic neuralgia: further post-mortem studies of cases with and without pain. *Pain* 1991;44:105–117.
26. Iadarola MJ, Max MB, Berman KF, et al. Unilateral decrease in thalamic activity observed with positron emission tomography in patients with chronic neuropathic pain. *Pain* 1995;63(1):55–64.
27. Arnold HL, Odom RB, James WD. Viral diseases. In: *Andrew's diseases of the skin. Clinical dermatology,* 8th ed. Philadelphia: Saunders, 1990:436–451.
28. Crosby DL. Varicella Zoster virus infections. In: Leppert PC, Howard FM, eds., *Primary care for women.* Philadelphia: Lippincott-Raven, 1997:859–863.
29. Galil K, Choo PW, Donahue JG, et al. The sequelae of Herpes Zoster. *Arch Intern Med* 1997;157:1209–1213.
30. Liesegang G. Varicella-zoster virus: systemic and ocular features. *J Am Acad Dermatol* 1984;11:165–191.
31. O'Doherty CJ. Dermatologic dyspnea. *Int J Dermatol* 1986;25: 58.
32. Tanikawa K, Kawamura N, Baba S. Urinary retention secondary to herpes zoster. *Hinyokika Kiyo-Acta Urologica Japonica* 1987; 33(8):1266–1271.
33. Jensen FS, Walter S. Herpes zoster induced reversible neurogenic bladder dysfunction. Urodynamic documentation of reversible bladder paralysis. *Ugeskrift for Laeger* 1991;153(3):197–199.
34. Persson C, Melchior H. Urinary retention in herpes zoster. *Urologe—Ausgabe A* 1986;25(5):286–287.
35. Jellinek EH, Tulloch WS. Herpes zoster with dysfunction of bladder and anus. *Lancet* 1976;2(7997):1219–1222.
36. Chen S-M, Chen J-T, Kuan T-S, et al. Myofascial trigger points in intercostal muscles secondary to herpes zoster infection of the intercostal nerve. *Arch Phys Med Rehabil* 1998;79:336–338.
37. Rowbowtham MC, Fields HL. Postherpetic neuralgia: the relation of pain complaint, sensory disturbance, and skin temperature. *Pain* 1989;39:129–144.
38. Dworkin RH, Hartstein G, Rosner HL, et al. A high risk method for studying psychosocial antecedents of chronic pain: the prospective investigation of herpes zoster.
39. Morton P, Thomson AN. Oral acyclovir in the treatment of herpes zoster in general practice. *NZ Med J* 1989;102:93–95.
40. Wood J, Ogan PH, McKendrick MW, et al. Efficacy of oral acyclovir treatment of acute herpes zoster. *Am J Med* 1988;85: 79–83.
41. Harding SP, Porter SM. Oral acyclovir in herpes zoster opthalmicus. *Curr Eye Res* 1991;10:177–182.
42. Beutner KR, Friedman DJ, Forszpaniak C, et al. Valaciclovir compared with acyclovir for improved therapy for herpes zoster in immunocompetent adults. *Antimicrob Agents Chemother* 1995; 39(7):1546–1553.
43. Herne K, Cirelli R, Lee P, et al. Antiviral therapy of acute herpes zoster in older patients. *Drugs Aging* 1996;8(2):97–112.
44. Jackson JL, Gibbons R, Meyer G, et al. The effect of treating herpes zoster with oral acyclovir in preventing postherpetic neuralgia. A meta-analysis. *Arch Intern Med* 1997;157(8):909–912.

45. Gelfand M. Treatment of herpes zoster with cortisone. *JAMA* 1954;154:911–912.

46. Keczkes K, Basheer AM. Do corticosteroids prevent post-herpetic neuralgia? *Br J Dermatol* 1980;102:551–555.

47. Whitley RJ, Weiss H, Gnann JW, et al. Acyclovir with and without prednisone for the treatment of herpes zoster. A randomized, placebo-controlled trial. *Ann Intern Med* 1996;125:376–383.

48. Peck RW, Crome P, Wood MJ, et al. Multiple dose netivudine, a potent anti-varicella zoster virus agent, in healthy elderly volunteers and patients with shingles. *J Antimicrob Chemother* 1996;37:583–597.

49. Peck RW, Weatherly BC, Wootton R, et al. Pharmacokinetics and tolerability of single doses of 882c87, a potent, new anti-varicella-zoster virus agent, in healthy volunteers. *Antimicrob Agents Chemother* 1995;39:20–27.

50. Fiddian AP, International Zoster Study Group. A randomised controlled trial of Zovirax (acyclovir, ACV) versus netivudine for the treatment of herpes zoster. *Antiviral Res* 1995;26(3):A297.

51. Stott GA. Famciclovir: a new systemic antiviral agent for herpesvirus infections. *American Family Physician* 1997;55(7):2501–2504.

52. Whitley RJ. Sorivudine: a potent inhibitor of varicella zoster virus replication. *Adv Experimental Medicine & Biol* 1996;394:41–44.

53. Wallace MR, Chamberlin CJ, Sawyer MH, et al. Treatment of adult varicella with sorivudine: a randomized, placebo-controlled trial. *J Infect Dis* 1996;174(2):249–255.

54. Whitley RJ. Sorivudine: a promising drug for the treatment of varicella-zoster virus infection. *Neurology* 1995;45(12 Suppl 8):73–75.

55. Woodforde JM, Dwyer B, McEwen BW. The treatment of postherpetic neuralgia. *Med J Aust* 1965;2:869–872.

56. Taub A. Relief of postherpetic neuralgia with psychotropic drugs. *J Neurosurg* 1973;39:235–239.

57. Watson CPN, Evans RJ, Reed K, et al. Amitriptyline versus placebo in postherpetic neuralgia. *Neurology* 1982;32:671–673.

58. Bowsher D. The effects of pre-emptive treatment of postherpetic neuralgia with amitriptyline: a randomized double-blind, placebo-controlled trial. *J Pain Symptom Manage* 1997;13(6):327–331.

59. Gobel H, Stadler T. Treatment of post-herpes zoster pain with tramadol. Results of an open pilot study versus clomipramine with or without levomepromazine. *Drugs* 1997;53(Suppl 2):34–39.

60. Manabe H, Dan K, Higa K. Continuous epidural infusion of local anesthetics and shorter duration of acute zoster-associated pain. *Clin J Pain* 1995;11(3):220–228.

61. Eide K, Stubhaug A, Oye I, et al. Continuous subcutaneous administration of the *N*-methyl-D-aspartic acid (NMDA) receptor antagonist ketamine in the treatment of postherpetic neuralgia. *Pain* 1995;61(2):21–28.

62. Hadzic A, Vloka JD, Saff GN, et al. The "Three-in-one" block for treatment of pain in a patient with acute herpes zoster infection. *Regional Anesthesia* 1997;22(6):575–578.

63. Rains C, Bryson HM. Topical capsaicin. A review of its pharmacological properties and therapeutic potential in postherpertic neuralgia, diabetic neuropathy and osteoarthritis. *Drugs Aging* 1995;7(4):317–328.

64. Meyerson BA. A electrostimulation procedures, effects, presumed rationale and possible mechanisms. *Advances Pain Res Ther* 1983;5:495–534.

65. Wolf SL, Gersh MR, Rao VR. Examination of electrode placements and stimulating parameters in treating chronic pain with conventional transcutaneous electrical nerve stimulation. *Pain* 1981;11:37–47.

66. Adapted from Staodyn TENS protocols. Http://www.staodyn.com.

54

SLEEP AND SLEEP DISTURBANCE

KEVIN M. KINBACK
JAMES E. CARTER

KEY TERMS AND DEFINITIONS

Electroencephalograph (EEG): An instrument for recording electrical activity of the brain, producing an electroencephalogram, or a recorded tracing; used to detect convulsive disorders, localize cerebral lesions, as well as measuring parameters of sleep.

Initial insomnia: Difficulty initiating sleep.

Insomnia: Inability to sleep, or sleep prematurely ended or interrupted by periods of wakefulness; may be a symptom of various diseases; most frequently is caused by anxiety or pain.

Middle insomnia: Difficulty in maintaining sleep.

Polysomnograph: Recording device using electrodes that measure brain waves, muscle activity, respiration, and other standard measures of sleep.

Rapid eye movement or REM sleep: A paradoxical sleep stage with low voltage, mixed frequency EEG waves, as well as intense autonomic activity including changes of heart rate, respiratory rate, and systolic blood pressure, and increased oxygen consumption, increased urine secretion, increased cerebral blood flow, increased brain temperature, and desynchronized neural firing with increased neural activity. Most dreaming occurs during REM sleep.

Sleep stages: Stage 0 is awake. Stage 1 is the least deep sleep, usually a transient stage of drowsiness between awake and actual sleep, and the stage from which the subject is most easily awakened. Stage 2 has EEG waves of various frequencies, with "sleep spindles" of 13 to 16 cycles per second and "K-complexes." Stage 3 is characterized by the appearance of high voltage, slow EEG waves (called delta), along with some sleep spindles. Stage 4 is the deepest sleep, when more than 50% of EEG waves are delta.

Somnifacient: A medicine producing sleep.

Somnolence: Prolonged drowsiness or sleepiness, or a condition resembling a trance, which may continue for a number of days.

Terminal insomnia: Early awakening from sleep, sometimes with inability to reinitiate sleep.

INTRODUCTION

There are wide variations in what may be considered "normal sleep." The nature of sleep and the amount of sleep required varies greatly across the lifespan of each individual. Sleep may be dysfunctional and there are a large number of well-defined disorders associated with disturbances of sleep. Sleep disorders are common, and clearly are closely associated with conditions of chronic pain, anxiety, and other medical problems.

Sleep has long been believed to be a state in which the body repairs itself, a time of anabolism. Others have theorized that it is a descent into a lower level of consciousness, often accompanied by complex dreams. Although sleep research has been going on for over 100 years, the electroencephalograph (EEG) was only available after 1935; it has revolutionized the field of sleep study. The EEG can distinguish between subtle stages of sleep, which previously could not be discerned by simple observation.

Normal sleep involves a process of lowered heart and respiratory rates, reduced systolic blood pressure, changes in electrical activity in the brain, and the presence or absence of muscle movement in various stages of sleep. There are generally five stages of sleep, which correspond to relative "depth" of sleep. Stage 0 is awake. Stage 1 is the least deep, usually a transient stage of drowsiness between awake (stage 0) and actual sleep, and the stage from which the subject is most easily awakened. It is marked by low voltage, mixed frequency EEG activity. Stage 2 has EEG waves of various frequencies, with "sleep spindles" of 13 to 16 cycles per second (CPS or HZ) and "K-complexes," which are single complex waves with excessively high amplitudes. Stage 3 is characterized by the appearance of high voltage, slow EEG waves (called delta), along with some sleep spindles. Less than 50% of EEG sleep waves are delta in stage 3. When more than 50% of waves are delta, stage 4, the deepest sleep, is reached. Efforts have been made to standardize these stages within various parameters including percentage of K-complexes and spindles, frequency, amplitude, and duration of various waves, eye movements, and instrument calibration (1).

Rapid eye movement, or REM sleep, is a paradoxical stage with low voltage, mixed frequency (stage 1), as well as intense autonomic activity including changes of heart rate, respiratory rate, and systolic blood pressure, and increased oxygen consumption, increased urine secretion, and desynchronized neural firing with increased neural activity. Cerebral blood flow is increased in REM sleep, as is brain temperature. Although no one is certain of the exact function of REM, most dreaming occurs during REM sleep. Dreaming in REM sleep has been thought of as a mechanism to "resolve emotional conflicts." However, in neonates more than 50% of sleep is REM, an unexpected finding given their apparent lack of emotional conflicts. It is unclear whether neonates dream.

Sleep patterns change with age and vary with gender. Women have fewer awakenings from sleep than men. Awakenings that usually are not recalled the following morning are normal. The percentage of awake time rapidly increases with age after 29 years of age, and awakenings occur earlier in the night. Slow wave sleep decreases with age, mostly in the twenties, as REM latency decreases to approximately 90 minutes. Men have less REM than women (1).

One study of 509 subjects without chronic pain showed an incidence of sleep disturbances of 10% in those 25 years old, but 100% in those over 95 years old, with 70% having initial insomnia and 40% having middle insomnia. Another study of 297 subjects from 15 to 91 years of age showed a 20% incidence of chronic sleep disturbance, and indicated that quality of sleep is important, as well as total amount of sleep. In this study only 3% used hypnotics, and only 2% used alcohol as a somnifacient (2). In a study comparing patients with CPP to asymptomatic patients, Nolan et al. found that 72% of patients with pelvic pain reported sleep disorders, of which 31% had initial insomnia, 51% had middle insomnia, and 18% reported both. Among the asymptomatic patients, only 4% had initial insomnia, 8% had middle insomnia, and 4% had both ($P < 0.0001$). There was also a statistically significant higher incidence of depression in the patients with chronic pelvic pain (CPP). This study included patients with either normal pelvic examinations or laparoscopy on enrollment. By the end of the study 4% of the patients were found to have mild endometriosis and the rest had CPP with no identified organic pathology (3).

In 1990 the Diagnostic Classification Committee of the American Sleep Disorders Association established the International Classification of Sleep Disorders (Table 54.1). The three major categories include dyssomnias, parasomnias, and sleep disorders associated with medical or psychiatric disorders. The dyssomnias may be important in CPP patients and include intrinsic disorders (e.g., narcolepsy, obstructive sleep apnea, restless leg syndrome), extrinsic disorders (e.g., environmental sleep disorder, inadequate sleep hygiene, alcohol-dependent sleep disorder), and circadian

TABLE 54.1. INTERNATIONAL CLASSIFICATION OF SLEEP DISORDERS

1. Dyssomnias
   A. Intrinsic sleep disorders
      1. Psychophysiological insomnia
      2. Sleep state misperception
      3. Idiopathic insomnia
      4. Narcolepsy
      5. Recurrent hypersomnia
      6. Idiopathic hypersomnia
      7. Posttraumatic hypersomnia
      8. Obstructive sleep apnea syndrome
      9. Central sleep apnea syndrome
      10. Central alveolar hypoventilation syndrome
      11. Periodic limb movement disorder
      12. Restless legs syndrome
      13. Intrinsic sleep disorder
   B. Extrinsic sleep disorders
      1. Inadequate sleep hygiene
      2. Environmental sleep disorder
      3. Altitude insomnia
      4. Adjustment sleep disorder
      5. Insufficient sleep syndrome
      6. Limit-setting sleep disorder
      7. Sleep-onset association disorder
      8. Food allergy insomnia
      9. Nocturnal eating (drinking) syndrome
      10. Hypnotic-dependent sleep disorder
      11. Stimulant-dependent sleep disorder
      12. Alcohol-dependent sleep disorder
      13. Toxin-induced sleep disorder
      14. Extrinsic sleep disorder NOS
   C. Circadian rhythm sleep disorders
      1. Time zone change (jet lag) syndrome
      2. Shift work sleep disorder
      3. Irregular sleep-wake pattern
      4. Delayed sleep phase syndrome
      5. Advanced sleep phase syndrome
      6. Non–24-hour sleep-wake disorder
      7. Circadian rhythm sleep disorder NOS
2. Parasomnias
   A. Arousal disorders
      1. Confusional arousals
      2. Sleepwalking
      3. leep terrors
   B. Sleep-wake transition disorders
      1. Rhythmic movement disorder
      2. Sleep starts
      3. Sleep talking
      4. Nocturnal leg cramps
   C. Parasomnias usually associated with REM sleep
      1. Nightmares
      2. Sleep paralysis
      3. Impaired–sleep-related penile erections
      4. Sleep-related painful erections
      5. REM–sleep-related sinus arrest
      6. REM sleep behavior disorder
   D. Other parasomnias
      1. Sleep bruxism
      2. Sleep enuresis
      3. Sleep-related abnormal swallowing syndrome
      4. Nocturnal paroxysmal dystonia
      5. Sudden unexplained nocturnal death syndrome
      6. Primary snoring

TABLE 54.1. *(Continued)*

    7. Infant sleep apnea
    8. Congenital central hypoventilation syndrome
    9. Sudden infant death syndrome
    10. Benign neonatal sleep myoclonus
    11. Other parasomnia NOS
3. Sleep disorders associated with medical-psychiatric disorders
  A. Associated with mental disorders
    1. Psychoses
    2. Mood disorders
    3. Anxiety disorders
    4. Panic disorder
    5. Alcoholism
  B. Associate with neurological disorders
    1. Cerebral degenerative disorders
    2. Dementia
    3. Parkinsonism
    4. Fatal familial insomnia
    5. Sleep-related epilepsy
    6. Electrical status epilepticus of sleep
    7. Sleep-related headaches
  C. Associated with other medical disorders
    1. Sleeping sickness
    2. Nocturnal cardiac ischemia
    3. Chronic obstructive pulmonary disease
    4. Sleep-related asthma
    5. Sleep-related gastroesophageal reflux
    6. Peptic ulcer disease
    7. Fibromyalgia (fibrositis) syndrome
4. Proposed sleep disorders
    1. Short sleeper
    2. Long sleeper
    3. Subwakefulness syndrome
    4. Fragmentary myoclonus
    5. Sleep hyperhidrosis
    6. Menstrual-associated sleep disorder
    7. Pregnancy-associated sleep disorder
    8. Terrifying hypnagogic hallucinations
    9. Sleep-related neurogenic tachypnea
    10. Sleep-related laryngospasm
    11. Sleep choking syndrome

rhythm sleep disorders (e.g., time zone change or jet lag syndrome, shift work sleep disorder). The sleep disorders associated with medical or psychiatric disorders are also important in CPP patients. They include disorders associated with mental disorders (e.g., anxiety disorders, mood disorders, alcoholism), neurological disorders (e.g., sleep-related epilepsy, sleep-related headaches), and other medical disorders (e.g., chronic obstructive pulmonary disease, peptic ulcer disease, fibromyalgia syndrome). The parasomnias are probably of less significance in CPP patients.

Sleep disorders have diverse etiologies and require various workups and different treatment modalities. In this chapter we will focus on "menstrual-associated sleep disorder" and on the perturbations of sleep caused by CPP. There is currently no specific category for sleep disorder caused by chronic pain.

ETIOLOGY

There are primary problems associated with sleep, such as sleep apnea, narcolepsy, restless legs syndrome, nocturnal myoclonus, sleep apnea, and periodic leg movements. Most primary childhood parasomnias, such as night terrors, are self-limited and resolve with time, usually without medication (4). The majority of disturbances of sleep, however, are not primary symptoms of other illnesses. With advancing age, sleep impairments such as unwanted arousals and awakenings and decreased slow wave sleep usually increase. Lack of deep, stage 4 sleep can contribute to cognitive disturbances, generalized joint and muscle pain, depression, and fatigue. Other causes of sleep disorders include drug use, chronic pain, cardiovascular disease, depression, diabetes, and psychiatric problems, especially stress and anxiety spectrum disorders. Poor sleep hygiene and other learned behaviors contribute significantly to sleep disorders. Chronic medical conditions, particularly arthritis, respiratory disorders such as e.g., chronic obstructive pulmonary disease (COPD), asthma, dermatological disorders, fibromyalgia, fibrocytis, chronic fatigue syndrome, and migraines, to name a few, contribute significantly to disturbances of sleep (5).

Chronobiological studies of circadian rhythms of sleep have discovered a link between disordered sleep physiology and fibromyalgia and chronic fatigue syndrome. They suggest interleukin-1 (IL-1) affects immune-neuroendocrine-thermal systems and hence the sleep-wake cycle. Age, menstruation, fibromyalgia, and chronic fatigue syndrome (CFS) affect these cycles. These apparent changes in hormonal cycles in CFS and fibromyalgia result in pain (usually of joints and muscles), fatigue, daytime somnolence, nonrestorative sleep, cognitive deficits, and mood changes. This is one example of medical illnesses directly affecting neuroendocrine and neurohormonal balance, and secondarily disrupting sleep (6).

PATHOLOGY

In CPP, it is often the sensation of pain itself that disrupts sleep. Patients often have difficulty remaining comfortable in one position, especially if lower back pain or radicular pain to the limbs is involved. Some patients with CPP who are also obese might suffer from obstructive sleep apnea (OSA) and related conditions, especially with increasing age. Upper airway occlusion, often accompanied by severe snoring, or periods of actual apnea, can lead to excess cardiovascular morbidity. Many advances have recently been made in treatment of these conditions (7).

There are also primary, idiopathic sleep problems. The system of sleep is complex, involving wide-ranging circuits that promote sleep, including solitary tract nuclei, raphe nuclei, and the medial forebrain area. Waking up is controlled by the reticular activating system (RAS). These two systems must be carefully tuned and balanced in order to produce restorative sleep. Some people seem to have disruptions in these systems from birth, and also tend to repress, deny, or minimize anxiety or emotional problems. This is greatly exacerbated during periods of stress, and many of these people display paradoxical reactions to hypnotics (2).

Hormonal changes associated with menopause can bring about changes in sleep patterns, as well as other somatic, behavioral, and psychological difficulties. This could be considered a subtype of the proposed menstrual-associated sleep disorder (8). A report of two cases of sleep-disordered breathing in climacteric showed a decrease in clinical symptoms with hormone replacement, but frequency of arousals was unchanged (9).

Temporal lobe dysfunction can result in disturbed sleep or dyssomnia. The limbic system helps organize sleep, with inputs into both sleep inducing, as well as arousal mechanisms. Experimental amygdala kindling, in an animal epilepsy model involving temporal structures, produced disturbed sleep patterns with frequent awakenings and light sleep. Epilepsy is associated with superficial, disrupted sleep patterns, even in the absence of observable seizures. Cognitive, affective, and behavioral sequelae often follow. Epilepsy must be carefully ruled out, because only treatment of the underlying seizure disorder will minimize the sleep disorder symptoms (10).

One form of severe insomnia, fatal familial insomnia (FFI), is characterized by severe, progressive degeneration of the thalamus. Sleep progressively decreases, and eventually ceases, with imbalances of sympathetic activation. The unchecked parasympathetic drive causes chronic secondary hypertension, with autonomic changes. Hypercortisolism with unchecked feedback suppression of adrenocorticotrophic hormone (ACTH) results in constantly elevated catecholamine levels, with high levels of growth hormone, prolactin, and melatonin. One study by Montagna et al. suggested that the thalamus plays a role as an integrative neural structure that modulates interaction between the limbic system (controlling emotions and mood), and the hypothalamus (controlling homeostatic balance). FFI is an autosomal dominant prion disease that is irreversible. This can serve as one model of neuropathology that has direct effects on sleep (11).

HISTORY

It seems that women with pelvic pain are more likely to have sleep disorders than women without pain. Based on this, seeking a history of sleep disorders should be a component of the comprehensive history in women with CPP. Most patients with sleep disorders present with vague complaints, such as, "I can't sleep," or even, "I'm not sleeping at all." A complete history of prior and current sleep patterns should be obtained. Careful attention should be paid to whether sleep problems are acute or were present to some degree before the onset of CPP. In some cases, a preexisting sleep disorder can be exacerbated by the pain. There is usually significant night-to-night variation of insomnia. A sleep log can help objectify the symptoms. This can prevent too much clinical emphasis being placed on specific instances, and can help pinpoint more complex etiologic factors (12).

One of the cardinal symptoms is excessive daytime sleepiness. Family members or coworkers can also be a source of history, especially if the patient is unaware of or fails to disclose having trouble staying awake at meetings or while driving, or going to bed early. Although sometimes, because of narcolepsy or obstructive sleep apnea, excessive daytime sleepiness plagues our society. Many people push to get more work and play done in decreasing amounts of time, staying up late, then trying to get up to start the next day on time. Detailed questioning about "sleep hygiene" should take place. Many of these patients will report high levels of job, family, or other types of stress.

Excessive snoring, reported either by the patient or other household members, may correspond to partial obstruction of the upper airway. This is practically always present in obstructive sleep apnea. Snoring increases with body weight. One large-scale study showed that 14% of women habitually snored, and another study from Finland showed a prevalence of 4%. The prevalence of snoring in Hispanic-American adult women, adjusted for age, was 15%. Snoring usually increases with age up to 65 years, but then decreases, probably with loss of body weight. Obesity is commonly associated with sleep disturbances, especially if the weight gain was accompanied by increased snoring. Other risk factors for sleep apnea include smoking and alcohol (owing to a central depressive effect), as well as hostility. There is also an association between habitual snoring and hypertension, as well as ischemic heart disease. Adenotonsillar hypertrophy in younger patients can obstruct the airway.

Mood changes or anxiety can be symptoms of a sleep disorder. Primary psychiatric problems may need to be ruled out, because sleep changes are secondary findings with many of these problems.

SIGNS

In addition to daytime somnolence, patients with disturbed sleep often show circles under their eyes, and may exhibit mood changes, either depressed or slightly euphoric. Other family members can often note that the patient with CPP may have an increased sleep latency or decreased total sleep time. It can be considered normal to have a sleep latency of up to 20 to 30 minutes, and a total sleep time as little as 6.5 hours (2).

DIAGNOSTIC STUDIES

Most sleep disorders, particularly narcolepsy and sleep apnea, are definitively diagnosed in the sleep lab. Polysomnography is used to measure many parameters of sleep. After several hours of measuring stages of sleep, muscle movement, and number of awakenings, and screening for apnea, a trial of continuous positive airway pressure (CPAP) may be given. CPAP is usually reserved for those who have significant oxygen saturation decreases associated with periods of apnea. Indices of apnea, such as the apnea-hypopnea index measure length of apnea, degree and number of desaturations, cardiac sequelae, and other parameters. Five or more apneic events per hour of sleep usually denote obstructive sleep apnea, although standardized criteria have not yet been developed or standardized. If the desaturations decrease significantly with the CPAP, then a small CPAP unit can be sent home with the patient. The sleep lab will also determine the ideal setting for the CPAP unit.

A relationship between HLA types and narcolepsy has been postulated. One study found 34% of Japanese are HLA-DR2 positive compared to 12% in Israel. The prevalence of narcolepsy is 0.26 per 1,000 in Japan, but only 0.004 in Israel. This may be a potential marker for at least one type of sleep disorder, but it is not in wide clinical use at this time (2).

DIFFERENTIAL DIAGNOSIS

Epilepsy can sometimes present as night terrors, nightmares, or paroxysmal nocturnal dystonia, and is also associated with significant insomnia, even in the absence of actual seizure activity (10,13). Many other neurologic disorders, such as Tourette's syndrome, various dystonias and choreas, muscular dystrophy, multiple sclerosis, and idiopathic autonomic insufficiency (Shy-Drager syndrome) cause sleep disturbances. Sleep apnea has been associated with obesity, as well as acromegaly.

Medications can profoundly disturb sleep. Many antidepressants, such as tricyclics, desyrel, mirtazepine, and the monoamine oxidase inhibitors (MAOIs) can produce excessive sleep and fatigue. Stimulants and pseudostimulants, including amphetamines, buproprion, and SSRIs in some patients may reduce sleep or cause insomnia. Some patients react paradoxically to antihistamines (including those in over-the-counter agents), and also desyrel, becoming acutely agitated, often with initial insomnia. Propranolol can disrupt sleep via an unknown mechanism and has been associated with severely vivid nightmares. Caffeine and sympathomimetics, such as theophylline and many other inhalers used for lung diseases, can cause unwanted stimulation, interfering with sleep. Other agents disrupting sleep include levodopa, methyldopa, diuretics, reserpine, and cimetidine. Nicotine has similar effects on sleep disruption as caffeine. Alcohol also causes profound problems with sleep, even in small amounts in certain susceptible individuals.

Menopause, whether natural or surgically induced, results in reduced estrogen and progesterone levels and can produce insomnia. Other endocrine abnormalities, such as thyroid and adrenal dysfunction, can disrupt sleep. In some patients, oral contraceptives and hormone replacement can actually have adverse affects on sleep as well.

Some infectious diseases, such as syphilis, acquired immunodeficiency syndrome (AIDS), and herpetic and other forms of encephalitis, can cause difficulty in maintaining sleep, as well as excessive sleepiness. Zidovudine (AZT) therapy can aggravate insomnia. These symptoms are usually greatest during the peak of infection. Syphilis and herpes can sometimes remain dormant for some time, or the initial infection may be forgotten while the central nervous system (CNS) effects slowly progress.

MANAGEMENT OR TREATMENT

Preliminary treatment in this patient population begins with good control of the pelvic pain itself, treatment of any underlying comorbid medical or psychiatric conditions, and elimination or reduction of any medications that could be associated with disrupted sleep. For example, hormone replacement can sometimes ameliorate insomnia caused by menopause or surgery. Subsequent treatment can then be broken down into three major areas: (a) sleep hygiene counseling, (b) behavioral techniques, and (c) pharmacotherapy.

Sleep Hygiene Counseling

Sleep hygiene relates to the patient's schedule of going to bed and arising, as well as the sleep environment. There is a wide variation in sensitivity to both noise and light. Often noises from outside the home, a snoring bed partner, or noise from household appliances can disrupt sleep. The patient may not be aware of the noise itself, but will still report the effects of sleep disruption, because events disrupting sleep may not necessarily be remembered on awakening. Women are more sensitive to noise than men, and this phenomenon increases with age. Noisy environments have been shown to produce increased arousals, sleep stage shifts, and increased body movements. Often ear plugs help, but can sometimes produce tinnitus. Some "white noise," such as a background sound generator, constant fan, or other low frequency source of sound, may mask other noises and thereby enable sound sleep.

The sleep surface must be comfortable, but has been shown to have only transient effects on sleep. Several objective studies failed to demonstrate differences in sleep owing to sleep surface (2). Sleep position may affect the quality of sleep. Horizontal sleeping is best, because polysomnographic studies have found that increasing back angles above horizontal has reduced total sleep time and increased wakefulness.

Good sleep hygiene also involves stabilization of the sleep schedule, minimizing "swing shift" working, and dealing assertively with the stress of life events. Major life events, such as tragic loss, financial problems, personal threats, or even beneficial events, produce transient insom-

TABLE 54.2. SLEEP HYGIENE INSTRUCTIONS

Avoid naps (but check with your physician first, because in some sleep disorders naps can be beneficial).

Restrict sleep period or time in bed to average number of hours you have actually slept in the preceding week. This is important to improve the quality of your sleep, and too much time in bed can actually decrease quality of sleep on the subsequent night.

Get regular exercise each day, preferably 40 minutes per day of an activity that causes you to sweat. It is best to finish exercising at least 6 hours before bedtime and avoid strenuous exercise after 6 PM.

Use stress management techniques in the daytime.

Keep a regular time out of bed 7 days a week.

Get at least one half hour of sunlight within 30 minutes of your out-of-bed time.

Limit caffeine use to no more than three cups no later than 10 AM. Also, avoid caffeine entirely for a 4-week trial period.

Limit alcoholic beverages to light or moderate use, if at all. Alcohol can fragment sleep over the second half of the sleep period.

List problems and one-sentence next steps for the following day before bedtime. Use this as time set aside as worry time. Forgive yourself and others.

Take a hot bath for 30 minutes within 2 hours of bedtime. The goal is to raise your temperature by 2°C. A hot drink may also warm you and help you relax as well.

Do not eat or drink heavily for 3 hours before bedtime. A light bedtime snack may be helpful.

If you have trouble with vomiting, acid reflux, or heartburn, be careful especially to avoid heavy meals and spices in the evening. Do not go to bed too full or too hungry. The head of the bed may need to be raised.

Use a bedtime ritual. For example, reading before lights-out may be helpful if it is not related to your work.

Use bedroom only for sleep; do not work or do other activities that lead to prolonged arousal.

Keep your room dark, quiet, well-ventilated, and at a comfortable temperature throughout the night. Ear plugs and eye shades are okay.

If possible, make arrangements for care-giving activities (children, pets, etc.) to be assumed by someone else.

Learn simple self-hypnosis or relaxation exercises to use if you wake up at night. Do not try too hard to sleep, but rather concentrate on the pleasant feeling of relaxation.

Avoid unfamiliar sleep environments as much as possible.

Be sure the mattress is not too soft or too firm, and the pillow is the right height and firmness.

Do not expose yourself to bright light if you have to get up at night.

Do not smoke to get yourself back to sleep. Do not smoke after 7 PM. Of course, it is best to give up smoking entirely.

Keep the clock face turned away and do not look to see what time it is if you wake up at night.

An occasional sleeping pill is probably all right.

---

nia that can last for up to 3 weeks. The most common complaint with these is initial insomnia. Daytime naps, extended "make up" bedtimes, alcohol, and caffeine must be avoided. Patients should be informed that the circadian rhythms are set by both total sleep time, and the awakening time; therefore, the most important factor is exposing the retinas to bright light on a consistent cycle. Sleeping too long or taking excessive daytime naps will sabotage this natural cycle. It is often helpful to point out the patients that often after 5 days of awakening at the exact same time, they will often awaken at the same hour on a nonworking day, even without setting an alarm. This is because their bodies have accepted this circadian rhythm, which will be subsequently disrupted if they continue to sleep past this time. Ignoring these rhythms often leads to a feeling of "jet lag," or in more severe cases feeling "like run over by a truck."

Table 54.2 is an example of instructional handout about sleep hygiene for patients (2).

Behavioral Techniques

There is good evidence that behavioral and relaxation interventions are effective treatments of chronic pain and insomnia. There is moderately good evidence that cognitive-behavioral techniques and biofeedback are effective for relief of chronic pain and insomnia (14).

For patients suffering delayed sleep phase syndrome (DSPS), in which they have difficulty falling asleep and difficulty arising at socially acceptable hours, there are a range of treatments. One treatment is schedule shifts, in which patients are sent to bed earlier and given a strict schedule for awakening. This schedule can be progressively tightened over time, to eventually produce the desired result. Medications, vitamins, and hormonal replacements have also been used, but one of the most effective techniques is bright light treatment. This potentially corrects the circadian abnormality of DSPS, and has proven to be ophthalmologically safe (15). Bright light treatment is usually given in the morning for at least 45 minutes. It is especially useful in the elderly population where poor tolerance of hypnotics is common (2). It has also been used in treatment of depression, especially the seasonal affective disorder subtype.

Because insomnia is partly a learned phenomenon, it can also be unlearned. Many insomniacs develop excessive anxiety about not being able to fall and stay asleep, with increasing apprehension toward bedtime. Assigning a "worry time" is often helpful. Patients can defer thoughts that increase tension and anxiety to a specific 30-minute period of the day. During this period, they are given permission to worry as much as they want. If they find themselves worrying at any other time, they simply tell themselves to stop, and then make a mental note to worry at the next daily worry time. In many cases, they will actually forget to worry during worry time, thus postponing their worries for another 24 hours! Deep breathing techniques are also helpful, as well as meditation. Hypnosis may be effective in some cases.

Anxiety can also be a learned phenomenon. The bedroom, and particularly the bed, should never be used for any activity other than sleeping, and perhaps intercourse. For some, even intercourse is associated with anxiety, and can lead to sleep disturbances. In these cases, the bed should be reserved for sleep only. Many patients who awaken during the night become anxious about falling back to sleep or become angry that they have awakened. These thoughts should be minimized with cognitive-behavioral therapy with a qualified professional therapist. Other techniques include relaxing music, imagery, and back massage.

Scheduling sleep hours is particularly important. Some women spend excessive hours in bed, unsuccessfully trying to sleep. They must be taught to get out of bed when they are not tired and to keep a rigid wake-up time, regardless of the amount of sleep they get. They may return to bed once they are sleepy. Often drinking some warm milk, reading a boring book, or performing some other task requiring sustained attention will induce sleep. "Paradoxical intention" can be useful, where the patient tries to stay as wide awake as possible, resisting becoming sleepy. This effort in itself produces fatigue, paradoxically promoting the onset of sleep.

Sleep state misperception is quite amenable to behavioral treatment. Sleep curtailment is often effective, in which a rigid time is set for getting out of bed, regardless of the quality or duration of the perceived sleep. This can be combined with limited, occasional hypnotic use, but only after several consecutive nights in which the patient experiences very poor sleep. Many of these patients perceive hypnotics to be helpful, but there is often a noticeable lack of polysomnographic evidence to confirm this (2).

Regular exercise has been found to have direct beneficial effects in sleep disorders. One randomized study, which included 403 women, demonstrated that vigorous activity and walking at a brisk pace for more than six blocks per day, with regular exercise, reduced the risk of disorders in maintaining sleep. A scheduled exercise program can be a powerful, nonpharmacologic tool in the therapeutic armamentarium (16).

In the case of menopause or other ovarian dysfunction, hormone replacement therapy (HRT) should be considered. If this is ineffective, pharmacotherapy should be instituted if the sleep disturbance is causing significant problems in daytime functioning. Dosage reduction should be attempted on regular intervals, especially immediately after the acute onset of menopause, because patients may adapt to the insomnia and may no longer require hypnotic agents.

Pharmacotherapy

Most physicians are appropriately cautious with sedative-hypnotic agents. They are indicated only for short-term use, except in cases such as restless legs syndrome (RLS) or nocturnal myoclonus, in which cases they seem to retain their effectiveness. Sedative-hypnotics, such as benzodiazepines (diazepam, chlordiazepoxide, and lorazepam), chloral hydrate, meprobamate, and the barbiturates are widely prescribed, but patients can quickly develop tolerance to these agents. Hypnotics increase arousal threshold, thereby decreasing arousals and wakefulness, causing increased sleep time. Close care is needed, because some patients find themselves in need of detoxification if they escalate their dosages without close medical supervision. These agents can also have detrimental effects on cognition, including access to memories, learning new information, and slowed reaction times. Driving and daytime alertness could become impaired, and addiction is also a risk. Hypnotics are associated with depression and can cause rebound anxiety on discontinuation. Withdrawal symptoms can include autonomic instability, tremors, severe anxiety, and seizures, especially if abruptly discontinued from chronic, higher dosages. These agents should only be used on an intermittent basis, for short periods of time (17). Triazolam has been associated with anterograde amnesia, and rebound insomnia. These agents should be avoided, or used with extreme caution, in patients with lung diseases such as asthma and chronic obstructive pulmonary disease (COPD), because they suppress the respiratory centers.

In the elderly population, one study found that use of long-acting benzodiazepines, such as flurazepam, diazepam, and chlordiazepoxide, for sleep disorders has been associated with increased risk of hip fracture. Nondrug interventions should be maximized in the elderly, and as a last resort only the short-acting benzodiazepines, such as temazepam and oxazepam, should be used (18).

Hormone replacement or augmentation should be considered in some patients, especially perimenopausal women. Progesterone receptor effects can regulate gene expression, which affects neurotransmitter-gated ion channels and "cross-talk" between membrane and nuclear hormone effects. The action of steroids influencing sleep may be mediated by enhanced τ-aminobutyric acid (GABA)-mediated chloride channels (19). An independent study showed that "neurosteroid" derivatives of steroid hormones, such as 3 α-OH DHP, a metabolite of progesterone, potentiates GABA responses of cerebellar Purkinje cells. The neurosteroid also enhanced GABA responses in the hippocampus, in a fashion similar to benzodiazepines. There is much less evidence of estrogen having similar effects that directly affect sleep; however, estrogens do alter responses to excitatory neurotransmitters or inputs. There is a lack of *in vivo* studies (20). A prospective, randomized, double-blind study of 63 postmenopausal women found that the severity of initial insomnia predicted a good response to estrogen that significantly diminished sleep complaints. Part of this benefit may have been from reduced climacteric symptoms overall by the estrogen (21). Sleep problems in younger women tend to increase perimenstrually, when plasma estrogen levels drop below 50 pg/mL. Most attempts to develop some standard unique dose of hormone replacement, when needed, have been confounded because of large individual variation in estrogen clearance rate—individual titration is mandatory. Sleep, as well as osteoporosis, headaches, asthenia, mood changes, bloating, and breast tenderness are often target symptoms of hormone replacement therapy (22). One pilot study of seven postmenopausal or posthysterectomy women with nocturnal diaphoresis and/or hot flashes showed a statistically significant decrease in overall number of hot flushes, as well as those associated with awakenings, with improved sleep efficiency and a reduction of cyclic alternating patterns of sleep. This study included a single-masked placebo arm (23).

Many of the antidepressants have admirable hypnotic properties. Desyrel is commonly used because it helps in sustaining sleep, preventing middle insomnia or frequent awakenings. A good starting dose is 25 to 50 mg, because the smallest tablet is 50 mg. Patients may be allowed to increase the dosage up to a few hundred milligrams, but a limited supply should be given to start. Patients with ventricular ectopy should not receive desyrel, because it can exacerbate arrhythmias. Dose-related orthostatic hypotension can occur in older women taking desyrel. Mirtazepine, a newer antidepressant, showed somnolence in 54% of the 453 patients in the initial 6-week study population. This side effect is said to be inversely related to dosage; therefore, so lower dosages should produce more sedation and higher doses should produce less. The usual starting dosage for the off-label purpose of sedation would be 7.5 or 15 mg, or one-half to one of the smallest tablet (15 mg). This agent has also been associated with increased appetite, so it should be used in caution if obesity is a concern. The package insert also describes some types of carcinoma in laboratory animals, as well as a few rare cases of agranulocytosis, and recommends that patients be advised of these findings. Cancer has not been associated in humans, however, and the agent does have FDA approval for depression. Although out of favor for use in depression, the tricyclic antidepressants, such as amitriptyline, imipramine, desipramine, and doxepin, are quite effective for inducing sleep, as well as prolonging sleep time. The dosage should be small to start, in the 10 to 25 mg range, and titrated upward to effect. If there are hangover-type effects, either reduce the dose or give it earlier in the evening. These agents are contraindicated in glaucoma and with monoamine oxidase inhibitors, and should be used with caution in patients on serotonin selective reuptake

inhibitors and antiarrhythmics. Patients over age 40 or those with known cardiac disease should have an electrocardiogram performed prior to starting a tricyclic agent.

Some patients want nonprescription medication and may use a variety of over-the-counter (OTC) agents. Most of these contain some type of antihistamine and many contain significant percentages of alcohol. Patients should be reminded that these can lead to drug interactions, cause daytime sedation, and produce tolerance. It may be preferable to simply prescribe an antihistamine alone, such as hydroxyzine or diphenhydramine, to eliminate the combination of agents sometimes found in OTC preparations. Many OTC agents include aspirin or acetaminophen, which can be toxic and lead to liver problems if used chronically or in excessive doses. These do not promote sleep in and of themselves and could be eliminated by prescribing antihistamines alone. A "hangover" effect is not uncommon with both antihistamines and tricyclics; therefore, patients often stop the medication on their own if this occurs. This may be helpful as a "self-taper" of the hypnotic, thereby avoiding prolonged use.

Barbiturates and strong agents such as chloral hydrate can be easily abused and have a narrow therapeutic index. These are rarely used anymore, because patients can inadvertently overdose on these agents because the effective dose is very close to the lethal dose.

Some of the antipsychotics, sometimes known as neuroleptics, such as chlorpromazine, prochlorperazine, and thioridizine are quite sedating, with anticholinergic and antihistiminergic properties, but should be avoided as routine hypnotics owing to the risk, of tardive dyskinesia (TD). TD is a potentially irreversible, involuntary movement disorder, usually of the mouth, lips, or tongue. The incidence of TD is higher in women and increases with age, duration of exposure, and total cumulative dose. Some of the newer atypical antipsychotics, such as olanzapine or risperidone, have a significantly lower incidence of TD, but still should be reserved for only the most refractory cases in off-label use as hypnotics for short periods only.

Treatment may also involve discontinuing agents that may disrupt sleep, or changing to alternative therapies, if available. For example, a hypertensive woman taking propranolol can be switched to an agent that does not cross the blood-brain barrier, such as atenolol, and is less likely to disrupt sleep. With the multitude of pharmacologic options currently available for a given disorder, medications likely to adversely affect sleep are more easily avoided. Stimulating agents, if absolutely necessary, should be given in the early morning to minimize the effect on sleep. Caffeine, diet pills, and other OTC agents, such as cold remedies, ephedrine, and herbs containing ma huang, should be discontinued.

After starting pharmacotherapy, the patient should be seen again within a short period of time, to ensure proper use of the agent. If the hypnotic is causing daytime sedation, the dose can be reduced or the medicine can be taken earlier in the day, as long as the onset of sleep is not so rapid as to disrupt the patient's evening schedule. If prolonged action remains a problem after these adjustments, the clinician can switch to a shorter-acting agent. If cognitive slowing, amnesia, or recall problems arise, then the dose should definitely be reduced. The next step would be changing from daily to intermittent use; and if this does not resolve the problem an alternate agent should be prescribed. Most patients should be given a "drug holiday" after several weeks of therapy to see if they can sleep on their own. They may have a few days of rebound insomnia, but then should settle into an acceptable pattern.

Newer agents are being considered, including partial agonists to benzodiazepine receptors, or agents binding to other specific receptor subtypes, such as zolpidem, which binds to the ω-benzodiazepine receptor. Zolpidem was found to produce neither physical dependence or withdrawal, nor tolerance to the effect, after 1 year of continuous use in test subjects. Like other hypnotics, however, zolpidem is still associated with cognitive difficulties, and can also produce anterograde amnesia. Patients should be cautioned that they may not be able to recall their actions after taking this agent, and they may misperceive stimuli if they awake after taking the medication. Zolpidem is best absorbed and most effective on an empty stomach, and patients should be directed to go *directly* to bed after ingesting the pill, because of possible abrupt onset of action. This agent has been effective in populations where long-term medication is often the only solution to chronic, intractable sleep disorders.

Another agent receiving increasing public attention is melatonin. Melatonin plays a role in the normal circadian sleep-wake cycle, and is thought to work by decreasing core temperature after acute administration. Studies show a dose-dependent, acute sleep-promoting effect, usually within 1 hour following treatment, regardless of time of melatonin administration. It is also postulated that melatonin can correct a circadian sleep rhythm that is out of phase. There is a high degree of interindividual variability in response, which also varies with age (24). One dose-finding study evaluated single evening doses of both 0.3 mg and 1 mg, with a placebo-controlled, double-blind, crossover method. The study was small, with only 15 healthy middle-aged volunteers, but showed the 1-mg dose of melatonin significantly increased sleep time, sleep efficiency, and both REM and non-REM sleep latency. This is consistent with the use of low dose melatonin as a mild hypnotic (25). A meta-analysis by Chase and Gidal noted that endogenous melatonin concentration is reduced with advancing age. It is also severely disrupted by blindness, shift work, jet lag, and depression. Melatonin appeared to induce sleep onset in patients with insomnia, but the optimal dosage, and best time to take

it remain unclear. Melatonin had modest efficacy in jet lag, as well as in neurologically impaired patients (26). One small study of melatonin given at 10AM showed shortened sleep onset latency at dosages of 1 mg, 10 mg, and 40 mg. Melatonin also completely suppressed the normal diurnal rise in core body temperature. This suggests the mechanism by which melatonin may be helpful to those needing to sleep at times other than their usual bedtime, such as travelers or shift workers (27). There is some evidence of action of melatonin on ovarian cells, and of antioxidant activity (28). For psychophysiological insomnia, one double-blind controlled study, using self-reported questionnaires, of melatonin 5 mg versus placebo failed to show improvement. Side effects were noted to be headache and a strange taste in the mouth (29). There is still a lack of date on long-term effects of melatonin, especially in pharmacologic doses, and some authors recommend caution with chronic, high dose administration, which may result in supraphysiologic circulating levels of the hormone (30). In Europe, melatonin is considered a neurohormone and is available only by prescription. Other side effects can include nightmares, hypotension, and abdominal pain. Because of the unknown long-term effects and uncertain pharmacologic profile, more research is needed into the possible toxic effects of melatonin. A literature review by Mendelson in 1997 concluded that the evidence is not convincing as to the efficacy of melatonin, except in circadian sleep disturbance (31).

Cessation of any medical treatment can be difficult, especially with longstanding use of longer acting agents. Rebound insomnia for several nights duration is common, with increased latency to sleep onset, more awakenings, reduced total sleep time, and daytime fatigue. This can also produce significant anxiety, irritability, or physical tremors. This is a dose-related phenomenon that worsens with tolerance to the hypnotic agent. It is important to educate the patient that rebound insomnia is not the same as withdrawal or addiction. She should be reassured that having two to three nights of disrupted sleep is to be expected, and should not result in a resumption of hypnotic use. Keeping dosages low and for brief periods will help prevent rebound effects. Intermittent use on an as-needed basis will also prevent tolerance from developing and may minimize rebound. For shorter-acting agents, tapering the dose can prevent rebound.

In obstructive sleep apnea (OSA), hypnotics must be used with extreme caution because they may further depress respiratory drive. Weight loss is often the first recommendation, as well as sleep hygiene. CPAP is effective in many cases. In some refractory patients, surgical ablation of the uvula and part of the soft palate is needed. Some newer laser techniques have reduced the morbidity of this procedure, although surgical intervention is the last resort in OSA.

KEY POINTS

Differential Diagnoses of Sleep Disorders with Chronic Pelvic Pain

- Epilepsy (with or without visible seizures)
- Sleep apnea
- Acromegaly
- Medications—some antidepressants (tricyclics, MAOIs, desyrel, mirtazepine), beta blockers, dopamine preparations, diuretics, reserpine, cimetidine, Zidovudine, oral contraceptives, and OTC stimulants such as caffeine, ephedrine, and herbs such as ma huang
- Menopause
- Breathing-related problems
- Infectious diseases—syphilis, AIDS, herpetic and other encephalitis
- Depression, anxiety, or other psychiatric disorders
- Substance abuse
- Thyroid or other endocrine abnormalities
- Neurological problems including multiple sclerosis, nocturnal myoclonus, restless legs syndrome, and primary parasomnias such as night terrors or sleep walking
- Chronic fatigue syndrome
- Fatal familial insomnia

Most Important Questions to Ask

- Do a complete sleep history, including subjective reports of sleep from the patient.
- Explore the patient's sleep hygiene, and sleep schedule in detail.
- Solicit information from other household members about actual sleep patterns (with consent of the patient first).
- Is there a history of loud snoring or periods where breathing apparently ceases?
- Is the sleep problem acute, or an exacerbation of a lifelong problem?
- How does the sleep problem affect functioning (i.e., is referral to a sleep specialist necessary?)
- Get a complete list of prescription and OTC medications currently in use.
- Is there a prior history of psychiatric illness?
- How does the sleep problem vary with the menstrual cycle?
- In what manner and to what degree does the pain affect the sleep problem?
- Which came first, the sleep problem or the onset of CPP?
- Is there a family history of sleep problems?
- Ask the patient to start keeping a sleep diary.

Most Important Examination Findings

- Changes in level of alertness
- Excessive daytime sleepiness
- Loud or congested daytime breathing (could suggest sleep apnea)
- Obesity (increases severity of sleep apnea)
- Visible anxiety or tension
- Problems concentrating or with memory
- Vegetative signs of depression (Chapter 50)

Most Important Diagnostic Studies

- Polysomnographic evidence of abnormal sleep patterns
- Polysomnographic response to CPAP if sleep apnea is suspected
- Oxygen saturation during sleep studies
- Possible relationship between HLA-DR2 positivity with narcolepsy

Treatments

- Good control of underlying cause of CPP
- Sleep hygiene counseling
  - Consistent schedule for bed and arising
  - Proper sleep environment (e.g., dark, quiet, right temperature)
  - Minimize shift work
  - Minimize stress and anxiety
  - Avoid daytime naps
  - Avoid alcohol and caffeine
  - Consider use of earplugs or white noise if needed
- Behavioral techniques
  - Hypnosis for pain control and sleep
  - Cognitive-behavioral therapy by a professional therapist
  - Biofeedback and relaxation training
  - Bright light therapy, especially if there's a seasonal component or depression
  - Assign a specific "worry time" daily and prohibit worry at any other time
  - Use the bed only for intercourse and sleep
  - Consider limiting total time in bed
  - Monitor compliance with CPAP usage
- Pharmacotherapy
  - Use sedative hypnotics in lowest possible dosages, for only a few weeks, unless long-term use is indicated
  - Avoid long-acting agents, especially in elderly women
  - Consider antidepressants for off-label use as hypnotics—tricyclics, desyrel and mirtazepine
  - Mirtazepine dosage is *inversely* proportional to somnolence (i.e., more sedating at lower doses)
  - OTC agents can be helpful, especially antihistamines such as diphenhydramine, but avoid combinations that contain other agents
  - Avoid herbal self-medication because of unknown dosages, drug interactions, and long-term effects
  - Avoid barbiturates because of rapid tolerance and narrow therapeutic index

- Use antipsychotics only as a last resort, for brief periods. Select alternative agents, such as antidepressants unless chronic psychosis is present
- Reduce the dosage or eliminate agents that disrupt sleep, such as propranolol, pulmonary inhalers, diet pills, and dopamine preparations
- Consider newer, atypical agents such as zolpidem, but be wary of possible side effects, including amnesia, and disturbed perception during the night

REFERENCES

1. Williams RL, Karacan I, Hursch CJ. *Electroencephalography (EEG) of human sleep: clinical applications.* New York: John Wiley & Sons, 1974.
2. Kryger MH, Roth T, Dement WC, eds. *Principles and practice of sleep medicine,* 2nd ed. Philadelphia: Saunders, 1994.
3. Nolan SE, Metheny WP, Smith RP. Unrecognized association of sleep disorders and depression with chronic pelvic pain. *So Med J* 1992;85(12):1181–1183.
4. Adair RH, Bauchner H. Sleep problems in childhood. *Curr Probl Pediatr* 1993;23(4):147–170.
5. Prinz PN. Sleep and sleep disorders in older adults. *J Clin Neurophysiol* 1995;12(2):139–146.
6. Moldofsky H. Sleep, neuroimmune and neuroendocrine functions in fibromyalgia and chronic fatigue syndrome. *Adv Neuroimmunol* 1995;5(1):39–56.
7. Grunstein RR, Wilcox I. Sleep-disordered breathing and obesity. *Baillieres Clin Endocrinol Metab* 1994;8(3):601–628.
8. Stone AB, Pearlstein TB. Evaluation and treatment of changes in mood, sleep, and sexual functioning associated with menopause. *Obstet Gynecol Clin N Am* 1994;21(2):391–403.
9. Watanabe T, Mikami A, Motonishi M, et al. Two cases of sleep-disordered breathing in climacteric. *Psychiatry Clin Neurosci* 1998;52(2):231–232.
10. Van Sweden B. Sleep and the temporal lobe. *Acta Neurologica Belgica* 1996;96(1):19–30.
11. Montagna P, Cortelli P, Gambetti P, et al. Fatal familial insomnia: sleep, neuroendocrine and vegetative alterations. *Adv Neuroimmunol* 1995;5(1):13–21.
12. Spielman AJ, Nunes J, Glovinsky PB. Insomnia. *Neurol Clin* 1996;14(3):513–543.
13. Scheffer IE, Bhatia KP, Lopes-Cendes I, et al. Autosomal dominant frontal epilepsy misdiagnosed as sleep disorder. *Lancet* 1994;343(8896):515–517.
14. Anonymous. Integration of behavioral and relaxation approaches into the treatment of chronic pain and insomnia. NIH Technology Assessment Panel on Integration of Behavioral and Relaxation Approaches into the Treatment of Chronic Pain and Insomnia. *JAMA* 1996;276(4):313–318.
15. Regestein QR, Pavolva M. Treatment of delayed sleep phase syndrome. *Gen Hosp Psychiatr* 1995;17(5):335–345.
16. Sherrill DL, Kotchou K, Quan SF. Association of physical activity and human sleep disorders. *Arch Intern Med* 1998;158(17):1894–1898.
17. Dingemanse J. Pharmacotherapy of insomnia: practice and prospects. *Pharm World Sci* 1995;17(3):67–75.
18. Grad RM. Benzodiazepines for insomnia in community-dwelling elderly: a review of benefit and risk. *J Fam Prac* 1995;41(5):473–481.
19. Rupprecht R, Hauser CA, Trapp T, et al. Neurosteroids: molecular mechanisms of action and psychopharmacological significance. *J Steroid Biochem Mol Biol* 1996;56(1–6 Spec No):163–168.
20. Wilson MA. GABA physiology: modulation by benzodiazepines and hormones. *Crit Rev Neurobiol* 1996;10(1):1–37.
21. Polo-Kantola P, Erkkola R, Helenius H, et al. When does estrogen replacement therapy improve sleep quality? *Am J Obstet Gynecol* 1998;178(5):1002–1009.
22. De Lignieres B. Hormone replacement therapy: clinical benefits and side effects. *Maturitas* 1996;23(Suppl):S31–36.
23. Scharf MB, McDannold MD, Stover R, et al. Effects of estrogen replacement therapy on rates of cyclic alternating patterns and hot-flash events during sleep in postmenopausal woman: a pilot study. *Clin Ther* 1997;19(2):304–311.
24. Zhdanova IV, Wurtman RJ. Efficacy of melatonin as a sleep-promoting agent. *J Biol Rhythms* 1997;12(6):644–650.
25. Attenburrow ME, Cowen PJ, Sharpley AL. Low dose melatonin improves sleep in healthy middle-aged subjects. *Psychopharmacology (Berlin)* 1996;126(2):179–181.
26. Chase JE, Gidal BE. Melatonin: therapeutic use in sleep disorders. *Ann Pharmacother* 1997;31(10):1218–1226.
27. Hughes RJ, Badia P. Sleep-promoting and hypothermic effects of daytime melatonin administration in humans. *Sleep* 1997;20(2):124–131.
28. Cagnacci A. Melatonin in relation to physiology in adult humans. *J Pineal Res* 1996;21(4):200–213.
29. Ellis CM, Lemmens G, Parkes JD. Melatonin and insomnia. *J Sleep Res* 1996;5(1):61–65.
30. Zhdanova IV, Lynch HJ, Wurtman RJ. Melatonin: a sleep-promoting hormone. *Sleep* 1997;20(10):899–907.
31. Mendelson WB. Efficacy of melatonin as a hypnotic agent. *J Biol Rhythms* 1997;12(6):651–656.

55

SOMATIC REFERRAL

C. PAUL PERRY

KEY TERMS AND DEFINITIONS

Antidromic activation: The mechanism by which chronic visceral nociception produces referred pain to distant somatic nerve endings by reversing the usual afferent flow of impulses in the somatic nerve fibers.

Dermatome: The area of skin supplied with a single afferent posterior spinal nerve root.

Head zones: Areas of cutaneous and muscular hypersensitivity to which pain from internal organs is referred in a reproducible pattern from patient to patient.

Referred pain: The perception of pain in a body region remote from the site of pathology.

Viscero-cutaneous reflex: Visceral pain referred to skin and soft tissue.

Viscero-muscular reflex: Visceral pain producing muscle spasm and referred pain.

Viscero-somatic convergence: The convergence of visceral and somatic afferent nerves on the same dorsal horn transmission cell of the spinal cord, thereby making it difficult for the cerebral cortex to discriminate between visceral and somatic pain.

Viscero-visceral reflex: Visceral pain producing alterations in function and sensitivity of other internal organs with subsequent pain.

INTRODUCTION

Chronic pelvic pain (CPP) is usually thought to be visceral in origin by patients and physicians alike. It is common for patients with low lateral pain to present with the chief complaints of "my ovary hurts," or "my endometriosis is back." Unfortunately, many physicians reinforce these assumptions without a critical analysis of the history. A careful physical examination also is necessary to rule out the possibility of somatic referral as a major cause of pain.

Many women with complex pelvic pain are treated with multiple surgeries, only to experience the same pain for which she originally sought relief. These patients are often found to have referred pain. This type of pain can be visceral or somatic in origin. Referred pain may persist long after the origin of visceral pain has been remedied. Proper recognition of referred pain may avoid many unnecessary diagnostic and surgical procedures. Even the most expert clinician may be doomed to failure if appropriate screening for referred pain is neglected before surgical treatment of chronic pelvic pain.

ETIOLOGY

Subjective discrimination of somatic and visceral pain is difficult because of a neurophysiologic phenomenon known as "convergence and projection" or "viscero-somatic convergence (1,2)." This occurs at the level of the dorsal horn neurons of the spinal cord (Fig. 55.1). The peripheral somatic nerves and the visceral nerves converge on the same dorsal horn transmission cell. These transmission cells relay the pain signal to the brain. The cortex interprets the signal as coming from the same dermatome level regardless of visceral or somatic origin. This makes it impossible for patients to distinguish internal organ pain from deep somatic pain. The origin of the pain may be "projected" by mental displacement to a site remote from the true source of pathology.

The pattern of referral has a distribution characteristic to a particular structure. This pattern of referred pain from internal organs to particular zones of muscle or skin (Head zones) varies little between individuals. These zones are determined by the dorsal roots through which primary afferents from an organ gain access to the spinal cord (3). They tend to be distributed to the skin in dermatomal fashion because the pain tends to be referred to a somatic region that is innervated by the spinal segment(s) that innervates the stimulated visceral organ. The general rule is that the further the stimulated organ is from the body surface, the more distant is the site to which pain is referred. Classic examples of this phenomenon are cardiac pain referred to the left arm or jaw or diaphragmatic pain referred to the shoulder and neck.

Those transmission cells sharing somatic and visceral nerves of the pelvis involve the dermatomes at the T12-L3

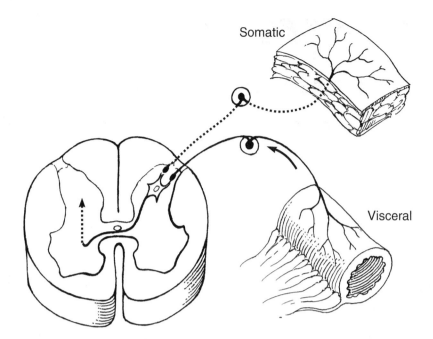

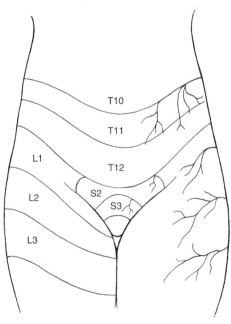

FIGURE 55.1. Visceral and somatic afferent fibers share dorsal horn transmission neurons. This produces the "convergence-projection" or "viscerosomatic convergence" phenomenon.

and S2–4 levels (Table 55.1). This permits pain from the uterus, tubes, ovaries, bladder, and rectum to be referred to the iliohypogastric, ilioinguinal, genitofemoral, and pudendal somatic nerve distributions. Their sensory innervation includes the skin, subcutaneous tissue, muscle, and parietal peritoneum. This comprises the dermatomes just below the umbilicus to the upper thigh (Figs. 55.2 and 55.3). Pelvic floor myalgia, abdominal wall trigger points, and vestibulitis may all be a result of referred pain.

PATHOLOGY

There is evidence that intraspinal neuronal reflexes contribute to remote pain produced by pathological processes in deep structures of the pelvis. These reflexes can be viscero-visceral (as in irritable bowel syndrome), viscero-muscular, or viscero-cutaneous.

Pelvic floor myalgia is an example of a viscero-muscular reflex. Input from visceral nociceptors is known to produce a powerful and sustained reflex muscle contraction (Fig. 55.4). Continued visceral nociceptive input produces muscle tenderness and the secondary source of muscle pain. This probably accounts for the strong association between

TABLE 55.1. PERIPHERAL SOMATIC NERVE DERMATOMES WITH CORRESPONDING VISCERAL SENSORY NERVE CONVERGENCE-PROJECTION FIELDS

Somatic Nerve	Dermatome	Visceral Field
Iliohypogastric	T12-L1	Ovary and distal fallopian tube
Ilioinguinal	L1–2	Proximal tube and uterine fundus
Genitofemoral	L1–2	Proximal tube and uterine fundus
Lateral femoral cutaneous	L2–3	Fundus and lower uterine segment
Pudendal	S2–4	Lower uterine segment, cervix, bladder, distal ureter, upper vagina, and rectum

FIGURE 55.2. Anterior abdominal and thigh distribution of pelvic nerve dermatomes.

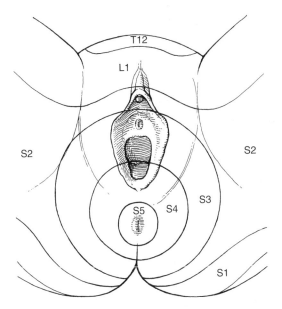

FIGURE 55.3. Perineal distribution of pelvic nerve dermatomes.

skin and soft tissue result. In this case, the brain correctly localizes the site of origin of the nociceptive message, but not the site of the original pathological process.

HISTORY

Initially visceral pain is usually dull, ill-defined, and episodic. Visceral pain may be aggravated by activity of the affected organ, such as painful intercourse, pain with evacuation of bowel, or pain with emptying of the bladder. Referred somatic pain is usually sharp, well localized, and aggravated by physical activity or position.

Patients with referred pain develop more complex pain patterns as the duration and severity of their visceral pain progresses. This is caused by greater and greater somatic nerve recruitment, which in turn produces greater and greater muscle spasm or soft tissue hyperalgesia.

Initially the patient relates the onset of pain to an inciting visceral tissue injury with its typical symptoms; for example, endometriosis, pelvic surgery, or interstitial cystitis. Over time, other manifestations such as vestibulitis, abdominal wall trigger points, and irritable bowel syndrome develop and become part of the patient's complaints. Patients who initially experience severe dysmenorrhea may go on to develop dyspareunia, back pain, abdominal tenderness, bloating, constipation or diarrhea, pain with exercise, and so on. They usually consider the entire pain complex to be from a single source.

These additional sources of referred pain may be just as confusing to the clinician as they are to the patient. Both try to explain all of the symptoms by one disease process, in accord with the "law of parsimony" (4). Clinicians are

CPP of visceral origin and the dyspareunia from pelvic floor myalgia (1).

Viscero-cutaneous reflexes are common findings in CPP patients. Referred pain can produce antidromic activation of skin and soft tissue receptors at distant secondary sites (Fig. 55.5). Vestibulitis and abdominal wall trigger points may be explained by this mechanism. According to this theory, chronic visceral pain stimulates the somatic nerve ending by reversing the usual afferent direction of impulse transmission. This releases pain-producing substances at the peripheral nerve terminals. Exquisitely sensitive spots of

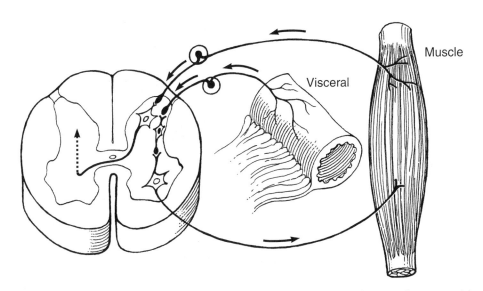

FIGURE 55.4. Viscero-muscular reflex. Visceral afferents can reflexly produce muscle spasms with resultant referred somatic pain.

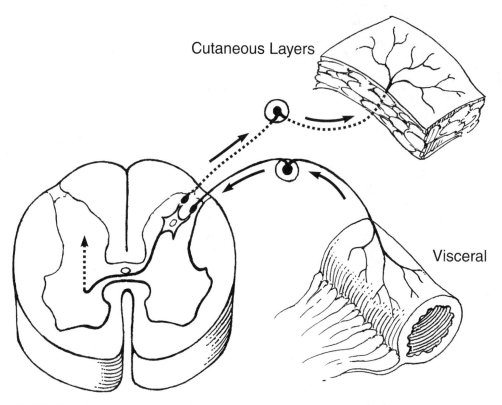

FIGURE 55.5. Viscero-cutaneous reflex. Visceral nociceptive impulses may be transmitted in an antidromic (reversal of normal direction), which could produce somatic trigger points.

taught to attribute the patient's symptoms and physical findings to the smallest number of identifiable disease processes and hence the fewest diagnostic labels. However, in CPP, several sources usually contribute to the pain complex. Each contribution must be accurately diagnosed and treated if maximum relief is to be obtained.

PHYSICAL EXAMINATION

Every patient with CPP should undergo a detailed physical examination specifically to identify all sources of pain, including referred pain. Referred pain must be sought by palpation with an effort to relate tender areas to dermatomal distributions. Correlation with the internal organ's referral pattern helps localize the source of visceral pain.

Palpation for trigger points in the abdomen, back, and pelvic floor should be performed. I find it most helpful to use a pencil eraser with light pressure along the course of those nerves known to be involved in referred pelvic pain (5). Fingertip pressure applied to the pelvic floor muscles distinguishes spasm (generalized tightness and tenderness) as opposed to muscle trigger points (localized spots of exquisite tenderness). Careful palpation of the pubococcygeus, piriformis, and obturator muscles must be performed to diagnose and treat pelvic floor myalgia. Addi-

tionally, localized trigger points may be present in some muscles, which may require treatment.

Vestibulitis should be ruled out by light touch of the minor vestibular glands with a cotton-tipped applicator or Q-tip. This is extremely important because many patients are not aware of allodynia in this area. Identification of this type of referred pain is one of the most frequently missed sources of CPP.

DIAGNOSTIC STUDIES

Appropriate studies to identify the original source of tissue injury should have priority. Laparoscopy, cystoscopy, and colonoscopy may all be indicated. Pain mapping under conscious sedation can be helpful. Imaging techniques such as pelvic ultrasound, CT, or MRI is sometimes necessary. These studies are discussed in detail in Chapters 4 and 5.

TREATMENT

Unless the source of chronic visceral pain is accurately identified and properly treated, referred pain may not be successfully eliminated. Therefore, every effort should be made

TABLE 55.2. MEDICATIONS EFFECTIVE FOR THE TREATMENT OF NEUROPATHIC PAIN

Medication	Dosage
Amitriptyline	10–75 mg at bedtime
Carbamazepine	200 mg b.i.d. (titrate with blood levels)
Doxepin	50–150 mg at bedtime
Gabapentin	100–400 mg t.i.d.
Lamotrigine	25 mg q.o.d. × 2 wks then q.d.
Mexiletine hydrochloride	200 mg t.i.d.
Nortriptyline	25 mg t.i.d. or q.i.d.
Phenytoin	100 mg t.i.d. (titrate with blood levels)
Trazodone	50–150 mg at bedtime

to reduce visceral nociception as soon as possible to obviate further peripheral nerve recruitment. Although the search for and the control of the original tissue injury is in progress, treatment should be instituted to reduce referred pain with analgesics, physical therapy, and psychological support. Abdominal wall trigger points can be treated with local anesthetics or "dry needling." Medications used to treat neuropathies are sometimes helpful (Table 55.2).

Vestibulitis may respond to certain oral, interstitially injected, or topical medications. Vestibulectomy should not be performed until all efforts to control visceral nociception are made. It has been my experience that control of chronic visceral nociception often eliminates the referred vestibulitis without further treatment.

Pelvic floor myalgia is treated most successfully with physical therapy techniques. Stretching exercises for the muscles involved in spasm is usually helpful. Injection of trigger points, with or without corticosteroids, may be necessary. Pelvic floor reeducation shows promise to alleviate pain in many patients (6).

KEY POINTS

Differential Diagnoses

- Primary musculoskeletal injury
- Peripheral neuropathies

Most Important Questions to Ask

- What is the quality of the pain: sharp or dull?
- What is the frequency of pain: intermittent or constant?
- What activities enhance the pain: intercourse, evacuating bowels or bladder, exercise, etc. and so on?
- Which came first, visceral or somatic pain?
- How did the various painful symptoms progress?

Most Important Physical Examination Findings

- Presence of trigger points
- Presence of muscle spasms
- Dermatomal distribution

Most Important Diagnostic Studies

- Endoscopic techniques to define the original source of pelvic pain
- Imaging studies to define the original source of pelvic pain
- Search for trigger points.
- Search for muscle spasm.
- Search for allodynia of the vestibule with the Q-tip test.

Treatments

- Surgical or medical treatments for the origin of visceral tissue injury
- Analgesics
- Neuropathic pain medications
- Injections of trigger points
- Physical therapy for alleviation of trigger points and muscle spasms
- Pelvic floor reeducation

REFERENCES

1. Fields HL. *Pain* New York: McGraw-Hill, 1987:79–97.
2. Rogers RM. Basic pelvic anatomy. In: Steege JF, Metzger DA, Levy BS, eds. *Chronic pelvic pain: an integrated approach.* Philadelphia: Saunders, 1998:31–58.
3. Head H. On disturbances of sensation with especial reference to the pain of visceral disease. *Brain* 1933:16:1–132.
4. Steege JF. Preface. In: Steege JF, Metzger DA, Levy BS, eds. *Chronic pelvic pain: an integrated approach.* Philadelphia: Saunders, 1998.
5. Slocumb JC. Neurological factors in chronic pelvic pain: trigger points in the abdominal pelvic pain syndrome. *Am J Obstet Gynecol* 1984;149:536–543.
6. Glazer HI, Rodke G, Swencionis C, et al. Treatment of vulvar vestibulitis syndrome with electromyographic biofeedback of pelvic floor musculature. *J Reprod Med* 1995;40:283–290.

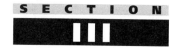

CHRONIC PAIN

56

CHRONIC PAIN AS A DIAGNOSIS

FRED M. HOWARD

KEY TERMS AND DEFINITIONS

Abstinence syndrome: The combination of symptoms that occur with acute termination of any drug capable of inducing physical dependence. The initial symptoms of opioid abstinence syndrome are yawning, diaphoresis, lacrimation, coryza, and tachycardia, followed by peak symptoms at 72 hours of abdominal cramps, nausea, and vomiting.

Addiction: A label that should probably be replaced by the term "psychological dependence."

Body-mind theory: A monistic theory that all diseases involve the mind and body as a single unit, in distinction to the traditional dualistic model of illness being either mental (psychologic) or physical (somatic) origin.

Cartesian pain theory: Postulates that perception of pain is the direct result of tissue trauma and that the severity of the pain is directly proportional to the severity of the traumatic insult. In this model pain unassociated with identifiable tissue injury is regarded as spurious or psychogenic.

Gate control pain theory: Proposes that neural mechanisms in the dorsal horn of the spinal cord act like a gate that can increase or decrease the flow of nerve impulses from peripheral fibers to the spinal cord cells that project to the brain.

Physical dependence: The appearance of an abstinence syndrome if the drug is withdrawn.

Placebo: Refers to an intervention designed to simulate medical treatment, but not believed by the clinician to be a specific treatment for the target condition. In clinical practice a placebo is used for its psychological effect. In research it is used to eliminate observer bias in the experimental setting.

Placebo effect: Refers to a change in the patient's condition or illness attributable to the symbolic importance of a treatment rather than a specific pharmacologic or physiologic property. The placebo effect does not require a placebo.

Placebo response: Refers to any change in the patient's condition following the administration of a placebo.

Psychological dependence: Refers to a set of aberrant behaviors consisting of drug craving, efforts to secure its supply, interference with physical health or psychological function, and recidivism after detoxification. It always includes a compulsion to take the drug on a continuous or periodic basis, in order to experience its psychic effects, and sometimes to avoid the discomfort of its absence.

Tolerance: The diminution of effectiveness over time from the same dose of drug.

Withdrawal syndrome: Same as abstinence syndrome.

INTRODUCTION

Although the etiology is not known, after 4 to 6 months' duration pain itself can become an illness (1). In other words, in such patients chronic pain is a disease, not a symptom (2). As a disease chronic pain probably represents a dysfunction of the psychoneurologic system. However, the question of whether chronic pain is "physical" (neurologic) or "mental" (psychologic) is not useful; somatogenic and psychogenic labels need not be and most often are not mutually exclusive (3,4). Trying to make such a distinction about pain is not useful in designing treatment, nor is it consistent with the current biologic understanding of pain.

Unfortunately, many physicians still hold to the classic Cartesian medical model that postulates that perception of pain is the direct result of tissue trauma and that the severity of the pain is directly proportional to the severity of the traumatic insult. In this model pain unassociated with identifiable tissue injury is regarded as spurious or psychogenic (5). Such a conclusion is not consistent with our current theories to explain pain. Melzack and Wall's gate control theory, although not entirely correct, represents a model closer to an accurate description of pain. This theory proposes that neural mechanisms in the dorsal horn of the spinal cord act like a gate that can increase or decrease the flow of nerve impulses from peripheral fibers to the spinal cord cells that project to the brain. The neurophysiologic events that gate or modulate the pain impulse may be influenced by numerous factors, both peripheral and central. The gates may be affected by: (a) the level of firing of the visceral afferent nerves, (b) afferent input from cutaneous and deep somatic structures, (c) endogenous opioid and nonopioid analgesic systems, and (d) various central excitatory and inhibitory influences from the brainstem, hypothalamus, and cortex (6). This theory provides a neurologic basis for the influence of both somatic and psychological factors on pain; that is, the perception of pain may increase or decrease with anxiety, depression, physical activity, mental concentration, marital discord, and so on. Although neurophysiologic and biochemical research have resulted in significant modifications of this theory since its original proposal, it still works as a good (but not only) model for the clinical observations in chronic pain patients and provides a more productive approach to therapy than the classic Cartesian model. The clinical relevance of current pain theories is that diagnosis and treatment must integrate many influences—the patient's personality and affect, cultural influences, stress, organic changes that may trigger nociceptive signals, sensory thresholds or gates, and the patient's cognition about pain. This model allows a possible understanding of how altered family roles and social supports, decreased activity, anxiety, and affective disturbances, especially depression, may influence nociception (1). Clearly, for chronic pain it is difficult to distinguish between psychological and physical causes of pain, nor are attempts to make such a distinction useful (7).

Care must be taken in explaining chronic pain to patients on the basis of such body-mind theories. Patients with CPP are characteristically resistant to any nonsomatic explanation or treatment for their pain (8). They are exquisitely sensitive to any innuendo that their pain may not be real (3). In fact, active, conscious feigning or simulation of a nonexistent pain complaint is rare, and it is important that the physician, in explaining the complexity of chronic pain, not give the patient the impression that her pain is not believed to be real (9).

Certainly there are a variety of pathological conditions that may cause, contribute to, or be associated with CPP (Chapter 1). A thorough evaluation often reveals a number of contributing disorders in any given patient, such as bladder irritability, irritable bowel syndrome, poor posture, emotional stresses, and endometriosis (1). Although "disquieting polypharmacy" may be instituted for each contributing factor, CPP often persists. In such cases it is often difficult to explain to the patient the concept of CPP as a diagnosis, not a symptom. If such a concept is introduced early in the course of the evaluation and treatment, rather than late, it is sometimes more readily accepted.

Therapy directed at the treatment of chronic pain as a diagnosis may be classified generally as:

- Pharmacologic
- Psychological
- Physical
- Neuroablative (10)

As treatment is undertaken it is important to recognize that chronic pain is distinctly different from acute pain both psychologically and physiologically (Table 56.1) Treatment of chronic pain, as opposed to treatment of acute pain, generally requires acceptance of the idea that managing rather than curing pain may be all that can be expected. The need for this acceptance by the patient argues for psychological involvement in care early in the course of the illness (11). Reasonable goals when treating chronic pain as a disease include:

1. To relieve suffering by treatment of identifiable symptoms and concurrent psychological morbidity
2. To restore normal function
3. To improve quality of life by managing symptoms and minimizing disability
4. To prevent recurrence of chronic symptoms and disability (5)

TABLE 56.1. THE CHARACTERISTICS OF ACUTE VERSUS CHRONIC PAIN

Acute Pain	Chronic Pain
Recent well-defined onset	Remote ill-defined onset
Expected to end in days or weeks	Duration unpredictable
Essential biologic warning function	No apparent biologic function
Impels rest and avoidance of further harm	Rest not helpful, nor does it avoid further pain
Variable intensity	Variable intensity
Anxiety common	Irritability or depression common
Pain behaviors are common when severe	Pain behaviors variable
Sympathetic hyperactivity signs when severe	Vegetative signs common
Monophasic or recurrent	Progressive or persistent
Symtom of injury or disease	Is a disease
	May be associated diseases that exacerbate or precipitate manifestations of chronic pain

PHARMACOLOGIC TREATMENT

Analgesics

Pharmacologic treatment of pain is based on the knowledge that pain reception, transmission, and perception involve a series of neural links from the periphery to the central nervous system (CNS) involving several neurotransmitters. This mosaic of neural elements and chemical mediators makes it possible for drugs with different pharmacologic profiles and mechanisms to interrupt or decrease the transmission of pain information and thereby decrease pain (10).

Optimization of oral analgesic therapy is sometimes overlooked in the initial treatment of CPP. Often this is best accomplished with a scheduled regimen, not a *prn* or as-needed regimen. Potential advantages of a scheduled regimen are both improved effectiveness by taking analgesics prior to severe pain symptoms and avoidance of the increased focus on pain symptoms that may actually increase pain severity with *prn* dosing (5). Scheduled dosing is consistent with operant conditioning principles, because it avoids a pain-contingent approach that has the tendency to use medication as a reinforcer of pain behaviors. However, a scheduled regimen also presents some hazards. For example, with nonsteroidal antiinflammatory drugs (NSAIDs) it may lead to gastric irritation or renal damage, and with opioids it may lead to constipation, sedation, habituation, addiction, or diminished analgesic potency (1).

Peripheral Acting Analgesics

Aspirin is a prototype peripheral-acting analgesic (Table 56.2) It acts to inhibit prostaglandin synthesis, which decreases inflammation and the activation of nociceptors, and blocks the action of bradykinin on pain receptors (10).

TABLE 56.2. PERIPHERAL-ACTING ANALGESICS

Generic	Proprietary	Usual Dosage (mg)	Comments
Aspirin	—	325–650 q4h	Prototype peripheral analgesic. Gastric irritation with chronic use. Inhibits platelet function.
Acetaminophen	Tylenol	325–650 q4h	Poor antiinflammatory activity. No gastric irritation. Overdosage can cause irreversible liver damage.
Diflunisal	Dolobid	500 q8–12h	NSAID. Effective analgesic, antiinflammatory, and antipyretic. GI bleeding, ulcers, nephrotoxicity, and hepatotoxicity possible.
Etodolac	Lodine	400 q8h	NSAID. Effective analgesic, antiinflammatory, and antipyretic. GI bleeding, ulcers, nephrotoxicity, and hepatotoxicity possible.
Fenoprofen	Nalfon	200–600 q4–6h	NSAID. Effective analgesic, antiinflammatory, and antipyretic. GI bleeding, ulcers, nephrotoxicity, and hepatotoxicity possible.
Flurbiprofen	Ansaid	50–100 q6–8h	NSAID. Effective analgesic, antiinflammatory, and antipyretic. GI bleeding, ulcers, nephrotoxicity, and hepatotoxicity possible.
Ibuprofen	Advil Motrin Nuprin	800 q8h	NSAID. Effective analgesic, antiinflammatory, and antipyretic. GI bleeding, ulcers, nephrotoxicity, and hepatotoxicity possible.
Ketoprofen	Orudis	25–75 q6–8h	NSAID. Effective analgesic, antiinflammatory, and antipyretic. GI bleeding, ulcers, nephrotoxicity, and hepatotoxicity possible.
Ketorolac	Toradol	10 q4–6h	Long-term use may have more risk of gastrointestinal adverse effects than aspirin or other NSAIDs.
Meclofenamate sodium	Meclomen	50–100 q6h	NSAID. Effective analgesic, antiinflammatory, and antipyretic. GI bleeding, ulcers, nephrotoxicity, and hepatotoxicity possible.
Mefenamic acid	Ponstel	250–500 q6h	NSAID. Effective analgesic, antiinflammatory, and antipyretic. GI bleeding, ulcers, nephrotoxicity, and hepatotoxicity possible.
Naproxen/Naproxen sodium	Naprosyn Anaprox Aleve	250–500 q6–8h (naproxen) 275–500 q8–12h (naproxen sodium)	NSAID. Effective analgesic, antiinflammatory, and antipyretic. GI bleeding, ulcers, nephrotoxicity, and hepatotoxicity possible.

The NSAIDs generally work via the same mechanisms, although potencies may vary significantly. However, not all peripheral-acting analgesics work this way. For example, acetaminophen has similar antipyretic and analgesic activity to aspirin, but has much weaker antiinflammatory activity and no significant effect on platelet function; exactly why it differs from aspirin in its activity has not been satisfactorily explained (10,12). Thus, aspirin and NSAIDs are the analgesics of choice when inflammation has caused sensitization of nociceptors and is an important component of pain (12). This is an important consideration when prescribing combined therapy with both central and peripheral acting analgesics. Because of the wide individual variations in response to different NSAIDs, even when the drugs are structurally similar and in the same chemical family, before abandoning or adding to NSAID therapy at least three different NSAID regimens should be tried (5).

The potential of side effects with NSAIDs is significant and their chronic use requires careful observation. Gastric or intestinal ulceration with chronic or acute gastrointestinal (GI) bleeding is the most common serious side effect. GI irritation may be less significant with only heartburn or dyspepsia, also. Nephropathy, although less common, represents a serious side effect that may be quite insidious in onset. NSAIDs also inhibit platelet function and with high doses or long-term use may lead to significant bleeding. They promote retention of salt and water and may cause edema in some patients. Certain individuals have intolerance to NSAIDs and display a "hyper-sensitivity reaction" to them that can manifest as vasomotor rhinitis, angioneurotic edema, urticaria, bronchial asthma, laryngeal edema, bronchoconstriction, or hypotension and shock. A history of hypersensitivity reaction to aspirin is an absolute contraindication to the use of any NSAID (12). Such hypersensitivity reactions do not appear to occur with acetaminophen.

Opioid Analgesics

Although the role of opioid analgesics is well recognized in acute pain management, their use in the treatment of chronic pain is controversial. Many authorities do not recommend opioid use for non–cancer-associated pain for more than 3 months because of (a) tolerance that results in increasing doses, (b) potent smooth muscle relaxing effects that cause exacerbation of dysmotility diseases (especially constipation), (c) sedation that limits restoration of normal function owing to debilitating side effects such as apathy, lethargy, and depression, and (d) the possibility of iatrogenic addiction and substance abuse (5,13).

However, others suggest that chronic low dose opioid therapy may allow the return of normal function without significant adverse side effects in those who have failed intensive pain clinic treatments (1). They have suggested the "ladder" approach recommended for cancer-associated pain may be used for non–cancer-associated pain, also (Fig. 56.1) For example, one observational study of 38 chronic pain patients

suggests that opioid maintenance therapy can be safely, and often effectively, continued for long periods of time after failed nonopioid therapy; 19 of these patients were on opioids for 4 or more years (14). Only two of the patients on opioids for more than 6 months had significant management problems. One, with a past history of polysubstance abuse and psychosis, had a rapid increase in medication use and required hospitalization and psychotropic treatment. Another required high doses of methadone and a check of plasma levels revealed no circulating drug, suggesting diversion of hoarding of methadone. Eleven (29%) of the patients reported adequate pain relief, 13 (34%) reported partial pain relief, and 14 (37%) reported episodic severe pain. None of the patients underwent a surgical procedure while on opioids for their chronic pain. However, the patients on opioids had significantly higher F and depression scores on MMPI testing than pain patients not on opioid medications. In this study all patients received treatment from a single physician, who took primary responsibility for overall management of the patients' medical problems as well as pain therapy.

Some of the *a priori* bias by physicians against opioid treatment of women with CPP stems from a lack of understanding of the difference between tolerance, dependence, and addiction. Tolerance is the diminution of effectiveness over time from the same dose of drug. Physical dependence is the appearance of an abstinence syndrome if the drug is withdrawn (14). The initial symptoms of the abstinence syndrome are yawning, diaphoresis, lacrimation, coryza, and tachycardia, followed by peak symptoms at 72 hours of abdominal cramps, nausea, and vomiting. Abstinence syndrome or withdrawal can be obviated by avoidance of antagonists and dosage taper prior to discontinuation of opioid medications. The label "addiction" should probably be replaced by the term "psychological dependence." This refers to a set of aber-

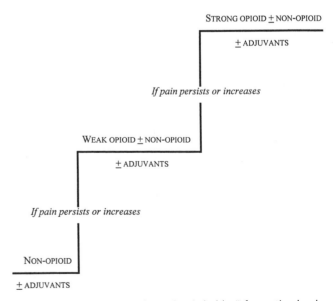

FIGURE 56.1. A suggested "analgesic ladder" for optimal pain management.

rant behaviors consisting of drug craving, efforts to secure its supply, interference with physical health or psychological function, and recidivism after detoxification (14). Although tolerance and dependence are significant problems with opioid treatment, for both the clinician and her patient, psychological dependence or addiction is the only complication that leads to unacceptable and illegal behavior by the patient. The majority of pain patients on chronic opioid maintenance never manifest addictive behavior. Estimates are that 3% to 16% of chronic pain patients experience addiction to opioids, whereas surveys show that 55% to 71% of patients referred to chronic pain centers are taking opioids regularly (15). True cases of iatrogenic addiction are sufficiently rare that it can generally be assumed that opioid treatment alone will rarely produce addiction without the presence of other risk factors. Clinical experience suggests that a prior history of addiction to legal or illegal substances is a major risk factor, and that patients with such histories are not good candidates for opioid treatment of CPP. Tables 56.3 and 56.4 list some of the factors and behaviors that suggest the need for evaluation for addiction. The diagnosis and treatment of addiction can be difficult because of a characteristic lack of insight or denial, and this is compounded by the patient's chronic pain and medically sanctioned drug use (15).

It can be difficult to discern addiction from pseudoaddiction, which is drug-seeking behavior when the patient cannot obtain tolerable pain relief on the prescribed dose and makes frequent requests for more analgesics or higher doses, or seeks medications from other sources. Pseudoaddiction is confirmed by the cessation of these behaviors once adequate opioid therapy is prescribed to obtain tolerable pain relief. Constant pain may lead to obsessive fixation on opioids and pain

TABLE 56.3. FACTORS PREDICTIVE OF ADDICTION

Multiple dose escalations or other noncompliance with treatment despite warnings
Ongoing pain complaints disproportionate to pathology
Repeatedly obtaining opioids from other prescribers without informing or after warnings by primary physician
Combining opioids with other medications for the additive intoxicant effects
Concurrent abuse of alcohol or illicit other drugs
Repeatedly visiting the emergency department with complaints of pain exacerbation
Frequent request for hospitalization and treatment with intravenous opioids
Family or friends' reports of compulsive medication use or intoxication
Selling prescription drugs
Prescription forgery
Multiple episodes of prescription "loss"
Stealing or borrowing drugs from others
Injecting oral formulations
Obtaining prescription from nonmedical sources
Evidence of deterioration in the ability to function at work, in the family, or socially that appears related to drug use

Suggest the need to evaluate for addiction in the chronic pain patient on opioid maintenance (15,60).

TABLE 56.4. FACTORS LESS PREDICTIVE OF ADDICTION

Requests for or aggressive complaining about the need for increasing amounts of medications
Drug hoarding during periods of decreased symptoms
Requesting specific drugs
Openly acquiring similar drugs from other medical sources
Unsanctioned increased dose or other noncompliance on one or two occasions
Unapproved use of the drug to treat other symptoms
Reporting psychic effects not intended by the clinician
Resistance to changes in treatment associated with "tolerable" adverse effects with expressions of anxiety related to the return of severe symptoms

May suggest the need to evaluate for addiction in the chronic pain patient on opioid maintenance (15,60).

patients may take what appear to take extraordinary steps or addictive behaviors to ensure adequate supply of medications, in the absence of addictive disease, because of fear of reemergence of pain and fear of withdrawal symptoms (15).

It seems most appropriate that opioid maintenance therapy for chronic pain should be considered only after all reasonable attempts at pain control have failed and persistent pain is the major impediment to improved function. Also it seems important that "the committed involvement of a single physician who will evaluate ongoing medical and psychological problems, as well as pain related issues, should be available before institution of opioid maintenance therapy is considered" (14). A formal written consent or a detailed notation in the chart that documents the patient has failed nonnarcotic treatment and has entered knowingly into a trial of opioid maintenance may be advisable. The risks of alcohol or other drug interactions, risks to pregnancy, and possible psychological dependence should be explained to the patient prior to initiating opioid maintenance. There should be a written or documented verbal contract or agreement with the patient that includes at least the following particulars:

1. The treating doctor is the sole provider of opioids.
2. The patient is seen by this physician before having her opioid prescription refilled.
3. Multiple-date prescriptions, each with small amounts, will be provided if the patient demonstrates she cannot responsibly take her medication as prescribed.
4. Lost medications or prescriptions will not be refilled.
5. The patient agrees that she will actively participate in strategies to develop alternative pain therapies.

Some physicians have advocated inclusion of random urine drug testing as a condition of opioid maintenance therapy (15).

Combining opioid treatment with centrally acting and peripherally acting medications may optimize efficacy with lower opioid doses, but use of commercially available formulations of opioids with acetaminophen, aspirin, or ibuprofen can lead to overdosage of the nonopioid drug. All medications are best given on a scheduled, not a *prn*, basis. In addition to the scheduled dosage, some clinicians suggest allowing transient escalation of medication on days of increased pain and prescribe an additional four to six "rescue doses" each month. Titration of the selected opioid should be done over several weeks with the goals of improvement in physical and social function and at least partial analgesia. Failure to achieve these goals at relatively low doses in the nontolerant patient should cause the clinician to question the feasibility of opioid maintenance therapy.

It is important to assess the extent of pain relief provided by the opioid medication and determine its role in restoring function and improving quality of life (15). When improved function and reasonable analgesia are achieved, close and regular follow-up is essential in CPP patients on opioid maintenance therapy. Most patients should be seen and drugs prescribed at least monthly. If doses escalate during opioid maintenance, hospitalization is recommended to evaluate the medication requirements and, if possible, return medications to their baseline level (14). If inappropriate use occurs, such as using the medication to treat depression or anxiety, drug diversion, or hoarding, this should be pursued and managed firmly. Use of the medication for symptoms other than prescribed (e.g., use for headaches in addition to pelvic pain) may lead to increased tolerance and dose escalation, and should be discouraged (15). If control cannot be maintained, then treatment with opioids should be discontinued (14).

Table 56.5 summarizes most of the opioids available in the United States as oral formulations, and gives doses that are equivalent to 10 mg of morphine administered intramuscularly. Side effects are common with opioid therapy. Opioids may cause drowsiness, difficulty in mentation, decreased physical activity, mood changes, respiratory depression, nausea, vomiting, dizziness, pruritus, constipation, increased biliary tract pressure, urinary retention, miosis, depression, and (rarely) convulsions. Considering this long list of untoward effects, as well as the risks of tolerance and addiction, it is again worth stating that opioid treatment should be initiated only after other treatments have been insufficient, the patient has been carefully counseled, and assurance of close follow-up is possible.

Tramadol is a synthetic centrally acting analgesic with a unique mode of action, displaying both weak opioid and nonopioid properties. Oral tramadol is a step 2 analgesic, that is, an alternative to codeine. Tramadol is usually administered in doses of 50 to 100 mg every 4 to 6 hours; experience with higher doses is limited. A typical daily dose for moderately severe pain is 200 mg. Tramadol causes much less constipation and respiratory depression than equianalgesic doses of other opioids. The likelihood of dependence is also considerably less. Although experience is limited, tramadol might be a reasonable alternative before progressing to opioids when NSAIDs are unsuccessful in the treatment of CPP.

Intrathecal Opioids

Opioids may be administered via intrathecal or epidural routes with significant analgesic effects and minimal side effects. The use of these modes of administration is common for postoperative pain. Continuous infusions for chronic pain have also been done. Intrathecal morphine utilizing an implantable pump has been used more than any other method thus far. Data are still insufficient to allow a conclusion as to efficacy and safety. There are published, uncontrolled trials for treatment of nonspecific chronic pain, neuropathic pain, failed back syndrome, and deafferention pain syndrome.

A retrospective evaluation of 120 chronic pain patients treated with 0.3 to 12 mg per day of intrathecal morphine showed decreased pain in 68% of patients with deafferention pain and in 62% with neuropathic pain (16). The average decrease in pain severity in all chronic pain patients was 67%, with 92% of patients satisfied with the treatment and 81% showing an improved quality of life. Seven patients developed opioid tolerance and 22 had their pumps removed for other reasons.

A small study of intrathecal morphine for failed back syndrome and neuropathic pain showed good to excellent response in six of nine failed back syndrome patients and two of two neuropathic pain patients, but two patients had bladder dysfunction that required removal of the pump (17).

A review of 10 reports consisting of 146 patients treated with intrathecal morphine revealed sufficient variation in the studies and the results that the authors concluded there are insufficient data to analyze as yet (18). They recommended that continuous intrathecal morphine infusion be considered experimental and only be done as part of an approved study protocol.

There are no published studies or series of cases of treatment of CPP with intrathecal opioids at this time. Although this therapy may be a rational option for women with CPP, several principles seem appropriate until more data are available. Patients should have intractable, incapacitating pain that has failed to respond to all other accepted treatment modalities. They should have psychological evaluations that confirm that no psychosis is present. Patients should not have a history of opioid addiction. There should be no medical contraindications to the treatment. The patients should understand the experimental nature of the treatment and be fully informed.

Antidepressants

Antidepressants, particularly tricyclic antidepressants (TCAs), have been used to treat a number of chronic pain syndromes including arthritis, diabetic neuropathy, headache, back pain, and cancer pain. They are generally thought to improve pain tolerance, restore sleep patterns, and reduce depressive symptoms. TCAs may result in improved pain levels at doses much lower than those typi-

TABLE 56.5. CENTRAL-ACTING ANALGESICS THAT CAN BE CONSIDERED FOR MAINTENANCE THERAPY OF CPP

Generic Name	Proprietary Names	Mean Duration (hrs)	Equianalgesic Dose (mg)	Metabolism and Comments
Butorphanol	Stadol	3–6	2–3 (intranasal)	Agonist-antagonist
Buprenorphine	Buprenex	5–6	0.8 (sublingual)	Agonist-antagonist
Codeine		4–6	200 (oral)	Very constipating; low abuse
Drocode (dihydrocodeine)	Synalgos-DC Compal	4–5	32 (oral)	Marketed in combination with additional ingredients
Fentanyl	Duragesic	72	25–100 µg/h (transdermal)	Transdermal delivery system
Hydrocodone	Hycodan, Vicodin, Lortab, Lorcet, others	4–5	5–10 (oral)	Most formulations are combined with acetaminophen
Hydromorphone	Dilaudid	4–5	6–7.5 (oral)	Severe pain; available in oral form
Levorphanol	Levo-Dromoran	4–8	4 (oral)	May exhibit cumulative effects with repeated dosing
				Significant CNS depression and abuse potential
				Nausea/vomiting/constipation
Meperidine	Demerol	2–5	300 (oral)	Normeperidine accumulates with repeated doses; is half as active as meperidine, but has greater convulsant activity
Methadone	Dolophine	4–6	20 (oral)	May accumulate with repeated doses; Minimal euphoria
Morphine	—	4–7	30–60 (oral)	Relatively short duration; significant side effects; 15% absorption orally
Oxycodone	Percodan Tylox Percocet Oxycontin	4–6	5–10 (oral)	Oxycontin is long-acting form with duration of 8-12 ties; most formulations are combined with acetaminophen or aspirin
Oxymorphone	Numorphan	3–6	5 (rectal)	
Pentazocine	Talwin	4–7	180 (oral)	Agonist-antagonist. Available with oral naloxone to avoid IV abuse.
Propoxyphene	Darvon	4–6	180–240 (po)	Usual available dose is 65 mg. Slightly better than placebo
	Darvocet			Dangerous with alcohol.

Equinanalgesic doses to 10 mg of morphine administered intramuscularly are given (C-2) (GG p535) (10).

cally used for the treatment of depression (5). However, substantive evidence for the efficacy of TCAs for chronic pain treatment does not necessarily demonstrate the magnitude of effect that is generally believed.

In a meta-analysis of 39 placebo controlled studies of antidepressants for chronic pain, patients treated with antidepressants had less pain than 74% of the placebo-treated patients. This suggests that antidepressants are effective for pain relief in some patients with chronic pain (19,20). However, another evaluation of 46 trials of antidepressants for chronic pain found methodological flaws in most and the authors were unable to substantiate efficacy of antidepressants for chronic pain except for the treatment of headache (19). A well-designed study of chronic unexplained chest pain showed that imipramine at 25 mg *qhs* for 1 week then 50 mg *qhs* decreased pain levels by more than 50% compared to a 1% decrease in a placebo group (21). However, another recent well-designed study of patients with chronic back pain showed small clinical effects of nortriptyline on pain levels (22% decrease in treated versus 9% decrease in placebo group) (22).

There has been little study of the use of antidepressants in women with CPP. In the only published study of TCA (nortriptyline) treatment of CPP in women (all had negative laparoscopies, pain of 6 or more months duration, and no specific diagnosis), some women reported a decreased intensity and duration of pain (13). However, this was a study of only 14 women, seven of whom dropped out of the study because of side effects of the nortriptyline. Doses were increased to 100 mg per day and six of the seven women remaining in the trial were pain free at 1 year.

Antidepressants may be helpful in treating CPP specifically because of their antidepressant effects, also. Pain patients with a family history of depression seem to derive the most benefit from TCAs and depression occurs with increased frequency in women with CPP (1). For example, a study by Hodgkiss and Watson compared 29 women undergoing laparoscopy for CPP to a control group of 33 women undergoing laparoscopy for sterilization or infertility (23). They found that 11 (38%) of the women with CPP were depressed by the Hospital Anxiety and Depression Questionnaire versus four (12%) of the control patients. This is consistent with the observed association of depression with other chronic pain syndromes. It may be that there is a shared neurochemical basis for depression and chronic pain, as suggested by psychological information and by responsiveness of chronic pain patients to antidepressant medications. Another hypothesis is that chronic pain is a psychobiological disease with characteristic clinical, psychodynamic, biographic, and genetic features that include depression (2).

There is a delayed response to antidepressants of 2 to 3 weeks usually when treating depression and the same is true in the treatment of CPP, too (13). Depression, its relationship to chronic pain, and its treatment are discussed more completely in the preceding chapter on depression (Chapter 50).

Antibiotics

Antibiotic treatment is often empirically tried in women with CPP because of the suspicion of "chronic pelvic inflammatory disease" or subclinical pelvic infection. There is no published evidence of efficacy for such empiric treatment. The relationship of pelvic inflammatory disease (PID) and subsequent CPP seems fairly clear (Chapter 19), but chronic pain seems to be a remote sequela of PID. Although there is some evidence of persistent presence of microorganisms in the uterus or tubes in some cases after PID, there is little evidence that persistent infection is the cause of the association of PID and CPP. Thus antibiotic treatment currently is recommended only for suspected acute or subacute upper genital tract infection based on positive cervical cultures in women not otherwise meeting criteria for the diagnosis of endometritis-salpingitis (5). Antibiotic therapy has also been suggested in women with chronic urethral syndrome and negative cultures, but efficacy is not well established (5). Generally, it is most appropriate to use antibiotics only to treat specific infections in women with CPP.

Combination Drug Therapy

Combination drug therapy that uses medications with different sites or mechanisms of action may improve the treatment of pain. For example, combining central-acting and peripheral-acting analgesics may improve the response owing to the action at two different sites (10). Such a combination might consist of an NSAID and an opioid, especially if significant inflammation were part of the pain syndrome. Combining two medications that are central-acting, but with different mechanisms, may also be appropriate, such as an antidepres-

sant and an opioid where depression or altered mood state is a part of the pain syndrome. If muscle spasm or tension is a contributor to pain then combining a tranquilizer or muscle relaxant with an opioid or NSAID may enhance the opioid or NSAID efficacy and decrease muscle spasm and pain. Combinations of medications may improve pain relief, but when combination drug therapy is necessary it is likely that the physician will need to pay compulsive attention to the patient's response and accept improvement as the goal; that is, in this circumstance no drug or combination of medications is a panacea for pelvic pain (11).

PSYCHOLOGICAL TREATMENT

There is no better argument for the fusion of pain and suffering than the fact that it requires a prefrontal lobotomy to disentangle them (24).

Ideally, psychological evaluation would be part of the initial evaluation and treatment of every patient with CPP. Even when there is no suspicion of a psychological diagnosis, it helps provide the physician with specific information about the patient that may be related to therapeutic responsiveness and prognosis, and can be used in treatment planning (25,26). For example, personality testing may assist in assessing the impact of pain on psychological functioning and vice versa. Objective tests, such as the MMPI or Pilowsky's Illness Behavior Questionnaire, are often used because they are easier to quantify than unstructured assessments of behavioral and cognitive function (4). Although in general CPP patients, with and without organic pathology, score higher on the hysteria, hyponchondriasis, and depressive scales of the MMPI than the normal population, specifically addressing individual problem areas in treatment planning may be more beneficial than a nonspecific approach (25).

Psychological evaluation and treatment of women with CPP is ideally done routinely, by a professional specializing in pain psychology, but this is not always possible. Furthermore, many women are unable to afford or reluctant to accept referral to a psychologist or psychiatrist for evaluation and treatment (13). However, there are women who clearly need the professional expertise of a psychologist or psychiatrist. For example, in a woman with the following criteria the clinician should insist she have psychological evaluation and treatment: (a) CPP, (b) thorough evaluation completed, including laparoscopy, with negative findings, (c) history of major psychosexual trauma, and (d) history of multiple consultations and treatments for multiple unrelated somatic symptoms (8).

Because in reality, routine psychological evaluation and treatment is not always possible, in practice psychological treatment is often initiated only when psychological problems have become apparent or other treatments have been inadequate. In the latter case psychological treatment is instituted as a nonspecific treatment; that is, treatment is directed to pain as a diagnosis, not to a psychiatric or psychological diagnosis. Patients may benefit from psychological support in the generic sense, because they exhibit tremendous anxiety over an undiagnosed and seemingly untreatable pain. This leads to helplessness, hopelessness, depression, and despair (26). In such cases the goals of psychological pain therapies are to:

1. Treat excess pain and disability.
2. Teach patients to live and cope better.
3. Teach patients to live well despite their pain (4).

Psychological pain therapies frequently used are hypnosis, individual psychotherapy, relaxation and biofeedback training, and cognitive-behavioral methods. The research on hypnosis for chronic pain is sparse and poor, but it is likely that in some patients it has been helpful (4). It has been suggested that hypnotherapy may be used for symptomatic relief of functional dysmenorrhea, pelvic congestion, dyspareunia, and bizarre pelvic pain syndromes (27). "Glove anesthesia," which follows no anatomical distribution, is a technique that may be used in hypnosis for treatment of pelvic pain.

Individual psychotherapy is generally not useful in CPP, as most women with chronic pain are not psychotic (8). In a study of women with "atypical" CPP and no objective findings of organic disease, only six (17%) of 35 had a diagnosis of a psychosis. In the nonpsychotic patients, only 12 would consent to individual psychotherapy and three (25%) had improvement, compared to improvement in four (24%) of those who refused psychotherapy (28). Behavioral programs with rehabilitation approaches, plus family dynamic interventions, are more useful (29).

The cognitive-behavioral approach to pain management teaches self-management techniques and active participation to lessen the impact of pain (30). Goals of cognitive-behavioral treatment for CPP are similar to those generically stated for psychological therapy.

1. To improve coping abilities and sense of control
2. To reduce disability and negative effects of pain on the patient's life
3. To promote behaviors that are incompatible with the chronic pain patient role (5)

The relevance of perceived control is that the person who sees herself having little control over physical and emotional events affecting her may be most vulnerable to developing and sustaining a chronic pain syndrome (1). Coping ability is believed to have similar significance. Also, for a subgroup of patients who had trouble coping before, CPP provides a sanctioned rationale for dropping out of a stressful and overwhelming life (26). Techniques that may increase the patient's coping ability and sense of control are relaxation techniques, attention diversion, decreased focusing on physical signals, and distraction techniques such as internal dialog, external focus, and activities (5). Table 56.6

lists some of the techniques that are used in treating patients with chronic pain.

Dealing with depression or anxiety may help to reduce disability and other negative effects of pain on the patient's life. The relationship of depression and pain, and the usefulness of antidepressive therapy have already been discussed earlier in this chapter and in Chapter 50. Anxiety and tension also are common in patients with chronic pain (e.g., patients with CPP have shown anxiety scores on Manifest Anxiety Scale evaluation that are double those of "normal" gynecological patients, and this may increase pain perception) (28,30). Even mild flare-ups are often made worse by anxious, excessive focus on the pain. In some cases pain significantly decreases with calming and relaxation. Relaxation exercises and stress management may be helpful in alleviating tension and anxiety (30). Biofeedback, self-hypnosis, and meditation, for example, may be taught for use at the first signs of a painful episode to help manage acute exacerbation of pain by decreasing muscle tension, achieving relaxation, and helping to gain control over bodily functions (3,26). Many women with LaMaze technique training for childbirth, which utilizes deep breathing exercises and progressive relaxation, can benefit by using some of this training to manage their pain (3). Whether or not pharmacologic treatment of anxiety in CPP patients is helpful is not clear. In patients with chronic pain secondary to malignancies and with significant anxiety, alprazolam (Xanax), a triazolobenzodiazepine with mixed anxiolytic and antidepressant effects, shows analgesic effects in moderate to high doses and appears to potentiate the anal-

TABLE 56.6. COGNITIVE-BEHAVIORAL PSYCHOLOGICAL PAIN MANAGEMENT TECHNIQUES (5,30)

Goal	Intervention
Control pain	Relaxation techniques
	Stress management
	"Self-talk"
	Pain coping strategies
	Pain attributions
	Distraction techniques
Reduce disability	Progressive activities
	Pain behavior modification
	Reemployment
	Treat substance abuse
Promote wellness and improve lifestyle	Eating behavior and nutrition
	Sleep hygiene
	Physical exercise
	Treat substance abuse
Treat psychological morbidity	Treat depression and anxiety
	Abuse survivors
	Couples and family counseling
	Sex therapy

From Milburn A, Reiter RC, Rhamberg AT. Multidisciplinary approach to chronic pelvic pain. *Obstet Gynecol Clin NA* 1993;20:643–661; Reiter RC, Milburn A. Exploring effective treatment for chronic pelvic pain. *Contemp OB/GYN* 1994;84–103, with permission.

gesic effect of narcotics. It is important to realize, however, that such medications cause significant effects on mentation and have significant dependence and addiction potential (1). Additionally, benzodiazepines often have rebound symptoms of anxiety, sleeplessness, and abdominal pain (5).

Cognitive and operant behavioral therapy utilizes many techniques to reduce reinforcers of pain and increase reinforces of well behavior and activity (Table 56.6) (3,26). Distraction techniques are used because awareness of all types of pain, including acute pain, can be decreased with cognitive distraction techniques. For example, this is often used in the focal point exercises in childbirth education preparation for labor. Return to work can serve as a powerful pain distractor and increase the patient's sense of competence and control. "Self-talk" refers to teaching patients to identify their negative self statements and replace them with more positive self statements. Self statements that emphasize loss of control and the catastrophic nature of pain episodes are associated with increased pain and distress (30). Patients sometimes balk at the suggestion that they can use their mind to affect their pain level. It is helpful to ask them why they find it so hard to imagine that the same brain capable of turning the face bluish-red at an indecent joke—the same brain that creates not only its own opioid analgesic, but also the more bewildering product known as human thought—might not on occasion be capable of suppressing pain (24).

The family dynamics of women with CPP may need to be specifically addressed. Family members often unwittingly sustain or reinforce illness and pain behaviors (15). Often the woman has diminished responsibilities in the family that initially are intended to be helpful, but in the long term lead to diminished self-esteem and decreased interactions with the family. Eventually the only interaction with the family relates to pain, with pain as the major means of maintaining communication within the family (1). In this setting reeducating the patient and her family concerning the development of pain problems and the perception of pain itself can be beneficial (11).

Unfortunately, after cognitive-behavioral psychological pain therapy about 25% of patients regress significantly within a few months of completion of treatment (5). This suggests there may be a good argument for long-term psychological treatment, but financial constraints rarely allow this option.

Although pain is usually the patient's chief concern, the majority of women with CPP have serious psychosocial problems that also need attention of their own accord (3). These psychosocial factors often appear to determine the extent of suffering and disability experienced (30). It is postulated that women with psychosocial problems, such as sexual abuse, marital discord, mild personality disorder, difficulty maintaining relationships, or distressed family of origin, may be more vulnerable to nociceptive signals and are ill-equipped to cope with uncomfortable somatic sensations accompanying any disease process (29). In some women their psychosocial problems result in unmet dependency needs that may lead them to seek external solutions via medical and surgical treatment (1). Certainly, CPP patients seem to have a higher incidence of marital distress and sexual dysfunction, especially dyspareunia. For example 56% of 220 CPP patients scored in the maritally distressed range on the Locke-Wallace Marital Adjustment Scale (1). Psychological treatment and support regarding psychosocial problems may decrease suffering and disability in CPP patients, which are worthwhile goals even if the severity of pain is not affected.

Patients with chronic pain develop psychological changes that maintain or increase the distress of their pain regardless of the degree of physical trauma or disease (11). Certainly there is evidence that patients with CPP have increased frequencies of psychiatric diagnoses compared to the general population (Table 56.7). When significant psychiatric diagnoses are present, the prognosis is worsened. For example, Reiter and Gambone found that of 38 patients with nongynecologic somatic diagnoses and no psychiatric diagnoses, 32 (84%) had long-term pain relief with treatment, compared to 11 (58%) of 19 patients with both somatic and psychiatric diagnoses (statistically different, $p < 0.05$) (31).

Personality disorders, especially borderline personality, are overrepresented in the severe, longstanding CPP patients who are seen in a referral center (1). However, in the primary care physician's practice, CPP patients with borderline personality disorders are less common and the label of personality disorder should not be applied to all angry or difficult patients. It is not unusual for CPP patients to be "difficult" patients. In this discussion a "difficult" patient refers to one who does not cooperate with her physician's and other healthcare provider's efforts toward optimal evaluation and treatment because of maladaptive personality reactions, traits, or a true psychiatric disorder. As such, they may evoke strong reactions in physicians, nursing staff, and other health care professionals. It is important to recognize and monitor emotional reactions to patients. These reactions are probably caused by an emotional problem being communicated by the patient (32).

TABLE 56.7. LIFETIME AND CURRENT HISTORIES OF PSYCHIATRIC DIAGNOSES IN 25 WOMEN WITH CPP

	(%) CPP	(%) Controls
Depression, lifetime	64	16
Depression, current	28	3
Phobias, current	32	10
Panic disorder, current	8	0
Alcohol dependence, lifetime	36	23
Alcohol dependence, current	20	20
Drug dependence, lifetime	56	20
Drug dependence, current	12	3

Compared to 30 controls undergoing laparoscopy for sterilization or infertility (61).

When emotional and psychological problems are present it is often difficult (and possibly a moot endeavor) to determine to what degree they preceded, developed as the result of, or are totally separate problems from CPP (1). Psychologic testing clearly shows typical and characteristic profiles, whether or not tissue pathology is present, with significant psychopathology in up to 50% of CPP patients (26). The fact that abnormal findings on psychometric tests sometimes revert to normal after successful treatment of pain suggests that, in some patients at least, these abnormalities are not permanent personality characteristics, but simply changes secondary to pain (11).

NEUROABLATIVE THERAPIES

Neurolytic therapies may be done by surgical transection or excision of nerves, injection of neurotoxic chemicals, or use of energy sufficient to destroy neural tissue (heat, cold, or laser). Although these therapies are most often used specifically to treat a particular nerve dysfunction, such as an entrapped iliohypogastric nerve, they may also be used more centrally to try to decrease pain even if there is no specific diagnosis or specific nerve dysfunction. In this chapter only neurolytic therapy used to treat CPP generally will be discussed. Therapies directed at specific diseases are discussed in the pertinent chapter on the disease, such as Chapter 44 and Chapter 21.

Surgical Neuroablation

The surgical procedures that are used to treat CPP are superior hypogastric plexus excision (presacral neurectomy), paracervical denervation (uterosacral neurectomy, uterine nerve ablation, or uterosacral ligament resection), and uterovaginal ganglion excision. All may be done via laparoscopy or laparotomy.

Presacral neurectomy (PSN) was first described independently by Jaboulay and Ruggi in 1899 (33,34). It consists of excision of the superior hypogastric plexus ("presacral nerve") just inferior to the bifurcation of aorta and confluence of vena cava, medial to the right common iliac artery and vein and right ureter on the right and medial to the inferior mesenteric vessels and sigmoid mesocolon on the left. The inferior margin of the dissection is the venous plexus of the sacral hollow. This procedure has been performed most often for severe dysmenorrhea or for endometriosis-associated pelvic pain. There are few reports of its use for CPP without associated pathology, that is, as treatment for CPP as a diagnosis (35,36). For dysmenorrhea, PSN gives pain relief in 60% to 90% of women, but for CPP the success appears to be lower (37).

For example, a retrospective study of experience with 6 years of laparoscopic presacral neurectomies in 655 patients, of whom 392 had dysmenorrhea and 135 had

CPP, shows that pain was decreased from moderate to severe preoperatively, to no pain or mild pain postoperatively in 284 (72%) of 392 with dysmenorrhea compared to 84 (62%) of 135 with CPP ($\chi2$ gives $p = 0.026$) (36). Not all studies have shown this difference, however (35).

There are only observational data regarding PSN for the treatment of CPP, with or without associated pathology, and the evidence is insufficient to show that presacral neurectomy is indicated in the treatment of pelvic pain in all women undergoing conservative surgery for pelvic pain. If it is efficacious, it appears to be so for patients with midline, not lateral, pain, and should be done only by a skillful surgeon (38).

It has been suggested that performing superior hypogastric nerve blocks prior to considering a presacral neurectomy might be predictive of surgical success. In a report by Bourke et al., 10 of 11 patients with pain relief after superior hypogastric plexus nerve blocks had greater than 50% pain relief with subsequent presacral neurectomies (39). Superior hypogastric plexus block is done by bilaterally inserting 7-in. 22G needles to the level of the L4–5 interspace, lateral to the vertebral bodies, then directing them medially and caudally to the anterolateral aspect of L5 vertebral body under fluoroscopy. Injection of 6 to 10 cc of 0.25% bupivicaine is then done through each needle (40). Superior hypogastric plexus nerve block at the time of conscious pain mapping has also been suggested as possibly predictive of success of presacral neurectomy (Chapter 5) (41). Possible complications of superior hypogastric plexus block are infection, bleeding, intramuscular, intravascular, subarachnoid or intraperitoneal injection, and nerve, renal, or ureteral injury.

Paracervical denervation techniques, usually performed by transecting the uterosacral ligaments, have also been performed primarily for relief of dysmenorrhea, not for CPP per se. Doyle and Des Rosiers performed abdominal paracervical denervations by elevating the uterosacral ligaments and placing a suture just above the point of insertion into the cervix (42). Their results in 102 patients with acquired dysmenorrhea were complete relief or pain in 90 (88%). Paracervical denervation can also be done vaginally and laparoscopically (it has been given the acronym "LUNA" for laparoscopic uterine nerve ablation) (43,44). Other have reported relief of dysmenorrhea in 70% to 80% of patients (43,44). There appear to be no published reports of paracervical denervation for the treatment of CPP without dysmenorrhea. The efficacy of laparoscopic uterosacral transection needs to be established through well-designed randomized clinical trials; its role in CPP treatment is currently controversial.

Uterovaginal ganglion excision involves excision of the inferior hypogastric plexus, a coalescence of parasympathetic and sympathetic nerves bilaterally at the base of the broad ligament lateral to the cervix, known by the eponym Frankenhauser's plexus. In an uncontrolled study by Perry, 17 (81%) of 21 patients with CPP experienced improvement after uterovaginal ganglion excision (45). Preoperative paracervical blocks were not predictive of surgical outcomes. Although these results are promising, more data are needed.

There are case reports of treatment of incapacitating pelvic pain via surgically created lesions of the central nervous system (46). Clearly, this represents a dramatic and potentially hazardous approach to treatment that requires extraordinary circumstances and a highly skilled neurosurgical team. It is not possible to speculate at this time as to the generalizability of these reports for treatment of CPP.

Although surgery is part of the management of CPP, its limitations must be recognized by both the surgeon and patient. A precaution is that, generally speaking, pain begins to return postoperatively in 6 to 18 months after surgical treatment, and particularly with neurosurgical procedures (4). Furthermore, in CPP patients without any apparent pathology, if surgery is done as a treatment for chronic pain as the diagnosis, there is a significant chance of increased pain and disability postoperatively because these patients respond poorly to invasive procedures (25). Because of this concern, the argument can be made that surgery for CPP should be scheduled only with a specific preoperative diagnosis in mind, not for CPP itself as the diagnosis. Certainly more studies and data would be useful before recommending any of the neuroablative surgical procedures as routine or common treatments for CPP.

Neurolytic Therapy

Neurolytic treatment can be done with cryoablation, thermocoagulation, or injection of chemical agents. Alcohol, phenol, and hypertonic saline are the most studied and successful chemical agents available in the United States. Capsaicin appears promising, but studies are limited even for nonpelvic chronic pain (47). Cryotherapy neuroablation is generally done using nitrous oxide at high pressures (700 psi) via a 15G Splembley-Lloyd cryoneedle. Commercial units are available for this purpose. Cryotherapy usually is not done on mixed nerves because there is loss of motor as well as sensory function (47). Generally speaking, neurolytic treatments show encouraging short-term results, but the success rates decline the longer the patients are followed.

Superior hypogastric plexus ablation with 10% phenol has been performed for intractable pelvic pain associated with cancer, with a 69% (18 of 26 patients) success rate of satisfactory pain relief at 6 months (48). Inferior hypogastric plexus or paracervical denervation by chemical ablation has been done using alcohol injections. In Davis' report of treatment of dysmenorrhea this technique yielded pain relief in 44 (61%) of 72 patients (49).

Neurolytic block of the ganglion impar (ganglion of Walther or sacrococcygeal ganglion) has been performed in cancer patients for intractable perineal and rectal pain. This unpaired ganglion lies anterior to the sacrococcygeal junction and is blocked by passing a needle through the anococcygeal ligament or the calcified sacrococcygeal ligament.

OTHER TREATMENTS OF CPP

There are many other treatments from many disciplines of healthcare, especially alternative or complementary medicine, that have been used in the management of women with CPP. Most patients use alternative treatments as adjuncts to conventional therapy, not as replacements. Thus, the name "complementary medicine" may be better terminology. Eisenberg found that one of three Americans use complementary medical treatments for a variety of illnesses with associated pain, and that 60% do so without any supervision by their conventional clinician or alternative practitioners (50). Most such treatments are not well-studied for chronic pain, let alone for CPP. Yet it is important to mention at least a few of them because they certainly seem helpful in the care of at least some women with CPP.

Relaxation therapy is well established as a psychogenic modality in the treatment of chronic pain. Most commonly, techniques such as progressive muscle relaxation are used to aid in treatment of chronic pain and especially for acute exacerbation of pain. Music therapy similarly has become relatively well established in the treatment of illness, including chronic pain. There appear to be no randomized clinical trials of its efficacy. One study of its use in the treatment of 30 patients with chronic pain secondary to rheumatoid arthritis showed decreased pain levels (51).

Transcutaneous electrical nerve stimulation (TENS) has been extensively used by physical medicine and pain physicians and by physical therapists with seemingly good results (52). About three-fourths of patients treated with TENS for chronic pain show improvement, although the degree of pain relief is not great (Tables 56.8 and 56.9).One might expect similar or better results with *acupuncture,* but not as much has been published. Rapkin has reported her preliminary results of treatment of women with CPP in a dedicated multidisciplinary clinic with a team consisting of a gynecologist, psychologist,

TABLE 56.8. THE EFFECTIVENESS OF NONMEDICAL TREATMENTS OF CHRONIC PAIN (NO STUDIES ARE OF CPP)

Treatment	Mean Effect Size	Std. Dev.	No. of Studies
Autogenic training	2.74	1.95	2
Hypnosis	2.67	—	1
Pill placebo	2.23	2.13	3
Package treatments	1.33	1.59	11
Biofeedback	0.95	1.16	24
Cognitive therapy	0.76	0.31	4
Relaxation	0.67	0.82	7
Operant conditioning	0.55	0.09	3
TENS	0.46	0.07	2

Based on mean effect size analysis. Data derived from meta-analysis of 48 valid studies from a total of 109 reviewed studies (62).
Effect size = (Mean$_{experimental group}$ − Mean$_{control group}$)/Standard deviation$_{control group}$.

TABLE 56.9. THE EFFECTIVENESS ON NONMEDICAL TREATMENT OF CHRONIC PAIN (NO STUDIES ARE OF CPP)

Treatment	Mean Percent	Std. Dev.	No. of Studies
Relaxation	95	12	4
Biofeedback	84	24	16
No therapy	77	23	14
TENS	74	18	4
Package treatment	72	33	15
Pill placebo	70	10	3
Autogenic training	68	12	4
Other	60	10	6
Hypnosis	13	—	1

Based on the percentage of patients improved as a function of the treatment. Data derived from meta-analysis of 48 valid studies from a total of 109 reviewed studies (62).

and anesthesiologist or acupuncturist (25). After three preliminary visits to complete psychological tests and assessment and examination by the pain manager and psychologist, women underwent 6 to 8 weeks of acupuncture treatments two times per week and trigger point injections (if indicated). However, they also had weekly therapy sessions with the psychologist with emphasis on coping skills, monthly evaluation by the pain manager, and some were treated with tricyclic antidepressants. Of 17 patients enrolled, 14 completed the program and 13 had significant improvement in their pain, based on daily pain diaries, a pelvic pain assessment form administered initially and at 1, 3, 6, and 12 months, symptoms recorded with visual analog scales, descriptive phrases, ratings of activities and records of medications, and measures of psychologic status at initial and follow-up visits (26). Obviously, it is difficult to discover how much the effectiveness of this program may be attributed to acupuncture. Helms has shown acupuncture to be an effective treatment for dysmenorrhea (53). There is sufficient evidence to conclude that acupuncture controls pain in at least some patients (52).

Bodywork of a less traditional nature than physical therapy, such as *massage therapy, chiropractic manipulation,* and *reflexology,* is suggested by many women as helpful in management of their CPP. There is no published research sufficient to reach a valid conclusion on such approaches as yet, although chiropractic therapy is widely accepted as useful in musculoskeletal and myofascial pain by the general public (52).

Magnetic therapy and *magnetic field therapy* have shown results in animal studies that suggest they decrease pain levels. No significant clinical studies have been published (52). There is also insufficient clinical evidence to reach a conclusion about the efficacy of hypnosis in the treatment of chronic pain.

Spiritual or religious treatments such as intercessionary prayer, healing, divine intercession, and meditation are important aspects of health care for many people, but have not been extensively studied with scientific techniques for pain treatment. One published study of 24 patients with chronic pain of idiopathic etiology, randomized to no treatment versus treatment by a spiritual healer, showed a small decrease of pain medication use, better sleep, and decreased feelings of helplessness in the treated patients (54).

General comfort measures should always be included in the treatment of CPP. Examples are heat packs, hot baths or whirlpools, ice packs, back rubs, enhanced empathy and attentive listening by clinicians, and compassionate interactions between doctor and patient (also see the subsequent discussion of the therapeutic relationship or placebo effect). For effectiveness on nonmedical treatment of chronic pain, see Tables 56.8 and 56.9.

MULTIDISCIPLINARY PAIN CENTERS

The goals of a specialized pain center are to give the patient responsibility for and control of her health care and to restore her to normal functioning (26). These goals reflect the fact that patients referred to a multidisciplinary pain center tend to have (a) severe disease, (b) limited psychological or environmental resources, or (c) limited social supports to provide the motivation needed to meet the challenges associated with functional living in the presence of chronic pain. Generally, pain centers do not set "cure" as a goal, but rather the achievement of reduced pain levels that allow return of normal activities (25). This goal is often incongruent with the goals of the woman with CPP, who remains focused on diagnosis and cure. She fears a disease that is continuously missed by her health care providers, and so seeks new physicians who will pay attention anew to her perception of a missed diagnosis and curable disease (13).

For women with CPP, a multidisciplinary clinic usually includes a gynecologist, anesthesiologist, psychologist, and physical therapist. Other disciplines that may be especially helpful in such a center are neurology, acupuncture, gastroenterology, urology, and pharmacology. It is not always practical to assemble such a multidisciplinary team in one clinic. If not, careful selection of a pool of consultants and the use of a multidisciplinary plan can still be useful and sufficient. The woman's primary physician can screen appropriately and look for possible diagnoses outside of her own discipline (55). If therapy is conducted in separate settings, constant flow of communication among practitioners is necessary to insure consistency of care (3,26). Efficiency of care may also be vital. Many women simply cannot spare the 3 to 5 hours per week that may be necessary in an ideal multidisciplinary clinic in a single site, or the even greater time required with a collaborative team at several different sites (26). The goal should not be to add to psychological stress by consuming time and resources beyond the means of the patient (26). Many women with CPP simply cannot afford the cost or time requirement of a multidisciplinary pain clinic (13).

Little has been reported about multidisciplinary clinics specifically for CPP. A randomized clinical trial by Peters et al. suggests multidisciplinary treatment is better than a traditional approach by a gynecologist alone, at least in women with a history of previous negative evaluations by a gynecologist (i.e., negative findings at the time of a prior laparoscopy or laparotomy) (56). They were able to show that an "integral approach" using gynecologists, psychologists, physiotherapists, and nutritionists for 6 months gave better outcomes in improved "general pain experience" (75% versus 41%), decreased "disturbance of daily activities" (68% versus 37%), and decrease of "associated symptoms" (75% versus 27%), compared to traditional gynecologic treatment with repeat laparoscopy.

After a CPP clinic was established that allowed extensive evaluations for various diagnoses, Reiter et al. noted a decrease in the number of referrals to the clinic with somatic pathologies. They speculated that this reflected an improved clinical expertise among the referring physicians and residents from working in and with the CPP clinic, allowing a fuller evaluation before patients were referred to the CPP clinic (31). As discussed previously, the multidisciplinary CPP clinic at UCLA reported by Rapkin achieved improvement in 13 of the 14 women that completed the program.

THE THERAPEUTIC RELATIONSHIP OR PLACEBO EFFECT

In general terms there are three reasons for clinical improvement in a patient's condition (57). First, the typical natural history of a chronic condition is fluctuation of symptom severity. Thus from severe symptom states the natural course is a regression to the mean, which is seen as improvement by the clinician (and patient). Patients tend to seek medical care when their symptoms are at their worst, so the next likely change is improvement. This improvement is likely to be attributed to the treatment prescribed by the clinician.

Second, the treatment may actually have specific therapeutic effects that result in improvement of the chronic disease. Most often a randomized, placebo-controlled clinical trial is necessary to estimate the actual therapeutic effect of any treatment.

Third, there may be nonspecific effects of the treatment that are attributable to factors other than any specific activity of the treatment; that is, a placebo effect (57). The term placebo is often used synonymously with nonspecific effects, but it should be distinguished from the term placebo effect. *Placebo* refers to an intervention designed to simulate medical treatment, but not believed by the clinician to be a specific treatment for the target condition. In clinical practice a placebo is used for its psychological effect. In research it is used to eliminate observer bias in the experimental setting. Placebo may also be applied to a treatment now believed ineffective, although previously it was believed to be effective. *Placebo response* refers to any change in the patient's condition following the administration of a placebo. *Placebo effect* refers to a change in the patient's condition or illness attributable to the symbolic importance of a treatment rather than a specific pharmacologic or physiologic property. The placebo effect does not require a placebo. Placebo effects are found with drugs, medical treatments, surgery, biofeedback, psychotherapy, and diagnostic tests. It may occur whenever the patient or physician perceives the "treatment" as effective. For example, it may occur simply owing to a visit with a physician.

It seems likely that a great deal of the response of the patient to a therapeutic relationship may be attributed to the placebo effect. From studies utilizing placebos it appears that placebo effects are likely to be strongest when (a) the patient is anxious, (b) the physician is perceived as having great expertise, (c) the patient and physician believe the treatment is powerful, and (d) the treatment is impressive and expensive (57). Clearly, to the extent that is ethical, physicians should use the placebo effect to their and their patients' advantage. An interesting study of nonspecific effects by a general practitioner showed that 64% of patients improved after a positive encounter with the physician compared to 39% after a negative encounter (statistically different, $p = 0.001$) (58). Patients' expectations also greatly influence response to treatment. For example, when a true bronchodilator is given, its effects are two times greater if patients are told it would produce this effect than if they were told the opposite. The expectation of improvement with treatment, active or placebo, may result in the patient's having a more positive attitude about pain treatment and viewing the pain as more controllable. This may lead to beneficial behavioral changes (57).

It is a gross error to use a placebo to assess whether a patient's pain is real or to dismiss or delegitimize the complaint on the basis of a placebo response. Patients suffering from organic pain respond to a more marked degree to placebo than those with nonorganic pain, indicating the importance of strong motivation (27). It is a clinical misconception that if a patient responds favorably to a placebo medication, then the pain must be of psychological origin. This is simply not true (2).

It is also a gross error and unethical to deliberately use placebo treatments in hopes of producing a placebo response. Doing so carries several risks. First, the patient may feel deceived if they discover the placebo treatment. Second, a placebo may make preexisting symptoms worse or produce adverse reactions. A review of 109 double-blind clinical trials showed a 19% incidence of adverse events owing to placebos. Third, failure to improve may lead to increased anxiety because of worry of a more serious problem by the patient. Finally, failure to improve with the placebo may psychologically condition the patient and increase the risk of not improving with subsequent treatments (57).

It is a common misconception that one-third of patients will have a placebo response or effect to any clinical treatment (57). In reality there is great variation in the placebo response, depending on the disease, the type of treatment, the characteristics of the patient and physician, and so on. In Beecher's classic review of 15 studies, including postoperative pain, cough, angina pectoris, headaches, drug-induced mood changes, seasickness, anxiety and tension, and the common cold, the average response to placebo was 35%, but the range was 15% to 58% (59).

SUMMARY

Although chronic pain may be difficult for the clinician and her patient to accept as a diagnosis, it is an important concept in the care of CPP. It allows the use of pain-directed therapies, that albeit not curative, permit the patient to progress toward a more normal life that is not dominated by pain. It also breaks the traditional hold of the Cartesian model of pain, so that if no organic lesion is found that leads to a cure the patient is not led to believe that her pain is not real or that it is "in her head." Finally, it offers hope that with future research the psychoneurologic dysfunctions responsible for chronic pain may be identified and lead to definitive, curative treatments.

REFERENCES

1. Steege JF. Assessment and treatment of chronic pelvic pain. *Telinde's Operative Gynecol Updates* 1992;1:1–10.
2. Grzesiak RC, Perrine KR. Psychological aspects of chronic pain. In: Ranaer M, ed. *Pelvic pain in women.* New York: Springer-Verlag, 1981.
3. Rosenthal RH. Psychology of chronic pelvic pain. *Obstet Gynecol Clin NA* 1993;20:627–642.
4. Sternbach RA. Clinical aspects of pain. In: Sternbach RA, ed. *The psychology of pain,* 2nd ed. New York: Raven Press, 1986:223–237.
5. Milburn A, Reiter RC, Rhamberg AT. Multidisciplinary approach to chronic pelvic pain. *Obstet Gynecol Clin NA* 1993;20:643–661.
6. Rapkin AJ. Neuroanatomy, neurophysiology, and neuropharmacology of pelvic pain. *Clin Obstet Gynecol* 1990;33:119–129.
7. Rosenthal RH. Psychology of chronic pelvic pain. *Obstet Gynecol Clin NA* 1993;20:627–642.
8. Reiter RC. A profile of women with chronic pelvic pain. *Clin Obstet Gynecol* 1990;33:130–136.
9. Ranaer M, ed. *Chronic pelvic pain in women.* New York: Springer-Verlag, 1981:25.
10. Condouris GA. Drug therapy in the treatment of chronic pain. In: Ranaer M, ed. *Chronic pelvic pain in women.* New York: Springer-Verlag, 1981.
11. Steege JF. The psychological component of chronic pelvic pain. *Female patient* 1986;11:139–147.
12. Insel PA. Analgesic-antipyretic and antiinflammatory agents and drugs employed in the treatment of gout. In: Hardman JG, Limbird LE, Molinoff PB, et al, ed. *Goodman and Gilman's the pharmacological basis of therapeutics,* 9th ed. New York: McGraw-Hill, 1996:617–657.
13. Walker EA, Sullivan MD, Stenchever MA. Use of antidepressants in the management of women with chronic pelvic pain. *Obstet Gynecol Clin NA* 1993;20:743–751.
14. Portenoy RK, Foley KM. Chronic use of opioid analgesics in non-malignant pain: report of 38 cases. *Pain* 1986;25:171–186.
15. Miotto K, Compton, Ling W, et al. Diagnosing addictive disease in chronic pain patients. *Psychosomatics* 1996;37:223–235.
16. Winkelmuller M, Winkelmuller W. Long-term effects of continuous intrathecal opioid treatment in chronic pain of nonmalignant etiology. *J Neurosurg* 1996;85:458–467.
17. Angel IF, Gould HJ Jr, Carey ME. Intrathecal morphine pump as a treatment option in chronic pain of nonmalignant origin. *Surg Neurol* 1998;49:92–98.
18. Maron J, Loeser JD. Spinal opioid infusions in the treatment of chronic pain of nonmalignant origin. *Clin J Pain* 1996;12:174–179.
19. Goodkin K, Guillon CM. Antidepressants for the relief of chronic pain: do they work? *Annals Behav Med* 1989;11:83–101.
20. Onghena P, Van Houdenhove BV. Antidepressant-induced analgesia in chronic non-malignant pain: a meta-analysis of 39 placebo controlled studies. *Pain* 1992;49:205–219.
21. Cannon RO III, Quyyumi AA, Mincemoyer R, et al. Imipramine in patients with chest pain despite normal coronary angiograms. *N Engl J Med* 1994;330:1411–1417.
22. Atkinson JH, Slater MA, Williams RA, et al. A placebo-controlled randomized clinical trial of nortriptyline for chronic low back pain. *Pain* 1998;76:287–296.
23. Hodgkiss AD, Watson JP. Psychiatric morbidity and illness behaviour in women with chronic pelvic pain. *J Psychosom Res* 1993;22:3–9.
24. Morris DB. *The culture of pain.* Berkeley and Los Angeles, CA: University of California Press, 1992:1444.
25. Rapkin AJ, Karnes LD. New hope for patients with chronic pelvic pain. *Female Patient* 1988;31:100–173.
26. Rapkin AJ, Kames LD. The pain management approach to chronic pelvic pain. *J Reprod Med* 1987;32:323–327.
27. Kroger WS. Hypnosis for the relief of pelvic pain. *Clin Obstet Gynecol* 1963;6:763–775.
28. Benson RC, Hanson KH, Matarazzo JD. Atypical pelvic pain in women: gynecologic-psychiatric considerations. *Am J Obstet Gynecol* 1959;77:806–825.
29. Steege JF, Stout AL. Resolution of chronic pelvic pain after laparoscopic lysis of adhesions. *Am J Obstet Gynecol* 1991;265:278–281.
30. Reiter RC, Milburn A. Exploring effective treatment for chronic pelvic pain. *Contemp OB/GYN* 1994;84–103.
31. Reiter RC, Gambone JC. Nongynecologic somatic pathology in women with chronic pelvic pain and negative laparoscopy. *J Reprod Med* 1991;36:253–259.
32. Thompson TL. Managing the "difficult" Ob/Gyn patient. *Female Patient* 1990;15:81–92.
33. Jaboulay M. Le traitement de la nevralgie pelvienne par la paralysie du sympathique sacre. *Lyon Med* 1899;90:102–108.
34. Ruggi C. Della sympatectamia al collo ed ale adome. *Policlinic* 1899:193.
35. Zulu F, Pellicano M, DeStafano R, et al. Efficacy of laparoscopic denervation in central-type chronic pelvic pain: a multicenter study. *J Gynecol Surg* 1996;12:35–40.
36. Chen F-P, Soong Y-K. The efficacy and complications of laparoscopic presacral neurectomy in pelvic pain. *Obstet Gynecol* 1997;90:974–977.
37. Lee RB, Stone K, Magelssen D, et al. Presacral neurectomy for chronic pelvic pain. *Obstet Gynecol* 1986;68:517–521.
38. Candiani GB, Fedele L, Vercellini P, et al. Presacral neurectomy for the treatment of pelvic pain associated with endometriosis: a controlled study. *Am J Obstet Gynecol* 1992;167:100–103.
39. Bourke DL, Foster DC, Valley MA, et al. Superior hypogastric

nerve block as predictive of presacral neurectomy success: a preliminary report. *Amer J Pain Manag* 1996;6:9–12.

40. Placante R, Amescua C, Patt RB, et al. Superior hypogastric plexus block for pelvic cancer pain. *J Anesthesiol* 1990;73:236–239.

41. Steege JF. Superior hypogastric block during microlaparoscopic pain mapping. *J Am Assoc Gynecol Laparosc* 1998;5:265–267.

42. Doyle JB, Des Rosiers JJ. Paracervical uterine denervation for relief of pelvic pain. *Clin Obstet Gynecol* 1963;6:742–753.

43. Lichten E, Bombard J. Surgical treatment of primary dysmenorrhea with laparoscopic uterine nerve ablation. *J Reprod Med* 1987;32:37–41.

44. Gurgan T, Urman B, Aksu T, et al. Laparoscopic CO2 laser uterine nerve ablation for treatment of drug resistant primary dysmenorrhea. *Fertil Steril* 1992;58:422–424.

45. Perry CP. Laparoscopic uterovaginal ganglion excision (LUVE) for chronic pelvic pain. *J Gynecol Surg* 1996;12:89–93.

46. Nauta HJ, Hewitt E, Westlund KN, et al. Surgical interruption of a midline dorsal column visceral pain pathway. Case report and review of the literature. *J Neurosurg* 1997;86:538–542.

47. Blum SL, Lubenow T. Neurolytic agents. *Curr Rev Pain* 1996; 1:70–78.

48. de Leon-Casasola OA, Kent E, Lema MJ. Neurolytic superior hypogastric plexus block for chronic pelvic pain associated with cancer. *Pain* 1993;54:145–151.

49. Davis A. Alcohol injection for relief of dysmenorrhea. *Clin Obstet Gynecol* 1963;6:754–762.

50. Eisenberg DM, Kessler RC, Foster C, et al. Unconventional medicine in the United States. *N Engl J Med* 1993;328:246–252.

51. Schorr JA. Music and pattern change in chronic pain. *Adv Nurs Sci* 1993;15:27–36.

52. Parris WCV. Alternative pain medicine:current modalities and principles. *Curr Rev Pain* 1996;1:54–60.

53. Helms JM. Acupuncture in the management of primary dysmenorrhea. *Obstet Gynecol* 1987;69:51–56.

54. Sundblom DM, Haikonen S, Niemi-Pynttari, et al. Effect of spiritual healing on chronic idiopathic pain: a medical and psychological study. *Clin J Pain* 1994;10:296–302.

55. Smith RP. Cyclic pain and dysmenorrhea. *Obstet Gynecol NA* 1993;20:753–764.

56. Peters AAW, van Dorst E, Jellis B, et al. A randomized clinical trial to compare two different approaches in women with chronic pelvic pain. *Obstet Gynecol* 1991;77:740–744.

57. Turner JA, Deyo RA, Loeser JD, et al. The importance of placebo effects in pain treatment and research. *JAMA* 1994; 271:1609–1614.

58. Thomas KB. General practice consultations: is there any point in being positive? *Br Med J* 1987;294:1200–1202.

59. Beecher HK. The powerful placebo. *JAMA* 1955;159:1602–1606.

60. Portenoy RK. Opioid therapy for chronic nonmalignant pain: current status. In: Fields HL, Liebeskind JC, eds. *Progress in pain research and management,* vol. 1. Seattle, WA: IASP Press, 1994: 247–287.

61. Harrop-Griffiths J, Katon W, Walker E, et al. The association between chronic pelvic pain, psychiatric diagnoses, and childhood sexual abuse. *Obstet Gynecol* 1988;71:589–594.

62. Malone MD, Strube MJ. Meta-analysis of non-medical treatments for chronic pain. *Pain* 1988;34:231.

57

ABUSE AND CHRONIC PAIN

FRED M. HOWARD

INTRODUCTION

Physical and sexual abuse are serious and pervasive problems. In the United States, domestic violence is the most common cause of injury to women, with a prevalence of physical abuse by a male partner of about 10% and of about 3% for severe abuse (1,2). Approximately 40% of adult women report that they have been abused by an intimate partner at some time in their lives (3). Childhood physical or sexual abuse is reported by 20% to 50% women (4). About 25% of women report a history of childhood sexual abuse, about 25% report a history of adulthood sexual abuse, and about 15% report both childhood and adulthood sexual abuse (5).

Abuse is related to a number of health problems, including chronic pain, depression, suicide attempts, and alcohol and substance abuse, and abusive experiences generally promote the chronicity of many different painful conditions. Women who are abused have more physician visits and increased somatic complaints than women who are not abused. They are more likely to have functional as opposed to organic diagnoses, to utilize health care resources, and to have pain in specific sites (e.g., pelvic pain and headaches) (6). There is a clear relationship between childhood sexual abuse and later alcohol and substance abuse, with 10 times the likelihood in those with a history of sexual abuse (7). Additionally, a past history of childhood sexual abuse has been found to greatly increase the occurrence of constipation in later years (8). Childhood sexual abuse is associated with sexual dysfunction, promiscuity, dependency, depression, and somatization in later life.

Of particular interest to this discussion, women who have been the victims of physical or sexual abuse appear to be significantly more likely to experience chronic pain, especially chronic pelvic pain (CPP) (9,10). In women with histories of abuse, the risk of having chronic pain appears to be at least double that of women with no histories of abuse. The prevalence of abuse in chronic pain patients ranges from 34% to 66% (11,12). In the general population the rate of abuse varies from 6% to as much as 62%, depending on the criteria used to define abuse (13). Similarly, women with CPP have a higher rate of abuse than pain-free

women. For example, in a comparison of women undergoing laparoscopy for CPP to women undergoing laparoscopy for sterilization or infertility, Walker et al. found that women with CPP were significantly more likely to have histories of abuse (Table 57.1) (14). Similar results were previously reported by Harrop-Griffiths et al. in a study comparing 25 women with CPP to 13 women for sterilization and 17 women with infertility undergoing laparoscopy (15). They found that more of the women with CPP had experienced some type of sexual abuse before 14 years of age and as an adult than the "control" women.

Jamieson and Steege found that sexual abuse only as a child or only as an adult did not correlate with significant pelvic pain, dysmenorrhea, or nonpelvic pain syndromes. However, both correlated with irritable bowel syndrome. A history of both child and adult sexual abuse correlated with significant pelvic pain, dyspareunia, irritable bowel syndrome, and other pain syndromes, but not dysmenorrhea (5).

It has been suggested that sexual abuse might in some way be specifically related to the development of CPP. A study by Rapken et al. specifically tried to evaluate this matter (11). They compared patients with chronic nonpelvic pain to patients with CPP regarding physical abuse as well as sexual abuse, both as a child and an adult (Table 57.2). Although the groups were not large, their data suggest that

TABLE 57.1. LIKELIHOOD OF ABUSE IN 50 WOMEN WITH CHRONIC PELVIC PAIN COMPARED TO 50 WOMEN WITH INFERTILITY OR DESIRING STERILIZATION

	Women with Pelvic Pain	Women without Pelvic Pain
Any childhood sexual abuse	29 (58%)	15 (30%)
Severe childhood sexual abuse	12 (24%)	2 (4%)
Any adulthood sexual abuse	26 (52%)	13 (26%)
Severe adulthood sexual abuse	19 (38%)	9 (18%)

Differences were statistically significant in all comparisons.

TABLE 57.2. WOMEN WITH CHRONIC PELVIC PAIN OR OTHER CHRONIC PAIN COMPARED TO CONTROLS IN REGARD TO PHYSICAL OR SEXUAL ABUSE

	Childhood Physical Abuse (%)	Childhood Sexual Abuse (%)	Adulthood Physical Abuse (%)	Adulthood Sexual Abuse (%)	Any Physical Abuse (%)	Any Sexual Abuse (%)	Any Abuse (%)
Chronic pelvic pain (n = 31)	39	19	10	6	39	26	55
Pathology (n = 19)	30	15	0	9	—	—	—
No pathology (n = 11)	54	27	27	5	—	—	—
Other chronic pain (n = 141)	18	16	16	8	28	19	36
Controls (n = 32)	9	12	3	0	9	12	16

sexual abuse occurred with equivalent frequency in CPP patients and chronic nonpelvic pain patients. Physical abuse in childhood, however, was more common in CPP patients. Their data also suggested that women with CPP and no pathology at the time of laparoscopy or laparotomy were more likely to have experienced abuse than those with pathology. They concluded, "it is unlikely that sexual abuse is specifically and, perhaps, psychodynamically related to pelvic pain. The experience of abuse in general, however, may promote the chronicity of painful conditions." I should add, however, that at this time no single theory or model has given an adequate explanation of why some persons become chronic pain patients.

A more recent study by Walling et al. concluded that their results "support a specific association between major sexual abuse and chronic pelvic pain and a more general association between physical abuse and chronic pain."(16) However, I do not think their data justify the conclusion that sexual abuse is any more specifically associated with CPP than physical abuse. Rather, their data suggest a strong association between a history of global abuse, including *both* physical and sexual abuse, and CPP (Table 57.3).

An uncontrolled study by Fry et al. found a prevalence of childhood sexual abuse of 30% in women with CPP, a prevalence not notably different from that in the general

British population (28%), and they questioned any specific etiologic role of childhood sexual abuse (17).

Thus, although it is intellectually tempting to etiologically link sexual abuse with pelvic pain, current data do not support an association with major sexual abuse any more specifically than they do an association with major physical (nonsexual) abuse. In other words, there appears to be an association between abuse, whether physical or sexual, and CPP. Patients with both physical and sexual abuse, especially during childhood, seem particularly at high risk of CPP, and it may be that a history of both serves as a marker for a greater magnitude of abuse, and that the greater the magnitude of abuse the stronger the correlation with CPP (16,18).

It is important in taking the history of a woman with CPP to ask about abuse. With the relatively high prevalence of abuse, the immediate concern is to assure that the woman is safe. Once it is clear that the patient is not currently being abused and not in imminent danger, then the history should be explored for prior abuse as an adult or child.

There are a number of ways that this history may be acquired. It is important that it be asked sensitively and that the patient's privacy be respected. Questions about abuse are often best explored in a private setting without the

TABLE 57.3. COMPARISON OF WOMEN WITH CHRONIC PELVIC PAIN TO WOMEN WITH CHRONIC HEADACHES OR WITH NO PAIN PROBLEMS

	Childhood Physical Abuse (%)	Childhood Sexual Abuse (%)	Adulthood Physical Abuse (%)	Adulthood Sexual Abuse (%)	Childhood and Adulthood Physical Abuse (%)	Childhood and Adulthood Sexual Abuse (%)	Major Sexual and Physical Abuse (%)
Chronic pelvic pain (n = 64)	39	36	36	33	25	16	42
Headache (n = 42)	29	17	14	17	5	0	19
Pain-free controls (n = 46)	15	20	20	17	4	9	20

According to prevalence of major sexual abuse and physical abuse.

spouse or significant other present. A standardized set of questions that are often used in research evaluations is summarized in Table 57.4. A more open-ended set of questions regarding abuse are:

1. *Childhood physical abuse.* Were you ever physically disciplined or punished as a child? What kind of discipline or punishment was used? Did the punishment ever lead to bruises, marks, welts, or other injury?
2. *Childhood sexual abuse.* When you were under 18 years old, was there ever a time when someone made any type of sexual contact with you, other than voluntary sexual activity with a same-aged boyfriend or girlfriend? Who? What was the nature of the sexual contact?
3. *Adult physical abuse.* As an adult, have you ever been hit or assaulted by your significant other, by a family member, or by some adult with whom you were having an ongoing relationship? Has this behavior resulted in marks, bruises, or signs of injury?
4. *Adult sexual abuse.* As an adult, has there been any occasion when someone you knew had any type of sexual contact with you against your will? What kind of contact and how often?

A history of abuse as a child or as an adult may not only be relevant in thinking about etiology, but also may help in the diagnostic evaluation and in treatment. Patients with chronic pain and a history of abuse, however, do not rate their pain severity any greater than those without a history

TABLE 57.4. SEXUAL-PHYSICAL ABUSE HISTORY QUESTIONNAIRE

Sexual abuse:

During your childhood (<14 years) has anyone ever:
  Exposed their sex organ(s) to you?
  Threatened to have sex with you?
  Touched your sex organ(s)?
  Made you touch their sex organ(s)?
  Tried forcefully or succeeded to have sex when you didn't want to?
  Tried any other unwanted sexual experiences not mentioned above?
During your adulthood has anyone ever:
  Threatened to have sex with you?
  Touched your sex organ(s) without your permission?
  Made you touch their sex organ(s)?
  Tried forcefully or succeeded to have sex when you didn't want to?
  Tried any other unwanted sexual experiences not mentioned above?

Physical abuse:

When you were a child did an older person hit, kick, or beat you?
  If *yes,* was this seldom, occasionally, or often?
Now that you are an adult does any other adult hit, kick, or beat you?
  If *yes,* was or is this seldom, occasionally, or often?

of abuse (13). Their rating of functional interference is also not any greater. Nor is it clear if women with CPP and histories of sexual abuse are any less likely to have positive laparoscopic findings than those women with CPP and no abuse history (19).

Patients with chronic pain and a history of physical or sexual abuse are more likely to use the emergency room for pain symptoms than those chronic pain patients without a history of abuse (13). A history of abuse may, therefore, lead the clinician to stress early in care that using the emergency department for care is not appropriate. Women with histories of childhood sexual abuse also are more likely to have histories of substance abuse (20). This can be important information early in the patient's care and may influence analgesic decisions. As an aside, of patients with chronic pain, 28% to 37% report childhood abuse, compared to reported childhood abuse in about 67% of nonpain patients that seek treatment for substance abuse. Such information suggests that childhood abuse leads to maladaptive coping skills in later life, not just chronic pain (21).

Confirming this, on psychological testing, patients with chronic pain and histories of abuse score lower on coping abilities than those without abuse histories. They also score higher on locus of control being attributed to chance and on psychological distress. The concept of perceived control holds that the person who sees herself having little control over physical and emotional events may be most vulnerable to developing a chronic pain syndrome. Such information can be helpful in designing treatment regimens. Additionally, CPP patients with abuse histories have higher dissociation and somatization scores on psychological tests. Women with CPP and no abuse history have dissociation scores within the normal range, whereas those with histories of abuse average scores two to three times higher than normal. Dissociation is a disruption in the usually integrated function of consciousness, memory, identity, or perception of the environment. It may be viewed as a means of splitting off from consciousness those frightening experiences that may not fit into existing cognitive schemes. As a defense mechanism, dissociation creates a psychological distance and serves as a normal adaptive coping skill in the face of traumatic events. It allows the victim to escape what in reality is inescapable. Dissociation becomes maladaptive if it continues throughout the victim's life.

Somatization is the presence of physical symptoms that are not fully accounted for by a general medical condition, the effects of a substance, or mental disorder, yet suggest the presence of a medical condition and cause clinically significant distress or impairment. Somatization in women with CPP suggests that they "convert" psychological difficulties into physical symptoms in favor of a somatic over a psychological representation of distress. Somatization is an avoidance coping strategy. Childhood physical abuse is strongly associated with later somatization (22). Sexual abuse may also be related to somatization and CPP. Reiter et al. suggest that nonsomatic CPP (they defined this as CPP with no apparent organic diagnosis) is one manifestation of somatization associated with sexual trauma (23). Women with both a history of sexual abuse and a somatization score of 8 or more (i.e., they had eight or more symptoms) were two times more likely to have a nonsomatic diagnosis than women with only one or no such risk factor. More specifically related to our discussion of abuse and somatization, they found that a history of sexual trauma and a high somatization score (i.e., eight or more somatic symptoms) were predictive of increased risk for nonsomatic pelvic pain, as opposed to somatic pelvic pain (Table 57.5).

There is information from pediatric pain research that may be relevant in mechanistically trying to explain the relationship of abuse to somatization and chronic pain. In a prospective study of extremely low birth weight (ELBW) children (<1,000 g) who were exposed to long neonatal intensive care unit courses with painful experiences, compared to control term infants without prolonged exposures to painful experiences, it was shown that at 4 to 5 years of age the infants from the ELBW group were significantly more likely to have somatization scores above the clinically significant level (9 of 36 versus 0 of 36, respectively, in the ELBW versus control infants) (24). ELBW infants have also been found to have significant differences as toddlers in their pain sensitivity, as rated by parental observations (25). These finding suggests that early pain experience may contribute to development of later somatization and pain sensitivity, and as previously discussed, these have significant relevance to pain syndromes.

Along a somewhat similar line, a study of infants' responses to painful stimuli at the time of DPT and HIB immunizations were significantly affected by an infant's earlier painful experiences associated with neonatal circumcision. Males who had undergone neonatal circumcision were observed to exhibit greater pain responses to childhood immunizations to DPT and then to HIB than did females. Taddio et al. were able to demonstrate that the gender difference was accounted for by a history of neonatal circumcision. Also, pain relief with eutectic mixture of local anesthetics (EMLA) for the immuniza-tions was less

effective in male infants who had neonatal circumcis-ions than in male infants who were not circumcised. These observations are suggestive that the circumcised infants were "conditioned" to pain, resulting in an augmented and exaggerated response in comparison to the uncircumcised infants. Furthermore, the observed pain reaction after the second immunization with HIB showed an even clearer association with circumcision status than the response after the first immunization with DPT. This may be interpreted as a "priming" effect in the circumcised infants, leading them to exhibit even more pain behavior after the HIB immunization (26). It is theoretically possible that repetitive childhood abuse has similar "priming" effects on the neurological and behavioral response to painful or potentially painful experiences, eventually resulting in a chronic pain syndrome.

CONCLUSION

Unfortunately, there is no consensus among mental health professionals as to the most appropriate treatment of victims of abuse. Treatment literature on the sequelae of abuse is disappointing, especially when the abuse occurred in the distant past. Because of this there are several points regarding a history of abuse that may be relevant and useful in diagnosis and treatment from the clinician's perspective. First, although women with pelvic pain should routinely be asked about sexual abuse, when an abuse history is elicited, clinicians are often unsure about what to do with this information. It is important to remember that a fundamental use of this information is to ensure that there is no ongoing abuse and that the patient is not in a dangerous environment. If, however, the abuse occurred at some point in the past, it is generally unclear to what degree, if any, the previous abuse is directly contributing to the current pain complaints and how helpful to the treatment of pain psychological counseling and treatment directed to the history of abuse will be. If it is clear that the patient's feelings about the prior abuse are preventing normal function, apart from her pelvic pain, then the decision about referral to psychotherapy and counseling is straightforward. Referral to investigate a potential causal rela-

TABLE 57.5. COMPARISON OF WOMEN WITH CHRONIC PELVIC PAIN AND HISTORY OF SEXUAL ABUSE TO THOSE WITH NO HISTORY OF SEXUAL ABUSE ACCORDING TO NUMBER OF SOMATIC COMPLAINTS AND SOMATIC DIAGNOSIS

	History of Sexual Abuse	No History of Sexual Abuse	p value
Somatic pain	13	34	
Number of somatic symptoms	8.6 ± 4.4	6.2 ± 3.6	NS
Nonsomatic pain	35	17	
Number of somatic symptoms	10.3 ± 4.8	5.9 ± 4.8	<0.002
Total patients	48	51	
Number of somatic symptoms	9.9 ± 4.8	6.1 ± 3.4	<0.001

NS, not significant.

tionship of the abuse to CPP does not seem to have therapeutic benefit (5). Victims of sexual and physical abuse have many negative emotional sequelae, and although pain problems may often occur after abuse, it is probably wisest that the clinician not assume that pain problems are directly caused by the abuse. It is likely that abuse is a marker for a psychological environment that was (or is) detrimental in many ways, leading to deficits of character and personality perhaps equal in importance to the terrible trauma of the abuse itself. Finally, it is important to remember that a large proportion of CPP patients have not been abused.

REFERENCES

1. Chez R. Woman battering. *Am J Obstet Gynecol* 1988;158:1–4.
2. Straus MA, Gelles RJ. Societal change and change in family violence from 1975 to 1985. *J Marriage Fam* 1986;48:465.
3. Hamberger K, Saunders D, Hovey M. Prevalence of domestic violence in community practice and rate of physician inquiry. *Fam Med* 1992;24:283–287.
4. McCauley J, Kern DE, Kolodner K, et al. Clinical characteristics of women with a history of childhood abuse. Unhealed wounds. *JAMA* 1997;27:1362–1368.
5. Jamieson DJ, Steege JF. The association of sexual abuse with pelvic pain complaints in a primary care population. *Am J Obstet Gynecol* 1997;17:1408–1412.
6. Drossman DA, Leserman J, Nachman G, et al. Sexual and physical abuse in women with functional or organic gastrointestinal disorders. *Ann Intern Med* 1990;113:828–833.
7. Singer MI, Petchers MK, Hussey D. The relationship between sexual abuse and substance abuse among psychiatrically hospitalized adolescents. *Child Abuse Negl* 1989;13:319–325.
8. Talley NJ, Helgeson S, Zinmeister AR. Are sexual and physical abuse linked to functional gastrointestinal disorders? *Gastroenterology* 1992;89:A523.
9. Haber J. Abused women and chronic pain. *Am J Nurs* 1985;85:1010–1016.
10. Chapman JD. A longitudinal study of sexuality and gynecologic health in abuse women. *J Am Osteopath Assoc* 1989;89:619–624.
11. Rapkin AJ, Kames LD, Darke LL, et al. History of physical and sexual abuse in women with chronic pelvic pain. *Obstet Gynecol* 1990;76:92–96.
12. Domino J, Haber J. Prior physical and sexual abuse in women with chronic headache: clinical correlates. *Headache* 1987;27:310–314.
13. Toomey TC, Seville JL, Mann D, et al. Relationship of sexual and physical abuse to pain description, coping, psychological distress, and health-care utilization in a chronic pain sample. *Clin J Pain* 1995;11:307–315.
14. Walker EA, Katon WJ, Hansom J, et al. Medical and psychiatric symptoms in women with childhood sexual abuse. *Psychom Med* 1992;54:658–664.
15. Harrop-Griffiths J, Katon W, Walker E, et al. The association between chronic pelvic pain, psychiatric diagnoses, and childhood sexual abuse. *Obstet Gynecol* 1988;71:589–594.
16. Walling MK, Reiter RC, O'Hara MW, et al. Abuse history and chronic pain in women: I. Prevalences of sexual abuse and physical abuse. *Obstet Gynecol* 1994;84:193–199.
17. Fry RPW, Crisp AH, Beard RW, et al. Psychological aspects of chronic pelvic pain, with special reference to sexual abuse. A study of 164 women. *Postgrad Med J* 1993;69:566–574.
18. Howard FM. Abuse history and chronic pain in women: I. prevalences of sexual and physical abuse. (Letter to the editor) *Obstet Gynecol* 1995;85:158–159.

SUBJECT INDEX

*Page numbers followed by f indicate figures;
those followed by t indicate tables.*

A

Abdominal epilepsy, 438–440
Abdominal migraines, 441–443
Abdominal muscle trigger points, 323, 328f,
    353, 355f
Abdominal wall tenderness test, 32–35,
    434, 434f
Accessory ovary. *See* Ovary, accessory
Acetaminophen, 495t, 496
Acetylcholine, in trigger point pathology,
    316
Activities of daily living
    musculoskeletal pain in pregnancy
        provoked by, 20t
    pelvic pain evaluation, 15f, 20–21
Acupuncture, 357, 501
    dysmenorrhea treatment, 104
Acute pelvic pain
    versus chronic pelvic pain, 493t
    diagnostic criteria, 3
Acyclovir, 118, 207
    herpes zoster infection treatment, 469
Addiction
    abstinence syndrome, 493, 496–497
    definition, 493
    predictors, 497t
    pseudoaddiction, 497
    risk, 496–497
Adductor muscle trigger points, 336–338,
    337f, 343–344
Adenocarcinoma
    versus adenomyosis, 90
    colon, 212
    in ovarian remnant syndrome, 165
    rectal, 212
Adenomatous polyp, 211
Adenomyoma
    definition, 86
    histopathology, 87
    imaging tests, 47
Adenomyosis
    associated pelvic pathology, 86, 87
    definition, 86
    differential diagnosis, 90
    dyspareunia and, 114
    endoscopic diagnosis, 55
    epidemiology, 86
    etiology, 86–87
    evaluation and diagnosis, 55, 88–90, 91
        imaging studies, 47, 50

histopathology, 87
hysterosalpingography, 48
menses-associated pain, 18
pain characteristics, 19f
pathology, 87
symptoms and signs, 87–88
treatment, 105
    medical, 90
    surgical, 90–91
Adhesiolysis, 60, 60t
    dyspareunia and, 118
    effectiveness in relieving CPP, 93, 93t, 96
    endometriosis surgery, 142
    indications, 96
    irritable bowel disease treatment, 244
    laparoscopy *versus* laparotomy, 95t
    in ovarian remnant syndrome surgery,
        167
    in ovarian retention syndrome surgery,
        160
    peritoneal cyst treatment, 248
    procedure, 95–96
Adhesive disease, 20
    chronic pelvic pain and, 55–57, 59, 93
    classification, 95, 95t
    definition, 93
    diagnosis, 94–95, 96
    dyspareunia and, 115
    endometriosis and, 157
    endoscopic findings, 55
    etiology, 93–94
    imaging studies, 50
    laparoscopic conscious pain mapping in
        diagnosis of, 71
    laparoscopic evaluation, 59–60
    laparoscopic surgery, 60, 60t
    ovarian remnant syndrome risk and, 163
    ovarian retention syndrome and,
        155–156, 156t
    pain characteristics, 13
    in pelvic inflammatory disease, 184,
        185t, 186
    postoperative peritoneal cysts, 62
    prevention, 60, 96
    staging, 95, 95t
    symptoms and signs, 94
    treatment, 95–96, 97
    See also Adhesiolysis
Adjustment disorder, 451–452
Adnexal cysts. *See* Cysts, adnexal
Adolescent patients
    dysmenorrhea in, 102, 103
    with endometriosis, 134

Affective disorders, 449
Aganglionosis, congenital, 220, 221
Age at onset or presentation
    abdominal migraine, 441
    chronic pelvic pain, 4f
    constipation, 223
    dysmenorrhea, 102
    endometrial polyps, 122
    endometriosis, 129
    herpes zoster infection, 466
    interstitial cystitis, 260
    multicystic peritoneal mesothelioma, 246
    ovarian remnant syndrome diagnosis,
        164, 165
    ovarian retention syndrome diagnosis,
        157, 157t, 159
    postherpetic neuralgia, 466
    postoperative peritoneal cysts, 246, 247t
    vestibulitis, 206
AIDS/HIV, 19
Algometry, pressure, 344
Allen-Masters syndrome, 171
Allodynia, 418
    definition, 204
    in peripheral nerve mononeuropathy, 422
    in postherpetic neuralgia, 468
Alternative therapies, 504–505
Amenorrhea, 109
δ-Aminolevulinic acid, in porphyria, 462,
    464
Amitriptyline, 207, 208
    depression therapy, 455
    dyspareunia management, 118
    interstitial cystitis treatment, 268
    peripheral nerve mononeuropathy
        treatment, 426
    postherpetic neuralgia therapy, 469
Anal examination, 39
    pelvic floor muscle dysfunction
        symptoms, 287
Anal sphincter trigger points, 326, 332f,
    342
Anatomic short leg. *See* Short leg syndrome
Androgen therapy, for endometriosis, 139
Anhedonia, 449
Anhidrosis in mononeuropathy, 423
Anismus, 222
    definition, 279
    in pelvic floor muscle dysfunction,
        290–291
    treatment, 293
Ankylotic joint, 359
Antibiotic therapy, 499